FOURTH EDITION

Essentials of Psychiatric-Mental Health Nursing

FOURTH EDITION

Essentials of Psychiatric-Mental Health Nursing

A Communication Approach to Evidence-Based Care

Elizabeth M. Varcarolis, RN, MA
Professor Emeritus, Formerly Deputy Chairperson
Department of Nursing
Borough of Manhattan Community College
Associate Fellow
Albert Ellis Institute for Rational Emotive Behavior Therapy (REBT)
New York, New York

Chyllia D. Fosbre, MSN, RN, PMHNP-BC
Psychiatric-Mental Health Nurse Practitioner
District Medical Group
Children's Rehabilitative Services
Phoenix, Arizona

Section Editor:
Lorraine Chiappetta, RN, MSN, CNE
Professional Faculty, Nursing & Health Sciences
Course Coordinator
Washtenaw Community College
Ann Arbor, Michigan

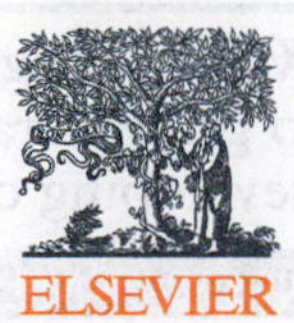

ELSEVIER

Elsevier
3251 Riverport Lane
St. Louis, Missouri 63043

ESSENTIALS OF PSYCHIATRIC-MENTAL HEALTH NURSING:
A COMMUNICATION APPROACH TO EVIDENCE-BASED CARE,
FOURTH EDITION

ISBN: 978-0-323-62511-1

Notice

Practitioners and researchers must always rely on their own experience and knowledge in evaluating and using any information, methods, compounds or experiments described herein. Because of rapid advances in the medical sciences, in particular, independent verification of diagnoses and drug dosages should be made. To the fullest extent of the law, no responsibility is assumed by Elsevier, authors, editors or contributors for any injury and/or damage to persons or property as a matter of products liability, negligence or otherwise, or from any use or operation of any methods, products, instructions, or ideas contained in the material herein.

Previous editions copyrighted 2017, 2013, 2009.

International Standard Book Number: 978-0-323-62511-1

Senior Content Strategist: Yvonne Alexopoulos
Senior Content Development Manager: Lisa P. Newton
Publishing Services Manager: Julie Eddy
Senior Project Manager: Jodi Willard
Design Direction: Maggie Reid

Printed in the United States of America

Last digit is the print number: 9 8 7 6 5 4 3

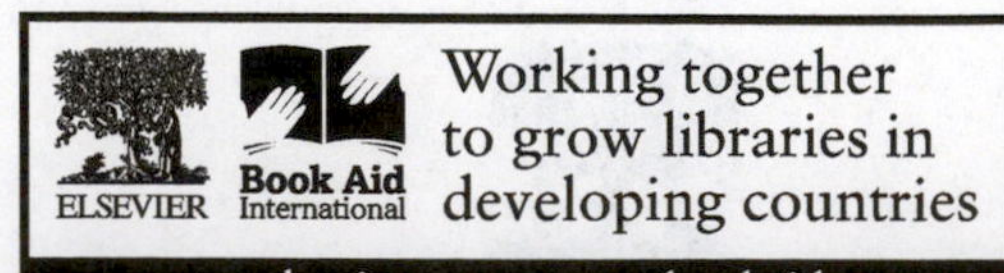

During the revision of this text, Elizabeth "Betsy" M. Varcarolis passed away.
Her husband, Paul, was by her side, supporting her to the very end.
Betsy has shaped the psychiatric nursing world through her numerous texts and years as a nursing instructor. Her fighting spirit and dedication to greatness will be missed.

To the memory of Josiah and Ruth Merrill, who gave me life and opportunity and whom I miss every day.

And especially to my husband, Paul, whose love and devotion become more and more evident as time passes. Thanks for the wonderful years. I love you dearly.

To the memory of Ruth Matheney and Suzanne Lego who, as mentors, made such a difference in my professional career.

And to a very much alive group of angels, Lydia, Presley, Julie, and Joanna.

Betsy M. Varcarolis

To Betsy M. Varcarolis, thank you for trusting me with your life's work and for giving me an opportunity to carry it forward.

To my husband, Jonathan, who picked up the slack and supported me in taking on a challenge that, as Betsy said, would change our lives forever.

To the patients and families who have allowed me to be a part of their lives and share what I have learned as I've walked with them and then turn around and share that knowledge to shape the future of nurses.

Chyllia D. Fosbre

Someone once said that life is a tragedy because it ends with death.
I believe that life becomes a tragedy only if it's not well spent.

Betsy M. Varcarolis spent her life contributing to our planet and to the people she connected with. She cared about our world and its citizens. She was a life enhancer and will be profoundly missed by all of the lives she touched. She left a positive, indelible footprint on our troubled globe.

Paul Varcarolis

ACKNOWLEDGMENTS

Elizabeth "Betsy" Merrill Varcarolis is a prolific author and respected leader in the field of psychiatric-mental health nursing. She published her first *Foundations of Psychiatric/Mental Health Nursing* in 1990, which is now carried forward by Margaret Halter with the eighth edition. With this text, she has written four editions of *Essentials of Psychiatric Mental Health Nursing*. There are also six editions of her *Manual of Psychiatric Nursing Care Plans*. In addition to these major works, she has also contributed to *The American Handbook of Psychiatric Nursing* and wrote the computer-assisted course Emotional Disorders in Adolescents and Children.

Elizabeth is Professor Emeritus and former deputy chairperson at Borough of Manhattan Community College. She graduated with her bachelor of science in nursing from Cornell University in 1964 and worked in a variety of settings, including hospitals in London, Bermuda, Glasgow, Nigeria, and New York. She worked in hospitals during times of famine and war and dedicated herself to a career of service. She volunteered at home and abroad and served as a Major in the United States Army Reserve–Army Nurse Corps.

Her dedication to the field of mental health nursing is reflected in the passion and hard work she has put into publishing over a dozen textbooks over the past 30 years. It is without a doubt that Elizabeth has touched the lives of a countless number of nurses as they have relied on her textbooks. It is with deep respect that her work is carried forward by Margaret Halter and Chyllia D. Fosbre.

It has been an honor to work with Elizabeth (Betsy) Varcarolis as her content strategist for the past three editions of *Essentials of Psychiatric Mental Health Nursing*. As a professional and educator, Betsy was a pioneer in the field of psychiatric mental health nursing, and her texts continue to lead the way in providing undergraduate nursing students with the very best of content. With sincere gratitude and thanks to Betsy for her many years of dedication and hard work, we will strive to keep Betsy's voice alive in future editions of this textbook.

Yvonne Alexopoulos
Senior Content Strategist
Elsevier–Traditional Education, Reference, and Continuity

I would like to express my heartfelt thanks to Betsy Varcarolis as her senior content development manager for the past three editions of *Essentials of Psychiatric Mental Health Nursing*. She not only provided me with the opportunity to develop such a wonderful textbook, but she also was always very collaborative in her approach and never hesitated to let me know how much she valued my opinions and feedback. It is my hope that this edition is the best edition yet, Betsy!

Lisa P. Newton
Senior Content Development Manager
Elsevier–Education, Reference, and Continuity

As is always the case, I owe a huge debt of gratitude to many for their contributions and support.

First, I would like to thank Chyllia D. Fosbre for working as my consultant and co-author on this edition. I would also like to thank Lorraine Chiappetta for her extensive review and updating of the clinical chapters.

I am also indebted to Dawn Scheick for the Applying the Art boxes found in all of the clinical chapters (Chapters 10–19). Dawn offered excellent examples of how a nurse can incorporate effective and insightful communication while working with patients who possess a variety of needs and display a wide range of behaviors.

Communication is one of the arts taught to all nursing students, and effective communication strategies are the cornerstone of psychiatric-mental health nursing. This text offers many pedagogical features that will benefit both cognitive learners and visual learners. It is hoped that the reader will gain fresh insights, attain a broader understanding, and learn effective tools for interactions with vulnerable individuals during their treatment toward a more mentally healthy quality of life.

I want to offer special thanks to the amazing authors who have contributed to this edition of *Essentials of Psychiatric-Mental Health Nursing* for their expertise and hard work. Sincere and profound thanks go to Peggy Halter, Jessica Gandy, Lois Angelo, Lorraine Chiappetta, Carol O. Long, and Lisa Baker, in order of the appearance of their chapters.

I have been fortunate to be part of a hardworking team. Those who work behind the scenes are always pivotal to the production of any successful text. These are the people who have provided support, kept the project on track, and solved myriad problems that are inherent to any production:

- Senior Content Strategist Yvonne Alexopoulos always provided support and everything needed to make the fourth edition of *Essentials* a success.
- Senior Content Development Manager Lisa P. Newton pulled together resources, provided support, and untangled dilemmas during the publication process.
- Senior Project Manager Jodi M. Willard managed consistency to the minutest detail and has made me look good throughout the process.
- Book Designer Maggie Reid created a vivid, exciting, and reader-friendly design.

Betsy M. Varcarolis

CONTRIBUTORS

Lois Angelo, MSN, APRN
Case Manager
Emergency Department
Newton-Wellesley Hospital
Newton, Massachusetts

Lisa M. Baker, DNP, PMHNP-BC
Outpatient Practice
DrLisaNP.com
Tucson, Arizona

Lorraine Chiappetta, RN, MSN, CNE
Professional Faculty (retired)
Nursing
Washtenaw Community College
Ann Arbor, Michigan

Chyllia D. Fosbre, MSN, PMHNP-BC
Psychiatric-Mental Health Nurse Practitioner
District Medical Group
Children's Rehabilitative Services
Phoenix, Arizona

Christina Fratena, MSN, PMHCNS-BC
Clinical Instructor of Nursing
Malone University
Canton, Ohio

Jessica Gandy, MEd, JD, Esquire
Professional Negligence Attorney
Las Vegas, Nevada

Margaret Jordan Halter, PhD, APRN
Editor, *Foundations of Psychiatric-Mental Health Nursing;*
Former APRN
Partial Hospitalization Program
Cleveland Clinic Akron General Medical Center
Akron, Ohio;
Former Adjunct Faculty
College of Nursing
Ohio State University
Columbus, Ohio

Carol O. Long, PhD, RN, FPCN, FAAN
Geriatric and Palliative Care Nursing Consultant
Fredericksburg, Virginia

Elizabeth M. Varcarolis, BSN, MSN
Professor Emeritus
Formerly Deputy Chairperson
Department of Nursing
Borough of Manhattan Community College
New York City, New York;
Associate Fellow
Albert Ellis Institute for Rational Emotive Behavior Therapy (REBT)
New York City, New York

Ancillary Writers

Linda Turchin, RN, MSN, CNE
Associate Professor of Nursing
Fairmont State University
Fairmont, West Virginia
Test Bank, NCLEX Review Questions, and Case Studies and Nursing Care Plans

Linda Wendling, MS, MFA
Learning Theory Consultant
University of Missouri–St. Louis
St. Louis, Missouri
TEACH for Nurses

REVIEWERS

Lisa M. Baker, DNP, PMHNP-BC
Outpatient Practice
DrLisaNP.com
Tucson, Arizona

Christina Flint, RN, MSN, MBA
Assistant Professor
Nursing
University of Indianapolis
Indianapolis, Indiana

Dianna Garza, MSN, RN
Assistant Professor
Nursing Education
Alamo College District, St. Philip's College
San Antonio, Texas

Linda Mollino, MSN, RN
Director, Career and Technical Education Programs:
Health and Human Services Career Instruction
Oregon Coast Community College
Newport, Oregon

Lisa J. Scott, DNP, MSN, BSN, RN
Instructor
Nursing and Allied Health
Norfolk State University
Norfolk, Virginia

Felisa Smith, RN, BSN, MSA, MSN/Ed, CNE
Acting Accelerated BSN Program Coordinator
Nursing and Allied Health
Norfolk State University
Norfolk, Virginia

The *Diagnostic and Statistical Manual of Mental Disorders,* 5th edition *(DSM-5)* is well represented in the fourth edition of *Essentials of Psychiatric-Mental Health Nursing: A Communication Approach to Evidence-Based Care,* as are medications recently approved by the U.S. Food and Drug Administration at this writing. The color plates depicting "The Neurobiology of Specific Disorders" come alive through animations on the Evolve website. This edition continues to provide the essential content for a shorter course without sacrificing either the current research or the nursing and psychotherapeutic interventions necessary for sound practice. In fact, all efforts have been made to ensure that research and psychotherapeutic interventions reflect current knowledge.

Essentials of Psychiatric-Mental Health Nursing, Fourth Edition, continues to provide a comprehensive but concise review of the prominent theorists and therapeutic modalities in use today, including milieu, group, and family therapies (Chapter 3, "Theories and Therapies"). Within each of the clinical chapters (Chapters 10–19), chapters that examine various psychiatric emergencies (Chapters 20–25), and chapters that address specific patient populations across the life span (Chapters 26–28), specific therapeutic modalities that have proven effective for each topic are covered thoroughly.

In addition to the overview of medication groups provided in Chapter 4 (Biological Basis for Understanding Psychopharmacology), specific medications are covered for each of the clinical disorders and include patient and family teaching guidelines. Integrative therapies are also included in each of the clinical chapters where they have proven effective.

To present the most essential base of knowledge for a shorter course, the pertinent information on some topics has been incorporated in the clinical chapters where applicable rather than discussed in a separate chapter. For example, rather than include a general chapter on culture, each of the clinical chapters incorporates relevant information on cultural aspects of the various clinical disorders, which can also help to give the reader a broader cultural perspective.

Forensic issues related to the nursing care of patients are included in specific chapters, especially Chapters 21 ("Child, Partner, and Elder Violence") and 22 ("Sexual Violence"). This discussion is in addition to Chapter 6 ("Legal and Ethical Basis for Practice").

THE SCIENCE AND ART OF PSYCHIATRIC-MENTAL HEALTH NURSING

The American Nurses Association's *Psychiatric-Mental Health Nursing: Scope and Standards of Practice* begins with the following statement that stresses the importance of both the art and the science employed by nurses caring for patients with mental health problems and psychiatric disorders:

> *Psychiatric-mental health nursing, a core mental health profession, employs a purposeful use of self as its art and a wide range of nursing, psychosocial, and neurobiological theories and research evidence as its science.*

In *Essentials of Psychiatric-Mental Health Nursing: A Communication Approach to Evidence-Based Care,* Fourth Edition, there is an effort to integrate and balance these two aspects of nursing care and to present all essential information on each so that students will be prepared to offer the best possible care when they enter practice.

The Science

Over the past few decades, we have seen remarkable scientific progress in our understanding of the workings of the brain and how abnormalities in the functioning of the brain are related to mental illness. As confidence in this research grew, the focus on scientific research expanded and led to more scientifically based treatment approaches, and the concept of *evidence-based practice* (EBP) became a dominant focus of mental health treatment.

While writing this text, great effort was made to provide the most current evidence-based information in the field while still keeping the material comprehensible and reader-friendly. Relevant information drawn from science is woven throughout the text.

Chapter 1 (Science and the Therapeutic Use of Self in Psychiatric-Mental Health Nursing) introduces the student to the evolution of EBP and its mechanics and provides guidelines for where and how to gather information for applying EBP in psychiatric nursing practice.

One of the unique features of this text is **Applying Evidence-Based Practice (EBP)**, which is introduced in Chapter 1 and runs throughout the clinical chapters. Each box poses a question, walks the readers through the process of gathering evidence-based data from a variety of sources, and presents a plan of care based on the evidence.

The Art

In comparison with the medical model, the **recovery model** is a more social, relationship-based model of care. The focus of the recovery model is a nurse–physician partner relationship. The recovery model began in the addiction field, in which the goal was for individuals to recover from substance abuse and addictions. Today the recovery model is gaining momentum in the larger mental health community. Its focus is on empowering patients by supporting hope, strengthening social ties, developing more effective coping skills, fostering the use of spiritual strength, and more.

By definition, nurses are primed to incorporate the biopsychosocial and cultural/spiritual approaches to care. Some nursing leaders express concern that the "art" of nursing is becoming marginalized by the emphasis on EBP. Chapter 1 covers some of these often minimized and uncharted interventions, such as the art of caring, the skill of attending, and patient advocacy. However, what also might be minimized and deemphasized is the tools that make nurses unique. Some of these tools include possessing effective communication skills, forming therapeutic relationships, and understanding ways of interviewing and assessing patients' needs. These areas are stressed in Chapters 8 ("Communication Skills: Medium for All Nursing Practice") and 9 ("Therapeutic Relationships and the Clinical Interview"). There is also a section in each of the clinical chapters on useful communication techniques for a specific disorder or situation.

Another unique feature that is included in the clinical chapters is **Applying the Art**, which depicts a clinical scenario demonstrating the interaction (both therapeutic and nontherapeutic) between a student and a patient, the student's perception of the interaction, and the identification of the mental health nursing concepts in play.

ORGANIZATION

Organized into five units, the chapters in the text have been grouped to emphasize the clinical perspective and to facilitate locating information. All clinical chapters are organized in a clear, logical, and consistent format, with the nursing process as the strong, visible framework. The basic outline for the clinical chapters is as follows:

- Prevalence and Comorbidity
  Knowing the comorbid disorders that are often part of the clinical picture of specific disorders helps students and clinicians to understand how to better assess and treat their patients.
- Theory
- Cultural Considerations
- Clinical Picture
- Application of the Nursing Process
  - **Assessment.** This section presents the appropriate assessments for specific disorders, including assessment tools and rating scales. The rating scales included help to highlight important areas in the assessment of a variety of behaviors and mental conditions. Because many of the answers are subjective, experienced clinicians use these tools in addition to their knowledge of their patients as a guide when planning care.
  - **Diagnosis.** This section includes the latest International Classification for Nursing Practice (ICNP) terminology.
  - **Outcomes Identification**
  - **Planning**
  - **Implementation.** Interventions follow the categories set by the American Nurses Association's *Psychiatric-Mental Health Nursing: Scope and Standards of Practice* (2014). Various interventions for each of the clinical disorders are chosen based on which most fit specific patient needs and include communication guidelines; health teaching and health promotion; milieu therapy; psychotherapy; and pharmacological, biological, and integrative therapies.
  - **Evaluation**

FEATURES

In addition to the **Applying Evidence-Based Practice (EBP)** and **Applying the Art** boxes described previously, the following features are included in the text to inform, heighten understanding, and engage the reader:

- Chapters open with **Objectives** and **Key Terms and Concepts** to orient the reader.
- Numerous **Vignettes** describing psychiatric patients and their disorders attract and hold the reader's interest.
- **Assessment Guidelines** are included in clinical chapters to familiarize readers with methods of assessing patients; these can also be used in the clinical setting.
- **Potential Nursing Diagnoses** tables based on ICNP terminology list several possible nursing diagnoses for a particular disorder, along with the associated signs and symptoms.
- **Nursing Interventions** tables list interventions for a given disorder or clinical situation, along with rationales for each intervention.
- ***DSM-5* criteria boxes** are provided for selected mental health disorders.
- **Neurobiology illustrations of selected mental health disorders and how medications help to mitigate classic symptoms** are included. These are also provided on the Student Resources of Evolve as Animations. See the Animation icon in the textbook.
- **Key Points to Remember** present the main concepts of each chapter in an easy-to-comprehend and concise bulleted list.
- **Applying Critical Judgment** questions at the end of all chapters introduce clinical situations in psychiatric nursing and encourage critical thinking processes essential for nursing practice.
- **NEW! Chapter Review Questions** at the end of each chapter reinforce key concepts.
- The Appendix provides the **Answers to Chapter Review Questions.**

LEARNING AND TEACHING AIDS

For Students

The Evolve Student Resources for this text include the following:

- ***Animations*** of the neurobiology illustrations for selected mental health disorders and how medications help to mitigate classic symptoms. You can also find these illustrations in the textbook with the icon next to them.
- ***Case Studies*** and ***Nursing Care Plans*** for clinical disorders
- ***Student Review Questions*** for each chapter

For Instructors

The Evolve Instructor Resources for this text include the following:

- ***TEACH for Nurses lesson plans,*** based on chapter Learning Objectives, serve as ready-made, modifiable lesson plans and a complete roadmap to link all parts of the educational package. These concise and straightforward lesson plans can be modified or combined to meet your particular scheduling and teaching needs.
- ***Test Bank*** in ExamView format, featuring approximately 800 test items, complete with correct answer, rationale, cognitive level, nursing process step, appropriate NCLEX® label, and corresponding text page reference. The ExamView program allows instructors to create new tests; edit, add, and delete test questions; sort questions by NCLEX® category, cognitive level, and nursing process step; and administer and grade tests online.
- ***PowerPoint Presentations*** with more than 600 customizable lecture slides
- ***Audience Response Questions*** for iClicker and other systems, with two to five multiple-answer questions per chapter to stimulate class discussion and assess student understanding of key concepts.

I hope all of you find that *Essentials of Psychiatric-Mental Health Nursing: A Communication Approach to Evidence-Based Care,* Fourth Edition, provides you with the information you need to be successful in your practice of nursing. Good luck to you all.

Betsy M. Varcarolis
Chyllia D. Fosbre

CONTENTS

UNIT V Age-Related Mental Health Disorders

UNIT I

Essential Theoretical Concepts for Practice

Dr. Hildegard E. Peplau (1909–1999) "Mother of Psychiatric Nursing"

Hildegard Peplau, known as the mother of psychiatric nursing, has had the most profound effect on the practice of nursing since Florence Nightingale. After earning her bachelor's degree in nursing and her master's degree and doctorate in psychology, she went on to become a certified psychoanalyst. She later joined the psychiatric nursing faculty at Rutgers University, where she developed the first program specifically for psychiatric nursing. She later worked with the World Health Organization (WHO), published extensively, served as executive director and president of the American Nurses Association, and was a visiting faculty and lecturer around the world (D'Antonio et al., 2014).

Peplau's theory of interpersonal relations, also known as psychodynamic nursing, was strongly influenced by Harry Stack Sullivan's interpersonal relationship theory and was the first to integrate concepts from other psychological and scientific fields into a nursing theory. Her interpersonal theory led to a paradigm shift in the nature of the nurse–patient relationship, now referred to as patient-centered care. Peplau's theory has been used as a framework for a wide variety of research topics, including patient education, depression, survivors of sexual violence, and research subject retention.

As you read through this textbook, you will learn about levels of anxiety, phases of the nurse–patient relationship, and the importance of observing your own thoughts and feelings within the context of the nurse–patient interaction. These indispensable tools used by competent nurses today are all contributions from Hildegard Peplau, and her theory continues to serve as a foundation for the development of therapeutic nursing interventions, including the therapeutic use of self, that positively affect patient outcomes. Peplau's influence goes beyond psychiatric nursing. She was a determined advocate of advanced practice nursing and the expansion of nursing from a job to a profession, which was a key aspect of the development of standards and credentialing. Every nurse is profoundly affected by the art and science that Peplau brought to nursing.

1

Science and the Therapeutic Use of Self in Psychiatric-Mental Health Nursing

Chyllia D. Fosbre, Elizabeth M. Varcarolis

http://evolve.elsevier.com/Varcarolis/essentials

OBJECTIVES

1. Explain what is meant by evidence-based practice (EBP), recovery model, and trauma-informed care models.
2. Identify the 5 A's used in the process of integrating EBP into the clinical setting.
3. Discuss at least three dilemmas nurses face when attempting to utilize EBP.
4. Identify four resources that nurses can use as guidelines for best-evidence interventions.
5. Identify basic principles of therapeutic self and apply them as an art of nursing.
6. Defend why the concept of caring should be a basic ingredient in the practice of nursing and how it is expressed while giving patient care.
7. Discuss what is meant by being a patient advocate.

KEY TERMS AND CONCEPTS

5 A's, p. 3
attending, p. 7
caring, p. 7
clinical algorithms, p. 4
clinical/critical pathways, p. 5
clinical practice guidelines, p. 4
evidence-based practice (EBP), p. 2
patient advocate, p. 7
psychiatric-mental health nursing, p. 2
Quality and Safety Education for Nurses (QSEN), p. 2
recovery model, p. 6
therapeutic use of self, p. 6
trauma-informed care, p. 6

CONCEPT: ADVOCACY: *Advocacy* is a signature aspect of professional identity among nursing and other professions and is a primary consideration for all decisions made within the health care environment. It involves a commitment to patients' health, well-being, and safety. The ability to speak out assertively and credibly on behalf of patients or families is critical to effective advocacy (Giddens, 2017). Psychiatric-mental health nurses also function as advocates when they advise patients of their rights, solve the prescription problems of the homeless patient engage in public speaking, write articles, and lobby congressional representatives to help improve mental health care, among other actions. It can take a great deal of courage to advocate for patients when we witness behaviors or actions of health care professionals that could have serious consequences.

INTRODUCTION

Psychiatric-mental health nursing is a specialized area of nursing based on evidence related to the neurobiology of psychiatric disorders, psychopharmacology and the effects of medications, and therapeutic relationships using evidence-based models like the recovery-based model and trauma-informed care. It is one of the few areas of nursing found in nearly every other specialty area. Having knowledge of psychiatric mental health will benefit every nurse.

Like all nursing specialties, psychiatric-mental health nursing employs both the *science* and the *art* of nursing. Included in the *science* of nursing are the major concepts of **evidence-based practice (EBP)**, the recovery model, trauma-informed care, and **Quality and Safety Education for Nurses (QSEN)**, as well as theories from a range of nursing, psychological, and neurobiological research. Concepts related to the *art* of nursing include caring, attending, and advocacy (American Nurses Association [ANA], 2017).

EVIDENCE-BASED PRACTICE

With the increased understanding of the biology of psychiatric illnesses beginning in the 1990s (termed the "decade of the brain"), treatment approaches rapidly evolved into more scientifically grounded methods, now known as EBP. In psychiatry, the evidence-based focus extends to treatment approaches in which there is scientific evidence for psychological and sociological modalities, as well as evidence related to the neurobiology of psychiatric disorders and psychopharmacology. The emergence of evidence-based nursing in the United States originated from the EBP movement in the medical community in England and Canada during the 1980s and 1990s. A noteworthy concept differentiating EBP in nursing from medicine is that the approach utilized in nursing incorporates more than clinical research. Evidence is not limited to what is found in research studies but also incorporates the nurse's clinical knowledge and experience, as well as the patient's preferences and desires (Disch, 2014; Melnyk & Fineout-Overholt, 2014).

Basing nursing practice on a systematic approach to care is not new. McDonald (2001) states that Florence Nightingale (1820–1910), the founder of modern nursing, had a philosophy reflecting an evidence-based framework, advocating for the "best possible research, access to the best available governmental statistics and expertise" (p. 2). In 1860, Nightingale made a proposal that resulted in "the first model for systematic collection of hospital data using a uniform classification of diseases and operations," eventually forming the basis of the coding system used worldwide, the *International Statistical Classification of Diseases and Related Health Problems (ICD)* (Centers for Disease Control and Prevention [CDC], 2011). Historically, mental health professionals in the United States have used the *Diagnostic and Statistical Manual of Mental Disorders (DSM)* classifications rather than the *ICD* system. However, in 2013, the *DSM* and the *ICD*, 10th Revision, Clinical Modification *(ICD-10)* codes were aligned.

Hildegard Peplau (1909–1999), considered the mother of psychiatric nursing, had a passion for clarifying and developing the art and science of professional nursing practice and believed that a scientific approach was essential to the practice of psychiatric nursing (D'Antonio et al., 2014). Her contributions went far beyond what she brought to the field of psychiatric nursing. She introduced the concept of advanced nursing practice and promoted professional standards and regulation through credentialing, among a multitude of other foundational contributions to nursing (D'Antonio et al., 2014).

It should be noted that psychiatry was one of the first medical specialties to extensively use randomized controlled trials. One of the founding principles of clinical psychology in the 1950s was that practice should be based on the results of experimental comparisons of treatment methods (Jackson, 2011). However, with limited scientific evidence for practice at that time, much of nursing care was based on tradition, personal experience, unsystematic trial and error, and the earlier experiences of nurses and others in the health care profession (Jackson, 2011). During that time, there was an increase in the publication of research-related journals.

Evidence-based practice (EBP) is the process of making clinical decisions based on available evidence, clinical experience, and patient preference. Melnyk and Fineout-Overholt (2014) state there is no magic bullet that provides a formula describing the weight of evidence that patient values and preferences and clinical expertise should take in making clinical decisions. Although EBP is equated with effective decision making, avoidance of habitual practice, and enhanced clinical performance, there may be a tendency to overlook practical knowledge that can provide useful information for individualized and effective practice.

Numerous definitions delineate the multistep process of integrating EBP into clinical practice. One that is simply stated and apt is referred to as the **5 A's** (Shaw-Kokot & Philpotts, 2015):

1. **Ask a question.** Identify a problem or need for change for a specific patient or situation.
2. **Acquire literature.** Search the literature for scientific studies and articles that address the issue(s) of concern.
3. **Appraise the literature.** Evaluate and synthesize the research evidence regarding its validity, relevance, and applicability using criteria of scientific merit.
4. **Apply the evidence.** Choose interventions that are based on the best available evidence with the understanding of the patient's preference and needs.
5. **Assess the performance.** Evaluate the outcomes, using clearly defined criteria and reports, and document the results.

Evaluating the evidence is done through a hierarchical rating system (Fig. 1.1 and Table 1.1). Systematic reviews or meta-analyses of randomized controlled studies and evidence-based clinical practice

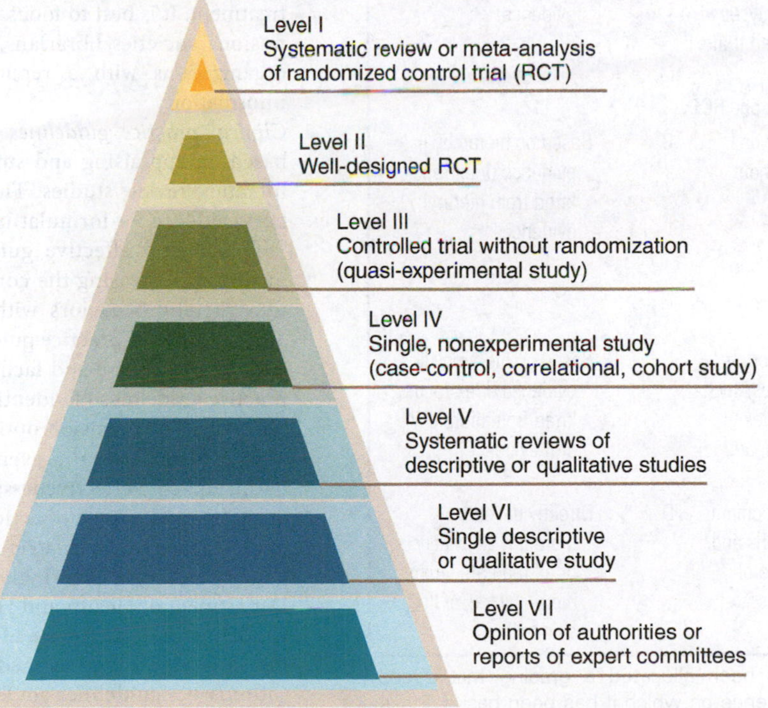

Fig. 1.1 Hierarchy of evidence. (From Melnyk, B. M., & Fineout-Overholt, E. [2014]. *Evidence-based practice in nursing & healthcare: A guide to best practice* [3rd ed.]. Philadelphia: Lippincott Williams & Wilkins; and Newhouse, R. P., Dearholt, S. L., Poe, S. S., et al. [2007]. *Johns Hopkins nursing: Evidence-based practice model and guidelines*. Indianapolis, IN: Sigma Theta Tau International.)

guidelines provide the strongest evidence on which to base clinical practice. In a randomized controlled trial (RCT), patients are chosen at random (by chance) to receive one of the clinical interventions or be in a control group with no treatment. One intervention would be the intervention under study, and another intervention might be the usual standard of care or a placebo. The weakest level of evidence includes expert committee reports, opinions, clinical experience, and descriptive studies. Although scientific evidence is ranked hierarchically, it is important to note the value of all types of evidence in clinical decision making.

The first Surgeon General's report published on the topic of mental health was in 1999 (U.S. Department of Health and Human Services [USDHHS], 1999). This landmark document was based on an extensive review of the scientific literature and created in consultation with mental health providers and consumers. The document concluded that there are numerous effective psychopharmacological and psychosocial treatments for most mental disorders. However, it raised some questions for psychiatric nurses, including the following:

- Are psychiatric nurses aware of the efficacy of the treatment and interventions they provide?
- Are they truly practicing evidence-based care?
- Is there documentation of the nature and outcomes of the care they provide?

TABLE 1.1 Hierarchy of Evidence and Grading of Recommendations[a]

HIERARCHY OF EVIDENCE		GRADING OF RECOMMENDATIONS	
Level	**Type of Evidence**	**Level**	**Type of Evidence**
Ia	Evidence from systematic reviews or meta-analyses of randomized controlled trials (RCTs)	A	Based on hierarchy I evidence
Ib	Evidence from at least one RCT		
IIa	Evidence from at least one controlled study without randomization	B	Based on hierarchy II evidence or extrapolated from hierarchy I evidence
IIb	Evidence from at least one other type of quasi-experimental study		
III	Evidence from nonexperimental descriptive studies, such as comparative studies, correlational studies, and case-control studies	C	Based on hierarchy III evidence or extrapolated from hierarchy I or II evidence
IV	Evidence from expert committee reports or opinions and/or clinical experience of respected authorities	D	Directly based on hierarchy IV evidence or extrapolated from hierarchy I, II, or III evidence

[a]Each recommendation has been allocated a grading that directly reflects the hierarchy of evidence on which it has been based. Please note that the hierarchy of evidence and the recommendation gradings relate the strength of the literature, not the clinical importance.
From Hierarchy of evidence and grading of recommendations. (2004). *Thorax, 59*(Suppl. 1), i13–i14.

The emphasis on EBP is expanding. However, this approach does not provide easy answers. For example, consider the following points:

- Who interprets "best evidence"?
- Not all nursing problems can be reduced to a clear issue that is solvable by scientific experiments.
- Relatively little higher-level nursing research addressing psychiatric nursing interventions and practice has been available.
- Despite the expectation to use EBP, little education is provided in undergraduate programs or in the workplace to prepare nurses for this process.
- How do nurses who are practicing in complex environments of reduced staffing and budgetary constraints find time to research and evaluate the literature and make decisions on "best evidence"?

Three basic aspects (or prongs) of EBP are the following:

- Evidence gleaned in review of the literature
- Clinical knowledge of the nurse from training and experience
- The desires of patients and the values for their care

Case-study examples of how evidence-based practice is applied are highlighted in the **Applying Evidence-Based Practice** boxes throughout the clinical chapters.

Resources for Clinical Practice

1. *Internet resources.* A number of websites provide mental health resources for information, treatment provisions, and the results of recent clinical studies. Some of the most extensive databases for psychiatric and medical resources include Cumulative Index to Nursing and Allied Health Literature (CINAHL), PubMed, and Cochrane reviews. There are self-tests for people to see if they may be experiencing symptoms of a specific disorder, such as depression, anxiety, or attention-deficit/hyperactivity disorder (ADHD). There are also resources for acquiring support and treatment. It is best to focus on sites that are maintained by professional societies, librarians, textbook publishers, or well-known organizations with a reputation for quality, evidence-based information.
2. *Clinical practice guidelines.* **Clinical practice guidelines** are based on appraising and summarizing the best evidence from literature review studies. They serve as tools for standardizing best evidence for formulating patient care and treatment plans. "Efficient and effective guidelines impact patient safety and quality by increasing the consistency of behavior and replacing idiosyncratic behaviors with best practices" (Keiffer, 2015, p. 328). The use of practice guidelines can increase the quality and consistency of care and facilitate outcome research. Essentially, practice guidelines (1) identify practice questions and explicitly identify all the decision options and outcomes; (2) identify the "best evidence" about prevention, diagnosis, prognosis, therapy, harm, and cost-effectiveness; and (3) provide decision points for deciding on a course of action. The *Clinical Practice Guidelines* of the American Psychiatric Association (APA) and the National Quality Measures Clearinghouse offer such guidelines. The U.S. Department of Health and Human Services sponsors a National Guidelines Clearinghouse of evidence-based guidelines pertaining to a wide range of medical and mental health conditions (http://www.guidelines.gov).
3. *Clinical algorithms.* **Clinical algorithms** are step-by-step guidelines prepared in a flowchart or decision-tree format. Alternative diagnostic and treatment approaches are described based on decision points using a large database relevant for the symptoms, diagnosis,

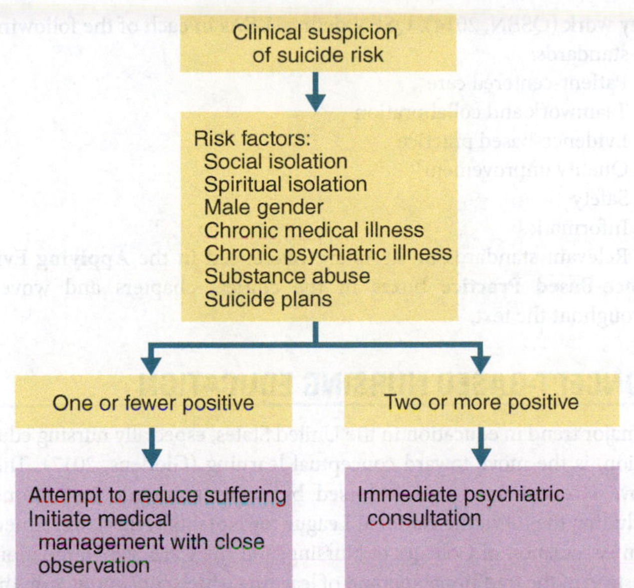

Fig. 1.2 Clinical algorithm for the suspicion of suicide risk. (Modified from Goldman, L., & Ausiello, D. [2008]. *Cecil medicine* [23rd ed.]. Philadelphia: Saunders.)

or treatment modalities. Fig. 1.2 depicts a clinical algorithm for the suspicion of suicide risk.

4. *Clinical/critical pathways.* **Clinical/critical pathways** are specific to the institution using them. These clinical pathways serve as a "map" for specified treatments and interventions to occur within specific time frames that have been shown to improve clinical outcomes. The interventions can include tests, health teaching, and medications. Each pathway lists the expected outcome using a measurable, time-specific format, and documentation is ongoing. Clinical pathways are one way that EBP can be integrated into clinical care.

The Research–Practice Gap

Unfortunately, there is a wide gap between the best-evidence treatments and their effective translation into practice. The need for continued research on how best to apply the findings of clinically relevant issues and their delivery into clinical practice has been the emphasis of the Institute of Medicine (IOM, 2006):

> ...Research that has identified the efficacy of specific treatments under rigorously controlled conditions has been accompanied by almost no research identifying how to make these same treatments effective when delivered in usual settings of care ... when administered by service providers without specialized education in the therapy. (p. 350)

A specialized area known as translational research looks at applying evidence to clinical or bedside practice.

Effective research is best reported in language that is understandable and free of unnecessary jargon:

- Simpler is better.
- Focus on what readers need to know.
- Reduce possible misinterpretations.

Despite the complexities and concerns that must be addressed when implementing best practice, evidence-based nursing is a standard and essential component of nursing practice.

To help the reader understand how best evidence is identified and applied to nursing interventions, this textbook contains a feature box titled **Applying Evidence-Based Practice.** It is hoped that this feature, presented in each of the clinical chapters, will underscore the importance of sound scientific inquiry and ignite the reader's interest in research.

APPLYING EVIDENCE-BASED PRACTICE (EBP)

Problem

A 63-year-old female patient was discharged from a psychiatric hospital. She was homeless and not enrolled in insurance or outpatient mental health services. The message number in the electronic health record (EHR) was no longer valid, so follow-up appointments were not scheduled. A week after discharge, the patient's medication was stolen, and she became suicidal and confused and called the crisis line at her community mental health clinic.

EBP Assessment

A. **What do you already know from experience?** Homeless patients have limited contact information and multiple health concerns.

B. **What does the literature say?** Some of the reasons cited for not attending follow-up appointments are illness, inadequate transportation, forgetting the appointment, and not feeling engaged with providers. Nurses can advocate for patients by addressing gaps in care.

C. **What does the patient want?** The patient wanted her medications and assistance with obtaining resources.

Plan

The crisis team assisted the patient in obtaining medications, finding transportation to a shelter, and enrolling in outpatient mental health services. The nurse practitioner (NP) developed a demographic page in the EHR designed to capture complex contact information for homeless patients, such as where they sleep and eat meals on specific days.

QSEN Prelicensure Knowledge, Skills, and Attitudes (KSAs) Addressed

Safety by minimizing the patient's risk through individual and system performance

Informatics by using technology to manage patient information and prevent error

From Batscha, C., McDevitt, J., Weiden, P., et al. (2011). The effect of an inpatient transition intervention on attendance at the first appointment post-discharge from a psychiatric hospitalization. *Journal of the American Psychiatric Nurses Association, 17*(5), 330–337; Cronenwett, L., Sherwood, G., Barnsteiner, J., et al. (2007). Quality and safety education for nurses. *Nursing Outlook, 55*(3), 122–131; Lamb, V., & Joels, C. (2014). Improving access to health care for homeless people. *Nursing Standard, 29*(6), 45–51; and National Healthcare for the Homeless Council. (2014). *Health reform & homelessness: Twelve key advocacy areas for the HCH community.* Retrieved from http://www.nhchc.org/wp-content/uploads/2011/10/2014-health-reform-policy-statement.pdf

Recovery Model

The mental health **recovery model** is more of a social model of disability than a medical model of disability. Therefore, the focus shifts from one of illness and disease to an emphasis on rehabilitation and recovery. The recovery model is focused on helping individuals develop the knowledge, attitudes, and skills they need to make good choices or change harmful behaviors (Substance Abuse and Mental Health Services Administration [SAMHSA], 2017). The underlying principle is that people can recover from mental illness and substance abuse to lead full, satisfying lives.

The recovery model originated from the 12-step program of Alcoholics Anonymous and a grassroots advocacy initiative called the consumer/survivor/ex-patient movement during the 1980s and 1990s. It is now one of the leading models promoted by SAMHSA (2017). The concept of recovery refers primarily to managing symptoms, reducing psychosocial disability, and improving role performance (SAMHSA, 2017). Holistic interventions, such as encouraging supportive relationships, are designed to promote recovery, as evidenced by functioning in work, engagement in community/social life, and a reduction of symptoms (SAMHSA, 2017). Empowering patients to realize their full potential and independence within the limitations of their illness is the main goal of this model. Recovering from a mental illness is viewed as a personal journey of healing.

The focus of the recovery model has the following mandates (Caldwell et al., 2010; Jacob, 2015):

- Mental health care is to be consumer and family driven, with patients being partners in all aspects of care.
- Care must focus on increasing consumer success in coping with life's challenges and building resilience, not just managing symptoms.
- An individualized care plan is to be at the core of consumer-centered recovery.

Trauma-Informed Care

Another model that is gaining momentum is **trauma-informed care**, a framework developed by the National Center for Trauma-Informed Care (NCTIC), a division of SAMHSA. Trauma-informed care recognizes that trauma is almost universally found in the histories of mental health patients and is a contributor to mental health issues, substance abuse, chronic health conditions, and contact with the criminal justice system. Trauma occurs in many forms, including physical, sexual, and emotional abuse; war; natural disasters; and other harmful experiences. Trauma-informed care provides guidelines for integrating an understanding of how trauma affects patients into clinical programming. A main concept of this approach is a change in paradigm from one that asks, "What's wrong with you?" to one that asks, "What has happened to you?" Key principles also include avoiding retraumatizing through restraints or coercive practices, an open and collaborative relationship between patient and provider, empowerment, and cultural respect.

The American Nurses Association (ANA, 2015), Institute of Medicine (IOM, 2006, 2011), and Quality and Safety Education for Nurses (QSEN, 2014) all support patient-centered care as best practice. Nurses are increasingly expected to understand and synthesize best practice from the literature, care models and theories, neurobiology of psychiatric disorders and medications, and other professional domains into clinical practice.

Quality and Safety Education for Nurses

There is a national initiative toward patient safety and quality, known as QSEN. The overall goal of QSEN is to prepare future nurses who will have the knowledge, skills, and attitudes (KSAs) necessary to continuously improve the quality and safety of the health care systems in which they work (QSEN, 2014). QSEN defines KSAs in each of the following six standards:

- Patient-centered care
- Teamwork and collaboration
- Evidence-based practice
- Quality improvement
- Safety
- Informatics

Relevant standards or KSAs are referenced in the **Applying Evidence-Based Practice** boxes in the clinical chapters and woven throughout the text.

CONCEPT-BASED NURSING EDUCATION

A major trend in education in the United States, especially nursing education, is the move toward conceptual learning (Giddens, 2017). This move is encouraged and endorsed by major academic institutions, including the IOM, the National League for Nursing (NLN), the American Association of Colleges of Nursing, and the Carnegie Foundation. "Instead of the traditional method of learning which concentrates on the ability to recall specific facts in isolation, concept-based learning concentrates on the understanding of broader principles (concepts) that can be applied to a variety of specific examples" (Lippincott Nursing Education, 2017).

According to Elsevier (2018), the following are some benefits of a concept-based curriculum:

- Encourages students to think at more elevated levels
- Facilitates collaborative and active learning
- Helps streamline content
- Focuses on problems across disease categories and populations
- Supports systematic observations about events or conditions that influence a problem
- Underscores the relationships among events or conditions that impact a situation
- Emphasizes nursing actions and interdisciplinary efforts
- Meets the needs of diverse learners
- Causes higher levels of retention

The Art of Nursing

Contemporary nursing relies on a scientific foundation and critical thinking. However, the art of nursing is equally important in delivering comprehensive and holistic care. Even the best evidence-based guidelines may not encompass the entire complexity of an individual patient, disorder, or situation. As Williams and Garner (2002, p. 8) conclude, "Too great an emphasis on evidence-based medicine oversimplifies the complex and interpersonal nature of clinical care." The arts of intuition, interpersonal skills, and cultural competence are indispensable parts of effective treatment.

Benner (2004) suggests that many of the attributes that fall under the art of nursing are invisible, intangible, rarely charted, and almost never suggested in a nursing care plan. Consequently, these attributes are often marginalized, undervalued, and demeaned. The arts of nursing are accomplished through the nurse's **therapeutic use of self**—"essentially, a healthcare provider's use of verbal and nonverbal communication, emotional exchange and other aspects of his or her personality to establish a relationship with the patient that promotes cooperation and healing" ("Therapeutic Use of Self," n.d.) that positively affects patient outcomes.

The health care professional uses self-reflection, self-awareness, and self-evaluation as tools in promoting cooperation, healing, and successful outcomes. It has long been noted that the deciding factor in therapy outcomes is not the theoretical basis of the clinician/nurse but, rather, the strength of the clinician–patient relationship. The relationship is strengthened when the patient has developed a sense of safety and respect and feels free to share his or her problems (Shea, 2017). Three areas inherent in the art of nursing addressed here are (1) caring, (2) attending, and (3) advocating.

Caring

Caring is a natural, essential, and fundamental aspect of human existence. An early survey by Schoenhofer and colleagues (1998) used a group process method to synthesize what was meant by *caring* to the participants. The following three themes emerged:

1. Caring is evidenced by empathic understanding, actions, and patience on another's behalf.
2. Caring for another through actions, words, and presence leads to happiness and touches the heart.
3. Caring is giving of self while preserving the importance of self.

The caring nurse is first and foremost a competent nurse. Without knowledge and competence, the demonstration of compassion and caring alone is powerless to help those under a nurse's care. Without a base of knowledge and skills, care alone cannot eliminate another person's confusion, grief, or pain, but a response of care can transform fear, pain, and suffering into a tolerable, shared experience (Smith et al., 2013).

Dr. Jean Watson founded the Watson Caring Science Institute. Watson's caring theory has a spiritual and existential underpinning (Watson Caring Science Institute, 2015). The theory integrates 10 *caritas* (loving principles) that encourage altruism, loving kindness toward self and others, faith and hope, honor, nurturing individual beliefs, helping and trusting relationships, accepting feelings while authentically listening, creative scientific problem solving, teaching and learning using individual styles, physical and spiritual healing environment, assisting with basic human needs, and openness to mystery and miracles.

Comforting as a part of caring includes providing social, emotional, physical, and spiritual support for a patient consistent with holistic nursing care. The provision of comfort measures can be lifesaving and is a basic component of good care. Economic strain and nursing shortages are barriers to the practice of caring and comforting because nurses are burdened with greater workloads and higher-acuity patients. However, caring is both an attitude that one communicates (a way of being with a patient) and also a set of skills that can be learned and developed. Listening to patients takes time, but with practice and experience, nurses can develop the ability to attend to emotional and spiritual needs and get to know their patients while completing an assessment or other tasks.

Attending

Attending refers to an *intensity of presence,* being there for and in tune with the patient. The experience of emotional or physical suffering can be isolating. When patients perceive that the nurse is there for them, a human connection is made, and the patient's sense of isolation is minimized or eliminated (Dossey & Keegan, 2013). Being present requires entering the patient's experience. Attending behaviors include active listening skills, such as body posture and eye contact, touching, or giving attentive physical care (Dossey & Keegan, 2013). It is through effective communication that we can fully understand another person's immediate experience, fears, perceptions, and concerns. Attending behaviors are learned and are inherent in a true therapeutic relationship. Chapter 9 discusses attending behaviors in more detail within the context of the nurse–patient relationship.

Advocating

Advocacy in nursing includes a commitment to patients' health, well-being, and safety across the life span; the alleviation of suffering; and the promotion of a peaceful, comfortable, and dignified death (ANA, 2017).

Patient advocacy can occur on many levels, including providing direct patient care; pleading for a course of action; and supporting change in institutional, global, and legislative arenas. The following are examples of patient advocacy activities:

- Providing informed consent, including refusal of treatment
- Respecting patient decisions, even those with which we disagree
- Protecting against threats to well-being
- Being informed about best practices

These are especially critical when patients lack the knowledge, skills, or ability to speak for themselves.

Patients are afforded protection through providing privacy and confidentiality during participation in research, using standards and reviews, and taking action against questionable or impaired practice.

Lawyers are often viewed as advocates for their clients; however, in nursing, being a **patient advocate** is not a legal role but, rather, an ethical one. Ethics is an integral part of the foundation of nursing. Refer to Chapter 6. The term *patient advocate* was first placed in the 1976 ANA *Code of Ethics for Nurses,* revision, and remains essentially unchanged up to the present. It reads:

> *The nurse must be alert to and take appropriate action regarding any instances of incompetent, unethical, illegal, or impaired practices(s) by any member of the health team or the health care system itself, or any action on the part of others that places the rights or best interest of the patient in jeopardy. (ANA, 2015, 3.5)*

It can take a great deal of courage to advocate for patients when we witness behaviors or actions of health care professionals that could have serious consequences.

Advocating demonstrates respect and value for human life while saving lives or bringing comfort to those who are dying. Psychiatric-mental health nurses also function as advocates when they engage in-public speaking, write articles, and lobby congressional representatives to help improve and expand mental health care (ANA, 2017). Throughout the text, a special feature titled **Applying the Art** gives the reader a glimpse of a nurse–patient interaction and the nurse's thought processes while attending to the patient's concerns.

KEY POINTS TO REMEMBER

- Nursing integrates both scientific knowledge and caring arts into a holistic practice.
- Evidence-based practice (EBP) is a process by which the best available research evidence, clinical expertise, and patient preferences are synthesized while making clinical decisions.
- The 5 A's process of integrating best evidence into clinical practice includes (1) asking, (2) acquiring, (3) appraising, (4) applying, and (5) assessing.
- Application of the recovery model assists people with psychiatric disabilities to effectively manage symptoms, reduce psychosocial disability, and find a meaningful life in a community of their choosing.
- Trauma-informed care recognizes that various traumas contribute to mental illness and substance abuse. Awareness of trauma can assist health care providers in giving appropriate care and avoiding retraumatization of patients.
- Some sources for obtaining research findings are (1) Internet resources, (2) clinical practice guidelines, (3) clinical algorithms, and (4) clinical/critical pathways.
- The art of nursing is accomplished through the *therapeutic use of self.*
- Three specific areas are inherent within the art of nursing: (1) caring, (2) attending, and (3) advocating.

APPLYING CRITICAL JUDGMENT

1. A friend of yours has recently returned from military service. You are startled when you encounter him on the street in a disheveled state. He appears frightened, seems to be talking to himself, and jumps when a car backfires nearby. You are astounded because there is such a change in his demeanor from the last time you saw him. When you approach him, he seems wary and guarded.
   A. How would the contribution of evidence-based practice (EBP) be helpful to learn about your friend's symptoms of posttraumatic stress disorder (PTSD)?
   B. What might be some specific needs that could be met under the recovery model?
   C. What insight could the trauma-informed care model provide into what your friend is experiencing?
   D. Discuss how nurses can incorporate EBP and care models in their practice.
2. A friend of yours says that he heard about a new practitioner in the area who is going to teach individuals with alcohol dependence how to safely drink in moderation. You state that from all you have read, and from what you know from your friends' experiences, controlled drinking is not thought to be an acceptable practice. Your friend contends that the practitioner has stories and testimonials from individuals with alcohol dependence who are able to drink in a controlled manner. You tell him that there is no strong evidence for this practice.
   A. How would you, as a nurse, evaluate this claim? Explain the five steps you would take to determne the strength of this claim.
   B. Using Table 1.1, what would you say about the quality of the evidence given?
   C. If your friend was in recovery and thinking of trying this treatment, what would you say that would make a strong argument against such a decision?
3. You are a new nursing student, and a friend of yours says, "What on earth is the 'art of nursing'? Isn't that some weird new-age stuff?"
   A. Discuss three components that are inherent in the art of nursing.
   B. Explain the concept of the therapeutic use of self in applying the art of nursing.
   C. Give your friend an example of how nurses demonstrate comfort or caring in the clinical area.
   D. Explain why patients need to have nurses act as their advocate. Can you think of an example from your clinical experience?
4. Go to the Centre for Evidence-Based Mental Health at http://www.cebmh.com and review at least one available clinical trial.

CHAPTER REVIEW QUESTIONS

1. In which scenario is it most urgent for the nurse to act as a patient advocate?
   a. An adult cries and experiences anxiety after a near-miss automobile accident on the way to work.
   b. A homeless adult diagnosed with schizophrenia lives in a community expecting a category 5 hurricane.
   c. A 14-year-old girl's grades decline because she consistently focuses on her appearance and social networking.
   d. The parents allow the prescription to lapse for 1 day for their 8-year-old child's medication for attention-deficit/hyperactivity disorder.
2. The nurse interacts with a veteran of World War II. The veteran says, "Veterans of modern wars whine and complain all the time. Back when I was in service, you kept your feelings to yourself." Select the nurse's best response.
   a. "American society in the 1940s expected World War II soldiers to be strong."
   b. "World War II was fought in a traditional way, but the enemy is more difficult to identify in today's wars."
   c. "We now have a better understanding of how trauma affects people and the importance of research-based, compassionate care."
   d. "Intermittent explosive devices (IEDs), which were not in use during World War II, produce traumatic brain injuries that must be treated."
3. A patient reports sleeplessness, fatigue, and sadness to the primary care provider. In our current health care climate, what is the most likely treatment approach that will be offered to the patient?
   a. Group therapy
   b. Individual psychotherapy
   c. Complementary therapy
   d. Psychopharmacological treatment
4. The nurse prepares outcomes to the plan of care for an adult diagnosed with mental illness. Which strategy recognizes the current focus of treatment services for this population?
   a. The patient's diagnoses are confirmed using advanced neuroimaging techniques.
   b. The nurse confers with the treatment team to verify the patient's most significant disability.

c. The nurse prioritizes the patient's problems in accordance with Maslow's hierarchy of needs.
d. The patient and family participate actively in establishing priorities and selecting interventions.

5. Which scenario best demonstrates empathic caring?
   a. A nurse provides comfort to a colleague after an error of medication administration.
   b. A nurse works a fourth extra shift in 1 week to maintain adequate unit staffing.
   c. A nurse identifies a violation of confidentiality and makes a report to an agency's privacy officer.
   d. A nurse conscientiously reads current literature to stay aware of new evidence-based practices.

REFERENCES

American Nurses Association (ANA). (2015). *Code of ethics for nurses with interpretive statements.* Silver Spring, MD: Nursebooks.org. Retrieved from www.nursingworld.org/MainMenuCategories/EthicsStandards/Revision-of-Code-of-Ethics-Panel.

American Nurses Association (ANA). (2017). *The voice of Nightingale on advocacy.* Retrieved May 13, 2018 from http://ojin.nursingworld.org/MainMenuCategories/ANAMarketplace/ANAPeriodicals/OJIN/TableofContents/Vol-17-2012/No1-Jan-2012/Florence-Nightingale-on-Advocacy.html.

Benner, P. (2004). Relational ethics of comfort, touch, and solace endangered arts? *American Journal of Critical Care, 13,* 346–349.

Caldwell, B. A., Sclasani, M., Swarbrick, M., et al. (2010). Psychiatric nursing practice & the recovery model of care. *Journal of PSN, 48*(7), 42–48.

Centers for Disease Control and Prevention. (2011). *History of the statistical classification of diseases and causes of death.* Retrieved from www.cdc.gov/nchs/data/misc/classification_diseases2011.pdf.

D'Antonio, P., Beeber, L., Sills, G., et al. (2014). The future in the past: Hildegard Peplau and interpersonal relations in nursing. *Nursing Inquiry, 21*(4), 311–317.

Disch, J. (2014). Using evidence-based advocacy to improve the nation's health. *Nurse Leader, 12*(4), 2831.

Dossey, B. M., & Keegan, L. (2013). *Holistic nursing: A handbook for practice* (6th ed.). Burlington, MA: Jones & Bartlett Learning.

Elsevier. (2018). *Why use conceptual learning in nursing?* Retrieved May 16, 2018 from https://evolve.elsevier.com/education/concept-based-curriculum/why-use-conceptual-learning/.

Giddens, J. F. (2017). *Concepts for nursing practice* (2nd.ed.). St. Louis: Elsevier.

Institute of Medicine (IOM). (2006). *Improving the quality of health care for mental and substance-use conditions.* Washington, DC: Institute of Medicine of the National Academies, National Academies Press.

Institute of Medicine (IOM). (2011). *Clinical practice guidelines we can trust.* Retrieved Sept 12, 2015, from http://iom.nationalacademies.org/Reports/2011/Clinical-Practice-Guidelines-We-Can-Trust.aspx.

Jackson, M. (2011). *The Oxford handbook of the history of medicine.* New York: Oxford University Press.

Jacob, K. S. (2015). Recovery model of mental illness: A complementary approach to psychiatric care. *Indian Journal of Psychological Medicine. 37*(2): 117–119.

Keiffer, M.R. (2015). Utilization of clinical practice guidelines: Barriers and facilitators. *The Nursing Clinics of North America 50*(2), 327-345. http://www.doi.org/10.1016/j.cnur.2015.03.007.

Lippincott Nursing Education. (2017). *Benefits of a concept-based curriculum in nursing education.* Retrieved May 5, 2018 from http://nursingeducation.lww.com/blog.entry.html/2017/01/28/benefits.of_a_concep-agYv.html.

McDonald, L. (2001). Florence Nightingale and the early origins of evidence-based nursing. *Evidence-Based Nursing, 4,* 68–69.

Melnyk, B. M., & Fineout-Overholt, E. (2014). *Evidence-based practice in nursing and healthcare: A guide to best practice* (3rd ed.). Philadelphia: Lippincott Williams & Wilkins.

Quality and Safety Education for Nurses (QSEN). (2014). *Competencies.* Retrieved from http://qsen.org/competencies/.

Schoenhofer, S., Bingham, V., & Hutchins, G. (1998). Giving of oneself on another's behalf: The phenomenology of everyday caring. *International Journal of Human Caring, 2*(2), 23–39.

Shaw-Kokot, J., & Philpotts, L. (2015). *Using evidence based nursing in practice.* Retrieved from http://guides.lib.unc.edu/ebn_practice.

Shea, S. C. (2017). *Psychiatric Interviewing E-Book: The art of understanding: A practical guide for psychiatrists, psychologists, counselors, social workers, nurses, and other mental health professionals* (p. 10). Elsevier Health Sciences. Kindle Edition.

Smith, M. C., Turkel, M. C., & Wolf, Z. R. (2013). *Caring in nursing classics: An essential resource.* New York: Springer.

Substance Abuse and Mental Health Services Administration (SAMHSA). (2017). *Prevention of substance abuse and mental health.* Retrieved May 2018 from https://www.samhsa.gov/prevention.

Therapeutic use of self. (n.d.). (2009). *Medical Dictionary.* Retrieved May 21 2018 from https://medical-dictionary.thefreedictionary.com/therapeutic+use+of+self.

U.S. Department of Health and Human Services (USDHHS). (1999). *Mental health: A report from the surgeon general.* Rockville, MD: National Institute of Mental Health.

Watson Caring Science Institute (WCSI). (2015). *Global translations-10 Caritas processes.* Retrieved from www.watsoncaringscience.org.

Williams, D. D. R., & Garner, J. (2002). The case against "the evidence": A different perspective on evidence-based medicine. *British Journal of Psychiatry, 180,* 8–12.

2

Mental Health and Mental Illness

Chyllia D. Fosbre

http://evolve.elsevier.com/Varcarolis/essentials

OBJECTIVES

1. Summarize factors that can affect the mental health of an individual, and explain how they influence a holistic nursing assessment.
2. Discuss dynamic factors (including social climate, politics, cultural beliefs, myths, and biases) that make it difficult to formulate a clear-cut definition of mental health.
3. Identify the processes leading to stigmatization of an individual or group, and discuss some of the effects that stigma can have on medical and psychological well-being.
4. Compare and contrast a *Diagnostic and Statistical Manual of Mental Disorders,* 5th edition *(DSM-5)* diagnosis with a nursing diagnosis.
5. Give examples of how cultural influences and norms can affect making an accurate *DSM-5* diagnosis.

KEY TERMS AND CONCEPTS

CONCEPT: FUNCTIONAL ABILITY: *Functional ability* refers to the individual's ability to perform the normal activities of life to meet basic needs; fulfill usual roles in the family, workplace, and community; and maintain health and well-being (Giddens, 2017). Mental illnesses are medical conditions that affect a person's thinking, feeling, mood, ability to relate to others, and daily functioning. Unfortunately, there is a myth about the mentally ill that they function in a different and odd way. Another misconception is that to be mentally healthy, a person must function logically and rationally at all times. There is no obvious, consistent line between mental illness and mental health functioning. As humans, we are far more similar than different, despite any diagnosis.

INTRODUCTION

Mental health and mental illness are not specific entities but, rather, they exist on a continuum. The mental health continuum is dynamic and shifting, ranging from mild to moderate to severe (Fig. 2.1). The diagnosis is an important factor; for example, schizophrenia is generally considered more impairing than anxiety. However, this is not always the case. An individual with schizophrenia with a good support system and treatment plan may be functioning at a higher level than someone with generalized anxiety who is in an abusive relationship with no mental health treatment. In addition, the same individual may function at different levels from week to week or year to year. Many biological and environmental factors influence mental health.

The U.S. Department of Health and Human Services (USDHHS, 2017) explains that **mental health** is multifaceted and involves our emotional, psychological, and social well-being. It can be affected by a variety of influences, such as genetics, brain chemistry, and life experiences (e.g., trauma or abuse or a family history of mental health issues). Positive mental health leads to reaching full potential, coping with stressors, increased productivity, and making meaningful contributions to society (USDHHS, 2017). According to the National Alliance on Mental Illness (NAMI, 2018a), **mental illnesses** affect a person's thinking, feeling, and mood, which can make it difficult to relate to others and maintain daily functioning. Basically, mental illness can be seen as the result of flawed biological, psychological, or social processes. Fortunately, mental illness is treatable, and individuals can experience symptom relief and a return to a high level of functioning (NAMI, 2018a).

In this chapter, the reader is introduced to the concepts of mental health and mental illness, the idea of mental disorders as medical conditions, the categorization of mental illness using the *Diagnostic and Statistical Manual of Mental Disorders*, and the use of cultural beliefs to determine the factors that constitute normal and abnormal behavior.

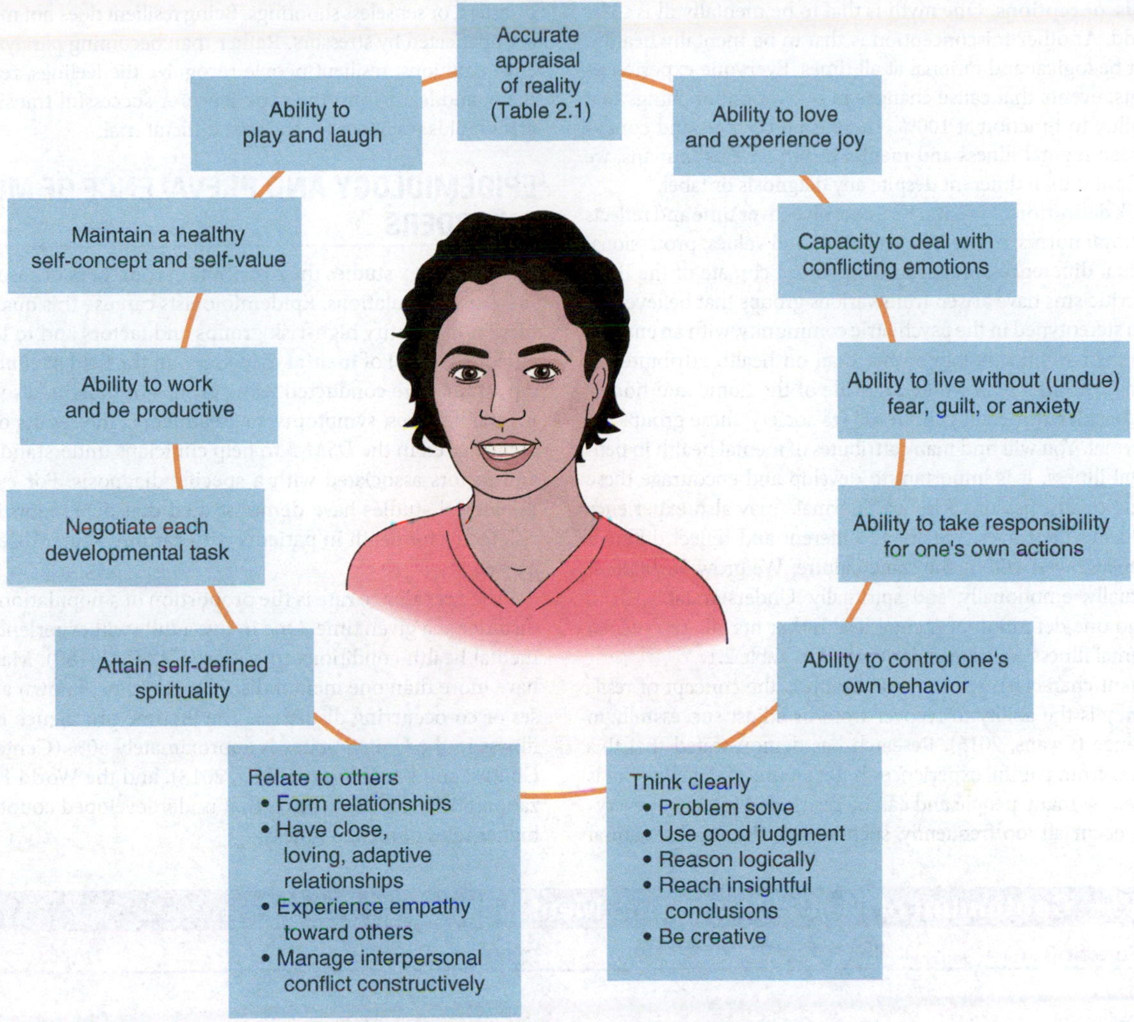

Fig. 2.1 Some attributes of mental health.

DIAGNOSTIC AND STATISTICAL MANUAL OF MENTAL DISORDERS

The ***Diagnostic and Statistical Manual of Mental Disorders*, 5th edition (*DSM-5*)** is the current official guidebook for categorizing and diagnosing psychiatric mental health disorders in the United States (American Psychological Association [APA], 2013). *The DSM-5 provides clinicians, researchers, regulatory agencies, health insurance companies, pharmacological companies, and policy makers with a standard language and criteria for the classification of mental disorders.* The *DSM-5* is used by psychiatrists, psychiatric nurse practitioners, therapists, and other clinicians as a guide for assessing, diagnosing, and planning care. The *DSM-5* lists specific diagnostic criteria for each mental disorder, which were developed using research and clinical observation. The *DSM-5* is the most recent edition, being published in 2013 after 10 years of professional discussion and debate, and some notable changes were made in this edition. One of these changes was the deletion of the five-axis system of diagnosis utilized in prior versions of the *DSM*. The intent of the axis system was to provide a global picture of an individual's functioning. Another significant change is that the coding system now mirrors, *International Statistical Classification of Diseases and Related Health Problems*, 10th Revision, Clinical Modification *(ICD-10)* codes, which are often used as part of the billing and tracking process. Although the axis system is no longer in use, it may be found in older medical documents, so a basic understanding may be helpful:

- **Axis I** lists the psychiatric diagnosis or diagnoses—for example, major depressive disorder, schizophrenia, and alcohol dependence.
- **Axis II** lists personality disorders and mental retardation to ensure long-standing issues that may co-occur with the Axis I disorders are considered, such as borderline personality disorder.
- **Axis III** lists any medical conditions the patient may have, which may or may not influence the mental health diagnosis (e.g., coronary artery disease and hypothyroidism).
- **Axis IV** lists psychosocial stressors in a brief narrative form (e.g., homelessness, going through divorce or job loss, parent–child relationship problems, or educational problems).
- **Axis V** contains the Global Assessment of Functioning (GAF). The GAF is rated on a scale of 1 to 100 and indicates the patient's level of functioning. The higher the score, the higher the level of functioning.

CONCEPTS OF MENTAL HEALTH AND ILLNESS

The Office of Disease Prevention and Health Promotion of the U.S. Department of Health and Human Services (2018) identifies mental illness as one of the leading causes of disability in the United States. Over 18% of years lost to disability are attributed to mental illness. Unfortunately, our understanding of mental illness is plagued by various

myths and misconceptions. One myth is that to be mentally ill is to be different or odd. Another misconception is that to be mentally healthy, a person must be logical and rational at all times. Everyone experiences stressing events, events that cause changes in our mood, or things that impair our ability to function at 100%. There is no obvious and consistent line between mental illness and mental health, and as humans, we are far more similar than different despite any diagnosis or label.

Psychiatry's definition of mental health evolves over time and reflects changes in cultural norms, society's expectations and values, professional biases, individual differences, and even the political climate of the time. For example, criticisms have arisen from various groups that believe that they have been stereotyped in the psychiatric community, with an emphasis on the group's psychopathology rather than on health attributes. At points in history, women who worked outside of the home and homosexuals were considered mentally ill. In today's society, these groups are considered normal. You will find many attributes of mental health in people with mental illness. It is important to develop and encourage these strengths. Additionally, persons who are "normal" may also experience dysfunction during their lives. We are all different and reflect different cultural influences, even within the same culture. We grow at different rates, intellectually, emotionally, and spiritually. Understandably, then, there can be no one definition of mental health that fits all. The mental health and mental illness continuum is depicted in Table 2.1.

An important characteristic of mental health is the concept of resiliency. **Resiliency** is the ability to recover from or adjust successfully to trauma or change (Ovans, 2015). Research has demonstrated that this ability to recover from painful experiences is not an unusual quality but is a trait possessed by many people and can be developed in almost everyone. Disasters occur all too frequently, such as terrorist attacks, natural disasters, or senseless shootings. Being resilient does not mean that people are unaffected by stressors. Rather than becoming paralyzed by the negative emotions, resilient people recognize the feelings, readily deal with them, and learn from the experience. A successful transition through a crisis builds resilience for the next difficult trial.

EPIDEMIOLOGY AND PREVALENCE OF MENTAL DISORDERS

Epidemiology studies the distribution (numbers of cases) of disorders in human populations. Epidemiologists can use this quantitative information to identify high-risk groups and factors and to learn about the etiology (cause) of **mental disorders**. In the field of *clinical* epidemiology, studies are conducted using groups of individuals with particular mental illnesses, symptoms, or treatments. The results of these studies are included in the *DSM-5* to help clinicians understand the frequency and factors associated with a specific diagnosis. For example, epidemiological studies have demonstrated that depression is a significant risk factor for death in patients with cardiovascular disease and breast cancer.

The **prevalence rate** is the proportion of a population with a mental disorder at a given time. One in five adults will experience one or more mental health conditions in a year (NAMI, 2018b). Many individuals have more than one mental disorder at a time, known as dual diagnoses or co-occurring disorders. The lifetime prevalence rate for mental illness in the United States is approximately 50% (Centers for Disease Control and Prevention [CDC], 2018), and the World Health Organization (WHO, 2018) reports that underdeveloped countries have even higher rates of mental illness.

TABLE 2.1 Continuum of Mental Health and Mental Illness

Ability to Function ⟷	Disability/Dysfunction
Happiness	
Finds life enjoyable	Loss of interest or pleasure
Optimistic about needs being met	Discouraged or hopeless mood
Control Over Behavior	
Ability to recognize cues and act appropriately	Aggressive or violent behaviors
Appraisal of Reality	
Sees environment accurately	Inaccurate perceptions of environment
Understands consequences	Hallucinations or delusions
Effectiveness in Work	
Performs within abilities	Deterioration in work performance
Recovery from minor failures	Inability to maintain steady employment
Healthy Self-Concept	
Reasonable self-confidence	Lacks self-confidence
Resourcefulness	Inability to function independently
Satisfying Relationships	
Stable, strong relationships	Unstable or intense relationships
Variety of social supports	Lack of support
Effective Coping Strategies	
Ability to problem solve and cope in ways that are not harmful (deep breathing, meditation)	Poor coping that creates further dysfunction (substance abuse, self-harm)

Modified from Redl, F., & Wattenberg, W. (1959). *Mental hygiene in teaching* (pp. 198–201). New York: Harcourt, Brace & World; Pierre, J. M. (2012). Mental illness and mental health: Is the glass half empty or half full? *Canadian Journal of Psychiatry, 57*(11), 651–658; and Winzer, R., Lindblad, F., Sorjonen, K., et al. (2014). Positive versus negative mental health in emerging adulthood: a national cross-sectional survey. *BioMed Central Public Health, 14*, 1238.

TABLE 2.2 Prevalence and Epidemiology of Psychiatric Disorders in the United States

Disorder	Prevalence Over 12 Months (%)	Estimated Number of People Affected by Disorder in the United States	Epidemiology
Schizophrenia	1.1	3.5 million	Affects men and women equally; appears earlier in men
Any affective (mood) disorder; includes major depression, dysthymic disorder, and bipolar disorder	9.5	30.0 million	Women affected at twice the rate as men; often co-occurs with anxiety and substance abuse
Major depressive disorder	6.7	21.1 million	Leading cause of disability in the United States; nearly twice as many women
Bipolar affective disorder	2.6	8.2 million	Affects men and women equally
Anxiety disorders; includes panic disorder, obsessive-compulsive disorder, posttraumatic stress disorder (PTSD), generalized anxiety disorder, and phobias	18.1	57.0 million	Frequently co-occurs with depressive disorders, eating disorders, and/or substance abuse
Panic disorder	2.7	8.5 million	Typically develops in adolescence or early adulthood; about one in three people develops agoraphobia
Obsessive-compulsive disorder	1.0	3.2 million	First symptoms begin in childhood or adolescence
PTSD	3.5	11.0 million	Can develop immediately or be delayed onset; approximately 30% of Vietnam veterans experienced PTSD; common after 9/11/01 terrorist attacks
Generalized anxiety disorder	3.1	9.8 million	Risk is highest between childhood and middle age
Social phobia	6.8	21.4 million	Typically begins in childhood or adolescence
Agoraphobia	0.8	2.5 million	
Specific phobia	8.7	27.4 million	
Any substance abuse	9.4	24.6 million	
Alcohol dependence	6.3	16.5 million	
Serious thoughts of suicide	3.8	8.7 million	

Data from National Alliance on Mental Illness. (2018). *Mental health conditions.* Retrieved from https://www.nami.org/Learn-More/Mental-Health-Conditions; and National Alliance on Mental Illness. (2018). *Mental health by the numbers.* Retrieved from https://www.nami.org/Learn-More/Mental-Health-By-the-Numbers; and Congressional Research Service. (2018). *Prevalence of mental illness in the United States: Data sources estimates.* Retrieved June 20, 2018 from https://www.fas.org/sgp/crs/misc/R43047.pdf.

Table 2.2 shows the epidemiology and prevalence rates of selected psychiatric disorders. Supported by the National Institute of Mental Health (NIMH), the study of epidemiology in mental health has progressed over the past 2 decades from simply counting the number of cases to delineating and understanding comorbidities, disease burden, and effective treatment.

Over a 12-month period, 60% of those with a mental illness received no treatment (APA, 2015). Delay to first treatment ranged from 6 to 23 years. Patients are more likely to receive help from a general medical professional or spiritual advisor than a psychiatrist because of already-established relationships and a shortage of psychiatric professionals. This illustrates that, as a nurse, you will encounter psychiatric components in your career regardless of the specialty area or clinical setting.

MENTAL ILLNESS POLICY AND PARITY

In 1996 the Mental Health Parity Act was passed by Congress, and a series of laws and commissions supporting parity followed over the next decade. This legislation required insurers to offer mental health benefits at the same level provided for medical coverage. In 2000 the Government Accountability Office found that although 86% of health plans complied with the 1996 law, they also imposed limits on mental health coverage. This has since improved with the implementation of the Affordable Care Act (ACA), which banned annual dollar limits on medical and mental health care and eliminated the lack of coverage for pre-existing conditions that had been put into effect by insurance companies during this time (USDHHS, 2015). At the writing of this text, there have been proposed budget changes that are causing some concern, with cuts in funding to the Substance Abuse and Mental Health Services Administration, a major government organization focused on the identification and treatment of mental illness and substance abuse. However, there are some additional budget items that target the opioid crisis and provide programs for people diagnosed with a serious mental illness (USDHHS, 2018).

Many of the most prevalent and disabling mental disorders have been found to have strong biological influences. Some of these include schizophrenia, bipolar disorder, depression, posttraumatic stress disorder, autism, and anorexia, among others. We can look at these disorders as "diseases" with an underlying biological component. However, this interpretation overlooks many other influences that affect the severity and progress of a mental illness and can affect a "normal" person's mental status as well. Some of these factors include support systems, family influences, developmental events, cultural beliefs and values, health practices, and negative influences impinging on an individual's life (Fig. 2.2).

The *DSM-5* cautions that the emphasis on the term *mental disorder* implies a distinction between "mental" disorder and "physical" disorder, which is an outdated concept, and stresses mind–body dualism. In physical health there is a component of mental health, and in mental health there is a physical component. The two cannot be separated as one versus another (APA, 2013).

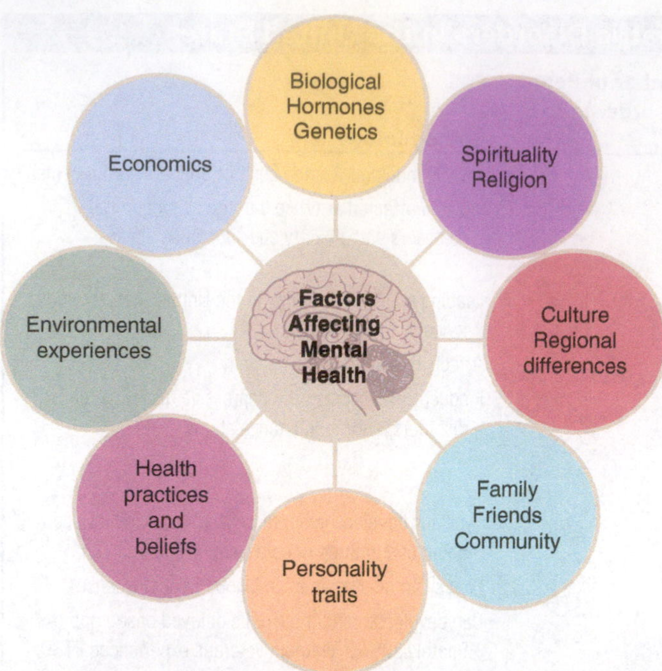

Fig. 2.2 Factors affecting mental health.

MEDICAL DIAGNOSIS AND NURSING DIAGNOSIS IN MENTAL ILLNESS

To perform their professional responsibilities, clinicians and researchers need clear and accurate guidelines for identifying and categorizing mental illness. Such guidelines help clinicians plan and evaluate treatment for their patients. A necessary element for categorization includes agreement regarding which constellation of symptoms indicate a mental illness.

Medical Diagnoses and the *DSM-5*

In the *DSM-5*, the mental disorders are clinically significant behavioral or psychological syndromes or patterns that occur in an individual and that are associated with **distress** (a painful symptom); **disability** (impairment in one or more important areas of functioning); or an increased risk of suffering death, pain, disability, or a loss of freedom or independence. This syndrome or pattern must not be merely an expected and culturally sanctioned response to a particular event, such as grief after the death of a loved one, but rather a manifestation of behavioral, psychological, or biological dysfunction in the individual as identified within the individual's cultural boundaries. Deviant behavior (e.g., political, religious, or sexual) and conflicts between the individual and society are not considered mental disorders according to the *DSM-5* unless the deviance or conflict is a symptom of a dysfunction in the individual.

It is important to stress that the *DSM-5* classifies disorders that people have, not the person. For this reason, the *DSM-5* avoids the use of expressions such as "a schizophrenic" or "an alcoholic" and instead uses the more accurate terms "an individual with schizophrenia" or "an individual with alcohol dependence." There is a recent movement in which people with an illness prefer to identify with that illness, such as individuals referring to themselves as an "Aspie" instead of a person with Asperger's. Terms like this should be used with caution and only when accepted by the individual being referred to by such a term. The *DSM* system began with the *DSM-I* in 1952 and included descriptions of 106 disorders called "reactions." The publication has progressed through extensive collaboration among experts to arrive at the current version, the *DSM-5* published in 2013. The revision process from the *DSM-IV* and *DSM-5* took a decade and brought together hundreds of international scientists during conferences supported by the National Institutes of Health (NIH). This current version delineates almost 300 diagnoses, with well-organized listings of diagnostic criteria, and is used for clinical assessment, teaching, and research purposes.

The *DSM-5* in Culturally Diverse Populations

Special efforts have been made in the *DSM-5* to incorporate an awareness that the manual is used in culturally diverse populations in the United States and internationally. Most anthropologists agree that culture includes traditions of thought, behavior, knowledge, and practices that are socially acquired, shared, and passed on to new generations (APA, 2013). The concept of culture is most often considered with racial or ethnic minority groups. However, the concept of culture also includes sexual orientation, age groups, physical abilities or disabilities, gender, religion, or socioeconomic status. Almost any group of persons with some type of shared belief can be included in the definition of culture. Therefore, clinicians are urged to consider these influences when evaluating individuals (Gopalkrishnan, 2018). Assessment can be especially challenging when a clinician from one ethnic/cultural group evaluates an individual from a different group. The *DSM-5* and prior versions are strongly biased toward a Western view of what is acceptable behavior. Some criteria considered as mental illness could, in fact, be normal in another culture. One way the *DSM-5* attempts to correct for this is through inclusion of the Cultural Formulation Interview (CFI). The CFI assesses the client's cultural perception of distress; social supports such as family and religion; and relationship factors between the patient and provider, including language and discrimination experiences in the societal majority. The *DSM-5* also provides a brief glossary of cultural concepts of distress, which includes culture-bound symptoms such as *ataque de nervios* ("attack of the nerves") or *sustos* ("fright") in Latino cultures and *shenjing shuairuo* ("weakness of the nervous system") in Mandarin Chinese culture.

Nursing Diagnoses

The psychiatric community uses the *DSM-5* to identify a common language for mental health providers and researchers. It is a way to describe and identify types of mental illness. The International Council of Nurses (2018) provides a common language called the International Classification for Nursing Practice (ICNP). This allows nurses to identify nursing diagnoses and interventions. Having a common language supports global communication, research, and policy making (International Council of Nurses, 2018). Terms are internationally accepted, which fosters communication between different regions or specialties. This text uses the ICNP terms and definitions as a reference to create a common language for the nursing process. This text will use the ICNP terms throughout, but it is good to keep in mind that, although this text is focused on mental health and appropriate nursing diagnoses within this specialty, there are terms that encompass any area of nursing. Many students may be familiar with NANDA International terms, which are very similar to those used by ICNP.

INTRODUCTION TO CULTURE AND MENTAL ILLNESS

As previously discussed, the *DSM-5* includes information related to culture in the discussion of each individual disorder, in the glossary of cultural concepts of distress, and by providing the CFI.

Health care providers must consider the influence of culture in determining the mental health or mental illness of the individual. Culture can influence how symptoms are viewed, the ability to cope with symptoms, and health-seeking behaviors (Gopalkrishnan, 2018). In developed countries, the culture supports the thought that a biological basis for mental illness and treatment is sought from health professionals such as therapists, nurse practitioners, and psychiatrists. In indigenous cultures, there is often a spiritual foundation to mental illness, and care is more likely to come from healers, such as curanderos, shaman, or other traditional practitioners. Eye contact can differ from culture to culture and should be considered during assessments. In some cultures, making eye contact is a sign of respect. In some Native American cultures, avoiding eye contact is a sign of respect. In Hispanic cultures, *mal de ojo* or the "evil eye" is caused by a look that inflicts injury, illness, or bad luck. In autism, delayed or impaired social skills, such as making eye contact, can be viewed as an indicator of the disorder. Something seemingly simple like eye contact can have a wide range of meanings.

A number of **culture-bound syndromes** (or **culture-related syndromes**) appear only in particular cultures and do not appear globally in all societies or parts of the world. For example, one form of mental illness recognized in parts of Southeast Asia is *running amok*, in which someone (usually a male) runs around engaging in furious, almost indiscriminate violent behavior. *Pibloktoq* is an uncontrollable desire to tear off one's clothing and expose oneself to severe winter weather; it is a recognized form of psychological disorder in parts of Greenland, Alaska, and the Arctic regions of Canada. In our own society, we recognize *anorexia nervosa* as a **psychobiological disorder** that entails voluntary starvation. This disorder is well known in Europe, North America, and Australia but is unheard of in many other societies.

What is to be made of the fact that certain disorders occur in some cultures but are absent in others? One interpretation is that the conditions necessary for causing a particular disorder occur in some places but are absent in others. Another interpretation is that people learn certain kinds of abnormal behavior by imitation. However, the fact that some disorders may be culturally determined does not prove that all mental illnesses are culturally based. The best evidence suggests that schizophrenia and bipolar affective disorders are found throughout the world. The symptom patterns of schizophrenia have been observed among indigenous Greenlanders and West African villagers, as well as in Western cultures. Schizophrenia could be interpreted as possession or even a positive spiritual connection in some societies.

PSYCHIATRY AND SPIRITUALITY/RELIGION

An important part of any culture is religious or spiritual beliefs. Historically, Western psychiatry tended to respect the medical approach while largely ignoring the importance of religion or spirituality in an individual's mental health. The profession of nursing has traditionally held a more holistic focus, which includes recognizing religious and/or spiritual needs of patients. Nursing leaders have contributed significantly to the body of research surrounding this concept. In more recent years, psychiatry has acknowledged and integrated the importance of religious and spiritual beliefs in the philosophy of health and healing.

Spirituality can include but is not limited to religion. Spirituality can be defined as a belief in a higher power, connection to the universe or universal energy, feeling "one" with nature, or calling on ancestors for wisdom and can include practices such as meditation, prayer, and helping others. There are many ways to achieve a spiritual connection that must be considered during assessment and diagnosis. For example, among certain cultural groups, hearing or seeing a deceased relative during bereavement is common and accepted, yet this may be misdiagnosed as a psychotic disorder by an unknowing clinician. These types of cultural misunderstandings have contributed to the distrust that minority or immigrant groups can hold toward psychiatric professionals.

Altered states of consciousness, such as those achieved through mysticism, meditation, and mindfulness, can be spiritually enriching and bring peace and serenity into people's lives but should not be confused with dissociative states caused by trauma. Meditation has many health benefits, is a valuable tool for dealing with chronic pain and stress, is a component of dialectic behavioral therapy (DBT) and stress-reduction programs, and plays a role in many other types of therapy.

Prayer is a widely used religious/spiritual ritual. Individuals pray for comfort, to make requests, and to offer praise. Prayer may incorporate singing, dancing, jumping, reciting prescribed words, and praying at certain locations or times. Prayer represents a way to connect with God or a supreme spiritual being or natural energy and to find support and meaning in life. A study on the effect of prayer on depression and anxiety showed improvement in symptoms when used in combination with medication management. Improvements were seen even a year after the study was conducted (Boelens et al., 2012).

A traditional helping strategy that is also identified as evidence-based practice is the use of storytelling. A tribal leader in indigenous cultures or a therapist in Western cultures can use a metaphor to offer a social message, create a narrative to help a child understand and cope with trauma, or help older adults reconnect with positive memories from the past.

APPLYING EVIDENCE-BASED PRACTICE (EBP)

Problem

An elementary school child is having difficulty focusing in class and turning in homework and is disruptive. The child was evaluated and diagnosed with attention-deficit/hyperactivity disorder (ADHD). The parents are refusing to have the child treated because they do not want the child to "be labeled or on medications that will cause him to be addicted."

EBP Assessment

A. **What do you already know from experience?** Parents can be reluctant to admit problems with their children because of embarrassment, fear, and lack of knowledge. Errors can occur in both overmedicating and undermedicating patients. When needed, medications can make a remarkable difference.

B. **What does the literature say?** Stigma and discrimination against people with mental illness are major barriers to success in relationships, treatment, and employment. Patients often avoid treatment as a result of stigma. Research shows that properly treated patients with ADHD are *less* likely to have addiction problems.

C. **What does the patient want?** The child in this case study wanted treatment because of decreasing self-esteem and performance at school. The parents are reluctant and refusing.

Plan

Educate the parents in a nonjudgmental fashion about the benefits of medication and therapy, including preserving the child's self-esteem, social functioning, and school performance. Ultimately, the parents understood the need to help their child and accepted treatment. Medication times were scheduled so that the child did not have to take medication at school, maintaining confidentiality. Unfortunately, stigma remains a concern for anyone receiving mental health treatment.

QSEN Prelicensure Knowledge, Skills, and Attitudes (KSAs) Addressed

Patient-Centered Care by seeing the situation through both the child's and parents' perspectives and maintaining confidentiality

Evidence-Based Practice by using current research to help educate the parents and develop a plan of care that addresses their concerns

STIGMA

Closely related to culture and spirituality is the concept of stigma. **Stigma** is a negative stereotype that leads to an attitude or belief that would cause one to view a person with mental illness as inferior, dangerous, or unstable (Mayo Clinic, 2017). Stigma has been acknowledged as a major barrier to mental health treatment and recovery. Stigma contributes to fear, rejection, and discrimination against the mentally ill. Stereotyping, labeling, and separating can occur on an individual or institutional level, resulting in an imbalance of power. Stigma can have harmful effects on an individual and family and result in social isolation and reduced opportunities. For example, the stigma of mental illness interferes with the person's ability to establish and maintain friendships, employment, and housing. It also leads to health care disparities, which affects the person's ability to obtain psychological and general medical treatment. Health care disparities are gaps in care for various subcultures.

An example of the cultural influence of stigmatizing in psychiatry is the inclusion of homosexuality as a disorder in earlier versions of the *DSM*, even though research consistently failed to demonstrate that people with a homosexual orientation were any more maladjusted than heterosexuals. Change occurred in the medical and psychiatric communities only through the efforts of gay rights' activists. Stigma and bias also affect minority groups, the elderly, children, and women.

Biases are often reflected in our organizational structures and political systems. Awareness of the dangers inherent in stereotyping and stigmatizing attitudes has enormous implications for nursing practice, especially in the field of mental health. It is important to remember that a patient is first and foremost a human being and not the patient's diagnosis. Although diagnoses are used to structure treatment and for billing purposes, labeling should be avoided whenever possible.

KEY POINTS TO REMEMBER

- Mental illness can be difficult to define. The *DSM-5* and cultural norms must be considered in evaluating mental health and illness.
- There are many myths surrounding mental illness, which contribute to the stigmatization of individuals. The stereotyping, discrimination, and rejection accompanying stigma contribute to poor self-image, isolation, and mental anguish. Stigma erects barriers to obtaining employment, housing, and health services. Nurses can use sensitivity and compassion to bridge the shame patients feel and encourage them to seek care.
- Mental health can be conceptualized along a continuum, from mild to moderate to severe to a profound degree of impairment in functioning.
- There are various components and influences that contribute to mental health, which are identified in Fig. 2.1.
- The study of epidemiology can help identify high-risk groups and behaviors and lead to enhanced understanding of causes and best treatment. Prevalence rates help us identify the proportion of a population with a mental disorder at a given time.
- With the current knowledge that many common mental disorders are biologically based, they are now recognized as medical diseases.
- Identifying a common language or set of terms, as has been done with the *DSM-5* and International Nursing Council definitions, helps to improve communication and coordination of care.

APPLYING CRITICAL JUDGMENT

1. A 23-year-old male was brought to the emergency department by ambulance after a suicide attempt. He has been extremely depressed since his girlfriend died in a car accident 5 months ago. He was the driver. Since the accident, he has not been attending college. He has also not shown up for his tutoring job. The patient's existing seizure disorder has worsened since the accident, but he refuses treatment. He states he deserves to be punished for "killing my girlfriend."
   - A. What evidence can you identify indicating a decline in the patient's level of functioning?
   - B. How might the patient's religious beliefs hinder and/or help his recovery?
   - C. Formulate one nursing diagnosis and two interventions reflective of his mental health needs.
   - D. Identify a concept from this chapter, such as stigma, support system, or culture, and relate it to this scenario.
   - E. Using the mental health continuum, would you rate this patient's symptoms as mild, moderate, or severe?
2. Reflect on an encounter you had with someone from an unfamiliar background in your personal or work life. What did you learn from the experience? How was the person's background similar to or different from your own? How could this affect the therapeutic nursing relationship?
3. Before your first day of clinical in the mental health setting, briefly describe in writing your current thoughts and attitudes about people with mental illnesses and working with them. Where or how do you think you developed these perceptions? After the clinical day, reflect upon the experience. Have your perceptions changed, and if so, in what way?

CHAPTER REVIEW QUESTIONS

1. A mentally ill gunman opens fire in a crowded movie theater, killing six people and injuring others. Which comment about this event by a member of the community most clearly shows the stigma of mental illness?
   a. "Gun control laws are inadequate in our country."
   b. "It's frightening to feel that it is not safe to go to a movie theater."
   c. "All these people with mental illness are violent and should be locked up."
   d. "These events happen because American families no longer go to church together."
2. The nurse presents a class about mental health and mental illness to a group of fourth graders. One student asks, "Why do people get mentally ill?" Select the nurse's best response.
   a. "There are many reasons why mental illness occurs."
   b. "The cause of mental illness is complicated and very hard to understand."
   c. "Sometimes a person's brain does not work correctly because something bad happens or he or she inherits a brain problem."
   d. "Most mental illnesses result from genetically transmitted abnormalities in cerebral structure; however, some are a consequence of traumatic life experiences."
3. An adult experienced a spinal cord injury resulting in quadriplegia 3 years ago and now lives permanently in a skilled care facility. Which comment by this person best demonstrates resiliency?
   a. "I often pray for a miracle that will heal my paralysis so I will be whole again."
   b. "I don't know what I did to deserve this fate or whether I am tough enough to endure it."
   c. "My accident was a twist of fate. I suppose there are worse things than being paralyzed."
   d. "Being paralyzed has taken things from me, but it hasn't kept me from being mentally involved in life."
4. A nursing assistant says to the nurse, "The schizophrenic in room 226 has been rambling all day." When considering the nurse's responsibility to manage the ancillary staff, which response should the nurse provide?
   a. "It is more respectful to refer to the patient by name than by diagnosis."
   b. "Thank you for informing me about that. I will document the behavior."
   c. "It is not unusual for schizophrenics to do that. It's just part of their illness."
   d. "You have a difficult job. I'm glad you are so accepting of our patients' behaviors."
5. Which scenario meets the criteria for "normal" behavior?
   a. An 8-year-old child's only verbalization is "No, no, no."
   b. A 16-year-old girl usually sleeps for 3 or 4 hours per night.
   c. A 43-year-old man cries privately for 1 month after the death of his wife.
   d. A 64-year-old woman has difficulty remembering the names of her grandchildren.

REFERENCES

American Psychological Association. (2013). *Diagnostic and statistical manual of mental disorders (DSM-5)* (5th ed.). Washington, DC: APA.

American Psychological Association. (2015). *Data on behavioral health in the United States.* Retrieved from www.apa.org/helpcenter/data-behavioral-health.aspx.

Boelens, P., Reeves, R. R., Replogle, W. H., & Koenig, H. G. (2012). The effect of prayer on depression and anxiety: Maintenance of positive influence one year after prayer intervention. *International Journal of Psychiatry in Medicine, 43*(1), 85–98. https://doi.org/10.2190/PM.43.1.f.

Centers for Disease Control and Prevention. (2018). *Mental health basics.* Retrieved from https://www.cdc.gov/mentalhealth/learn/index.htm.

Giddens, J. F. (2017). *Concepts for nursing practice* (2nd ed). St. Louis: Elsevier.

Gopalkrishnan, N. (2018). Cultural diversity and mental health: Considerations for policy and practice. *Frontiers in Public Health, 47*(2010), 610–628. https://doi.org/10.3389/fpubh.2018.00179.

International Council of Nurses. (2018). *International Classification for Nursing Practice (ICNP) information sheet.* Retrieved from http://www.icn.ch/images/stories/documents/pillars/Practice/icnp/ICNP_FAQs.pdf.

Mayo Clinic. (2017). *Mental health: Overcoming the stigma of mental health.* Retrieved from http://www.mayoclinic.org/diseases-conditions/mental-illness/in-depth/mental-health/art-20046477.

National Alliance on Mental Illness (NAMI). (2018a). *Mental health conditions.* Retrieved June 29, 2018 from https://www.nami.org/Learn-More/Mental-Health-Conditions.

National Alliance on Mental Illness (NAMI). (2018b). *Mental health by the numbers.* Retrieved June 29, 2018 from https://www.nami.org/Learn-More/Mental-Health-By-the-Numbers.

Office of Disease Prevention and Health Promotion (ODPHP) and the United States Department of Health and Human Services (USDHHS). (2018). *Mental health and mental disorders.* Retrieved June 29, 2018 from https://www.healthypeople.gov/2020/topics-objectives/topic/mental-health-and-mental-disorders.

Ovans, A. (2015). *What resilience means, and why it matters.* Harvard Business Review. Retrieved from https://hbr.org/2015/01/what-resilience-means-and-why-it-matters.

U.S. Department of Health and Human Services (USDHHS). (2015). *Key concepts of the Affordable Care Act.* Retrieved from http://www.hhs.gov/healthcare/facts-and-features/key-features-of-aca-by-year/index.html#.

U.S. Department of Health and Human Services. (2017). *What is mental health?* Retrieved June 29, 2018 from https://www.mentalhealth.gov/basics/what-is-mental-health.

U.S. Department of Health and Human Services. (2018). *FY 2019 budget in brief.* Retrieved June 29, 2018 from https://www.hhs.gov/sites/default/files/fy-2019-budget-in-brief.pdf.

World Health Organization. (2018). *Mental disorders: Key facts.* Retrieved from https://www.who.int/en/news-room/fact-sheets/detail/mental-disorders.

3

Theories and Therapies

Margaret Jordan Halter

http://evolve.elsevier.com/Varcarolis/essentials

OBJECTIVES

1. Discuss the contributions of theories and therapies from a variety of disciplines and areas of expertise.
2. Choose two of the major theories that you believe are among the most relevant to psychiatric and mental health nursing care and defend your choice, giving examples.
3. Identify the origins and progression of dominant theories and treatment modalities.
4. Discuss the relevance of these theories and treatments to the provision of psychiatric and mental health care.
5. Demonstrate comprehensive understanding of Peplau's theoretical base for practice that is beneficial to all settings.
6. Identify three different theoretical models of mental health care, and demonstrate how each could be used in specific circumstances.
7. Distinguish models of care used in clinical settings, and cite benefits and limitations of these models.

KEY TERMS AND CONCEPTS

autocratic leader, p. 28
automatic thoughts, p. 24
aversion therapy, p. 22
behavioral therapy (or behavior modification), p. 22
biofeedback, p. 22
boundaries, p. 30
cognitive-behavioral therapy (CBT), p. 24
cognitive distortions, p. 24
community meetings, p. 30
conscious, p. 19
conservation, p. 25
countertransference, p. 21
curative factors, p. 29
democratic leader, p. 29
ego, p. 19
egocentric thinking, p. 25
group, p. 28
group content, p. 28
group development, p. 28
group process, p. 28
id, p. 19
interpersonal therapy (IPT), p. 22
laissez-faire leader, p. 29
leadership style, p. 28
Maslow's hierarchy of needs theory, p. 22
object permanence, p. 25
person-centered therapy, p. 23
preconscious, p. 19
psychotherapy, p. 19
psychoanalytic therapy, p. 19
psychodynamic therapy, p. 21
recovery model, p. 27
schemata, p. 24
self-actualization, p. 23
self-transcendence, p. 23
superego, p. 19
systematic desensitization, p. 22
transference, p. 21
unconscious, p. 19

CONCEPT: FAMILY DYNAMICS: *Family dynamics* is defined as the forces at work within a family that produce particular behaviors or symptoms. The dynamic is created by the way in which family members live and interact with one another. That dynamic, whether positive or negative, supportive or destructive, nurturing or damaging, changes who people are and influences how they view and interact with the world outside of the family (Giddens, 2017). Family therapy is an adjunct to individual treatment and refers to the treatment of the family as a whole. The major goals of family therapy are to improve family communication skills, heighten awareness and sensitivity to other family members' emotional needs, and strengthen the family's ability to cope with major life stressors and traumatic events.

INTRODUCTION

We expect others (and ourselves) to behave in certain ways, and we seek explanations for behavior that deviates from what we believe to be normal. What causes excessive sadness or extreme happiness? How do we explain mistrust, anxiety, confusion, or apathy—degrees of which may range from mildly disturbing to incapacitating? It is by understanding a problem that we can begin to devise solutions to treat or eradicate it. Mental illness has long defied explanation, even as other so-called physical illnesses were being quantified and often controlled.

It was not until the late 1800s that psychological models and theories were conceived, developed, and disseminated into mainstream

TABLE 3.1 Major Theories of Psychiatric Care

Theory	Theorist	Tenets	Therapeutic Model
Psychoanalytic	Freud	Unconscious thoughts; psychosexual development.	Psychoanalysis to learn unconscious thoughts; therapist is nondirective and interprets meaning.
Interpersonal	Sullivan	Relationships are the basis for mental health or illness.	Therapy focuses on here and now and emphasizes relationships; therapist is an active participant.
Behavioral	Pavlov, Watson, Skinner	Behavior is learned through conditioning.	Behavioral modification addresses maladaptive behaviors by rewarding adaptive behavior.
Cognitive	Beck	Negative and self-critical thinking cause depression.	Cognitive-behavioral therapists assist in identifying negative thought patterns and replacing them with rational ones; therapy often involves homework.
Biological	Many	Psychiatric disorders are heavily influenced by and/or cause changes to the brain and/or neurotransmitter(s), resulting in changes in thinking and behavior.	Neurochemical imbalances are corrected through medication and talk therapy (e.g., cognitive-behavioral therapy).

thinking. They provided structure for considering developmental processes and possible explanations for our thoughts, feelings, and behaviors. The theorists believed that if complex workings of the mind could be understood, they could also be treated, and from these models and theories, therapies evolved.

Early practitioners used various forms of talk therapy, formally known as **psychotherapy**, that focused on the complexity and inner workings of the mind. These early talk therapies emphasized environmental influences on mental health and illness. Beginning in the early 20th century, biological explanations for mental alterations began to gain acceptance. Currently, the dominant belief is that psychiatric disorders and conditions are the result of both genetic variables and environmental factors.

Mental health professionals continue to rely on theoretical models as a basis for treating psychiatric alterations. This chapter provides an overview of therapeutic models and related treatments and discusses the potential connection between them and the provision of psychiatric nursing care. Table 3.1 provides a snapshot of the major theories.

PROMINENT THEORIES AND THERAPEUTIC MODELS

Psychoanalytic Theory

Sigmund Freud (1856–1939), an Austrian neurologist, is considered the "father of psychiatry." His work was based on psychoanalytic theory, in which Freud claims that most psychological disturbances are the result of early trauma or incidents that are often not remembered or recognized.

Freud (1961) identified three layers of mental activity: the conscious, the preconscious, and the unconscious mind. The **conscious** mind is your current awareness—thoughts, beliefs, and feelings. However, most of the mind's activity occurs outside of this conscious awareness, like an iceberg with its bulk hidden under the water. The **preconscious** mind lies immediately below the surface. Although its content is not currently the subject of our attention, it is accessible with conscious effort. The deepest and biggest chunk of the iceberg is referred to as the unconscious mind. The **unconscious** is where our most primitive feelings, drives, and memories reside, especially those that are unbearable and traumatic. The conscious mind is then influenced by the preconscious and unconscious mind (Fig. 3.1).

One of Freud's later and widely known constructs concerns the interactive agents within the brain known as the id, the ego, and the superego (see Fig. 3.1).

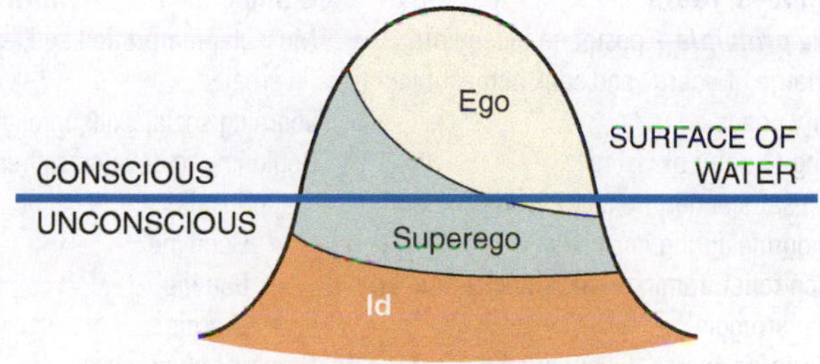

Fig. 3.1 The mind as an iceberg.

- The **id** is the primitive, pleasure-seeking, and impulsive part (according to Freud, predominantly sexual pleasure) of our personalities that lurks in the unconscious mind.
- The **ego** is the problem solver and reality tester that navigates in the outside world. It acts as an intermediary between the id and reality by using ego defense mechanisms, such as repression, denial, and rationalization (see Chapter 11).
- The **superego** represents the moral component of the personality that Freud referred to as our conscience (our sense of what is right or wrong). The superego is greatly influenced by parents' or caregivers' moral and ethical stances.

In healthy individuals, the three systems of the personality work together under the administrative leadership of the ego. The ego is able to realistically evaluate situations, limit the id's primitive impulses, and keep the superego from becoming too rigid and obsessive.

Freud believed that personality development is based on stages. During these stages, the id focuses on an erogenous zone of the body. These zones are oral, anal, and phallic. Fixation through overindulgence or frustration results in pathological conditions and personality disorders. Freud's work has been criticized for a variety of reasons. One of the harshest criticisms stems from the concept of penis envy, in which females suffer from feelings of inferiority for not having male genitalia. Table 3.2 provides a summary of Freud's developmental stages, along with Sullivan's and Erikson's, two other models that are discussed later in this chapter.

Therapeutic Model

Psychoanalytic therapy was Freud's answer for a scientific method to relieve emotional disturbances. An often time-consuming (e.g., three to five times a week for many years), expensive, and emotionally painful process, the goal of this therapy is to know and understand what is happening at the unconscious level in order to uncover the truth.

TABLE 3.2 Development of Personality According to Freud, Sullivan, and Erikson[a]

Freud	Sullivan	Erikson
Oral: Birth to 1½ Years ***Pleasure–pain principle*** ***Id,*** the instinctive and primitive mind, is dominant Demanding, impulsive, irrational, asocial, selfish, trustful, omnipotent, and dependent Primary thought processes Unconscious instincts—source–energy–aim–object Mouth—primary source of pleasure Immediate release of tension/anxiety and immediate gratification through oral gratification ***Task***—develop a sense of trust that needs will be met	**Infancy: Birth to 1½ Years** Mothering object relieves tension through empathic intervention and tenderness, leading to decreased anxiety and increased satisfaction and security; mother becomes symbolized as "good mother" Goal is biological satisfaction and psychological security Denial of tension relief creates anxiety, and mother becomes symbolized as "bad mother" Anxiety in mother yields anxiety and fear in child via empathy These states are experienced by the child in a diffuse and undifferentiated manner ***Task***—learn to count on others for satisfaction and security to trust	**Infancy: Birth to 1½ Years** ***Trust vs. mistrust*** Egocentric ***Danger***—during second half of first year, an abrupt and prolonged separation may intensify the natural sense of loss and may lead to a sense of mistrust that may last throughout life ***Task***—develop a basic sense of trust that leads to hope Trust requires a feeling of physical comfort and a minimal experience of fear or uncertainty; if this occurs, the child will extend trust to the world and self
Anal: 1½–3 Years ***Reality principle***—postpone immediate discharge of energy and seek actual object to satisfy needs Learning to defer pleasure Gaining satisfaction from tolerating some tension-mastering impulses Focus on toilet training—retaining/letting go; power struggle ***Ego development***—functions of the ego include problem-solving skills, perception, ability to mediate id impulses ***Task***—delay immediate gratification	**Childhood: 1½–6 Years** Muscular maturation and learning to communicate verbally Learning social skills through consensual validation Beginning to develop self-esteem via reflected appraisals: • Good me • Bad me • Not me Levels of awareness: • Awareness • Selective inattention • Dissociation ***Task***—learn to delay satisfaction of wishes with relative comfort	**Early Childhood: 1½–3 Years** ***Autonomy vs. shame/doubt*** Develop confidence in physical and mental abilities that leads to the development of an autonomous will ***Danger***—development of a deep sense of shame/doubt if child is deprived of the opportunity to rebel; learns to expect defeat in any battle of wills with those who are bigger and stronger ***Task***—gain self-control of and independence within the environment
Phallic: 3–7 Years ***Superego develops*** via incorporating moral values, ideals, and judgments of right and wrong that are held by parents; superego is primarily unconscious and functions on the **reward and punishment principle** (sexual identity attained via resolving oedipal conflict) Conflict differs for boy and girl; masturbatory activity ***Task***—develop sexual identity through identification with same-sex parent		**Play Age: 3–6 Years** ***Initiative vs. guilt*** Interest in socially appropriate goals leads to a sense of purpose Imagination is greatly expanded because of increased ability to move around freely and increased ability to communicate Intrusive activity and curiosity and consuming fantasies, which lead to feelings of guilt and anxiety Establishment of conscience ***Danger***—may develop a deep-seated conviction that he or she is essentially bad, with a resultant stifling of initiative or a conversion of moralism to vindictiveness ***Task***—achieve a sense of purpose and develop a sense of mastery over tasks
Latency: 7–12 Years Desexualization; libido diffused Involved in learning social skills, exploring, building, collecting, accomplishing, and hero worship Peer-group loyalty begins Gang and scout behavior Growing independence from family ***Task***—sexuality is repressed during this time; learn to form close relationship(s) with same-sex peers	**Juvenile: 6–9 Years** Absorbed in learning to deal with ever-widening outside world, peers, and other adults Reflections and revisions of self-image and parental images ***Task***—develops satisfying interpersonal relationships with peers that involve competition and compromise **Preadolescence: 9–12 Years** Develop intimate interpersonal relationship with person of same sex who is perceived to be much like oneself in interests, feelings, and mutual collaboration ***Task***—learn to care for others of same sex who are outside the family; Sullivan called this the "normal homosexual phase"	**School Age: 6–12 Years** ***Industry vs. inferiority*** Develops a healthy competitive drive that leads to confidence In learning to accept instruction and to win recognition by producing "things," the child opens the way for the capacity of work enjoyment ***Danger***—the development of a sense of inadequacy and inferiority in a child who does not receive recognition ***Task***—gain a sense of self-confidence and recognition through learning, competing, and performing successfully

Continued

TABLE 3.2 Development of Personality According to Freud, Sullivan, and Erikson[a]—cont'd

Freud	Sullivan	Erikson
Genital Phase (Adolescence): 13–20 Years Fluctuation regarding emotional stability and physical maturation Very ambivalent and labile, seeking life goals and emancipation from parents Dependence vs. independence Reappraisal of parents and self; intense peer loyalty ***Task***—form close relationships with members of the opposite sex based on genuine caring and pleasure in the interaction	**Adolescence: 12–20 Years** *Early adolescence: 12–14 years* Establishing satisfying relationships with opposite sex *Late adolescence: 14–20 years* Interdependent and establishing durable sexual relations with a select member of the opposite sex ***Task***—form intimate and long-lasting relationships with the opposite sex and develop a sense of identity	**Adolescence: 12–20 Years** ***Identity vs. role confusion*** Diffusion Differentiation from parents leads to fidelity (sense of self) Physiological revolution that accompanies puberty (rapid body growth and sexual maturity) forces the young person to question beliefs and to refight many of the earlier battles ***Danger***—temporary identity diffusion (instability) may result in a permanent inability to integrate a personal identity ***Task***—integrate all the tasks previously mastered into a secure sense of self
		Young Adulthood: 20–30 Years ***Intimacy and solidarity vs. isolation*** Maturity and social responsibility result in the ability to love and be loved As people feel more secure in their identity, they are able to establish intimacy with themselves (their inner lives) and with others, eventually in a love-based, satisfying sexual relationship with a member of the opposite sex ***Danger***—fear of losing identity may prevent intimate relationship and result in a deep sense of isolation ***Task***—form intense long-term relationships and commit to another person, cause, institution, or creative effort
		Adulthood: 30 to 65 Years ***Generativity vs. self-absorption*** Interest in nurturing subsequent generations creates a sense of caring, contributing, and generativity ***Danger***—lack of generativity results in self-absorption and stagnation ***Task***—achieve life goals and obtain concern and awareness of future generations
		Senescence: 65 Years to Death ***Integrity vs. despair*** Acceptance of mortality and satisfaction with life loads to wisdom Satisfying intimacy with other human beings and adaptive response to triumphs and disappointments Marked by a sense of what life is and was and its place in the flow of history ***Danger***—without this "accrued ego integration," there is despair, usually marked by a display of displeasure and distrust ***Task***—derive meaning from one's whole life and obtain/maintain a sense of self-worth

[a]Developed from original sources by Freud, Sullivan, and Erikson.

The analyst is nondirective but does give his or her interpretations of symbols, thoughts, and dreams. *Free association* is used to search for forgotten and repressed memories. The patient is encouraged to say anything that comes to mind in response to a word or phrase. For example, "What do you think of when I say 'water'?" A patient may respond, "Warm … June … darkness … can't breathe," revealing a long-forgotten and traumatic near-drowning incident.

Psychodynamic therapy is theoretically related to psychoanalytic therapy and views the mind in essentially the same way. It tends to be shorter, about 10 to 12 sessions. The therapist takes a more active role because the therapeutic relationship is part of the healing process.

Transference occurs as the patient projects intense feelings onto the therapist related to unfinished work from previous relationships. Safe expression of these feelings is crucial to successful therapy. An example of this would be a when a patient acts more immature when in the presence of a therapist who reminds the patient of his or her mother. Psychodynamic therapists are taught to recognize that they, too, have unconscious emotional responses to the patient. This **countertransference** must be scrutinized in order to prevent damage to the therapeutic relationship.

Interpersonal Theory

Interpersonal theory focuses on what occurs between people, as opposed to psychoanalytic theory, which is rooted in what occurs in the mind. Herbert "Harry" Stack Sullivan (1892–1949), an American psychiatrist, believed that social forces and interpersonal problems were the cause of psychiatric alterations.

According to Sullivan (1953), human beings are driven by the need for interaction. In fact, loneliness is considered the most painful human experience. He emphasized the early relationship with the *significant other* (primary parenting figure) as crucial for personality development and believed that healthy relationships are necessary for a healthy personality.

Despite our need for human interaction, Sullivan believed that interaction is the source of anxiety. In the earliest relationship, anxiety is transmitted from the significant other to the child. The child's anxiety is also based on perceived degrees of approval or disapproval of the primary caregiver. According to Sullivan, all behavior is aimed at avoiding anxiety and threats to self-esteem.

One of the ways that we avoid anxiety is by focusing on positive attributes, or the *good me* ("I'm a good skier"), and hiding the negative aspects, the *bad me* ("I failed an exam"), of ourselves from others and maybe even from ourselves. The *not me* is used to separate us from parts of ourselves that we cannot bear to acknowledge that are pushed deep into the unconscious and disassociated from our sense of self. An example is a female adolescent from a strict and conservative family who begins to have stirrings of attraction toward girls, yet firmly maintains (and believes) that she has feelings for and interest in boys.

Sullivan's theory of development echoes that of Freud's in that personalities are influenced by the social environment as children, particularly as adolescents. He believed that personality is most influenced by the mother but that personality can be molded even in adulthood. Table 3.2 summarizes Sullivan's interpersonal theory of development.

Therapeutic Model

Interpersonal therapy (IPT) is a hands-on system in which therapists actively guide and challenge maladaptive behaviors and distorted views. The premise for this work is that if people are aware of their dysfunctional patterns and unrealistic expectations, they can modify them. The focus is on the here and now, with an emphasis on the patient's life and relationships at home, at work, and socially. The therapist becomes a "participant observer" and reflects the patient's interpersonal behavior, including responses to the therapist.

Behavioral Theories

As the psychoanalytic movement was developing in the 20th century, so, too, was the behaviorist school of thought. Ivan Pavlov (1927) is famous for investigating *classical conditioning,* in which involuntary behavior or reflexes can be conditioned to respond to neutral stimuli. Pavlov's dogs became accustomed to receiving food after a bell was rung. Later, these dogs salivated in response to the sound of the bell alone. For human beings, classical conditioning can occur under such circumstances as when a baby's crying induces a milk-letdown reflex or when a rape victim begins to hyperventilate and sweat when she hears footsteps behind her.

John B. Watson (1930) rejected psychoanalysis and sought an objective therapy that did not focus on unconscious motivations. He contended that personality traits and responses, adaptive and maladaptive, are learned. In a famous and ethically awful experiment, Watson conditioned Little Albert, a 9-month-old child, to be terrified at the sight of white fur or hair. He concluded that through behavioral techniques, anyone could be trained to be anything, from a beggar to a merchant.

B. F. Skinner (1938) conducted research on operant conditioning in which voluntary behaviors are learned through consequences of positive reinforcement (a consequence that causes the behavior to occur more frequently) or negative reinforcement or punishment (a consequence that causes the behavior to occur less frequently). An example of positive reinforcement is studying hard, which results in good grades and increases the chances that studying will continue to occur. An example of negative reinforcement is driving too fast, which may result in a speeding ticket. This ticket should decrease the chances that speeding will occur in the future.

Therapeutic Models

Behavioral therapy, or **behavior modification**, uses basic tenets from each of the behaviorists described previously. It attempts to correct or eliminate maladaptive behaviors or responses by rewarding and reinforcing adaptive behavior.

Systematic desensitization is based on classical conditioning. The premise is that learned responses can be reversed by first promoting relaxation and then gradually facing a particular anxiety-provoking stimulus. This method has been particularly successful in extinguishing extreme fears, or phobias. Agoraphobia, the fear of open places, can be treated by initially visualizing trips outdoors while using relaxation techniques. Later, the individual can practice actual excursions that gradually increase in length, thereby eliminating or reducing agoraphobia.

Aversion therapy is based on both classical and operant conditioning. It is used to eradicate unwanted habits by associating unpleasant consequences with them. One pharmacologically based aversion therapy is disulfiram (Antabuse). People who take this medication and then ingest alcohol become extremely ill, with nausea, vomiting, and dizziness. Aversion therapy has also been used with sex offenders, who may, for example, receive electric shocks in response to arousal from child pornography.

Biofeedback is a technique in which individuals learn to control physiological responses such as breathing rates, heart rates, blood pressure, brain waves, and skin temperature. This control is achieved by providing visual or auditory biofeedback of the physiological response and then using relaxation techniques such as slow, deep breathing or meditation. There is a recent emergence of smartphone apps and wearable devices that provide this immediate physiological feedback.

Humanistic Theory

Humanists rejected the psychoanalysts' focus on unconscious conflicts, which they considered too pessimistic. They also rejected the behaviorists' focus on learning, which they considered too scientific. The humanists developed a psychological science concerned with the human potential for development, knowledge attainment, motivation, and understanding.

Maslow's hierarchy of needs theory was introduced by the American psychologist Abraham Maslow (1971). Needs are placed conceptually on a pyramid, with the most basic and important needs on the lower level (Fig. 3.2). The higher levels, the more distinctly human needs, occupy the top sections of the pyramid. According to Maslow, when deficiencies at the lower levels are fulfilled, higher-level needs can emerge.

- *Physiological needs.* The most basic needs are the physiological drives, including the need for food, oxygen, water, sleep, sex, and a constant body temperature. If all levels in the pyramid were deprived, this level would take priority.
- *Safety needs.* Once physiological needs are met, safety needs take precedence. Safety needs include security, protection, and freedom from fear and chaos. Safety needs include seeking law, order, and limits.

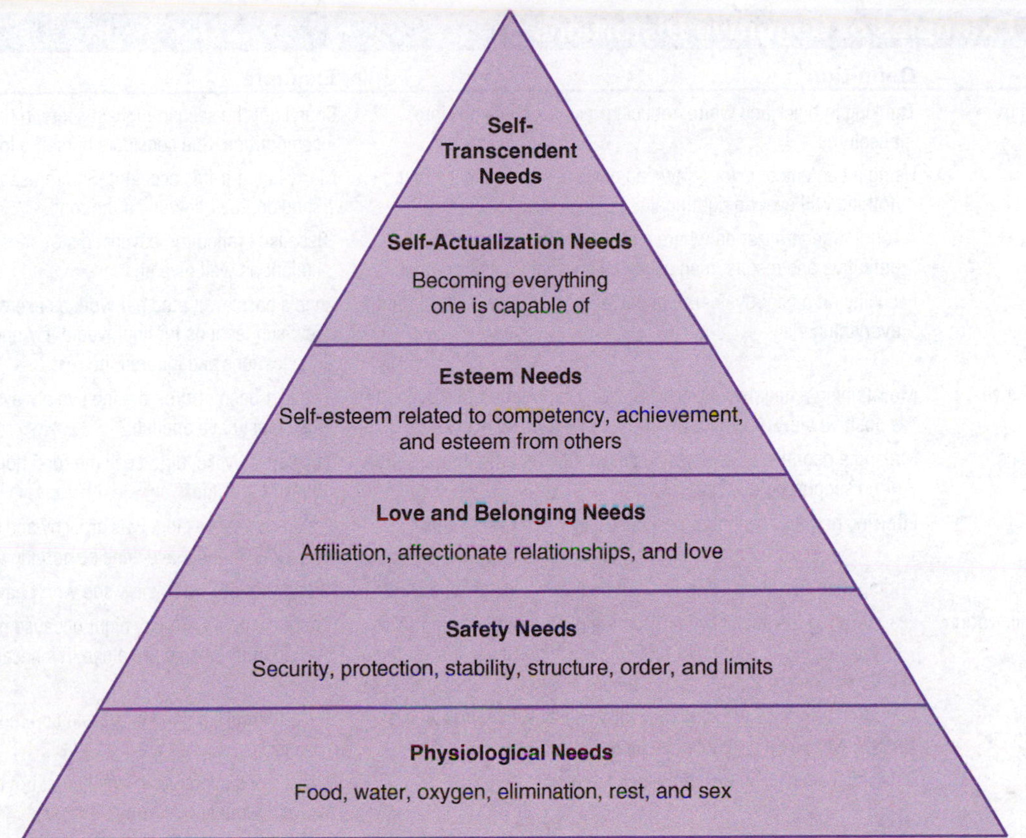

Fig. 3.2 Maslow's hierarchy of needs. (Adapted from Maslow, A. H. [1971]. *The farther reaches of human nature.* New York, NY: Viking.)

- *Belonging and love needs.* People seek belonging, intimate relationships, love, and affection to overcome loneliness and alienation. Maslow stresses the importance of having a family, having a home, and being part of identifiable groups.
- *Esteem needs.* People need to have a positive self-regard and have it reflected to them from others. If self-esteem needs are met, we feel confident, valued, and valuable. When self-esteem is compromised, we feel inferior, worthless, and helpless.
- ***Self-actualization.*** According to Maslow, we are hard-wired to be everything that we are capable of becoming, to fulfill our own potential. He said, "What a man *can* be, he *must* be." What we are capable of becoming is highly individual—an artist must paint, a writer must write, and a healer must heal. The drive to satisfy this need is felt as a sort of restlessness, a sense that something is missing.
- ***Self-transcendence.*** Self-transcendence refers to the drive to go beyond the personal self. This moving beyond oneself is evident in mystical, aesthetic, and emotional peak experiences of seeking a higher truth, often in the service of other people, other species, nature, and the cosmos.

Maslow later added two other interrelated needs: cognitive and aesthetic. The acquisition of knowledge and the need to understand are inborn and essential drives. Human beings are hard-wired to be curious, explore, and find meaning. In much the same way, aesthetic needs result in a craving and a search for beauty and symmetry and the contemplation of these qualities.

Therapeutic Model

Carl Rogers, an American psychologist, popularized **person-centered therapy** in the 1940s. Rogers, unlike Freud, saw people as basically healthy and good. He identified people and all living organisms as having innate self-actualizing tendencies to grow, develop, and realize their full potential (Rogers, 1986). He believed that clients (he did not call them patients) were in the best position to explore, understand, and identify solutions to their own problems. He uses the analogy of teaching a child to ride a bicycle. It is not enough to tell the child how to ride; it is imperative that the child tries to ride the bike. (See Chapter 9 for further discussion on Rogers's use of therapeutic relationships.)

Patient-centered therapy is an existentially based therapy. The emphasis is on self-awareness and the present because the past has already happened, and the future has not yet occurred. The role of the therapist is that of a nondirective facilitator who seeks clarification and provides encouragement in this process. Three essential qualities in the therapist are congruence (genuineness), empathy, and respect. If these three qualities are present, the patient will improve; without them, there is little chance that the therapy will be successful.

Cognitive Theory

Aaron T. Beck was convinced that depressed people generally have standard patterns of negative and self-critical thinking (Beck, 1963). He believed that cognitive appraisals of events lead to emotional responses—it is not the event itself that causes the response but, instead, one's evaluation of the event. An example of the stimulus–appraisal–response relationship would be a woman whose sister had been depressed since their tumultuous and unsteady childhoods. In response to a question about how she and her sibling handled their parents' divorce and subsequent move to a small apartment, one of the siblings observed: "My sister fell apart. She retreated, barely talked.

TABLE 3.3 Examples of Cognitive Distortions

Distortion	Definition	Example
All-or-nothing thinking	Thinking in black and white, reducing complex outcomes into absolutes	Cheryl got the second-highest score in the cheerleading competition. She considers herself a loser.
Overgeneralization	Using a bad outcome (or a few bad outcomes) as evidence that nothing will ever go right again	Marty had a traffic accident. She refuses to drive and says, "I shouldn't be allowed on the road."
Labeling	A form of generalization where a characteristic or event becomes definitive and results in an overly harsh label for self or others	"Because I failed the advanced statistics exam, I am a failure. I might as well give up."
Mental filter	Focusing on a negative detail or bad event and allowing it to taint everything else	Anne's boss evaluated her work as exemplary and gave her a few suggestions for improvement. Anne obsessed about the suggestions and ignored the rest.
Disqualifying the positive	Maintaining a negative view by rejecting information that supports a positive view as being irrelevant, inaccurate, or accidental	"I've just been offered the job I've always wanted. No one else must have applied."
Jumping to conclusions	Making a negative interpretation despite the fact that there is little or no supporting evidence	"My fiancé, Mike, didn't call me for 3 hours; therefore, he doesn't love me."
a. Mind reading	Inferring negative thoughts, responses, and motives of others	The grocery store clerk was grouchy and barely made eye contact. "I must have done something wrong."
b. Fortune-telling error	Anticipating that things will turn out badly as an established fact	"I'll ask her out, but I know she won't have a good time."
Magnification or minimization	Exaggerating the importance of something (e.g., a personal failure or the success of others) or reducing the importance of something (e.g., a personal success or the failure of others)	"I'm alone on a Saturday night because no one likes me. When other people are alone, it's because they want to be."
a. Catastrophizing	An extreme form of magnification in which the very worst is assumed to be a probable outcome	"If I don't make a good impression on the boss at the company picnic, she will fire me."
Emotional reasoning	Drawing a conclusion based on an emotional state	"I'm nervous about the exam. I must not be prepared. If I were, I wouldn't be afraid."
"Should" and "must" statements	Rigid self-directives that presume an unrealistic amount of control over external events	"My patient is worse today. I should give better care so that she will get better."
Personalization	Assuming responsibility for an external event or situation that was likely out of personal control	"I'm sorry that your party wasn't more fun. It's probably because I was there."

Adapted from Burns, D. D. (1989). *Feeling good: The new mood therapy.* New York, NY: William Morrow.

Mom asked me how I was doing. I told her I was excited to get a new bedroom and make new friends. And I was telling the truth."

Therapeutic Model

Cognitive-behavioral therapy (CBT) is a popular, effective, and well-researched therapeutic tool. It is based on both cognitive and behavioral theory and seeks to modify negative thoughts that lead to dysfunctional emotions and actions. Several concepts underlie this therapy. One is that we all have **schemata**, or unique assumptions about ourselves, others, and the world around us. For example, if someone has a schema that no one can be trusted, this person will question everyone's motives and expect deception in relationships. Other dominant forms of negative schemata include incompetence, abandonment, evilness, and vulnerability.

Typically, people are unaware of their basic assumptions. However, their beliefs and attitudes will make the assumptions apparent. Rapid, unthinking responses based on these schemata are known as **automatic thoughts**. These responses are particularly intense and frequent in psychiatric disorders such as depression and anxiety. Often these automatic thoughts, or **cognitive distortions**, are irrational because people make false assumptions and misinterpretations. Common cognitive distortions are listed in Table 3.3.

The goal of CBT is to identify the negative patterns of thought that lead to negative emotions. Once the maladaptive patterns are identified, they can be replaced with rational thoughts. A particularly useful technique in CBT is to use a four-column format to record the precipitating event or situation, the resulting automatic thought, the ensuing feeling(s) and behavior(s), and finally, a challenge to the negative thoughts based on rational evidence and thoughts. This is sometimes referred to as the *ABCs of irrational beliefs* and is a good exercise for you to try for yourself (Box 3.1).

BOX 3.1 Example of ABCs of Irrational Beliefs

Activating Event
Jack has been in counseling for depression. His therapist's administrative assistant called and canceled this week's appointment.

Belief
My therapist is disgusted with me and wants to avoid me.

Consequence
Sadness, rejection, and hopelessness. Decides to call off work and just go back to bed.

Reframing
There is no evidence to believe the therapist finds me disgusting. Would the therapist have called to reschedule if he really didn't want to see me again?

Biological Theory

Psychiatric care is dominated by the biological model, in which mental disorders are believed to have physical causes. If mental disorders have physical causes, then they will respond to physical treatment. Sigmund Freud himself researched neurological causes for mental illness and considered cocaine a possible treatment.

In the 1950s a surgeon noticed that surgical patients were calmed by the administration of chlorpromazine (Thorazine) as a preanesthetic agent. It soon became widely used for the treatment of schizophrenia and dramatically reduced the use of restraint and seclusion. This discovery spurred the development of other drug-based treatments and the adoption of a chemical-imbalance theory of psychiatric disorders.

If chemical imbalances exist, how do they develop? Twin studies have been useful to support the genetic transmission of certain disorders. Whereas only 1% of the population has schizophrenia, among identical twins, the concordance rate (the percentage of the time that both twins will be affected) is about 40% to 50% (Sadock, Sadock, & Ruiz, 2015). Although this indicates genetic involvement, it cannot be the whole story. If it were, the concordance rate of schizophrenia in identical twins would be 100%. It is likely that the environment exerts an influence on the developing embryo or child. Research has proposed toxins, viruses, hostile environments, and brain trauma as possible catalysts for the development of psychiatric disorders (see Chapter 4).

Biological Therapy

Psychopharmacology is the primary biological treatment for mental disorders. (Refer to Chapter 4 for a full discussion of the biological basis for understanding psychopharmacology.) Major classifications of medications are antidepressants, antipsychotics, antianxiety agents, mood stabilizers, and psychostimulants. Clinicians recognize the importance of optimizing other biological variables, such as correcting hormone levels (as in hypothyroidism), regulating nutritionally deficient diets, and balancing inadequate sleep patterns. (Refer to Chapters 10 to 19 for relevant uses of psychopharmacology.)

Electroconvulsive therapy (ECT) has proven to be an effective treatment for severe depression and other psychiatric conditions. ECT is a procedure that uses electrical current to induce a seizure and is thought to work by affecting neurotransmitters and neuroreceptors (see Chapter 15 for more discussion regarding ECT).

Besides ECT, other brain-stimulation therapies are increasingly being used in psychiatry. Repetitive transcranial magnetic stimulation (rTMS) uses an electromagnetic device to deliver a rapidly pulsed magnetic field to the cerebral cortex to activate neurons. Magnetic seizure therapy (MST) uses higher-frequency electronic pulses instead of electricity to induce a seizure. Vagus nerve stimulation (VNS) works by stimulating the vagus nerve, which results in improved levels of neurotransmitters. Deep-brain stimulation (DBS) relies on surgically implanted electrodes stimulating a specific area of the brain.

Most mental health professionals combine biological approaches with talk therapy. Research indicates that the use of medication and CBT is an extremely effective treatment for many psychiatric disorders, especially major depression (Sadock et al., 2015). If a hostile environment can trigger negative brain chemistry or transmission, then a positive environment may reverse and improve the process.

A Note on How Psychotherapy Changes the Brain

Numerous studies have indicated that all mental processes are derived from the brain. Therefore, psychotherapeutic outcomes, such as changes in symptoms, psychological abilities, personality, or social functioning, are generally accepted to be attributed to brain changes brought about either by medication or psychotherapy. Numerous studies compiled by Karlsson (2011) substantiate positive treatment responses with various psychotherapies resulting in brain changes for the following disorders: major depressive disorder (MDD), anxiety disorders (panic disorder, social anxiety disorder, specific phobias), posttraumatic stress disorder (PTSD), borderline personality disorder, and obsessive-compulsive disorder (OCD). These studies suggest that currently, the most effective therapies for treating the aforementioned disorders resulting in brain changes are cognitive behavioral therapy (CBT), dialectic behavior therapy (DBT), psychodynamic psychotherapy, and interpersonal psychotherapy (IP).

OTHER MAJOR THEORIES

Theory of Cognitive Development

Jean Piaget (1896–1980) was a Swiss psychologist and researcher. Piaget noticed that children consistently gave wrong answers on intelligence tests that revealed a maturational pattern of cognitive processing. He concluded that cognitive development was a progression from primitive awareness to complex thought and responses (Piaget & Inhelder, 1969).

An understanding of cognitive development assists nurses in tailoring care to suit the cognitive level of the patient. For example, the concept of dying is difficult to grasp for the 5-year-old child who has lost a parent. Support for a child of this age will require different skills than those required for a 10-year-old child, who can understand the permanence of death. A summary of developmental stages is provided in Table 3.4.

Theory of Psychosocial Development

German-born American Erik Erikson (1902–1994) was a child psychoanalyst who described development as occurring in eight predetermined life stages, whose levels of success are related to the preceding stage (see Table 3.2).

Developmental tasks during these stages ideally result in a successful resolution. For example, from the ages of 7 to 12, the child's task is to understand his or her own abilities and competence and expand relationships beyond the immediate. The attainment of this task *(industry)* brings about confidence. The inability to gain a mastery of age-appropriate tasks and make connections with peers results in failure *(inferiority)*.

TABLE 3.4 Stages of Cognitive Development

Stage	Features
Sensorimotor (birth to 2 years)	Begins with basic reflexes and culminates with purposeful movement, spatial abilities, and hand–eye coordination. Around 9 months, **object permanence** is achieved, and the child can conceptualize objects that are no longer visible.
Preoperational (2–7 years)	Language develops, yet children think in a concrete fashion. Expecting others to view the world as they do is called **egocentric thinking**. Children begin to think in images and symbols and engage in such activities as playing house.
Concrete operational (7–11 years)	The child is able to think logically and use abstract problem solving. He or she is able to see another's point of view and is able to see a variety of solutions to a problem. **Conservation** is possible. For example, two small cups of liquid can be seen to equal a tall glass. The child is able to classify by characteristics, order objects in a pattern, and understand the concept of reversibility.
Formal operational (11 years to adulthood)	Conceptual reasoning begins at approximately the same time as puberty. At this stage, the child's basic abilities to think abstractly and problem solve are similar to those of an adult.

Each stage does not depend on completely integrating the positive characteristic and completely abandoning the negative. Ideally, harmony is achieved between the two characteristics. For example, we would not want a person to be 100% trusting—a degree of mistrust is essential for safety.

Theory of Object Relations

The theory of object relations was developed by interpersonal theorists who emphasize past relationships in influencing a person's sense of self as well as the nature and quality of relationships in the present. The term *object* refers to another person, particularly a significant person.

Margaret Mahler (1897–1985) was a Hungarian-born child psychologist who developed a framework for studying how an infant transitions from complete self-absorption, with an inability to separate from its mother, to a physically and psychologically differentiated toddler. Mahler believed that psychological problems were largely the result of a disruption of this separation.

During the first 3 years, the significant other (e.g., the mother) provides a secure base of support that promotes enough confidence for the child to separate. This confidence is achieved through a balance of holding (emotionally and physically) the child enough to feel safe while encouraging independence and natural exploration.

Problems may arise in this process. For example, if a toddler leaves his mother on the park bench and wanders off to the sandbox, the child should be encouraged with smiles and reassurance, such as, "Go on, honey; it's safe to go away a little." The mother should be reliably present when the child returns, thereby rewarding his efforts. Mahler notes that raising healthy children does not require that parents never make mistakes and that "good-enough parenting" will promote successful separation and individuation.

Theories of Moral Development

Lawrence Kohlberg (1927–1987) was an American psychologist who applied Piaget's theory to moral development. Based on interviews with youths, Kohlberg developed a theory of how people progressively develop a sense of morality (Kohlberg & Turiel, 1971). His theory helps us understand the progression from black-and-white thinking to a context-dependent decision-making process regarding the rightness or wrongness of an action.

Carol Gilligan (born in 1936) is an American psychologist, ethicist, and feminist who worked with Kohlberg. She later criticized his work for being male based. Gilligan also believed that the scoring method favored males' methods of reasoning. Based on Gilligan's critique, Kohlberg revised his scoring methods, which resulted in a greater similarity between girls' and boys' scores.

Gilligan's ethics of care theory emphasizes the importance of forming relationships and putting the needs of those for whom we care above the needs of strangers. Like Kohlberg, Gilligan asserts that moral development progresses through three major divisions: pre-conventional, conventional, and post-conventional. These transitions are dictated by personal development and changes in the sense of self. Kohlberg's and Gilligan's stages of moral development are summarized in Table 3.5.

NURSING MODELS

We have been examining theories and therapies developed by professionals from a variety of disciplines that date back to the late 1800s. It was not until the 1950s that the profession of nursing began to develop, record, and test theories (Alligood, 2013). The drive to create these theories began as a result of nursing education being moved from hospital-based programs to college- and university-based programs where nurses became involved in research. This research became the impetus for nurses to develop theories and a strong scientific body of knowledge.

Hildegard Peplau's work in the early 1950s is most often associated with psychiatric nursing, and her work will be presented in the following section. However, most nursing theories are applicable and of value to psychiatric nursing because interpersonal relations, caring, and communication are key aspects of the foundation of nursing. A summary of selected nursing theorists, the focus of their theoretical works, and examples of how their contributions can be utilized in psychiatric nursing is provided in Table 3.6. It is worth noting that among all the nurse theorists, psychiatric nurses are well represented.

Interpersonal Relations in Nursing

Hildegard Peplau's (1909–1999) seminal work *Interpersonal Relations in Nursing* was first published in 1952 and has served as a foundation for understanding and conducting therapeutic nursing relationships ever since. Peplau based her work on Sullivan's interpersonal theory and emphasized that the nature of the nurse–patient relationship strongly influenced the outcome for the patient.

Peplau made an extremely useful contribution to understanding anxiety by conceptualizing the four levels still in use today:

1. Mild anxiety is a day-to-day alertness (e.g., "I'm awake and taking care of business"). Stimuli in the environment are perceived and understood, and learning can easily take place.

TABLE 3.5 Stages of Moral Development According to Kohlberg and Gilligan

Level	Kohlberg's Stages	Gilligan's Stages
Pre-conventional	Stage 1: Obedience and punishment—a focus on rules and listening to authority to avoid punishment. Stage 2: Individualism and exchange—growing awareness that not everyone thinks the same. Breaking rules is a personal choice.	The goal is individual survival. Characterized by selfishness.
Conventional	Stage 3: Good interpersonal relationships—rightness or wrongness is based on individual motivations, personality, or the goodness or badness of the person. People should get along and have similar values. Stage 4: Maintaining the social order—rules are rules. Listening to authority maintains the social order.	Self-sacrifice is good. A responsibility for others develops.
Post-conventional	Stage 5: Social contract and individual rights—social order is important, but it also must be *good*. A corrupt social order should be changed. Stage 6: Universal ethical principles—actions should create unbiased results for everyone. We are obliged to break unjust laws.	The principle of nonviolence and not hurting others or self is essential. A balance of caring for self with caring for others emerges.

TABLE 3.6 Nursing Theoretical Works Relevant to Psychiatric Nursing

Theorist	Model/Theory	Focus of Nursing	Example
Dorothy Johnson	Behavioral system	Helping a patient return to a state of equilibrium when exposed to stressors by reducing or removing them and by supporting adaptive processes (Johnson, 1980)	Providing prn antianxiety medication and encouraging slow, deep breathing for a patient who is experiencing panic attacks
Imogene King	Goal attainment	Developing an interpersonal relationship and helping the patient to achieve his or her goals based on the patient's roles and social contexts (King, 1981)	Sitting with a new mother who is experiencing depression and developing a discharge plan in the context of childcare and financial deficits
Madeleine Leininger[a]	Culture care	Promoting health and helping people to cope with illness while recognizing cultural issues and their importance to health (Leininger, 1995)	Including the family in the plan of care for an Amish man who has recently attempted suicide
Betty Neuman[a]	System model	Developing a nurse–patient relationship; assessing and intervening with the person's response to stress (Neuman, 1982)	Considering the impact of shingles and graduate school stressors on a person diagnosed with generalized anxiety disorder
Dorothea Orem	Self-care deficit	Addressing self-care deficits and encouraging patients to be actively involved in their own care (Orem, 2001)	Temporarily helping a person with an exacerbation of paranoia to meet his or her hygiene needs
Ida Orlando[a]	Dynamic nurse–patient relationship	Addressing the patient's immediate need for help; the longer the unmet need, the more stress will be experienced (Orlando, 1990)	Asking, "Would you like to talk?" to a man who has begun pacing in the hallway and shaking his head
Hildegard Peplau[a]	Interpersonal relations	Using the interpersonal environment as a therapeutic tool for healing and in reduction of anxiety (Peplau, 1992)	Sitting quietly beside a new father who has recently lost his job and attempted suicide and does not want to talk
Jean Watson[a]	Transpersonal caring	Caring is as important as procedures and tasks; developing a nurse–patient relationship that results in a therapeutic outcome (Watson, 2007)	Taking time from a busy assignment to meet a patient's husband

[a]Psychiatric nursing background.

2. Moderate anxiety is felt as a heightened sense of awareness, such as when you are about to take an exam. The perceptual field is narrowed, and an individual hears, sees, and understands less. Learning can still take place, although it may require more direction.
3. Severe anxiety interferes with clear thinking, and the perceptual field is greatly diminished. Nearly all behavior is directed at reducing the anxiety. An example of this is your response to your car skidding on wet pavement.
4. Panic anxiety is overwhelming and results in either paralysis or dangerous hyperactivity. An individual cannot communicate, function, or follow directions. This is the sort of anxiety that is associated with the terror of panic attacks.

Refer to Chapter 11 for application of these levels to the nursing process.

One of the most useful constructs of Peplau's theory is in providing structure for how we view the therapeutic relationship, which she divided into four phases. Each of these overlapping and interlocking phases includes tasks, the expression of needs by the patient, and the interventions facilitated by the nurse. Refer to Chapter 9 for more information on the phases of the nurse–patient relationship.

Influence of Theories and Therapies on Nursing Care

Other theories and therapies presented earlier in this chapter are also relevant to nursing care. Nurses constantly borrow concepts and carry out interventions that are supported by these models. Some examples of how they may be used are as follows:

- **Behavioral:** Promoting adaptive behaviors through reinforcement can be valuable and important in working with patients, especially when working with a pediatric population. These patients look forward to positive reinforcement for good behavior and will work hard for gold stars or other privileges.
- **Cognitive:** Helping patients identify negative thought patterns is a worthwhile intervention in promoting healthy functioning and improving neurochemistry. Workbooks are available to aid in the process of identifying these cognitive distortions.
- **Psychosocial development:** Erikson's theory provides a structure for understanding critical junctures in development. The older adult who has suffered a stroke may be depressed and despairing because he can no longer take care of his house. In this case, the nurse and patient could explore ways of optimizing the patient's remaining strengths and talents, such as by nurturing and tutoring young people or by developing attainable goals such as getting the mail, taking out the trash, and so forth.
- **Hierarchy of needs:** Maslow's theory is useful in prioritizing nursing care. When working with actively suicidal patients, students sometimes think it is rude to ask if the patients are thinking about killing themselves. However, safety supersedes this potential threat to self-esteem. Although the "must dos" in nursing begin with physical care (e.g., providing medication and hydration through intravenous [IV] fluids), the goal should also include higher-level needs, which can be obtained by listening, observing, and collaborating with the patient in the development of the plan of care.

The Mental Health Recovery Model in Psychiatric Nursing

Although we tend to think of recovery as regaining health or being cured from an episode of illness, the term *recovery* in this model has a different meaning. The mental health **recovery model** is not a focus on a cure but, instead, emphasizes living adaptively with chronic mental illness. It is viewed as both an overarching philosophy of life for people with mental illness and an approach to care for use by those who treat, finance, and support mental health care. It is also an effective approach to dealing with substance abuse.

A diagnosis of mental illness once meant that you listened to health care professionals and relied upon them to chart your course in treatment. This medical model approach often results in apathy and discouragement: "They want me to take medication for the rest of my life; I don't like it and won't take it." The recovery model shifts the responsibility for care from the provider to the individual: "I will discuss the medication side effects with my friends who have similar problems and then talk to my nurse practitioner about my options and preferences."

This model emphasizes hope, social connection, empowerment, coping strategies, and meaning in life. A recovery approach to care has been embraced by the American Psychiatric Association from a service perspective. The U.S. Department of Health and Human Services uses recovery concepts to guide federal and state initiatives, particularly as they relate to empowering mental health consumers (people with mental illness) and in campaigns to reduce mental illness stigma. Illness management and recovery (IMR) programs are becoming popular and are increasingly supported by research (McGuire et al., 2014).

The use of the recovery model in psychiatric nursing is a natural extension of what we have traditionally done. Peplau (1952) set the standard by providing a structure for developing a therapeutic interpersonal relationship with a patient. The recovery model moves this relationship from a nurse–patient relationship to a nurse–patient partnership.

Therapies for Specific Populations

Group Therapy

This therapeutic method is commonly derived from interpersonal theory. It operates under the assumption that interaction within the group can provide support or bring about desired change among individual participants.

A **group** is defined as "a gathering of two or more individuals (b) who share a common purpose and (c) meet over a substantial time period (d) in face-to-face interaction (e) to achieve an identifiable goal" (Arnold & Boggs, 2016, p. 525). Experts disagree on the ideal size of the group, but it is usually somewhere between 6 and 10 members. A group that is too small will limit diversity of opinion and put pressure on members to participate. Overly large groups reduce the members' ability to share, especially if some members dominate the group.

Setting. Settings for groups are important. The room should be private, and the seating should be comfortable and arranged so that people can see one another. Using tables is discouraged because they can be psychological barriers between group members. One of the worst arrangements for discussion is the traditional classroom seating with everyone facing a central speaker, thereby limiting free interaction among participants.

Groups possess both content and process dimensions. **Group content** refers to the actual dialogue between members or the type of information that can be transcribed (written or recorded) in minutes of meetings. **Group process** includes all the other elements of human interaction, such as nonverbal communication, adaptive and maladaptive roles, energy flow, power plays, conflict, hidden agendas, and silence. Although the content is essential to the group's work, it is the process that becomes the real challenge for leaders as well as participants.

Group development tends to follow a sequential pattern of growth and requires less leadership with time. Understanding this pattern is especially helpful to the leader in order to anticipate distinct phases and provide guidance and interventions that are most effective. Tuckman's (1965) model of group development has four stages: forming, storming, norming, and performing. A fifth stage, adjourning (mourning), was later added (Tuckman & Jensen, 1977). These stages are comparable to human development from infancy into old age, accompanied by varying levels of maturity, confidence, and need for direction (Table 3.7).

TABLE 3.7 Tuckman's Stages of Group Development and Comparable Life Phases

Stage	Comparable Life Phase	Description
Forming	Infancy	The task and/or purpose of the group is defined. Connecting with others, desiring acceptance, and avoiding conflict define early groups. Members gather commonalities and differences as they attempt to know one another. The leader is the main connection and necessary for direction.
Storming	Adolescence	Important issues are being addressed, and conflict begins to surface. Personal relations may interfere with the task at hand. Some members will dominate, and some will be silent. Rules and structure are helpful. Members may challenge the role of the leader, who has the opportunity to model adaptive behavior.
Norming	Early adulthood	Members know one another, and rules of engagement (norms) are evident. There is a sense of group identity and cohesion. Members resist change, which could lead to a group breakup or a return to the discomfort of storming. Leadership is shared.
Performing	Mature adulthood	Groups who reach this stage are characterized by loyalty, flexibility, interdependence, and productivity. There is a balance between focus on work and focus on the welfare of group members.
Adjourning (mourning)	Older adult years	Groups in this stage are ready to disband, tasks are terminated, and relationships are disengaged. Accomplishments are recognized, and members are pleased to have been part of the group. A sense of loss is an inevitable consequence.

From Tuckman, B. W., & Jensen, M. A. (1977). Stages of small-group development revisited. *Group & Organization Management, 2*, 419–427.

Roles of Group Members. Studies of group dynamics have identified informal roles of members that are necessary to develop a successful group. The most common descriptive categories for these roles are task, maintenance, and individual roles (Benne & Sheats, 1948). Task roles serve to keep the group focused and attend to the business at hand. Maintenance roles function to keep the group together and provide interpersonal support. Individual roles are not related to group goals but, rather, to specific personalities. These roles can interfere with the group's functioning. Table 3.8 describes the roles of group members.

Roles of the Group Leader. The group leader has multiple responsibilities in starting, maintaining, and terminating a group. In the initial forming phase, the leader defines the structure, size, composition, purpose, and timing for the group. The leader facilitates communication and ensures that meetings start and end on time. In the adjourning phase, the leader ensures that each member summarizes individual accomplishments and gives positive and negative feedback regarding the group experience.

Leadership style depends on group type. A leader should select the style that is best suited to the needs of a particular group. The **autocratic leader** exerts control over the group and does not

TABLE 3.8 Roles of Group Members

Role	Function
Task Roles	
Coordinator	Connects various ideas and suggestions
Initiator-contributor	Offers new ideas or a new outlook on an issue
Elaborator	Gives examples and follows up on meaning of ideas
Energizer	Encourages group to make decisions or take action
Evaluator	Measures group's work against a standard
Information/opinion-giver	Shares opinions, especially to influence group values
Orienter	Notes progress of the group toward goals
Maintenance Roles	
Compromiser	In a conflict, yields to preserve group harmony
Encourager	Praises and seeks input from others; warm and accepting
Follower	Attentive listener and integral to the group
Gatekeeper	Ensures participation, encourages participation, points out commonality of thought
Harmonizer	Mediates conflicts constructively among members
Standard setter	Assesses explicit and implicit standards for group
Individual Roles	
Aggressor	Criticizes and attacks others' ideas and feelings
Blocker	Disagrees with group issues, opposes others, stalls the process
Help seeker	Asks for sympathy of group excessively, self-deprecating
Playboy/playgirl	Distracts others from the task; jokes, introduces irrelevant topics
Recognition seeker	Seeks attention by boasting and discussing achievements
Monopolizer	Dominates conversation, thereby preventing equal input
Special-interest pleader	Advocates for a special group, usually with own prejudice or bias

Data from Benne, K. D., & Sheats, F. (1948). Functional roles of group members. *Journal of Social Issues, 4*(2), 41.

encourage much interaction among members. In contrast, the **democratic leader** supports extensive group interaction in the process of problem solving. A **laissez-faire leader** allows the group members to behave in any way they choose and does not attempt to control the direction of the group. For example, the staff leading a community meeting with a fixed, time-limited agenda may tend to be more autocratic. In an educational group, the leader may be more democratic to encourage members to share their experiences. In a creative group, such as an art or horticulture group, the leader may choose a laissez-faire style, giving minimal direction to allow for a variety of responses.

Types of Groups. Educational groups form for the purpose of imparting information and require active expert leadership and careful planning. Task groups are typically time limited and have a common goal, and the role of the leader is to facilitate team building and cooperation. Support groups bring together people with common concerns and may be facilitated by a supportive leader or by group members. Therapy groups are led by professional group therapists whose styles may range from a directive and confrontational approach to a more hands-off approach in which the therapist lets the group members learn from one another.

TABLE 3.9 Yalom's Curative Factors of Group Membership

Curative Factor	Definition	Example
Altruism	Giving appropriate help to other members	"We've spent all this time talking about me. Lou needs to talk about his visit with his dad. Let's focus on him."
Cohesiveness	Feeling connected to other members and belonging to the group	"People in our group always listen to each other. We've been polite since the first day."
Interpersonal learning	Learning from other members	"Sammi said it takes 2 weeks for Prozac to really work. I should give it more time."
Guidance	Receiving help and advice	"I've also had that feeling where I just had to have a drink, Don. Just pick up the phone and call me next time it happens."
Catharsis	Releasing feelings and emotions	A new mother of twins begins to cry and says, "It sounds terrible, but sometimes I wish I'd never had children."
Identification	Modeling after member or leader	David notices that the leader projects confidence by speaking clearly, making good eye contact, and sitting up straight. David does the same.
Family reenactment	Testing new behaviors in a safe environment	"I learned to always smile and agree so that Dad wouldn't go off on me. I don't have to be cheery, and I can speak my mind here."
Self-understanding	Gaining personal insights	Dale realizes that his negativity has kept him from getting the friends he wants.
Instillation of hope	Feeling hopeful about one's life	"Sue has managed to stay sober for 2 years. I think I can do this."
Universality	Feeling that one is not alone	Aaron, a quiet group member, finally comments, "My son has schizophrenia, too, and it helps to hear that other people have the same worries I do."
Existential factors	Coming to understand what life is about	"I guess I've been obsessing about being a perfect housekeeper and haven't noticed that my children are growing up without me."

From Yalom, I. D. (1985). *The theory and practice of group psychotherapy*. New York, NY: Basic Books.

Benefits of Group Therapy. One of the benefits of group therapy is that it is more efficient, both pragmatically and financially, than individual therapy. This efficiency is due to the fact that many people can engage in therapy at once. However, it is the nature of the interaction between people with common concerns and frames of references that seems to provide the greatest benefit to members. Yalom (1985) identified 11 benefits, or **curative factors**, of group membership (Table 3.9).

Roles of Nurses. Psychiatric-mental health nurses are involved in a variety of therapeutic groups in acute care and long-term treatment settings. For all group leaders, a clear theoretical framework provides a structure for understanding group interaction. Co-leadership of groups is a common practice and has several benefits:

- Provides training for less experienced staff
- Allows for immediate feedback between the leaders after each session
- Gives two role models for teaching communication skills to members

Basic-level registered nurses have biopsychosocial educational backgrounds. Psychiatric mental health registered nurses (PMH-RNs) gain experience and expertise in caring for individuals who have physical, psychological, mental, and spiritual distress (American Psychiatric Nurses Association, International Society of Psychiatric-Mental Health Nurses, & American Nurses Association, 2014). PMH-RNs are ideally suited to teach a variety of health subjects. *Psychoeducational groups* are established to support and teach patients and families ways to help prevent relapse. These groups may be time limited or may be supportive for long-term treatment. Generally, written handouts or audiovisual aids are used to focus on specific teaching points. Psychiatric-mental health nurses commonly lead the following psychoeducational groups:

- **Medication education groups** allow patients to hear the experiences of others who have taken medication and to have an opportunity to ask questions without the fear of being judged; these groups also allow patients to learn to take the medications correctly.
- **Dual-diagnosis groups** focus on co-occurring psychiatric illness and substance abuse. The PMH-RN may co-lead this group with a dual-diagnosis specialist (master's level clinician).
- **Symptom management groups** are designed for patients to share coping skills regarding a common problem, such as cognitive distortions or substance use. New and alternate skills can be learned to help patients develop more effective strategies for reducing symptoms and preventing relapse.
- **Stress management groups** teach members about various relaxation techniques, including deep breathing, exercise, music, and spirituality.
- **Self-care groups** focus on activities of daily living, such as bathing and grooming.

Psychiatric mental health advanced practice registered nurses (PMH-APRNs) may lead any of the groups described earlier as well as psychotherapy groups. Psychotherapy groups require specialized training in techniques that allow for deep self-reflection, disclosure, sharing, confrontation, and healing among participants.

Therapeutic Milieu

A therapeutic milieu (mil-yoo), or healthy environment, combined with a healthy social structure within an inpatient setting or structured outpatient clinic is essential to supporting and treating those with mental illness. Within these small versions of society, people are safe to test new behaviors and increase their ability to interact adaptively with the outside community.

Community meetings or goal-setting meetings are frequently held at the beginning of the day. They usually include all patients and the treatment team. Functions include orienting new members to the unit, encouraging patients to engage in treatment, and evaluating the treatment program. Nursing staff often lead these groups and are in a strong position to give valuable feedback to the team about group interactions.

Other therapeutic milieu groups aim to help increase patients' self-esteem, decrease social isolation, encourage appropriate social behaviors, and educate patients in basic living skills. These groups are often led by occupational or recreational therapists, although nurses frequently co-lead them. Examples of therapeutic milieu groups are recreational groups, physical activity groups, creative arts groups, and storytelling groups.

BOX 3.2 Central Concepts to Family Therapy

- **Boundaries:** ***Clear boundaries*** maintain distinctions among individuals within the family and between the family and the outside world. Clear boundaries allow for a balanced flow of energy among members.
    - ***Diffuse*** or ***enmeshed boundaries*** are those in which there is a blending of the roles, thoughts, and feelings of the individuals so that clear distinctions among family members fail to emerge.
    - ***Rigid*** or ***disengaged boundaries*** are those in which the rules and roles are followed in spite of the consequences.
- **Triangulation:** The tendency, when two-person relationships are stressful and unstable, to engage a third person to stabilize the system through the formation of a coalition in which two members are pitted against the third.
- **Scapegoating:** A form of displacement in which a family member (usually the least powerful) is blamed for another family member's distress. The purpose is to keep the focus off the painful issues and the problems of the blamers.
- **Double bind:** A double bind is a no-win situation in which you are "darned if you do, darned if you don't."
- **Hierarchy:** The function of power and its structures in families, differentiating parental and sibling roles and generational boundaries.
- **Differentiation:** The ability to develop a strong identity and sense of self while maintaining an emotional connectedness with one's family of origin.
- **Sociocultural context:** The framework for viewing the family in terms of the influence of gender, race, ethnicity, religion, economic class, and sexual orientation.
- **Multigenerational issues:** The continuation and persistence from generation to generation of certain emotional interactive family patterns (e.g., reenactment of fairly predictable patterns; repetition of themes or toxic issues; and repetition of reciprocal patterns such as those of overfunctioner and underfunctioner).

Family Therapy

Family therapy developed around the mid-20th century. It is used as an adjunct to individual treatment and refers to the treatment of the family as a whole. Family therapists are trained at the graduate level. They use a variety of theoretical models to reduce or eliminate dysfunctional patterns of behavior and interaction. Some therapists may focus on the present, whereas others may rely more heavily on the family's history and reports of interactions between sessions. Terms related to family therapy are listed in Box 3.2.

Although therapists may use a wide variety of therapeutic methods, the goals of family therapy are basically the same. These goals include the following (Nichols, 2012):

- To reduce the dysfunctional behavior of individual family members
- To resolve or reduce intrafamily relationship conflicts
- To mobilize family resources and encourage adaptive family problem-solving behaviors
- To improve family communication skills
- To heighten awareness and sensitivity to other family members' emotional needs and help family members meet their needs
- To strengthen the family's ability to cope with major life stressors and traumatic events, including chronic physical or psychiatric illness
- To improve integration of the family system into the societal system (e.g., school, medical facilities, workplace, and especially the extended family)

Complementary and Alternative Treatments

Alternative treatments for psychiatric conditions and disorders have grown in popularity over recent decades. The National Center for Complementary and Integrative Health (NCCIH) is part of the National Institutes of Health and is the lead organization for research on practices and products that are not generally considered part of conventional medicine. The terminology used in the NCCIH name refers to:

- Complementary approaches in which nontraditional treatments are provided in addition to conventional medical treatments
- Integrative health care in which conventional and complementary approaches are brought together in a coordinated way

These approaches are often helpful and have the potential for even more benefits in the future. However, nurses need to recognize that, unlike prescription medications, the U.S. Food and Drug Administration (FDA) does not review or approve most of them. See Appendix A for a summary of complementary and integrative health care treatments and their uses in treating psychiatric disorders.

KEY POINTS TO REMEMBER

- Theoretical models and therapeutic strategies provide a useful framework for the delivery of psychiatric nursing care.
- The psychoanalytic model is based on unconscious motivations and the dynamic interplay between the primitive brain (id), the sense of self (ego), and the conscience (superego). The focus of psychoanalytic theory is on understanding the unconscious mind.
- The interpersonal model maintains that the personality and mental health disorders are created by social forces and interpersonal experiences. Interpersonal therapy aims to provide positive and repairing interpersonal experiences.
- The behavioral model suggests that because behavior is learned, behavioral therapy should improve behavior through rewards and reinforcement of adaptive behavior.
- The humanist model is based on human potential, and therapy is aimed at maximizing this potential. Maslow developed a theory of personality that is based on the hierarchical satisfaction of needs. Rogers's person-centered theory uses self-actualizing tendencies to promote growth and healing.
- The cognitive model posits that disorders, especially depression, are the result of faulty thinking. Cognitive-behavioral therapy is empirically supported and focuses on the recognition of distorted thinking and its replacement with more accurate and positive thoughts.
- The biological model is currently the dominant model and focuses on physical causation for personality problems and psychiatric disorders. Medication is the primary biological therapy.
- Various nursing theories are useful in psychiatric nursing. Hildegard Peplau developed an important interpersonal theory for the provision of psychiatric nursing care.
- Group therapy offers the patient significant interpersonal feedback from multiple people.
- Groups transition through predictable stages, benefit from therapeutic factors, and are characterized by members filling specific roles.
- The therapeutic milieu refers to the safe and therapeutic physical and social environment in which psychiatric care is provided.
- Family therapy is based on various theoretical models and aims to decrease emotional reactivity among family members and encourage differentiation among individual family members.

APPLYING CRITICAL JUDGMENT

1. How could the theorists discussed in this chapter influence your nursing care? Specifically:
   A. How do Freud's concepts of the conscious, preconscious, and unconscious affect your understanding of patients' behaviors?
   B. What are the implications of Sullivan's focus on the importance of interpersonal relationships for your interactions with patients?
   C. Can you think of anyone who seems to be self-actualized or self-transcendent? What is your reason for this conclusion?
   D. How do you utilize Maslow's hierarchy of needs in your nursing practice?
   E. What do you think about the behaviorist point of view that to change behaviors is to change personality?
2. Which of the therapies described here do you think can be the most helpful to you in your nursing practice? What are your reasons for this choice?

CHAPTER REVIEW QUESTIONS

1. A nurse plans a group meeting for adult patients in a therapeutic milieu. Which topic should the nurse include?
   a. Coping with grief and loss
   b. The importance of hand washing
   c. Strategies for money management
   d. Staffing shortages expected over the next 3 days
2. Considering Maslow's pyramid, which comment indicates that an individual is motivated by one of the higher levels of need?
   a. "Even though I'm 40 years old, I have returned to college so that I can get a better job."
   b. "I help my community by volunteering at a thrift shop that raises money for the poor."
   c. "I recently applied for public assistance in order to feed my family, but I hope it's not forever."
   d. "My children tell me I'm a good parent. I feel happy being part of a family that appreciates me."
3. Which patient is likely to achieve maximum benefit from cognitive-behavioral therapy (CBT)?
   a. Older adult diagnosed with stage 3 Alzheimer's disease
   b. Adult diagnosed with schizophrenia and experiencing delusions
   c. Adult experiencing feelings of failure after losing the fourth job in 2 years
   d. School-age child diagnosed with attention-deficit/hyperactivity disorder (ADHD)
4. An adult plans to attend an upcoming 10-year high school reunion. This person says to the nurse, "I am embarrassed to go. I will not look as good as my classmates. I haven't been successful in my

career." Which comment by the nurse addresses this cognitive distortion?
a. "You look fine to me. Do you think you will have fun at your reunion?"
b. "Everyone ages. Other classmates have had more problems than you."
c. "Do you think you are the only person who has aged and faced difficulties in life?"
d. "I think you are doing well in the face of the numerous problems you have endured."

5. A distraught 8-year-old girl tells the nurse, "I had a horrible nightmare and was so scared. I tried to get in bed with my parents, but they said, 'No.' I think I could have gone back to sleep if I had been with them." Which family dynamic is likely the basis of this child's comment?
a. Boundaries in the family are rigid.
b. The family has poor differentiation of roles.
c. The girl is enmeshed in part of a family triangle.
d. Generational boundaries in the family are diffuse.

REFERENCES

Alligood, M. R. (2013). *Nursing theorists and their work* (8th ed.). St. Louis: Mosby.

American Psychiatric Nurses Association, International Society of Psychiatric-Mental Health Nurses, & American Nurses Association. (2014). *Psychiatric-mental health nursing: Scope and standards of practice* (2nd ed.). Silver Spring, MD: American Nurses Association.

Arnold, E., & Boggs, K. U. (2016). *Interpersonal relationships: Professional communication skills for nurses* (7th ed.). St. Louis: Saunders.

Beck, A. T. (1963). Thinking and depression. *Archives of General Psychiatry, 9*, 324–333.

Benne, K. D., & Sheats, F. (1948). Functional roles of group members. *Journal of Social Issues, 4*(2), 41–49.

Freud, S. (1961). The ego and id. In J. Strachey (Ed.), *The standard edition of the complete psychological works of sigmund freud* (Vol. 19) (pp. 3–66). London: Hogarth Press (Original work published 1923).

Giddens, J. F. (2017). *Concepts for nursing practice* (2nd ed.). St. Louis: Elsevier.

Johnson, D. E. (1980). The behavioral system model for nursing. In J. P. Riehl, & C. Roy (Eds.), *Conceptual models for nursing practice* (2nd ed.). New York: Appleton-Century-Crofts.

Karlsson, H. (2011). How psychotherapy changes the brain. *Psychiatric Times, 28*(8). Retrieved from www.nwmedicalhypnosis.com/documents/How%20Psychotherapy%20Changes%20the%20Brain.pdf.

King, I. M. (1981). *A theory for nursing: Systems, concepts, process*. New York: Wiley.

Kohlberg, L., & Turiel, E. (1971). Moral development and moral education. In G. Lesser (Ed.), *Psychology and educational practice*. Glenville, IL: Scott, Foresman and Company.

Leininger, M. (1995). Culture care theory, research, and practice. *Nursing Science Quarterly, 9*(2), 71–78.

Maslow, A. H. (1971). *The farther reaches of human nature*. New York: Viking.

McGuire, A. B., Kukla, M., Green, A., et al. (2014). Illness management and recovery: A review of the literature. *Psychiatric Services, 65*(2), 171–179.

Neuman, B. (1982). *The Neuman systems model: Application to nursing education and practice*. New York: Appleton-Century-Crofts.

Nichols, M. P. (2012). *Family therapy: Concepts and methods* (10th ed.). Upper Saddle River, NJ: Prentice Hall.

Orem, D. E. (2001). *Nursing: Concepts of practice* (6th ed.). St. Louis: Mosby.

Orlando, I. J. (1990). *The dynamic nurse-patient relationship: Function, process, and principles* (Pub. No. 15–2341). New York: National League for Nursing.

Pavlov, I. P. (1927). *Conditioned reflexes*. London: Routledge and Kegan Paul.

Peplau, H. E. (1952). *Interpersonal relations in nursing: A conceptual frame of reference for psychodynamic nursing*. New York: Putnam.

Peplau, H. E. (1992). *Interpersonal relations in nursing*. New York, NY: Putnam.

Piaget, J., & Inhelder, B. (1969). *The psychology of the child*. New York: Basic Books.

Rogers, C. R. (1986). Carl Rogers on the development of the person-centered approach. *Person-Centered Review, 1*(3), 257–259.

Sadock, B. J., Sadock, V. A., & Ruiz, P. (2015). *Synopsis of psychiatry* (11th ed.). Philadelphia: Walters Kluwer.

Skinner, B. F. (1938). *The behavior of organisms*. New York: Appleton-Century-Crofts.

Sullivan, H. S. (1953). *The interpersonal theory of psychiatry*. New York: Norton.

Tuckman, B. W. (1965). Developmental sequence in small groups. *Psychological Bulletin, 63*, 384–399.

Tuckman, B. W., & Jensen, M. A. (1977). Stages of small-group development revisited. *Group & Organization Management, 2*, 419–427.

Watson, J. (2007). *Watson caring science Institute*. Retrieved from www.watsoncaringscience.org/caring_science/index.html.

Watson, J. B. (1930). *Behaviorism* (rev. ed.). Chicago: University of Chicago.

Yalom, I. D. (1985). *The theory and practice of group psychotherapy*. New York: Basic Books.

4

Biological Basis for Understanding Psychopharmacology

Chyllia D. Fosbre

http://evolve.elsevier.com/Varcarolis/essentials

OBJECTIVES

1. Identify at least three major brain structures and eight major brain functions that can be altered by mental illness and psychotropic medications.
2. Describe how evidence-based neuroimaging is helpful in understanding abnormalities of brain function, structure, and receptor pharmacology. **QSEN: Evidence-Based Practice**
3. Explain the basic process of neurotransmission and synaptic transmission using Figs. 4.5, 4.6, and 4.7.
4. Identify the main neurotransmitter systems affected by the following psychotropic drugs:
   a. Antidepressants
   b. Antianxiety agents
   c. Sedative-hypnotics
   d. Mood stabilizers
   e. Antipsychotic agents
   f. Anticholinesterase drugs
5. Explain the relevance of psychodynamic and psychokinetic drug interactions in the delivery of safe, effective nursing care. **QSEN: Safety**
6. Discuss safety concerns related to dietary and drug restrictions with monoamine oxidase inhibitors (MAOIs).
7. Compare and contrast typical and atypical antipsychotic drugs with regard to side-effect profile and quality of life.
8. Discuss the relationship between the immune system and the nervous system in mental health and mental illness.
9. Describe how genes and culture affect an individual's response to psychotropic medication.

KEY TERMS AND CONCEPTS

acetylcholine, p. 39
acetylcholinesterase (AChE) inhibitors, p. 40
agonist, p. 40
agranulocytosis, p. 46
α_1-receptors, p. 46
amygdala, p. 34
antagonist, p. 40
antianxiety or anxiolytic drugs, p. 34
autonomic nervous system, p. 36
basal ganglia, p. 34
bupropion, p. 43
buspirone, p. 45
carbamazepine, p. 46
circadian rhythms, p. 36
corticotropin-releasing hormone, p. 36
cross-cultural psychopharmacology, p. 48
divalproex sodium, p. 46
dopamine, p. 40
dopamine receptor agonists (DRAs), p. 46
extrapyramidal symptoms (EPSs), p. 35
first-generation antipsychotics (FGAs)/typical agents, p. 35
5-HT_2 receptors, p. 46
fluphenazine, p. 46
γ-aminobutyric acid (GABA), p. 39
glutamate, p. 39
H_1 receptors, p. 46
hippocampus, p. 34
histamine, p. 42
hypertensive crisis, p. 44
hypnotic, p. 45
hypothalamus, p. 35
lamotrigine, p. 46
limbic system, p. 34
lithium, p. 45
monoamine oxidase (MAO), p. 37
monoamine oxidase inhibitors (MAOIs), p. 44
monoamines, p. 37
muscarinic cholinergic receptors, p. 46
neurohormones, p. 36
neuroimaging, p. 37
neuroleptics, p. 46
neurons, p. 34
neurotransmission, p. 37
neurotransmitter, p. 37
norepinephrine (NE), p. 42
paliperidone, p. 47
parasympathetic nervous system, p. 36
pharmacodynamic interactions, p. 42
pharmacokinetic interactions, p. 42
plasticity, p. 34
psychoneuroimmunology (PNI), p. 48
psychotropic, p. 42
receptors, p. 37
reticular activating system (RAS), p. 34
reuptake, p. 37
second-generation antipsychotics (SGAs)/atypical agents, p. 35

CONCEPT: INTRACRANIAL REGULATION: *Intracranial regulation* (ICR) includes normal and abnormal processes of intracranial function. Nurses care for individuals experiencing a wide variety of ICR issues in both community and inpatient settings.

ICR functioning depends on a consistent supply of blood delivering oxygen and nutrients, with carbohydrates as the main source of fuel for the brain (Giddens, 2017). Alterations in these basic processes can lead to mental disturbances and physical manifestations. Unfortunately, agents used to treat mental disease can cause a variety of undesired effects, such as sedation or excitement, motor disturbances, sexual dysfunction, and weight gain. There is a continuing effort to develop new drugs that are effective, safe, and well tolerated.

INTRODUCTION

One of the goals of psychiatric-mental health nursing is to understand the neurobiology of psychiatric disorders and how psychotropic medications help manage a constellation of symptoms and reduce the risk of relapse. Because all brain functions are carried out by similar mechanisms (interactions of **neurons**), often in similar locations, it is not surprising that mental disturbances are frequently associated with alterations in other brain functions. The drugs used to treat mental disturbances can provide symptom relief but can also interfere with other activities of the brain. Box 4.1 summarizes some of the major brain functions.

BRAIN STRUCTURES AND FUNCTIONS

The basic architecture of the brain is genetically programmed; however, plasticity occurs throughout life. **Plasticity** is a process of adapting and changing as gray matter shrinks and thickens and connections are pruned or forged (Kania, Wronska, & Zieba, 2017). The connections between neurons can change with mental illness or psychotropic medications.

Cerebrum

The cerebrum or cerebral cortex is made up of the four different lobes of the brain. It is also called the human brain or higher brain and is responsible for higher cognitive skills, self-awareness, and executive functions. The four lobes are the frontal, parietal, occipital, and temporal lobes (Fig. 4.1). The frontal lobe is responsible for conscious movement, problem-solving skills, and speech production. The prefrontal cortex (PFC) is the most anterior part of the frontal cortex and is involved in moderating social behaviors, goal setting and planning, and personality. The parietal lobes are involved in tactile sensation and spatial awareness. The occipital lobe is primarily responsible for vision and visual processing. The temporal lobe is responsible for hearing, language reception, and language comprehension.

BOX 4.1 Functions of the Brain

- Monitor changes in the external world
- Monitor the composition of body fluids
- Regulate the contractions of the skeletal muscles
- Regulate the internal organs
- Initiate and regulate the basic drives: hunger, thirst, sex, aggressive self-protection
- Mediate conscious sensation
- Store and retrieve memories
- Regulate mood (affect) and emotions
- Think and perform intellectual functions
- Regulate the sleep cycle
- Produce and interpret language
- Process visual and auditory data

Brainstem

Basic vital life functions occur through the brainstem, composed of the midbrain, pons, and medulla (Fig. 4.2).

Through projections called the **reticular activating system (RAS)**, the brainstem sets the level of consciousness and regulates the cycle of sleep and wakefulness. Unfortunately, drugs used to treat psychiatric conditions may interfere with the regulation of sleep and alertness; thus, the warning to take sedating drugs at bedtime and to use caution while driving is found on many psychotropic medications.

Cerebellum

The cerebellum (see Fig. 4.2) contributes to both motor control and cognitive processing. Alterations in cerebello-thalamo-cortical circuits are associated with the development of positive symptoms (hallucinations, delusions, and altered perception) in people with schizophrenia (Bernard, Orr, & Mittal, 2017). There have been cases of long-term movement abnormalities associated with cerebellar dysfunction when lithium toxicity occurs (Banwari et al., 2016).

Limbic Brain

In addition to the gray matter forming the cortex, there are pockets of gray matter lying deep within the cerebrum: the hippocampus, the amygdala, and the basal ganglia. The **hippocampus** interacts with the PFC in making new memories. The **amygdala** plays a major role in processing fear and anxiety. The hippocampus and amygdala, along with the hypothalamus and thalamus, are a group of structures called the **limbic system** or "emotional brain." Chronic stress triggers shrinkage of the hippocampus, which may lead to higher levels of depression and cognitive impairment (Lin et al., 2018). Structural plasticity of both the hippocampus and the amygdala is induced by electroconvulsive therapy in major depressive disorder (MDD), especially in individuals with smaller hippocampal volumes at baseline (Joshi et al., 2016). Amygdala hyperactivity is common in trauma and may underlie paranoia in schizophrenia (Pinkham et al., 2015). Amygdala hypoactivity predicts a general capacity to respond to antidepressants (Williams et al., 2015).

Linking the frontal cortex, basal ganglia, and upper brainstem, the limbic system mediates thought and feeling through complex, bidirectional connections. **Antianxiety drugs (anxiolytics)** slow the limbic system. Subcortical **basal ganglia** play a major role in motor responses via the extrapyramidal motor system, which relies on the neurotransmitter dopamine to maintain proper muscle tone and motor stability. Neuroimaging shows that haloperidol can reduce striatal volume within hours, temporarily changing brain structure and producing abnormal involuntary motor symptoms (**extrapyramidal symptoms [EPSs]**). In the basal ganglia, two types of movement disturbances may occur: (1) acute EPS, which develops early in treatment, and (2) tardive dyskinesia (TD), which usually occurs much later. **First-generation antipsychotics (FGAs) (typical agents)** and high doses of **second-generation antipsychotics (SGAs) (atypical agents)** such as risperidone are most likely to cause EPSs.

It is important to remember that movement is regulated by the basal ganglia, including the diaphragm (essential for breathing) and the muscles of the throat, tongue, and mouth (essential for speech). Thus, drugs that affect brain function can stimulate or depress respiration or affect speech patterns (e.g., slurred speech).

Thalamus

The thalamus filters sensory information before it reaches the cerebral cortex. Disrupted sensory filtering in schizophrenia is associated with altered connections between the thalamus and prefrontal cortex (PFC). Deep-brain stimulation (DBS) changes electrical impulses in the cortico-basal ganglia-thalamic loops and is being investigated in treating chronic, severe depression; obsessive-compulsive disorder (OCD); anorexia nervosa; and other psychiatric disorders (Graat, Figee, & Denys, 2017).

Hypothalamus

The **hypothalamus** maintains homeostasis. It regulates temperature, blood pressure, perspiration, libido, hunger, thirst, and

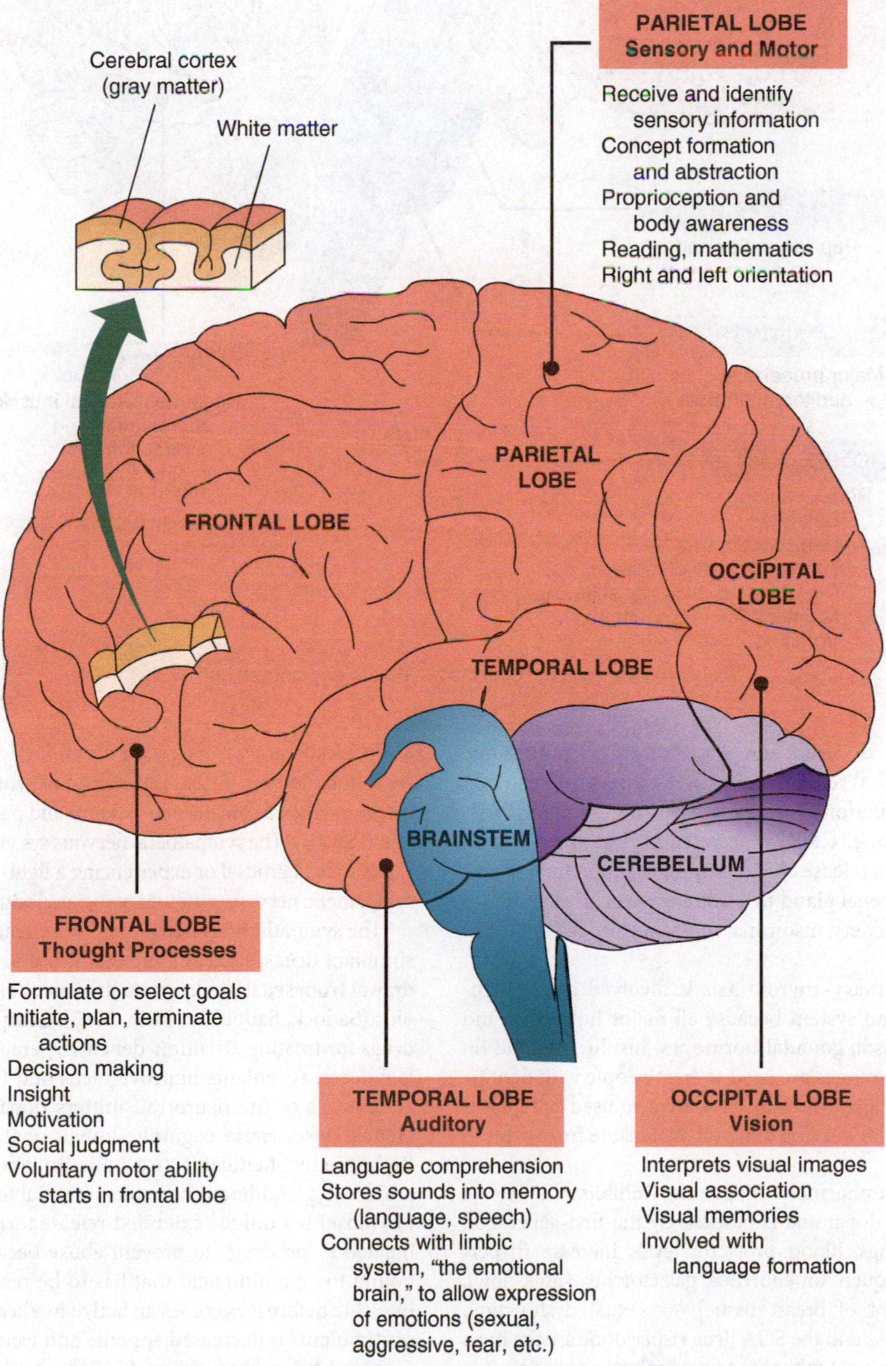

Fig. 4.1 Functions of the cerebral lobes: frontal, parietal, temporal, and occipital.

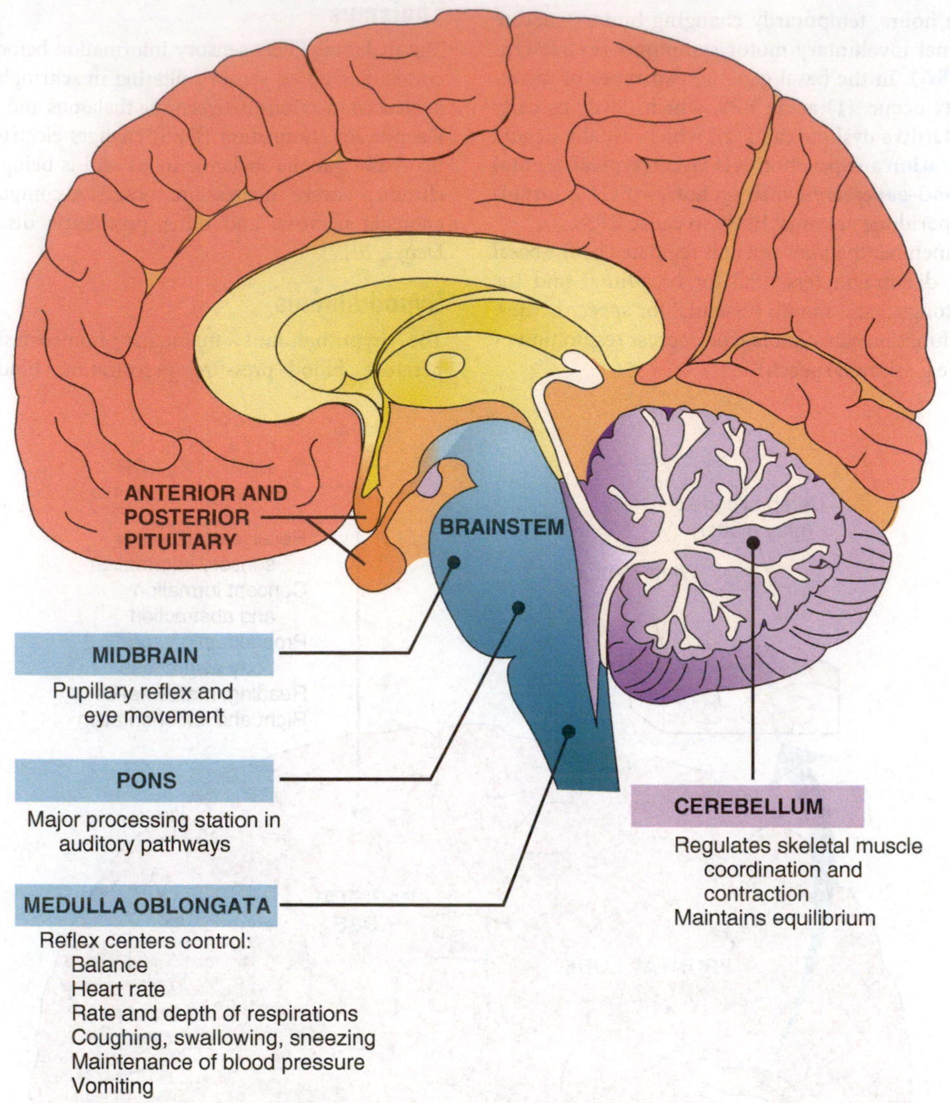

Fig. 4.2 Functions of the brainstem and cerebellum.

circadian rhythms, such as sleep and wakefulness. Hypothalamic **neurohormones**, often called releasing hormones, direct the secretion of hormones from the anterior pituitary gland. For example, **corticotropin-releasing hormone (CRH)** is secreted in response to stress. It stimulates the pituitary to release corticotropin, which in turn stimulates the cortex of each adrenal gland to secrete cortisol. This system is disrupted in depression, anxiety, insomnia, substance use disorder, and Alzheimer's dementia.

The hypothalamic–pituitary–thyroid axis is involved in the regulation of nearly every organ system because all major hormones and catecholamines (e.g., cortisol, gonadal hormones, insulin) depend on thyroid status. Thyroid hormones are used to treat people with depression or rapid-cycling bipolar I disorder. They are also used as replacement therapy for people who develop a hypothyroid state from lithium treatment (Gitlin, 2018).

The hypothalamic neurohormone dopamine inhibits the release of prolactin. When excess dopamine is blocked by the first-generation (typical) antipsychotic drugs, blood prolactin levels increase (hyperprolactinemia), with subsequent amenorrhea, galactorrhea (milk flow), gynecomastia (development of breast tissue), or sexual dysfunction. Among antipsychotics, FGAs and the SGA drug risperidone are the most frequent offenders, whereas most other SGAs are prolactin sparing.

In addition to working with the endocrine system, the hypothalamus sends instructions to the **autonomic nervous system**, which is divided into the **sympathetic nervous system** and **parasympathetic nervous system** (Fig. 4.3). The sympathetic nervous system is activated when someone is in a state of arousal or experiencing a fight-or-flight response. The parasympathetic nervous system is associated with a calm and relaxed state.

The sympathetic system is highly activated by sympathomimetic or stimulant drugs, such as amphetamine and cocaine, as well as by withdrawal from sedating drugs, such as alcohol, benzodiazepines, and opioids (Sadock, Sadock, & Ruiz, 2015). Sympathomimetics are first-line drugs for treating attention-deficit/hyperactivity disorder (ADHD). In low doses, stimulants improve focus and thinking by increasing synaptic levels of the neurotransmitters dopamine and norepinephrine. Higher doses cause cognitive impairment and locomotor activation. Both methylphenidates (e.g., Ritalin and Concerta) and amphetamines (e.g., Adderall) have the potential for abuse. Lisdexamfetamine (Vyvanse) is a unique extended-release formulation that has been designated a "prodrug" to prevent abuse because its active ingredient is bound to an amino acid that has to be removed by an enzyme in the intestine before it becomes an active medication. A common side effect of stimulants is decreased appetite and weight loss, which can often be managed by eating before taking the medication and by maximizing

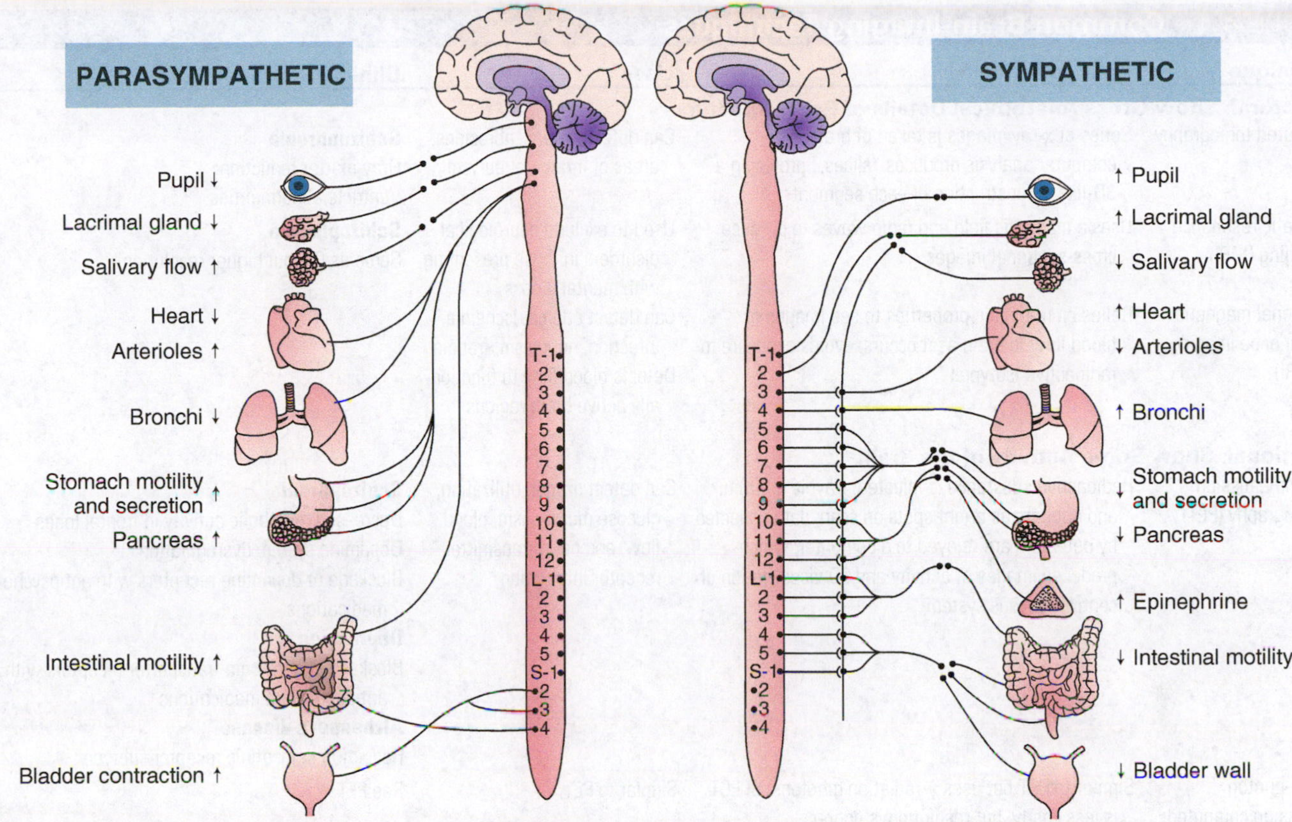

Fig. 4.3 The autonomic nervous system has two divisions: sympathetic and parasympathetic. The sympathetic division is dominant in stress situations, such as fear and anger—known as the fight-or-flight response.

caloric intake with snacks when "off" medications (e.g., at breakfast or a bedtime snack).

Visualizing the Brain

Neuroimaging visualizes a brain that is structurally and functionally interconnected. Some common brain-imaging techniques that measure structure and function are identified in Table 4.1.

Functional neuroimaging with positron emission tomography (PET) and single-photon emission computed tomography (SPECT) use ionizing radiation to localize brain regions associated with perceptual, cognitive, emotional, and behavioral functions. Based on the increase in blood flow to the local vasculature that accompanies neural activity, PET scans have provided evidence of decreased metabolism in unmedicated individuals with depression or schizophrenia and increased metabolism in OCD (Fig. 4.4). PET and SPECT have also shown dopamine system dysregulation in schizophrenia and loss of monoamines in depression.

Functional magnetic resonance imaging (fMRI) measures how well two regions of the brain communicate with each other. In patients suffering from first-episode schizophrenia, fMRI demonstrates that individual differences in striatal functional connectivity predict the response to antipsychotic drug treatment. Researchers hope that this striatal connectivity index (SCI) will eventually predict who will respond to medications and who will not (Sarpal et al., 2016).

CELLULAR COMPOSITION OF THE BRAIN

Neurons

The brain is composed of a vast network of more than 100 billion interconnected nerve cells (neurons) and supporting cells. An essential feature of neurons is their ability to initiate signals and conduct an electrical impulse from one end of the cell to the other, called **neurotransmission** (Fig. 4.5). Electrical signals within neurons are then converted at synapses into chemical signals through the release of molecules called **neurotransmitters**, which then elicit electrical signals on the other side of the synapse.

Synaptic Transmission

Once an electrical impulse reaches the end of a neuron, the neurotransmitter is released from the axon terminal at the presynaptic neuron and diffuses across a **synapse** to a postsynaptic neuron. Here it attaches to specialized **receptors** on the cell surface and either inhibits or excites the postsynaptic neuron. It is the interaction between neurotransmitter and receptor that is a major target of psychotropic drugs. Fig. 4.6 shows how an insufficient degree of transmission may be caused by a deficient release of neurotransmitters from the presynaptic cell or by a decrease in receptors. Fig. 4.7 illustrates how excessive transmission may be due to the excessive release of a transmitter or to increased receptor responsiveness, as occurs in schizophrenia.

After attaching to a receptor and exerting its influence on the postsynaptic cell, the transmitter separates from the receptor and is destroyed. Some transmitters (e.g., acetylcholine) are destroyed by specific enzymes (e.g., acetylcholinesterase). In the case of **monoamine** transmitters, the destructive enzyme is **monoamine oxidase (MAO)**. Other transmitters are taken back into the cell from which they were originally released by a process called cellular **reuptake**. The transmitters are then either reused or destroyed by intracellular enzymes. The two basic mechanisms of destruction are described in Box 4.2.

Neurotransmitters

A neurotransmitter is a chemical messenger between neurons by which one neuron triggers another. Four major groups of neurotransmitters in the brain are monoamines (biogenic amines), amino acids, peptides,

TABLE 4.1 Common Brain-Imaging Techniques

Technique	Description	Uses	Clinical Research Examples
Structural: Show Gross Anatomical Details of Brain Structures			
Computed tomography (CT)	Series of x-ray images is taken of brain, and computer analysis produces "slices," providing a 3D-like reconstruction of each segment	Can detect lesions, abrasions, areas of infarct, aneurysm	**Schizophrenia** Gray-matter reduction Ventricle abnormalities
Magnetic resonance imaging (MRI)	Uses a magnetic field and radio waves to produce cross-sectional images	Used to exclude neurological disorders in those presenting with mental illness	**Schizophrenia** Same as CT (but higher resolution)
Functional magnetic resonance imaging (fMRI)	Relies on magnetic properties to see images of blood flow in brain as it occurs; avoids exposure to radioactive isotypes	Can detect edema, ischemia, infection, neoplasm, trauma Detects blood flow to functionally active brain regions	
Functional: Show Some Activity of the Brain			
Positron emission tomography (PET)	Radioactive substance is injected, travels to brain, and appears as bright spots on scan; data collected by detectors are relayed to a computer, which produces images of activity and 3D visualization of central nervous system	Can detect oxygen utilization, glucose metabolism, blood flow, and neurotransmitter–receptor interaction	**Schizophrenia** Decreased metabolic activity in frontal lobes Dopamine system dysregulation Blockade of dopamine receptors with antipsychotic medications **Depression** Blockade of serotonin transporter receptors with antidepressant medications **Alzheimer's disease** Reduction in nicotinic receptor subtype
Single-photon emission computed tomography (SPECT)	Similar to PET but uses γ-radiation (photons) SPECT is less costly, but resolution is poorer	Similar to PET	See PET

3D, Three-dimensional.

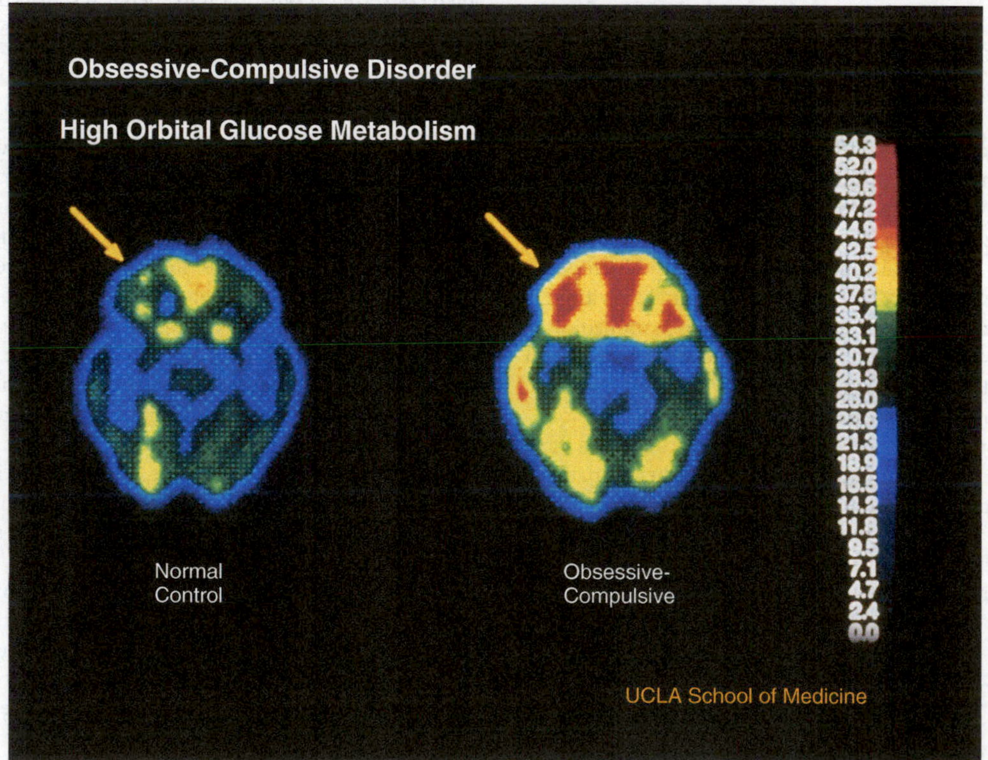

Fig. 4.4 Positron emission tomographic scans show increased brain metabolism *(brighter colors)*, particularly in the frontal cortex, in a patient with obsessive-compulsive disorder (OCD), compared with a normal control. This suggests altered brain function in OCD. (From Lewis Baxter, MD, University of California, Los Angeles; courtesy National Institute of Mental Health.)

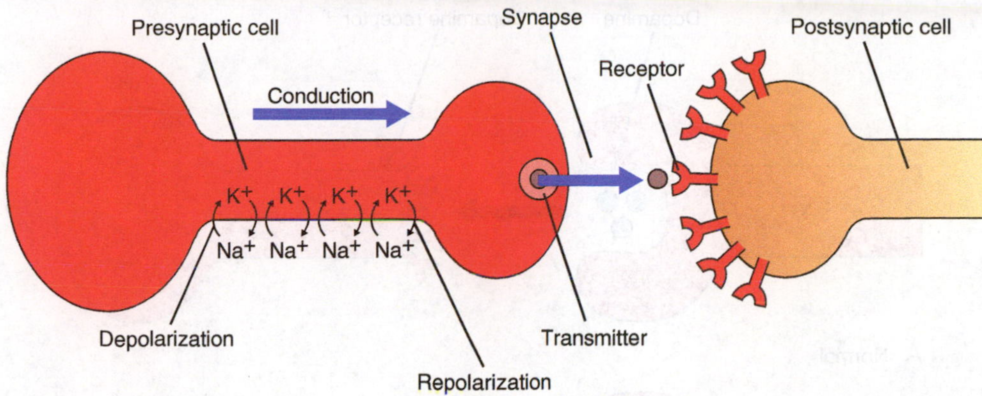

Fig. 4.5 Activities of neurons. Conduction along a neuron involves the inward movement of sodium ions (Na^+) followed by the outward movement of potassium ions (K^+). When the current reaches the end of the cell, a neurotransmitter is released. The transmitter crosses the synapse and attaches to a receptor on the postsynaptic cell. The attachment of a transmitter to a receptor either stimulates or inhibits the postsynaptic cell.

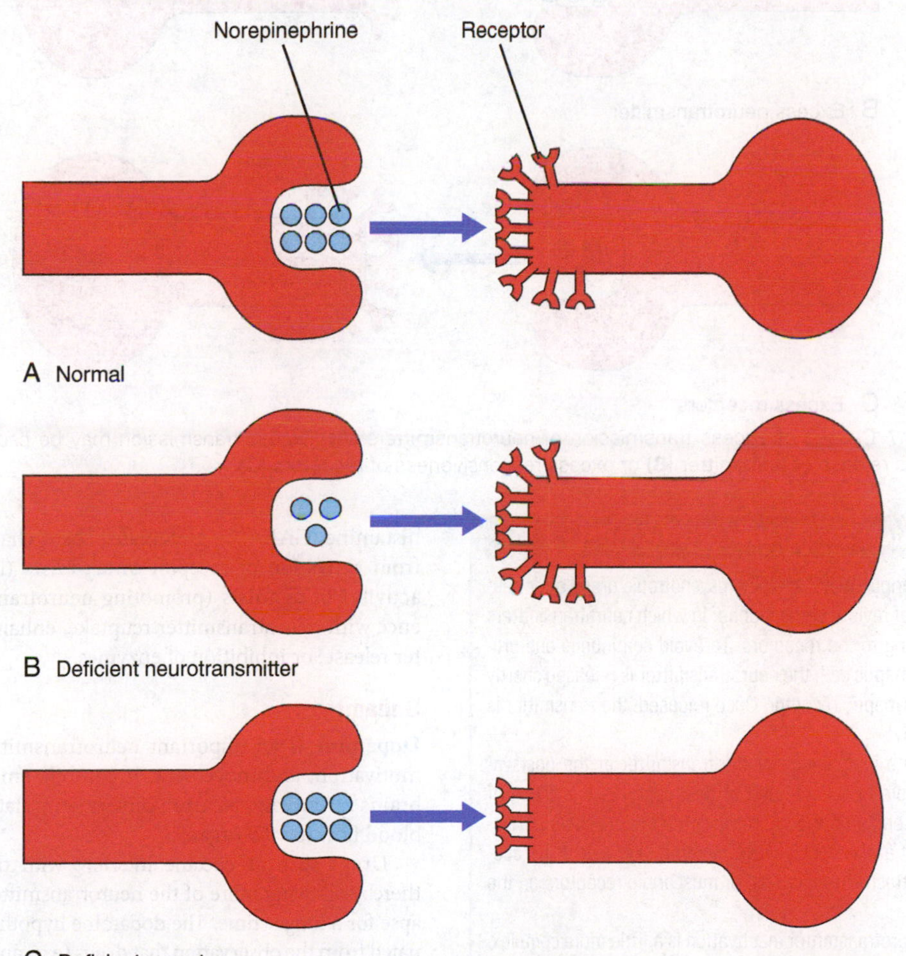

Fig. 4.6 Normal transmission of neurotransmitters **(A)**. Deficiency in transmission may be caused by a deficient release of transmitter **(B)** or by a reduction in receptors **(C)**.

and cholinergics (e.g., acetylcholine). Monoamine neurotransmitters (dopamine, norepinephrine, serotonin) and acetylcholine are implicated in a variety of neuropsychiatric disorders.

Amino acid neurotransmitters, such as the inhibitory γ-aminobutyric acid (GABA) and the excitatory glutamate, balance brain activity. Peptide neurotransmitters such as hypothalamic CRH modulate or adjust general brain function. Table 4.2 lists important neurotransmitters, types of receptors to which they attach, and mental disorders that are associated with an increase or decrease in the levels of neurotransmitters.

Interaction of Neurons, Neurotransmitters, and Receptors

Most psychotropic drugs produce effects by altering synaptic concentrations of dopamine, acetylcholine, norepinephrine, serotonin,

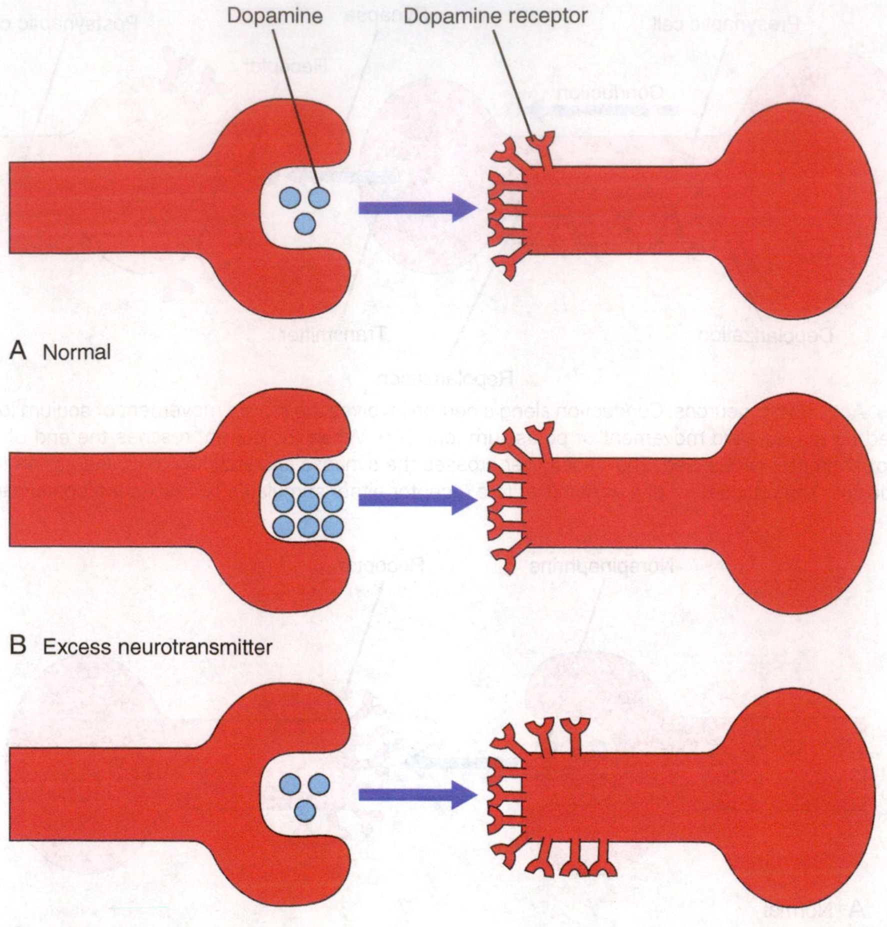

Fig. 4.7 Causes of excess transmission of neurotransmitters **(A)**. Excess transmission may be caused by excess release of transmitter **(B)** or excess responsiveness of receptors **(C)**.

BOX 4.2 Destruction of Neurotransmitters

A full explanation of the various ways in which psychotropic drugs alter neuronal activity requires a brief review of the manner in which neurotransmitters are destroyed after attaching to the receptors. To avoid continuous and prolonged action on the postsynaptic cell, the neurotransmitter is released shortly after attaching to the postsynaptic receptor. Once released, the transmitter is destroyed in one of two ways.

One way is the immediate inactivation of the transmitter at the postsynaptic membrane. An example of this method of destruction is the action of the enzyme acetylcholinesterase on the neurotransmitter acetylcholine. Acetylcholinesterase is present at the postsynaptic membrane and destroys acetylcholine shortly after it attaches to nicotinic or muscarinic receptors on the postsynaptic cell.

The *second* method of neurotransmitter inactivation is a little more complex. After interacting with the postsynaptic receptor, the transmitter is released and taken back into the presynaptic cell, the cell from which it was released. This process, referred to as the reuptake of neurotransmitter, is a common target for drug action. Once inside the presynaptic cell, the transmitter is either recycled or inactivated by an enzyme within the cell. The monoamine neurotransmitters norepinephrine, dopamine, and serotonin are all inactivated in this manner by the enzyme monoamine oxidase.

In looking at this second method, one might naturally ask what prevents the enzyme from destroying the transmitter before its release. The answer is that before release, the transmitter is stored within a membrane and is thus protected from the degradative enzyme. After release and reuptake, the transmitter is either destroyed by the enzyme or reenters the membrane to be reused.

histamine, GABA, or glutamate. These changes are thought to result from activation of receptor **antagonists** (blocking neurotransmitter activity) or **agonists** (promoting neurotransmitter activity), interference with neurotransmitter reuptake, enhancement of neurotransmitter release, or inhibition of enzymes.

Dopamine

Dopamine is an important neurotransmitter involved in cognition, motivation, and movement. It controls emotional responses and the brain's reward and pleasure centers, stimulates the heart, and increases blood flow to vital organs.

Drugs such as cocaine interfere with the reuptake of dopamine, thereby allowing more of the neurotransmitter to stay active in the synapse for a longer time. The dopamine hypothesis of schizophrenia originated from the observation that drugs (e.g., amphetamines) that stimulate dopamine activity can induce psychotic symptoms, whereas drugs that block dopamine receptors (e.g., haloperidol) have antipsychotic activity.

Acetylcholine

Dopamine is balanced by acetylcholine, which is released by cholinergic neurons. Acetylcholine plays a role in skeletal muscle movement, arousal, memory, and the sleep–wake cycle. Because acetylcholine is deficient in Alzheimer's disease, drugs have been developed to inhibit the enzyme that degrades acetylcholine (i.e., acetylcholinesterase). **Acetylcholinesterase (AChE) inhibitors** such as donepezil (Aricept), galantamine (Razadyne), and rivastigmine (Exelon) are prescribed to delay cognitive decline in Alzheimer's disease.

TABLE 4.2 Transmitters and Receptors

Transmitters	Receptors	Functions	Clinical Relevance
Monoamines			
Dopamine (DA)	D_1, D_2, D_3, D_4, D_5	Fine muscle movement Integration of emotions and thoughts Decision making Stimulates hypothalamus to release hormones (sex, thyroid, adrenal)	**Increase:** Psychosis Mania **Decrease:** Parkinson's disease Depression
Norepinephrine (NE) (noradrenaline)	α_1, α_2, β_1, β_2	Mood Attention and arousal Stimulates sympathetic branch of autonomic nervous system for "fight or flight" in response to stress	**Increase:** Mania Anxiety Psychosis **Decrease:** Depression
Serotonin (5-HT)	5-HT, 5-HT_2, 5-HT_3, 5-HT_4	Mood Sleep regulation Hunger Pain perception Aggression and libido Hormonal activity	**Increase:** Anxiety states **Decrease:** Depression
Histamine	H_1, H_2	Alertness Inflammatory response Stimulates gastric secretion	**Decrease:** Sedation Weight gain
Amino Acids			
γ-Aminobutyric acid (GABA)	$GABA_A$, $GABA_B$	**Inhibitory neurotransmitter:** Reduces anxiety, excitation, aggression May play a role in pain perception Anticonvulsant and muscle-relaxing properties May impair cognition and psychomotor functioning	**Increase:** Reduction of anxiety **Decrease:** Mania Anxiety Psychosis
Glutamate	NMDA, AMPA	**Excitatory neurotransmitter:** AMPA plays a role in learning and memory	**Increased NMDA:** Prolonged increase can kill neurons (neurotoxicity) Neurodegeneration in Alzheimer's disease **Decreased NMDA:** Psychosis **Increased AMPA:** Improvement of cognitive performance in behavioral tasks
Cholinergics			
Acetylcholine (ACh)	Nicotinic, muscarinic (M_1, M_2, M_3)	Plays a role in learning, memory Regulates mood: mania, sexual aggression Affects sexual and aggressive behavior Stimulates parasympathetic nervous system	**Decrease:** Alzheimer's disease Huntington's chorea Parkinson's disease **Increase:** Depression
Peptides (Neuromodulators)			
Substance P (SP)	SP	Centrally active SP antagonist has antidepressant and antianxiety effects in depression Promotes and reinforces memory Enhances sensitivity to pain receptors to activate	Involved in regulation of mood and anxiety Role in pain management
Somatostatin (SRIF)	SRIF	Altered levels associated with cognitive disease	**Decrease:** Alzheimer's disease Decreased levels of SRIF in spinal fluid of some depressed patients **Increase:** Huntington's chorea
Neurotensin (NT)	NT	Endogenous antipsychotic-like properties	Decreased levels in spinal fluid in patients with schizophrenia

AMPA, α-Amino-3-hydroxy-5-methyl-4-isoxazolepropionic acid; *NMDA*, *N*-methyl-D-aspartate; *SRIF*, somatotropin release-inhibiting factor.

Although all acetylcholine receptors respond to acetylcholine, they also respond to other molecules. For example, nicotinic acetylcholine receptors are particularly responsive to nicotine. People with schizophrenia and attention problems may be more likely to smoke as a way of normalizing cognitive and sensory deficits. Because these individuals are also more likely to suffer adverse effects, scientists are trying to develop drugs that target nicotine receptors without the carcinogenic, cardiovascular, and addictive effects.

Norepinephrine

Norepinephrine (NE) is released from noradrenergic neurons. Low levels of NE are linked to low arousal (e.g., sedation) and depression. High levels can create a feeling of hyperarousal. NE is primarily an activator of α-receptors, subdivided into α_1- and α_2-receptors. Prazosin, an antihypertensive drug, blocks excessive responsiveness to NE at postsynaptic α_1-adrenergic receptors and is used for treating nightmares in posttraumatic stress disorder (PTSD; Stahl, 2017). Many FGA (conventional) antipsychotic drugs act as antagonists at the α_1-receptor for NE. Blockage of these receptors can cause vasodilation and a consequent drop in blood pressure, or orthostatic hypotension. Blockage of α_1-receptors on the vas deferens can lead to a failure to ejaculate.

Serotonin

Serotonin (5-HT), found in the brain and spinal cord, helps regulate mood, arousal, attention, behavior, and body temperature. When some antidepressants are combined with other drugs or supplements that increase serotonin production (e.g., St. John's wort or over-the-counter cough and cold medications containing dextromethorphan), serotonin syndrome may occur. Symptoms of high levels of serotonin range from mild (restlessness, shivering, and diarrhea) to severe (muscle rigidity, fever, and seizures). These symptoms can be alleviated by muscle relaxants and drugs that block serotonin production. Research is shifting from antidepressants that elevate serotonin levels to new drugs that strengthen serotonergic signaling.

Regulation of the serotonin transporter (SERT), a protein that facilitates the transport of serotonin into the cell, is a key action for major antidepressants. Blockade of SERT by a selective serotonin reuptake inhibitor leads to a decreased concentration of serotonin within platelets and slight inhibition of platelet aggregation. Therefore, the risk of bleeding should be mentioned to patients taking nonsteroidal anti-inflammatory drugs (NSAIDs), aspirin, warfarin, or antiplatelet drugs.

Histamine

Many FGA (conventional) antipsychotic agents, as well as a variety of other psychiatric drugs, block the H_1 receptors for **histamine**. Two significant side effects of blocking these receptors are sedation and substantial weight gain. Sedation may be beneficial in severely agitated patients, and weight gain can be preferred in someone with decreased appetite or low body weight.

γ-Aminobutyric Acid

The major inhibitory neurotransmitter γ-aminobutyric acid (GABA) modulates neuronal excitability and is associated with the regulation of anxiety. Most antianxiety (anxiolytic) drugs act by increasing the effectiveness of GABA, primarily by increasing receptor responsiveness. Because GABA neurons suppress dopamine release, a novel antipsychotic drug targeting dopamine hyperactivity and GABA hypoactivity might lead to a new and better option for treating schizophrenia.

Glutamate

Glutamate, a potent excitatory neurotransmitter, activates the *N*-methyl-D-aspartate (NMDA) receptor. Any disruption in this pathway leading to either enhanced or decreased activity may result in neuropsychiatric symptoms. High concentrations of glutamate or overly sensitive receptors can lead to cell death, as occurs in neurodegenerative conditions such as Alzheimer's disease. As a corollary, NMDA receptor antagonists, such as the drug memantine, decrease excitability and neurotoxicity. Glutamate acts on several receptor types in addition to NMDA, and it is the balance between these receptors as well as the balance between glutamate and GABA that may be critical in slowing the progression of psychosis. Lumateperone (Caplyta) is a new medication approved by the U.S. Food and Drug Administration and has a unique serotonergic-dopaminergic-glutametergic profile for treating schizophrenia (FDA, 2020). Both NMDA and α-amino-3-hydroxy-5-methyl-4-isoxazolepropionic acid (AMPA) receptors are binding sites for glutamate, and the interplay of the two receptors is being explored in developing ketamine-like drugs to rapidly reverse depressive symptoms.

PSYCHOTROPIC DRUGS AND INTERACTIONS

Psychotropic drugs work by mechanisms not yet fully understood, and understanding their action becomes more challenging when drug interactions alter or modify their effects.

Pharmacokinetic interactions occur when one drug alters the absorption, distribution, metabolism, or elimination of another, thereby affecting plasma concentrations. Most pharmacokinetic interactions result from inhibition or induction of cytochrome P450 (CYP450) enzymes. Potent CYP450 inhibitors added to drugs metabolized by CYP450 enzymes increase drug concentrations and the risk for toxicity. CYP450 inducers decrease concentrations and result in decreased efficacy unless the dose is increased. With the exception of paliperidone, all SGA (atypical) antipsychotics undergo extensive hepatic metabolism and can be altered by CYP450 inducers or inhibitors.

Pharmacogenetic tests provide information on which medications each individual can metabolize properly, primarily focusing on pharmacokinetic genes from the CYP450 family and pharmacodynamic genes related to the regulation of neurotransmitters. For example, GeneSight pharmacogenomics technology covers FDA-approved medications for people diagnosed with behavioral health conditions such as schizophrenia, depression, anxiety, bipolar disorder, PTSD, and ADHD (Assurex Health, 2018).

Pharmacodynamic interactions occur when drugs act at the same or interrelated receptor sites, resulting in synergistic or antagonistic effects. For example, using two medications with sedative effects caused by two different receptors, such as a benzodiazepine and an antihistamine, will have an additive effect, causing an increase in sedation over what would be seen with either medication if taken alone (DeVane & Nemeroff, 2018). Managing drug interactions is complicated by comorbid conditions and polypharmacy, especially in older adults.

ANTIDEPRESSANT DRUGS

Several hypotheses of depression have been proposed for the action of antidepressants:

1. The monoamine hypothesis suggests a lack of three monoamines (dopamine, norepinephrine, or serotonin) in various brain regions. However, there is no clear evidence that monoamine deficiency accounts for depression.
2. The monoamine receptor hypothesis suggests that low levels of neurotransmitters cause increased receptor sensitivity (up-regulation) over time; thus, it may take several weeks for patients to feel better when they are taking antidepressants.

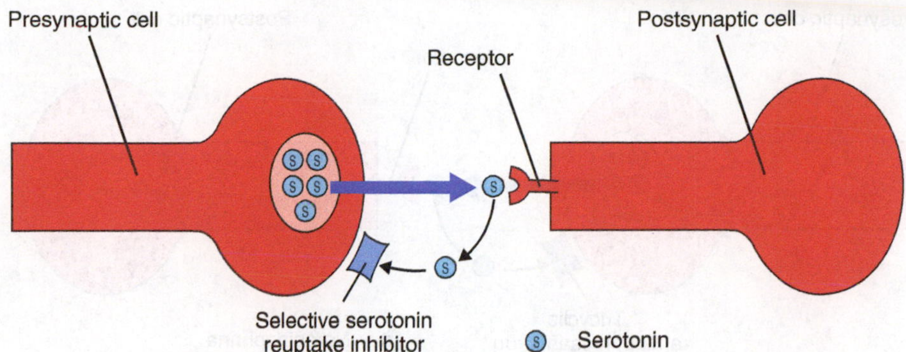

Fig. 4.8 Mechanism of action of selective serotonin reuptake inhibitors (SSRIs).

3. More recent hypotheses focus on the "downstream molecular events" that the receptors trigger, including the regulation of genes. For example, one hypothesis is that the gene for brain-derived neurotrophic factor (BDNF) is repressed in depression and may be activated by antidepressants.

Selective Serotonin Reuptake Inhibitors

As the name implies, **selective serotonin reuptake inhibitors (SSRIs)** inhibit the reuptake of serotonin, making it stay longer in the synapse. Examples include fluoxetine (Prozac), sertraline (Zoloft), paroxetine (Paxil), citalopram (Celexa), and escitalopram (Lexapro). Vilazodone (*Vilbryd Medication Guide*, 2018) offers a novel combination of selective serotonin reuptake inhibition and serotonergic (5-HT$_{1A}$) receptor partial agonist activity. The idea behind a partial agonist is that it will effectively block the negative feedback caused by higher levels of serotonin and increase serotonin release even more.

The new SSRI vortioxetine (Trintellix) displays agonist activity at the 5-HT$_{1A}$ receptor as well as partial agonist activity at 5-HT$_{1B}$ and antagonist activity at 5-HT$_3$, 5-HT$_{1D}$, and 5-HT$_7$ receptors. These multimodal actions may benefit patients for whom first-line therapy was not effective.

Refer to Fig. 4.8 for an explanation of the mechanism of action of SSRIs. For a more detailed description of how SSRIs work, visit the Evolve website at http://evolve.elsevier.com/Varcarolis/essentials.

Selectivity results in fewer side effects because SSRIs do not inhibit receptors for other neurotransmitters (e.g., acetylcholine, histamine, norepinephrine). However, too much serotonergic activity can result in *anxiety, insomnia, sexual dysfunction,* and *gastrointestinal disturbances*. Serotonin toxicity may occur with coadministration of other serotonergic drugs (e.g., monoamine oxidase inhibitor [MAOIs], SSRIs, serotonin-norepinephrine reuptake inhibitors [SNRIs], lithium, triptan, buspirone, tramadol, over-the-counter cough and cold medications containing dextromethorphan) or antidopaminergic drugs such as tetrabenazine (Xenazine) and first- and second-generation antipsychotics. Similarly, the risk of serotonin toxicity may be increased by pharmacokinetic interactions because serotonergic antidepressants are metabolized by CYP450 enzymes, and any drug that inhibits a CYP450 enzyme increases serotonin levels. For example, metabolism by CYP3A4 is a major elimination pathway for SSRIs, so doses should be reduced with co-administered CYP3A4 inhibitors (e.g., ketoconazole). On the other hand, CYP34A inducers (e.g., rifampin) can result in inadequate plasma concentrations and diminished effectiveness.

Adverse events can occur upon discontinuation of serotonergic antidepressants, particularly when discontinuation is abrupt. The discontinuation syndrome is most likely to occur with SSRIs or SNRIs having a short half-life. Thus, it is more common with paroxetine (Paxil) than with fluoxetine (Prozac).

Serotonin-Norepinephrine Reuptake Inhibitors

Serotonin-norepinephrine reuptake inhibitors (SNRIs) block the reuptake of both serotonin and norepinephrine, but it remains controversial whether the dual action of SNRIs, such as **venlafaxine** (Effexor), duloxetine (Cymbalta), and desvenlafaxine (Pristiq), results in greater efficacy than SSRIs. SNRIs are also used to treat other conditions, such as anxiety and neuropathic pain.

Serotonin-Norepinephrine Disinhibitors

Serotonin-norepinephrine disinhibitors (SNDIs), represented by only mirtazapine (Remeron), increase norepinephrine and serotonin transmission by blocking presynaptic α_2-noradrenergic receptors. Mirtazapine is often combined with SSRIs to augment antidepressant response or counteract the serotonergic side effects of nausea, anxiety, or insomnia.

Norepinephrine-Dopamine Reuptake Inhibitors

Unlike other currently used antidepressants, **bupropion** (Wellbutrin) does not act on the serotonin system. It is a norepinephrine-dopamine reuptake inhibitor (NDRI), and it also inhibits nicotinic acetylcholine receptors to reduce the addictive action of nicotine. Thus, the bupropion preparation Zyban is also prescribed for smoking cessation.

Serotonin Antagonists/Reuptake Inhibitors

High doses are required for the serotonergic action of the serotonin antagonist/reuptake inhibitor (SARI) **trazodone** (Desyrel). At lower doses, it loses its antidepressant action while retaining hypnotic effects through histamine receptor antagonism (Stahl, 2017). Although useful for insomnia, trazodone's potent α-adrenergic blocking properties can cause priapism (painful prolonged penile erections).

Selective Norepinephrine Reuptake Inhibitors

Norepinephrine reuptake inhibitors (NRIs) block presynaptic norepinephrine transporters (NETs), thereby inhibiting the reuptake of

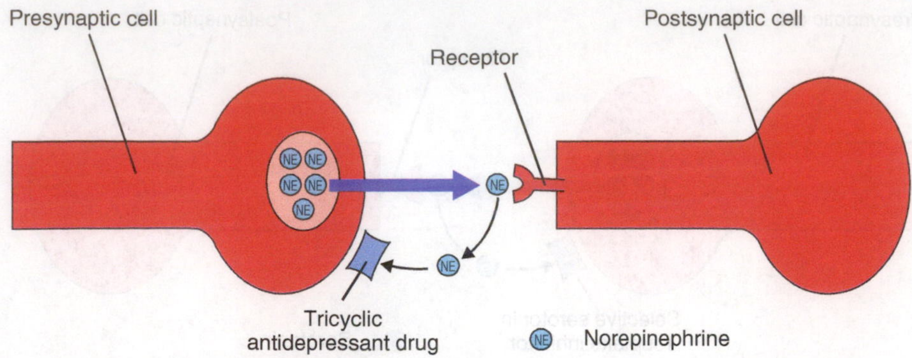

Fig. 4.9 Mechanism by which tricyclic antidepressant drugs block the reuptake of norepinephrine.

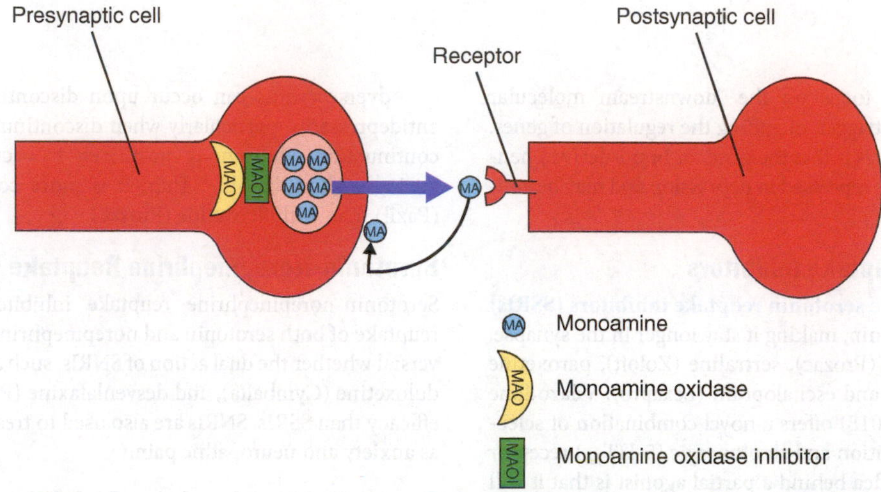

Fig. 4.10 Blocking of monoamine oxidase (MAO) by inhibiting agents (MAOIs) prevent the breakdown of monoamine (MA) by MAO.

norepinephrine. The first truly selective noradrenergic reuptake inhibitor marketed in the United States was atomoxetine (Strattera). It is used to treat ADHD when stimulants cannot be tolerated, but it does not show a significant benefit for depression. Refer to Chapter 15 for more information on antidepressant medications, nursing considerations, and patient and family teaching.

Tricyclic Antidepressants

Originally termed tricyclic antidepressants (TCAs), these agents are more accurately called *cyclic antidepressants (CAs)* because newer members of this class have a four-ring structure. TCAs, such as amitriptyline (Elavil) and nortriptyline (Pamelor), act primarily by blocking the presynaptic transporter protein receptors for norepinephrine and, to a lesser degree, serotonin (Fig. 4.9). This blocking prevents norepinephrine from coming into contact with its degrading enzyme, MAO, and thus increases the level of norepinephrine at the synapse.

Multiple pharmacological mechanisms of TCAs have proven beneficial in treating difficult cases of depression and chronic pain. However, multiple actions on several receptors also earned TCAs the name "dirty drugs" because of their many side effects. For example, to varying degrees, TCAs block muscarinic receptors that normally bind acetylcholine, leading to anticholinergic effects. Again to varying degrees, TCAs block H_1 receptors, causing sedation and weight gain. Strong binding at adrenergic receptors causes dizziness and hypotension, thereby increasing the risk of falls. Pharmacokinetics must be considered in TCA overdose fatalities because TCAs are highly lipid soluble and rapidly absorbed. This may result in cardiotoxicity and death before the patient can reach a hospital, especially if the patient is an older adult with a slower rate of drug elimination. For a more detailed description of how TCAs work, visit the Evolve website at http://evolve.elsevier.com/Varcarolis/essentials.

Monoamine Oxidase Inhibitors

To understand the action of **monoamine oxidase inhibitors (MAOIs)**, keep in mind the following definitions:

- **Monoamines:** a type of organic compound, including the neurotransmitters, that is further divided into subgroups called catecholamines (e.g., norepinephrine, epinephrine, dopamine) and indolamines (e.g., serotonin) and many different drugs and food substances
- **Monoamine oxidase (MAO):** an enzyme that destroys monoamines
- **Monoamine oxidase inhibitors (MAOIs):** drugs that increase concentrations of monoamines by inhibiting the action of MAO (Fig. 4.10)

Because MAOIs block the enzyme that metabolizes monoamines, they may occasionally be used to increase the levels of serotonin and norepinephrine in intractable depression. However, SSRIs and SNRIs are the more commonly used antidepressants because of the vasopressor effects that occur when MAOIs are combined with other sympathomimetics (amines that stimulate the sympathetic nervous system). The most feared vasopressor effect is the **hypertensive crisis** that can result if a patient takes over-the-counter medications with pseudoephedrine or consumes the adrenergic monoamine tyramine, commonly found in aged foods, fermented foods, and certain beverages. Dietary restriction of tyramine must be maintained for 2 weeks after stopping MAOIs to allow the body

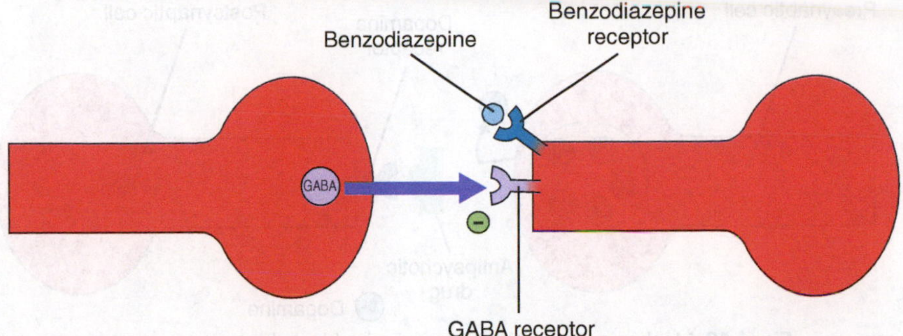

Fig. 4.11 Action of the benzodiazepines. Drugs in this group attach to receptors adjacent to the receptors for the neurotransmitter γ-aminobutyric acid (GABA). Drug attachment to these receptors results in strengthening of the inhibitory effects of GABA. In the absence of GABA, there is no inhibitory effect of benzodiazepines.

to resynthesize the MAO enzyme. The EMSAM patch delivers the MAOI selegiline through the skin and has diminished hypertensive effects compared with the oral preparations phenelzine (Nardil) and tranylcypromine (Parnate). However, dietary precautions are still required. Chapter 15 contains a list of foods and beverages to avoid while taking MAOIs and gives nursing measures and instructions for teaching patients who are taking MAOIs. For a more detailed description of how MAOIs work, visit the Evolve website at http://evolve.elsevier.com/Varcarolis/essentials.

ANTIANXIETY OR ANXIOLYTIC DRUGS

Treating Anxiety Disorders With Antidepressants

Antidepressants have been found effective in treating anxiety disorders because of many shared symptoms, neurotransmitters, and circuits. SSRIs are commonly used to treat panic disorder, generalized anxiety disorder (GAD), OCD, PTSD, and social phobia. The SNRIs venlafaxine (Effexor) and duloxetine (Cymbalta) are also used to treat GAD.

Buspirone (BuSpar)

Buspirone (BuSpar) reduces anxiety without causing the immediate sedative and mildly euphoric effects of benzodiazepines. Its mechanism of action is unknown, but it has a high affinity for serotonin 5-HT_{1A} receptors, which mediate its antidepressant effects. Concomitant use of higher doses of buspirone and alcohol should be avoided, but the potential for addiction that exists with benzodiazepines does not exist for buspirone.

Benzodiazepines

Benzodiazepines were previously one of the most commonly used pharmacological agents for anxiety, but due to tolerance, high levels of abuse, and recent connections to dementia, they are losing favor among providers. They are now being recommended for only short-term use and should be avoided with opioid medications. Benzodiazepines promote the activity of GABA by binding to a specific receptor on the $GABA_A$ receptor complex. Fig. 4.11 shows that benzodiazepines such as diazepam (Valium), clonazepam (Klonopin), and alprazolam (Xanax) bind to $GABA_A$ receptors with different α-subunits.

The fact that benzodiazepines do not inhibit neurons in the absence of GABA limits their potential toxicity. However, sedative/hypnotic effects put patients at risk for developing tolerance and withdrawal. Some benzodiazepines, such as flurazepam (Dalmane) and triazolam (Halcion), have a predominantly **hypnotic** (sleep-inducing) effect, whereas others, such as lorazepam (Ativan) and alprazolam (Xanax), reduce anxiety without being as **soporific** (sleep-producing).

The ability of benzodiazepines to potentiate GABA could account for their ability to reduce neuronal excitement in seizures and alcohol withdrawal. When used alone, benzodiazepines rarely inhibit the brain to the degree that respiratory depression, coma, and death result. However, when combined with other central nervous system (CNS) depressants, such as alcohol, opiates, or TCAs, the inhibitory actions of the benzodiazepines can lead to life-threatening respiratory depression.

Any drug that inhibits electrical activity in the brain can interfere with motor ability and judgment. Therefore, patients must be cautioned about engaging in activities that could be dangerous if reflexes and attention are impaired (e.g., driving) and should avoid making legal decisions. Ataxia is a common side effect secondary to the abundance of GABA receptors in the cerebellum.

Short-Acting Sedative-Hypnotic Sleep Agents

Nonbenzodiazepine hypnotic agents, such as zolpidem (Ambien), zaleplon (Sonata), and eszopiclone (Lunesta), demonstrate selectivity for $GABA_A$ receptors containing α_1-subunits. Termed the "Z-hypnotics," they have sedative effects without the antianxiety, anticonvulsant, or muscle-relaxant effects of benzodiazepines.

Melatonin Receptor Agonists

Ramelteon (Rozerem), a hypnotic, acts much the same way as endogenous melatonin. It has a high selectivity at the melatonin-1 receptor site, which is thought to regulate sleepiness, and at the melatonin-2 receptor site, which is thought to regulate circadian rhythms.

MOOD STABILIZERS

Lithium

The precise action of **lithium** as a mood stabilizer has not been established, but a common theme is that lithium affects multiple steps in cellular signaling. It appears to exert therapeutic actions through second-messenger systems, causing alterations in calcium and protein kinase C–mediated processes.

Primarily because of its effects on electrical conductivity, lithium has a low **therapeutic index** (the ratio of the lethal dose to the effective dose); therefore, it is important to monitor blood lithium levels, which are dependent on kidney function. Changes in sodium and hydration can affect the amount of lithium salts excreted. When sodium is depleted, the kidneys attempt to retain lithium, and this may result in toxicity. Conversely, excessive sodium lowers lithium. Long-term use of lithium increases the risk of both kidney and thyroid disease. Chapter 16 considers lithium treatment in more detail.

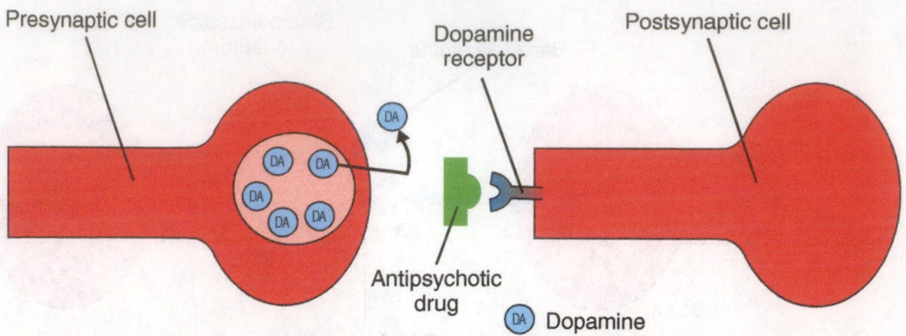

Fig. 4.12 Mechanism by which antipsychotics block dopamine receptors.

Anticonvulsant Mood Stabilizers

Valproate, available as **divalproex sodium** (Depakote) and **valproic acid** (Depakene), is helpful in patients with bipolar disorder who are unresponsive to lithium. It possibly works by inhibiting enzymes involved in GABA catabolism, thereby inhibiting neuronal excitability. Black Box warnings include hepatotoxicity, teratogenicity, and pancreatitis. Because of the potential for causing birth defects, women of childbearing age should use effective birth control methods while taking valproate.

Valproate increases the concentrations of another mood stabilizer, **lamotrigine** (Lamictal). Effective in bipolar depression, lamotrigine inhibits the release of glutamate and aspartate. Lamotrigine may trigger a severe skin reaction called Stevens–Johnson syndrome (SJS).

Carbamazepine (Tegretol) is less effective than lithium and causes more side effects than valproate, but it may be better in rapid-cycling bipolar disorder. It makes neurons less excitable in acute mania by stabilizing the inactive state of sodium channels in neurons (Stahl, 2017). A complete blood count (CBC) must be done periodically because of rare but serious blood dyscrasias (e.g., aplastic anemia and agranulocytosis).

Other Agents

Off-label mood stabilizers include oxcarbazepine (Trileptal), gabapentin (Neurontin), and topiramate (Topamax). Benzodiazepines may be used for their calming effects during mania, and sometimes antipsychotics and antidepressants are used along with a mood stabilizer. Refer to Chapter 16 for nursing considerations and patient and family teaching for the mood-stabilizing drugs.

ANTIPSYCHOTIC DRUGS

First-Generation Antipsychotics/Conventional Antipsychotics

First-generation antipsychotics (FGAs) were once called **neuroleptics** because they cause significant neurological effects. They are also referred to as **dopamine receptor agonists (DRAs)** because they bind to dopamine type 2 (D_2) receptors and reduce dopamine transmission, as illustrated in Fig. 4.12.

D_2 blockade achieves the therapeutic effect of decreasing positive symptoms in schizophrenia, but it can also lead to extrapyramidal side effects, such as dystonia (muscle stiffness), akathisia (restlessness), tardive dyskinesia (TD), and drug-induced parkinsonism. Anticholinergic agents such as benztropine (Cogentin) may be used to manage drug-induced parkinsonism, but anticholinergic therapy is itself linked to confusion, memory problems, and dementia in older adults (Gray et al., 2015).

D_2 blockade also may lead to a rare but life-threatening complication called neuroleptic malignant syndrome (NMS) involving autonomic, motor, and behavioral symptoms. The antipsychotic agent should be stopped immediately if the patient develops signs of NMS, such as severe muscle rigidity; confusion; agitation; and increased temperature, pulse, and blood pressure.

In addition to adverse effects occurring with D_2 blockade, unpleasant effects also result from antipsychotics blocking other receptors, such as those identified in Fig. 4.13. For example, blocking **muscarinic cholinergic receptors** can result in blurred vision, dry mouth, constipation, and urinary hesitancy. Antagonism of the **H_1 receptors** causes sedation and weight gain. Blockage at the **α_1-receptors** for norepinephrine can affect vasodilation and result in a consequent drop in blood pressure, or orthostatic hypotension. Antagonism of either α_1-receptors or **5-HT_2 receptors** may result in ejaculatory dysfunction. For a more detailed description of how the antipsychotic drugs block specific receptors, visit the Evolve website at http://evolve.elsevier.com/Varcarolis/essentials.

FGAs are further classified as high potency or low potency to indicate the drug's affinity for the D_2 receptor, which, in turn, influences the adverse-effect profile of the drug. Although high-potency haloperidol (Haldol) and **fluphenazine** (Prolixin) have less sedation and fewer anticholinergic effects than low-potency chlorpromazine (Thorazine), they cause more EPSs. An acute dystonic reaction (ADR) is more likely to occur early in treatment with a high-potency neuroleptic, especially if the patient uses cocaine.

In a large government-sponsored trial called the CATIE Project, the moderate-potency conventional antipsychotic perphenazine (Trilafon) was found to be comparable in efficacy to newer atypical agents. This finding, as well as the cost-effectiveness of FGAs, has renewed interest in their use.

Second-Generation/Atypical Antipsychotic Agents

Atypicals are known as serotonin-dopamine antagonists (SDAs) because they have a higher ratio of serotonin (5-HT_2) to dopamine D_2-receptor blockade than first-generation DRAs. They are prescribed more frequently because their different receptor-binding profile accounts for fewer EPSs. Abnormal functioning of brain circuits involving serotonin is believed to be linked to bipolar disorder and depression. Therefore, several SGAs are FDA approved for treating these disorders.

In addition to being potent 5-HT_{2A} receptor antagonists, some SGAs have significant anticholinergic and antihistaminic activity.

Clozapine (Clozaril)

Clozapine, the first of the atypical antipsychotics, is several times more potent in blocking 5-HT_2 receptors than D_2 receptors. It also has binding activity at a variety of other receptors, which may account for its advantages in treating patients who respond poorly to other antipsychotics. Clozapine is not a first-line treatment because it may suppress the bone marrow, resulting in **agranulocytosis**, a rare but serious decrease in granulated white blood cells (WBCs). Patients on clozapine will have weekly blood draws to monitor the absolute neutrophil count (ANC) for the first 6 months of treatment. If the ANC does not indicate agranulocytosis, blood work is spaced out to every 2 weeks for 6 months, and after a

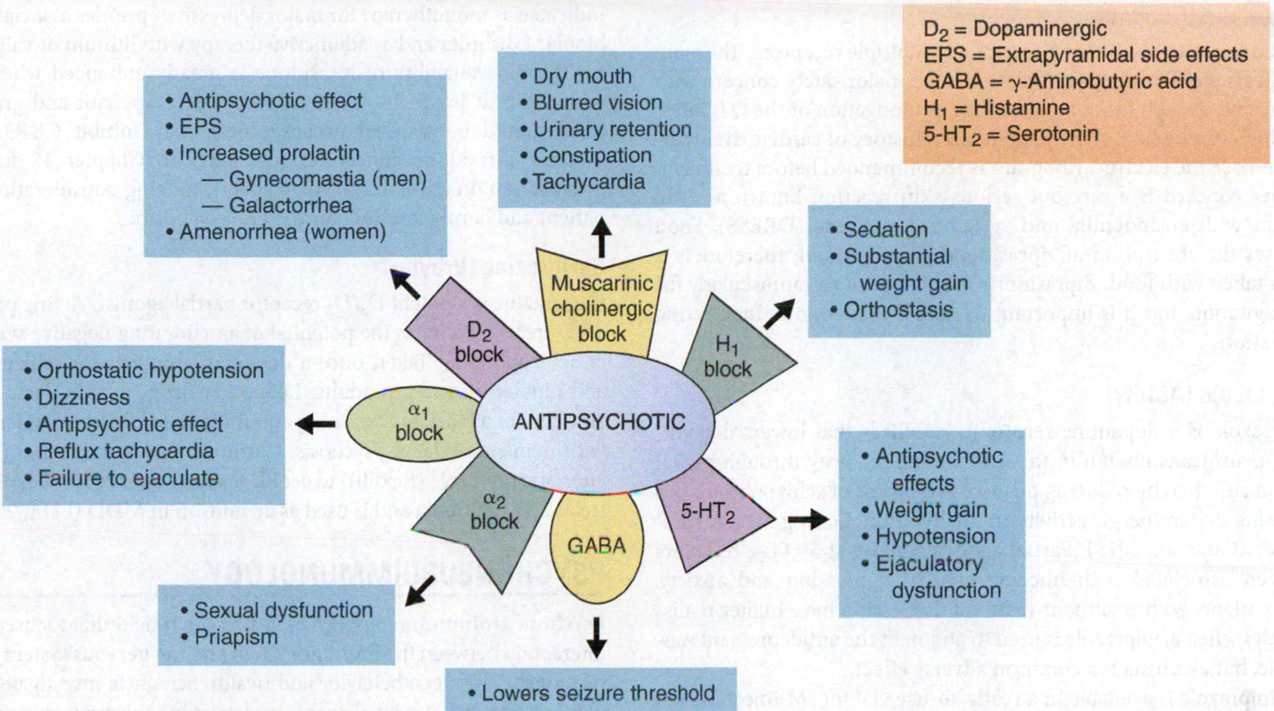

Fig. 4.13 Adverse effects of receptor blockage of antipsychotic agents. (From Varcarolis, E. [2015]. *Manual of psychiatric nursing care plans* [5th ed.]. St. Louis: Elsevier.)

year of monitoring, the ANC is measured every month for as long as the patient is on clozapine. Prescribers must document the ANC in an online database. The pharmacy must verify that the ANC is documented in the database before the medication can be refilled.

Seizures are a dose-related side effect of clozapine, so caution should be used with the co-administration of drugs such as SSRIs that elevate clozapine concentrations. Drooling, a paradoxical side effect, can cause social discomfort or speech problems. Hypersalivation may be relieved by sublingual drops of atropine ophthalmic solution.

Olanzapine (Zyprexa)

Olanzapine, a derivative of clozapine, has comparable receptor occupancies and similar metabolic side effects, such as weight gain. Metabolic monitoring for all patients receiving SGAs (atypicals) is recommended, although risperidone (Risperdal) and quetiapine (Seroquel) have a lower weight gain and ziprasidone (Geodon) and aripiprazole (Abilify) are considered weight neutral. Metabolic monitoring usually includes measurements of body weight, body mass index (BMI), waist circumference, fasting plasma glucose level, and fasting lipid profile.

Metformin—a medication used to regulate blood glucose level—reduces weight gain and waist circumference when used as an adjunct to SGAs. Although the metabolic effects are unhealthy, these adverse effects are often more tolerable than the neurological adverse effects of conventional antipsychotics.

Olanzapine is sedating because of its antagonism of H_1 receptors, so it is common practice to administer the medication at bedtime. It was the first antipsychotic available as orally disintegrating tablets. Olanzapine pamoate (Zyprexa Relprevv) is an extended-release injectable suspension that carries a warning for post-injection delirium/sedation. Thus, it requires at least 3 hours of continuous observation in a certified health care facility.

Risperidone (Risperdal)

Risperidone exhibits high levels of D_2-receptor blockade and a very high affinity for 5-HT_2 receptors. EPSs may occur if the dosage is only slightly higher than the effective dose. Therefore, the patient should be carefully monitored for motor difficulties if the dosage exceeds 4 to 6 mg/day. Because risperidone blocks α_1 and H_1 receptors, it can cause orthostatic hypotension and sedation, which can lead to falls—a serious problem for older adults. Weight gain and sexual dysfunction also are adverse effects that may affect medication adherence. It is also known to increase the prolactin level, which can cause gynecomastia, even in males. Patients on risperidone should have prolactin levels monitored periodically.

Risperidone (Risperdal Consta) was the first atypical antipsychotic available as a long-acting injectable (LAI) with intramuscular (IM) administration every 2 weeks. It is useful with nonadherent patients when it is necessary to keep the dosage regimen constant, particularly in patients with schizophrenia under court-ordered treatment. A longer-acting risperidone LAI (Perseris) is newly available and requires administration just once a month.

Paliperidone is the principal active metabolite of risperidone in Invega extended-release tablets. Paliperidone is used in schizophrenia and schizoaffective disorder and as an adjunct to mood stabilizers or antidepressants. Unlike its parent compound, paliperidone is eliminated almost independently of the CYP2D6 pathway and is cleared through the kidneys. Due to the osmotic release oral system (OROS) providing 24-hour release, morning administration is recommended. Paliperidone palmitate (Invega Sustenna) is offered as a once-monthly deltoid or gluteal injection.

Quetiapine (Seroquel)

Quetiapine has a broad receptor-binding profile with low binding at D_2 receptors and a low risk of EPSs. Its strong blockage of histamine-1 receptors accounts for somnolence, making quetiapine a preferred choice in patients with poor sleep onset or duration (Stahl, 2017). The combination of histamine-1 and serotonin-receptor blockage leads to weight gain and moderate risk for metabolic syndrome. Orthostatic hypotension is explained by antagonism of adrenergic α_1-receptors.

Ziprasidone (Geodon)

Ziprasidone is an SNRI that also binds to multiple receptors. The main side effects are dizziness and sedation. One major safety concern with ziprasidone, as with other atypicals, is a prolongation of the QT_c interval, which can be fatal if the patient has a history of cardiac dysrhythmias. A baseline electrocardiogram is recommended before treatment. Another concern is a rare but serious skin reaction known as drug reaction with eosinophilia and systemic symptoms (DRESS). Food increases the absorption of ziprasidone up to twofold; therefore it is always taken with food. Ziprasidone may be given intramuscularly for acute agitation, but it is important to note that it is not a long-acting preparation.

Aripiprazole (Abilify)

Aripiprazole is a dopamine-serotonin stabilizer that lowers dopaminergic neurotransmission in the mesolimbic pathway through partial D_2 agonism, thereby reducing positive symptoms of schizophrenia but increasing dopaminergic activity in the hypofunctioning mesocortical pathway (Guzman, 2015). Partial agonist activity at 5-HT_{1A} receptors has been associated with improvement of depression and anxiety. Older patients with treatment-resistant depression have higher remission rates when aripiprazole is used to augment the antidepressant venlafaxine, but akathisia is a common adverse effect.

Aripiprazole is available in a ready-to-use vial for IM injection and control of agitation in schizophrenia or bipolar disorder. Abilify Maintena is a once-monthly IM injection for the maintenance treatment of schizophrenia in adult patients stabilized with oral aripiprazole. An oral solution and oral disintegrating tablets (Abilify Discmelt) are also available. In addition, a new oral tablet (Abilify MyCite) allows users to wear a transdermal patch on the abdomen. A signal within the pill is transmitted when it comes in contact with digestive enzymes. The patch then communicates with a smartphone app that allows prescribers to track if and when the medication has been taken.

Iloperidone (Fanapt)

Although iloperidone is like the other SGAs in having a high affinity for both D_2 and 5-HT_{2A} receptors, it also has a high affinity for the D_3 receptor and noradrenergic receptor. Although orthostatic hypotension related to noradrenergic A1 antagonism is problematic, it tends to abate with time.

Lurasidone Hydrochloride (Latuda)

Lurasidone HCl has a high affinity for D_2 and 5-HT_{2A} receptors in addition to other serotonergic receptors. It exerts its effect in bipolar depression through agonistic activity at 5-HT_{1A} and antagonism at α_1-noradrenergic and 5-HT_{2A} receptors (Fountoulakis et al., 2015). It is indicated as monotherapy for major depressive episodes associated with bipolar I disorder and as adjunctive therapy with lithium or valproate.

The bioavailability of lurasidone is greatly enhanced when taken with food (at least 350 calories). However, grapefruit and grapefruit juice should be avoided because these may inhibit CYP3A4 and increase lurasidone concentrations. Refer to Chapter 17 for more information on adverse and toxic effects, nursing considerations, and patient and family teaching for the antipsychotics.

Cariprazine (Vraylar)

Cariprazine is a potent D_3/D_2 receptor partial agonist. Acting primarily on D_3 receptors, it has the potential of ameliorating negative symptoms of schizophrenia. Taken once a day, it is approved for schizophrenia and bipolar disorder in adults. Like other drugs in this class, cariprazine carries a black box warning about increased death in older people with dementia-related psychosis. Cariprazine was the second atypical after brexpiprazole (Rexulti) to get FDA approval in 2015. Brexpiprazole treats schizophrenia and is used as an add-on in MDD (FDA, 2015).

PSYCHONEUROIMMUNOLOGY

Psychoneuroimmunology (PNI) is a research field that focuses on the interaction between the immune system and the nervous system and the relationship between behavior and health. Scientists investigate molecular, cellular, and neuronal events to determine their role in psychiatric disorders. Chronic inflammation releases cytokines and pro-inflammatory chemicals. These cytokines can change the neuroplasticity of and reduce neurogenesis in the hippocampus. When this occurs, patients may experience a decrease in cognitive skills and display learning delays and mood changes (Chesnokova, Pechnick, & Wawrowsky, 2016). Neuroimmunopharmacology focuses on drugs modulating neuroimmune processes and is beginning to explore highly advanced technologies such as nanotechnology to develop approved nanodrugs.

CONSIDERING CULTURE

Cross-cultural psychopharmacology explores different responses that exist among ethnic groups and the reasons for these effects. Ethnic variations are influenced by genetic predisposition as well as cultural beliefs surrounding mental illness and pharmacotherapy. A patient's perception of the need for treatment, aversion to certain side effects, and preference for alternative or complementary therapies must be considered.

Genes are considered "plastic" because the dynamic pattern of gene regulation is a response to internal cues (e.g., neurotransmitters) as well as external cues (e.g., psychotropic drugs, psychotherapies). Monitoring the effects of integrated methods of treatment and empowering patients to make informed treatment decisions are at the heart of psychiatric nursing.

KEY POINTS TO REMEMBER

- All actions of the brain—sensory, motor, intellectual—are carried out through the interactions of nerve cells involving impulse conduction, transmitter release, and receptor response. Alterations in these basic processes can lead to mental disturbances and physical manifestations.
- In particular, it seems that excess activity of dopamine, among other factors, is involved in the thought disturbances of schizophrenia, and deficiencies of norepinephrine, serotonin, or both underlie depression and anxiety. Insufficient activity of γ-aminobutyric acid (GABA) also plays a role in anxiety.
- Pharmacological treatment of mental disturbances is directed at the suspected transmitter–receptor problem. Antipsychotic drugs decrease dopamine levels, antidepressant drugs increase synaptic levels of norepinephrine and/or serotonin, and antianxiety drugs increase the effectiveness of GABA or increase 5-HT and/or norepinephrine levels.
- Because the immediate target activity of a drug can result in many downstream alterations in neuronal activity, drugs with a variety of chemical actions may show efficacy in treating the same clinical condition. Thus, newer drugs with novel mechanisms of action are being used in the treatment of mental illness.
- Unfortunately, agents used to treat mental disease can cause various undesired effects. Prominent among these can be sedation or excitement, motor disturbances, muscarinic blockage, α-adrenergic antagonism, sexual dysfunction, and weight gain. There is a continuing effort to develop new drugs that are effective, safe, and well tolerated.

APPLYING CRITICAL JUDGMENT

1. No matter where you practice nursing, individuals under your care will be taking psychotropic drugs. Consider the importance of understanding normal brain structure and function as they relate to mental disturbances and psychotropic drugs by addressing the following questions:
   A. How can you use your knowledge of normal brain function (control of peripheral nerves, skeletal muscles, the autonomic nervous system, hormones, and circadian rhythms) to better understand how a patient can be affected by psychotropic drugs or psychiatric illness?
   B. What information from the various brain-imaging techniques can you use to understand and treat patients with mental disorders and provide support to their families? How might you use that information for patient and family teaching?
2. Based on your understanding of symptoms that may occur when the following neurotransmitters are altered, what specific information would you include in medication teaching?
   A. Dopamine D_2 (as with the use of antipsychotic drugs)
   B. Blockage of muscarinic receptors (as with the use of phenothiazines and other drugs)
   C. B_1-receptors (as with the use of phenothiazines and other drugs)
   D. Histamine (as with the use of phenothiazines and other drugs)
   E. Monoamine oxidase (MAO) (as with the use of a monoamine oxidase inhibitor [MAOI])
   F. γ-Aminobutyric acid (GABA) (as with the use of benzodiazepines)
   G. Serotonin (as with the use of selective serotonin reuptake inhibitors [SSRIs] and other drugs)
   H. Norepinephrine (as with the use of serotonin-norepinephrine reuptake inhibitors [SNRIs])

CHAPTER REVIEW QUESTIONS

1. A patient is diagnosed with an abscess in the cerebellum. Which nursing diagnosis has priority for the plan of care?
   a. Risk for falls related to loss of balance and equilibrium
   b. Unilateral neglect related to impairment in perception
   c. Impaired physical mobility related to spasticity and changes in muscle tone
   d. Risk for impaired cerebral tissue perfusion related to obstruction secondary to infection
2. A patient begins a new prescription for risperidone (Risperdal). Which intervention should the nurse include in the plan of care?
   a. Monitor intake and output daily.
   b. Educate patient about foods that contain tyramines.
   c. Assess sitting, standing, and lying blood pressure daily.
   d. Administer with food to reduce gastrointestinal irritation.
3. Systematic measurement of body weight, body mass index (BMI), waist circumference, and glucose levels would be most important for a patient beginning a new prescription for which medication?
   a. Aripiprazole (Abilify)
   b. Olanzapine (Zyprexa)
   c. Ziprasidone (Geodon)
   d. Quetiapine (Seroquel)
4. A patient tells the community mental health nurse, "I told my health care provider I was having trouble sleeping, and he prescribed trazodone 50 mg every night. I read on the Internet that the drug is an antidepressant, but I'm not depressed. What should I do?" Which response by the nurse is correct?
   a. "I will help you contact your health care provider for clarification regarding this new prescription."
   b. "Insomnia and depression usually go hand in hand. If your depression is relieved, your sleep will improve."
   c. "In low doses, trazodone helps relieve insomnia. Higher doses are needed for antidepressant effects to occur."
   d. "Information on the Internet is often misleading and incorrect. It's more important to trust the judgment of your health care provider."
5. Which patient would the nurse expect to have the most difficulty with problem solving and decision making?
   a. An 18-year-old diagnosed with bulimia nervosa at age 14; has taken oral doses of fluoxetine (Prozac) daily for 3 years
   b. A 46-year-old diagnosed with schizophrenia at age 24; has taken oral doses of clozapine (Clozaril) daily for 18 years
   c. A 62-year-old diagnosed with bipolar disorder at age 28; has taken oral divalproex sodium (Depakote) daily for 16 years
   d. A 52-year-old diagnosed with schizophrenia at age 21; has taken monthly injections of haloperidol (Haldol decanoate) for 12 years

REFERENCES

Assurex Health. (2018). *GeneSight: For clinicians*. Retrieved April 27, 2018 from https://genesight.com/for-clinicians/.

Banwari, G., Chaudhary, P., Panchmatia, A., & Patel, N. (2016). Persistent cerebellar dysfunction following acute lithium toxicity: A report of two cases. *Indian Journal of Pharmacology*, *48*(3), 331–333. https://doi.org/10.4103/0253-7613.182896.

Bernard, J. A., Orr, J. M., & Mittal, V. A. (2017). Cerebello-thalamo-cortical networks predict positive symptom progression in individuals at ultra-high risk for psychosis. *NeuroImage: Clinical*, *14*(2017), 622–628. https://doi.org/10.1016/j.nicl.2017.03.001.

Chesnokova, V., Pechnick, R. N., & Wawrowsky, K. (2016). Chronic peripheral inflammation, hippocampal neurogenesis, and behavior. *Brain, Behavior and Immunity*, *58*, 1–8. https://doi.org/10.1016/j.bbi.2016.01.017.

DeVane, C. L., & Nemeroff, C. B. (2018). *The 2018 handbook of psychotropic drug interactions*. Los Angeles: Medworks Media Inc.

Fountoulakis, K. N., Gazouli, M., Kelsoe, J., et al. (2015). *The pharmacodynamics properties of lurasidone and their role in its antidepressant efficacy in bipolar disorder*. Retrieved April 29, 2015, from www.ncbi.nlm.nih.gov/pubmed/25596883.

Giddens, J. F. (2017). *Concepts for nursing practice* (2nd. ed.). St. Louis: Elsevier.

Gitlin, M. (2018). *Unipolar depression in adults: Augmentation of antidepressants with thyroid hormone*. Retrieved April 27, 2018 from www.UpToDate.com.

Graat, I., Figee, M., & Denys, D. (2017). The application of deep brain stimulation in the treatment of psychiatric disorders. *International Review of Psychiatry*, *29*(2), 178–190. https://doi.org/10.1080/09540261.2017.1282439.

Gray, S. L., Anderson, M. L., Dublin, S., et al. (2015). Cumulative use of strong anticholinergics and incident dementia. *JAMA Internal Medicine*. Retrieved April 28, 2015, from www.ncbi.nlm.nih.gov/pubmed/25621434.

Guzman, F. (2015). *Mechanism of action of aripiprazole*. Psychopharmacology Institute. Retrieved April 21, 2015, from http://psychopharmacologyinstitute.com/antipsychotics/aripiprazole/mechanism-of-action-aripiprazole/.

Joshi, S. H., Espinoza, R. T., Pirnia, T., et al. (2016). Structural plasticity of the hippocampus and amygdala induced by electroconvulsive therapy in major depression. *Biological Psychiatry, 79*(4), 282–292.

Kania, B. F., Wronska, D., & Zieba, D. (2017). Introduction to neural plasticity mechanism. *Journal of Behavioral and Brain Science, 7*(2), 41–49. https://doi.org/10.4236/jbbs.2017.72005.

Lin, M., Hou, G., Zhao, Y., & Yuan, T. (2018). Recovery of chronic stress-triggered changes of hippocampal glutamatergic transmission. *Neural Plasticity.* https://doi.org/10.1155/2018/9360203.

Pinkham, A. E., Liu, P., Lu, H., et al. (2015). Amygdala hyperactivity at rest in paranoid individuals with schizophrenia. *American Journal of Psychiatry, 172*(8), 784–792.

Sadock, B. J., Sadock, V. A., & Ruiz, P. (2015). *Kaplan & Sadock's synopsis of psychiatry: Behavioral sciences/clinical psychiatry* (11th ed.). Philadelphia: Wolters Kluwer.

Sarpal, D. K., Argyelan, M., Robinson, D. G., et al. (2016). Baseline striatal functional connectivity as a predictor of response to antipsychotic drug treatment. *American Journal of Psychiatry, 173*(1), 69–77.

Stahl, S. M. (2017). *Stahl's essential psychopharmacology: Prescriber's guide* (6th ed.). New York: Cambridge University Press.

U.S. Food and Drug Administration (FDA). (2015). *FDA News Release: FDA approves new drug to treat schizophrenia and as an add on to an antidepressant to treat major depressive disorder.* Retrieved September 24, 2015, from www.fda.gov/NewsEvents/Newsroom/PressAnnouncements/ucm454647.htm.

U.S. Food and Drug Administration (FDA). (2020). Drug trial snapshots: Caplyta. Retrieved from https://www.fda.gov/drugs/drug-approvals-and-databases/drug-trials-snapshots-caplyta.

Viibryd Medication Guide. (2018). Retrieved April 28, 2018, from https://www.viibryd.com/.

Williams, L. M., Korgaonkar, M. S., Song, Y. C., et al. (2015). Amygdala reactivity to emotional faces in the prediction of general and medication-specific responses to antidepressant treatment in the randomized iSPOT-D Trial. *Neuropsychopharmacology, 40*(10), 2398–2408.

5

Settings for Psychiatric Care

Margaret Jordan Halter

http://evolve.elsevier.com/Varcarolis/essentials

OBJECTIVES

1. Describe the evolution of treatment settings for psychiatric care.
2. Compare and contrast inpatient and outpatient treatment environments in which psychiatric care is provided.
3. Discuss the role of mental health professionals in assisting people with mental illness symptoms or mental illnesses.
4. Explain methods for financing psychiatric care.

KEY TERMS AND CONCEPTS

Affordable Care Act (ACA), p. 57
collaboration, p. 54
community mental health centers (CMHCs), p. 53
comorbid conditions, p. 54
consumers, p. 57
crisis intervention, p. 55
elopement, p. 54
intensive outpatient programs (IOPs), p. 53
least restrictive environment, p. 52
mental health parity, p. 58
partial hospitalization programs (PHPs), p. 53
patient-centered medical homes (PCMHs), p. 52
primary care providers (PCPs), p. 52
psychiatric home care, p. 53
psychiatric mental health advanced practice registered nurses, p. 53
psychiatric rehabilitation services, p. 53
recovery, p. 57
residential treatment programs, p. 55
stigma, p. 51
teamwork, p. 54
therapeutic milieu, p. 54

CONCEPT: HEALTH DISPARITIES: *Health disparities* is defined as health care differences that occur by gender, race or ethnicity, education or income, disability—physical or mental, living in rural localities, or sexual orientation. Both implicit and explicit attitudes of health care providers significantly shape interactions with patients, guide expectations, and can affect clinical outcomes (Giddens, 2017). Compared with obtaining treatment for physical disorders, entry into the health care system for the treatment of mental health problems can be stigmatizing. Negative attitudes toward the mentally ill may have harmful effects on an individual and family and result in social isolation and reduced opportunities. Having a psychiatric illness is often hidden as a result of embarrassment or concern over stigma, shame, or perceptions of being flawed.

INTRODUCTION

Most people know what to do when they experience physical health problems. For example, if you wake up with a sore throat, you know what to do and basically what will happen. It is likely that if you feel bad enough, you will see your primary care provider (PCP), which may be a nurse practitioner or a physician. You will then be examined and maybe get a throat culture. If the cause is determined to be bacterial, you will probably be prescribed an antibiotic. If you do not improve in a certain period of time, your PCP may order more tests or recommend that you see an ear, nose, and throat specialist.

Compared with physical disorders, entry into the health care system for the treatment of psychiatric problems may be challenging. There are several challenges in accessing and navigating this care system. One reason is that we just do not have much of a frame of reference for the treatment of psychiatric problems. We are unlikely to benefit from the experience of others because having a psychiatric illness is often hidden. Hiding these experiences is due to embarrassment or concern over the stigma, or a sense of responsibility, shame, and being flawed, associated with these disorders (refer to Chapter 2 for more on stigma). You may know that when your grandmother had heart disease, she saw a cardiac specialist and had coronary artery bypass surgery. You may not know that she was also treated for a "nervous breakdown" by a psychiatrist.

Obtaining treatment for mental health problems is also complicated by the nature of mental illness. At the most extreme, disorders with a psychotic component, such as schizophrenia, may disorganize thoughts and impair a person's ability to recognize the need for care. There is a word for this inability: anosognosia (uh-no-sog-NOH-zee-uh). Major depressive disorder, a common psychiatric condition, may interfere with the motivation to seek care because the illness often causes feelings of apathy, hopelessness, and anergia (lack of energy).

Psychiatric symptoms are also confused with other conditions. For example, anxiety disorders are often accompanied by somatic symptoms such as racing heartbeat, sweaty palms, and dizziness, which could be symptoms of cardiac problems. Because psychiatric illness is largely based on symptoms and not on objective measurements such as electrocardiograms (ECGs) and blood counts, ruling out other physical illnesses is important. However, ruling out other illnesses often results in further treatment delay.

Another complication in treating mental illness is the unique nature of the system of care, which is rooted in the public as well as private sectors. The purpose of this chapter is to provide an overview of this system, briefly examine the evolution of mental health care, and explore different venues in which people receive treatment for mental health problems. Treatment options are presented in order of acuteness, beginning with those in the **least restrictive environment**—the setting that provides the necessary care while allowing the greatest personal freedom. This chapter also explores how mental health care is funded and describes the challenges in securing adequate funding.

BACKGROUND

Although people with financial resources have a variety of psychiatric treatment options, state or county governments coordinate a separate care system for uninsured individuals, often for those with the most serious and persistent illnesses. This separate system of care has its roots in asylums that were created in most existing states before the Civil War. These asylums were created with good intentions in an environment of optimism about recovery. The dominant belief was that states had a special responsibility to care for people who were then called "insane" (Latin *insanus*, from *in-* "not" + *sanus* "healthy").

Effective treatments were not yet developed, and community care was virtually nonexistent. By the early 1950s, there were only two real options for psychiatric care—a private psychiatrist's office or a mental hospital. At that time, there were 550,000 patients in state hospitals. A majority were individuals with disabling conditions who had become institutionalized in the asylums.

The number of people in state-managed psychiatric hospitals began to decrease with the creation of Medicare and Medicaid during the 1960s Great Society reform period. Medicaid had an especially potent effect because it paid for short-term hospitalization in general hospitals and medical centers and for long-term care in nursing homes. However, it did not cover care for most patients in psychiatric hospitals. These incentives stimulated the development of general hospital psychiatric units and also led states to transfer geriatric patients from 100% state-paid psychiatric hospitals to Medicaid-reimbursed nursing facilities.

In the 1999 *Olmstead* decision, the Supreme Court decreed that institutionalizing people in psychiatric hospitals was considered unjustified isolation. The opinion of the court was that mental illness is a disability, that institutionalization is in violation of the Americans with Disabilities Act, and that all people with disabilities have a right to live in the community.

These forces combined to lead to the gradual and incomplete creation of state- and county-financed community care systems. These systems served to complement, and largely replace, the functions of state hospitals. The number of state psychiatric hospitals continues to be cut and has been reduced from 322 in 1950 to 188 in 2015 (National Association of State Mental Health Program Directors, 2017).

The management of state- and county-financed community care systems varies depending on where you live. In Ohio, for example, a state agency—the Ohio Department of Mental Health and Addictions Services—certifies, monitors, and funds agencies that provide services. These agencies may be for profit or nonprofit. County boards (depending on whether alcohol/substance use disorders and mental health boards are combined) provide more local oversight and management of these agencies.

Related to the shift from hospital to community care were the pharmacological breakthroughs in the second half of the 20th century that led to dramatic changes in the provision of psychiatric care. The introduction of chlorpromazine (Thorazine), the first antipsychotic medication, in the early 1950s contributed to hospital discharges. Gradually, more psychopharmacological agents were added to treat psychosis, depression, anxiety, and other disorders. Treatment could be provided not only by specialists in psychiatry but also by general practitioners.

Our current system of psychiatric care includes outpatient and inpatient settings. Decisions for the level of care tend to be based on the condition being treated and the acuteness of the problem. However, these are not the only criteria. Levels of care may be influenced by such factors as a concurrent psychiatric or substance use problems, medical problems, acceptance of treatment, social supports, and disease chronicity or potential for relapse.

OUTPATIENT CARE SETTINGS

Primary care providers (PCPs) are the first choice for most people when they are ill, but what do people do when they suspect they may have a psychiatric problem? Imagine that you are feeling depressed, so depressed, in fact, that you are miserable and cannot carry out your normal activities. You recall that a friend who was depressed saw a psychiatrist (or was that a psychologist?), but that seems too drastic. You do not feel *that* bad. Perhaps you are coming down with something. After all, you have been tired, and you are not eating very well. You decide to visit your PCP, a general health care provider who may be a physician, an advanced practice nurse, or a physician assistant in an office, hospital, or clinic.

This is not an unusual choice. Seeking help for psychiatric problems from PCPs rather than from mental health specialists is common and similar to seeking help for other medical disorders. This is especially true because most psychiatric disorders are accompanied by unexplained physical symptoms. Most people treated for psychiatric disorders will not go beyond this level of care and may feel more comfortable being treated in a familiar setting. Furthermore, being treated in primary care rather than in the mental health system may lessen the degree of stigma, self-perceived or societally, attached to getting psychiatric care.

Disadvantages to being treated by PCPs include time constraints—a 15-minute appointment is usually inadequate for a mental and physical assessment. Because PCPs typically have limited training in psychiatry, they may lack expertise in the diagnosis and treatment of psychiatric disorders. Whereas this may be the only source many people use for receiving mental health services, sometimes PCPs refer people to specialty mental health care.

Patient-centered medical homes (PCMHs) received strong support from the Affordable Care Act of 2010. These health homes were developed in response to fragmented care that resulted in some services never being delivered while others were duplicated. The focus of care is patient centered and provides access to physical health, behavioral health, and supportive community and social services. Services range from preventive care and acute medical problems to chronic conditions and end-of-life issues. According to the Agency for Healthcare Research and Quality (n.d.), these homes have five key characteristics:

1. **Comprehensive care**—All levels (preventive, acute, and chronic) of mental and physical care are addressed. Physicians or advanced practice nurses lead teams that include nurses, physician assistants, pharmacists, nutritionists, social workers, educators, and care coordinators.
2. **Patient centered**—Care is relationship based and focused on the patient (family) and takes into account the unique needs of the

whole person. The patient is a core member of the team that manages and organizes the care.

3. **Coordinated care**—Care is coordinated with the broader health system, such as hospitals, specialty care, and home health.
4. **Accessible service**—Patients do not wait until Monday through Friday from 9 AM to 5 PM to get the care they need. In addition to extended hours of service, these homes provide email and phone support.
5. **Quality and safety** —Evidence-based care is provided with a continuous feedback loop of evaluation and quality improvement. Sharing data publicly is an essential part of a commitment to quality and safety in primary care medical homes.

The treatment of psychiatric disorders and mental health alterations can be addressed as part of a comprehensive approach to care. Electronic communication (e.g., follow-up emails and reminders) and record keeping are viewed as essential to this process.

Community mental health centers (CMHCs) were developed from President John F. Kennedy's Community Mental Health Centers Act of 1963. These centers signaled a policy preference for community care as opposed to institutionalization. Although only about 700 of the anticipated 2800 CMHCs were funded, the legislation marked a change in direction and led to state laws and budgets favoring community care.

CMHCs are regulated through state mental health departments and funded by the state. Some areas may provide local funding. Because of this limited government funding, financial support services may be restricted to those whose income and medical expenses make them eligible. Typically, fees are determined using a sliding scale based on income and ability to pay.

Community-based facilities provide comprehensive services to prevent and treat mental illness. These services include assessment, diagnosis, individual and group counseling, case management, medication management, education, rehabilitation, and vocational or employment services. Some centers may provide an array of services across the life span, whereas others may be population specific, such as adult, geriatric, or children.

People with serious mental illness are often isolated, impoverished, and regressed. They may benefit from **psychiatric rehabilitation services** that are provided through the community mental health system or other organizations. Psychiatric rehabilitation is a social model that emphasizes and supports recovery and integration into society rather than accepting a medical model of dysfunction. The development of social skills, the ability to access resources, and the acquisition of optimal social, working, living, and learning environments are the focus of this treatment method.

Psychiatric home care can be provided by any mental health professional. However, nurses who have inpatient experience and are able to provide biologically based and psychotherapeutic care usually take the lead. The care may be coordinated by the community mental health system or through other agencies such as Visiting Nurse Services. Home care may reduce the need for costly and disruptive hospitalizations and may provide a more comfortable and safer alternative to clinical settings.

To qualify for reimbursement, patients must have a psychiatric diagnosis, be under the care of a PCP, and be homebound. The designation of homebound generally is given when patients cannot safely leave home, if leaving home causes undue stress, if the nature of the illness results in a refusal to leave home, or if they cannot leave home unaided. However, one major insurer, Medicare, does allow the covered person to leave home once a week for religious services and once a week for hair care.

Intensive outpatient programs (IOPs) and **partial hospitalization programs (PHPs)** function as intermediate steps between inpatient and outpatient care. The primary difference between the two groups is the amount of time that patients spend in them. Both groups tend to operate Monday through Friday, but IOPs are usually half a day, whereas PHPs are longer (about 6 hours because they are "partially hospitalized"). These programs provide structured activities with nursing and medical supervision, intervention, and treatment. They tend to be located within general hospitals, in psychiatric hospitals, and as part of community mental health.

A multidisciplinary team facilitates group therapy, individual therapy, other therapies (e.g., art and occupational), and pharmacological management. Coping strategies that are learned during the program can be applied and practiced in the outside world and then explored and discussed later. Patients who are admitted to IOPs and PHPs are closely monitored to determine the need for admission or readmission to inpatient care.

Role of Nurses in Outpatient Care Settings

Psychiatric mental health registered nurses who work in outpatient settings provide nursing care for individuals with psychiatric disorders, substance use disorders, and intellectual disabilities, along with their families or caretakers. These community mental health nurses work to develop and implement a plan of care along with the multidisciplinary treatment team. They may choose to be certified in psychiatric-mental health nursing.

Community mental health nurses need to be knowledgeable about community resources such as shelters for abused women, food banks for people with severe financial limitations, and agencies that provide employment options for people with mental illnesses. Nurses may also assess the patient and living arrangements in the home, provide teaching, refer to community supports, and supervise unlicensed care staff. An important concept for community mental health nurses is viewing the entire community as a patient. This perspective promotes community interventions, such as conducting stress reduction classes and facilitating grief support groups.

Psychiatric mental health advanced practice registered nurses are valuable outpatient care providers. These master's level or doctorate-prepared nurse practitioners and clinical nurse specialists provide assessment, diagnosis, and treatment in all outpatient treatment settings (American Psychiatric Nurses Association, International Society of Psychiatric-Mental Health Nurses, & American Nurses Association, 2014). In fact, in many community health centers, psychiatric mental health advanced practice registered nurses far outnumber their medically prepared colleagues, psychiatrists. They are also instrumental in providing preventive care to individuals in the community. The focus of this care is on teaching patients to pay attention to symptoms, seek help when necessary, and be mindful of overall health.

INPATIENT CARE SETTINGS

Inpatient care has undergone significant change over the past 40 years. During the 1980s, inpatient stays were at their peak as private and nonfederal general hospital psychiatric units proliferated. During the mid-1990s, the number of patient days, psychiatric beds, and psychiatric facilities dipped sharply (Table 5.1). This decline was caused by improvements brought about by managed care, tougher limitations of covered days by insurance plans, and alternatives to inpatient hospitalization such as partial hospitalization programs and residential facilities.

Inpatient care is the most intensive. These facilities provide 24-hour nursing care in a safe and structured setting. Such a setting is essential to caring for those who are in need of protection from suicidal ideation, aggressive impulses, medication adjustment and monitoring, crisis

TABLE 5.1 **Number and Rate of 24-Hour Hospital and Residential Treatment Beds by Type of Mental Health Organization**

Type of Organization	1980	1990	2000	2010	2014
All organizations	274,713	325,529	214,186	181,622	182,516
State and county mental hospitals	156,482	102,307	61,833	48,069	37,953
Private psychiatric hospitals	17,157	45,952	26,402	28,672	31,918
Nonfederal general hospitals with separate psychiatric services	29,384	53,576	40,410	37,460	36,782
Veterans Administration (VA) medical centers[a]	33,796	24,799	8,989	6,746	7,877
Residential treatment centers for emotionally disturbed children	20,197	35,170	33,508	31,895	23,555
Residential treatment centers for emotionally disturbed adults	—	—	—	14,980	23,476

[a]Department of Veterans Affairs medical centers (VA general hospital psychiatric services and VA psychiatric outpatient clinics) were dropped from the survey in 2004.

Data from Substance Abuse and Mental Health Services Administration. (2014). *Mental health facilities data.* Retrieved from https://www.samhsa.gov/data/mental-health-facilities-data-nmhss/reports.

stabilization, substance use detoxification, and behavior modification. Referrals for inpatient treatment may come from a PCP or mental health provider, agencies, another hospital unit, emergency facilities, or nursing homes. Hospital admissions are made under the services of a psychiatrist, although a PCP also may have admitting privileges.

Patients may be admitted voluntarily or involuntarily (see Chapter 6). Units may be unlocked or locked. Locked units provide privacy and prevent **elopement**—leaving before being discharged (also referred to as being "away without leave" or AWOL). There may also be psychiatric intensive care units (PICUs) within the general psychiatric units to provide better monitoring of those who display an increased risk for danger to self or others.

The **therapeutic milieu** is essential to successful inpatient treatment. *Milieu* refers to the environment in which holistic treatment occurs and includes all members of the treatment team in a positive physical setting, with interactions among those who are hospitalized and activities that promote recovery.

Teamwork and **collaboration** are essential elements of interprofessional teams in acute care inpatient settings. *Teamwork* refers to a group of people working together to improve patient health, with each member of the team performing specialized functions (Box 5.1). There may be a leader of the team—often this is the registered nurse. Collaboration is a type of teamwork that requires team members (including the patient) to work directly together to make decisions and develop strategies to optimize care and achieve successful outcomes. Communication is central to this process. A formal structure for collaboration is a multidisciplinary team meeting where patients are discussed and care is planned. As a student, you may have a chance to attend team meetings and witness the level of interprofessional collaboration that, ideally, occurs in psychiatric care settings.

Inpatient care provides a structure in which patients eat meals, receive medication (if necessary), attend activities, and participate in individual and group therapies on a schedule. For those younger than the age of 18, school attendance is required. Patients are active participants in their plans of care and have the right to refuse treatments as long as they have not been declared incompetent. Advocates are usually available to provide advice and counsel for people who have doubts, and most facilities distribute a patient's bill of rights on admission or have it clearly posted. Box 5.2 provides a sample list of patient's rights.

Inpatient rooms are usually less institutional-looking than other hospital rooms and tend to resemble hotel rooms. Showers may be in the individual rooms or dorm-style, with one or two per hallway. Rooms are private, semiprivate, or occasionally, wards. Units may be made up solely of males or of females or may be co-ed.

Rooms are designed with safety in mind. Hanging is the most common method of inpatient suicide, and strict measures are taken to prevent it. Closet rods and hooks, towel bars, and shower rods are constructed to break if subjected to more than a minimal amount of weight. Sprinklers and showerheads tend to be flush-mounted, and utility pipes are enclosed. Other safety measures include locked windows, platform beds rather than mechanical hospital beds to prevent possible crushing, and furniture with rounded corners to reduce intentional injury. Furniture for inpatient rooms tends to be heavy and durable so that it cannot be thrown or dismantled and used as a weapon.

Inpatient care begins with a medical assessment to rule out or consider **comorbid conditions**—one or more disorders that occur along with another condition in the same person at the same time. A multidisciplinary treatment team conducts comprehensive assessments, and a plan of care is developed, monitored, evaluated, and refined (see Box 5.1). Crisis intervention and stabilization and patient safety are the goals of inpatient care. Psychotropic medication evaluation, prescription, and management are usually part of the plan of care, as is individual therapy.

Group therapy is an important facet of inpatient care. Coping skills are taught and enhanced through cognitive-behavioral groups. Occupational therapy provides an opportunity to practice life skills that have been delayed, hampered, or eroded. Psychoeducational groups focus on specific psychiatric disorders, medication, symptom management, goal setting, life planning, and recovery.

The length of stay varies depending on the severity of the illness and symptoms. Nationwide, the mental health average length of stay is 8 days, and for substance use, the average length of stay is 4.8 days (Piper Report, 2011). Therapeutic passes may be helpful so that the patient may go home for limited periods. In some cases, especially with children and people with severe mental illness, privileges and rewards, such as recreational outings, walks on the hospital grounds, and tokens to buy items from a unit "store," may be earned in order to reinforce adaptive behaviors.

Discharge planning begins on the first day of admission based on the patient's unique needs. Case management and collaboration with the patient's outpatient clinician, PCP, family, and community agencies such as the visiting nurse agency facilitate an integrated approach and establish comprehensive transition plans from inpatient to the community setting. This allows the patient to live effectively and safely in the community. Effective case management and collaboration also reduce recidivism.

BOX 5.1 Members of the Treatment Team

- **Psychiatric mental health registered nurses (PMH-RNs)** are registered nurses with specialized skills gained through education and experience in caring for individuals with mental health problems, psychiatric disorders, and substance use disorders. They may or may not have certification in psychiatric-mental health nursing.
- **Psychiatric mental health advanced practice registered nurses (PMH-APRNs)** are registered nurses who have completed a master's or doctoral degree. They can assess, diagnose, and treat patients. The two advanced practice roles in psychiatry are clinical nurse specialist (CNS) and nurse practitioner (NP). Unlike other specialty areas, there is no significant difference between these roles. Both assess health and psychiatric disorders, provide psychotherapy, and prescribe medications. Only one—the Psychiatric-Mental Health Nurse Practitioner-Board Certified (PMHNP-BC)—is available for national certification.
- **Psychiatrists** are state-licensed medical doctors who have at least 4 years of additional training in diagnosing and treating psychiatric disorders. The dominant treatment method used by psychiatrists includes medication prescribing and monitoring.
- **Psychologists** are licensed by individual states. They hold a doctoral degree in clinical, educational, counseling, or research psychology. Their expertise lies in evaluation, psychological testing, psychotherapy, and counseling. Some states may allow prescriptive authority for psychologists.
- **Social workers** are licensed by the state and may enter general practice with a bachelor's degree in social work. They may provide counseling and plan for supportive services such as housing, health care, and treatment after the patient is returned to the community. Social workers who hold a master's and doctoral degree are also able to provide assessment and treatment (usually psychotherapy) of psychiatric illness.
- **Licensed professional counselors** possess a master's or doctoral degree in counseling and are licensed by the state. They are trained to assess and diagnose psychiatric conditions and to provide individual, family, and group counseling.
- **Occupational therapists** are usually state regulated and are prepared at the master's and doctoral levels. They assist individuals in developing or regaining independent living skills, activities of daily living, and role performance that have been affected by psychiatric conditions and disorders.
- **Physical therapists** are educated with practice doctoral degrees and are accredited by the state. Their role is to rehabilitate individuals with physical disabilities that may be present concurrently with psychiatric disabilities.
- **Art therapists** are prepared at the master's level in art therapy and are credentialed at the national level. A minority of states requires licensing. Art therapists use creative expression to help people understand their problems, enhance healthy development, and reduce the effects of their illnesses.
- **Recreation therapists** are typically bachelor's prepared and are nationally certified. A small number of states require licensing. Recreational activities are used to improve emotional, physical, cognitive, and social well-being.
- **Pharmacists** are state licensed and prepared through 6 years of secondary education for a doctor of pharmacy (PharmD) degree. They provide distribution and centralized monitoring of drug regimens. Board Certified Psychiatric Pharmacists possess advanced training and skills in working with psychotropic medications.
- **Medical personnel** are physicians whose focus is the provision of nonpsychiatric care for comorbid conditions.
- **Mental health workers** or psychiatric aides are nonprofessional staff who may be state certified. They have extensive contact with patients while assisting with hygiene and meals and participating in unit activities. Mental health workers communicate important information concerning the patient's condition to professional staff.
- **Pastoral counselors** are clergy who have clinical pastoral education and are certified through the American Association of Pastoral Counselors. They provide individual and group counseling.
- **Peer specialists** are paid or volunteer individuals with serious mental illness who are trained and nationally certified. Some areas require state-specific certification. They use their experiences to provide recovery-oriented services and to support others with mental illness.

At discharge, patients should be stabilized. Discharge instructions include follow-up appointments, medication directions, education, prescriptions, and if necessary, assistance with living arrangements that may include a private residence, shelter, halfway house, or group home.

Crisis intervention is provided in emergency departments of general hospitals or in community-based *crisis intervention centers*. Crisis care may be initiated by the individual, friends, family, health care provider, or law enforcement personnel. Some patients are involuntarily committed. Psychiatric emergencies may include suicidal or homicidal ideation, acute psychosis, or behavioral responses to drugs. The stay in such facilities tends to be short, usually less than 24 hours. At that point the patient may be discharged to home, referred for inpatient care, or transferred to another community facility such as a shelter.

Residential treatment programs are structured short- or long-term 24-hour living environments in which individuals are provided with varying levels of supervision and support. Psychoeducation is provided for symptom management and medications. Vocational training and even training for daily activities of living may also be part of the program. The residents learn to access community support as an alternative to hospitalization and are encouraged to achieve maximal independence.

State Acute Care System

Today's state-operated psychiatric hospitals are an extension of what remains of the old system, although the quality of care in state hospitals has improved dramatically. The clinical role of state hospitals is to serve the most seriously ill patients, but this role varies widely, depending on available levels of community care and on payments by state Medicaid programs. In some states, state hospitals primarily provide intermediate treatment for patients unable to be stabilized in short-term general hospital units, and long-term care for individuals judged too ill for community care. In other states, the emphasis is on acute care that is reflective of gaps in the private sector, especially for the uninsured or for those who have exhausted limited insurance benefits.

In most states, the state hospitals provide forensic (court-related) care and monitoring as part of their function for those found *not guilty by reason of insanity* (NGRI). The state or county system also advises the courts as to defendants' sanity who may be judged to have been so ill when they committed the criminal act that they cannot be held responsible but require treatment instead. One tragic example is that of Andrea Yates, the Texas woman who in 2001 drowned her five young children under the delusional belief that she was saving them from their sinfulness. She was found NGRI and was committed to a Texas state psychiatric facility.

BOX 5.2 Typical Items Included in Hospital Statements of a Patient's Rights

- Right to be treated with dignity
- Right to be involved in treatment planning and decisions
- Right to refuse treatment, including medications
- Right to request to leave the hospital, even against medical advice
- Right to be protected against the possible impulse to harm oneself or others that might occur as a result of a mental disorder
- Right to the benefit of the legally prescribed process of an evaluation occurring within a limited period (in most states, 72 hours) in the event of a request for discharge against medical advice that may lead to harm to self or others
- Right to legal counsel
- Right to vote
- Right to communicate privately by telephone and in person
- Right to informed consent
- Right to confidentiality regarding one's disorder and treatment
- Right to choose or refuse visitors
- Right to be informed of research and to refuse to participate
- Right to the least restrictive means of treatment
- Right to send and receive mail and to be present during any inspection of packages received
- Right to keep personal belongings unless they are dangerous
- Right to lodge a complaint through a plainly publicized procedure
- Right to participate in religious worship

General Hospital Psychiatric Units and Private Psychiatric Hospital Acute Care

Acute care general hospital psychiatric units tend to be housed on a floor or floors of a general hospital. Private psychiatric hospitals are free-standing facilities. As noted, the dramatic growth of acute care psychiatric hospitals and hospital units is the result of a shift away from institutionalization in state-managed hospitals. Since that time, reduced reimbursement, increased managed care, enhanced outpatient options, and expanded availability of outpatient and partial hospitalization programs have resulted in the steady decline of these facilities.

Role of Psychiatric Nurses in Inpatient Care Settings

As professional care providers available around the clock every day of the week, nurses are at the center of any acute care inpatient facility. Management of these units, ideally, is by nurses with backgrounds in psychiatric-mental health nursing. Staff nurses tend to be nurse generalists, that is, nurses who have basic training as registered nurses. Some registered nurses obtain national certification in psychiatric-mental health nursing through the American Nurses Credentialing Center. The psychiatric mental health registered nurse carries out the following nursing responsibilities:

- Completing comprehensive data collection that includes the patient, family, and other health care workers
- Developing, implementing, and evaluating plans of care
- Assisting or supervising mental health care workers (e.g., nursing assistants with or without additional training in working with people who have mental illnesses)
- Maintaining a safe and therapeutic environment
- Facilitating health promotion through teaching
- Monitoring behavior, affect, and mood
- Maintaining oversight of restraint and seclusion
- Coordinating care by the treatment team

Medication administration is an essential skill for psychiatric nurses. In this specialty area, nurses often exert a strong influence on medication decisions and adjustments. This influence is due to nurses' continual observation of the expected, interactive, and adverse effects of medications. For example, feedback about a patient's excessive sedation or increased agitation may lead to a decision to decrease or increase the dosage of an antipsychotic medication.

A common misperception regarding psychiatric nurses in acute care settings is that because they "just talk," they lose their skills, including physical tasks such as starting and maintaining intravenous (IV) lines and changing dressings. First, therapeutic communication itself is a skill that people are not born with and must learn. Second, patients on the psychiatric unit are not limited to *Diagnostic and Statistical Manual of Mental Disorders,* 5th edition *(DSM-5)* diagnoses and often have complex health care needs. For example, an older adult male with brittle diabetes and a recent foot amputation may become actively suicidal. In this case, it is likely he will be transferred to the psychiatric unit, where his blood glucose level will be monitored and wound care completed.

Psychiatric mental health advanced practice registered nurses are also represented in inpatient care settings. These master's level or doctoral-prepared nurses are trained to provide much of the same care as psychiatrists. Assessment of mental health, diagnosis of mental health disorders, and prescription of psychiatric medication fall under the job description, with varying levels of state-mandated supervision by a physician. Advanced practice psychiatric nurses are qualified to engage in talk therapy (psychotherapy), group therapy, and managing patient care across the life span.

SPECIALTY TREATMENT SETTINGS

Treatment options are available that provide specialized care for specific groups of people. These options include inpatient, outpatient, and residential care.

Pediatric Psychiatric Care

Children with mental illnesses have the same range of treatment options as do adults but receive them apart from adults in pediatric settings. Inpatient care may be necessary if the child's symptoms become severe. Parental or guardian—including Department of Children and Families—involvement in the plan of care is integral so that they understand the illness, the treatment, and the family's role in supporting the child. Additionally, hospitalized children, if able, attend school for several hours a day.

Geriatric Psychiatric Care

The older adult population may be treated in specialized mental health settings that take into account the effects of aging on psychiatric symptoms. Physical illness and loss of independence can be strong precipitants in the development of depression and anxiety. Dementia is a particularly common problem that is addressed in geriatric psychiatry. Treatment is aimed at careful evaluation of the interaction of mind and body and provision of care that optimizes strengths, promotes independence, and focuses on safety.

Veterans Administration Centers

Active military personnel and veterans who were not dishonorably discharged may receive federally funded inpatient or outpatient care and medication for psychiatric and alcohol or substance use disorders. One of the greatest challenges veterans face is dealing with the aftereffects of the traumas of active combat. During Civil War times, these late effects were termed "soldier's heart." After World War I, soldiers had "shell shock," and after World War II, it was termed "battle fatigue." Currently, mental health services are inundated by people suffering from posttraumatic stress disorder (PTSD). There is a prevalence of PTSD in the general population of about 7%. Among male and female soldiers aged 18 years or older returning from Iraq and Afghanistan, rates range from 9% shortly after returning from deployment to 31% a year after deployment (Veterans Statistics, 2015). This creates a tremendous need for strong psychiatric services for this population.

Forensic Psychiatric Care

Incarcerated populations, both adult and juvenile, have higher-than-average incidences of mental health or substance use disorders. In 44 of the 50 states and the District of Columbia, prisons or jails hold more people with serious mental illness than the state's largest state psychiatric hospital (Treatment Advocacy Center, 2014). Treatment may be provided within the prison system, where inmates are often separated from the general prison population. State hospitals also treat forensic patients. Most facilities provide psychotherapy, group counseling, medication management, and assistance with transition to the community.

Alcohol and Drug Use Disorder Treatment

All the mental health settings that were previously described may provide treatment for alcohol and substance use disorders, although specialized treatment centers exist apart from the mental health care system. Although an estimated 22.7 million people older than age 12 needed treatment for an illicit drug or alcohol use problem in 2013, only 2.5 million received treatment at a specialty facility (Substance Abuse and Mental Health Services Administration [SAMHSA], 2014). This treatment is typically outpatient and includes counseling, education, medication management, and 12-step programs. Because alcohol detoxification can be life-threatening, inpatient care may be required for medical management. Drug rehabilitation facilities provide inpatient care for detoxification of drugs, including opiates and alcohol, and offer all levels of outpatient care.

Self-Help Options

Obtaining sufficient sleep, meditating, eating right, exercising, abstaining from smoking, and limiting the use of alcohol are healthy responses to a variety of illnesses such as diabetes and hypertension. As with other medical conditions, lifestyle choices and self-help responses can have a profound influence on the quality of life and the course, progression, and outcome of psychiatric disorders.

If we accept the notion that psychiatric disorders are usually a combination of biochemical interactions, genetics, and environment, then it stands to reason that by providing a healthy living situation, we are likely to fare better. If, for example, a person has a family history of anxiety and has demonstrated symptoms of anxiety, then a good first step (or an adjunct to psychiatric treatment) could be to learn yoga and balance the amounts of life's obligations with relaxation.

A voluntary network of self-help groups operates outside the formal mental health care system to provide education, contacts, and support. Since the introduction of Alcoholics Anonymous in the early 20th century, self-help groups have multiplied and have proven to be effective in the treatment and support of psychiatric problems. Groups specific to anxiety, depression, loss, caretakers' issues, bipolar disorder, posttraumatic stress disorder, and almost every other psychiatric issue are widely available in most communities.

Consumers, people who use mental health services, and their family members have successfully united to shape the delivery of psychiatric care. Nonprofit organizations such as the National Alliance on Mental Illness (NAMI) encourage self-help and promote the concept of **recovery**, or the self-management of mental illness. Introduced in Chapter 1 and discussed further in Chapters 3 and 19, these grassroots groups also confront social stigma, influence policies, and support the rights of people experiencing mental illness.

PAYING FOR MENTAL HEALTH CARE

On March 23, 2010, President Barack Obama signed into law the **Affordable Care Act (ACA)**. This groundbreaking piece of legislation helped millions of people who could not previously afford health care insurance. The ACA added millions of children and adults with mental health conditions who would no longer be denied health care because of pre-existing conditions. Some other provisions under this law include the following:

- Inability of insurance companies to deny a person coverage because of pre-existing conditions or rescind or take away insurance for health/mental health–related reasons
- Expansion of coverage for young adults up to the age of 26 under the parents' family policy
- A provision for people over 65 on Medicare—a 50% discount for name-brand drugs that reach the Medicare "donut hole"
- Tax credits for small businesses that offer insurance
- Affordable coverage for millions of Americans who are not able to afford care
- Insurance to cover preventive services such as depression screening and behavioral assessment for children
- Expanded integration between primary care and behavioral health care

In addition to the ACA and state and private insurance coverage, public assistance is available for mental health care and costs of living. Four assistance programs are Medicare, Medicaid, Social Security, and the Veterans Administration (VA). Medicare is a national program that provides benefits to people who are 65 years of age or older and to individuals who have become totally disabled. Medicaid operates under federal guidelines and state regulations and pays mental health care costs for people who have extreme financial need.

States vary widely in how they fund mental health care, but all states must provide benefits for inpatient care, PCP services, and treatment for those younger than age 21. Social Security has two federal programs designed to help people with disabilities. Social Security Disability Insurance (SSDI) may be provided to individuals who have worked a required length of time, have paid into Social Security, and are disabled for 12 months or more. In 2016, 6 out of 10 recipients of SSDI under the age of 65 were diagnosed with a psychiatric disorder (Social Security Administration, 2017).

Supplemental Security Income (SSI) is a federal income supplement program that is funded by general tax revenues. It provides benefits to older adults, those who are blind, and people with disabilities who have little or no income for basic needs such as food, clothing, and shelter.

A VISION FOR MENTAL HEALTH CARE IN AMERICA

Despite the availability and variety of community psychiatric treatments in the United States, many patients in this country in need of services are not receiving them. In addition to stigma, there are geographic, financial, and systems factors that limit access to psychiatric care. For example, mental health services are scarce in some rural areas, and many American families cannot afford health insurance even if they are working.

A vision for mental health care in the future includes the following:

- Americans understand that mental health is essential to overall health.
- Mental health care is consumer and family driven.

- Disparities in mental health services are eliminated.
- Early mental health screening, assessment, and referral to services are common practice.
- Excellent mental health care is delivered, and research is accelerated.
- Technology is used to access mental health care and information.

Psychiatric registered nurses are uniquely qualified to address each of the goals just mentioned due to an integrated educational background that includes biology, psychology, and the social sciences. Nurses specializing in this area will increasingly be in demand. As the population ages, more geropsychiatric nurses will be needed to work with older adult psychiatric patients with complex health problems. Advanced practice psychiatric nurses may collaborate more with primary health care practitioners or in independent practice to fill the gap in existing community services.

KEY POINTS TO REMEMBER

- Compared with seeking care for physical disorders, finding care for psychiatric disorders can be complicated by a two-tiered system of care provided in the private and public sectors.
- Nonspecialist primary care providers treat a significant portion of psychiatric disorders.
- Psychiatric care providers are specialists who are licensed to prescribe medication and conduct therapy. They include psychiatrists, advanced practice psychiatric nurses, physicians' assistants, and in some states, psychologists.
- Community mental health centers are state-regulated and state-funded facilities that are staffed by a variety of mental health care professionals.
- Other outpatient settings include psychiatric home care, intensive outpatient programs, and partial hospitalization programs.
- Inpatient care is used when less restrictive outpatient options are insufficient in dealing with symptoms. It can be provided in general medical centers, private psychiatric centers, crisis units, and state hospitals.
- Nurses provide the basis for inpatient care and are part of the overall unit milieu that emphasizes the role of the total environment in providing support and treatment.
- Specific populations such as children, veterans, geriatric patients, and forensic patients benefit from treatment geared to their unique needs.
- Financing psychiatric care has been complicated by lack of parity, or equal payment for physical as compared to psychiatric disorders. Legislation has been proposed and passed to improve mental health parity.

APPLYING CRITICAL JUDGMENT

1. You are a community psychiatric-mental health nurse working at a local mental health center. A single, 45-year-old patient reports that his thoughts seem to be "all tangled up." He states that he does not know how much longer he can go on, but he makes no direct reference to suicidal intent. He is disheveled and has been sleeping poorly at shelters. He becomes agitated when you suggest that it might be helpful for you to contact his family. He refuses to sign any release-of-information forms. He admits to recent hospitalization at the local veterans' hospital and reports previous treatment at a dual-diagnosis facility even though he denies substance misuse. In addition to his mental health problems, he says that he has tested positive for human immunodeficiency virus and should be taking multiple medications that he cannot name.
   - A. What are your biopsychosocial and spiritual concerns about this patient?
   - B. What is the highest-priority problem to address before he leaves the clinic today?
   - C. Do you feel that you need to consult with any other members of the multidisciplinary team today about this patient?
   - D. In your role as case manager, what systems of care will you need to coordinate to provide quality care for this patient?
   - E. How will you start to develop trust with the patient to gain his cooperation with the treatment plan?

CHAPTER REVIEW QUESTIONS

1. A patient diagnosed with major depressive disorder tells the community mental health nurse, "I usually spend all day watching television. If there's nothing good to watch, I just sleep or think about my problems." What is the nurse's best action?
   - a. Refer the patient for counseling with a recreational therapist.
   - b. Ask the patient, "What kinds of program do you like to watch?"
   - c. Suggest to the patient, "Are there some friends you could call instead?"
   - d. Advise the patient, "Watching television and thinking about problems makes depression worse."
2. The nurse admits a patient experiencing hallucinations and delusional thinking to an inpatient mental health unit. The plan of care will require that which service occurs first?
   - a. Social history
   - b. Psychiatric history
   - c. Medical assessment
   - d. Psychological evaluation
3. A nurse working in an acute care unit for adolescents diagnosed with mental illness says, "Our patients have so much energy. We need some physical activities for them." In recognition of needs for safety and exercise, which activity could the treatment team approve?
   - a. Badminton tournament
   - b. Competitive soccer matches
   - c. Intramural basketball games
   - d. Line dancing to popular music
4. As Election Day nears, a psychiatric nurse studies the position statements of various candidates for federal offices. Which candidate's commentary would the nurse interpret as supportive of services for persons diagnosed with mental illness?
   - a. Full-parity insurance coverage for mental illness
   - b. Coverage for biologically based mental illnesses
   - c. Reimbursement for initial treatment of addictions
   - d. Managed care oversight for mental illness services

5. An experienced nurse in a major medical center requests a transfer from a general medical unit to an acute care psychiatric unit. Which organizational feature would best support this nurse's successful transition?
   a. Assignment to medication administration for the first 6 months
   b. Working with a seasoned mental health technician for the first month
   c. Co-assignment with a knowledgeable psychiatric nurse for an extended orientation
   d. Staff development activities focused on developing therapeutic communication skills

REFERENCES

Agency for Healthcare Research and Quality. (n.d.). Defining the PCMH. Retrieved from www.pcmh.ahrq.gov/page/defining-pcmh.

American Psychiatric Nurses Association, International Society of Psychiatric-Mental Health Nurses, & American Nurses Association. (2014). *Psychiatric-mental health nursing: Scope and standards of practice* (3rd ed.). Silver Spring, MD: American Nurses Association.

Giddens, J. F. (2017). *Concepts for nursing practice* (2nd ed). St. Louis: Elsevier.

National Association of State Mental Health Program Directors. (2017). *Trends is psychiatric inpatient capacity, United States and each state 1970 to 2014.* Retrieved from https://www.nri-inc.org/media/1319/tac-paper-10-psychiatric-inpatient-capacity-final-09-05-2017.pdf.

Piper Report. (2011). *Hospitalizations for mental health and substance abuse disorders: Costs, length of stay, patient mix, and payor mix.* Retrieved from www.piperreport.com/blog/2011/06/25/hospitalizations-for-mental-health-and-substance-abuse-disorders.

Social Security Administration. (2017). SSDI annual statistical report, 2016. Retrieved from https://www.ssa.gov/policy/docs/statcomps/ssi_asr/.

Substance Abuse and Mental Health Services Administration. (2014). *Substance use and mental health estimates from the 2013 national survey on drug use and health.* Retrieved from www.samhsa.gov/data/sites/default/files/NSDUH-SR200-RecoveryMonth-2014/NSDUH-SR200-RecoveryMonth-2014.htm.

Treatment Advocacy Center. (2014). *The treatment of persons with mental illness in prisons and jails: A state survey.* Retrieved from http://www.treatmentadvocacycenter.org/storage/documents/treatment-behind-bars/treatment-behind-bars.pdf.

Veterans Statistics. (2015). *PTSD, depression, TBI, suicide. Veterans and PTSD.* Retrieved September 20, 2015 from www.veteransandptsd.com/PTSD-statistics.html.

6

Legal and Ethical Basis for Practice

Jessica Gandy

http://evolve.elsevier.com/Varcarolis/essentials

OBJECTIVES

1. Compare and contrast the different admission procedures, including admission criteria.
2. Summarize patients' rights as they pertain to the patient's (a) right to treatment, (b) right to refuse treatment, and (c) right to informed consent.
3. Delineate the steps nurses are advised to take to ensure patient safety if they suspect negligence or illegal activity on the part of a professional colleague or peer. **QSEN: Safety**
4. Discuss the legal considerations of patient privilege (a) after a patient has died, (b) if the patient tests positive for human immunodeficiency virus, or (c) if the patient's employer states a "need to know." **QSEN: Patient-Centered Care**
5. Summarize situations in which health care professionals have a duty to break patient confidentiality. **QSEN: Safety**
6. Discuss a patient's civil rights, and describe how they pertain to restraint and seclusion.
7. Discuss in detail the balance between the patient's rights and the rights of society with respect to the following legal concepts relevant in nursing and psychiatric nursing: (a) duty to intervene, (b) documentation and charting, and (c) confidentiality.

KEY TERMS AND CONCEPTS

abandonment, p. 69
administrative determination, p. 63
agency determination, p. 63
assault, p. 67
autonomy, p. 62
battery, p. 67
beneficence, p. 62
bioethics, p. 61
breach of duty, p. 67
bullying, p. 67
cause in fact, p. 68
child abuse reporting statutes, p. 66
civil rights, p. 61
commitment, p. 63
conditional release, p. 63
confidentiality, p. 65
damages, p. 68
defamation of character, p. 69
discharge, p. 63
due process, p. 62
duty to protect, p. 66
duty to warn, p. 66
elder abuse reporting statutes, p. 67
ethical dilemma, p. 61
ethics, p. 61
false imprisonment, p. 67
fidelity, p. 62
foreseeability of harm, p. 68
Health Insurance Portability and Accountability Act (HIPAA), p. 64
implied consent, p. 64
informed consent, p. 63
intentional torts, p. 67
involuntary admission, p. 62
involuntary outpatient commitment, p. 63
judicial determination, p. 63
justice, p. 62
least restrictive alternative doctrine, p. 62
legal guardian, p. 64
negligence, p. 67
proximate cause, p. 68
punitive damages, p. 68
right to privacy, p. 65
right to refuse treatment, p. 63
right to treatment, p. 63
tort, p. 67
veracity, p. 62
voluntary admission, p. 62
writ of habeas corpus, p. 62

CONCEPT: ETHICS: *Ethics* is the study of morality through a variety of different approaches. Technical proficiency in nursing is important, but it is not enough to guarantee a sense of integrity. To achieve professional integrity, one needs the skills and abilities of moral sensitivity and reflection. Moral courage enables us to act on our decisions even under the most challenging circumstances (Giddens, 2017). A goal of psychiatric care is to balance the rights of the individual patient and the rights of society at large. At times, a nurse's values may be in conflict with the value system of the institution. For example, a nurse may experience a conflict of values when adults are routinely sedated to a degree that may seem excessive. Some nurses respond by working to change the system or advocating for legislation related to a particular issue.

INTRODUCTION

This chapter introduces current legal and ethical issues that may be encountered in the practice of psychiatric nursing. A fundamental goal of psychiatric care is to strike a balance between the rights of the individual patient and the rights of society at large. This chapter is designed to assist you in understanding the implications of ethical and legal issues on the provision of care in a psychiatric setting.

An **ethical dilemma** results when there is a moral conflict between two or more courses of action, with each potential choice carrying similarly favorable and unfavorable consequences. How we respond to these dilemmas is based largely on our own morals and values. Suppose you are caring for a pregnant woman with schizophrenia who wants to carry the baby to term but whose family insists she must get an abortion. In order to promote fetal safety, her antipsychotic medication would need to be reduced, putting her at risk of exacerbation of her mental health symptoms. Furthermore, there is a question as to whether she can safely care for the child. If you relied on the ethical principle of autonomy, you might conclude that she has the right to decide. Would other ethical principles be in conflict with autonomy in this case?

At times, your values may conflict with those of the patient, state law, or institutional policy. This further complicates the decision-making process and necessitates careful consideration of the patient's desires and controlling law. For example, you may experience a moral conflict in a setting where patients are tranquilized to a degree that you find excessive. Whenever one's value system is challenged, increased stress results.

LEGAL AND ETHICAL CONCEPTS

Ethics is the study of philosophical beliefs about what is considered right or wrong in a society. **Bioethics** is a more specific term that refers to the ethical questions that arise in health care. The five basic principles of bioethics are shown in Table 6.1.

Law and ethics may be closely related because laws tend to reflect the ethical values of society. Legal obligations can be found in federal or state statutes, Board of Nursing ("Board") regulations, or administrative code. You should familiarize yourself with all sources of nursing law in your state because they vary depending on the jurisdiction. Although they come from a variety of sources, we refer to them collectively as "laws" because there are legal consequences for violating them.

It should be noted that although you may feel personally obligated to follow ethical guidelines, these guidelines should never override laws. For example, if you are aware of a law that prohibits a certain action (e.g., restraining patients against their will) and you feel you have an ethical obligation to protect the patient by engaging in such an action (e.g., using restraints), you would be wise to follow the law. If you feel you cannot breach your ethical standards to remain within the bounds of the law, you must immediately notify your supervisor.

MENTAL HEALTH LAWS

Specific laws have been enacted to regulate the care and treatment of a person with mental illness. Many of these laws have undergone major revision since 1963, which reflects a shift in emphasis from state or institutional care to community-based care. This shift was heralded by the enactment of the Community Mental Health Center Act of 1963 under President John F. Kennedy (Box 6.1). Along with this shift in emphasis has come the more widespread use of psychotropic drugs in the treatment of mental illness—which has enabled many people to integrate more readily into the larger community—and an increasing awareness of the need to provide patients with humane care that respects their civil rights. Parity in health insurance coverage for mental health treatment was addressed in 2010 by two separate laws. The Paul Wellstone and Pete Domenici Mental Health Parity and Addiction Equity Act (MHPAEA) states that if mental health or substance abuse care is covered by a private insurance plan, then these conditions must receive coverage equitable to other physical medical conditions. The 2010 Health Insurance Exchanges program requires that each state must offer mental health care and substance use services equal to other medical services (Bazelon, 2010).

In providing coverage for mental health and substance abuse, the Affordable Care Act (ACA) built upon the MHPAEA, which provided rehabilitative support services for behavioral health needs. The MHPAEA was signed into law on October 3, 2008, and became effective on January 1, 2010 (Beronio et al., 2013). Mental health coverage and substance abuse coverage are included in the "essential health benefits" provision of the ACA. Mental health coverage must be at parity with medical and surgical benefits, meaning coverage cannot be more restrictive than coverage for general medical benefits. It is projected that the ACA has expanded mental health and substance abuse benefits with parity protections to between 60 and 62 million Americans. Most health plans must now cover preventive mental services at no cost. Screening for depression and other adult mental health conditions as well as behavioral assessments for children are covered by the ACA. Additionally, as of 2014, insurance plans cannot charge more or deny coverage for pre-existing mental health conditions (Beronio et al., 2013).

However, disparities in state-by-state coverage affect access to mental health care. More than 21 states initially refused the ACA provisions to expand Medicaid coverage following the 2012 U.S. Supreme Court decision to allow states to opt out. Homeless and low-income persons are affected by Medicaid coverage. Sixteen states and the District of Columbia set up their own insurance exchanges and thus determine their own "essential benefits," which may not include mental health care (Brink, 2014). Nurses working with mental health and substance abuse patients should be aware of the benefits of coverage in their own jurisdiction.

In 2017, Congress and President Donald Trump expressed plans to either repeal the ACA and, with it, the federal and state Health Insurance Exchanges or enact significant amendments to the existing ACA. As of this writing, those plans have been unsuccessful; however, any changes to the ACA have the potential to reduce access to mental health or substance abuse care or reduce the number of insured Americans (Appleby, 2017).

Civil Rights

People with mental illness are guaranteed the same rights under federal and state laws as any other citizen. Most states specifically prohibit any person from depriving an individual receiving mental health services of his or her **civil rights**, including the right to vote; the right to civil

TABLE 6.1 The Five Basic Principles of Bioethics

Concept	Definition	Example
Beneficence	The duty to act so as to benefit or promote the good of others	Spending extra time to help calm an extremely anxious patient
Autonomy	Respecting the rights of others to make their own decisions	Acknowledging the patient's right to refuse medication
Justice	The duty to distribute resources or care equally, regardless of personal attributes	Devoting equal attention to both a friendly patient and a patient who will not speak or make eye contact
Fidelity (nonmaleficence)	Maintaining loyalty and commitment to the patient and doing no wrong to the patient	Maintaining expertise in nursing skill through nursing education
Veracity	One's duty to communicate truthfully	Describing the purpose and side effects of psychotropic medications in a truthful and nonmisleading way

BOX 6.1 The Legacy of Rosemary Kennedy

Rosemary Kennedy, the younger sister of President John F. Kennedy, was born with an intellectual disability, and some believe she was epileptic. As a child, her family routinely hid her away and sent her to "special" schools in an attempt to maintain the family reputation. As Rosemary became a young adult in the 1930s, she became increasingly frustrated with her exclusion and her inability to participate in family functions. In an attempt to improve her mental health, her parents forced her to undergo a lobotomy. The procedure was a disaster, leaving her physically and mentally incapacitated. The Kennedys attempted to hide the horrific results, virtually scrubbing Rosemary from the family history and moving her to a secluded cottage in Wisconsin.

In the 1960s, Rose Kennedy, the family matriarch, began speaking openly about Rosemary and became a vocal advocate for mental health care. Rose influenced President Kennedy to enact some of the first federal mental health care legislation. The Kennedy family also created a foundation to care for children with mental disabilities and founded the Special Olympics and Best Buddies.

service ranking; the rights related to granting, forfeit, or denial of a driver's license; the right to make purchases and to enter contractual relationships, including marriage (unless the patient has lost legal capacity by being deemed legally incompetent); the right to press charges against another person; and the right to personal and religious expression. The patient's rights also include the right to humane care and treatment. The medical, dental, and psychiatric needs of the patient must be met in accordance with the prevailing standards accepted in these professions. Individuals in prisons and jails are afforded the same protections.

In recent years, many states have established mental health courts to process nonviolent criminal cases involving defendants with mental illnesses to curb the growing population of mental health patients in jail and prison. According to a Department of Justice study, over 40% of inmates self-report a history of a mental health condition, with over 20% self-reporting "serious psychological condition" (Bronson, 2017). To combat this statistic, mental health courts attempt to direct their defendants to treatment and services in the community.

ADMISSION AND DISCHARGE PROCEDURES

Due Process in Civil Commitment

In 1972, the Supreme Court held that involuntary civil commitment to a mental hospital is a "massive curtailment of liberty" (*Humphrey v. Cady*, 1972), requiring due process protections in the civil commitment procedure. **Due process** is a legal term referring to the requirement of state and federal governments to follow fair procedures before depriving someone of "life, liberty, or property." The right to due process derives from the Fifth and Fourteenth Amendments of the U.S. Constitution. The Fifth Amendment applies exclusively to actions of the federal government; the Fourteenth Amendment extends due process to state actors. In 2001, the Supreme Court extended those rights to non-citizens (*Zadvydas v. Davis*).

State civil commitment statutes, if challenged in the courts on constitutional grounds, must afford minimal due process protections to pass the court's scrutiny (*Zinermon v. Burch*, 1990). In most states, a patient can challenge involuntary commitments through a **writ of habeas corpus**, which is a formal written request to "deliver the body" to a court of law to challenge continued confinement.

The writ of habeas corpus and the least restrictive alternative doctrine are two of the most important concepts applicable to civil commitment cases. The **least restrictive alternative doctrine** mandates that the least drastic means be taken to achieve a specific purpose. For example, if someone can safely be treated for depression on an outpatient basis, hospitalization would be too restrictive and disruptive, and thus unnecessary.

Admission to the Hospital

All students are encouraged to become familiar with the important provisions of the laws in their own states regarding admissions, discharges, patients' rights, and informed consent.

A medical standard or justification for admission should exist. The presenting illness should also be of such a nature that it causes an immediate crisis situation or that other, less restrictive alternatives are inadequate or unavailable. There should also be a reasonable expectation that the hospitalization and treatment will improve the presenting problems.

In the case of *Olmstead v. L.C.* (1999), the Supreme Court ruled that states are required to place patients with mental health needs in less restrictive community settings, rather than institutions, when the treatment profession has determined that a community setting is appropriate and the patient is not opposed.

Voluntary Admission

Generally, **voluntary admission** is sought by a patient or a patient's guardian through a written application to the facility. Voluntarily admitted patients have the right to demand and obtain release at any time. However, few states require voluntarily admitted patients to be notified of the rights associated with their status. In addition, many states require that a patient submit a written release notice to the facility staff, who then reevaluate the patient's condition for possible conversion to involuntary status according to criteria established by state law.

Involuntary Admission (Commitment)

Involuntary admission is made without the patient's consent. Generally, involuntary admission is necessary when a person is in need of psychiatric treatment, presents a danger to self or others, or is unable to meet his or her own basic needs due to mental illness. Involuntary commitment requires that the patient retain freedom from unreasonable bodily restraints as well as the right to informed consent and the right to refuse medications, including psychotropic or antipsychotic medications.

Three different commitment procedures are commonly available: **judicial determination**, **administrative determination**, and **agency determination**. In addition, a specified number and type of physicians must certify that a person's mental health status justifies detention and treatment. Involuntary hospitalization can be further categorized by the nature and purpose of the involuntary admission: emergency hospitalization, observational or temporary hospitalization, long-term or formal commitment, or outpatient commitment.

Emergency Involuntary Hospitalization. Most states provide a mechanism for emergency involuntary hospitalization or civil **commitment** for a specified period of hours or days to prevent dangerous behavior that is likely to cause harm to self or others. Police officers, physicians, and mental health professionals may be designated by law to authorize the detention of individuals believed to have mental illness who present a danger to themselves or others.

Long-term or Formal Commitment. Long-term commitment for involuntary hospitalization has, as its primary purpose, extended care and treatment of a patient with mental illness. Those who undergo extended involuntary hospitalization are committed through medical certification, judicial, or administrative action. Some states do not require a judicial hearing before commitment, but they often provide the patient with an opportunity for a judicial review after commitment procedures. This type of involuntary hospitalization generally lasts 60 to 180 days but may be for an indeterminate period.

Involuntary Outpatient Commitment. Beginning in the 1990s, states began to pass legislation that permitted outpatient commitment as an alternative to forced inpatient treatment. Recently, states have begun using **involuntary outpatient commitment** as a preventive measure, allowing a court order before the onset of a psychiatric crisis that would result in an inpatient commitment. The order for involuntary outpatient commitment is usually tied to the receipt of goods and services provided by social welfare agencies, including disability benefits and housing. To access these goods and services, the patient is mandated to participate in treatment and may face inpatient admission for failure to participate (Zilber, 2016). The American Psychological Association (APA, 2013) adopted the position that this type of intervention is appropriate only for individuals with severe illness but who are unwilling or unable to participate in voluntary outpatient care. Ideally, this should be a temporary condition, with the individual converting to voluntary therapy within weeks or months. Forced treatment raises ethical dilemmas regarding autonomy versus paternalism, privacy rights, duty to protect, and right to treatment and has been challenged on constitutional grounds.

Discharge From the Hospital

Release from hospitalization depends on the patient's admission status. Patients who sought informal or voluntary admission, as previously discussed, have the right to request and receive release. Some states, however, do allow for a temporary hold of a voluntary patient so safety concerns can be assessed by the psychiatrist or psychiatric nurse practitioner before the patient is discharged. States may also provide for the conditional release of voluntary patients, which enables the treating physician or administrator to order continued treatment on an outpatient basis if the clinical needs of the patient warrant further care.

Conditional release usually requires outpatient treatment for a specified period to determine the patient's adherence to medication protocols, ability to meet basic needs, and ability to reintegrate into the community. Unconditional release, or **discharge**, is the termination of a patient–institution relationship. This release may be court ordered or administratively ordered by the institution's officials. Generally, the administrative officer of an institution has the discretion to discharge patients.

PATIENTS' RIGHTS UNDER THE LAW

Inpatient psychiatric facilities usually provide patients with a written list of basic patient rights. These rights are derived from a variety of sources, especially legislation that was developed during the 1960s. Since then, they have been modified to some degree, but most lists share commonalities, as stated in the following sections.

Right to Treatment

With the enactment of the Hospitalization of the Mentally Ill Act in 1964, the federal statutory right to psychiatric treatment in public hospitals was created. The act requires that medical and psychiatric care and treatment be provided to all public hospital patients.

Although state courts and lower federal courts have decided that there may be a federal constitutional right to treatment, the U.S. Supreme Court has never firmly defined the **right to treatment**. The evolution of these cases in the courts provides a history of the development and shortcomings of our mental health delivery system. Based on several early decisions, treatment must meet the following criteria:

- The environment must be humane.
- Staff must be qualified and sufficient to provide adequate treatment.
- The plan of care must be individualized.

The first cases pondering the psychiatric patient's right to treatment questioned the constitutionality of involuntary commitment. In 1975, the Supreme Court held in *O'Connor v. Donaldson* (1975) that a state cannot confine a nondangerous individual to a psychiatric facility if that individual can survive safely in freedom by himself or herself or with the help of willing and responsible family members or friends.

Right to Refuse Treatment

A companion to the right to consent to treatment is the right to withhold consent. A patient may withdraw consent at any time. Retraction of consent previously given must be honored, whether it is verbal or written. However, the mentally ill patient's **right to refuse treatment** with psychotropic drugs has been debated in the courts, based partly on the issue of patients' competency to give or withhold consent to treatment and their status under the civil commitment statutes. These early cases, initiated by state hospital patients, considered medical, legal, and ethical considerations, such as basic treatment problems, the doctrine of informed consent, and the bioethical principle of autonomy. For a summary of the evolution of one landmark set of cases regarding the patient's right to refuse treatment, see Table 6.2.

The notion of refusing treatment becomes especially important if we consider medication a "chemical restraint." If it is, the infringement on a person's liberty is equal to involuntary commitment. As such, the noninstitutionalized, competent, mentally ill patient has the right to determine whether to be involuntarily committed or to be medicated.

Cases involving the right to refuse psychotropic drug treatment are still evolving. Without clear direction from the Supreme Court, individual states can continue to follow their own laws. The numerous cases involving the right to refuse medication have illustrated the complex and difficult task of translating social policy concerns into a clearly articulated legal standard.

Right to Informed Consent

The principle of **informed consent** is based on a person's right to self-determination, as established in *Canterbury v. Spence* (1972). The Washington, DC, Appellate Court determined that a medical

TABLE 6.2 Right to Refuse Treatment: Evolution of Massachusetts Case Law to Present Law

Case	Court	Decision
Rogers v. Okin, 478 F. Supp. 1342 (D. Mass. 1979)	Federal District Court	Ruled that involuntarily hospitalized patients with mental illness are competent and have the right to make treatment decisions. Forcible administration of medication is justified in an emergency if needed to prevent violence and if other alternatives have been ruled out. A guardian may make treatment decisions for an incompetent patient.
Rogers v. Okin, 634 F. 2nd 650 (1st Cir. 1980)	Federal Court of Appeals	Affirmed that involuntarily hospitalized patients with mental illness are competent and have the right to make treatment decisions. The staff has substantial discretion in an emergency. Forcible medication is also justified to prevent the patient's deterioration. A patient's rights must be protected by judicial determination of competency or incompetency.
Mills v. Rogers, 457 U.S. 291 (1982)	U.S. Supreme Court	Set aside the judgment of the Court of Appeals with instructions to consider the effect of an intervening state court case.
Rogers v. Commissioner of the Department of Mental Health, 458 N.E.2d 308 (Mass. 1983)	Massachusetts Supreme Judicial Court answering questions certified by the Federal Court of Appeals	Ruled that involuntarily hospitalized patients are competent and have the right to make treatment decisions unless they are judicially determined to be incompetent.

provider has an affirmative duty to disclose all of the known risks and complications of a proposed treatment to allow the patient to make an informed decision as to whether to proceed with that treatment. This standard was soon adopted nationwide.

As a result, proper orders for specific therapies and treatments are required and must be documented in the patient's chart. Consent for surgery, electroconvulsive treatment, or the use of experimental drugs or procedures must be obtained. In some state institutions, consent is required for every medication addition or change. Patients have the right to refuse participation in experimental treatments or research and the right to voice grievances and recommend changes in policies or services offered by the facility, without fear of punishment or reprisal.

For consent to be legally effective, it must be informed. Patients must be informed of the nature of their problem or condition, the nature and purpose of a proposed treatment, the risks and benefits of that treatment, the alternative treatment options available, the probability that the proposed treatment will be successful, and the risks of not consenting to treatment. It is important for psychiatric nurses to know that the presence of psychotic symptoms does not mean that the patient is incompetent or incapable of understanding.

Neither voluntary nor involuntary admission to a mental facility determines whether patients are capable of making informed decisions about the health care they may need. Patients must be considered legally competent until they have been declared incompetent through a legal proceeding. Competency is related to the capacity to understand the consequences of one's decisions. The determination of legal competency is made by the courts. If found incompetent, the court may appoint a **legal guardian** to be responsible for giving or refusing consent for a person the court has found to be incompetent (a "ward").

Guardians have a duty to act in their wards' best interests. Courts appoint guardians to care for people who cannot take care of themselves due to age or mental disability. It is important to recognize that a power of attorney (or POA) is not a substitute for a guardian. A POA may make decisions on behalf of an individual but generally cannot override that individual's decisions. Conversely, a guardian has control over all medical, financial, and personal decision making. However, where appropriate, courts may appoint guardians with limited authority (National Association for Court Management [NACM], 2014).

Guardians are usually selected from among family members. If a family member is either unavailable or unwilling to serve as guardian, the court may appoint a court-trained and court-approved social worker representing the county or state or a member of the community. In recent years, due to rampant guardianship abuses, states have become more cautious when appointing non–family member guardians (Ardanowski, 2018).

Many procedures that nurses perform have an element of implied consent attached. For example, if you approach the patient with a medication in hand and the patient indicates a willingness to receive the medication, **implied consent** has occurred. It should be noted that many institutions, particularly state psychiatric hospitals, have a requirement to obtain informed consent for every medication given. As a general rule, the more intrusive or risky the procedure, the higher the likelihood that informed consent must be obtained. The fact that you may not have a *legal* duty to inform patients of the associated risks and benefits of a procedure does not eliminate your professional duty to clarify the procedure to patients and ensure their expressed or implied consent.

Rights Surrounding Involuntary Commitment and Psychiatric Advance Directives

Patients concerned that they may be subject to involuntary psychiatric commitment can prepare an advance psychiatric directive document that will express their treatment choices. The advance directive for mental health decision making should be followed by health care providers when patients are not competent to make informed decisions for themselves. This document can clarify the patient's choice of a surrogate decision maker and instructions about hospital choices, medications, treatment options, and emergency interventions. Identification of individuals who are to be notified of the patient's hospitalization and who may have visitation rights is especially helpful given the privacy demands of the **Health Insurance Portability and Accountability Act (HIPAA)**.

Rights Regarding Restraint and Seclusion

The use of the least restrictive means of restraint for the shortest duration is always the general rule and even the law. Verbal interventions or enlisting the cooperation of patients are examples of first-line interventions. Recent changes in state laws regarding the use of restraints and seclusion have prompted agencies to revise their policies and procedures, further limiting these practices. The current trend is toward "restraint-free" environments and alternative methods of therapy and cooperation with the patient, which is proving successful.

Typically, medication is considered if verbal or environmental interventions fail. Chemical interventions are usually considered less restrictive than mechanical, but they can have a greater effect on the patient's ability to relate to the environment. When used judiciously, psychopharmacology is extremely effective and helpful as an alternative to other physical methods of restraint.

The history of mechanical restraint and seclusion is one that is marked by abuses and overuse. This was especially true before the 1950s, when there were no effective chemical treatments. Legislation has dramatically reduced this problem by mandating strict guidelines. The newest guidelines of the Centers for Medicare and Medicaid Services (CMS) and The Joint Commission (2008) guidelines read as follows:

A-0154 (Rev. 37, Issued: 10-17-08; Effective/Implementation Date: 10-17-08) §482.13(e) Standard: **Restraint or seclusion.** All patients have the right to be free from physical or mental abuse, and corporal punishment. All patients have the right to be free from restraint or seclusion, of any form, imposed as a means of coercion, discipline, convenience, or retaliation by staff. Restraint or seclusion may only be imposed to ensure the immediate physical safety of the patient, a staff member, or others and must be discontinued at the earliest possible time.

(Rev. 37, Issued: 10-17-08; Effective/Implementation Date: 10-17-08) §482.13(e)(8)—Unless superseded by State law that is more restrictive—(i) Each order for restraint or seclusion used for the management of violent or self-destructive behavior that jeopardizes the immediate physical safety of the patient, a staff member, or others may only be renewed in accordance with the following limits for up to a total of 24 hours:

A. 4 hours for adults 18 years of age or older;
B. 2 hours for children and adolescents 9 to 17 years of age; or
C. 1 hour for children under 9 years of age.

In an emergency, *an appropriately trained staff member for the proper and safe use of seclusion and restraint interventions* may place a patient in seclusion or restraint and obtain a written order within an hour. With the exception of a patient-initiated request to be placed in seclusion, federal laws require an emergency situation to exist in which an immediate risk of harm to the patient or others can be documented. While in restraints, the patient must be protected from all sources of harm. The behavior leading to restraint or seclusion and the time the patient is placed in and released from the restraint must be documented; the patient in restraint must be assessed at regular and frequent intervals (e.g., every 15–30 minutes) for physical needs (e.g., food, hydration, toileting), safety, and comfort, and these observations also must be documented (every 15 to 30 minutes). The patient must be removed from restraints when safer and quieter behavior is observed. Although state laws may be *more* restrictive than federal law, they cannot be *less* restrictive.

Maintenance of Patient Confidentiality

Confidentiality of care and treatment is an important right for all patients, particularly psychiatric patients. Any discussion or consultation involving a patient should be conducted discreetly and only with individuals who have a need and a right to know this privileged information. The American Nurses Association's (ANA) *Code of Ethics for Nurses With Interpretive Statements* (2015) asserts the duty of the nurse to protect confidential patient information (Box 6.2). Failure to provide this protection may harm the nurse-patient relationship, as well as the patient's well-being. However, the code clarifies that this duty is not absolute. In some situations, disclosure may be mandated to protect the patient, other people, or public health.

BOX 6.2 *Code of Ethics for Nurses*

The House of Delegates of the American Nurses Association approved these nine provisions at its June 30, 2001, meeting in Washington, DC. In July 2001, the Congress of Nursing Practice and Economics voted to accept the new language of the interpretive statements, resulting in a fully approved revised *Code of Ethics for Nurses With Interpretive Statements.*

1. The nurse, in all professional relationships, practices with compassion and respect for the inherent dignity, worth, and uniqueness of every individual, unrestricted by considerations of social or economic status, personal attributes, or the nature of health problems.
2. The nurse's primary commitment is to the patient, whether an individual, family, group, or community.
3. The nurse promotes, advocates for, and strives to protect the health, safety, and rights of the patient.
4. The nurse is responsible and accountable for individual nursing practice and determines the appropriate delegation of tasks consistent with the nurse's obligation to provide optimum patient care.
5. The nurse owes the same duties to self as to others, including the responsibility to preserve integrity and safety, to maintain competence, and to continue personal and professional growth.
6. The nurse participates in establishing, maintaining, and improving health care environments and conditions of employment conducive to the provision of quality health care and consistent with the values of the profession through individual and collective action.
7. The nurse participates in the advancement of the profession through contributions to practice, education, administration, and knowledge development.
8. The nurse collaborates with other health professionals and the public in promoting community, national, and international efforts to meet health needs.
9. The profession of nursing, as represented by associations and their members, is responsible for articulating nursing values, for maintaining the integrity of the profession and its practice, and for shaping social policy.

Health Insurance Portability and Accountability Act

The psychiatric patient's right to receive treatment and have confidential medical records is legally protected. The fundamental principle underlying the ANA *Code of Ethics for Nurses* on confidentiality is a person's constitutional **right to privacy**. Generally, your legal duty to maintain confidentiality is to protect the patient's right to privacy. HIPAA became effective on April 14, 2003. Therefore, you may not, without the patient's consent, disclose information obtained from the patient or information in the medical record to *anyone* except those individuals for whom it is necessary for implementation of the patient's treatment plan without appropriate written authorization. HIPAA requires that notes used in psychotherapy are kept separate from the patient's health information. Discussions about a patient in public places, such as elevators and the cafeteria, even when the patient's name is not mentioned, can lead to inadvertent disclosures of confidential information and liabilities for you and the facility. Any release of information to a third party, including the patient's family or employer, about the patient's condition, without the patient's express consent, is a breach of confidentiality that subjects you and the facility to tort liability as well as a HIPAA violation.

In general, for information to be considered privileged, a patient–health professional relationship must exist and the information must concern the care and treatment of the patient. The health professional may refuse to disclose information to protect the patient's privacy. However, the right to privacy is the *patient's right*, and health professionals cannot invoke confidentiality for their own defense or benefit.

Rights After Death

A person's right to privacy continues after death. Nurses may not divulge information after a person's death that could not have been legally shared before the death, except with proper legal authorization. HIPAA protects confidential information about people, even when they are not alive to speak for themselves.

A legal privilege of confidentiality exists to protect the confidentiality of professional communications (e.g., nurse–patient). The theory behind such privileged communications is that patients will not be comfortable or willing to disclose personal information about themselves if they fear that nurses will repeat their confidential conversations. There are, however, exceptions to privilege, and a health care provider may be compelled to provide testimony under subpoena.

Furthermore, privilege does not apply in cases where a health care provider has a duty to report past, present, or future abuse or criminal activity. If a duty to report exists, you may be required to divulge private information shared by the patient.

Patient Privilege and Sexually Transmitted Disease

Some states have enacted mandatory or permissive statutes that direct health care providers to warn a spouse if a partner tests positive for human immunodeficiency virus (HIV) or other sexually transmitted diseases. Nurses must understand the laws in their jurisdiction of practice regarding privileged communications and warnings of infectious disease exposure.

Exceptions to Confidentiality

Duty to Warn and Protect Third Parties

The California Supreme Court, in its 1974 landmark decision *Tarasoff v. Regents of University of California,* ruled that a psychotherapist has a **duty to warn** a patient's intended victim of potential harm. A university student, Prosenjit Poddar, was in counseling at a California university after being romantically rejected by Tatiana Tarasoff. Poddar told his doctor that he was upset by the breakup and planned to stab Tarasoff. The psychologist notified police verbally and in writing that the young man may be dangerous to Tarasoff and recommended civil commitment. The police questioned the student, found him to be rational, and secured his promise to stay away from his love interest. The supervising psychologist stated that commitment was not appropriate and that Poddar should not be detained.

Poddar stopped seeing his therapist and befriended Tarasoff's brother to gain insight into her activities, eventually becoming his roommate. Poddar killed Tarasoff 2 months later in the same manner he described to his doctor. This case created much controversy and confusion in the psychiatric and medical communities over breach of patient confidentiality and its effect on the therapeutic relationship in psychiatric care and over the ability of the psychotherapist to predict when a patient is truly dangerous. This trend continues as other jurisdictions have adopted or modified the California rule despite the objections of the psychiatric community. These jurisdictions view public safety to be more important than privacy in narrowly defined circumstances.

The *Tarasoff* case acknowledged that generally, there is no common-law duty to aid third parties. An exception is when special relationships exist, and the court found the patient–therapist relationship sufficient to create a duty of the therapist to aid Ms. Tarasoff, the victim. The duty to protect the intended victim from danger arises when the therapist determines—or should have determined—that the patient presents a serious danger to another person. The California Supreme Court held "the protective privilege ends where public peril begins," signaling the concern for public safety. Any action reasonably necessary under the circumstances, including notification of the potential victim, the victim's family, and the police, discharges the therapist's duty to the potential victim.

In 1976, the California Supreme Court issued a second ruling in the case of *Tarasoff v. Regents of University of California* (now known as *Tarasoff II*). This ruling broadened the earlier ruling, the duty to warn, to include the **duty to protect**.

Most states have similar laws regarding the duty to warn third parties of potential life threats. Currently, 33 states have an affirmative duty to warn or protect, with an additional 11 states permitting a health care professional to break privilege to warn intended victims (Johnson, Persad, & Sisti, 2014). The duty to warn usually includes the following:

- Assessing and predicting the patient's danger of violence toward another
- Identifying the specific individual(s) being threatened
- Taking appropriate action to protect the identified victims

Nursing Implications

As this trend toward making it the therapist's duty to warn third parties of potential harm continues to gain wider acceptance, it is important for students and nurses to understand its implications for nursing practice. Although none of these cases has dealt with nurses, it is fair to assume that in jurisdictions that have adopted the *Tarasoff* doctrine, the duty to warn third parties will be applied to *advanced practice psychiatric-mental health health nurses* (PMH-APRNs) in private practice who engage in individual therapy.

If, however, a staff nurse who is a member of a team of psychiatrists, psychologists, psychiatric social workers, and other psychiatric nurses does not report patient threats of harm against specified victims or classes of victims, this failure is likely to be considered substandard (negligent) nursing care and may lead to legal liability.

The failure to communicate and record relevant information from police, relatives, or previous records might also be deemed negligent. Breach of patient–nurse confidentiality should not pose ethical or legal dilemmas for nurses in these situations because a team approach to the delivery of psychiatric care presumes communication of pertinent information to other staff members to develop a treatment plan in the patient's best interest.

Child and Elder Abuse Reporting Statutes

Because of their interest in protecting children, all 50 states and the District of Columbia have enacted **child abuse reporting statutes**. Although these statutes differ from state to state, they generally include a definition of child abuse, a list of individuals required or encouraged to report abuse, and the governmental agency designated to receive and investigate the reports. Most statutes include civil penalties for failure to report. Many states specifically require nurses to report cases of suspected abuse.

There is a conflict between federal and state laws with respect to child abuse reporting when the health care professional discovers child abuse or neglect during the suspected abuser's alcohol or drug treatment. Federal laws and regulations governing the confidentiality of patient records, which apply to almost all substance use and alcohol treatment providers, prohibit any disclosure without a court order. In this case, federal law supersedes state reporting laws, although compliance with the state law may be maintained under the following circumstances:

- If a court order is obtained, pursuant to the regulations
- If a report can be made without identifying the abuser as a patient in an alcohol or drug treatment program
- If the report is made anonymously (some states, to protect the rights of the accused, do not allow anonymous reporting)

As reported incidents of abuse to other persons in society surface, states may require health professionals to report other kinds of abuse. A growing number of states have **elder abuse reporting statutes**, which require nurses to report cases of abuse of older adults. Agencies that receive federal funding (i.e., Medicare or Medicaid) must follow strict guidelines for reporting and preventing elder abuse. Older adults are defined as adults 65 years of age and older. These laws also apply to dependent adults—that is, adults between 18 and 64 years of age whose physical or mental limitations restrict their ability to carry out normal activities or to protect themselves—when the nurse has actual knowledge that the person has been the victim of abuse.

Under most state laws, a person who is required to report suspected abuse, neglect, or exploitation of a disabled adult and who willfully does not do so is guilty of a misdemeanor crime. Most state statutes declare that anyone who makes a report in good faith is immune from civil liability in connection with the report.

Nurses may also report knowledge of, or reasonable suspicion of, mental or emotional abuse. Dependent adults and older adults are protected by the law from purposeful physical or fiduciary neglect or abandonment. **Because state laws vary, students are encouraged to become familiar with the reporting requirements of their states.**

TORT LAW APPLIED TO PSYCHIATRIC SETTINGS

Torts are a category of civil law that commonly applies to health care practice. A **tort** is a civil wrong for which money damages may be collected by the injured party (the plaintiff) from the wrongdoer (the defendant). The injury can be to person, property, or reputation. Because tort law has general applicability to nursing practice, this section may contain a review of material previously covered elsewhere in your nursing curriculum.

Violence

Bullying has become a recognized form of violence in our society. Nurses may encounter bullying behaviors from nursing supervisors, peers, patients, and even family members of patients. There is some legal precedent for holding professionals liable if they are aware of bullying behavior that is within their sphere of control and do not take affirmative steps to protect the known victim. For example, if a patient is bullying staff or other patients at an inpatient facility or during group therapy sessions, the professional has a duty to minimize those harms.

When nurses in psychiatric settings encounter provocative, threatening, or violent behavior from patients, the use of restraint or seclusion might be required until a patient demonstrates safer behavior. Accordingly, the nurse in the psychiatric setting should understand the **intentional torts** of **battery**, **assault**, and **false imprisonment** (described in Boxes 6.3 and 6.4). More on the use of restraints and seclusion is found in Chapters 16 and 24.

Negligence/Malpractice

Most legal issues in medical care stem from allegations of **negligence**, commonly referred to as "malpractice." Negligence or malpractice is an act or failure to act that breaches the duty owed to a patient by a provider. The four elements required to prove negligence are (1) duty, (2) breach, (3) causation, and (4) damages. The foreseeability or likelihood of harm may also be evaluated to determine civil liability but is not typically a factor in professional discipline investigations.

As professionals, nurses owe patients a duty to provide a specific level of care at all times. Nurses employed in specialized fields, such as psychiatric care, are required to have the requisite education, training, and experience in order to understand the theory, treatments, and medications used in the specialty care of these patients. Providers who represent themselves as possessing superior knowledge and skill, such as psychiatric nurse specialists, are held to a higher standard of care in the practice of their profession.

If a nurse is not willing or able to provide the requisite standard of care that other nurses would be expected to provide under the same or similar circumstances, that nurse has breached the duty of care. **Breach of duty** is the conduct that exposes the patient to an unreasonable risk of harm, through either actions or failure to act by the nurse.

BOX 6.3 Contraindications to Seclusion and Restraint

- Extremely unstable medical and psychiatric conditions[a]
- Delirium or dementia leading to inability to tolerate decreased stimulation
- Severe suicidal tendencies
- Severe drug reactions or overdoses or need for close monitoring of drug dosages
- Desire for punishment of patient or convenience of staff

[a]Unless close supervision and direct observation are provided.
From Simon, R. I. (2001). *Concise guide to psychiatry and law for clinicians* (3rd ed., p. 117). Washington, DC: American Psychiatric Press.

BOX 6.4 False Imprisonment and Negligence: *Plumadore v. State of New York* (1980) 427 N.Y.S. 2d 90 (New York Supreme Court, Appellate Division)

Mrs. Plumadore was admitted to Saranac Lake General Hospital for a gallbladder condition. Her medical workup revealed emotional problems stemming from marital difficulties, which had resulted in suicide attempts several years before her admission. After a series of consultations and tests, she was advised by the attending surgeon that she was scheduled to have gallbladder surgery later that day. After the surgeon's visit, a consulting psychiatrist who examined Mrs. Plumadore directed her to dress and pack her belongings because he had arranged to have her admitted to a state hospital at Ogdensburg.

Subsequently, two uniformed state troopers handcuffed Mrs. Plumadore and strapped her into the back seat of a patrol car. She was also accompanied by a female hospital employee and was transported to the state hospital. On arrival, the admitting psychiatrist recognized that the referring psychiatrist lacked the requisite authority to order her involuntary commitment. He therefore requested that she sign a voluntary admission form, which she refused. Despite Mrs. Plumadore's protests regarding her admission to the state hospital, the psychiatrist assigned her to a ward without physical or psychiatric examination and without the opportunity to contact her family or her medical physician. The record of her admission to the state hospital noted an "informed admission," which is patient-initiated voluntary admission in New York.

The court awarded $40,000 to Mrs. Plumadore for false imprisonment, negligence, and malpractice.

Causation is determined through "cause in fact" and "proximate cause." **Cause in fact** is typically evaluated through the "but for" test: "But for what the nurse did, would this injury have occurred?" **Proximate cause**, or legal cause, is more complicated. A finder of fact will evaluate whether there were any unforeseeable, intervening actions or inactions that were the actual cause of harm to the patient. For example: Nurse A dispensed the wrong medication, which fell below the standard of care, but when delivering the medication, Nurse B inadvertently left the patient's door unsecured, which resulted in the patient leaving the unit, falling down the stairs, and breaking a leg. Although both nurses fell below the standard of care, Nurse B was the *proximate cause* of the patient's injury. Even though the incorrect medication may have contributed to the patient's actions or led to harm, the unsecured door was an unrelated, unforeseeable, and negligent action that directly led to the injury. **Foreseeability of harm** evaluates the likelihood of the outcome under the circumstances.

Damages include actual damages (e.g., loss of earnings, medical expenses, and property damage) and pain and suffering to the injured party as well as immediate family members. A number of states have enacted legislation to limit (or cap) noneconomic, or pain and suffering, damages in civil litigation; however, amounts vary from state to state. If a litigation alleges that a nurse acted fraudulently, maliciously, or outside the scope of his or her employment, a court may award additional **punitive damages** as "punishment" for egregious behavior.

DETERMINATION OF A STANDARD OF CARE

Professional standards of practice determined by professional associations are not equivalent to the standards embodied in the minimum qualifications established by state licensure for entry into the profession of nursing. The ANA has established standards for psychiatric-mental health nursing practice and credentialing for the psychiatric mental health registered nurse (PMH-RN) and the psychiatric mental health advanced practice nurse (PMH-APRN) in psychiatric mental health nursing (ANA, 2015).

Standards for psychiatric-mental health nursing practice differ markedly from minimal state requirements. The state's qualifications for practice provide consumer protection by ensuring that all practicing nurses have successfully completed an approved nursing program and passed the national licensing examination. The ANA's primary focus is to elevate the practice of its members by setting standards of excellence.

Nurses are held to the standard of care provided by other nurses possessing the *same degree of skill or knowledge in the same or similar circumstances*. In the past, community standards existed for urban and rural agencies. However, with greater mobility and expanded means of communication, national standards have evolved, with limited exceptions for remote areas. Psychiatric patients have the right to the standard of care recognized by professional bodies governing nursing, whether they are in a rural or an urban facility. Nurses must participate in continuing education courses to stay current with existing standards of care.

Hospital policies and procedures establish institutional criteria for care, and these criteria, such as the frequency of rounds, may be introduced to allege a standard that the nurse met or failed to meet. States vary as to whether policies may be substituted for a standard of care because policies may be more or less stringent than the standard of care. For example, the state licensing laws for institutions might set a minimum requirement for staffing or frequency of rounds for certain patients, and the hospital policy might fall below that minimum. **Substandard institutional policies do not absolve the individual nurse of responsibility to practice on the basis of professional standards of nursing care.**

Like hospital policy and procedures, customs of practice may be used as evidence of a standard of care. This is typically provided through the written opinions or testimony of a recognized expert in the field. In the absence of a written policy on the use of restraint, testimony might be offered regarding the customary use of restraint in emergency situations in which the combative, violent, or confused patient poses a threat of harm to self or others. Using traditions to establish a standard of care may result in the same defect as in using hospital policies and procedures: customs may not comply with the laws, recommendations of the accrediting body, or other recognized standards of care. Customs must be carefully and *regularly* evaluated to ensure that substandard routines have not developed.

Protection of Patients

Legal issues common in psychiatric nursing often relate to the failure to protect the safety of patients:

- If a suicidal patient is left alone with the means to harm him- or herself, the nurse who has a duty to protect the patient may be held legally responsible for the resultant injuries.
- Precautions to prevent harm must be taken whenever a patient is restrained.
- Precautions must be taken to protect patients from those who exhibit violent or abusive behaviors. A facility or provider may be held legally liable if one patient is injured by another.
- Miscommunication and medication errors are common in all areas of nursing, including psychiatric care.
- A common area of liability in psychiatry is abuse of the therapist–patient relationship. Issues of sexual misconduct during the therapeutic relationship have become a source of concern in the psychiatric community.

Misdiagnosis or failure to timely diagnose a medical condition is also frequently charged in legal suits. See Table 6.3 for common liability issues.

Guidelines for Nurses Who Suspect Negligence

It is not unusual for a student or practicing nurse to suspect negligence on the part of a peer. In most states, nurses have a legal duty to report such risks of harm to the patient. It is also important to document the evidence clearly and accurately before making accusations against a peer. If you question the appropriateness of physician's orders or actions or those of a fellow nurse, it is wise to communicate these concerns directly to the person involved. If the questioned behavior continues, you have an obligation to communicate these concerns to a supervisor, who should then intervene to ensure that the patient's rights and well-being are protected. If there is not a supervisor on-site, it is your duty to communicate your concerns to the appropriate person as soon as possible.

If you suspect a peer of being chemically impaired or of practicing irresponsibly, you have an obligation to protect not only the rights of the peer but also the rights of all patients who could be harmed. Reporting also allows impaired health care workers to receive treatment, and in many states, they can retain their license to work (although not necessarily their jobs) under certain circumstances. However, if you have reported the suspected behavior of concern to a supervisor and the danger persists, you have a duty to report the concern to the next level of authority. It is important to follow the channels of communication in an organization, but it is also important to protect the safety of the patients. If the supervisor's actions or inactions do not rectify the

TABLE 6.3 Common Liability Issues

Issue	Definition	Examples
Patient safety	Any action or inaction that results in decreased patient safety or security	Suicide risks Elopement Miscommunication
Defamation of character • Slander (spoken) • Libel (written)	Publishing knowingly false information to third parties, resulting in reputational harm	Blog or social media posts Gossiping Media interviews
Supervisory liability (vicarious liability)	A strict liability tort that holds a supervisor responsible for the negligent acts of the subordinate	Supervisory liability is often triggered by: Inappropriate delegation of duties Lack of supervision Improper or incomplete training methods
Intentional torts • May also carry criminal penalties • Punitive damages may be awarded • Not covered by professional insurance • Self-defense or protection of others may serve as a defense to charges of an intentional tort.	Intentional acts that lead to the harm of a third party It is important to note that the consequence (harm) does not need to be intentional, only the underlying act.	Physical assault Bullying Sexual misconduct Theft
Negligence or malpractice	Action or inaction with foreseeable harm to a third party	Carelessness Purposeful action that falls below the standard of care
Assault	Verbal or physical action that causes a third party reasonable belief of immediate harm	Threatening harm if a patient does not comply with treatment or instruction
Battery	Purposeful touching of another person resulting in (physical or emotional) harm	Any unwanted or offensive physical contact Treatment without patient's consent
False imprisonment	Intentional restriction of movement without justification or consent	Indefensible use of seclusion or restraints Refusal to discharge a patient without appropriate legal justification

dangerous situation, you have a continuing duty to report the behavior of concern to the appropriate regulatory authority, such as the Board of Nursing.

A useful reference for nurses is the ANA's *Code of Ethics for Nurses With Interpretive Statements*:

> Nurses must be alert to and must take appropriate action regarding all instances of **incompetent, unethical, illegal, or impaired practices(s) or actions that place the rights** or best interests of the patient in jeopardy. (ANA, 2015, 3.5 p. 12)
>
> Nurses must protect the patient, the public, and the profession from potential harm when practice appears to be impaired. The nurse's duty is to take action to protect patients and to ensure the impaired individual receives assistance. (ANA, 2015, 3.6 p. 13)

Duty to Intervene and Duty to Report

The psychiatric-mental health nurse has a duty to intervene when the safety or well-being of the patient or another person is obviously at risk. A nurse who follows an order that is known to be incorrect or that the nurse believes will harm the patient may be held legally responsible for the harm that results to the patient. **If a nurse believes that a physician's orders need to be clarified or changed, it is his or her duty to intervene and protect the patient.** It is important to communicate with the physician who has ordered the treatment and explain the concern. If the treating physician does not appear willing to consider those concerns, a nurse should carry out the duty to intervene by bringing those concerns to the next level of authority.

It is important to express concerns to the supervisor to allow the supervisor to communicate with the appropriate medical staff for any necessary intervention in the physician's treatment plan. *As the patient's advocate*, a nurse has a duty to intervene to protect the patient; at the same time, a nurse does not have the right to interfere with the physician–patient relationship.

It is also important to follow agency policies and procedures for communicating differences of opinion. If a nurse fails to intervene in conduct a nurse knows or should have known would reasonably lead to patient injury and the patient is injured, that nurse may be partly liable for the injuries that result.

Another, less considered, type of negligence is patient abandonment. The legal concept of **abandonment** may also arise when a nurse does not leave a patient safely reassigned to another health professional before discontinuing treatment. When a nurse is given an assignment to care for a patient, the nurse must provide the care or ensure that the patient is safely reassigned to another nurse for the continuation of care. Abandonment issues arise when accurate, timely, and thorough reporting has not occurred or when follow-through of patient care, on which the patient is relying, has not occurred. The same principles apply for the psychiatric-mental health nurse who is working in a community setting. For example, if a suicidal patient refuses to go to the hospital for treatment, a nurse cannot abandon the patient but must take the necessary steps to ensure the patient's safety. These actions may include enlisting the assistance of the legal system or emergency medical providers or providing a recommendation to temporarily involuntarily commit the patient.

The duty to intervene on the patient's behalf poses many legal and ethical dilemmas for nurses in the workplace. Institutions that have a chain-of-command policy or other reporting mechanisms offer some assurance that the proper administrative authorities are consistently notified. Most patient care issues regarding physicians' orders or treatments can be settled fairly early in the process by discussing concerns with the physician. If further intervention by the nurse is required to protect the patient, the next step in the chain of command can be followed. Generally, the nurse then notifies the immediate nursing supervisor; the supervisor then discusses the problem with the physician, then with the chief of staff of a particular service, until a resolution is reached. If there is no time to resolve the issue through the normal process because of the life-threatening nature of the situation, the nurse must act to protect the patient's life.

Unethical or Illegal Practices

The issues become more complex when a professional colleague's conduct, including that of a student nurse, is criminally unlawful. Specific examples of this may include the diversion of drugs from the hospital or sexual misconduct with patients. Increasing media attention and the recognition of substance abuse as an occupational hazard for health professionals have led to the establishment of mandatory substance abuse education programs in many states, as well as rehabilitation programs for health care workers. These programs provide appropriate treatment for impaired professionals to protect the public from harm and to rehabilitate the professional in an appropriate way.

The problem previously discussed—of reporting impaired colleagues—becomes a difficult one, particularly when no direct harm has occurred to the patient. Concern for professional reputations, damaged careers, and personal privacy rather than public protection has generated a code of silence regarding substance abuse among health professionals.

To combat this misconception, several states now *require* reporting of impaired or incompetent colleagues to the professional licensing boards. In the absence of such a legal mandate, the questions of whether to report and to whom to report become ethical ones. Chapter 19 deals more fully with issues related to the chemically impaired nurse.

The duty to intervene includes the duty to report known abusive behavior. Most states have enacted statutes to protect children and older adults from abuse and neglect. Psychiatric-mental health nurses working in the community may be required by law to report unsafe relationships they discover. It is important that nurses become familiar with their state's mandatory reporting requirements.

DOCUMENTATION OF CARE

Purpose of Medical Records

The purpose of the medical record is to provide accurate and complete information about the care and treatment of patients and to give health care personnel responsible for that care a means of communicating with one another. The medical record allows for continuity of care. A record's usefulness is determined by evaluating, when the record is read later, how accurately and completely it portrays the patient's behavioral status at the time it was written. The patient has the right to see the chart, but the chart belongs to the institution. The patient must follow appropriate protocol to view his or her records.

If a psychiatric patient describes to a nurse a plan to harm himself or herself or another person and that nurse fails to appropriately and timely document the information, including the need to protect the patient or the identified victim, the information will be lost when the nurse leaves work, and the patient's plan may be executed. The harm caused could be linked directly to the nurse's failure to communicate this important information. Even though documentation takes time away from the patient, the importance of communicating and preserving the nurse's memory through the medical record cannot be overemphasized. Keep in mind that when a new provider or outside agency reviews medical records, the writer is not present to explain or elaborate on his or her notes; therefore, documentation must be thorough.

Facility Use of Medical Records

The medical record has many other uses aside from providing information on the course of the patient's care and treatment to health care professionals. A retrospective chart review can provide valuable information to the facility on the quality of care provided and on possible ways to improve that care. A facility may conduct reviews for risk management purposes to determine areas of potential liability for the facility or providers and to evaluate methods used to reduce the facility's exposure to liability. Documentation of the use of restraints and seclusion for psychiatric patients may be reviewed by risk managers. Accordingly, the chart may be used to evaluate care for quality assurance or peer review. Utilization review analysts review the chart to determine appropriate use of hospital and staff resources consistent with reimbursement schedules. Insurance companies and other reimbursement agencies rely on the medical record in determining what payments they will make on the patient's behalf.

Medical Records as Evidence

From a legal perspective, the chart is a recording of data, opinions, and decisions made in the normal course of the patient's care. It is deemed to be good evidence because it is presumed to be true and is contemporaneous with treatment. Accordingly, the medical record finds its way into litigation for a variety of reasons. Some examples of its use include determining (1) adherence to standards of care and the extent of the patient's damages and/or pain and suffering in personal injury or professional negligence cases, (2) the nature and extent of injuries in child abuse or elder abuse cases, (3) the nature and extent of physical or mental disability in disability cases, and (4) the nature and extent of injury and rehabilitative potential in workers' compensation cases.

Medical records may also be used in police investigations, civil conservatorship proceedings, competency hearings, and commitment procedures. In states that mandate mental health legal services or a patients' rights advocacy program, regular audits may be performed to determine the facility's compliance with state laws or violations of patients' rights. Finally, medical records will be used in professional and hospital negligence cases.

During the discovery phase of litigation, the medical record is a pivotal source of information for attorneys in determining whether a cause of action exists in a professional negligence or hospital negligence case. Evidence of the nursing care rendered will be found in the notes charted by the nurse. Nurse charting will often be analyzed to determine (1) the timeline of events (because nurse charting is often more frequent that physician charting, nursing notes are often used to create the most thorough timeline of events), (2) whether nursing staff carried out the physician's orders in a timely manner, and (3) whether changes in patient status were acted on and/or reported to physicians in a timely manner.

Nursing Guidelines for Computerized Charting

Accurate, descriptive, and legible nursing notes serve the best interests of the patient, the nurse, and the institution. As computerized charting becomes the standard of care, it is important for psychiatric-mental health nurses to understand how to protect the confidentiality of these records. Institutions must also protect against intrusions into the privacy of the patient record systems.

Concerns for the privacy of the patient's records have been addressed legally by federal laws that provide guidelines for agencies that use computerized charting. These guidelines include the recommendation that staff be assigned a password for entering patients' records in order to identify staff who have accessed patients' confidential information. There are penalties, including termination, if staff enter a record for which they are not authorized to have access. Only those staff who have a legitimate need to know about the patient are authorized to access a patient's computerized chart.

Nurses must keep their passwords private and never allow someone else to access a record under their password. Nurses are responsible for all entries into records using their password. The various systems allow specific time frames within which the nurse must make any necessary corrections if a charting error is made. However, facilities often have policies regarding when to correct a charting error and when an addendum should be made. These policies are put in place to protect facilities and providers from allegations that charting is changed to "cover up" mistakes.

Any charting method that improves communication between care providers should be encouraged. Courts assume that nurses and physicians read one another's notes on patient progress. Legally, if something is not charted, it becomes difficult to prove. Charting also serves as a valuable memory refresher because lawsuits often take place months or years after the care is rendered. In providing complete and timely information on the care and treatment of patients, the medical record enhances communication among health professionals. Internal institutional audits of the record can improve the quality of care rendered. Chapter 7 describes common charting forms and gives examples as well as the pros and cons of each.

FORENSIC NURSING

Forensic nurses work with crime victims or perpetrators to gather evidence or provide expert testimony in court. This is a specialized field for which a nurse must have the proper training and experience to meet a state's guidelines for expert testimony. The nurse acts as an advocate, educating the court about the science of nursing, in the courtroom-based practice of forensic nursing. Examples of psychiatric forensic nursing may include cases related to patient competency, fitness to stand trial, and commitment or responsibility for a crime. The relevance of nursing facts is presented and applied to the legal facts. Forensic cases also pertain to personal injury and murder proceedings.

KEY POINTS TO REMEMBER

- States' power to enact laws for public health and safety and for the care of those unable to care for themselves often pits the rights of society against the rights of the individual.
- Psychiatric nurses frequently encounter problems requiring ethical choices.
- The nurse's privilege to practice nursing carries with it the responsibility to practice safely, competently, and in a manner consistent with state and federal laws.
- Knowledge of the law, the American Nurses Association's (ANA) *Code of Ethics for Nurses With Interpretive Statements*, and the ANA's standards of care from *Psychiatric–Mental Health Nursing: Scope and Standards of Practice* is essential to provide safe, effective psychiatric nursing care and will serve as a framework for decision making when the nurse is presented with complex problems involving competing interests.
- Psychiatric records are subject to even more stringent HIPAA regulation and may require additional authorization of release from the patient and psychiatric providers.

APPLYING CRITICAL JUDGMENT

1. Two nurses, Joe and Beth, have worked on the psychiatric unit for 2 years. During the past 6 months, Beth has confided to Joe that she has been experiencing a particularly difficult marital situation. Joe has observed that over those 6 months, Beth has become increasingly irritable and difficult to work with. He notices that tranquilizers are frequently missing from the unit dose cart on the evening shift. He complains to the pharmacy and is informed that the drugs were stocked as ordered. Several patients state that they have not been receiving their usual drugs. Joe finds that Beth has recorded that the drugs have been given as ordered. He also notices that Beth is diverting the drugs.
   - **A.** What action, if any, should Joe take?
   - **B.** Should Joe confront Beth with his suspicions?
   - **C.** If Beth admits that she has been diverting the drugs, should Joe's next step be to report Beth to the supervisor or to the Board of Nursing?
   - **D.** Should Joe make his concern known to the nursing supervisor directly by identifying Beth, or should he state his concerns in general terms?
   - **E.** Legally, must Joe report his suspicions to the Board of Nursing? To the police?
   - **F.** Does the fact that harm to the patients is limited to increased agitation affect your responses?
2. A 40-year-old man who is admitted to the emergency department for a severe nosebleed has both nares packed. Because of his history of alcoholism and the probability of ensuing delirium tremens, the patient is transferred to the psychiatric unit. He is admitted to a private room, placed in restraints, and checked by a nurse every hour per physician's orders. While unattended, the patient suffocates, apparently by inhaling the nasal packing, which had become dislodged from the nares. On the next 1-hour check, the nurse finds the patient without pulse or respiration. A state statute requires that a restrained patient on a psychiatric unit be assessed by a nurse every hour for safety, comfort, and physical needs.
   - **A.** If standards are not otherwise specified, do statutory requirements set forth minimal or maximal standards?
   - **B.** Does the nurse's compliance with the state statute relieve him or her of liability in the patient's death?
   - **C.** Does the nurse's compliance with the physician's orders relieve him or her of liability in the patient's death?
   - **D.** Was the order for the restraint appropriate for this type of patient?
   - **E.** What factors did you consider in making your determination?
   - **F.** Was the frequency of rounds for assessment of patient needs appropriate in this situation?
   - **G.** Did the nurse's conduct meet the standard of care for psychiatric nurses? Why or why not?
   - **H.** What nursing action should the nurse have taken to protect the patient from harm?
3. Assume that there are no mandatory reporting laws for impaired or incompetent colleagues in the following clinical situation. In a private psychiatric unit in California, a 15-year-old boy is admitted at

the request of his parents because of violent, explosive behavior that seems to stem from his father's recent remarriage after his parents' divorce. A few days after admission, while in group therapy, he has an explosive reaction to a discussion about weekend passes for Mother's Day. He screams that he has been abandoned and that nobody cares about him. Several weeks later, on the day before his discharge, he elicits from the nurse a promise to keep his plan to kill his mother confidential. Consider the American Nurses Association's (ANA) *Code of Ethics for Nurses* on patient confidentiality, the principles of psychiatric nursing, the statutes on privileged communications, and the duty to warn third parties in answering the following questions.

A. Did the nurse use appropriate judgment in promising confidentiality?
B. Does the nurse have a legal duty to warn the patient's mother of her son's threat?
C. Is the duty owed to the patient's father and stepmother?
D. Would a change in the admission status from voluntary to involuntary protect the patient's mother without violating the patient's confidentiality?
E. Would your response be different depending on the state in which the incident occurred? Why or why not?
F. What nursing action, if any, should the nurse take after the disclosure by the patient?

CHAPTER REVIEW QUESTIONS

1. A nurse's sibling happily says, "I want to introduce you to my fiancé. We're getting married in 6 months." The nurse has encountered the fiancé in a clinical setting and is aware of the fiancé's diagnosis of schizophrenia. What is the nurse's best response?
   a. In private, tell the sibling about the fiancé's diagnosis.
   b. Encourage the sibling to postpone the wedding for at least a year.
   c. Ask the fiancé, "Have you told my sibling about your mental illness?"
   d. Say to the sibling and fiancé, "I hope you will be very happy together."
2. A patient has been disruptive to the therapeutic milieu for 2 days. A certified nursing assistant says to the nurse, "We need to seclude this patient because this behavior is upsetting everyone on the unit." Considering patients' rights, how should the nurse respond?
   a. "Seclusion is not part of this patient's plan of care."
   b. "Let's think of some new ways to help this patient be less disruptive."
   c. "Thank you for that suggestion. I will discuss it with the health care provider."
   d. "Disruptive behavior is expected with mental illness. We must respond therapeutically."
3. A day-shift nurse contacts a nurse scheduled for the night shift at home and says, "Our unit is full, and there are eight patients in the emergency department waiting for a bed." The night-shift nurse replies, "Thanks for telling me. I am calling in sick." Which type of problem is evident by the night-shift nurse's reply?
   a. Ethical problem of fidelity
   b. Legal problem of negligence
   c. Legal problem of an intentional tort
   d. Violation of the patients' right to treatment
4. In a staff meeting at an inpatient mental health facility for individuals, the administrator announces that psychiatric technicians will now be supervised by the milieu director rather than by nurses. What is the nurse's best action?
   a. Confer with colleagues about their opinions regarding the proposed change.
   b. Volunteer to participate on a committee charged with defining the job responsibilities of unlicensed assistive personnel.
   c. Ask the administrator to delay implementation of this change until the decision can be reviewed by an interdisciplinary team.
   d. Advise the administrator of regulations in the state nurse practice act regarding supervision of unlicensed assistive personnel.
5. A colleague tells the nurse, "I have not been able to sleep for the past 3 days. I feel like a robot." What is the nurse's best action?
   a. Direct the colleague to leave the facility immediately.
   b. Observe the colleague closely for evidence of impaired practice.
   c. Offer to administer medications to patients assigned to the colleague.
   d. Confer with the supervisor about the nurse's ability to safely deliver care.

REFERENCES

American Nurses Association (ANA). (2015). *Code of ethics for nurses with interpretive statements.* Washington, DC: APA.

American Psychiatric Association (APA). (2013). *Diagnostic and statistical manual of mental disorders (DSM-5)* (5th ed.). Washington, DC: APA.

Appleby, J. (2017). Analysis: What you need to know about Trump's changes to the health law. Retrieved July 4, 2018, from https://www.pbs.org/newshour/health/need-know-trumps-changes-health-law.

Ardanowski, E. (2018). Developments in guardianship law and increased difficulty in establishing guardianships. Texas Lawyer. Retrieved July 7, 2018 from https://www.law.com/texaslawyer/2018/03/01/developments-in-guardianship-law-and-increased-difficulty-establishing-guardianships/?slreturn=20180607181024.

Bazelon, D. L. (2010). *Mental health parity.* Washington, DC: Bazelon Center for Mental Health Law. Retrieved March 4, 2011, from http://www.bazelon.org/Where-We-Stand/Access-to-Services/Mental-Health-Parity.aspx. http://www.bazelon.org/Where-We-Stand/access-to-Services/diversion-from-incarceration.

Beronio, K., Po, R., Skopec, L., & Glied, S. (2013, February 20). Office of the Assistant Secretary for Planning and Evaluation. *Affordable Care Act expands mental health and substance use disorder benefits and federal parity protections for 62 million Americans.* Retrieved from https://aspe.hhs.gov/report/affordable-care-act-expands-mental-health-and-substance-use-disorder-benefits-and-federal-parity-protections-62-million-americans.

Brink, S. (2014, April 29). *Mental health now covered under ACA, but not for everyone.* U.S. News & World Report. Retrieved from http://www.usnews.com/news/articles/2014/04/29/mental-health-now-covered-under-aca-but-not-for-everyone.

Bronson, J. (2017, June). *Indicators of mental health problems reported by Prisoners and jail inmates, 2011–12.* U.S. Department of Justice. Retrieved July 4, 2018 from https://www.bjs.gov/content/pub/pdf/imhprpji1112.pdf.

Canterbury v. Spence, 464 F.2d 772 (D.C. Cir. 1972), quoting *Schloendorff v. Society of N.Y. Hosp.*, 211 N.Y. 125, 105 N.E. 92, 93 (1914).

Centers for Medicare and Medicaid Services and The Joint Commission. (2008). *State operations manual. Provider certification (U.S. Department of Health and Human Services Pub. 100-07).* Baltimore, MD: Centers for Medicare and Medicaid Services.

Giddens, J. F. (2017). *Concepts for nursing practice* (2nd ed.). St. Louis: Elsevier.

Health Insurance Portability and Accountability Act (HIPAA). U.S.C, 45, (2003) C.F.R § 164.501.

Humphrey v. Cady. (1972). 405 U.S. 504.

Johnson, R., Persad, G., & Sisti, D. (December 2014). The Tarasoff rule: The implications of interstate variation and gaps in professional training. *Journal of the American Academy of Psychiatry and the Law, 42*(4), 469–477.

National Association for Court Management (NACM). (2014). Adult guardianship guide: A guide to plan, develop, and sustain a comprehensive court guardianship and conservatorship program. Retrieved July 7, 2018 from https://nacmnet.org/sites/default/files/publications/AdultGuardianship-Guide_withCover.pdf.

O'Connor v. Donaldson. (1975). 422 U.S. 563.

Olmstead v. L.C. (98–536). (1999). 527 U.S. 581.

Plumadore v. State of New York. (1980). 427 N.Y.S.2d 90.

Tarasoff v. Regents of University of California. (1974). 529 P.2d 553, 118 Cal Rptr 129.

Tarasoff v. Regents of University of California. (1976). 551 P.2d 334, 131 Cal Rptr 14.

Zadvydas v. Davis. (2001) 533 U.S. 678 185 F.3d 279 and 208 F.3d 815.

Zilber, C. (2016, November 26). Ethics considerations of involuntary outpatient treatment. *Psychiatric News*. Retrieved July 5, 2018 from https://psychnews.psychiatryonline.org/doi/full/10.1176/appi.pn.2016.12a16.

Zinermon v. Burch. (1990). 494 U.S. 113, 108 L.Ed.2d 100, 110 S. Ct. 975.

UNIT II

Tools for Practice of the Art

Madeleine Leininger, PhD, RN, LhD, FAAN (1925–2012)
Founder of Transcultural Nursing

Even during the 1950s, long before "transcultural nursing" became a buzzword in nursing practice, Madeleine Leininger was an adamant supporter of health care workers understanding cultural nuances for the purpose of providing authentic, holistic, patient-centered care.

Leininger was a nurse pioneer in transcultural nursing as well as a scientist, anthropologist, researcher, theorist, leader, certified transcultural nurse specialist, and author and editor of more than 27 books. Leininger developed her theory of cultural care and universality based on her observations in the 1950s and 1960s of the people of New Guinea, where she lived for 2 years. She recognized the need for nurses to deliver care that combined both humanism and scientific knowledge and that would be meaningful to people from culturally diverse backgrounds.

She was the first graduate-prepared nurse to earn a PhD in cultural and social anthropology. In 1954, Leininger obtained a master's degree in psychiatric nursing from the Catholic University of America in Washington, DC. Soon afterward, she developed the first master's level clinical specialist program in child psychiatric nursing at the University of Cincinnati. She subsequently developed the first graduate transcultural nursing program in psychiatric nursing, also at the University of Cincinnati.

Simply stated, transcultural nursing is the practice of nursing that provides culturally congruent, competent, and equitable care practices in a world that has become increasingly multicultural in nature.

Leininger (1998) states that when nurses do not take into account a patient's spiritual and religious beliefs, family ties, and economic and educational factors, they are at risk for demonstrating a noncaring attitude that may result in nonbeneficial outcomes. Human care and caring are defined within the context of culture. Leininger's transcultural nursing theory has "caring" as its focus. She believed a caring focus should be the dominant focus in all areas of nursing. Caring is the most holistic, complete, and creative way to help others. (Leininger, 1981).

The 21st century has ushered in cultural neuroscience, which studies the differences in brain functions among people of different cultures (e.g., Western and East Asian cultures) and how these differences affect emotions, psychopathology, and cognition. Evidence exists that neurobiological processes underlie social behaviors. Shared cultural meaning and cultural experiences trigger a neurobiological, psychological, and behavioral chain of events (Kim & Sasaki, 2014). Understanding neuroscience and ethnopharmacology can enhance cultural competence in psychiatric nursing.

Kim, H. S., & Sasaki, J. Y. (2014). Cultural neuroscience: Biology of the mind in cultural contexts. *Annual Review of Psychology, 65*, 487–514.

Leininger, M. M. (1981). *Caring: An essential human need.* Thorofare, NJ: Charles B. Slack.

Leininger, M. M. (1998). *What is transcultural nursing?* Livonia, MI: Transcultural Nursing Society.

7

The Nursing Process in Psychiatric-Mental Health Nursing

Lois Angelo

http://evolve.elsevier.com/Varcarolis/essentials

OBJECTIVES

1. Identify the main differences and similarities between a psychiatric and medical nursing care plan.
2. Conduct a mental status examination (MSE).
3. Perform a psychosocial assessment, including cultural and spiritual components.
4. Explain three principles a nurse follows in planning actions to reach approved outcome criteria.
5. Develop a holistic plan of care for a patient with a mental or emotional health problem.
6. Describe how adverse childhood events (ACEs) may impact the needs of an adult.
7. Explain how the concepts of self-awareness and assertiveness affect patient outcomes for both the nurse and patient.

KEY TERMS AND CONCEPTS

evidence-based practice (EBP), p. 83
health teaching, p. 83
holistic approach to care, p. 75
mental status examination (MSE), p. 78
milieu therapy, p. 84
nonadherent, p. 84
outcomes criteria, p. 83
psychiatric mental health advanced practice registered nurse (PMH–APRN), p. 83
psychiatric mental health registered nurse (PMH–RN), p. 83
psychosocial assessment, p. 79
self-care activities, p. 83

CONCEPT: LEADERSHIP: *Leadership* is defined as an interactive process that provides needed guidance and direction. There are three dynamic elements involved: a leader, a follower, and a situation. Registered nurses (RNs) are summoned to be leaders as part of their daily work throughout the delivery of the nursing process (Giddens, 2017). Leadership is particularly important in utilizing clinical-based opportunities. For example, during a clinical assessment interview, a patient becomes upset, defensive, or uncomfortable with a particular topic; the nurse then leads by suggesting that it would be best discussed when the client feels more comfortable. Leadership attributes, such as professionalism and honesty, effectively and positively support patients and other staff in the delivery of care in mental health nursing (Ennis, 2015).

INTRODUCTION

Psychiatric-mental health nursing practice bases nursing judgments and behaviors on the nursing process. The nursing process is the framework for nursing practice and has been identified as nursing's scientific methodology in the delivery of patient care. The nursing process is a problem-solving method that encourages clinical care based on systematic decision making and can be utilized by larger systems to solve problems in organizations, facilities, and communities. The nursing process helps to distinguish nursing as a profession. It is the common knowledge thread uniting different types of nurses who work in varied areas and is the essential core of practice for the nurse to deliver patient-focused care. The nursing process, utilized at any point in the health–illness continuum, is the basis for all significant action taken by nurses in providing safe, evidence-based, holistic, and individualized psychiatric care to all patients.

The six steps in the nursing process—assessment, nursing diagnosis, outcome, planning, implementation, and evaluation—are also integrated throughout the test plan for the National Council Licensure Examination for registered nurses (NCLEX®) relating nursing behaviors and client situations (Fig. 7.1).

STANDARDS OF PRACTICE FOR PSYCHIATRIC-MENTAL HEALTH NURSING

STANDARD 1: ASSESSMENT

The psychiatric mental health registered nurse collects and synthesizes comprehensive health data that are pertinent to the health care consumer's health and/or situation (ANA et al., 2014, p. 44).

A view of the individual as a complex blend of many parts is consistent with nurses' **holistic approach to care**. Nurses who care for people with physical illnesses ideally maintain a holistic view that involves an awareness of psychological, social, cultural, environmental, functional, and spiritual issues as well as ethnicity, sexual orientation, and age (e.g., child, teenager, older adults). Likewise, nurses who work in the mental health field need to assess, or have access to, past

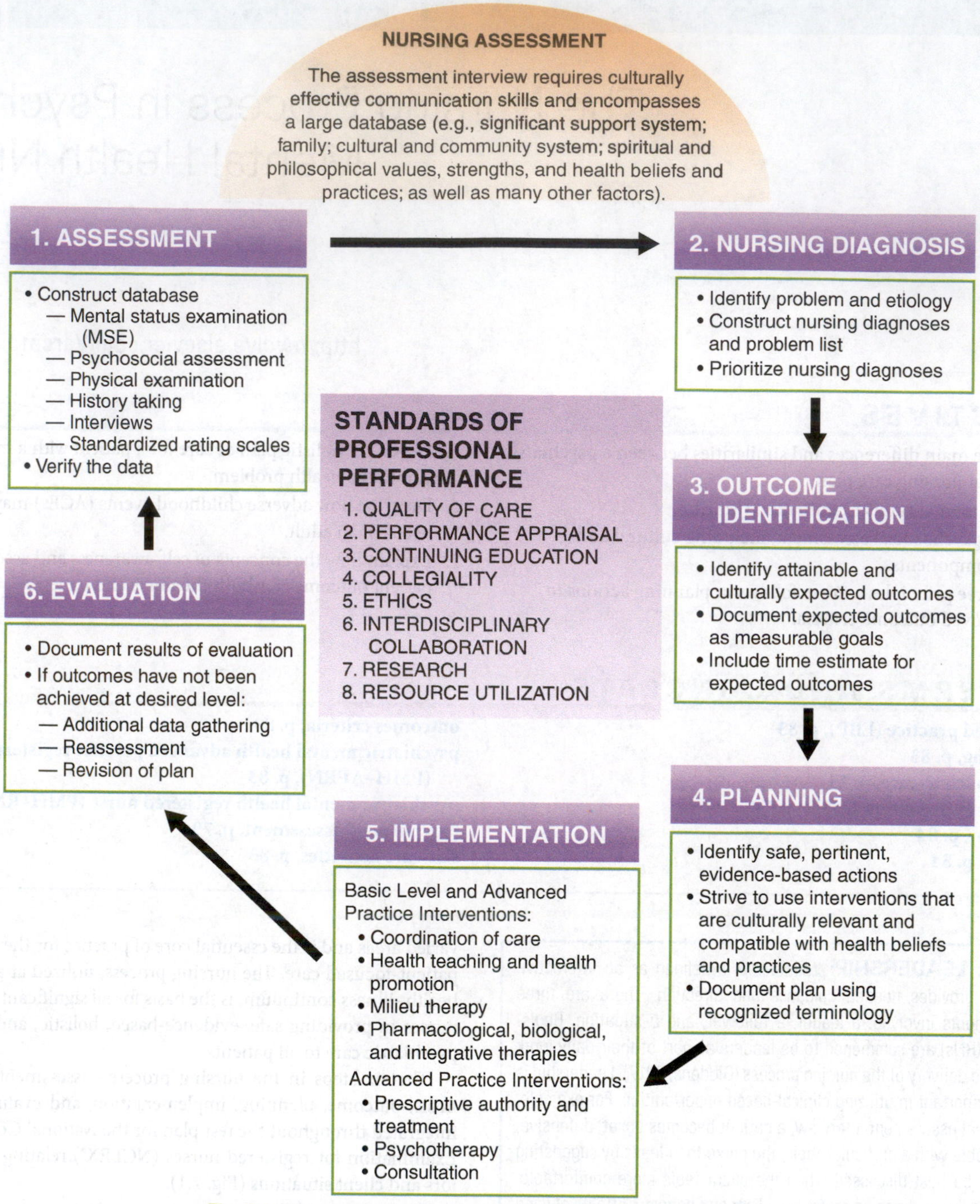

Fig. 7.1 The nursing process in psychiatric-mental health nursing.

and present medical history, a recent physical examination, and any physical complaints the patient is experiencing, as well as document any observable physical conditions or behaviors (e.g., unsteady gait, abnormal breathing pattern, facial grimacing, or changing position to relieve discomfort). It is important to note that the nursing process is cyclical. Assessment is ongoing and continues throughout the planning, intervention, and evaluation phases. The initial assessment often identifies the client's immediate needs. As the nurse continues to work with the patient, the assessment is evolving, and other problems may become evident. There is progress toward a more "strengths-based" approach to assessment. Patients find this approach to be more affirming rather than listing all of the problems that need to be solved (Coombs & Crookes, 2013).

An unintended consequence of frequently obtaining information from the electronic medical record instead of from the patient has been the atrophy of the powers of observation (Gupta, 2017). Particularly in the area of psychiatric nursing, observation is not only important for clinical diagnosis, but it is also a first step in being empathetic. To be able to empathize, one must be able to recognize emotions, which inherently requires the skill of observation (Gurwin & Revere, 2018). The nurse observes the person's physical behavior, verbal and nonverbal communications, appearance, speech, thought content, and cognitive ability and makes observations centering on the presenting problem(s), current lifestyle, and strength of resources such as family, friends, education, and work experiences (Box 7.1).

BOX 7.1 Florence Nightingale on "Observation"

In her 1860 classic book *Notes on Nursing*, Florence Nightingale stated, "What you want are facts, not opinions—for who can have any opinion of any value as to whether the patient is better or worse, excepting the constant attendant, or the really observing nurse?"

The most important practical lesson that can be given to nurses is to teach them what to observe, how to observe, what symptoms indicate improvement, which indicate the reverse, which are of importance, which are of none, and which are the evidence of neglect and of what kind of neglect. She added, "If you cannot get the habit of observation one way or other, you had better give up nursing, it is not your calling, however kind you may be."

BOX 7.2 Professional Curiosity

Professional curiosity is defined as "[t]he cornerstone of learning and growth. ... What makes me question, know, act, ask again, recognize" (Freire, 1998, p. 79). Curiosity in working with the mentally ill means to be open to the unexpected and to welcome information that may not support the initial assumptions. The way that the first assessment is carried out can influence the first connection between the nurse and the patient. Nonjudgmental professional curiosity is an approach that emphasizes empathy and partnership. Early therapeutic alliance appears to be a consistent predictor of engagement and retention in both mental health and substance abuse treatment. The qualities and skills of the individual nurse are key. In a multicultural society, professional curiosity means also exploring the client's treatment culture. For example, how are substance abuse and mental health problems defined by clients' parents, peers, and other clients; what do they think should be done to remedy these problems; and what kinds of treatment settings do they feel most comfortable with (Milani, 2017)?

The nurse collects comprehensive data using therapeutic techniques employing evidence-based assessment. Assessments are conducted by a variety of professionals, including nurses, psychiatrists, social workers, dietitians, and other therapists. Every patient should have a thorough and formal nursing assessment on entering treatment to develop a basis for the plan of care in preparation for discharge. Subsequent to the formal assessment, data are collected continually and systematically as the patient's condition changes.

Particularly in the process of data collection, it is important for the nurse to engage in continuing "professional curiosity," which delves into data that might initially seem minimal but upon exploration open up more realization and understanding of the patient situation. It is important for the nurse to be alert to ongoing, multiple cues in the patient's internal and external environment (Box 7.2).

Mental health nursing assessments also involve engaging patients and putting them at ease. This can be seen as normalizing the process of assessment to demonstrate empathy and to relax patients so that they feel comfortable discussing often-difficult issues (Coombs & Crookes, 2013).

Document relevant data in a retrievable format. Virtually all facilities have standardized nursing assessment forms to aid in organization and consistency among reviewers. These forms will most likely be computerized, although some institutions may still use hardcopy assessments according to the resources and preferences of the institution. The time required for the nursing interview varies, depending on the assessment form and on the patient's response pattern (e.g., a lengthy or rambling historian, a patient prone to tangential thoughts, or a patient having memory disturbances or markedly slowed responses). In emergency situations, immediate intervention is essential and may be based on a minimal amount of data. Refer to Chapter 9 for guidelines for setting up and conducting a clinical interview.

Whenever possible, involve the patient, family, other health care providers, and other support systems in holistic data collection. The nurse's *primary source* for data collection is the patient; however, there may be times when it is necessary to supplement or rely completely on another source for the assessment information. These *secondary sources* can be invaluable when caring for a patient experiencing psychosis, muteness, agitation, or catatonia. Such secondary sources include family, friends, neighbors, police, health care workers, and previous medical records.

Age Considerations

Assessment of Children

Assess interpersonal relationships among all age groups, including a history of adverse childhood experiences (ACEs). ACEs include physical and emotional abuse and/or neglect, sexual abuse, violent experiences, substance abuse within the household, and parental/significant loss, among others. ACEs can contribute to chronic and toxic stress as well as physical and mental illnesses. Asking about ACEs can help with efforts to prevent negative impacts on development for the patient and family (Bethell & Carle, 2017). ACEs will be discussed in many chapters. There is a connection between negative childhood experiences and a future risk of physical or mental health consequences.

In North America, one out of every five children experiences a mental health concern, such as depression, anxiety, attention-deficit/hyperactivity disorder, or conduct problems. The stability, persistence, and adverse long-term outcomes of childhood illness and trauma are evident across the life span. Over 50% to 75% of adult mental health issues have their onset in childhood or adolescence, and children who experience mental health issues are at increased risk for academic underachievement, underemployment, criminal activity, and risk for suicide. There is a need for ongoing assessments of both internalizing behaviors (e.g., depression, anxiety) and externalizing behaviors (e.g., aggressive symptoms). Over 75% of children who experience mental health issues do not have access to appropriate treatment (Stewart & Hamza, 2017).

An effective interviewer working with children should have familiarity with basic cognitive and social/emotional developmental theory and have some exposure to applied child development (Sommers-Flanagan & Sommers-Flanagan, 2012–2013). The role of the caregiver is central in the interview.

When assessing children, it is important to gather data from a variety of sources. Although the child is the best source in determining inner feelings and emotions, the caregivers (parents or guardians) can often best describe the behavior, performance, and conduct of the child. Caregivers are also often helpful in interpreting the child's words and responses. However, a separate interview is advisable when an older child is reluctant to share information, especially in cases of suspected abuse (Arnold & Boggs, 2016). School personnel such as teachers, counselors, or nurses may also be able to provide pertinent data.

As mentioned, developmental levels should be considered in the evaluation of children. One of the hallmarks of psychiatric disorders in children is the tendency to regress—that is, to return to a previous level of development. Although it is developmentally appropriate for toddlers to suck their thumbs, such a gesture is unusual in an older child.

Assessment of children should be accomplished by a combination of interview and observation. Watching children at play provides important clues to their functioning. Using age-appropriate storytelling, playing with dolls, drawing, and playing games can be useful as assessment tools when determining critical concerns and painful issues a child may have difficulty expressing. When assessing the child, be sure to position yourself at the child's level and avoid towering over him or her. Always use familiar words and age-based vocabulary. Usually, a clinician/nurse clinician with special training in child and adolescent psychiatry works with young children. Refer to Chapter 26 for further discussion on the assessment of children.

Assessment of Adolescents

All patients are concerned with confidentiality. This is especially true for adolescents. Adolescents may fear that anything they say to the nurse will be repeated to their parents. At least part of the interview should be conducted without the parent/caregiver present. Adolescents need to be told right from the very beginning that their records are private and should receive an explanation as to how information will be shared among the treatment team. Questions related to sensitive issues such as substance abuse or sexual abuse demand confidentiality (Arnold & Boggs, 2016). However, threats of suicide or homicide, use of illegal drugs, or issues of abuse must be shared with other professionals as well as with the parent(s). Because identifying risk factors is one of the key objectives when assessing adolescents, it is helpful to use a brief structured interview technique called the HEADSSS interview (Box 7.3). Refer to Chapter 26 for more information on the assessment of adolescents.

Assessment of the Older Adult

Older adults often need special attention. Pre-existing mental health disorders can significantly contribute to the development of chronic disease over time, and pre-existing chronic disease(s) can significantly contribute to the development of mental health disorders. In addition to assessing and treating chronic disease(s) in older people, it is also important to monitor and treat their mental health disorders. Doing so will result in overall better health outcomes and will facilitate a better quality of life as they age (Chun-Min, 2017).

The nurse needs to be aware of any physical limitations—any sensory condition (vision or hearing deficits), motor condition (difficulty walking or maintaining balance), or medical condition (cardiac condition)—that could cause increased anxiety, stress, or physical discomfort for the patient while attempting to assess mental and emotional needs.

It is wise to identify any physical deficits the patient may have at the onset of the assessment and make accommodations for them. For example, if the patient is hard of hearing, speak a little more slowly and in clear, louder tones (but not too loud), and seat the patient close to you without invading his or her personal space. Refer to Chapter 28 for more on communicating with the older adult.

BOX 7.3 The HEADSSS Psychosocial Interview Technique

H Home environment (e.g., relations with parents and siblings)
E Education and employment (e.g., school performance)
A Activities (e.g., sports participation, afterschool activities, peer relations)
D Drug, alcohol, or tobacco use
S Sexuality (e.g., whether the patient is sexually active, practices safe sex, uses contraception, or practices alternative sexual lifestyles)
S Suicide risk or symptoms of depression or other mental disorder
S "Savagery" (e.g., violence or abuse in home environment or in neighborhood)

Psychiatric Nursing Assessment

The psychiatric nursing assessment has many goals, including the following:

- Establish rapport.
- Obtain an understanding of the current problem or chief complaint.
- Review physical status and obtain baseline vital signs.
- Assess for risk factors affecting the safety of the patient or others (suicide/homicide).
- Assess mental status.
- Assess psychosocial status.
- Identify mutual goals for treatment.
- Formulate a plan of care that prioritizes the patient's immediate condition and needs.
- Document data in a retrievable format.

Gathering Data

Review of Systems

The mind–body connection is significant in the understanding and treatment of psychiatric disorders. Many patients who are admitted for treatment of psychiatric conditions also are given a thorough physical examination by a primary care provider. Likewise, most nursing assessments include a physical component, such as obtaining a baseline set of vital statistics, a historical and current review of body systems, and documentation of allergic responses.

People with severe mental illness (SMI)—including schizophrenia, bipolar disorder, major depressive disorder, and their related spectrum disorders—have a life expectancy that is shortened by 10 to 17.5 years compared with the general population. Although suicide explains some of this reduced life expectancy, it is now established that physical diseases account for the overwhelming majority of premature mortality. Among physical conditions, cardiovascular disease (CVD) is the main potentially avoidable contributor to early deaths in patients with severe mental illness (Correll, 2017). *There are many medical conditions that can mimic psychiatric illnesses* (Box 7.4). By the same token, when depression is secondary to a known medical condition, it may go unrecognized and thus untreated. *Conversely, psychiatric disorders can result in physical or somatic symptoms, such as abdominal pain, headaches, lethargy, insomnia, and intense fatigue.* Therefore, all patients presenting to the health care system need to have both a medical and a psychological health assessment to ensure a correct diagnosis and appropriate care.

Laboratory Data

Disorders such as hypothyroidism may have the clinical appearance of depression, and hyperthyroidism may appear to be a manic phase of bipolar disorder; a simple blood test can usually differentiate between a mood disorder and thyroid disorders. Abnormal liver enzyme levels can explain irritability, depression, and lethargy. People who have chronic renal disease often suffer from the same symptoms when their blood urea nitrogen and electrolyte levels are abnormal. Results of a toxicology screen for the presence of either legal (e.g., prescription pain medication, Adderall) or illegal drugs (e.g., designer drugs, hallucinogenic, heroin) also may provide useful information.

Mental Status Examination

Fundamental to the assessment is a **mental status examination (MSE)**. In fact, an MSE is part of the assessment in all areas of medicine. The MSE in psychiatry is analogous to the physical examination in general medicine. The mental status examination is also useful in differentiating between a variety of systemic conditions, as well as neurologic

BOX 7.4 Some Medical Conditions That May Mimic Psychiatric Illness

Depression

Neurological disorders:

- Cerebrovascular accident (stroke)
- Alzheimer's disease
- Brain tumor
- Huntington's disease
- Epilepsy (seizure disorder)
- Multiple sclerosis
- Parkinson's disease
- Cancer

Infections:

- Mononucleosis
- Encephalitis
- Hepatitis
- Tertiary syphilis
- Human immunodeficiency virus (HIV) infection

Endocrine disorders:

- Hypothyroidism and hyperthyroidism
- Cushing's syndrome
- Addison's disease
- Parathyroid disease

Gastrointestinal disorders:

- Liver cirrhosis
- Pancreatitis

Cardiovascular disorders:

- Hypoxia
- Congestive heart failure

Respiratory disorders:

- Sleep apnea

Nutritional disorders:

- Thiamine deficiency
- Protein deficiency
- B_{12} deficiency
- B_6 deficiency
- Folate deficiency

Collagen vascular diseases:

- Lupus erythematosus
- Rheumatoid arthritis

Anxiety

Neurological disorders:

- Alzheimer's disease
- Brain tumor
- Stroke
- Huntington's disease

Infections:

- Encephalitis
- Meningitis
- Neurosyphilis
- Septicemia

Endocrine disorders:

- Hypothyroidism and hyperthyroidism
- Hypoparathyroidism
- Hypoglycemia
- Pheochromocytoma
- Carcinoid

Metabolic disorders:

- Low calcium level
- Low potassium level
- Acute intermittent porphyria
- Liver failure

Cardiovascular disorders:

- Angina
- Congestive heart failure
- Pulmonary embolus

Respiratory disorders:

- Pneumothorax
- Acute asthma
- Emphysema

Drug effects:

- Stimulants
- Sedatives (withdrawal)
- Lead or mercury poisoning

Psychosis

Medical conditions:

- Temporal lobe epilepsy
- Migraine headaches
- Temporal arteritis
- Occipital tumors
- Narcolepsy
- Encephalitis
- Hypothyroidism
- Addison's disease
- HIV infection

Drug effects:

- Hallucinogens (e.g., LSD)
- Phencyclidine
- Alcohol withdrawal
- Stimulants
- Cocaine
- Corticosteroids

and psychiatric disorders ranging from delirium and dementia to bipolar disorder and schizophrenia (Norris, 2016). For acutely disturbed patients, it is typical for the mental health clinician to administer the MSE every day. Box 7.5 lists the elements of a basic MSE.

Generally, the MSE aids in collecting and organizing *objective data*. The nurse observes the patient's physical behavior, nonverbal communication, appearance, speech patterns, mood and affect, thought content, perceptions, cognitive ability, and insight and judgment.

Psychosocial Assessment

A **psychosocial assessment** provides additional information from which to develop a plan of care beyond the MSE. It includes obtaining the following information about the patient:

- Central or chief complaint (in the patient's own words)
- History of violent, suicidal, or self-mutilating behaviors
- Alcohol and/or substance abuse
- Family psychiatric history
- Personal psychiatric treatment including medications and complementary therapies
- Current stressors and coping methods
- Quality of activities of daily living
- Personal background
- Social background, including support system
- Weaknesses, strengths, and goals for treatment
- Racial, ethnic, and cultural beliefs and practices
- Spiritual beliefs or religious practices

BOX 7.5 Content of a Mental Status Examination

Personal Information
- Age
- Gender
- Marital status
- Religious preference
- Race
- Ethnic background
- Employment
- Living arrangements

Appearance
- Grooming and dress
- Level of hygiene
- Pupil dilation or constriction
- Facial expression
- Height, weight, nutritional status
- Presence of body piercing or tattoos, scars, other
- Relationship between appearance and age

Behavior
- Excessive or reduced body movements
- Peculiar body movements (e.g., scanning of the environment, odd or repetitive gestures, level of consciousness, balance and gait)
- Abnormal movements (e.g., tardive dyskinesia, tremors)
- Level of eye contact (keep cultural differences in mind)

Speech
- Rate: slow, rapid, normal
- Volume: loud, soft, normal
- Disturbances (e.g., articulation problems, slurring, stuttering, mumbling)
- Cluttering (e.g., rapid, disorganized, tongue-tied speech)

Affect and Mood
- Affect: flat, bland, animated, angry, withdrawn, appropriate to context
- Mood: sad, labile, euphoric

Thought
- Thought process (e.g., disorganized, coherent, flight of ideas, neologisms, thought blocking, circumstantiality)
- Thought content (e.g., delusions, obsessions, suicidal thought)

Perceptual Disturbances
- Hallucinations (e.g., auditory, visual)
- Illusions

Cognition
- Orientation: time, place, person
- Level of consciousness (e.g., alert, confused, clouded, stuporous, unconscious, comatose)
- Memory: remote, recent, immediate
- Fund of knowledge
- Attention: performance on serial sevens, digit span tests
- Abstraction: performance on tests involving similarities, proverbs
- Insight
- Judgment

The patient's psychosocial history is most often the *subjective* part of the assessment. The focus of the history is the patient's perceptions and recollections of his or her current lifestyle and life in general (e.g., family, friends, education, work experience, coping styles, and spiritual and cultural beliefs) (Box 7.6).

Spiritual and/or Religious Assessment

The importance of spirituality and religious beliefs is an often-overlooked element of patient care, although numerous empirical studies have suggested that being part of a spiritual community is helpful to people coping with illness and recovering from surgery. Spirituality and religious beliefs have the potential to exert an influence on how people understand meaning and purpose in their lives and how they use critical judgment to solve problems (e.g., crises of illness).

The terms *spirituality* and *religion* are different, although not mutually exclusive. Spirituality refers to how we find meaning, hope, purpose, and a sense of peace in our lives. Spirituality is more of an internal phenomenon centering on universal personal questions and needs. It is the part of us that seeks to understand life. The term *spirituality* is more about the believer's faith being more personal, less dogmatic, and more inclusive, considering that there are many spiritual paths and no one "real path." A person's spiritual beliefs may or may not be connected with the community or with religious rituals.

Religion is an external system that includes beliefs, patterns of worship, and symbols. Religious affiliation is a choice to connect personal spiritual beliefs with a larger organized group or institution and typically involves rituals. Belonging to a religious community can provide support during difficult times. For many individuals, prayer is a source of hope, comfort, and support in healing.

Spiritual and religious practices have been determined to enhance healthy behaviors, social support, and a sense of meaning in people's lives, all of which are linked to decreased overall mental and physical stress, which in turn relate to a decreased incidence of illness in many people. A recent study of the "baby boomer" generation, born during the years 1946 to 1964, showed that higher levels of spirituality were related to better mental and physical health, resulted in lower anxiety about and fear of aging, and buffered the impact of negative life events where they occurred (MacKinlay & Burns, 2017). (Refer to Chapter 10 for the effects of stress on health and illness.)

Cultural and Social Assessment

Because nurses are increasingly faced with caring for culturally diverse populations, there is a growing need for nursing assessment, nursing diagnoses, and subsequent care to be planned around unique cultural health care beliefs, values, and practices. It is becoming more evident that all mental health professionals, and perhaps especially nurses, must have an increased understanding of the complexity of the cultural and social factors that influence health and illness. Knowledge of individual cultural beliefs and health care practices can mitigate against stereotyping, stigmatizing, and labeling of patients.

In fact, it seems that patients from culturally diverse backgrounds respond better when nurses incorporate the clients' individual needs, values, and social circumstances into their plan of care (Arnold & Boggs 2016; Knoerl et al., 2011). Unfortunately, there are many opportunities for misunderstandings when assessing a patient from a different cultural or social background, particularly if the interview is conducted in English and the patient speaks a different language. Often health care professionals require an interpreter to understand

BOX 7.6 Psychosocial Assessment

A. Previous hospitalizations
B. Educational background
C. Occupational background
   1. Employed? Where? What length of time?
   2. Special skills
D. Social patterns
   1. Describe family.
   2. Describe friends.
   3. With whom does the patient live?
   4. To whom does the patient go in time of crisis?
   5. Who makes the decisions in your family?
   6. Describe a typical day.
E. Sexual patterns
   1. Sexually active? Practices safe sex? Practices birth control?
   2. Sexual orientation
   3. Sexual difficulties
F. Interests and abilities
   1. What does the patient do in his or her spare time?
   2. In which sport, hobby, or leisure activity does the patient participate?
   3. Does the patient excel in any particular activity or hobby?
   4. What gives the patient pleasure?
G. Substance use and abuse
   1. What medications does the patient take? How often? How much?
   2. What herbal or over-the-counter drugs does the patient take? How often? How much?
   3. What psychotropic drugs does the patient take? How often? How much?
   4. How many drinks of alcohol does the patient take per day? Per week?
   5. What recreational drugs does the patient take? How often? How much?
   6. Does the patient identify the use of drugs as a problem?
H. Coping abilities
   1. What does the patient do when he or she gets upset?
   2. To whom can the patient talk?
   3. What usually helps to relieve stress?
   4. What did the patient try this time?
I. Spiritual assessment
   1. Does the patient have a spiritual or religious affiliation?
   2. What gives the patient strength and hope?
   3. Does the patient participate in any spiritual/religious activities?
   4. What role does religion/spiritual practice play in the patient's life?
   5. Do the patient's spiritual or religious beliefs help him or her in stressful situations?
   6. Are there any restrictions on diet or medical interventions within the patient's religious, spiritual, or cultural beliefs?
J. Cultural assessment
   1. Does the patient need an interpreter?
   2. What is the first thing the patient does when he or she becomes ill to address the illness?
   3. How has the patient been treating this illness?
   4. How is this condition (medical or mental) viewed in the patient's culture?
   5. Are there special health care practices within the patient's culture that address his or her medical/mental problem?
   6. What are the attitudes toward mental illness in the patient's culture?
   7. Does the patient have culture-specific beliefs that help him or her cope (with racism, prejudice, or discrimination)?
   8. Does the patient's diet consist of culture-specific foods? If so, what foods should not be part of the patient's diet?

the patient's history and health care needs. Federal law mandates the use of a trained professional interpreter in health care settings when language is a barrier to communication. A professionally trained translator needs to be proficient in both English and the patient's spoken language and dialect and be familiar with the culture and mores of the patient's background. In addition, he or she is expected to maintain confidentiality and follow specific guidelines (Arnold & Boggs, 2016). Therefore it is strongly recommended to not use untrained interpreters (e.g., family members, friends, neighbors), who may easily misinterpret or try to "translate" the patient's intent. Unfortunately, professional interpreters are not always readily available in many health care facilities.

After the assessment, it is useful to summarize pertinent data with the patient. This summary provides the patient with reassurance that the health care provider understands his or her message, and it gives the patient an opportunity to clarify any misinformation. The patient should be told what will happen next. For example, if the initial assessment takes place in the hospital, you should tell the patient whom he or she will be seeing next. If the initial assessment was conducted by a psychiatric nurse in a mental health clinic, the individual will be informed of the future schedule for therapy with a clinician/psychiatric advanced practice nurse. If a referral is necessary, this should be discussed with the patient. For individuals with severe mental health requiring long-term care, some specific assessment guidelines can be helpful. Refer to Chapter 27.

Self-Awareness Assessment

Self-awareness is a positive trait, and a competent and effective interviewer needs to possess a high degree of psychological, emotional, and social/cultural self-awareness to perform optimally. We all have personal biases and "off days" (i.e., days we feel sad or upset), and we all hold our own expectations of the outcome of the interview. In addition, we all come from a specific culture/subculture with inherent expectations, traditions, and well-ingrained social beliefs. Being consciously aware of our personal biases and emotional states can help us become cognizant of how these traits can influence and distort our understanding of the individual before us.

It is a good idea to be aware of your personal cultural and social beliefs that may influence your interactions with a person from another background with inherently different cultural, social, and spiritual/religious beliefs. Also examine how you are feeling at the moment before an interview. We are not always aware of personal feelings or how they are affecting us when we first begin an interview. Some anxiety while conducting an interview, especially as a student, is a normal response. How do we obtain a good picture of ourselves in relationship to our interviewing skills? One way is clinical supervision from a seasoned and effective psychiatric nurse or clinician. Another effective way is through the use of videotapes of ourselves during an interview (usually a very painful experience, initially). Even seasoned interviewers can be shocked and surprised by their videotapes. Although these insights may be painful, they are enormously helpful in becoming more self-aware, and they increase our awareness of our patients as well. Taking notes shortly after an interview of what the patient said and what you said (process recordings) is a useful exercise because these "verbatim" notes provide an overall evaluation of your interaction, which may help you reevaluate and review not only what you missed but also what you could have done differently to be more effective. Although these assessment methods are not as popular as they were in the past in nursing education, they offer the opportunity for important learning experiences in improving communication skills.

Positive work environments can provide a safe place for both nurses and patients to discuss and assess their stressors and receive support. Nurses and other health care professionals who have a history of adverse childhood experiences (ACEs) may, like their patients, experience physical, social, emotional, and behavioral effects that could hinder/help patient–staff relationships. Research suggests that nursing and other health care professional work, given its often-stressful nature, exacerbates the stress of ACEs and that ACEs may negatively affect performance in the work setting (Girouard & Bailey, 2017).

Assertiveness

Assertiveness is one of the most important skills for nurses to demonstrate while utilizing the nursing process and is especially important in the assessment portion of the nursing process. Being assertive and confident when building a professional relationship with patients will improve communication. In the workplace, assertiveness reduces interpersonal stress, builds effective team relationships, and provides thorough, holistic nursing care. Assertiveness is typically defined in terms of the honest and legitimate expression of one's personal opinions, needs, wants, and feelings without denying or violating the rights of others. Previous studies have indicated that poor assertiveness in nurses is related to burnout, less commitment to work, and less effective utilization of the nursing process. Assertive communication also enables nurses to build effective team relationships because collaboration with other health care professionals requires a high level of both assertiveness and cooperation. Further, poor or ineffective communication is a major cause of medical errors. A nurse's ability to be assertive is key not only to preventing medical errors but also to reducing patients' risk and improving nursing care because nurses are able to observe and act on early signs of unsafe conditions in the provision of care (Yoshinaga & Nakamura, 2017).

It is important that the nurse understands and utilizes assertive communication skills in order to teach those much-needed skills to patients with mental illness who may have difficulty with passivity and/or aggressiveness in personal relationships and communication.

STANDARD 2: DIAGNOSIS

The psychiatric mental health registered nurse analyzes the assessment data to determine diagnoses, problems, and areas of focus for care and treatment, including level of risk (ANA et al., p 46). This text uses the International Classification for Nursing Practice (ICNP) nursing diagnoses, although other systems with their own terminology exist. ICNP classifies patient data and clinical activity in nursing and can be used for decision making and policy development aimed at improving health status and health delivery (International Council of Nurses, 2020). ICNP nursing diagnoses allow inclusion of positive aspects of a person's behaviors, which enhances self-esteem and reinforces successful behaviors. The team can view the patient more holistically with both positive areas and those areas needing improvement.

Formulating a Nursing Diagnosis

A nursing diagnosis is a clinical judgment about a patient's response, needs, mental health problems, level of risk, and potential comorbid (co-occurring) physical illnesses. An actual or potential problem can be related to a psychiatric disorder (e.g., self-mutilation, hopelessness), a medical disorder (e.g., ineffective breathing pattern), or a potential co-occurring physical illness (e.g., impaired physical mobility). Nursing diagnoses help us determine appropriate nursing interventions and outcomes.

Standard Nursing Diagnosis

A standard nursing diagnosis has three structural components: the **problem** (the unmet need), the **etiology** (the probable cause), and the **supporting data** (the signs and symptoms supporting the stated problem).

The Problem

The problem or unmet need describes the state of the patient at present. Problems that are within the nurse's domain to treat are termed *nursing diagnoses*. An example is *Self-mutilation*.

The Etiology

The etiology includes factors that contribute to or are related to the development or maintenance of a nursing diagnosis title. The related factors tell us what needs to be done to effect change and identify what needs to be targeted through nursing interventions. An example is *Self-mutilation related to disturbed body image*.

Note that the difference in identifying a plan of care for someone with the same nursing diagnoses is related to a patient's individual and unique "cause and supporting data."

Defining Characteristics (Supporting Data)

Supporting signs and symptoms are the "defining characteristics" that make up the patient's objective and measurable signs, plus the more subjective symptoms that reflect the patient's present situation. The defining characteristics may be linked to the diagnosis and probable cause with the words *as evidenced by*.

Supporting data that would validate the diagnosis *Self-mutilation related to disturbed body image* might include the following:

- Poor impulse control
- Self-inflicted cutting
- Ineffective coping skills
- Statements like "I'm so ugly, and when I cut myself, I feel better about myself."

Therefore, a completed nursing diagnosis includes (1) the **problem,** which is the area that needs intervention; (2) the **etiology,** which is what is responsible for aggravating the problem; and (3) the **defining characteristics,** which are the objective and subjective data that support the validity of the diagnosis (the problem):

Self-mutilation + related to disturbed body image + as evidenced by self-cutting, impulsivity, and statements that cutting helps relieve painful feelings of inadequacy.

Risk Diagnoses

Risk diagnoses are employed when there is a high probability that a future event may occur in a vulnerable individual. "Risk for" diagnoses are made to help prevent a potential unwanted or dangerous future event in an effort to ensure patient safety. For example, assessment in an elderly patient with a recent hip replacement might warrant a nursing diagnosis of *Risk for fall-related injury + related to (risk factors) postoperative condition and unsteady gait*. For a suicidal individual, the diagnosis *Risk for suicide* would be appropriate. For someone who has recently lost a spouse, *Risk for loneliness* and *Risk for dysfunctional grief* are possible nursing diagnoses.

Health Promotion Diagnoses

Health promotion diagnoses are used when clinical observations and/or patient (family, group, etc.) statements indicate a willingness and a wish to enhance specific health behaviors. Health promotion diagnoses are always stated in the form of "readiness for enhanced" and supported by the data/defining characteristics. In cases of health promotion diagnoses, the "related to" factors are already known (motivation to improve health status), so they are not listed in the problem statement. An example is *Readiness for effective coping + (defining characteristics) as evidenced by willingness to enhance self-concept and accept limitations and strengths.*

STANDARD 3: OUTCOMES IDENTIFICATION

The psychiatric mental health registered nurse identifies expected outcomes, and the health care consumer's goals are planned and individualized to the health care consumer or to the situation (ANA et al., 2014, p. 48).

Determining Outcomes

Outcomes criteria are the optimal goal outcomes that reflect the maximal level of patient health that can realistically be achieved through evidence-based nursing interventions. Whereas nursing diagnoses identify nursing problems, outcomes reflect the desired change. The expected outcomes provide direction for continuity of care and are culturally appropriate. Outcomes are stated in measurable terms and are achievable through evidence-based interventions and include a time estimate for attainment. Therefore, outcomes criteria are patient centered, geared to each individual, and documented as obtainable goals (ANA et al., 2014).

STANDARD 4: PLANNING

The psychiatric mental health registered nurse develops a plan that prescribes strategies and alternatives to assist the health care consumer in the attainment of expected outcomes (ANA et al., 2014, p. 50).

Inpatient and community-based facilities may use standardized tools (e.g., care plans, flowcharts, clinical pathways) for patients with specific diagnoses. Standard tools allow for the inclusion of evidence-based practice (EBP) and newly tested interventions as they become available. Although these tools may be more time efficient, they may not be appropriately focused on the individual's needs. Whatever the care planning procedures in a specific institution, the nurse considers the following specific principles when planning care:

- *Safety.* They must be safe for the patient as well as for other patients, staff, and family.
- *Appropriate.* They must be compatible with other therapies and with the patient's personal goals and spiritual and cultural values, as well as with institutional rules.
- *Individualized to the patient* (patient centered). They should be realistic (1) within the patient's capabilities given the patient's age, physical strength, condition, and willingness to change; (2) consider the patient's preferences, health practices, coping styles, and developmental level and the individual's recovery goals (to name a few); and (3) reflective of the actual available community resources and technology.
- *Evidence based.* The plan should integrate current scientific evidence, trends, and research. Using best-evidence interventions and treatments as they become available is being stressed in all areas of medical and mental health care. Evidence-based practice essentially means "a conscientious, explicit, and judicious use of current best evidence in making decisions about the care of individual patients" (Sackett et al., 2000) (refer to Chapter 1). Evidence-based practice (EBP) for nurses is a combination of clinical skills and the use of clinically relevant research in the delivery of effective patient-centered care. Therefore, the use of the best available research coupled with patient preferences and sound clinical judgment and skills makes an optimal patient-centered nurse–patient partnership (Sackett et al., 2000). Keep in mind that any interventions that are chosen to be used need to be acceptable and appropriate to the individual patient.

STANDARD 5: IMPLEMENTATION

The psychiatric-mental health nurse implements the identified plan (ANA et al., 2014, p. 52).

Recent graduates and practitioners new to the psychiatric setting will participate in many of these activities with the guidance and support of more experienced health care professionals. The psychiatric mental health registered nurse (PMH–RN), who has earned a baccalaureate degree, practices on the basic level of intervention, whereas the psychiatric mental health advanced practice registered nurse (PMH–APRN), prepared at the master's level or above, is prepared to function at an advanced level.

The basic level for psychiatric-mental health nursing practice is accomplished through the nurse–patient partnership and the use of therapeutic intervention skills. The nurse implements the plan using evidence-based interventions whenever possible, utilizing community resources and collaborating with nursing colleagues. Provision of care implies that interventions are age appropriate and culturally and ethnically sensitive. Nursing's contribution to the interdisciplinary team focuses on establishing trust and giving positive feedback for day-to-day accomplishments in an effort to boost self-esteem and encourage independence.

Basic Level Interventions

Basic Level: Psychiatric Mental Health Registered Nurse

Standard 5A: Coordination of Care. **The nurse coordinates care delivery** (ANA et al., 2014, p. 54).

The nurse coordinates and implements the plan, maximizing quality of life, independence, and optimal recovery. The nurse communicates among family and other health care workers and advocates respectable care for the individual by the interprofessional team. The nurse assists the patient and family to find alternatives to care and documents the coordination of care.

Standard 5B: Health Teaching and Health Promotion. **The psychiatric mental health registered nurse employs strategies to promote health and safe environment** (ANA et al., 2014, p. 55).

Psychiatric-mental health nurses use a variety of health teaching methods adaptive to the patient's special needs (e.g., age, culture, ability to learn, readiness) and recovery goals, integrating current knowledge and evidence-based psychoeducational strategies in their interventions.

Health teaching includes identifying the health education needs of the patient and providing health care teaching, such as coping skills, self-care activities, stress management, problem-solving skills, relapse prevention, conflict management, and giving information about coping with interpersonal relationships. Among the most vital parts of health promotion is identifying resources for prevention and recovery mental health care services in the community.

Standard 5E: Pharmacological, Biological, and Integrative Therapies. **The psychiatric mental health registered nurse incorporates knowledge of pharmacological, biological, and complementary interventions with applied clinical skills to restore the consumer's health and prevent further disability** (ANA et al., 2014).

The nurse is knowledgeable regarding the current research findings, intended action, therapeutic dosage, adverse reactions, and safe blood levels of medications being administered and monitors the patient for any untoward effects. The nurse is expected to discuss and provide health care teaching regarding medication to the patient and family for any drug action, adverse side effects, dietary restrictions, and drug interactions and to provide time for questions. The nurse's assessment of the patient's response to psychobiological interventions is communicated to other members of the mental health team.

Standard 5F: Milieu Therapy. **The psychiatric mental health registered nurse provides, structures, and maintains a safe, therapeutic, recovery-oriented environment in collaboration with health care consumers, families, and other health care clinicians** (ANA et al., 2014, p. 60).

Among other things, ***milieu therapy*** includes orienting patients to their rights and responsibilities. Milieu therapy also includes informing patients in a culturally competent manner about the need for structure, maintenance of a safe environment, and limits set on the unit. The nurse selects activities (both individual and group) that meet the patient's physical and mental health needs. The patient should always be maintained in the least restrictive environment.

Standard 5G: Therapeutic Relationship and Counseling. **The nurse uses the therapeutic relationship and counseling interventions to assist health care consumers in their individual recovery journeys by improving and regaining their previous coping abilities, fostering mental health, and preventing mental disorder and disability** (ANA et al., 2014, p. 62).

Advanced Practice Interventions: Psychiatric Mental Health Advanced Practice Registered Nurse

Prescriptive Authority and Treatment

The psychiatric mental health advanced practice nurse has additional education and the authority to prescribe medication and provide therapies and referrals for the treatment of mental health conditions. An APRN can also provide group, couples, individual, and family psychotherapy and may consult with the treatment team to provide guidance for care. The full extent of an APRN's ability to practice independently depends on state and national laws (ANA et al., 2014).

STANDARD 6: EVALUATION

The psychiatric mental health registered nurse enhances progress toward attainment of expected outcomes (ANA et al., 2014, p. 65).

Unfortunately, evaluation of patient outcomes is often the most neglected part of the nursing process. Evaluation of the individual's response to treatment should be systematic, ongoing, and criterion based. Supporting data are included to clarify the evaluation. Ongoing assessment of data allows for revisions of nursing diagnoses, changes to more realistic outcomes, or identification of more appropriate interventions when outcomes are not met.

DOCUMENTATION

Documentation could be considered the seventh step in the nursing process. Keep in mind that patient records are legal documents and may be used in a court of law. Besides the evaluation of stated outcomes, the notes of all health care workers should record changes in patient condition, informed consent (for medications and treatments), reaction to medication, documentation of symptoms (verbatim when appropriate), concerns of the patient, and any untoward incidents in the health care setting. Documentation of patient progress is the responsibility of the entire mental health team. Box 7.7 lists the key points that should be documented in a mental health plan.

Documentation of "Nonadherence"

When patients do not follow medication and treatment plans, they are often labeled as "noncompliant." Applied to patients, the term *noncompliant* often has negative connotations because *compliance* traditionally referred to the extent that a patient obediently and faithfully followed the health care providers' instructions. "That patient is noncompliant" often translates into he or she is "bad" or "lazy," subjecting the patient to blame and criticism. Crane (2012) cautions nurses and physicians not to blame noncompliance on a patient's stubbornness or bad mood; this can leave both the nurse and the patient frustrated and angry. The term *noncompliant* is invariably judgmental. A much more useful term would be **nonadherent**. It now invites us to find out what is going on in the patient's life that is influencing the client's ability or willingness to take medication.

Crane (2012) also emphasizes that under the Affordable Care Act, documenting "noncompliance" no longer protects the physician, nurse, manager, or hospital for bad outcomes that have led to further illness or injury. A finding of noncompliance may void Medicaid or Medicare reimbursements, which can lead to financial losses to the institution and damage to the facility's reputation (Scudder, 2013).

Furthermore, "patient did not comply" does not protect nurses, physicians, or health care workers from malpractice lawsuits. Crane (2012) advises that meticulous records that document the doctor's or nurse's "rationale for treatment, clear explanations of what he or she wants the patient to do, and whether the patient actually complied with that advice" will help protect health care workers in the event of lawsuits. The lesson is to treat noncompliance/nonadherence seriously. "Each compliance issue, large and small, must be recognized as an indicator of potential trouble and must be addressed early and appropriately" (Scudder, 2013). Probably the biggest issue involved in a malpractice verdict is if the patient was given instructions or printed information sheets, it is possible that the patient did not understand the instructions or didn't realize how important the treatment (medication, a follow-up, etc.) was to their health.

Systems of Charting

Although communication among team members and coordination of services are the primary goals when choosing a system for charting, practitioners in all settings must also consider professional standards, legal issues, requirements for reimbursement by insurers, and accreditation by regulatory agencies.

Information also must be in a format that is retrievable for quality assurance monitoring, utilization management, peer review, and research. Documentation, using the nursing process as a guide, is reflected in many of the different formats that are commonly used in health care settings. Computerized clinical documentation is preferred in today's medical settings. Nurses need to be trained to use these technologies, and the medical setting should be prepared to provide further training for nurses in the use of terminology, progress notes relating to needs assessment, nursing interventions, and nursing diagnoses (Hayrinen, 2010). Any documentation format used by a health care facility must be focused, organized, and pertinent and must conform to certain legal and other generally accepted principles. Refer to Box 7.8 for more details on the do's and don'ts of documentation. Table 7.1 compares narrative charting to SOAPIE charting (two structures used in documentation). The structure used is often determined by the electronic health record and the forms created to capture information.

The nursing process appears as a linear process, but it is important to note that all phases of the nursing process are in motion at any given time. A nurse should be assessing patient status and evaluating progress toward the goals at all times. Documentation is critical to the plan of care so progress can be observed and the plan of care can be adjusted accordingly.

BOX 7.7 Documentation Outline for an Initial Mental Health Plan

- Name
- Demographics: age, marital status, living situation, employment present/past
- History of mental illness/substance abuse
- Presenting problem(s)
- "Why now" stressor(s)
- Lethality assessment and risk factors—include firearms assessment
- Treatment history
- Quality of activities of daily living
- Patient strengths
- Medical diagnoses/current vital signs/medications and adherence
- *Diagnostic and Statistical Manual of Mental Disorders,* 5th edition *(DSM-5)* diagnoses
- Nursing diagnoses
- Short- and long-term goals
- Suggested interventions related to goals
- Supports available for safety
- Discharge plan

BOX 7.8 Legal Considerations for Documentation of Care

Do's

- Chart in a timely manner all pertinent and factual information.
- Be familiar with the nursing documentation policy in your facility and make your charting conform to this standard. The policy generally states the method, frequency, and pertinent assessments, interventions, and outcomes to be recorded. If your agency's policies and procedures do not encourage or allow for quality documentation, bring the need for change to the administration's attention.
- Chart legibly in ink.
- Chart facts fully, descriptively, and accurately.
- Chart what you see, hear, feel, and smell.
- Chart pertinent observations: psychosocial observations, physical symptoms pertinent to the medical diagnosis, and behaviors pertinent to the nursing diagnosis.
- Chart follow-up care provided when a problem has been identified in earlier documentation. For example, if a patient has fallen and injured a leg, describe how the wound is healing.
- Chart fully the facts surrounding unusual occurrences and incidents.
- Chart all nursing interventions, treatments, and outcomes (including teaching efforts and patient responses), and safety and patient protection interventions.
- Chart the patient's expressed subjective feelings.
- Chart each time you notify a physician and record the reason for notification, the information that was communicated, the accurate time, the physician's instructions or orders, and the follow-up activity.
- Chart physicians' visits and treatments.
- Chart discharge medications and instructions given for use, as well as all discharge teaching performed, and note which family members were included in the process.

Don'ts

- Do *not* chart opinions that are not supported by the facts.
- Do *not* defame patients by calling them names or by making derogatory statements about them (e.g., "an unlikable patient who is demanding unnecessary attention").
- Do *not* chart before an event occurs.
- Do *not* chart generalizations, suppositions, or pat phrases (e.g., "patient in good spirits").
- Do *not* obliterate, erase, alter, or destroy a record. If an error is made, draw one line through the error, write "mistaken entry" or "error," and initial. Follow your agency's guidelines closely.
- Do *not* leave blank spaces for chronological notes. If you must chart out of sequence, chart "late entry." Identify the time and date of the entry and the time and date of the occurrence.
- If an incident report/occurrence is filed, *do not note in the chart that one was filed.* This form is generally a privileged communication between the hospital and the hospital's attorney. Describing it in the chart may destroy the privileged nature of the communication. The incident as it occurred should be documented in the patient's records.

TABLE 7.1 Narrative Versus Problem-Oriented Charting[a]

Narrative Charting	Problem-Oriented Charting: SOAPIE
Characteristics	
A descriptive statement of patient status written in chronological order throughout a shift. Used to support assessment finding from a flow sheet. In charting by exception, narrative notes are used to indicate significant symptoms, behaviors, or events that are exceptions to norms identified on assessment flow sheet.	Developed in the 1960s for physicians to reduce inefficient documentation. Intended to be accompanied by a problem list. Originally SOAP, with IE added later. Emphasis is on problem identification, process, and outcome. **S:** Subjective data (patient statement) **O:** Objective data (nurse observations) **A:** Assessment (nurse interprets S and O and describes either a problem or a nursing diagnosis) **P:** Plan (proposed intervention) **I:** Interventions (nurse's response to problem) **E:** Evaluation (patient outcome)
Example	
Date/time/discipline: Patient was agitated in the morning and pacing in the hallway. Blinked eyes, muttered to self, and looked off to the side. Stated heard voices. Verbally hostile to another patient. Offered 2 mg of haloperidol (Haldol) prn and sat with staff in quiet area for 20 minutes. Patient returned to community lounge and was able to sit and watch television.	Date/time/discipline: **S:** "I'm so stupid. Get away, get away." "I hear the devil telling me bad things." **O:** Patient paced the hall, mumbling to self and looking off to the side. Shouted derogatory comments when approached by another patient. Watched walls and ceiling closely. **A:** Patient was having auditory hallucinations and increased agitation. **P:** Offered patient haloperidol prn. Redirected patient to less stimulating environment. **I:** Patient received 2 mg of haloperidol PO prn. Sat with patient in quiet room for 20 minutes. **E:** Patient calmer. Returned to community lounge, sat, and watched television.
Advantages	
Uses a common form of expression (narrative writing). Can address any event or behavior. Explains flow sheet findings. Provides multidisciplinary ease of use.	Structured. Provides consistent organization of data. Facilitates retrieval of data for quality assurance and utilization management. Contains all elements of the nursing process. Minimizes inclusion of unnecessary data. Provides multidisciplinary ease of use.
Disadvantages	
Unstructured. May result in different organization of information from note to note. Makes it difficult to retrieve quality assurance and utilization management data. Frequently leads to omission of elements of the nursing process. Commonly results in inclusion of unnecessary and subjective information.	Requires time and effort to structure the information. Limits entries to problems. May result in loss of data about progress. Not chronological. Carries negative connotation.

KEY POINTS TO REMEMBER

- The nursing process is a six-step problem-solving approach to patient care to help secure safety and quality care for patients.
- The *primary source* of assessment is the patient. *Secondary sources* of information include the family, neighbors, friends, police, and other members of the health care team.
- The assessment interview includes gathering objective data (mental or emotional status) and subjective data (psychosocial assessment). A number of tools are provided in this textbook for the evaluation of cultural, spiritual/religious, and mental status.
- The medical examination, history, and systems review provide complete a comprehensive assessment.
- An important part of planning patient-centered care is to understand how spiritual/religious beliefs play a part in a person's life and how he or she deals with stress.
- Caregivers should also have an awareness of the person's cultural background and social attachments and how these issues affect the way a person experiences healing in his or her culture.
- Assessment tools and standardized rating scales may be used to evaluate and monitor a patient's progress. Emphasis needs to be placed on further evaluation of progress and sharing of this information with other members of the health care team.
- Self-assessment is an important part of the assessment process. There are a number of ways that novice interviewers can gain valuable feedback, support, and supervision.
- Determination of the nursing diagnosis defines the practice of nursing, improves communication between staff members, and assists in accountability for care.
- A nursing diagnosis consists of (1) an unmet need or problem and/or progress toward goal, (2) an etiology or probable cause, and (3) supporting data.
- Outcomes are variable, measurable, and stated in terms that reflect a patient's actual state.
- Behavioral goals support outcomes. Short- and long-term outcomes are measurable, indicate the desired patient behavior(s), include a set time for achievement, and are short and specific.

- Planning nursing actions to achieve the stated outcomes include the use of the following specific principles: the plan should be (1) safe, (2) evidence based whenever possible, (3) realistic, and (4) compatible with other therapies.
- Practice in psychiatric nursing encompasses basic-level interventions: coordination of care; health teaching and health promotion; milieu therapy; and pharmacological, biological, and integrative therapies.
- Advanced practice interventions are carried out by a nurse who is educated at the master's level or higher. Nurses certified for advanced practice psychiatric mental-health nursing may be additionally prepared to practice psychotherapy, prescribe certain medications, and perform consulting work.
- The evaluation of care is a continual process of determining to what extent the outcome criteria have been achieved. The plan of care may be revised on the basis of the evaluation.
- Documentation of patient progress through evaluation of outcome criteria is crucial. The patient's record is a legal document and should accurately reflect the patient's condition, medications, treatment, tests, responses, and any untoward incidents.
- Simply documenting a patient's noncompliance/nonadherence to medical treatment no longer protects nurses, doctors, other health care professionals, and/or institutions from lawsuits when further harm to the patient presents itself. Careful documentation of what has been done to help the individual understand the instructions, understand the reasons behind the medical advice, and follow up on compliance issues should be included.

APPLYING CLINICAL JUDGMENT

1. A 37-year-old Hispanic man arrived by ambulance from a supermarket, where he had fallen. He remains lethargic. On his arrival to the emergency department (ED), his breath smelled "fruity." He appears confused and anxious, saying that "they put the 'evil eye' on me, they want me to die, they are drying out my body … it's draining me dry … they are yelling, they are yelling … no, no I'm not bad … oh God, don't let them get me." When his mother arrives in the ED, she tells the staff, through the use of an interpreter, that Pedro is a severe diabetic and has a diagnosis of paranoid schizophrenia, and this happens when he does not take his medications. In a group or in collaboration with a classmate, respond to the following:
   - **A.** A number of nursing diagnoses are possible in this scenario. Formulate in writing at least two nursing diagnoses (problems) given the preceding information, and include "related to" and "as evidenced by."
   - **B.** For each of your nursing diagnoses, list one long-term outcome (e.g., the problem, what should change). Include a time frame, desired change, and three criteria that will help you evaluate if the outcome has been met, not met, or partially met.
   - **C.** For each long-term outcome, list two short-term outcomes (goals) (the steps that need to be taken in order for the goal to be accomplished), including time frame, desired outcomes, and evaluation criteria.
   - **D.** What are the four basic principles for planning nursing interventions?
   - **E.** What specific needs might you take into account when planning nursing care for Mr. Gonzales?
   - **F.** Using informatics, evaluate optimal outcomes for Mr. Gonzalez at your current health care setting, or use the charting method employed by the institution.
   - **G.** Give an example of the QSEN competencies you might stress when planning care for Mr. Gonzalez.

CHAPTER REVIEW QUESTIONS

1. A new patient whose chief concern is, "I'm tired of crying every day." Which comment from the patient would prompt the nurse to suspect that a medical reason is causing the problem rather than depression?
   - **a.** "I usually drink two or three cups of coffee in the morning."
   - **b.** "I often have headaches, especially when the pollen count is high."
   - **c.** "Years ago I had thyroid problems, but they cleared up and I stopped the medicine."
   - **d.** "I recently had three moles removed because my doctor thought they were suspicious."
2. A 55-year-old lives 100 miles from her parents and mother-in-law. In the past year, her father had back surgery, her mother broke her hip, and her mother-in-law had a cardiac event. Which nursing diagnosis is most applicable to the 55-year-old?
   - **a.** Risk for dysfunctional grief related to impending deaths of parents
   - **b.** Risk for injury related to frequent long drives to care for aging parents
   - **c.** Risk for situational low self-esteem related to overwhelming responsibilities
   - **d.** Risk for caregiver stress related to responsibilities for care of aging parents
3. A patient asks the psychiatric mental health registered nurse, "I'm having so much anxiety. I think hypnosis would help me. Will you do that for me?" When determining a response, which factor should the nurse consider?
   - **a.** The patient's current medication regime
   - **b.** State regulations regarding scope of practice
   - **c.** The patient's level of participation within the therapeutic milieu
   - **d.** The plan of care the multidisciplinary team has developed for the patient
4. The nurse plans care for a newly hospitalized patient experiencing panic-level anxiety after an automobile accident. The patient has no physical injuries. When selecting goals and outcomes, the nurse will:
   - **a.** select outcomes related to patient learning.
   - **b.** focus first on the long-term goals for the patient.
   - **c.** individualize outcomes based on the patient's needs.
   - **d.** confer with the patient about which outcomes the patient wants to achieve.
5. On an inpatient unit, one patient assaults another patient, resulting in a small laceration. Considering the patients' right to confidentiality, how will the nurse effectively document this event?
   - **a.** Ensure unit safety by documenting the hostile and combative characteristics of the assaulting patient.
   - **b.** Document in each patient's medical record the events and actions taken, using the initials of the other patient involved.
   - **c.** Document in both patients' medical records that an occurrence (incident) report was prepared according to agency policy.
   - **d.** Verbally report the events to other team members and minimize written documentation in order to reduce potential legal consequences.

REFERENCES

American Nurses Association (ANA), American Psychiatric Nurses Association, & International Society of Psychiatric-Mental Health Nurses. (2014). *Psychiatric-mental health nursing: Scope and standards of practice*. Washington, DC: Nursebooks.org.

Arnold, E. C., & Boggs, K. U. (2016). *Interpersonal relationships: Professional communication skills for nurses* (6th ed.). St. Louis: Saunders.

Bethell, C., & Carle, A. (2017). Methods to assess adverse childhood experiences of children and families: Toward approaches to promote child well-being in policy and practice. *Academic Pediatrics,. 17*(7), S51–S69.

Chen, C. M. (2017). The longitudinal relationship between mental health disorders and chronic disease for older adults: A population-based study. *International Journal of Geriatric Psychiatry, 32*(9), 1017–1026.

Coombs, T., & Crookes, P. (2013). What is the process of a comprehensive mental health nursing assessment? Results from a qualitative study. *International Nursing Review, 60*, 96–102.

Correll, C. (2017). Prevalence, incidence and mortality from cardiovascular disease in patients with pooled and specific severe mental illness: A large-scale meta-analysis of 3,211,768 patients and 113,383,368 controls. *World Psychiatry, 16*(2), 163–180.

Crane, M. (2012). Documenting noncompliance won't protect you anymore. Retrieved February 18, 2013, from www.Medscape.com/viewarticle/773918.

Ennis, G. B. (2015, May). Enabling professional development in mental health nursing: the role of clinical leadership. *Journal of Psychiatric and Mental Health Nursing.*

Freire, P. (1998). *Pedagogy of freedom: Ethics, democracy, and civil courage*. New York: Roman and Littlefield.

Giddens, J. F. (2017). *Concepts for nursing practice (2nd ed)*. St. Louis: Elsevier.

Girouard, S., & Bailey, N. (2017). ACEs implications for nurses, nursing education, and nursing practice. *Academy of Pediatrics, 17*(7s), S16–S17. https://doi:10.1016/j.acap.2016.08.008.

Gupta, S. (2017). Hiding in plain sight: Resurrecting the power of inspecting the patient. *JAMA Internal Medicine, 177*(6), 757–758.

Gurwin J, Revere KE, Niepold S, et al. (2018). A randomized controlled study of art observation training to improve medical student ophthalmology skills. Ophthalmology, 125, 8–14.

Hayrinen, K. (2010). Evaluation of electronic nursing documentation—nursing process model and standardized terminologies as key to visible and transparent nursing. *International Journal of Medical Informatics, 79*(8), 554–564.

International Council of Nurses. (2020). *What we do.* Retrieved from https://www.icn.ch/what-we-do.

Knoerl, A. M., Esper, K., Hasenau, S., et al. (2011). Cultural sensitivity in patient health education. *Nursing Clinics of America, 46*(3), 335–340.

MacKinlay, E., & Burns, R. (2017). Spirituality promotes better health outcomes and lowers anxiety about aging: The importance of spiritual dimensions for baby boomers as they enter older adulthood. *Journal of Religion, Spirituality and Aging, 29*(4).

Milani, R. M. (2017, October 24). Substance misuse assessment in mental health services: The importance of professional curiosity. *International Journal of Psychological Research, 2*(4).

Norris, D., & Clark, M. (2016). The mental status examination. *American Family Physician, 94*(8), 635–641.

Sackett, D. L., Straus, S., Richardson, W., et al. (2000). *Evidence-based medicine: How to practice and teach EBM*. London: Churchill Livingstone.

Scudder, L. (2013). Nurses and noncompliance: A primer. Retrieved March 18, 2013, from www.medscape.com/viewarticle/779149_print.

Sommers-Flanagan, J., & Sommers-Flanagan, R. (2012–2013). *Clinical interviewing* (5th ed.). Hoboken, NJ: John Wiley & Sons.

Stewart, S., & Hamza, C. (2017, January 26). The Child and Youth Mental Health Assessment (ChYMH): An examination of the psychometric properties of an integrated assessment developed for clinically referred children and youth. *BMC Health Services Research.*

Yoshinaga, N., & Nakamura, Y. (2017, July 25). Is modified brief assertiveness training for nurses effective? A single group study with long-term follow-up. *Journal of Nursing Management.*

8

Communication Skills: Medium for All Nursing Practice

Elizabeth M. Varcarolis, Chyllia D. Fosbre

http://evolve.elsevier.com/Varcarolis/essentials

OBJECTIVES

1. Discuss three personal and two environmental factors that can impede accurate communication.
2. Discuss the differences between verbal and nonverbal communication, and demonstrate at least five areas of nonverbal communication.
3. Demonstrate two attending behaviors that you will work on to increase your communication skills.
4. Relate problems that can arise when nurses are insensitive to cultural differences in patients' communication styles.
5. Compare and contrast the range of verbal and nonverbal communication of your cultural groups with those of another cultural group in your community in the areas of (a) communication style, (b) eye contact, and (c) touch.
6. State rationales for four techniques that can obstruct communication, highlighting what makes them ineffective.
7. Role-play with a classmate the techniques of "what if" and the "miracle question," and then switch roles. Identify what new information you might have learned about your classmate and what new insight you might have about yourself.
8. Identify the advantages and the use of telehealth technologies in the community in which you live.

KEY TERMS AND CONCEPTS

active listening, p. 93
clarifying techniques, p. 94
complementary relationship, p. 91
congruent message, p. 92
cues, p. 92
cultural competence, p. 98
cultural filters, p. 100
disapproving, p. 98
double messages, p. 92
excessive questioning, p. 96
exploring, p. 94
feedback, p. 90
giving advice, p. 98
giving approval, p. 97
incongruent message, p. 92
information communication technologies (ICTs), p. 100
media, p. 90
message, p. 90
miscommunication, p. 98
mobile medical apps, p. 101
nontherapeutic techniques, p. 93
nonverbal communication, p. 92
paraphrasing, p. 94
receiver, p. 90
reflecting, p. 94
restating, p. 94
sender, p. 90
sharing observations, p. 94
silence, p. 93
stimulus, p. 90
symmetrical relationship, p. 91
telehealth technologies, p. 100
therapeutic communication, p. 90
therapeutic techniques, p. 93
verbal communication, p. 92
"why" questions, p. 98

CONCEPT: COMMUNICATION: As defined, *communication* simply describes the transmission of ideas between people. Communication becomes very complex when studied and is therefore a major field for academics and professionals. Miscommunication is a frequently cited cause of errors in the delivery of health care (Giddens, 2017). In psychiatric nursing, communication skills assume a new emphasis because psychiatric disorders can cause emotional symptoms that affect a person's ability to relate to others. When stress or negative feelings occur within the relationship, effective communication has a higher potential to falter, and there is a greater chance for miscommunication. Being an effective communicator is not just a matter of knowing what techniques to use. Genuine respect for the individual and the ability to listen compassionately and empathetically are the essence of psychological healing.

INTRODUCTION

Humans have a fundamental need to relate to others. Our advanced ability to communicate gives our lives sustenance and meaning. We also share a need to be understood and form satisfying relationships with others. This is usually accomplished through effective communication skills. On the other hand, when stress or negative feelings occur within a relationship, effective communication has a higher potential to break down, and there is a greater chance for miscommunication. All of our actions, words, and expressions convey meaning to others. It is even said that we cannot *not* communicate. Silence, for example, can communicate acceptance, anger, or thoughtfulness. In the provision of nursing care, however, communication has a new emphasis. Just as social relationships are different from therapeutic relationships, basic communication is different from the professional, goal-directed, and scientifically based communication we call **therapeutic communication**.

COMMUNICATION

The ability to form patient-centered therapeutic relationships/partnerships is essential to effective nursing care, and therapeutic communication is crucial to the therapeutic relationship. Determining levels of pain in the postoperative patient; listening as parents express feelings of fear concerning their child's diagnosis; or understanding, without words, the needs of the intubated patient in the intensive care unit are essential skills in providing quality nursing.

Ideally, therapeutic communication is a professional skill you learn and practice early in your nursing curriculum. But in psychiatric nursing, communication skills assume a different and new emphasis because psychiatric disorders cause not only physical symptoms (e.g., fatigue, loss of appetite, and insomnia) but also emotional symptoms (e.g., sadness, anger, hopelessness, euphoria, as well as sensory distortions) that affect a person's very ability to communicate effectively with others.

It is often in the psychiatric rotation that students discover the importance of communication and increase their ability to utilize "therapeutic communication" and begin to rely on techniques they once considered artificial. **Note:** There is a fundamental difference between performing an *assessment* and the use of *therapeutic communication. Assessment* is an information-gathering approach designed to meet the nurse's needs, whereas *therapeutic communication* meets the patient's needs.

With continued practice, you will develop your own style and rhythm, and eventually these techniques will become a part of the way you communicate with others. With time and practice, the nurse will begin to relate to the person behind the diagnoses and to experience, to some extent, the world through the eyes of another individual.

WILL I SAY THE WRONG THING?

Novice psychiatric practitioners are often concerned that they may say the wrong thing, *especially* when learning to apply therapeutic techniques. Will you say the "wrong" thing? The answer is, yes, you probably will. That is how we all learn to find more useful and effective ways of helping individuals reach their goals. Your challenge is to work with your instructor/supervisor and find more useful responses.

Will saying the "wrong" thing be harmful to the patient? Hardly, especially if your intent is honest, your approach is respectful, and you have a genuine concern for the patient. Communication is up to 90% nonverbal, and surprisingly, most individuals pay attention to nonverbal cues, such as what they perceive as your intent. Scientific investigations have identified special skills and methods that can aid people in becoming more effective helpers. However, knowledge of skills and techniques is not enough. Being an effective communicator, whether in nursing or in any other area of life, is not just a matter of knowing what techniques to use. *Genuine respect for the individual and the ability to listen compassionately and empathetically are the essence of psychological healing.*

THE COMMUNICATION PROCESS

For our purposes here, we will use Berlo's communication model as an example of a classic communication model (Berlo, 1960). It was developed in 1960; however, it remains relevant today.

1. One person has a need to communicate with another (**stimulus**). For example, the stimulus for communication can be a need for information, comfort, or advice.
2. The person sending the message (**sender**) initiates interpersonal contact.
3. The **message** is the information sent or expressed to another. The clearest messages are those that are well organized and expressed in a manner familiar to the receiver.
4. The message can be sent through a variety of **media**, including auditory (hearing), visual (seeing), tactile (touch), olfactory (smell), or any combination of these senses.
5. The person receiving the message (**receiver**) then interprets the message and responds to the sender by providing **feedback**. The nature of the feedback often indicates whether the meaning of the message sent has been correctly interpreted by the receiver. Validating the accuracy of the sender's message is extremely important. An accuracy check may be obtained by simply asking the sender, "Is this what you mean?" or "I notice you turn away when we talk about your going back to college. Is there a conflict there?"

Fig. 8.1 shows this simple model of communication, along with some of the many factors that affect communication.

Communication is complex and involves a variety of personal and environmental factors that can distort both the sending and the receiving of messages.

Factors That Affect Communication

Personal Factors

Personal factors that can impede accurate transmission or interpretation of messages include *emotional factors* (e.g., mood, responses to stress, personal bias, relationship misunderstandings), *social factors* (e.g., previous experience, cultural differences, language differences, lifestyle differences), and *cognitive factors* (e.g., problem-solving ability, knowledge level, language use).

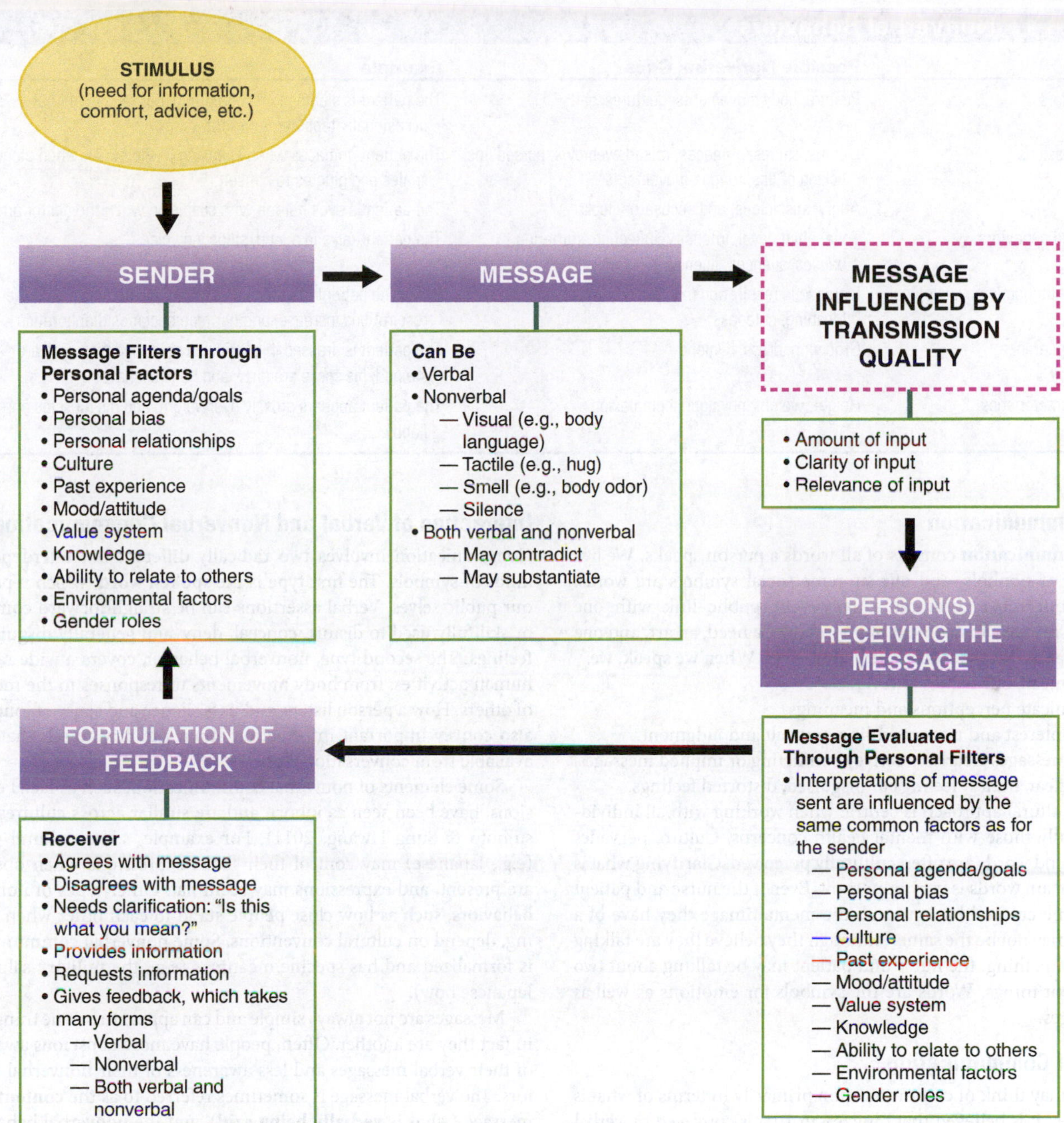

Fig. 8.1 Operational definition of communication. (Adapted from Ellis, R. B., Gates, B., & Kenworthy, N. [2003]. *Interpersonal communication in nursing: Theory and practice*. London, England: Churchill Livingstone Elsevier.)

Environmental Factors

Environmental factors that may affect communication include *physical factors* (e.g., background noise, lack of privacy, uncomfortable accommodations) and *societal determinants* (e.g., sociopolitical, historical, or economic factors; the presence of others; the expectations of others).

Relationship Factors

Here, relationship factors refer to whether the participants are equal or unequal. When the two participants are equal, such as friends or colleagues, the relationship is said to be a **symmetrical relationship**. However, when there is a difference in status or power, such as between nurse and patient or teacher and student, the relationship is characterized by inequality (one participant is "superior" to the other) and is called a **complementary relationship**. For example, social status, age, gender differences, financial status, and educational differences can be influential in the communication process.

We all have prejudices. Our duty to our patients is to guard against negative feelings toward others who seem different from us (e.g., color of skin, sexual orientation, religious beliefs, country of origin, etc.) from leading to demeaning or devaluing behavior toward another. Our duty toward ourselves as professionals is to our personal growth. Personal growth is a lifelong journey. However, the more we grow and learn, the more human we become, and the more effective we become with people under our care. Despite our differences, we are all more alike than different (Sommers-Flanagan & Sommers-Flanagan, 2017).

TABLE 8.1 Nonverbal Behaviors

Behavior	Possible Nonverbal Cues	Example
Body behaviors	Posture, body movements, gestures, gait	The patient is slumped in a chair, puts her face in her hands, and occasionally taps her right foot.
Facial expressions	Frowns, smiles, grimaces, raised eyebrows, pursed lips, licking of lips, tongue movements	The patient grimaces when speaking to the nurse; when alone, he smiles and giggles to himself.
Eye cast	Angry, suspicious, and accusatory looks	The patient's eyes harden with suspicion when the doctor arrives.
Voice-related behaviors	Tone, pitch, level, intensity, inflection, stuttering, pauses, silences, fluency	The patient talks in a loud, singsong voice.
Observable autonomic physiological responses	Increase in respirations, diaphoresis, pupil dilation, blushing, paleness	When the patient mentions discharge, she becomes pale, her respirations increase, and her face becomes diaphoretic.
Personal appearance	Grooming, dress, hygiene	The patient is dressed in a wrinkled shirt, and his pants are stained; his socks are dirty, and he is unshaven.
Physical characteristics	Height, weight, physique, complexion	The patient appears grossly overweight, and his muscles appear flabby.

Verbal Communication

Verbal communication consists of all words a person speaks. We live in a society of symbols, and our supreme social symbols are words. Talking is our most common activity—our public link with one another, the primary instrument of instruction, a need, an art, and one of the most personal aspects of our private lives. When we speak, we:

- Communicate our beliefs and values.
- Communicate perceptions and meanings.
- Convey interest and understanding *or* insult and judgment.
- Convey messages clearly *or* convey conflicting or implied messages.
- Convey clear, honest feelings *or* disguised, distorted feelings.

A multicultural approach is central when working with all individuals, especially those with mental health concerns. Culture pervades everything, and words are often culturally perceived. Clarifying what is meant by certain words is very important. Even if the nurse and patient have the same cultural background, the mental image they have of a given word may not be the same. Although they believe they are talking about the same thing, the nurse and patient may be talking about two quite different things. Words are the symbols for emotions as well as mental images.

Nonverbal Communication

Many of us may think of communication primarily in terms of what is said; however, it is believed that only 5% to 10% is conveyed by verbal means and that nonverbal behaviors comprise from 65% to 95% of a sent message. Therefore, it comes as no surprise that nonverbal behaviors and cues drastically influence communication. Effective communicators pay attention to both the verbal and nonverbal cues.

Nonverbal communication refers to any body gestures, such as facial expressions, body posture, hand movements, and so forth. The tone and pitch of a person's voice and the way a person paces speech are also examples of nonverbal communication. It is important to keep in mind, however, that culture influences the pitch and the tone a person uses. For example, the tone and pitch of a voice used to express anger can vary widely within cultures and families. Other common examples of nonverbal communication (often called cues) are physical appearance, facial expressions, body posture, amount of eye contact, eye cast (i.e., emotion expressed in the eyes), sighs, fidgeting, and yawning. Table 8.1 identifies key components of nonverbal behaviors. Nonverbal behaviors need to be observed and interpreted while considering a person's culture, class, gender, age, sexual orientation, and spiritual norms.

Interaction of Verbal and Nonverbal Communication

Communication involves two radically different but interdependent kinds of symbols. The first type is the **spoken word**, which represents our public selves. Verbal assertions can be straightforward comments or skillfully used to distort, conceal, deny, and generally disguise true feelings. The second type, nonverbal behavior, covers a wide range of human activities, from body movements to responses to the messages of others. How a person listens and uses silence and sense of touch may also convey important information about the private self that is not available from conversation alone.

Some elements of nonverbal communication, such as facial expressions, have been seen as inborn and are similar across cultures (Matsumoto & Sung Hwang, 2011). For example, some cultural groups (e.g., Japanese) may control their facial expressions when observers are present, and expressions may seem flat. Other types of nonverbal behaviors, such as how close people stand to each other when speaking, depend on cultural conventions. Some nonverbal communication is formalized and has specific meanings (e.g., the military salute, the Japanese bow).

Messages are not always simple and can appear to be one thing when in fact they are another. Often, people have more conscious awareness of their verbal messages and less awareness of their nonverbal behaviors. The verbal message is sometimes referred to as the **content** of the message (**what is verbally being said**), and the nonverbal behavior is called the **process** of the message.

When the substance of the message is the same as what is meant (content same as process), we refer to the communication as being congruent with the process; it is a congruent message. With congruent communication, the message is more clearly understood and is considered healthy. For example, if a student says, "It's important that I get good grades in this class," that is *content.* If the student is browsing through social media, that is *process.* In this situation, the content and process are incongruent and send a mixed message. If the student had been skimming through a nursing textbook (process), the message would have been congruent. Conflicting messages are known as double messages or incongruent messages. One way a nurse can respond to verbal and nonverbal incongruity is to reflect and validate the patient's feelings. "You say you are upset that you did not pass this semester, but I notice that you look more relaxed and less conflicted than you have all term. What do you see as some of the pros and cons of not passing the course this semester?"

Messages are sent to create meaning but can also be used defensively to hide what is occurring, create confusion, and adversely affect relatedness. An incongruent or mixed message is a mix of content (what is said) and process (what is transmitted nonverbally) and can have a nurturing or harmful aspect, which is often implied, as shown in the following vignette.

VIGNETTE: A 17-year-old female who lives at home with her mother wants to go out for an evening with her friends. She is told by her chronically ill but not helpless mother: "Oh, that's okay, go ahead, have fun. I'll just sit here by myself, and I can always call 911 if I don't feel well, but you go ahead and have fun." The mother says this while looking sad, slumped in her chair, and letting her cane drop to the floor.

The recipient of this mixed or incongruent message is caught between contradictory statements implying that she cannot do the right thing. If she goes out for the evening, the implication is that she is being selfish by leaving her sick mother alone. If she stays, the mother could say, "I told you to go have fun." If she does go out, the chances are she will not have much fun. No matter what the daughter does, she cannot win. The daughter can clarify the message by reflecting what her mother is saying, both verbally and nonverbally, and asking for clarification by stating, "I hear you say that you want me to go out and have fun, but when you say 'I'll just sit here by myself' while looking sad, I don't know if you mean what you say." A similar technique can be used with patients to address incongruent messages.

With experience in making observations, nurses become increasingly aware of the verbal and nonverbal communication of the patient/person. Nurses can compare patients' dialogue with their nonverbal communication to gain important clues about the real message. What individuals do either expresses and reinforces or contradicts what they say. As in the saying "Actions speak louder than words," actions often reveal the true meaning of a person's intent, whether it is conscious or unconscious.

EFFECTIVE COMMUNICATION SKILLS FOR NURSES

The art of communication was emphasized by Peplau (1952) to highlight the importance of nursing interventions in facilitating the achievement of quality patient care and quality of life. Therefore, as stated, the goal of the nurse in the mental health setting is to provide a place of safety and hope where the patient can feel comfortable and understood. Eventually, the long-term goals are to help the patient:

- Identify and explore problems relating to others.
- Discover healthy ways of meeting emotional needs.
- Experience satisfying interpersonal relationships.

Once specific needs and problems have been identified, the nurse can work with the patient on increasing critical thinking skills, learning new coping behaviors, and experiencing more appropriate and satisfying ways of relating to others. To do this, the nurse needs to have a sound knowledge of communication skills. Therefore, nurses best serve their patients when they become more aware of their own interpersonal methods and work on eliminating obstructive **nontherapeutic techniques** and developing additional responses that maximize nurse–patient interactions and increase the use of helpful **therapeutic techniques.**

Useful tools for nurses when communicating with their patients are (1) silence, (2) active listening, and (3) clarifying techniques.

Use of Silence

When used properly, the use of silence can be an effective tool in encouraging individuals to open up. However, silence can be uncomfortable for nurses and patients (Sommers-Flanagan & Sommers-Flanagan, 2017). In our society, and in nursing, there is an emphasis on action. In communication, we tend to expect a high level of verbal activity. Many students and practicing nurses find that when the flow of words stops, they become uncomfortable. **Silence** is not the absence of communication; it is a specific channel for transmitting and receiving messages. The practitioner needs to understand that silence is a significant means of influencing and being influenced by others, and if used judiciously, it can be a powerful listening response.

In the initial interview, the patient may be reluctant to speak because the newness of the situation may be overwhelming; the fact that the nurse is a stranger may cause unease; or the patient may feel self-conscious, embarrassed, or shy. Talking is highly individualized; some find the telephone a nuisance, but others talk/text on their cell phones almost constantly (e.g., shopping, in a restaurant with friends, and sitting in a classroom or meeting). The nurse must recognize and respect individual differences in styles and tempos of responding. People who are quiet, those who have a language barrier or speech impediment, older adults, and those who lack confidence in their ability to express themselves may communicate a need for support and encouragement through their silence. Although there is no universal rule concerning how much silence is too much, silence has been said to be worthwhile only when it serves a function and is not frightening for the individual. Knowing when to speak during the interview largely depends on the nurse's perception about what is being conveyed through the silence. Icy silence may be an expression of anger and hostility. Being ignored or given the silent treatment is recognized as an insult and is a harmful form of communication. Silence may relate to anger, insulted feelings, or a lack of trust. Conversely, therapeutic silence may provide meaningful moments of reflection for both participants. It gives each individual an opportunity to contemplate thoughtfully what has been said and felt, weigh alternatives, formulate new ideas, and gain a new perspective on the matter under discussion. If the nurse waits to speak and allows the patient to break the silence, the patient may share thoughts and feelings that would otherwise have been withheld.

Nurses who feel compelled to fill every void with words often do so because of their own anxiety, self-consciousness, and embarrassment. When this occurs, the nurse's need for comfort tends to take priority over the needs of the patient. Or conversely, prolonged and frequent silences by the nurse may hinder an interview that requires verbal articulation. Although the untalkative nurse may be comfortable with silence, this mode of communication may make the patient feel uncomfortable and withhold information. Therefore, the nurse needs to check with the patient from time to time because, without feedback, patients have no way of knowing whether they are being understood.

Active Listening

People want more than just a physical presence in human communication. Most people want the other person to be there for them psychologically, socially, and emotionally. **Active listening** includes the following:

- Observing the patient's nonverbal behaviors
- Listening to and understanding the patient's verbal message
- Listening to and understanding the person in the context of the social and cultural setting of his or her life
- Listening for "false notes" (i.e., inconsistencies or things the patient says that need more clarification)
- Providing the patient with feedback about himself or herself of which the patient might be unaware

Sommers-Flanagan and Sommers-Flanagan (2017) advise students, as well as experienced clinicians, to learn to quiet themselves in order to help reduce their stress. Students and nurses alike need to minimalize any sudden natural, although distracting, urges to help, to meet personal needs, to start thinking of the next question they wish to ask, and so forth. Relaxation techniques may help before an interview with the patient (e.g., closing one's eyes and breathing slowly for a few minutes or using mindfulness techniques). This usually results in more concentration on the patient and less distraction by personal worries or thoughts of what to say next.

Effective interviewers must become accustomed to silence, but it is just as important for effective interviewers to learn to become active listeners when the patient is talking, as well as when the patient becomes silent. During active listening, nurses carefully note what the patient is saying verbally and nonverbally, as well as monitor their own nonverbal responses. Using silence effectively and learning to listen on a deeper, more significant level—to the patient as well as to your own thoughts and reaction—are both key ingredients of effective communication. Both skills take time to develop but can be learned; you will become more proficient with guidance and practice.

Some principles important to *active listening* are always relevant, such as the following:

- Everything you hear is modified by the patient's filters.
- Everything you hear is modified by your own filters.
- Therefore every piece of communication must pass through two filters.
- It is okay to feel confused and uncertain.
- Listen to yourself, too.

Active listening helps strengthen the patient's ability to use critical thinking in order to solve problems. By giving the patient undivided attention, the nurse communicates that the patient is not alone. This kind of intervention enhances self-esteem and encourages the patient to direct energy toward finding ways to deal with problems. Serving as a sounding board, the nurse listens as the patient tests thoughts by voicing them aloud. This form of interpersonal interaction often enables the patient to clarify thinking, link ideas, and tentatively decide what should be done and how best to do it. Active listening is an art that develops with practice over time.

Clarifying Techniques

Understanding depends on clear communication, which is aided by verifying with the patient the nurse's interpretation of the patient's messages. The nurse must request feedback on the accuracy of the message received from verbal as well as nonverbal cues. For example, "I'm not quite sure what you were saying. Did you say you are not going to group tonight?" The use of **clarifying techniques** helps both participants identify major differences in their frame of reference, giving them the opportunity to correct misperceptions before they cause any serious misunderstandings. The patient who is asked to elaborate on or to clarify vague or ambiguous messages needs to know that the purpose is to promote mutual understanding.

Paraphrasing (Reflection of Content)

For clarity, the nurse might use **paraphrasing**, which means restating in different (often fewer) words the basic content of a patient's message. Using simple, precise, and culturally relevant terms, the nurse may readily confirm his or her interpretation of the patient's previous message before the interview proceeds. By prefacing statements with a phrase such as, "I'm not sure I understand" or "In other words, you seem to be saying …," the nurse helps the patient form a clearer perception of what may be a bewildering mass of details. After paraphrasing, the nurse must validate the accuracy of the restatement and its helpfulness to the discussion. The patient may confirm or deny the perceptions through nonverbal cues or by direct response to a question such as, "Was I correct in saying …?" As a result, the patient is made aware that the interviewer is actively involved in the search for understanding.

Restating

In **restating**, the nurse mirrors the patient's overt and covert messages; thus, this technique may be used to echo feelings as well as content. Restating differs from paraphrasing in that it involves repeating the same key words the patient has just spoken. If a patient remarks, "My life is empty … It has no meaning," additional information may be gained by restating, "Your life has no meaning?" The purpose of this technique is to explore subjects that may be significant. However, too frequent and indiscriminate use of restating might be interpreted by patients as inattention, disinterest, or worse.

It is easy to overuse this tool so that its application becomes mechanical. Parroting or mimicking what another has said may be perceived as poking fun at the person, in which case the use of this nondirective approach can become a definite barrier to communication. To avoid overuse of restating, the nurse can combine restatements with direct questions that encourage descriptions: "What does your life lack?" "What kind of meaning is missing?" "Describe one day in your life that appears empty to you."

Reflecting of Feelings

Reflection is a means of assisting people to better understand their own thoughts and feelings. **Reflecting** may take the form of a question or a simple statement that conveys the nurse's observations of the patient when sensitive issues are being discussed. The nurse might then describe briefly to the patient the apparent meaning of the emotional tone of the patient's verbal and nonverbal behavior. For example, to reflect a patient's feelings about his or her life, a good beginning might be, "You sound as if you have had many disappointments."

Sharing observations with a patient shows acceptance. The nurse helps make the patient aware of feelings and encourages the patient to own them. For example, the nurse may tell a patient, "You look sad." Perceiving the nurse's concern may allow a patient spontaneously to share feelings. The use of a question in response to the patient's question is another reflective technique (Arnold & Boggs, 2016). For example:

Patient: "Nurse, do you think I really need to be hospitalized?"
Nurse: "What do you think, Jane?"
Patient: "I don't know; that's why I'm asking you."
Nurse: "I'll be willing to share my impression with you at the end of this first session. However, you've probably thought about hospitalization and have some feelings about it. I wonder what they are."

Exploring

A technique that enables the nurse to examine important ideas, experiences, or relationships more fully is **exploring**. For example, if a patient tells the nurse that he does not get along well with his wife, the nurse will want to further explore this area. Possible openers include the following:

- "*Tell me* more about your relationship with your wife."
- "*Describe* your relationship with your wife."
- "*Give me an example* of how you and your wife don't get along."

Asking for an example can greatly clarify a vague or generic statement made by a patient.

Patient: "No one likes me."
Nurse: "Give me an example of one person who doesn't like you."
or
Patient: "Everything I do is wrong."

Nurse: "Give me an example of one thing you do that you think is wrong."

Table 8.2 lists more examples of techniques that enhance communication.

Projective Questions: The "What if" Question

Projective questions can help people imagine the conflicts, thoughts, values, feelings, and behaviors they might have in certain situations (Sommers-Flanagan & Sommers-Flanagan, 2017).

Projective questions usually start with a *"what if"* to help people articulate, explore, and identify thoughts and feelings. For example:

- If you had three wishes, what would you wish for?
- What if you could go back and change how you acted in (X situation/significant life event); what would you do differently now?
- What would you do if you were given $1 million, no strings attached?

Presupposition Questions: The "Miracle Question"

Suppose you woke up in the morning and a miracle happened and this problem had gone away. What would be different? How would it change your life?

These two questions can reveal a lot about a person and can be used to identify goals that the patient may be motivated to pursue, and they often get to the crux of what might be the most important issues in a person's thinking/life.

NONTHERAPEUTIC TECHNIQUES

Although people may use nontherapeutic techniques in their daily lives, they can become problematic when working with patients. Table 8.3 offers samples of nontherapeutic techniques and suggestions for more helpful responses.

TABLE 8.2 Techniques That Enhance Communication

Technique	Discussion	Examples
Using silence	Gives the person time to collect thoughts or think through a point.	Encourage a person to talk by waiting for the answers.
Accepting	Indicates that the person has been understood. The statement does not necessarily indicate agreement but is nonjudgmental. However, nurses should not imply that they understand when they do not understand.	"Yes." "Uh-huh." "I follow what you say."
Giving recognition	Indicates awareness of change and personal efforts. Does not imply good or bad, or right or wrong.	"Good morning, Mr. James." "You've combed your hair today." "I notice that you shaved today."
Offering self	Offers presence, interest, and a desire to understand. Is not offered to get the person to talk or behave in a specific way.	"I would like to spend time with you." "I'll stay here and sit with you for a while."
Offering general leads	Allows the other person to take direction in the discussion. Indicates that the nurse is interested in what comes next.	"Go on." "And then?" "Tell me about it."
Giving broad openings	Clarifies that the lead is to be taken by the patient. However, the nurse discourages pleasantries and small talk.	"Where would you like to begin?" "What are you thinking about?" "What would you like to discuss?"
Placing the events in time or sequence	Puts events and actions in better perspective. Notes cause-and-effect relationships and identifies patterns of interpersonal difficulties.	"What happened before?" "When did this happen?"
Offering observations	Calls attention to the person's behavior (e.g., trembling, nail biting, restless mannerisms). Encourages the person to notice the behavior to describe thoughts and feelings for mutual understanding. Helpful with mute and withdrawn people.	"You appear tense." "I notice you're biting your lips." "You appear nervous whenever John enters the room."
Encouraging description of perception	Increases the nurse's understanding of the patient's perceptions. Talking about feelings and difficulties can lessen the need to act them out inappropriately.	"What do these voices seem to be saying?" "What is happening now?" "Tell me when you feel anxious."
Encouraging comparison	Reveals recurring themes in experiences or interpersonal relationships. Helps the person clarify similarities and differences.	"Has this ever happened before?" "Is this how you felt when …?" "Was it something like …?"
Restating	Repeats the main idea expressed. Gives the patient an idea of what has been communicated. If the message has been misunderstood, the patient can clarify it.	*Patient:* "I can't sleep. I stay awake all night." *Nurse:* "You have difficulty sleeping?" *Patient:* "I don't know … He always has some excuse for not coming over or keeping our appointments." *Nurse:* "You think he no longer wants to see you?"
Reflecting	Directs questions, feelings, and ideas back to the patient. Encourages the patient to accept his or her own ideas and feelings. Acknowledges the patient's right to have opinions and make decisions and encourages the patient to think of self as a capable person.	*Patient:* "What should I do about my husband's affair?" *Nurse:* "What do you think you should do?" *Patient:* "My brother spends all of my money and then has the nerve to ask for more." *Nurse:* "You feel angry when this happens?"

Continued

TABLE 8.2 Techniques That Enhance Communication—cont'd

Technique	Discussion	Examples
Focusing	Concentrates attention on a single point. It is especially useful when the patient jumps from topic to topic. If a person is experiencing a severe or panic level of anxiety, the nurse should not persist until the anxiety lessens.	"This point you are making about leaving school seems worth looking at more closely." "You've mentioned many things. Let's go back to your thinking of 'ending it all.'"
Exploring	Examines certain ideas, experiences, or relationships more fully. If the patient chooses not to elaborate by answering no, the nurse does not probe or pry. In such a case, the nurse respects the patient's wishes.	"Tell me more about that." "Would you describe it more fully?" "Could you talk about how it was that you learned your mom was dying of cancer?"
Giving information	Makes available facts the person needs. Supplies knowledge from which decisions can be made or conclusions drawn. For example, the patient needs to know the role of the nurse; the purpose of the nurse–patient relationship; and the time, place, and duration of the meetings.	"My purpose for being here is …" "This medication is for …" "The test will determine …"
Seeking clarification	Helps patients clarify their own thoughts and maximize mutual understanding between nurse and patient.	"I am not sure I follow you." "What would you say is the main point of what you just said?" "Give an example of a time you thought everyone hated you."
Presenting reality	Indicates what is real. The nurse does not argue or try to convince the patient, just describes personal perceptions or facts in the situation.	"That was Dr. Todd, not a terrorist stalking and trying to harm you." "That was the sound of a car backfiring." "Your mother is not here; I am a nurse."
Voicing doubt	Undermines the patient's beliefs by not reinforcing the exaggerated or false perceptions.	"Isn't that unusual?" "Really?" "That's hard to believe."
Seeking consensual validation	Clarifies that both the nurse and the patient share mutual understanding of communications. Helps the patient become clearer about what he or she is thinking.	"Tell me whether my understanding agrees with yours."
Verbalizing the implied	Puts into concrete terms what the patient implies, making the patient's communication more explicit.	*Patient:* "I can't talk to you or anyone else. It's a waste of time." *Nurse:* "Do you feel that no one understands?"
Encouraging evaluation	Aids the patient in considering people and events from the perspective of the patient's own set of values.	"How do you feel about …?" "What did it mean to you when he said he couldn't stay?"
Attempting to translate into feelings	Responds to the feelings expressed, not just the content. Often termed *decoding*.	*Patient:* "I am dead inside." *Nurse:* "Are you saying that you feel lifeless? Does life seem meaningless to you?"
Suggesting collaboration	Emphasizes working with the patient, not doing things for the patient. Encourages the view that change is possible through collaboration.	"Perhaps you and I can discover what produces your anxiety." "Perhaps by working together we can come up with some ideas that might improve your communications with your spouse."
Summarizing	Combines the important points of the discussion to enhance understanding. Also allows the opportunity to clarify communications so that both nurse and patient leave the interview with the same ideas in mind.	"Have I got this straight?" "You said that …" "During the past hour, you and I have discussed …"
Encouraging formulation of a plan of action	Allows the patient to identify alternative actions for interpersonal situations the patient finds disturbing (e.g., when anger or anxiety is provoked).	"What could you do to let anger out harmlessly?" "The next time this comes up, what might you do to handle it?" "What are some other ways you can approach your boss?"

Asking Excessive Questions

Excessive questioning, or asking multiple questions at the same time, especially closed-ended questions, casts the nurse in the role of interrogator, raising a demand for information without respect for the patient's willingness or readiness to respond. This approach conveys a lack of respect for and sensitivity to the patient's needs. Excessive questioning or asking multiple questions at the same time controls the range and nature of the response and can easily result in a therapeutic stall or termination of an interview. It is a controlling tactic and may reflect the interviewer's lack of security in letting the patient tell his or

TABLE 8.3 **Nontherapeutic Communication**

Nontherapeutic Technique	Examples	Discussion	More Helpful Response
Giving premature advice	"Get out of this situation immediately."	Assumes the nurse knows best and the patient cannot think for self. Inhibits problem solving and fosters dependency.	*Encouraging problem solving:* "What are the pros and cons of your situation?" "What were some of the actions you thought you might take?" "What are some of the ways you have thought of to meet your goals?"
Minimizing feelings	*Patient:* "I wish I were dead." *Nurse:* "Everyone gets down in the dumps." "I know what you mean." "You should feel happy you're getting better." "Things get worse before they get better."	Indicates that the nurse is unable to understand or empathize with the patient. The patient's feelings or experiences are being belittled, which can cause the patient to feel small or insignificant.	*Empathizing and exploring:* "You must be feeling very upset. Are you thinking of hurting yourself?"
Falsely reassuring	"I wouldn't worry about that." "Everything will be all right." "You will do just fine; you'll see."	Underrates the patient's feelings and belittles the patient's concerns. May cause the patient to stop sharing feelings if the patient thinks he or she will be ridiculed or not taken seriously.	*Clarifying the patient's message:* "What specifically are you worried about?" "What do you think could go wrong?" "What are you concerned might happen?"
Making value judgments	"How come you still smoke when your wife has lung cancer?"	Prevents problem solving. Can make the patient feel guilty, angry, misunderstood, not supported, or anxious to leave.	*Making observations:* "I notice you are still smoking even though your wife has lung cancer. Is this a problem?"
Asking "why" questions	"Why did you stop taking your medication?"	Implies criticism; often has the effect of making the patient feel defensive.	*Asking open-ended questions; giving a broad opening:* "Tell me some of the reasons that led up to you not taking your medications."
Asking excessive questions	*Nurse:* "How's your appetite? Are you losing weight? Are you eating enough?" *Patient.* "No."	Results in the patient's not knowing which question to answer and possibly being confused about what is being asked.	*Clarifying:* "Tell me about your eating habits since you've been depressed."
Giving approval; agreeing	"I'm proud of you for applying for that job." "I agree with your decision."	Implies that the patient is doing the *right* thing—and that not doing it is wrong. May lead the patient to focus on pleasing the nurse or clinician; denies the patient the opportunity to change his or her mind or decision.	*Making observations:* "I noticed that you applied for that job." "What factors led you to change your mind about applying for that job?" *Asking open-ended questions; giving a broad opening:* "What led to that decision?"
Disapproving; disagreeing	"You really should have shown up for the medication group." "I disagree with that."	Can make a person defensive.	*Exploring:* "What was going through your mind when you decided not to come to your medication group?" "That's one point of view. How did you arrive at that conclusion?"
Changing the subject	*Patient:* "I'd like to die." *Nurse:* "Did you go to Alcoholics Anonymous like we discussed?"	May invalidate the patient's feelings and needs. Can leave the patient feeling alienated and isolated and increase feelings of hopelessness.	*Validating and exploring:* *Patient:* "I'd like to die." *Nurse:* "This sounds serious. Have you thought of harming yourself?"

From Hays, J. S., & Larson, K. (1963). *Interacting With Patients.*

her own story. It is better to ask more open-ended questions and follow the patient's lead. For example:

Excessive questioning: "Why did you leave your wife? Did you feel angry at her? What did she do to you? Are you going back to her?"

More therapeutic approach: "Tell me about the situation between you and your wife."

Although you may end up with a lot of facts about a person if you use excessive questioning, it does not mean you understand an individual or the individual's concerns.

Giving Approval or Disapproval

"You look great in that dress." "I'm proud of the way you controlled your temper at lunch." "That's a great quilt you made." What could be bad about giving someone a pat on the back once in a while? Nothing, if it is done without carrying a judgment (positive or negative) by the nurse. We often give our friends and family approval when they do something well. However, in a nurse–patient situation, giving approval often becomes much more complex. A patient may be feeling overwhelmed, experiencing low self-esteem, or feeling unsure of where his or her life is going and consequently feel very needy for recognition, approval, and attention. Yet when people are feeling vulnerable, a value comment might be misinterpreted. For example:

Giving approval: "You did a great job in group telling John what you thought about how rudely he treated you."

Implied in this message is that the nurse was pleased by the way the patient talked to John. The patient then sees such a response as a way to please the nurse by doing the right thing. To continue to please the nurse (and get approval), the patient may continue the behavior. The behavior might be useful for the patient, but when a behavior is being done to please another person, it is not coming from the individual's own volition or conviction.

Also, when the other person whom the patient needs to please is not present, the motivation for the new behavior might not be there either. Thus, the new response really is not a change in behavior as much as a ploy to win approval and acceptance from another person. Giving approval also stops further communication. It is a statement of the observer's (nurse's) judgment about another person's (patient's) behavior. A more useful comment would be the following:

More therapeutic approach: "I noticed that you spoke up to John in group yesterday about his rude behavior. How did it feel to be more assertive?"

This opens the way for finding out if the patient was scared or comfortable, wants to work more on assertiveness, or has other issues to discuss. It also suggests that this was a self-choice the patient made. The patient is given recognition for the change in behavior, and the topic is also opened for further discussion.

Disapproving is moralizing and implies that the nurse has the right to judge the patient's thoughts or feelings. Again, an observation should be made instead.

Disapproving: "You really should not cheat, even if you think everyone else is doing it."

More therapeutic approach: "Can you give me two examples of how cheating could negatively affect your goal of graduating?"

Advising

Although we ask for and give advice all the time in daily life, **giving advice** to a patient is rarely helpful. Often when we ask for advice, our real motive is to discover if we are thinking along the same lines as someone else or if he or she would agree with us. When the nurse gives advice to a patient who is having trouble assessing and finding solutions to conflicted areas in his or her life, the nurse is interfering with the patient's ability to make personal decisions. Giving a person a solution robs the patient of self-responsibility. When the nurse offers the patient solutions, the patient eventually begins to think that the nurse does not view the patient as capable of making effective decisions.

People often feel inadequate when they are given no choices over decisions in their lives. Giving advice to patients can foster dependency ("I'll have to ask the nurse what to do about ...") and can undermine their sense of competence and adequacy. However, people do need information to make informed decisions. Often the nurse can help the patient define a problem and identify what information might be needed to attain an informed decision. A more useful approach would be, "What do you see as some possible actions you can take?" It is much more constructive to encourage critical thinking. At times the nurse can suggest several alternatives that a patient might consider (e.g., "Have you ever thought of telling your friend about the incident?"). The patient is then free to say yes or no and make a decision from among the suggestions.

Asking "Why" Questions

"Why did you come late?" "Why didn't you go to the funeral?" "Why didn't you study for the exam?" Very often, **"why" questions** imply criticism. We may ask our friends or family such questions, and in the context of a solid relationship, the "why?" may be understood more as "what happened?" With people we do not know—especially an anxious person who may be feeling overwhelmed—a "why" question from a person in authority (nurse, physician, teacher) can be experienced as intrusive and judgmental, which serves only to make the person defensive.

It is much more useful to ask *what* is happening rather than *why* it is happening. Questions that focus on who, what, where, and when often elicit important information that can facilitate problem solving and further the communication process.

GUARDING AGAINST MISCOMMUNICATION

Because we know that there are a number of barriers that can impede accurate communication, we need to stress the need for accurate communication. **Death from miscommunication is currently the third leading cause of medical deaths behind heart disease and cancer** (Makary, 2016).

Communication errors are often silent and can be invisible. However, when there's a breakdown in communication, **miscommunication** can set the stage for potential errors. Those medical errors can lead to upward of 1,000 deaths per day and cost trillions of dollars in health care costs each year (Noguchi, 2014–2018). Poor communication skills (nontherapeutic) are responsible for 210,000 to 440,000 preventable deaths a year (Makary, 2016). A study from UC San Francisco and eight other institutions found that increasing the accuracy of communication between health care workers can result in up to a 30% reduction in injuries from medical errors (Noguchi, 2014–2018).

COMMUNICATING ACROSS CULTURES

Cultural competence means being respectful of and responsive to the health beliefs and practices—and cultural and linguistic needs—of diverse population groups. Developing cultural competence is also an evolving, dynamic process that takes time and occurs along a continuum (Substance Abuse and Mental Health Services Administration [SAMHSA], 2016). Communicating across culture poses many challenges for health care workers. We all need a frame of reference to help us function in our world. The trick is to understand that other people use many other frames of reference to help them function in their world. Acknowledging that others view the world quite differently and trying to understand other people's ways of experiencing and living in the world can go a long way toward minimizing our personal distortions in listening and miscommunication. Building acceptance and understanding of those culturally different from ourselves is a skill, too.

Awareness of the cultural meaning of certain verbal and nonverbal communications in initial face-to-face encounters with individuals from cultures different from our own can lead to the formation of a positive therapeutic alliance (or lead to frustration and misunderstanding).

Unrecognized differences between aspects of the cultural identities of patient and nurse can result in assessments and interventions that are ineffective and can appear disrespectful and/or prejudiced. By the same token, nurses should also have a strong understanding and awareness of their own cultural identities and biases. Especially important are nurses' attitudes and beliefs from their own cultural background toward those from ethnically diverse populations and subcultures (e.g., alternate lifestyles, different socioeconomic groups, those with disabilities, different ethnic backgrounds, lifestyle differences, the elderly). Unawareness of personal bias invariably affects communication and relationships.

SAMHSA's Center for Substance Abuse Prevention has identified the following principles of cultural competence when setting up a program for specific communities (SAMHSA, 2016):

- Ensure community involvement in all areas.
- Use a population-based definition of community (let the community define itself).
- Stress the importance of relevant, culturally appropriate prevention approaches.
- Employ culturally competent evaluators.
- Promote cultural competence among program staff members that reflects the community they serve.
- Include the target population in all aspects of prevention planning.

Four areas that may prove problematic for the nurse interpreting the specific verbal and nonverbal messages of the patient include the following:

1. Communication styles
2. Use of eye contact
3. Perception of touch
4. Cultural filters

One caveat: It is important to recognize that there are varying degrees of diversity among and within most cultural groups. For the following discussions, we will use generally accepted common, although stereotypical, frames of reference to illustrate the four problematic areas.

Communication Styles

Some ethnic backgrounds may communicate in an intense and highly emotional manner. For example, from the perspective of a non-Hispanic person, many Hispanic Americans may appear to use dramatic body language when describing their emotional problems. Such behavior may be perceived as out of control and thus viewed as having a degree of pathology that is not actually present. Within the Hispanic culture, however, intensely emotional styles of communication are culturally appropriate and often expected. French and Italian Americans also show animated facial expressions and expressive hand gestures during communication that can be mistakenly interpreted by others.

Conversely, in other cultures, a calm facade may mask severe distress. For example, in Asian cultures, expression of either positive or negative emotions is a private affair, and open expression of emotions is considered to be in bad taste and possibly a weakness. A quiet smile by an Asian American may signal a variety of emotions. A smile might be an expression of joy, an apology, stoicism in the face of difficulty, or even anger. In general, Asian individuals exercise emotional restraint in communication, and interpersonal conflicts are not directly addressed or even allowed (Arnold & Boggs, 2016). German and British Americans also highly value the concept of self-control and may show little facial emotion in the presence of great distress or emotional turmoil.

It is important to understand an ethnic minority in light of the historical context in which it evolved and its relationship to the dominant culture. For example, African Americans, whose historical background in the United States is one of slavery and oppression, are likely to be aware of a basic need for survival. Some African Americans have become highly selective and guarded in their communication with those outside their cultural group. This may explain the distrust that many African Americans have about the American health care system (American Nurses Association [ANA], 2018). Stigma, religious beliefs, and distrust of the medical profession are all communication barriers to forming alliances between African Americans and health care workers from the dominant American culture.

Eye Contact

The presence or absence of eye contact should not be used to assess attentiveness, to judge truthfulness, or to make assumptions on the degree of engagement one has with the patient. Culture dictates a person's comfort or lack of comfort with direct eye contact. Some cultures consider direct eye contact disrespectful and improper. For example, in some Hispanic subcultures, individuals have traditionally been taught to avoid eye contact with authority figures such as nurses, physicians, and other health care professionals. Avoidance of direct eye contact is seen as a sign of respect to those in authority. To nurses or other health care workers, lack of eye contact may be wrongly interpreted by the interviewer as disinterest in the interview or even as a lack of respect.

Similarly, in Asian cultural subgroups, respect is shown by avoiding eye contact. For example, in Japan, direct eye contact is considered to show lack of respect and to be a personal affront; the preference is for shifting or downcast eyes or a focus on the speaker's neck. Among many Chinese, gazing around and looking to one side when listening to another is considered polite. Philippine Americans may try to avoid eye contact; however, once it is established, it is important to return and maintain eye contact.

Many Native American groups believe it is disrespectful or even a sign of aggression to engage in direct eye contact, especially if the speaker is younger. Direct eye contact by members of the dominant culture in the health care system can and does cause discomfort for some patients and is considered a sign of disrespect, whereas listening is considered a sign of respect and is essential to learning about the other individual.

Among German Americans, direct and sustained eye contact indicates that the person listens or trusts, is somewhat aggressive, or may be sexually interested. Russians also find direct, sustained eye contact the norm for social interactions. French, British, and many African Americans maintain eye contact during conversation; avoidance of eye contact by another person may be interpreted as being disinterested, not telling the truth, or avoiding the sharing of important information. In some Arab cultures, for a woman to make direct eye contact with a man may imply a sexual interest or even promiscuity. In Greece, staring in public is acceptable.

Touch

A great number of cultural expressions are achieved through touch. There are also widely ranging cultural viewpoints on the appropriate rules regarding physical contact between both similar and opposite genders.

The therapeutic use of touch is a basic aspect of the nurse–patient relationship, and touch is normally perceived as a gesture of warmth and friendship. However, in some cultures, touch can be perceived as an invasion of privacy or an invitation to intimacy by some patients. The response to touch is often culturally defined. For example, many Hispanic Americans are accustomed to frequent physical contact. Holding the patient's hand in response to a distressing situation or giving the patient a reassuring pat on the shoulder may be experienced as supportive and thus help facilitate openness early in the therapeutic relationship; however, this might not always be the case.

When the nurse is working with a Mexican American, often the touch of the nurse is welcome because in the minds of some Mexican Americans, this action can both prevent and treat illness (Giger & Davidhizar, 2007). People of Italian and French backgrounds may also be accustomed to frequent touching during conversation. In Russia, touch is often an important part of nonverbal communication used freely with intimate and close friends (Giger & Davidhizar, 2007). However, the degree of comfort conveyed by touch in the nurse–patient relationship depends on the patient's country of origin.

Within the context of an interview, touch might easily be experienced as patronizing, intrusive, aggressive, or sexually inviting. For example, among German, Swedish, and British Americans, touch practices are infrequent, although a handshake may be common at the beginning and end of an interaction. In India, men may shake hands with other men but not with women; an Asian Indian man may greet a woman by nodding and holding the palms of his hands together but not touching the woman. In Japan, handshakes are acceptable; however, a pat on the back is not. Chinese Americans may not like to be touched by strangers. Some Native Americans extend their hand and lightly touch the hand of the person they are greeting rather than shake hands.

Even among people of the same culture, the use of touch has different interpretations and rules when the touch is between individuals of different genders and classes. Students are urged to check the policy manual of their facility because some facilities have a "no-touch" policy, particularly with adolescents and children who may have experienced inappropriate touch and may misinterpret the intention behind the touch.

Lesbian, Gay, Bisexual, Transgender

Lesbian, gay, bisexual, and transgender individuals (LGBT) are used to being judged harshly and experiencing rejection, contributing to a distrust of mental health professionals. Many have endured loneliness, physical violence, and verbal abuse and have been severely marginalized in the dominant culture and cultural subgroups. More recently, "affirmative psychotherapy" is a dominant trend for LGBT individuals and has become a major movement within the counseling and psychotherapy community; this approach validates and advocates for the needs of these individuals (Sommers-Flanagan & Sommers-Flanagan, 2017).

Cultural Filters

It is important to recognize that it is impossible to listen to people in an unbiased way. In the process of socialization, we develop **cultural filters** through which we listen to ourselves, others, and the world around us. Cultural filters are a form of cultural bias or cultural prejudice that determines what we notice and what we ignore.

We need these cultural filters to provide structure for ourselves and to help us interpret and interact with the world. However, unavoidably, these cultural filters also introduce various forms of bias into our listening because they are bound to influence our personal, professional, familial, and sociological values and interpretations. If the cultural filters are strong, the likelihood for bias is increased. Bias builds a distorted understanding and a tendency to pigeonhole a person because of factors like race, sexual orientation, nationality, social status, religious persuasion, or lifestyle (Egan, 2013).

COMMUNICATION THROUGH TECHNOLOGIES

Telehealth is the use of electronic information and telecommunication technologies to support long-distance clinical health care in order to eliminate barriers from the delivery of health care services. **Telehealth technologies** include such electronic means of communication as video conferencing, the Internet, telephone/cell phone consultation and counseling, image transmission, and interactive video sessions. These techniques allow for establishing and maintaining therapeutic relationships. However, "particular attention must be directed to confidentiality, informed consent, documentation, maintenance of records, and the integrity of the transmitted information" (ANA, 2014, p. 37).

Over 90% of hospitals allow patients online access to their health care records (American Hospital Association, 2018). Informatics and information technology are increasingly being adopted in medical and mental health care in the United States. The adoption of sophisticated **information communication technologies (ICTs)** is associated with greater use of pre-established medical protocols and higher patient satisfaction. ICTs are used as live interactive mechanisms, to track clinical progress, and provide access to people who otherwise might not receive medical or psychosocial help (e.g., those in rural areas and chronically ill, home-bound, and underserved individuals).

It is estimated that about one in four adults could be diagnosed with a mental health issue. Mental health issues range from anxiety, stress, marital issues, and depression to substance abuse. Most of these mental health issues are not addressed because of the fear of stigma, the scarcity of health care providers in remote areas, or problems with transportation (e.g., because of anxiety, physical limitations, or lack of transportation). The consequences of not seeking help can be significant and can range from problems at work to domestic violence, increased depression, and suicide—consequences that can result in a host of other ramifications

The U.S. Department of Defense (DOD) is expanding its ability to deliver telehealth services to active-duty military personnel in international settings and to veterans and their families by designating a provider of telemedicine services to operate on its networks through the use of GlobalMed, an international provider of telehealth services (Bazzoli, 2018). These technologies are used for telepsychiatric appointments ranging from treating posttraumatic stress disorder and depression to providing wellness and resiliency interventions, especially in rural areas. These technologies also help facilitate health assessments, diagnoses, treatments and interventions, and clinical consultations to all DOD members (Bazzoli, 2018).

As ICTs advance, it is possible that electronic house calls, Internet support groups, and virtual health examination may well be the wave of the future, eliminating office visits altogether (Arnold & Boggs, 2016). It is a valuable tool for patients as well as practitioners to access current psychiatric and medical breakthroughs, diagnoses, and treatment options (Arnold & Boggs, 2016).

Besides providing better health care for those in rural areas or for those who cannot travel, telehealth may help to relieve the impending nursing shortage. Nursing schools are having a difficult time meeting the nursing shortage because of a decrease in financial resources and retiring faculty. The use of telehealth/tele-home care technologies allows nurses to monitor patients' vital signs, including lung sounds, and identify changes in patients' physiological states. Clinicians can conduct remote physical assessment and consults, which are especially helpful in facilities that have limited nursing resources, including schools, prisons, health clinics, and rural hospitals.

Mobile Apps

According to Peek (2015):

1. Mobile phones are the most quickly adopted consumer technology in human history. From 2013 to 2016, the share of adults 65 and older who report owning a smartphone rose from 18% to 42% in the United States (Raine & Perrin, 2017).
2. Psychiatric patients own smartphones at high rates and are interested in using them to monitor their mental health, based on published surveys.
3. There are thousands of apps that target psychiatric conditions; however, there is less clinical research on these apps. For depression and bipolar disorder, one review found less than 15 published studies. There are also concerns for unintended adverse effects in app usage.
4. There is growing interest in using "passive data" information.

SAMHSA has resources that can help address some of the toughest mental health and substance use challenges, including suicide prevention, bullying prevention, behavioral health following a disaster, and underage drinking prevention.

- **Suicide Safe** helps health care providers integrate suicide prevention strategies into their practice and address suicide risk among their patients.

FACILITATIVE SKILLS CHECKLIST

Instructions: Periodically during your clinical experience, use this checklist to identify areas where growth is needed and progress has been made. Think of your clinical client experiences. Indicate the extent of your agreement with each of the following statements by marking the scale: *SA*, strongly agree; *A*, agree; *NS*, not sure; *D*, disagree; *SD*, strongly disagree.

1. I maintain good eye contact.	SA	A	NS	D	SD
2. Most of my verbal comments follow the lead of the other person.	SA	A	NS	D	SD
3. I encourage others to talk about feelings.	SA	A	NS	D	SD
4. I am able to ask open-ended questions.	SA	A	NS	D	SD
5. I can restate and clarify a person's ideas.	SA	A	NS	D	SD
6. I can summarize in a few words the basic ideas of a long statement made by a person.	SA	A	NS	D	SD
7. I can make statements that reflect the person's feelings.	SA	A	NS	D	SD
8. I can share my feelings relevant to the discussion when appropriate to do so.	SA	A	NS	D	SD
9. I am able to give feedback.	SA	A	NS	D	SD
10. At least 75% or more of my responses help enhance and facilitate communication.	SA	A	NS	D	SD
11. I can assist the person to list some alternatives available.	SA	A	NS	D	SD
12. I can assist the person to identify some goals that are specific and observable.	SA	A	NS	D	SD
13. I can assist the person to specify at least one next step that might be taken toward the goal.	SA	A	NS	D	SD

Fig. 8.2 Facilitative skills checklist. (Adapted from Myrick, D., & Erney, T. [2000]. *Caring and sharing* [2nd ed., p. 168]. Copyright ©2000 by Educational Media Corp., Minneapolis, MN.)

- **KnowBullying** provides information and guidance on ways to prevent bullying and build resilience in children. A great tool for parents and educators, KnowBullying is meant for kids ages 3 to 18.
- **SAMHSA Disaster App** provides responders with access to critical resources—like psychological first aid and responder self-care—and SAMHSA's behavioral health treatment services locator to help responders provide support to survivors after a disaster.
- **Talk. They Hear You** is an interactive game that can help parents and caregivers prepare for conversations about underage drinking.

Look up SAMHSA's mobile apps at SAMHSA.gov. Ten more approved mental health apps can be found at http://www.psychiatryadvisor.com/top-10-mental-health-apps/slideshow/2608/.

As previously mentioned, significant concerns with mobile medical apps remain unresolved, including potential privacy and confidentiality issues, lack of current clinical data for efficacy, safety of specific mobile apps, and liability issues. Quality clinical trials and evaluation of risks and benefits are sparse. Other issues include ensuring privacy and safety, reviewing legal policies, and creating professional and ethical guidelines (Peek, 2015).

EVALUATION OF CLINICAL SKILLS

After you have had some introductory clinical experience, you may find the facilitative skills checklist in Fig. 8.2 useful for evaluating your progress in developing interviewing skills. Note that some of the items might not be relevant for some of your patients (e.g., numbers 11 through 13 may not be possible when a patient is highly psychotic). Self-evaluation of clinical skills is a way to focus on therapeutic improvement. Role-playing can be a useful tool in preparation for the clinical experience and can provide practice in acquiring more effective and professional communication skills.

KEY POINTS TO REMEMBER

- Developing competent communication and interviewing techniques is the foundation for a patient-centered partnership. Goal-directed, professional communication is referred to as therapeutic communication.
- Communication is a complex process. Berlo's communication model has five parts: stimulus, sender, message, medium, and receiver. Feedback is a vital component of the communication process for validating the accuracy of the sender's message.
- A number of factors can minimize or enhance the communication process. For example, differences in culture, language, and knowledge levels; noise; lack of privacy; the presence of others; and expectations can all influence communication.
- There are verbal and nonverbal elements in communication; the nonverbal elements often play the larger role in conveying a person's message. Verbal communication consists of all words a person speaks. Nonverbal communication consists of the behaviors displayed by an individual, in addition to the actual content of speech.
- Communication has two levels: the content level (verbal) and the process level (nonverbal behavior). When content is congruent with process, the communication is said to be healthy. When the verbal message is not reinforced by the communicator's actions, the message is ambiguous; we call this a double (or mixed) message.
- Cultural background (as well as individual differences) has a great deal to do with what nonverbal behavior means to different individuals. The degree of eye contact and the use of touch are two nonverbal aspects that can be misunderstood by individuals of different cultures.

KEY POINTS TO REMEMBER—CONT'D

- There are a number of communication techniques that nurses can use to enhance their nursing practices. Many widely used communication enhancers are cited in Table 8.2.
- There are a number of nontherapeutic techniques that nurses can learn to avoid in order to enhance their effectiveness with people. Some are cited in Table 8.3 along with suggestions for more helpful responses.
- Nurses are more effective when they use nonthreatening and open-ended communication techniques.
- Effective communication is a skill that develops over time and is integral to the establishment and maintenance of a therapeutic alliance.
- The application of information communication technologies in the psychosocial sciences is relatively new, but it is viewed as a tool for helping people with mental health needs. It is particularly well suited for individuals in rural areas and for those individuals for whom accessing health care/mental health clinics is not possible either physically or financially.
- The use of apps for those with anxiety, depression, and other mental health issues (e.g., posttraumatic stress disorder, bipolar, etc.) can provide greater accessibility to psychiatric care. The one caveat is that an app should be approved and well accepted within the mental health community.

APPLYING CRITICAL JUDGMENT

1. Keep a log for 30 minutes a day of your communication pattern (a tape recorder is ideal). Name four effective techniques that you notice you use frequently. Identify two techniques that are obstructive. In your log, rewrite these nontherapeutic communications and replace them with statements that would better facilitate discussion of thoughts and feelings. Share your log and discuss the changes you are working on with one classmate.
2. Role-play with a classmate at least five nonverbal communications, and have your partner identify the message he or she was receiving.
3. Using touch and eye contact, act out how the nurse would use the nonverbal messages with three different cultural groups.
4. When interviewing Tom shortly after his return from Afghanistan, he makes the following statement to you. Reply to this statement using each of the techniques indicated:
   "I am so afraid to go to sleep at night since I came back from Afghanistan. The nightmares are so real, I can hear the screams of the wounded, and the visions in my mind are terrifying."
   Restating:
   Rephrasing:
   Giving information:
   Reflecting feelings:
5. Answer the following questions as honestly as you can in a conversation with a good friend or partner (Sommers-Flanagan & Sommers-Flanagan, 2012–2013):
   A. Has there ever been a time in your life when you experienced racism or discrimination? What were your thoughts and feelings related to this experience?
   B. Can you relate a time when your own thoughts about people who are different from you affected how you treated them? Would you do anything differently now?
   C. How would you describe the "American culture"? What part of this culture do you embrace? What parts do you reject? How does your internalization of the "American culture" impact what you think constitutes a "mentally healthy individual"?
6. How would information communication technologies (ICTs) be best used in your community? Specifically, which ICTs would you choose if you were opening a telehealth communication center in your community?

CHAPTER REVIEW QUESTIONS

1. An adult experiencing a recent exacerbation of ulcerative colitis tells the nurse, "I had an accident while I was at the grocery store. It was so embarrassing." Select the nurse's therapeutic response.
   a. "Most grocery stores have public restrooms available."
   b. "Tell me more about how you felt when that happened."
   c. "People usually have compassion about those types of events."
   d. "Your disease is now in remission so that is not likely to happen again."
2. A nurse counsels a widow whose husband died 5 years ago. The widow says, "If I'd done more, he would still be alive." Select the nurse's therapeutic response.
   a. "I understand how you feel after such a terrible loss."
   b. "That was a long time ago. Now it's time to move on with your life."
   c. "You did a very good job of caring for him, especially because he was sick for so long."
   d. "Your husband was 82 years old with severe chronic obstructive pulmonary disease."
3. A patient has been out of work for 3 weeks with a major illness and anticipates another month of recovery. The patient tells the nurse, "I'm trying to keep up with my work email from home. They hired a new person in my department, but that person has no experience." Select the nurse's therapeutic response.
   a. "It sounds like you're saying you are worried about your job security."
   b. "No one expects you to keep pace with your job while you're recovering."

CHAPTER REVIEW QUESTIONS—CONT'D

c. "Your employer is required to hold your job for you while you're on sick leave."
d. "Don't worry about your job right now. It's more important for you to recover."

4. In which nurse–patient interaction might it be appropriate for the nurse to consider using touch?
   a. Comforting a tearful patient of Japanese heritage
   b. Counseling a child who was physically abused by a parent
   c. Welcoming a person of Hispanic heritage to a new group session
   d. Interacting with a Native American who has a hearing impairment

5. A nurse prepares a patient in a rural community for an initial telehealth visit with the health care provider. Select the nurse's priority action.
   a. Ensure that the patient's rights to privacy are respected.
   b. Ask the patient, "How much do you know about the Internet?"
   c. Inform the patient, "This experience will be like appearing on television."
   d. Advise the patient, "You will be able to hear, but not see, your health care provider."

REFERENCES

American Hospital Association. (2018, March). American Hospital Association annual survey IT supplement brief #1. Expanding electronic patient engagement. Retrieved from https://www.aha.org/system/files/2018-03/expanding-electronic-engagement.pdf.

American Nurses Association (ANA), American Psychiatric Nurses Association, & International Society of Psychiatric-Mental Health Nurses. (2014). *Psychiatric-mental health nursing: Scope and standards of practice.* Washington, DC: Nursebooks.org.

Arnold, E. C., & Boggs, K. U. (2016). *Interpersonal relationships: Professional communication skills for nurses* (7th ed.). St. Louis: Elsevier Saunders.

Bazzoli, F. (2018). DOD takes steps to expand use of telehealth services. Retrieved from https://www.healthdatamanagement.com/.

Berlo, D. K. (1960). *The process of communication.* San Francisco: Reinhart Press.

Egan, G. (2013). *The skilled helper: A problem-management approach and opportunity-development approach to helping* (10th ed.). Belmont, CA: Brooks/Cole, Cengage Learning.

Giddens, J. F. (2017). *Concepts for nursing practice* (2nd ed.). St. Louis: Elsevier.

Giger, J. N., & Davidhizar, R. E. (2007). *Transcultural nursing: Assessment and intervention* (5th ed.). St. Louis: Mosby Elsevier.

Makary, M. A. (2016). Medical error-the third leading cause of death in the US. Retrieved from https://www.ncbi.nlm.nih.gov/pubmed/271.

Matsumoto, D., & Sung Hwang, H. (2011). Reading facial expressions of emotion. Retrieved from www.apa.org/science/about/psa/2011/05/facial-expressions.aspx.

Noguchi, I. (2014–2018). Miscommunication a major cause of medical error, study shows. Retrieved from ttps://www.kqed.org/stateofhealth/22697/miscommunication-a-major-cause-of-medical-error-study-shows.

Peek, H. (2015). Evolving potential of mobile psychiatry: Current barriers and future solutions. Retrieved from http://www.psychiatrictimes.com/telepsychiatry/technology-psychiatry-year-review?GUID=67CBCF91-8666-442D-9DDD-0FED4DF8E580&rememberme=1&ts=26122015#sthash.0Yr4YTpt.dpuf.

Peplau, H. E. (1952). *Interpersonal relations in nursing: A conceptual frame of reference for psychodynamic nursing.* New York: Putnam.

Raine, L, & Perrin, A. (2017). 10 facts about smartphones as the iPhone turns 10. Retrieved from http://www.pewresearch.org/fact-tank/2017/06/28/10-facts-about-smartphones/.

Sommers-Flanagan, J., & Sommers-Flanagan, R. (2012–2013). *Clinical interviewing* (5th ed.). Hoboken, NJ: Wiley.

Sommers-Flanagan, J., & Sommers-Flanagan, R. (2017). *Clinical interviewing* (6th ed.). Hoboken, NJ: Wiley.

Substance Abuse and Mental Health Services Administration (SAMHSA). (2016). *Cultural competence.* Retrieved from https://www.samhsa.gov/capt/applying-strategic-prevention/cultural-competence.

9

Therapeutic Relationships and the Clinical Interview

Elizabeth M. Varcarolis

http://evolve.elsevier.com/Varcarolis/essentials

OBJECTIVES

1. Compare and contrast the three phases of the nurse–patient relationship.
2. Compare and contrast a social relationship and a therapeutic relationship regarding purpose, focus, communication styles, and goals.
3. Identify at least four patient behaviors a nurse may encounter in the clinical setting.
4. Explore aspects that foster a therapeutic nurse–patient relationship and those that are inherent in a nontherapeutic nursing interactive process.
5. Define and discuss the role of empathy, genuineness, and positive regard on the part of the nurse in a nurse–patient relationship.
6. Role-play with a classmate or group two attitudes and four actions that may reflect the nurse's positive regard for a patient.
7. Explain how the influence of transference and countertransference can cause boundary blurring.
8. Act out the use of attending behaviors (eye contact, body language, vocal qualities, and verbal tracking) with a classmate or friend.
9. Discuss the influences of different values and cultural beliefs on the therapeutic relationship.

KEY TERMS AND CONCEPTS

boundaries, p. 106
clinical supervision, p. 116
confidentiality, p. 111
contract, p. 109
countertransference, p. 107
empathy, p. 113
genuineness, p. 113
intimate distance, p. 115
modeling, p. 108
narcissism, p. 106
orientation phase, p. 109
paralinguistics, p. 116
patient-centered partnership, p. 105
personal distance, p. 115
process recordings, p. 116
public distance, p. 116
rapport, p. 109
social distance, p. 116
social relationship, p. 105
termination phase, p. 112
therapeutic encounter, p. 106
therapeutic relationship/partnership, p. 105
therapeutic use of self, p. 105
transference, p. 106
values, p. 108
working phase, p. 111

CONCEPT: COLLABORATION: *Collaboration* in nursing is the development of partnerships to achieve the best possible outcomes that reflect the particular needs of the patient, family, and community. Collaborative relationships include nurse–nurse, nurse–patient, and interprofessional relationships (Giddens, 2017). The nurse–patient relationship is the basis of all psychiatric-mental health treatment approaches, regardless of specific goals. The very first connections between nurse and patient are to establish an understanding that the nurse is safe, confidential, reliable, and consistent and that the relationship will occur within appropriate and clear boundaries.

INTRODUCTION

Psychiatric-mental health nursing is based on the principles of *science*. A background in anatomy, physiology, and chemistry is the basis for the safe and effective provision of biological treatments. For example, it is assumed the nurse has knowledge of the effects of medications, the indications for use, and the adverse effects based on best-evidence studies and trials. However, it is the caring relationship and the development of the skills needed to enhance and maintain these relationships that include aspects of the *art* of psychiatric nursing. This human relationship can allow a place for caring and healing to occur. The nurse's uniqueness (therapeutic use of self) is a critical way that nurses make themselves available to their patients.

It is helpful to remember that basic level psychiatric-mental health nurses do not practice psychotherapy because this is an advanced skill. They do, however, use counseling techniques in the context of the therapeutic relationship. Counseling is a supportive process that helps individuals problem solve, resolve personal conflicts, and feel supported (Halter, 2018).

Nurse–Patient Partnership/Relationship

Nurses have been using the concepts of *nurse–patient relationship* and *patient-centered care* since Hildegard Peplau introduced these concepts into nursing. A newer way to look at the relationship between health care provider and patient in light of the recovery model might be *patient centered partnership.*

The core concepts of patient- and family-centered care consist of (1) dignity and respect, (2) information sharing, (3) patient and family participation, and (4) the patient's feeling of being heard and understood. These tenants have long been identified as factors in the nurse–patient relationship, more recently referred to as the *nurse–patient partnership.* A **patient-centered partnership** implies a patient's participation in his or her health care decisions, hence the term *collaborative patient-centered treatment planning.* For our purposes here, the term *nurse–patient relationship/partnership* implies collaboration with the patient and family regarding health care goals, plans to meet those goals, and appropriate interventions within the framework of the patient's/family's cultural and ethnic background and comfort levels.

The therapeutic nurse–patient relationship is the basis of all psychiatric nursing treatment approaches regardless of the specific aim. The very first connections between nurse and patient are to establish an understanding that the nurse is safe, reliable, and consistent and will keep the individual's information private. The patient-centered relationship is conducted within appropriate and clear boundaries.

It is true that many disorders, such as schizophrenia and mood disorders, have strong biochemical and genetic components. However, many accompanying emotional problems, such as poor self-image, low self-esteem, and difficulties with adherence to treatment, can be significantly improved through a therapeutic patient-centered alliance. All too often, individuals who enter treatment have taxed or exhausted their familial and social resources and have found themselves in a position of isolation from people who will listen for more than a few minutes.

The nurse–patient relationship is a creative process and unique to each nurse. Each person brings his or her own uniqueness to this relationship. Each of us has unique gifts that we can learn to use creatively to form positive bonds with others. Historically this has been referred to as the **therapeutic use of self.** Therapeutic use of self is an example of the practice of the "art of nursing." *It is important to remember* that the efficacy of this therapeutic use of self has been scientifically substantiated as an evidence-based intervention. A positive therapeutic alliance that is collaborative and respectful is one of the best predictors of positive outcomes in therapy (Gordon & Beresin, 2016). On the other hand, nonadherence with treatment and poor outcomes in therapy are related to a patient feeling unheard, disrespected, or otherwise unconnected with the clinician/health care worker (Gordon & Beresin, 2016). Research suggests that therapeutic success is a result of the personal characteristics of the clinician and the patient, not necessarily a result of the particular process employed. Furthermore, there is evidence that psychotherapy (talk therapy) and a therapeutic alliance can *actually change brain chemistry* in much the same way as medication. There is great support for the practice of a combination of medication and psychotherapy for the treatment of many psychiatric problems. Cognitive-behavioral therapy, in particular, has met with great success in the treatment of depression, phobias, obsessive-compulsive disorders, posttraumatic stress disorder (PTSD), and others.

Establishing a therapeutic alliance or patient-centered partnership with an individual takes time. Skills in this area gradually improve with guidance from those with more skill and experience. When patients do not engage in a therapeutic alliance, chances are that no matter what interventions are made, nothing significant will happen except mutual frustration and mutual withdrawal.

WHAT IS A THERAPEUTIC RELATIONSHIP?

The nurse–patient relationship is often loosely defined, but a therapeutic relationship incorporating principles of mental health nursing is more clearly defined and differs from other relationships. A therapeutic nurse–patient relationship has specific goals and functions. Goals in a therapeutic relationship include the following:

- **Facilitating** communication of distressing thoughts and feelings
- **Assisting** patients with problem solving to help facilitate activities of daily living
- **Helping** patients examine self-defeating behaviors and test alternatives
- **Promoting** self-care and independence

A relationship is an interpersonal process that involves two or more people. Throughout life, we meet people in a variety of settings and share a variety of experiences. We develop long-term relationships with some individuals; with others, the relationship lasts only a short time. Naturally, the kinds of relationships we enter vary from person to person and from situation to situation. Generally, relationships can be defined as (1) social or (2) therapeutic.

Social Relationships Versus Therapeutic Relationships

A **social relationship** can be defined as a relationship that is primarily initiated for the purpose of friendship, socialization, enjoyment, or accomplishment of a task. Mutual needs are met during social interaction (e.g., participants share ideas, feelings, and experiences). Communication skills used in social relationships may include giving advice and (sometimes) meeting basic dependency needs, such as lending money and helping with jobs. Often the content of the communication remains superficial. During social interactions, roles may shift. Within a social relationship, there is little emphasis on the evaluation of the interaction:

Patient: "Oh, gosh, I hate to be alone. It gets me down and hurts so much."

Nurse: "I know just how you feel. I don't like it either. What I do is get a friend and go to a movie or something. Do you have someone to hang with?" *(In this response, the nurse is minimizing the patient's feelings and giving advice prematurely.)*

Patient: "No, not really. I don't even feel like going out. I just sit at home feeling scared and lonely."

Nurse: "Most of us feel like that at one time or another. Maybe if you took a class or joined a group, you could meet people. I know of some great groups you could join. It's not good to be by yourself all of the time." *(Again, the nurse is not "hearing" the patient's distress and, in so doing, is again minimizing her pain and isolation. The nurse goes on to give the patient banal advice, thus closing off the patient's feelings and experience.)*

Therapeutic Relationships

The **therapeutic relationship/partnership** (patient-centered partnership) between nurse and patient differs from both a social and an intimate relationship in that the nurse maximizes his or her communication skills, understanding of human behavior, and personal strengths to enhance the patient's growth. Patients more easily engage in the relationship when the clinician's interactions address their concerns, respect the patient as a partner in decision making, and use language that is straightforward (Gordon & Beresin, 2016). That suggests the focus of the relationship needs to be on the patient's ideas, experiences, and feelings. Inherent in a therapeutic relationship is the nurse's focus on significant personal issues introduced by the patient during the clinical interview. The nurse and the patient identify areas that need exploration and periodically evaluate the degree of change in the patient.

Although the nurse may assume a variety of roles (e.g., teacher, counselor, socializing agent, liaison), the relationship is consistently focused on the patient's problem and needs. Nurses must meet their own needs outside of the therapeutic relationship. When nurses begin to want the patient to "like them," "do as they suggest," "be nice to them," or "give them recognition," the needs of the patient cannot be adequately met, and the interaction could be detrimental (nontherapeutic) to the patient.

Working under supervision (i.e., more experienced nurse, nursing instructor, therapist) is an excellent way to keep the focus and boundaries clear. Communication skills and knowledge of the stages of and phenomena occurring in a therapeutic relationship are crucial tools in the formation and maintenance of that relationship. Within the context of a helping relationship, the following occur:

- The needs of the patient are identified and explored.
- Alternate problem-solving approaches are taken.
- New coping skills may develop.
- Behavioral change is encouraged.

Staff nurses and students may struggle with the boundaries between social and therapeutic relationships. There is a fine line. In fact, students often feel more comfortable "being a friend" to a patient because it is a more familiar role, especially with people close to their own age. However, when this occurs, nurses or students need to make it clear (to themselves and the patient) that the relationship is a therapeutic one. This does *not* mean that the nurse is not friendly toward the patient, and it does *not* mean that talking about innocuous topics (e.g., television, weather, children's pictures) is forbidden. It does mean, however, that the nurse follows the prior stated guidelines regarding a therapeutic relationship; essentially, the focus is on the patient, and the relationship is not designed to meet the nurse's needs. The patient's problems and concerns are explored, potential solutions are discussed by both patient and nurse, and solutions are implemented by the patient:

Patient: "Oh, gosh, I hate to be alone. It gets me down and hurts so much."

Nurse: "Loneliness can be painful. What is going on now that you are feeling so alone?"

Patient: "Well, my mom died 2 years ago, and last month, my—oh, I am so scared." *(Patient takes a deep breath, looks down, and looks like she might cry.)*

Nurse: (Sits in silence while the patient recovers.) "Go on …"

Patient: "My boyfriend left for an overseas assignment. I haven't heard from him, and I can't get any answers from his boss. He was my best friend, and we were going to get married. If something happens to him, I don't want to live."

Nurse: "Have you thought of killing yourself?"

Patient: "Well, if he dies, I will. I can't live without him."

Nurse: "Have you ever felt like this before?"

Patient: Yes, when my mom died. I was depressed for about a year until I met my boyfriend."

Nurse: "It sounds like you are going through a very painful and scary time. Perhaps you and I can talk some more and come up with some ways for you to feel less anxious, scared, and overwhelmed. Would you be willing to work on this together?"

The ability of the nurse to engage in interpersonal interactions in a goal-directed manner for the purpose of assisting this young woman with her emotional and, if needed, physical health needs is the foundation of patient-centered care. The nurse–patient relationship is synonymous with a professional helping relationship. Behaviors that have relevance to nurses are as follows:

- **Accountability:** Nurses assume responsibility for their conduct and the consequences of their actions.
- **Focus on patient needs:** The interest of the patient, rather than the nurse, other health care workers, or the institution, is given first consideration. The nurse's role is that of patient advocate.
- **Clinical competence:** The criteria on which the nurse bases his or her conduct are principles of knowledge and conduct that is appropriate to the specific situation. This involves awareness and incorporation of the latest knowledge made available from research (evidence-based practice).
- **Delaying judgment:** Ideally, nurses refrain from judging patients and avoid transferring their own values and beliefs to others.
- **Supervision** by a more experienced clinician or team is essential to developing one's competence in this area.

The nurse–patient relationship may be informal and brief, such as when the nurse and patient meet for only a few sessions. However, even though it is brief, the relationship may be substantial, useful, and important for the patient. This limited relationship is often referred to as a **therapeutic encounter**. When the nurse shows true concern for another's circumstances (has positive regard, empathy), even a short encounter with the individual can have a powerful effect on that individual's life.

At other times, the encounters may be longer and more formal, such as in inpatient settings, mental health units, crisis centers, and mental health outpatient facilities, and in private practice. This longer time span allows greater development of an effective therapeutic nurse–patient relationship.

Establishing Relationship Boundaries

A well-defined therapeutic relationship allows for the establishment of clear patient **boundaries** that provide a safe space through which the patient can explore feelings and treatment issues. The nurse's role in the therapeutic relationship is theoretically rather well defined. The patient's needs are separated from the nurse's needs, and the patient's role is different from that of the nurse. Therefore the boundaries of the relationship seem to be well stated. In reality, boundaries are at risk of blurring, and a shift in the nurse–patient partnership may lead to nontherapeutic dynamics. Examples of circumstances that can produce blurring of boundaries include the following:

- When the relationship slips into a social context
- When the nurse's needs are met at the expense of the patient's needs

The following are some warning signals that indicate a nurse may be blurring boundaries:

- **Overhelping:** Doing for patients what they are able to do themselves or going beyond the wishes or needs of patients
- **Controlling:** Asserting authority and assuming control of patients "for their own good"
- **Narcissism:** Needing to find weakness, helplessness, and/or disease in patients to feel helpful, at the expense of recognizing and supporting patients' healthier, stronger, and more competent features

When situations such as these arise, the relationship has ceased to be a helpful one, and the phenomenon of control becomes an issue. Role blurring is often a result of unrecognized transference or countertransference.

Self-Check on Boundary Issues

It is helpful for all of us to take time to be reflective and try to be aware of our thoughts and actions with patients, as well as with colleagues, friends, and family. Fig. 9.1 is a helpful self-test you can use throughout your career, no matter what area of nursing you choose.

Transference

Transference is a phenomenon originally identified by Sigmund Freud. Transference is the process whereby a person unconsciously

NURSING BOUNDARY INDEX SELF-CHECK

Please rate yourself according to the frequency with which the following statements reflect your behavior, thoughts, or feelings within the past 2 years while providing patient care.*

1. Have you ever received any feedback about your behavior being overly intrusive with patients and their families?	Never ____	Rarely ____	Sometimes ____	Often ____
2. Do you ever have difficulty setting limits with patients?	Never ____	Rarely ____	Sometimes ____	Often ____
3. Do you ever arrive early or stay late to be with your patient for a longer period?	Never ____	Rarely ____	Sometimes ____	Often ____
4. Do you ever find yourself relating to patients or peers as you might to a family member?	Never ____	Rarely ____	Sometimes ____	Often ____
5. Have you ever acted on sexual feelings you have for a patient?	Never ____	Rarely ____	Sometimes ____	Often ____
6. Do you feel that you are the only one who understands the patient?	Never ____	Rarely ____	Sometimes ____	Often ____
7. Have you ever received feedback that you get "too involved" with patients or families?	Never ____	Rarely ____	Sometimes ____	Often ____
8. Do you derive conscious satisfaction from patients' praise, appreciation, or affection?	Never ____	Rarely ____	Sometimes ____	Often ____
9. Do you ever feel that other staff members are too critical of "your" patient?	Never ____	Rarely ____	Sometimes ____	Often ____
10. Do you ever feel that other staff members are jealous of your relationship with your patient?	Never ____	Rarely ____	Sometimes ____	Often ____
11. Have you ever tried to "match-make" a patient with one of your friends?	Never ____	Rarely ____	Sometimes ____	Often ____
12. Do you find it difficult to handle patients' unreasonable requests for assistance, verbal abuse, or sexual language?	Never ____	Rarely ____	Sometimes ____	Often ____

* Any item that is responded to with "Sometimes" or "Often" should alert the nurse to a possible area of vulnerability. If the item is responded to with "Rarely," the nurse should determine whether it is an isolated event or a possible pattern of behavior.

Fig. 9.1 Nursing boundary index self-check. (From Pilette, P. C., Berck, C. B., & Achber, L. C. [1995]. Therapeutic management of helping boundaries. *Journal of Psychosocial Nursing and Mental Health Services, 33*[1], 45.)

and inappropriately displaces (transfers) patterns of behaviors and emotional reactions toward another person that originated in relation to significant figures in childhood. The patient may even say, "You remind me of my . . . . " (e.g., mother, sister, father, brother). For example:

Patient: "Oh, you are so high and mighty. Did anyone ever tell you that you are a cold, unfeeling machine, just like others I know?"

Nurse: "Tell me about one person who is cold and unfeeling toward you." *(In this example, the patient is experiencing the nurse in the same way she did with a significant other[s] during her formative years. It turns out that the patient's mother was very aloof, leaving her with feelings of isolation, worthlessness, and anger.)*

Although the transference phenomenon occurs in all relationships, transference seems to be intensified in relationships of authority. Because the process of transference is accelerated toward a person in authority, physicians, nurses, and social workers are all potential objects of transference. It is important to realize that the patient may experience thoughts, feelings, and reactions toward a health care worker that are realistic and appropriate; these are *not* transference phenomena.

Common forms of transference include the desire for affection or respect and the gratification of dependency needs. The transferential feelings the patient might experience are hostility, jealousy, competitiveness, and love. Requests for special favors (e.g., cigarettes, water, extra time in the session) are concrete examples of transference phenomena.

Countertransference

Countertransference refers to the tendency of the nurse to displace onto the patient feelings related to people in his or her past. Frequently, the patient's transference to the nurse evokes countertransference feelings in the nurse. For example, it is normal to feel angry when persistently attacked, annoyed when unreasonably frustrated, or flattered when idealized. A nurse might feel extremely important when depended on exclusively by a patient. If the nurse does not recognize his or her own omnipotent feelings as countertransference, encouragement of independent growth in the patient can be minimized at best. Recognizing our countertransference reactions maximizes our ability to *empower* our patients. When we fail to recognize our countertransference toward our patients, the therapeutic relationship stalls, and essentially, we *disempower* our patients by experiencing them not as individuals but, rather, as inner projections. For example:

Patient: "Yeah, well, I decided not to go to that dumb group. 'Hi, I'm so and so, and I'm an alcoholic.' Who cares?" *(Patient sits slumped in a chair, chewing gum, nonchalantly looking around.)*

Nurse: (in a very impassioned tone) "You always sabotage your chances. You need AA to get in control of your life. Last week you were going to go, and now you have disappointed everyone." *(Here the nurse is reminded of her mother, who was an alcoholic. The nurse had tried everything to get her mother into treatment and took it as a personal failure and deep disappointment that her mother never sought recovery. After the nurse sorts out her thoughts and feelings, she realizes the frustration and feelings of disappointment and failure come from feelings toward her mother and not the patient. The nurse starts the next session with the following approach.)*

Nurse: "Look, I was thinking about last week, and I realize the decision to go to AA or find other help is solely up to you. It is true that I would like you to live a fuller and more satisfying life, but it is your decision. I am wondering, however, what happened to change your mind to not go to AA."

If the nurse feels either a strongly positive or a strongly negative reaction to a patient, the feeling most often signals countertransference in the nurse. Another sign of countertransference is overidentification with the patient. In this situation, the nurse may have difficulty recognizing or understanding problems the patient has that are similar to the nurse's own. For example, a nurse who is struggling with an alcoholic family member may feel disinterested, cold, or disgusted toward an alcoholic patient. Other indications of countertransference occur when the nurse becomes involved in power struggles, competition, or arguments with the patient.

Identifying and working through various transference and countertransference issues are crucial if the nurse is to achieve professional and clinical growth and allow for positive change in the patient. These issues are best handled through the use of supervision by either the peer group or the therapeutic team. Regularly scheduled supervision sessions provide the nurse with the opportunity to increase self-awareness, clinical skills, and growth, as well as allow for the continued growth of the patient.

Values, Beliefs, and Self-Awareness

Relationships are complex. We bring into our relationships a multitude of thoughts, feelings, beliefs, and attitudes (cultural filters)—some rational and some irrational. We form these from families or cultures, our spiritual beliefs and experiences, and our "heroes." From those, we form our values. **Values** are abstract standards and represent an ideal, either positive or negative. Our values are usually culturally oriented and influenced in a variety of ways through our parents, teachers, religious institutions, workplaces, peers, and political leaders, as well as through films and the media. All these influences attempt to instill their values and to form and influence our values.

Modeling is perhaps one of the most potent means of value education because it presents a vivid example of values in action. We all need role models to guide us in negotiating life's many choices. Young people in particular are hungry for role models and will find them among peers as well as adults. As nurses, parents, bosses, coworkers, friends, lovers, teachers, spouses, and singles, we are constantly (in either a positive or a negative manner) being a role model to others.

Our culture—and more precisely our own subculture—defines the guidelines that provide structure to our lives. It is through this that our beliefs, thoughts, behaviors, and feelings are interpreted (Sommers-Flanagan & Sommers-Flanagan, 2017). Our cultural values and beliefs provide meaning to our lives and our environment in the form of an operating system or interpretive system. How we view the world and how we are supposed to behave, think, believe, and live are influenced by this interpretive system.

Most often, problems arise when the interpretive system of the clinician and that of the individual seeking guidance are glaringly different. When the nurse is working with an individual from a culturally distinct environment, the interpretive system between them might be so different at times that it is difficult for the patient and the clinician to connect in a clinically meaningful way (Hays, 2008). According to Sommers-Flanagan and Sommers-Flanagan (2017, p. 35), "Developing cultural self-awareness begins with acceptance of differences as normal, interesting, and even desirable aspects of being human."

It is helpful, even crucial, for us to have an understanding of our *own* values and attitudes so that we may become aware of personal beliefs or attitudes that may interfere with a working or therapeutic relationship.

When working with patients, it is important for nurses to understand that our values and beliefs are not necessarily the right ones—and certainly are not right for everyone. It is helpful to realize that our values and beliefs (1) reflect our own culture/subculture, (2) are derived from a range of choices, and (3) are those we have chosen for ourselves from a variety of influences and role models. These chosen values (religious, cultural, societal) guide us in making decisions and taking actions that we hope will make our lives meaningful, rewarding, and fulfilled.

Interviewing and even working with others whose values, beliefs, cultures, or lifestyles are radically different from our own can be a challenge. Several topics that cause controversy in society in general—including religion, gender roles, abortion, war, politics, money, drugs, alcohol, sex/sexual orientation, and the practice of corporal punishment—can cause conflict between nurses and their patients. Although we emphasize that the patient and the nurse should identify outcomes together, what happens when the nurse's values, beliefs, and interpretive system are very different from the patient's? Consider the following possible conflicts:

- The patient wants an abortion, which is against the nurse's values.
- The nurse believes the patient who was raped and became pregnant should get an abortion, but the patient refuses.
- The patient engages in unsafe sex with multiple partners, which is against the nurse's concern for safety and values.
- The nurse cannot understand a patient who refuses life-saving treatment on religious grounds.
- The patient puts material gain and objects far ahead of loyalty to friends and family, in direct contrast to the nurse's values.
- The patient is deeply religious, whereas the nurse has difficulty with organized religion related to an experience with a religious cult.
- The patient's lifestyle includes taking illicit drugs, which is against the nurse's values.

How can nurses develop working relationships and help patients solve problems when patients' values, goals, and interpretive systems are so different from their own? Self-awareness requires that we understand what we value and those beliefs that guide our behaviors. It is critical that, as nurses, we not only understand and accept our own values and beliefs but also are sensitive to and accepting of the unique and different values and beliefs of others. This is another area in which supervision by an experienced colleague can prove invaluable.

Personal values may change over time; indeed, they may change many times over the course of a lifetime. The values you held as a child are different from those you held as an adolescent, and so forth.

Cultural Competence Self-Test

A cultural competence self-test can assist care providers in identifying areas in which they might improve the quality of their services to culturally diverse populations. Go to YouTube and search the phrase "Cultural Competence, Self-Test" for a fun, informative, and short instruction video.

PHASES OF THE NURSE–PATIENT RELATIONSHIP

Hildegard Peplau introduced the concept of the nurse–patient relationship in 1952 in her ground-breaking book *Interpersonal Relations in Nursing*. This model of the nurse–patient relationship (patient-centered relationship) is well accepted in the United States and Canada and has become an important tool for all nursing practice. Peplau (1952, p. 12) proposed that the nurse–patient relationship "facilitates forward movement" for both the nurse and the patient. Peplau's interactive nurse–patient process is designed to facilitate the patient's boundary management, independent problem solving, and decision making that promotes autonomy.

It is most likely that in the brief period you have for your psychiatric nursing rotation, all phases of the nurse–patient relationship will not have time to develop. However, it is important for you to be aware of these phases because you must be able to recognize and use them later if you will be spending long periods with a specific patient/individual. It is also important to remember that any contact that is caring and respectful and demonstrates concern for the situation of another person can have an enormous positive impact.

Peplau (1952, 1999) described the nurse–patient relationship as evolving through interlocking, overlapping phases. The distinctive phases of the nurse–patient relationship are generally recognized as follows:

- Orientation phase
- Working phase
- Termination phase

Although various phenomena and goals are identified for each phase, they often overlap. Even before the first meeting, the nurse may have many thoughts and feelings related to the first clinical session. This is sometimes referred to as the *preorientation phase.*

Preorientation Phase

Novice health care professionals usually have many concerns and experience a mild to moderate degree of anxiety on their first clinical day. Commonly, nursing instructors will encourage students to identify concerns about working with psychiatric patients in preconference on the first clinical day. These concerns focus on being afraid of people with psychiatric problems, saying "the wrong thing," and being unaware of the proper responses to certain patient behaviors. There really are no magic words. Talking with the instructor and supervised peer-group discussion will add confidence by providing feedback and suggestions. Chapter 8 discusses the use of communication strategies in clinical practice.

Often, students new to the mental health setting are concerned about being in situations that they may not know how to handle. These concerns are universal and often arise in the clinical setting. Table 9.1 identifies common patient behaviors (e.g., crying, asking the nurse to keep a secret, threatening to commit suicide, giving a gift) and gives examples of an appropriate response, the rationale for the response, and a possible verbal statement. The exact words depend on the situation, but understanding the rationale will aid you in applying the information in future interactions.

Most experienced psychiatric nursing faculty and staff monitor the unit atmosphere and have a sixth sense pertaining to behaviors that indicate escalating tension. They are trained in crisis interventions, and formal security is often available onsite to give the staff support. Your instructor will set the ground rules for safety during the first clinical day. For example, do not enter a patient's room alone, know if there are any patients who should not be engaged, stay in open areas that have other health care personnel, and recognize the signs and symptoms of escalating anxiety. There are certain rules of thumb regarding actions a nurse can take if a patient's anger begins to escalate (see Chapter 24). You should always trust your own instincts. If you feel uncomfortable for any reason, excuse yourself for a moment and discuss your feelings with your instructor or a staff member. In addition to obtaining reassurance and support, students can often provide valuable information about the patient's condition by sharing these perceptions.

Orientation Phase

The **orientation phase** can last for a few meetings or can extend over a longer period. It is the first time the nurse and the patient meet, and they are strangers to each other. When strangers meet, they interact according to their own backgrounds, standards, values, and experiences. This fact—that each person has a unique frame of reference—underlies the need for self-awareness on the part of the nurse. The initial interview includes the following:

- An atmosphere is established in which rapport can grow.
- The nurse's role is clarified, and the responsibilities of both the patient and the nurse are defined.
- The contract containing the time, place, date, and duration of the meetings is discussed.
- Confidentiality is discussed and assumed.
- The terms of termination are introduced (these are also discussed throughout the orientation phase and beyond).
- The nurse becomes aware of transference and countertransference issues.
- Patient problems are articulated, and mutually agreed goals are established.

Establishing Rapport

The major emphasis during the first few encounters with the patient is on providing an atmosphere in which trust and understanding can grow and facilitating the establishment of **rapport.** As in any relationship, rapport can be nurtured by demonstrating genuineness and empathy, developing positive regard, showing consistency, and offering assistance in problem solving and in providing support. It is important for the nurse to first identify how the patient wants to be addressed. In some countries, it is very important that people are addressed by their professional title if they have one. To some people, calling them by their first name, such as a young person addressing an older person by "John" or "Phoebe," would be insulting and likely stall the process. The health care worker simply asks, "What do people call you?" or "How should I address you?"

Parameters of the Relationship

The patient needs to know about the nurse (who the nurse is and the nurse's background) and the purpose of the meetings. For example, a student might furnish the following information:

Student: "Hello, Mrs. Rodriquez. I am Jim from Scottsdale Community College. I am in my psychiatric rotation and will be coming here for the next six Thursdays. I would like to spend time with you each Thursday while you are here. I'm here to be a support person for you as you work on your treatment goals."

Formal or Informal Contract

A **contract** emphasizes the patient's participation and responsibility because it shows that the nurse does something *with* the patient rather than *for* the patient. The contract, either verbal or written, contains the place, time, date, and duration of the meetings. During the orientation phase, the patient may begin to express thoughts and feelings, identify problems, and discuss realistic goals. Therefore mutual agreement on goals is also part of the contract:

Student: "Mrs. Rodriquez, we will meet at 10 AM each Thursday in the consultation room at the clinic for 45 minutes from September 15 to October 27. We can use that time for further discussion of your feelings of loneliness and anger and explore some things you could do to make the situation better for yourself."

TABLE 9.1 Common Patient Behaviors and Nurse Responses

Possible Reactions by Nurse	Useful Responses by Nurse
What to Do if the Patient Says He or She Wants to Kill Himself or Herself	
The nurse may feel overwhelmed or responsible for "talking the patient out of it." The nurse may pick up some of the patient's feelings of hopelessness.	The nurse assesses whether the patient has a plan and the lethality of the plan. The nurse tells the patient that this is serious, that the nurse does not want harm to come to the patient, and that this information needs to be shared with other staff. "This is very serious, Mr. Lamb. I do not want any harm to come to you. I will have to share this with the other staff." The nurse can then discuss with the patient the feelings and circumstances that led up to this decision. (Refer to Chapter 23 for strategies in suicide intervention.)
What to Do if the Patient Asks the Nurse to Keep a Secret	
The nurse may feel conflict because the nurse wants the patient to share important information but is unsure about making such a promise.	The nurse *cannot* make such a promise. The information may be important to the health or safety of the patient or others. "I cannot make that promise. It might be important for me to share it with other staff." The patient then decides whether to share the information.
What to Do if the Patient Asks the Nurse a Personal Question	
The nurse may think that it is rude not to answer the patient's question. A new nurse might feel relieved to delay the start of the interview. The nurse may feel uneasy and want to leave the situation. New nurses are often manipulated by a patient into changing roles. This keeps the focus off the patient and prevents the creation of a relationship.	The nurse may or may not answer the patient's query. If the nurse decides to answer a natural question, he or she answers in a word or two, then refocuses back on the patient. *Patient:* Are you married? *Nurse:* Yes. Do you have a spouse? *Patient:* Do you have any children? *Nurse:* This time is for you—tell me about yourself. *Patient:* You can just tell me if you have any children. *Nurse:* This is your time to focus on your concerns. Tell me something about your family.
What to Do if the Patient Makes Sexual Advances	
The nurse feels uncomfortable but may feel conflicted about "rejecting" the patient or making him or her feel "unattractive" or "not good enough."	The nurse needs to set clear limits on expected behavior. "I am not comfortable having you touch (kiss) me. This time is for you to focus on your problems and concerns." Frequently restating the nurse's role throughout the relationship can help maintain boundaries. If the patient does not stop the inappropriate behavior, the nurse might say, "If you can't stop this behavior, I'll have to leave. I'll be back at [time] to spend time with you then." Leaving gives the patient time to gain control. The nurse returns at the stated time.
What to Do if the Patient Cries	
The nurse may feel uncomfortable and experience increased anxiety or feel somehow responsible for making the person cry.	The nurse should stay with the patient and reinforce that it is all right to cry. Often it is at that time that feelings are closest to the surface and can be best identified. "You seem ready to cry." "You are still upset about your brother's death." "What are you thinking right now?" The nurse offers tissues when appropriate.
What to Do if the Patient Leaves Before the Session Is Over	
The nurse may feel rejected, thinking it was something that he or she did. The nurse may experience increased anxiety or feel abandoned by the patient.	Some patients are not able to relate for long periods without experiencing an increase in anxiety. On the other hand, the patient may be testing the nurse. "I will wait for you here for 15 minutes, until our time is up." During this time, the nurse does not engage in conversation with any other patient or even with the staff. When the time is up, the nurse approaches the patient, says the time is up, and restates the day and time the nurse will see the patient again.
What to Do if the Patient Says He or She Does Not Want to Talk	
The nurse new to this situation may feel rejected or ineffectual.	At first, the nurse might say something to this effect: "It's all right. I would like to spend time with you. We don't have to talk." The nurse might spend short, frequent periods (e.g., 5 minutes) with the patient throughout the day. "Our 5 minutes is up. I'll be back at 10 AM and stay with you for 5 more minutes." This gives the patient the opportunity to understand that the nurse means what he or she says and is back on time consistently. It also gives the patient time between visits to assess how he or she feels and what he or she thinks about the nurse, and perhaps to feel less threatened. Or… The nurse could suggest other activities, such as walking with him or her down the hall, seeing what is going on in the activities room or seeing what activities are being scheduled, or sitting in a quiet space and quietly look at magazines together.

TABLE 9.1 Common Patient Behaviors and Nurse Responses—cont'd

Possible Reactions by Nurse	Useful Responses by Nurse
What to Do if the Patient Gives the Nurse a Present	
The nurse may feel uncomfortable when offered a gift. The meaning needs to be examined. Is the gift (1) a way of getting better care, (2) a way to maintain self-esteem, (3) a way of making the nurse feel guilty, (4) a sincere expression of thanks, or (5) a cultural expectation?	Possible guidelines: If the gift is expensive, the only policy is to graciously refuse. If it is inexpensive, then: (1) if it is given at the end of hospitalization when a relationship has developed, graciously accept; (2) if it is given at the beginning of the relationship, graciously refuse and explore the meaning behind the present. "Thank you, but it is our job to care for our patients. Are you concerned that some aspect of your care will be overlooked?" If the gift is money, it is always graciously refused. However, if the gift is candy, flowers, or something similar, thank the patient and let him or her know that you will be sharing the gift with the staff at the nursing station.
What to Do if Another Patient Interrupts During Time With Your Selected Patient	
The nurse may feel a conflict. The nurse does not want to appear rude. Sometimes the nurse tries to engage both patients in conversation.	The time the nurse has contracted with a selected patient is that patient's time. By keeping his or her part of the contract, the nurse demonstrates that he or she means what is said and views the sessions as important. "I am with Mr. Rob for the next 20 minutes. At 10 AM, after our time is up, I can talk to you for 5 minutes."

Confidentiality

The patient has a right to know who else will be given the information shared with the nurse and that the information may be shared with specific people, such as a clinical supervisor, the physician, the staff, or other students in conference. The patient also needs to know that the information will *not* be shared with relatives, friends, or others outside the treatment team, except in extreme situations. Safeguarding the privacy and confidentiality of individuals is not only the nurse's ethical obligation but also a legal responsibility.

Extreme situations include (1) child or elder abuse, (2) threats of self-harm or harm to others, or (3) intention not to follow through with the treatment plan. If information must be given to others, this is usually done by the physician, according to legal guidelines (refer to Chapter 6). The nurse must be aware of the patient's right to confidentiality and must not violate that right:

Student: "Mrs. Rodriquez, I will be sharing some of what we discuss with my nursing instructor, and at times, I may discuss certain concerns with my peers in conference or with the staff. However, I will *not* be sharing this information with your husband or any other members of your family or anyone outside the hospital without your permission."

Termination

Termination begins in the orientation phase. It also may be mentioned when appropriate during the working phase if the nature of the relationship is time limited (e.g., six or nine sessions). The date of the termination phase should be clear from the beginning. In some situations, the nurse–patient contract may be renegotiated when the termination date has been reached. In other situations, when the therapeutic nurse–patient relationship is an open-ended one, the termination date is not known:

Student: "Mrs. Rodriquez, as I mentioned earlier, our last meeting will be on October 27. We will have three more meetings after today."

Working Phase

The promotion of a strong working relationship develops over time and allows for the patient to experience anxiety and demonstrate dysfunctional behaviors in a safe setting while experimenting with new and more adaptive coping behaviors. Specific tasks of the working phase of the nurse–patient relationship in current clinical practice are as follows:

- Maintain the relationship.
- Gather further data.
- Promote the patient's problem-solving skills, self-esteem, and use of language.
- Facilitate behavioral change.
- Overcome resistance behaviors.
- Evaluate problems and goals, and redefine them as necessary.
- Promote practice and expression of alternative adaptive behaviors.

During the working phase, the nurse and patient together identify and explore areas in the patient's life that are causing problems. Often, a patient's present ways of handling situations stem from his or her earlier means of coping devised to survive in a chaotic and dysfunctional family environment. Although certain coping methods may have worked for the patient at an earlier age, they now interfere with the patient's interpersonal relationships and prevent him or her from attaining current goals. The patient's dysfunctional behaviors and basic assumptions about the world are often defensive, and the patient is usually unable to change the dysfunctional behavior at will. Therefore most of the problem behaviors or thoughts continue because of unconscious motivations and needs that are beyond the patient's awareness.

The nurse can work with the patient to identify these unconscious motivations and assumptions that keep the patient from finding satisfaction and reaching his or her potential. Describing, and often reexperiencing, old conflicts generally awakens high levels of anxiety in the patient. Patients may use various defenses against anxiety and displace their feelings onto the nurse. Therefore during the working phase, intense emotions such as anxiety, anger, self-hatred, hopelessness, and helplessness may surface. Defense mechanisms, such as acting out anger inappropriately, withdrawing, intellectualizing, manipulating, and denying, are to be expected.

During the working phase, the patient may unconsciously transfer strong feelings into the present and onto the nurse that belong to significant others from the past (transference). The emotional responses and behaviors in the patient may also awaken strong countertransference feelings in the nurse. The nurse's awareness of personal feelings and reactions to the patient are vital for effective interaction with the patient.

Termination Phase

The termination phase is the final, integral phase of the nurse–patient relationship. Termination is discussed during the first interview and again during the working stage at appropriate times. Termination may occur when the patient is discharged or when the student's clinical rotation ends. Basically, the tasks of termination are as follows:

- Summarizing the goals and objectives achieved in the relationship
- Discussing ways for the patient to incorporate into daily life any new coping strategies learned during the time spent with the nurse
- Reviewing situations that occurred during the time spent together
- Exchanging memories, which can help validate the experience for both nurse and patient and facilitate closure of that relationship

Termination often awakens strong feelings in both the nurse and patient. Termination of the relationship signifies a loss for both, although the intensity and meaning of termination may be different for each. If a patient has unresolved feelings of abandonment, loneliness, or rejection, these feelings may be reawakened during the termination process. This process can be an opportunity for the patient to express these feelings, perhaps for the first time.

Important reasons for the student or nurse to address the termination phase are as follows:

- Feelings are aroused in both the patient and the nurse with regard to the experience they have shared; when these feelings are recognized and shared, patients learn that it is acceptable to feel sadness and loss when they lose someone for whom they care.
- Termination can be a learning experience; patients can learn that they are important to at least one person.
- By sharing the termination experience with the patient, the nurse demonstrates caring for the patient.
- This may be the first successful termination experience for the patient.

When a nurse/advanced practice nurse has been working with a patient for a while, it is important for the nurse to help the patient acknowledge any feelings and reactions he or she may be experiencing related to separations. If a patient denies that the termination is having an effect (assuming the nurse–patient partnership was strong), the nurse may say something like, "Goodbyes are difficult for people. Often they remind us of other goodbyes. Tell me about another separation in the past." If the patient appears to be displacing anger, either by withdrawing or by being overtly angry at the nurse, the nurse may use generalized statements such as, "People may experience anger when saying goodbye. Sometimes they are angry with the person who is leaving. Tell me how you feel about my leaving." New practitioners, as well as students in the psychiatric setting, need to consider their last clinical experience with their patient and work with their supervisor or instructor to facilitate communication during this time.

A common response of beginning practitioners, especially students, is feeling guilty about terminating the relationship. These feelings may, in rare cases, be manifested by the student giving the patient his or her telephone number, making plans to get together for coffee after the patient is discharged, continuing to see the patient afterward, or exchanging letters. Maintaining contact after discharge is not acceptable and is in opposition to the goals of a therapeutic relationship. Often this is in response to the student's need to (1) feel less guilty for "using the patient for learning needs," (2) maintain feelings of being

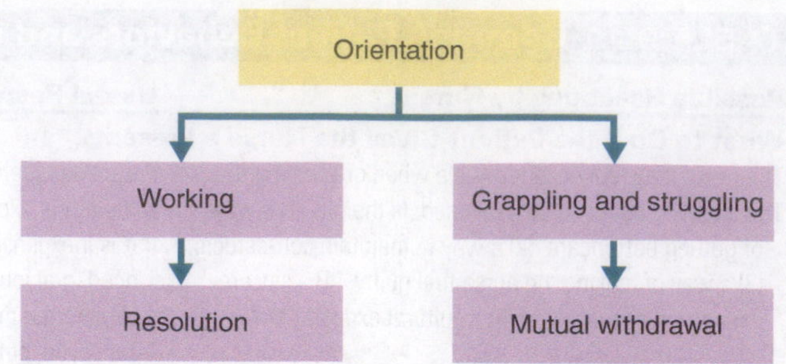

Fig. 9.2 Phases of therapeutic and nontherapeutic relationships. (From Forchuk, C., Westwell, J., Martin, M., et al. [2000]. The developing nurse-client relationship: Nurses' perspectives. *Journal of the American Psychiatric Nurses Association, 6*[1], 3–10.)

"important" to the patient, or (3) sustain the illusion that the student is the only one who "understands" the patient, among other student-centered rationales.

Indeed, part of the termination process may be to explore, after discussion with the patient's case manager, the patient's plans for the future: where the patient can go for help, which agencies to contact, and which people may best help the patient find appropriate and helpful resources.

WHAT HINDERS AND WHAT HELPS

Not all nurse–patient relationships follow the classic phases as outlined by Peplau. Some nurse–patient relationships start in the orientation phase but move to a mutually frustrating phase and finally to mutual withdrawal (Fig. 9.2).

A classic study by Forchuk and associates (2000) is still relevant today. Forchuk and her associates conducted a qualitative study of the nurse–patient relationship. They examined the phases of both the therapeutic and the nontherapeutic relationship. From the data, they identified certain behaviors that were beneficial to the progression of the nurse–patient relationship as well as those that hampered the development of this relationship. The study emphasized the importance of consistent, regular, and private interactions with patients as essential to the development of a therapeutic alliance as well as the importance of listening, pacing, and consistency.

Data findings that enhance the nurse–patient relationship, allowing it to progress in a mutually satisfying manner, include the following:

- **Consistency** includes ensuring that a nurse is always assigned to the same patient and that the patient has a regular routine for activities. Interactions are facilitated when they are frequent and regular in duration, format, and location. Consistency also refers to the nurse being honest and consistent (congruent) in what is said to the patient.
- **Pacing** includes letting the patient set the pace and letting the pace be adjusted to fit the patient's moods. A slow approach helps reduce pressure, and at times, it is necessary to step back and realize that developing a strong relationship may take a long time.
- **Listening** includes letting the patient talk when needed. The nurse becomes a sounding board for the patient's concerns and issues. Listening is perhaps the most important skill for nurses to master. Truly listening to another person, attending to what is behind the words, is a learned skill.
- **Initial impressions,** especially positive initial attitudes and preconceptions, are significant considerations in how the relationship will progress. Preconceived negative impressions and feelings toward the patient usually bode poorly for the positive growth of the relationship. In contrast, the nurse's feeling that the patient is

"interesting" or "a challenge" and a positive attitude about the relationship are usually favorable signs for the developing therapeutic alliance.

- **Comfort and control,** that is, promoting patient comfort and balancing control, usually reflect caring behaviors. Control refers to keeping a balance in the relationship: not too strict and not too lenient.
- **Patient factors** that seem to enhance the relationship include trust on the part of the patient and the patient's active participation in the nurse-patient relationship.

Two Major Factors That Hamper the Development of Positive Relationships

In the study by Forchuk and associates (2000), there seemed to be evidence that **inconsistency** and **unavailability** (e.g., lack of contact, infrequent meetings, meetings in the hallway) on the part of the nurse, patient, or both, hindered the progress of the nurse–patient relationship. When nurse and patient are reluctant to spend time together and meeting times become sporadic and/or superficial, the term *mutual avoidance* is used. This is clearly a lose-lose situation.

The nurse's feelings and lack of self-awareness are major elements that contribute to the lack of progression of positive relationships. Negative preconceived ideas about the patient and negative feelings (e.g., discomfort, dislike, fear, and avoidance) seem to be a constant in relationships that end in frustration and mutual withdrawal. Sometimes these feelings are known, and sometimes the nurse is only vaguely aware of them.

Factors That Enhance Growth

Rogers and Truax (1967) in their classic text identified three personal characteristics that help promote change and growth in patients, which are classic guidelines for establishing a therapeutic alliance or relationship: (1) genuineness, (2) empathy, and (3) positive regard. These are some of the intangibles that are at the heart of the art of nursing.

Genuineness

Genuineness, or self-awareness of one's feelings as they arise within the relationship and the ability to communicate them when appropriate, is a key ingredient in building trust. When a person is genuine, one gets the sense that what is displayed on the outside of the person is congruent with the internal processes. It is conveyed by listening to and communicating with others without distorting their messages and by being clear and concrete in communications with patients. Being genuine in a therapeutic relationship implies the ability to use therapeutic communication tools in an appropriately spontaneous manner, rather than rigidly or in a parrot-like fashion.

Empathy

Empathy is a complex multidimensional concept that has moral, cognitive, emotional, and behavioral components. Perhaps Carl Rogers (1980), in his classic writing, defined empathy the most clearly:

> It means entering the private perceptual world of the other and becoming thoroughly at home with it. It involves being sensitive, moment by moment, to the changing felt meanings which flow in this other person, to the fear or rage or tenderness or confusion or whatever that he or she is experiencing. It means temporarily living in the other's life, moving about in it delicately without making judgments. (p. 142)

Therefore empathy signifies a central focus and feeling with and within the patient's world.

Empathy Versus Sympathy. There is much confusion regarding empathy versus sympathy. A simple way to distinguish them is that in empathy, we *understand* the feelings of others. In sympathy, we *feel* the feelings of others. When a helping person is feeling sympathy for another, objectivity is lost, and the ability to assist the patient in solving a personal problem ceases. Furthermore, sympathy is associated with feelings of pity and commiseration. Although these are considered nurturing human traits, they may not be particularly useful in a therapeutic relationship. When people express sympathy, they express agreement with another, which in some situations may discourage further exploration of a person's thoughts and feelings.

The following examples are given to clarify the distinction between empathy and sympathy. A friend tells you that her mother was just diagnosed with inoperable cancer. Your friend then begins to cry and pounds the table with her fist.

> *Sympathetic response:* "I know exactly how you feel. My mother was hospitalized last year, and it was awful. I was so depressed. I still get upset just thinking about it." *(You go on to tell your friend about the incident.)*

Sometimes when nurses try to be sympathetic, they are apt to project their own feelings onto those of the patient, which thus limits the patient's range of responses. A more useful response might be as follows:

> *Empathic response:* "How upsetting this must be for you. Something similar happened to my mother last year, and I had so many mixed emotions. What thoughts and feelings are you having?" *(You continue to stay with your friend and listen to his or her thoughts and feelings.)*

In the practice of psychotherapy or counseling, empathy is an essential ingredient in a therapeutic relationship, both for the better-functioning patient and for the patient who functions at a more primitive level.

Positive Regard

Positive regard implies respect. It is the ability to view another person as being worthy of caring about and as someone who has strengths and achievement potential. Positive regard is usually communicated indirectly by actions rather than directly by words.

Attitudes

One attitude through which a nurse might convey respect is a willingness to work with the patient. That is, the nurse takes the patient and the relationship seriously. The experience is viewed not as "a job," "part of a course," or "time spent talking," but as an opportunity to work with patients to help them develop personal resources and actualize more of their potential in living.

Actions

Some actions that manifest an attitude of respect are attending, suspending value judgments, and helping patients develop their own resources.

Attending

Attending behavior is a crucial element in a successful interview. To succeed, nurses must pay attention to their patients in culturally and individually appropriate ways. *Attending* is a special kind of listening that refers to an intensity of presence or being with the patient. At times, simply being with another person during a painful time can make a difference.

Body posture, eye contact, and body language are nonverbal behaviors that reflect the degree of attending and are highly culturally influenced. The cultural components of body posture, eye contact, and body language are covered in more detail in Chapter 8.

Suspending Value Judgments

Although we will always have personal opinions, nurses are more effective when they guard against using their own value systems to judge patients' thoughts, feelings, or behaviors. For example, if a patient is taking drugs or is involved in risky sexual behavior, you might recognize that these behaviors are hindering the patient from living a more satisfying life, posing a potential health threat, or preventing the patient from developing satisfying relationships. However, labeling these activities as good or bad is not useful. Rather, focus on exploring the behavior of the patient, and work toward identifying the thoughts and feelings that influence this behavior. Judgmental behavior on the part of the nurse will most likely interfere with further exploration and hinder communication.

The first steps in eliminating judgmental thinking and behaviors are to (1) recognize their presence, (2) identify how or where you learned these responses to the patient's behavior, and (3) construct alternative ways to view the patient's thinking and behavior. Denying judgmental thinking will only compound the problem (Sommers-Flanagan & Sommers-Flanagan, 2017). Refer to the following example:

Patient: I am really sexually promiscuous, and I love to gamble when I have money. I have sex whenever I can find a partner and spend most of my time in the casino. This has been going on for at least 3 years."

A judgmental response would be the following:

Nurse A: "So your promiscuous sexual and compulsive gambling behaviors really haven't brought you much happiness, have they? You are running away from your problems and could end up with AIDS, broke, or even dead."

A more helpful response would be the following:

Nurse B: "So, your sexual and gambling activities are part of the picture also. You sound as if these activities are not making you happy."

In this example, Nurse B focuses on the patient's behaviors and the possible meaning they might have to the patient. Nurse B does not introduce personal value statements or prejudices regarding promiscuous behavior. Empathy and positive regard are essential qualities of a successful nurse–patient relationship.

Helping Patients Develop Resources

Through therapeutic communication, the nurse becomes aware of patients' strengths and encourages patients to work at their optimal level of functioning. The nurse does not act *for* patients unless absolutely necessary, and then only as a step toward helping them act on their own. It is important that patients remain as independent as possible to develop new resources for problem solving.

Patient: "This medication makes my mouth so dry. Could you get me something to drink?"

Nurse: "There is juice in the refrigerator. I'll wait here for you until you get back."

or

Nurse: "I'll walk with you while you get some juice from the refrigerator."

or

Patient: "Could you ask the doctor to let me have a pass for the weekend?"

Nurse: "Your doctor will be on the unit this afternoon. I'll let her know that you want to speak with her."

Consistently encouraging patients to use their own resources helps minimize feelings of helplessness and dependency and validates the potential for change.

THE CLINICAL INTERVIEW

The content and direction of the clinical interview are decided by the patient. The patient leads. The nurse employs communication skills and active listening to better understand the patient's situation. During the clinical interview, the nurse provides the opportunity for the patient to reach specific goals, including the following:

- To feel safe
- To feel understood and comfortable
- To identify and explore problems relating to others
- To discuss healthy ways of meeting emotional needs
- To experience a satisfying interpersonal relationship

Preparing for the Interview

Helping a person with an emotional or medical problem is rarely a straightforward task. The goal of assisting a patient to regain psychological or physiological stability can be difficult to achieve. Extremely important to any kind of counseling is permitting the patient to set the pace of the interview, no matter how slow the progress may be (Arnold & Boggs, 2016).

Setting

Effective communication can take place almost anywhere. However, because the quality of the interaction—whether in a clinic, an inpatient unit, an office, or the patient's home—depends on the degree to which the nurse and patient feel safe, establishing a setting that enhances feelings of security can be important to the helping relationship. A health care setting, a conference room, or a quiet part in the unit that has relative privacy but is within view of others is ideal. When the interview takes place in the home, it offers the nurse a valuable opportunity to assess the person in the context of everyday life.

Seating

In all settings, chairs need to be arranged so that conversation can take place in normal tones of voice and eye contact can be comfortably maintained or avoided. For example, a nonthreatening physical environment for nurse and patient would involve the following:

- Assuming the same height, either both sitting or both standing.
- Avoiding a face-to-face stance when possible; a 90- to 120-degree angle or side-by-side position may be less intense, and the patient and nurse can look away from each other without discomfort.
- Providing safety and psychological comfort in terms of exiting the room. The patient should not be positioned between the nurse and the door, nor should the nurse be positioned in such a way that the patient feels trapped in the room.
- Avoiding a desk barrier between the nurse and the patient.

Introductions

In the orientation phase, students tell the patient who they are, what the purpose of the meeting is, and how long and at what time they will be meeting with the patient. The issue of confidentiality is addressed during the initial interview. Please remember that all health care professionals must respect the private, personal, and confidential nature of the patient's communication except in specific situations as outlined earlier (e.g., harm to self or others, child abuse, elder abuse). What is discussed with staff and your clinical group in conference should not be discussed outside with others, no matter who they are (e.g., patient's relatives, news media, friends). The patient needs to know that whatever is discussed will stay confidential unless permission is given for it to be disclosed.

The nurse can then ask the patient how he or she would like to be addressed. This question accomplishes a number of tasks (Arnold & Boggs, 2016). For example:

- It conveys respect.
- It gives the patient direct control over an important ego issue. (Some patients like to be called by their last names; others prefer being on a first-name basis with the nurse.)

Initiating the Interview

Once introductions have been made, the nurse can turn the interview over to the patient by using one of a number of open-ended statements, such as the following:

- "Where should we start?"
- "Tell me a little about what has been going on with you."
- "What are some of the stresses you have been coping with recently?"
- "Tell me a little about what has been happening in the past couple of weeks."
- "Perhaps you can begin by letting me know what some of your concerns have been recently."
- "Tell me about your difficulties."

Communication can be facilitated by appropriately **offering leads** (e.g., "Go on"), making **statements of acceptance** (e.g., "Uh-huh"), or otherwise conveying interest.

Tactics to Avoid

The nurse needs to avoid certain behaviors, as outlined by Moscato (1988); they still serve as important guidelines today. For example:

Do Not:	Try To:
Argue with, minimize, or challenge the patient.	Keep the focus on facts and the patient's perceptions.
Give false reassurance.	Make observations of the patient's behavior. "Change is always possible."
Interpret to the patient or speculate on the dynamics.	Listen attentively, use silence, and try to clarify the patient's problem.
Question or probe patients about sensitive areas that they do not wish to discuss.	Pay attention to nonverbal communication. Strive to keep the patient's anxiety decreased.
Try to sell the patient on accepting treatment.	Encourage the patient to look at pros and cons.
Join in attacks patients launch on their mates, parents, friends, or associates.	Focus on facts and the patient's perceptions. Be aware of nonverbal communication.
Participate in criticism of another nurse or any other staff member.	Focus on facts and the patient's perceptions. Check out serious accusations with the other nurse or staff member. Have the patient meet with the nurse or staff member in question and senior staff or clinician and clarify perceptions.

Helpful Guidelines

Classic guidelines for conducting the initial interviews are as follows:

- Speak briefly.
- When you do not know what to say, say nothing.
- When in doubt, focus on feelings.
- Avoid advice.
- Avoid relying on questions.
- Pay attention to nonverbal cues.
- Keep the focus on the patient.

Attending Behaviors: The Foundation of Interviewing

Engaging in attending behaviors and listening well are two key principles of counseling on which just about everyone can agree (Sommers-Flanagan & Sommers-Flanagan, 2017). Attending behaviors were addressed earlier but are covered more thoroughly here as they relate to the clinical interview. The nurse/counselor strives to be culturally relevant and individually appropriate in terms of the use of eye contact, body language, vocal qualities, and verbal tracking. Sommers-Flanagan and Sommers-Flanagan (2017) state that positive attending behaviors can open up communication and encourage free expression. However, negative attending behaviors are more likely to inhibit expression. These behaviors need to be evaluated in terms of the cultural patterns and past experiences of both the interviewer and the interviewee. There are no universals; however, there are guidelines that students can follow.

Eye Contact

Even among people from similar cultural backgrounds, there may be variation in what an individual is personally comfortable with in terms of eye contact. For some patients and interviewers, sustained eye contact is normal and comfortable, whereas for other patients and interviewers, it may be more comfortable and natural to make brief eye contact but look away or down much of the time. Sommers-Flanagan and Sommers-Flanagan (2017) state that it is appropriate for most nurse clinicians to maintain more eye contact when the patient speaks and less constant eye contact when the nurse speaks. However, in general, Caucasian patients are more comfortable with more sustained eye contact much of the time; Native Americans, African Americans, and Asian patients often prefer less eye contact.

Body Language

Body language involves two elements: kinesics and proxemics. *Kinesics* is associated with physical characteristics such as body movements and postures. The way someone holds the head, legs, and shoulders; facial expressions; eye contact or lack thereof; and so on convey a multitude of messages. For example, a person who slumps in a chair, rolls the eyes, and sits with arms crossed in front of the chest can be perceived as resistant and unreceptive to what another wants to communicate.

On the other hand, positive body language may include leaning in slightly toward the speaker, maintaining a relaxed and attentive posture, making direct eye contact, making hand gestures that are unobtrusive and smooth while minimizing the number of other movements, and matching one's facial expressions to one's feelings or to the patient's feelings.

Proxemics refers to personal space and what distance between oneself and others is comfortable for an individual. Proxemics takes into account that these distances may be different for different cultural groups. **Intimate distance** in the United States is 0 to 18 inches and is reserved for those we trust most and with whom we feel most safe. **Personal distance** (18 to 40 inches) is for personal communications, such as those with friends or colleagues. **Social distance** (4 to 12 feet) is applied to strangers or acquaintances, often in public places or formal social gatherings. **Public distance** (12 feet or more) relates to public space (e.g., public speaking). In public space, one may hail another, and the parties may move about while communicating with one another.

Vocal Qualities

Vocal quality, or **paralinguistics**, encompasses voice loudness, pitch, rate, and fluency. Sommers-Flanagan and Sommers-Flanagan (2017, p. 56) believe that effective interviewers use vocal qualities to "enhance rapport, communicate interest and empathy, and emphasize special issues or conflicts." Therefore "*It's not what you say, but how you say it.*" Speaking in soft and gentle tones is apt to encourage a person to share thoughts and feelings, whereas speaking in a rapid, high-pitched tone may convey anxiety and create it in the patient. Consider, for example, how tonal quality can affect communication in a simple sentence like "I will see you tonight."

1. "*I* will see you tonight." (I will be the one who sees you tonight.)
2. "I *will* see you tonight." (No matter what happens, or whether you like it or not, I will see you tonight.)
3. "I will see *you* tonight." (Even though others are present, it is you I want to see.)
4. "I will see you *tonight.*" (It is definite; tonight is the night we will meet.)

Verbal Tracking

Verbal tracking is just that: tracking what the patient is saying. Individuals cannot know if you are hearing or understanding what they are saying unless you provide them with cues. Verbal tracking is giving neutral feedback in the form of restating or summarizing what the patient has already said. It does *not* include personal or professional opinions of what the patient has said (Sommers-Flanagan & Sommers-Flanagan, 2017). For example:

Patient: "I don't know what the fuss is about. I smoke marijuana to relax, and everyone makes a fuss."

Nurse: "Do you see this as a problem for you?"

Patient: "No, I don't. It doesn't affect my work … well, most of the time, anyway. I mean, of course, if I have to think things out and make important decisions, then obviously it can get in the way. But most of the time, I'm cool."

Nurse: "So when important decisions have to be made, then it interferes; otherwise, you don't see it affecting your functioning."

Patient: "Yeah, well, most of the time, I'm cool."

Verbal tracking involves pacing the interview with the patient by sticking closely with the patient's speech content (as well as speech volume and tone, as discussed earlier). It can be difficult to know which leads to follow if the patient introduces many topics at once.

Clinical Supervision and Process Recordings

Communication and interviewing techniques are acquired skills. Nurses learn to increase their ability to use communication and interviewing skills through practice and clinical supervision. In **clinical supervision**, the focus is on the nurse's behavior in the nurse–patient relationship. The nurse and the supervisor examine and analyze the nurse's feelings and reactions to the patient and the way they affect the relationship.

> And I would emphasize that, no matter how good we become at being our own inner supervisor, professional help and support from experienced (external) supervisor is essential to good practice. (Fox, 2008, p. 21)

Clinical supervision can also be a therapeutic process for the nurse. During the process, feelings and concerns are validated as they relate to the developing nurse–patient relationship. The opportunity to examine interactions, obtain insights, and devise alternative strategies for dealing with various clinical issues enhances clinical growth and minimizes frustration and burnout. Clinical supervision is a necessary professional activity that fosters professional growth and helps minimize the development of nontherapeutic nurse–patient relationships.

The best way to increase communication and interviewing skills is to review clinical interactions exactly as they occur. This process offers students the opportunity to identify themes and patterns in their own, as well as their patients', communications. Students also learn to deal with the variety of situations that arise in the clinical interview.

In some clinics, institutes, and other places of learning, there is increased use of taping and videotaping of interactions or role-playing for the purpose of learning. However, if taping or videotaping the interaction is not available, the use of process recordings is a good mechanism to identify patterns in the student's and the patient's communication. **Process recordings** are written records of a segment of the nurse–patient session that reflect as closely as possible the verbal and nonverbal behaviors of both patient and nurse, which were introduced in Chapter 7.

KEY POINTS TO REMEMBER

- The nurse–patient relationship/partnership is well defined, and the roles of the nurse and the patient must be clearly stated.
- It is important that the nurse be aware of the differences between a therapeutic relationship and a social or intimate relationship. In a therapeutic nurse–patient relationship, the focus is on the patient's needs, thoughts, feelings, and goals. The nurse is expected to meet personal needs outside this relationship in other professional, social, or intimate arenas.
- Genuineness, positive regard, and empathy are personal strengths in the helping person that foster growth and change in others.
- Although the boundaries of the nurse–patient relationship generally are clearly defined, they can become blurred; this blurring can be insidious and may occur on an unconscious level. Usually, transference and countertransference phenomena are operating when boundaries are blurred.
- It is important to have a grasp of common countertransferential feelings and behaviors and of the nursing actions to counteract these phenomena.
- Supervision aids in promoting the professional growth of the nurse as well as in the nurse–patient relationship, allowing the patient's goals to be addressed and met.
- The phases of the nurse–patient relationship include the orientation, working, and termination phases, which are in reality very fluid.
- The clinical interview is a key component of psychiatric-mental health nursing. Consideration is needed for establishing a safe setting and planning for appropriate seating, introduction, and initiation of the interview.

- Attending behaviors (e.g., eye contact, body language, vocal qualities, and verbal tracking) are key elements in effective communication.
- Cultural background (as well as individual values and beliefs) has a great deal to do with what nonverbal behavior means to different individuals. The degree of eye contact and the use of touch are two nonverbal aspects that can be misunderstood by individuals of different cultures.
- A meaningful therapeutic relationship is facilitated when values and cultural influences are considered. It is the nurse's responsibility to seek to understand the patient's perceptions.

APPLYING CRITICAL JUDGMENT

1. On your first clinical day, you spend time with an older woman, Mrs. Schneider, who is very depressed. Your first impression is, "Oh, my, she looks like my mean Aunt Helen. She even sits like her." Mrs. Schneider asks you, "Who are you, and how can you help me?" She tells you that "a student" could never understand what she is going through. She then says, "If you really wanted to help me, you could get me a good job after I leave here."
   - **A.** Identify transference and countertransference issues in this situation. What is your most important course of action? What, from the classic study of Forchuk and associates, indicates that this is a time for you to exercise self-awareness and self-insight to establish the potential for a therapeutic encounter or relationship?
   - **B.** How could you best respond to Mrs. Schneider's question about who you are? What other information will you give her during this first clinical encounter? Be specific.
   - **C.** What are some useful responses you could give her regarding her legitimate questions about ways you could be of help to her?
   - **D.** Analyze Mrs. Schneider's request that you find her a job. How does this request relate to boundary issues, and how can this be an opportunity for you to help Mrs. Schneider develop resources? Keeping in mind the aim of Peplau's interactive nurse–patient process, describe some useful ways you could respond to this request.
2. You are attempting to conduct a clinical interview with a very withdrawn patient. You have tried silence and open-ended statements, but all you get is one-word answers. What other actions could you take at this time?

CHAPTER REVIEW QUESTIONS

1. Which comment by the nurse would be appropriate to begin a new nurse–patient relationship?
   - **a.** "Which of your problems is most serious?"
   - **b.** "I want you to tell me about your problems."
   - **c.** "I'm an experienced nurse. You can trust me."
   - **d.** "What would you like to tell me about yourself?"
2. A neighbor telephones the nurse daily, giving lengthy details about multiple somatic complaints and relationship problems. Which limit-setting strategy should the nurse employ?
   - **a.** Suggest the neighbor call other people in the community.
   - **b.** Say to the neighbor, "I can talk to you for 15 minutes twice a week."
   - **c.** Use the telephone's caller identification to screen calls from the neighbor.
   - **d.** Tell the neighbor, "You should discuss these concerns with your personal physician rather than me."
3. A patient has been oppositional, demanding, and resistant to working on goals. A mental health nurse tells the nursing supervisor, "We finally had a serious talk. I let that patient know it's time to get right with God and stop this behavior." Recognizing the nurse's actions were not acceptable, select the supervisor's responding action.
   - **a.** Review the facility policies regarding patient's rights with the nurse.
   - **b.** Ask the nurse about documentation related to this patient interaction.
   - **c.** Schedule the nurse for a staff development activity on cultural sensitivity.
   - **d.** Work with the nurse to prepare and analyze a process recording of the interaction.
4. A nurse participating in a community health fair interviews an adult who has had no interaction with a health care professional for more than 10 years. The adult says, "I like to keep to myself. Crowds make me nervous." Which action should the nurse employ?
   - **a.** Refer the adult for a full health assessment.
   - **b.** Explore the adult's family and social relationships.
   - **c.** Ask the adult, "How do you feel about the quality of your life?"
   - **d.** Explain to the adult, "We can help you feel better about yourself."
5. A few nurses are privately discussing patients under their care. Which nurse's comment indicates the need for clinical supervision regarding countertransference?
   - **a.** "My patient is always asking my permission to do something, just like a child."
   - **b.** "When our unit is understaffed, it seems like we have more incidents of disruptive behavior."
   - **c.** "My patient tries to tell me what to do all the time. I got a divorce because my spouse used to do that."
   - **d.** "Our patients have had so many traumatic life experiences. I find myself feeling sympathetic sometimes."

REFERENCES

Arnold, E. C., & Boggs, K. U. (2016). *Interpersonal relationships: Professional communication skills for nurses* (6th ed.). St. Louis: Saunders.

Forchuk, C., Westwell, J., Martin, M., et al. (2000). The developing nurse-client relationship: Nurse's perspectives. *Journal of the American Psychiatric Nurses Association*, *6*(1), 3–10.

Fox, S. (2008). *Relating to clients: The therapeutic relationship for complementary therapists.* London and Philadelphia: Jessica Kingsley Publishers.

Giddens, J. F. (2017). *Concepts for nursing practice* (2nd ed.). St. Louis: Elsevier.

Gordon, C., & Beresin, E. V. (2016). The doctor-patient relationship. In T. Stern, M. Fava, T. Wilens, et al. (Eds.), *Massachusetts general hospital: Comprehensive clinical psychiatry* (2nd ed.). Philadelphia: Saunders/Elsevier.

Halter, M. J. (2018). *Varcarolis' foundations of psychiatric-mental health nursing - E-book: A clinical approach.* (p. 125). St. Louis: Elsevier.

Hays, P. (2008). *Addressing cultural complexities in practice* (2nd ed.). Washington, DC: American Psychological Association.

Moscato, B. (1988). The one-to-one relationship. In H. S. Wilson, & C. S. Kneisel (Eds.), *Psychiatric nursing* (3rd ed.). Menlo Park, CA: Addison-Wesley.

Peplau, H. E. (1952). *Interpersonal relations in nursing: A conceptual frame of reference for psychodynamic nursing*. New York: Putnam.

Peplau, H. E. (1999). *Interpersonal relations in nursing: A conceptual frame of reference for psychodynamic nursing*. New York: Springer.

Rogers, C. R. (1980). *A way of being*. Boston: Houghton Mifflin.

Rogers, C. R., & Truax, C. B. (1967). The therapeutic conditions antecedent to change: A theoretical view. In C. R. Rogers (Ed.), *The therapeutic relationship and its impact*. Madison: University of Wisconsin Press.

Sommers-Flanagan, J., & Sommers-Flanagan, R. (2017). *Clinical interviewing* (5th ed.). Hoboken, NJ: Wiley.

UNIT III

Caring for Patients With Psychobiological Disorders

Sheila Rouslin Welt, MS, APN
Pioneering the Process of Certification in Psychiatric-Mental Health Nursing

Sheila Rouslin Welt is a clinical specialist in psychiatric nursing. She established the first position for clinical specialists in community mental health centers in the state of New Jersey and was among the first private practice nurses in psychotherapy. A longtime editor of *Perspectives in Psychiatric Care*, Rouslin Welt was the first nurse to co-author a book on group psychotherapy and has authored more than 15 articles and book chapters. For 12 years she taught in the graduate psychiatric nursing program at Rutgers University. In addition to being a national and international lecturer, Rouslin Welt has maintained a private psychotherapy, supervision, and consultation practice in New Jersey for the past 30 years.

Although graduate education in the early 1970s permitted a nurse to attain the title of clinical specialist in psychiatric nursing and act as a psychotherapist, the practice of nurse psychotherapy was unprotected by existing nurse practice acts or specialty certification. In the state of New York, anyone could practice as a psychotherapist at that time, but in New Jersey, the Psychology Practice Act specified psychotherapy as within the purview of some disciplines, but not nursing. With the help of psychologist Allan Williams, the New York State Psychological Association's executive director, Rouslin Welt, Marcia Stachyra, and other nurse leaders began the process of certification that would legitimize advanced practice.

The process began within the New York State Nurses Association by revising the Nurse Practice Act to include regulations guiding practice that would legitimize psychotherapy by a properly prepared nurse. This led to the development of post-degree certification through a designated process of clinical supervision and testing. The process became a model for New Jersey and, later, a prototype for national certification.

10

Trauma and Stress-Related Disorders and Dissociative Disorders

Lorraine Chiappetta, Elizabeth M. Varcarolis

http://evolve.elsevier.com/Varcarolis/essentials

OBJECTIVES

1. Differentiate between eustress and distress.
2. Describe some of the common symptoms displayed by people when they experience stress.
3. Describe the fight-or-flight or freeze response of the autonomic nervous system when triggered by an acute stressor.
4. Describe the hypothalamus–pituitary–adrenal (HPA) axis and its role in acute and chronic stress responses.
5. Describe the cluster of symptoms associated with posttraumatic stress disorder (PTSD) and dissociative disorders and the evidence-based treatments of these disorders. **QSEN: Evidence-Based Practice [EBP]**
6. Identify populations that are at greater risk of experiencing trauma and developing dissociative disorders and PTSD.
7. Explain how traumatic brain injury (TBI) is frequently a co-occurring syndrome for those who experience a traumatic injury that leads to PTSD and how this can complicate treatment.
8. Compare and contrast the differences between PTSD and acute stress disorder and dissociative disorders.
9. Describe components of interprofessional and intraprofessional teamwork and collaboration that facilitate safe and effective care for individuals with PTSD, other stress-related disorders, and dissociative disorders. **QSEN: Teamwork and Collaboration; Safety**
10. Describe symptoms associated with secondary traumatic stress/compassion fatigue, why health care workers are especially at risk for developing these symptoms, and ways to mitigate its occurrence.

KEY TERMS AND CONCEPTS

acute stress disorder, p. 124
alternate personality (alter), p. 129
compassion fatigue/secondary traumatic stress, p. 124
depersonalization/derealization disorder, p. 128
dissociative amnesia, p. 128
dissociative amnesia with fugue, p. 129
dissociative disorders, p. 128
dissociative identity disorder (DID), p. 128
distress, p. 120
eustress, p. 120
flashbacks, p. 122
posttraumatic stress disorder (PTSD), p. 121
stress response, p. 121

CONCEPT: STRESS: *Stress* can be conceptualized as "a process with physical, psychological, behavioral and cognitive components in response to an individual's perception of the physical, environmental and psychosocial demands placed on the individual" (Giddens, 2017, pp. 301). Stress has the potential for positive and negative effects on health and well-being.

We do not know if severe stress is a risk factor for the development of a mental illness or if having a mental illness influences the likelihood of adverse stress responses. The nurse helps individuals reduce stress by providing a healing environment and helping the patient develop successful coping strategies.

INTRODUCTION

The *Stress in America* survey of the American Psychological Association examines sources and impacts of stress on the health and well-being of Americans living in the United States. The results of the January 2017 poll showed a statistically significant increase in perceived stress for the first time since the survey was first conducted in 2007. In an August 2017 survey, 3 in 10 Americans said that their stress had increased in the past year, and 20% reported experiencing extreme stress (a rating of 8, 9, or 10 on the 10-point scale) (American Psychological Association, 2017).

We all experience stress, and some stress is "good" stress. **Eustress** is considered normal and beneficial stress. It motivates people to develop the skills they need to solve problems and meet personal goals. However, **distress** causes problems, both emotionally and physically. When individuals feel "stressed out," they often have trouble sleeping or eating, experience physical aches and pains, lose interest in favorite activities, feel tense and become irritable, and often feel powerless. Long-term chronic stress can cause physiological harm and chronic emotional difficulties.

Stressors, the triggers of stress, can be real or perceived. Stressors can be found in the environment, such as loud noises, extreme heat or cold, or other disturbing physical conditions. Stress can be psychosocial, including threats to self-esteem, low social status, and feeling disrespected or stigmatized. Stress can also be spiritual, such as when a person experiences an existential crisis: "What should I be doing with my life?" "Where am I going in life?" "Is there a God? What does God want of me?" Socioeconomic status also plays a role. Wahowiac (2015) contends that poverty is one of the major risk factors in stress and mental health.

We all have individual thresholds for how well we tolerate stress. Some people are more resilient than others, but stress is a part of everyday life for everyone. Responses to stress can be operationally defined (Fig. 10.1).

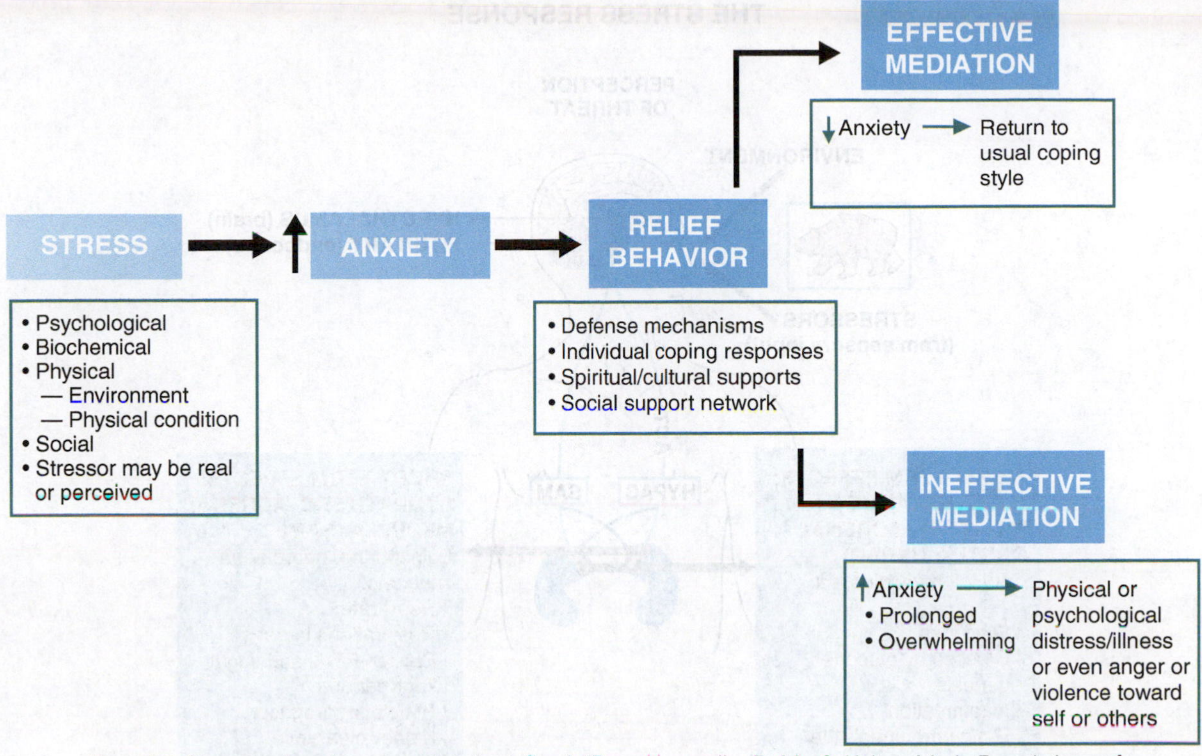

Fig. 10.1 Stress and anxiety operationally defined. (From Varcarolis, E. M., & Halter, M. J. *Foundations of psychiatric mental health nursing.* [6th ed.]. St Louis: Elsevier.)

Physiological and Psychological Responses to Stress

The **stress response** is also referred to as the "fight-or-flight response." This response is a survival mechanism by which the body and mind become immediately ready to meet a threat (or stressor).

When someone is confronted by danger, information is sent to the amygdala, the emotional processing part of the brain. When the amygdala perceives a threat, it instantly sends a distress signal to the hypothalamus.

The hypothalamus acts like a command center by communicating with the rest of the body through the **autonomic nervous system**. This system controls involuntary body functions such as breathing, blood pressure, and heartbeat. The **autonomic nervous system** has two components, the **sympathetic nervous system** and the **parasympathetic nervous system**. The **sympathetic nervous system** triggers the fight-or-flight response, providing the body with a burst of energy so that it can respond to perceived dangers.

Signals are sent to the **adrenal glands**, which respond by pumping the hormone epinephrine (or adrenaline) into the bloodstream. Circulating epinephrine increases the heart rate, elevates blood pressure, increases blood flow to the skeletal muscles, and increases muscle tension. Respirations increase, bringing more oxygen to the lungs, which is then sent to the brain, increasing alertness. These responses happen so quickly that people aren't consciously aware of them.

As the initial rush of epinephrine subsides, the hypothalamus stimulates the hypothalamus–pituitary–adrenal (HPA) axis. If the stress is prolonged, the hypothalamus releases corticotropin-releasing hormone (CRH), which in turn travels to the pituitary gland and triggers the release of adrenocorticotropic hormone (ACTH). ACTH then travels to the adrenal glands, stimulating the release of cortisol. Cortisol helps to supply cells with amino acids and fatty acids for energy and diverts glucose from muscles to the brain to maintain vigilance.

An alternative autonomic stress response that can be added to the fight-or-flight response is called freeze. Clinically, a "freeze" state may look like the person goes blank and stops responding (like a deer in headlights). In the context of an overwhelming trauma in which a person has no hope of escape, like a car accident or an assault, a person may "freeze." Understanding this phenomenon helps to make sense of some of the symptoms exhibited by a traumatized patient.

As the threat passes, the **parasympathetic branch** of the autonomic nervous system promotes the "rest-and-digest" response that calms the body down. Cortisol levels drop as the body returns to a more normal and healthier state.

When stress is prolonged, the body does not return to the relaxed state. A sustained increase in the chemicals produced by the stress response can have damaging effects on the body, causing psychological and physical diseases. It is believed that as many as 90% of diseases are stress related. Stress alone does not cause disease, but it does contribute to it (Harvard Health Publishing, 2016).

The stress response is presented in Fig. 10.2.

POSTTRAUMATIC STRESS DISORDER

The diagnosis of **posttraumatic stress disorder (PTSD)** and its deleterious effects have received increased awareness over the past decade related to the large number of military personnel exposed to war. PTSD is not limited to military personnel. It can occur in *any individual who has had exposure to a trauma severe enough to be outside the range of normal human experience* (American Psychiatric Association [APA], 2013). Specific examples of trauma include physical abuse, torture/kidnap, sexual assault, natural disasters, accidents, and crime-related and terrorist events. PTSD can also occur in people who have *witnessed* an unbearable event, such as a first responder answering a call to a violent incident. The common element in all these experiences is the individual's feelings of

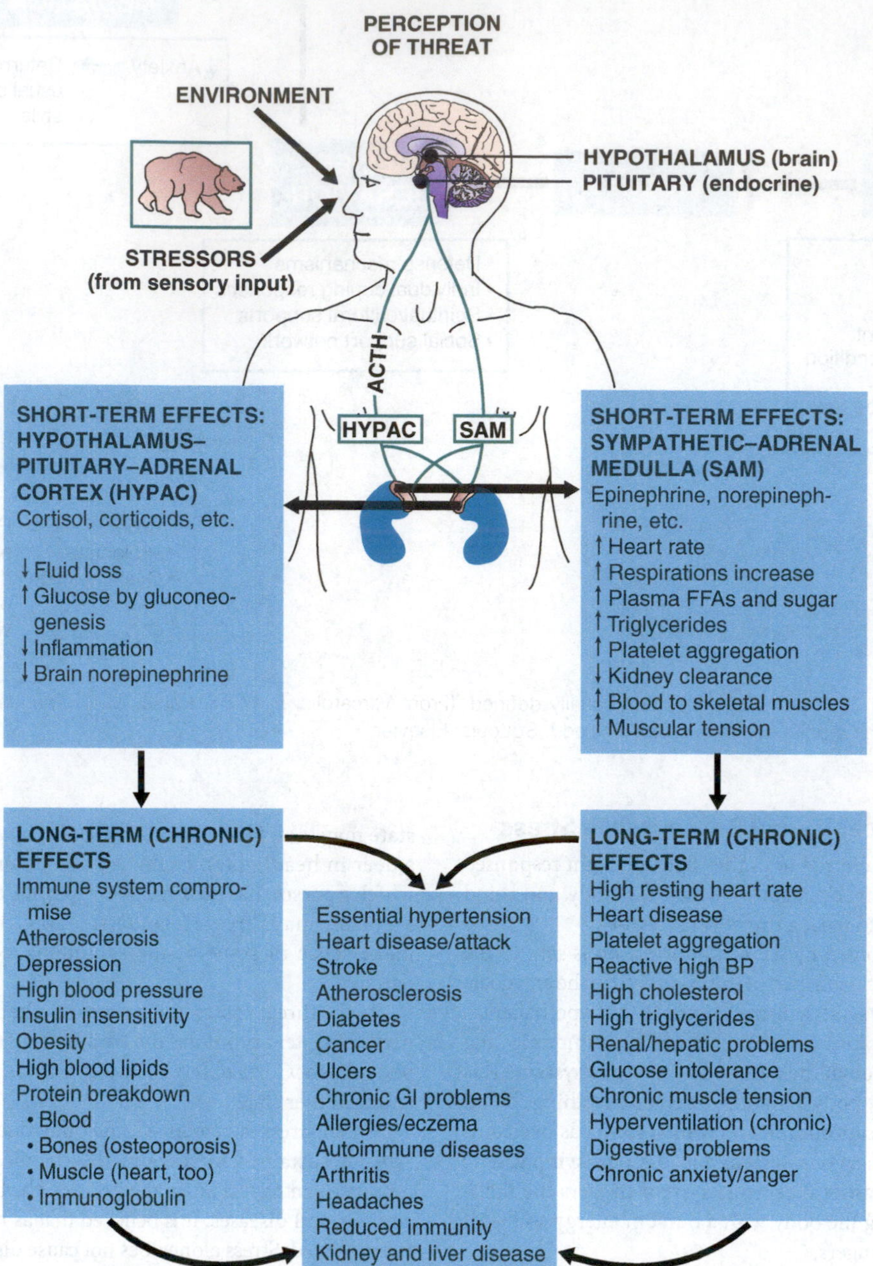

Fig. 10.2 The stress response. (*BP,* Blood pressure; *FFAs,* free fatty acids; *GI,* gastrointestinal.) (From Brigham, D.D. [1994]. *Imagery for getting well: clinical applications for behavioral medicine.* Copyright © 1994 by Deirdre Davis Brigham. Used by permission of W. W. Norton & Company, Inc.)

extraordinary helplessness or powerlessness in the face of overwhelming circumstances.

In addition to experiencing a traumatic event, the four categories of symptoms of PTSD are as follows (APA, 2013):

- Intrusive reexperiencing of the initial trauma
  - Flashbacks—acting or feeling as though the traumatic event is happening again
  - Recurrent nightmares
  - Unwanted distressing memories of the event
  - Having strong physical and emotional responses of distress when reminded of the traumatic event
- **Avoidance:** attempting to avoid anything that might cause recall of the event
- **Alteration in arousal:** includes increased irritability, angry outbursts, self-destructive behavior, exaggerated startle response, hypervigilance, sleep difficulties
- **Persistent negative alterations in cognition and mood:** includes distorted cognitions about self and others leading to excessive fear, guilt, and feelings of detachment

People who have been diagnosed with PTSD may also experience **dissociative symptoms**, or recurrent feelings of being detached. This can include a *flashback*, feeling you are losing touch with events going on around you, and *"blanking out,"* or being unable to remember a period of time.

The symptoms of PTSD are terrifying and often disrupt a person's ability to carry out daily activities. The symptoms must last longer than a month for a diagnosis to be made (APA, 2013).

DSM-5 DIAGNOSTIC CRITERIA

Posttraumatic Stress Disorder

Note: The following criteria apply to adults, adolescents, and children older than 6 years. For children 6 years and younger, see the corresponding criteria that follow.

A. Exposure to actual or threatened death, serious injury, or sexual violence in one (or more) of the following ways:
   1. Directly experiencing the traumatic event(s).
   2. Witnessing, in person, the event(s) as it (they) occurred to others.
   3. Learning that the traumatic event(s) occurred to a close family member or close friend. In cases of actual or threatened death of a family member or friend, the event(s) must have been violent or accidental.
   4. Experiencing repeated or extreme exposure to aversive details of the traumatic event(s) (e.g., first responders collecting human remains; police officers repeatedly exposed to details of child abuse).

   Note: Criterion A4 does not apply to exposure through electronic media, television, movies, or pictures, unless this exposure is work related.

B. Presence of one (or more) of the following intrusion symptoms associated with the traumatic event(s), beginning after the traumatic event(s) occurred:
   1. Recurrent, involuntary, and intrusive distressing memories of the traumatic event(s).

   Note: In children older than 6 years, repetitive play may occur in which themes or aspects of the traumatic event(s) are expressed.

   2. Recurrent distressing dreams in which the content and/or effect of the dream is/are related to the traumatic event(s).

   Note: In children, there may be frightening dreams without recognizable content.

   3. Dissociative reactions (e.g., flashbacks) in which the individual feels or acts as if the traumatic event(s) were recurring. (Such reactions may occur on a continuum, with the most extreme expression being a complete loss of awareness of present surroundings.)

   Note: In children, trauma-specific reenactment may occur in play.

   4. Intense or prolonged psychological distress at exposure to internal or external cues that symbolize or resemble an aspect of the traumatic event(s).
   5. Marked physiological reactions to internal or external cues that symbolize or resemble an aspect of the traumatic event(s).

C. Persistent avoidance of stimuli associated with the traumatic event(s), beginning after the traumatic event(s) occurred, as evidenced by one or both of the following:
   1. Avoidance of or efforts to avoid distressing memories, thoughts, or feelings about or closely associated with the traumatic event(s).
   2. Avoidance of or efforts to avoid external reminders (people, places, conversations, activities, objects, situations) that arouse distressing memories, thoughts, or feelings about or closely associated with the traumatic event(s).

D. Negative alterations in cognitions and mood associated with the traumatic event(s), beginning or worsening after the traumatic event(s) occurred, as evidenced by two (or more) of the following:
   1. Inability to remember an important aspect of the traumatic event(s) (typically due to dissociative amnesia and not to other factors such as head injury, alcohol, or drugs).
   2. Persistent and exaggerated negative beliefs or expectations about oneself, others, or the world (e.g., "I am bad," "No one can be trusted," "The world is completely dangerous," "My whole nervous system is permanently ruined").
   3. Persistent, distorted cognitions about the cause or consequences of the traumatic event(s) that lead the individual to blame himself or herself or others.
   4. Persistent negative emotional state (e.g., fear, horror, anger, guilt, or shame).
   5. Markedly diminished interest or participation in significant activities.
   6. Feelings of detachment or estrangement from others.
   7. Persistent inability to experience positive emotions (e.g., inability to experience happiness, satisfaction, or loving feelings).

E. Marked alterations in arousal and reactivity associated with the traumatic event(s), beginning or worsening after the traumatic event(s) occurred, as evidenced by two (or more) of the following:
   1. Irritable behavior and angry outbursts (with little or no provocation) typically expressed as verbal or physical aggression toward people or objects.
   2. Reckless or self-destructive behavior.
   3. Hypervigilance.
   4. Exaggerated startle response.
   5. Problems with concentration.
   6. Sleep disturbance (e.g., difficulty falling or staying asleep or restless sleep).
   7. Duration of the disturbance (Criteria B, C, D, and E) is more than 1 month.
   8. The disturbance causes clinically significant distress or impairment in social, occupational, or other important areas of functioning.
   9. The disturbance is not attributable to the physiological effects of a substance (e.g., medication, alcohol) or another medical condition.

Specify Whether:

With dissociative symptoms: The individual's symptoms meet the criteria for posttraumatic stress disorder, and in addition, in response to the stressor, the individual experiences persistent or recurrent symptoms of either of the following:
1. Depersonalization: Persistent or recurrent experiences of feeling detached from, and as if one were an outside observer of, one's mental processes or body (e.g., feeling as though one were in a dream; feeling a sense of unreality of self or body or of time moving slowly).
2. Derealization: Persistent or recurrent experiences of unreality of surroundings (e.g., the world around the individual is experienced as unreal, dreamlike, distant, or distorted).

Note: To use this subtype, the dissociative symptoms must not be attributable to the physiological effects of a substance (e.g., blackouts, behavior during alcohol intoxication) or another medical condition (e.g., complex partial seizures).

Specify If:

With delayed expression: If the full diagnostic criteria are not met until at least 6 months after the event (although the onset and expression of some symptoms may be immediate).

From the American Psychiatric Association. (2013). *Diagnostic and statistical manual of mental disorders* (5th ed.). Washington, DC: Author.

Symptoms of PTSD can be hard to identify, especially when the symptoms occur months after the initial trauma. A simple way to remember the general symptoms of PTSD is the use of the memory tool **TRAUMA:**

- Traumatic event
- Re-experiencing the trauma (intrusive memories and nightmares)
- Avoiding things associated with the trauma; and emotional numbing
- Unable to function
- For 1 Month
- Increased Arousal (hypervigilance, startle response)

During the assessment process, the generalist nurse can play a significant role in the recognition of symptoms that suggest PTSD so that appropriate referrals for a more comprehensive assessment can be facilitated.

Prevalence

About 60% of men and 50% of women will experience at least one trauma in their lives. Women are more likely to experience sexual assault, child sexual abuse, domestic violence, or the sudden loss of a loved one. Men are more likely to experience accidents, physical assault, combat, or disasters and to witness death or injury.

The incidence of PTSD is as follows:

- About 7% to 8% of the population will develop PTSD at some point in their lives.
- About 8 million adults have PTSD during a given year.
- About 10% of women and 4% of men develop PTSD sometime in their lives.

The incidence of PTSD varies across different studies and populations (Chang et al., 2017).

PTSD and the Military

The number of veterans with PTSD varies by service era:

- Operations Iraqi Freedom (OIF) and Enduring Freedom (OEF): 11% to 20% experience PTSD in a given year.
- Gulf War (Desert Storm): 12% experience PTSD in a given year.
- Vietnam War (estimated): 30% of Vietnam veterans have had PTSD in their lifetime.

Another source of PTSD in the military population is related to military sexual trauma (MST), defined as sexual harassment or sexual assault that occurs while you are in the military. The incidence of MST is as follows:

- Twenty-three percent of women reported sexual assault when in the military.
- Fifty-five percent of women and 38% of men have experienced sexual harassment when in the military.
- At least half of all veterans who experience military sexual trauma are men (U.S. Department of Veterans Affairs, 2016).

Risk Factors and Comorbid Conditions

There are factors that predispose individuals to develop PTSD in the context of a traumatic event(s): age at traumatic event, female gender, personal or family history of psychiatric illness, and lower education level are all reported as pre-traumatic risk factors across trauma types (Chang et al., 2017).

Cardiovascular disease, bipolar disorder, and major depressive disorder are the disorders that most significantly increase the risk of developing PTSD (Chang et al., 2017).

In the veteran population, factors that increase the risk of PTSD include some of the ones listed previously: younger age, female gender, and lower education. Other factors specific to veterans include racial minority status, lower socioeconomic status, lower military rank, higher number of deployments, longer deployments, prior psychological problems, and lack of social support from family, friends, and community (Reisman, 2016).

Multiple studies indicate a wide range of common comorbidities associated with PTSD. PTSD may lead to poor health through a complex interaction between biological and psychological mechanisms. The current thinking is that the experience of trauma brings about neurochemical changes in the brain that potentially affect all body systems. Both gamma-aminobutyric acid (GABA) and glutamate play a role in encoding fear memories and are implicated in PTSD.

An increased incidence of cardiovascular diseases in those with PTSD is the most substantiated comorbid condition. Cancer, diabetes, obesity, angina, hypertension, gastrointestinal disorders, and arthritis are also associated with PTSD (Chang et al., 2017). Musculoskeletal disorders, abnormalities in thyroid and other hormone functions, and increased susceptibility to infections and immunologic disorders have all been associated with PTSD. The risk of developing dementia later in life is higher for those with PTSD (Jankowsi, 2017).

The most prevalent comorbid mental illnesses are depressive disorders, anxiety disorders, and substance-related disorders. Comorbid depression is very common in PTSD, with a prevalence as high as 50%. PTSD is also associated with sleep disturbances, including nightmares and insomnia.

A body of research indicates that there is an increased risk of suicide in all trauma survivors (Hudenko et al., 2018). Specifically, childhood abuse and a history of MST both increase the risk of suicide and intentional self-harm. Studies show that trauma from exposure to suicide (e.g., witnessing a suicide) can also contribute to PTSD. Finally, PTSD has been found to be a potential risk factor for suicide for all combat veterans (Hudenko et al., 2018).

Several studies indicate that 40% to 50% of individuals with lifetime PTSD also met criteria for substance use disorders (SUDs) (U.S. Department of Veterans Affairs, 2017). Misuse of substances may begin as an attempt to decrease anxiety, depression, and some of the other symptoms associated with PTSD. Responses to chronic stress in PTSD, such as increased substance misuse, poor diet, and inactivity, have the potential to further harm health (McLeay et al., 2017). Difficulty with interpersonal, social, or occupational relationships nearly always accompanies PTSD.

Traumatic brain injuries (TBIs) can be a complicating comorbid condition for some individuals with PTSD. These two disorders may coexist because brain injuries are often sustained during a traumatic experience. An accurate diagnosis is further complicated because there is an overlapping of symptoms of these two disorders. It has been estimated that up to 20% of our combat veterans suffer some degree of TBI related to blast injuries. Even when accounting for predeployment symptoms, prior TBI, and combat intensity, TBI during the most recent deployment is the strongest predictor of postdeployment PTSD symptoms (Yurgil et al., 2014).

Professional athletes who are involved in contact sports, such as boxing and football; individuals who have been involved in accidents or falls; and children exposed to shaken baby syndrome are examples of civilian populations that can potentially develop TBI. High-risk individuals should be screened for this complicating condition, especially when the brain injury is associated with a traumatic event.

PTSD symptoms can begin within a few months after the trauma, but a delay of months or more is not uncommon. Early intervention leads to better outcomes. Most people who go through a traumatic event have stress-related symptoms initially, but the symptoms do not necessarily lead to the development PTSD.

According to Scheier and colleagues (2014), factors predictive of positive outcomes for individuals with PTSD include a solid social support system, good premorbid psychiatric and physical health, and the rapid onset of symptoms.

Acute Stress Disorder

Acute stress disorder can occur after experiencing a traumatic event or repeatedly witnessing a violent or traumatic event. Precipitating traumatic events are the same as those discussed under PTSD. However, in an acute stress disorder, the symptoms resolve within 1 month.

Compassion Fatigue/Secondary Traumatic Stress

Nurses should be alert to **compassion fatigue**, sometimes also called **secondary traumatic stress**. These terms describe a phenomenon in which nurses and other health care workers become *indirectly*

APPLYING EVIDENCE-BASED PRACTICE (EBP)

Problem

A 29-year-old nurse is called in by the director of nursing (DON) to discuss an increase in recent sick days and patient complaints of rudeness. The nurse begins crying and says, "I don't know what's wrong; I just don't feel good lately. I wanted to be a nurse so badly, and now I dread coming to work." The DON suspects compassion fatigue (CF) because this is a new nurse who graduated just about a year ago. Further discussion reveals the nurse has recently cared for several patients who died. The nurse reports not feeling supported by coworkers, and a mentor recently left the company.

EBP Assessment

A. **What do you already know from experience?** The workload on this unit has been high. New nurses do better with support and ongoing mentoring. Demands on nurses are higher than ever.

B. **What does the literature say?** Symptoms of CF may include impaired job performance, absenteeism, and high turnover, with physical or mental exhaustion. Perceived lack of support by peers and supervisor can contribute to CF. Higher staff turnover rates within the first 1 to 3 years of a nurse's career may be related to CF.

C. **What does the patient want?** The nurse wants to:
- Feel good about work again and feel like she is making a difference.
- Feel supported in the job.
- Feel confident in her abilities and not be overwhelmed by the workload.

Plan

- The DON recognized that the nurse had not received her full orientation when hired. The DON also recognized that the nurse did not have a mentor.
- The DON acknowledged that the nurse wanted to do a good job and had an appropriate skill set for her experience level.
- Plan:
  - Complete the orientation program.
  - Assign a new mentor.
  - Meet periodically with DON to make sure the nurse is feeling supported and confident.
  - DON will schedule training for the entire staff on self-care and recognizing compassion fatigue.

QSEN Prelicensure Knowledge, Skills, and Attitudes (KSAs) Addressed

Evidence-Based Practice: DON recognized compassion fatigue and used findings from the literature to assist the nurse and the entire team.

Teamwork and Collaboration: By listening to the nurse's concerns and providing a mentor, the nurse feels more supported, and staff conflict is lessened.

Sheppard, K. (2015). Compassion fatigue among registered nurses: Connecting theory and research. *Applied Nursing Research, 28*(1), 57–59.

traumatized when trying to help a person who has experienced primary traumatic stress. The American Bar Organization (2018) summarizes some of the symptoms of secondary traumatic stress:

- Feeling overwhelmed, physically and mentally exhausted
- Inability to function
- Intrusive thoughts/images of another's critical experience
- Difficulty separating work from personal life
- Becoming pessimistic, critical, irritable, prone to anger
- Dread of working with certain individuals
- Depression
- Ineffective and/or destructive self-soothing behaviors
- Withdrawing socially and becoming emotionally disconnected from others
- Becoming demoralized and questioning one's professional competence and effectiveness
- Becoming easily frustrated
- Insomnia
- Lowered self-esteem in nonprofessional situations
- Loss of hope

Nurses who work with and hear the personal stories of patients who have experienced trauma may be vulnerable to compassion fatigue or secondary traumatic stress. Those who are at high risk are nurses who work in hospice care, pediatrics, emergency departments (EDs), oncology, and forensic nursing. Nurses who have unrealistic self-expectations, are overinvolved with the patient, are inexperienced, or are having a personal crisis are also at risk.

Nurses need to practice self-care. Some guidelines include the following:

- Make a concerted effort to put activities in your schedule that add an experience of joy, pleasure, and diversion.
- Allow for mini escapes to relieve the intensity of your work.
- Make an effort to take scheduled breaks during your shift.
- Get medical care to relieve symptoms that interfere with your daily functioning.
- Refrain from the use of alcohol or drugs to self-medicate.
- Reframe the negative aspects of your work by challenging the negativity, finding meaning, and finding aspects in your life for which you are grateful.

Trauma-Informed Care

According to the U.S. Department of Health and Human Services Office on Women's Health (2018), 55% to 99% of women in substance use treatment and 85% to 95% of women in the mental health system report a history of trauma. The Adverse Childhood Experiences (ACE) study conducted by the U.S. Centers for Disease Control and Prevention identified that almost two-thirds of the participants (both men and women) reported at least one childhood experience of physical or sexual abuse, neglect, or family dysfunction in their lifetimes. High ACE scores were associated with increased physical and psychiatric disorders (Withers, 2017).

Trauma-informed care is an approach to treatment that includes an awareness of the prevalence of trauma, an understanding of the impact of trauma on physical, emotional, and mental health, how trauma can impact behaviors around *seeking treatment*, and an understanding that current service systems can potentially retraumatize individuals.

APPLICATION OF THE NURSING PROCESS

ASSESSMENT

PTSD has many comorbid conditions, both physical and psychological. The nursing assessment should first be focused on safety. Because there is a higher risk for suicide in someone who has experienced trauma, the potential for suicide should be assessed. Substance use disorder and withdrawal from substances can also pose life-threatening risks and should be evaluated by nurses and other health care providers. Nurses should also ensure the traumatizing event is not currently a risk. If someone is coming from an abusive relationship, safety procedures should be implemented, such as not disclosing where patients are discharged if the potential abuser calls.

DIAGNOSIS

Table 10.1 lists some of the nursing diagnoses that can be considered for PTSD.

OUTCOMES IDENTIFICATION

The following are the optimal outcomes for the individual with PTSD. The patient will:

- Remain safe
- Recognize the need to keep significant others safe
- Receive treatment for co-occurring conditions
- Attend support groups
- Expand social support network
- Exhibit an increase in restful sleep
- Have fewer nightmares and flashbacks
- Express decreased irritability
- Demonstrate effective anxiety reduction techniques

(Refer to Chapters 20 and 22 for more information about PTSD.)

PLANNING AND IMPLEMENTATION

Psychotherapeutic Treatment Strategies

Although one in five U.S. military personnel serving in combat will suffer some form of PTSD, only half of those who do get diagnosed get treatment. Barriers to treatment include the social stigma associated with mental illness, feeling shame and embarrassment about seeking treatment, perceiving mental illness as a sign of weakness, or feeling that it is possible to "tough it out." Access to timely evidence-based care is also considered to be another significant barrier (PBS News Hour, 2017). The Veterans Affairs (VA) system has initiated programs to destigmatize treatment for mental disorders and to increase access through the use of innovative programs, such as telecommunication systems to provide care to rural areas (Reisman, 2016).

Psychotherapy

The use of psychological interventions is a first-line treatment approach for PTSD. Cognitive-behavioral therapy (CBT) has the strongest evidence for reducing the symptoms of PTSD in veterans. (Refer to Chapter 15 for a detailed explanation of CBT.) Two of the most studied types of CBT are as follows:

- **Cognitive processing therapy (CPT):** teaches the person how to evaluate and change upsetting thoughts experienced since the trauma. Changing thoughts can change how you feel.
- **Prolonged exposure (PE) therapy:** teaches the patient to gradually approach trauma-related memories, feelings, and situations that have been avoided since the trauma. By confronting these challenges, PTSD symptoms decrease (Reisman, 2016).

Eye movement desensitization and reprocessing (EMDR) is an evidence-based psychotherapy for this disorder. EMDR helps to change the way those with PTSD react to memories of their trauma. While thinking of or talking about the traumatic memories, the individual focuses on other stimuli, such as eye movements, hand taps, and sounds.

The VA's National Center for PTSD developed a smartphone application called **PTSD Coach** as a self-management adjunct to psychotherapy. It features reliable information on PTSD and treatments that work; tools for screening, tracking, and handling PTSD symptoms; and direct links to support and help. Nearly 90% of surveyed veterans who used the app were "moderately to extremely satisfied" with it (U.S. Department of Veterans Affairs, 2018). There is a similar version online: https://www.ptsd.va.gov/apps/ptsdcoachonline/default.htm

Psychopharmacology

There are two medications approved by the U.S. Food and Drug Administration (FDA) for PTSD: sertraline and paroxetine. Discontinuation symptoms associated with paroxetine can be problematic and therefore need careful monitoring. Although used off-label, the selective serotonin reuptake inhibitor (SSRI) fluoxetine and the serotonin–norepinephrine reuptake inhibitor (SNRI) venlafaxine are recommended as first-line treatments in the VA/Department of Defense (DoD) Clinical Practice Guideline for PTSD. Second-line treatment includes other antidepressants. The antidepressant vortioxetine, which modulates GABA and glutamate neurotransmission, has shown some initial promise. Anticonvulsants, such as topiramate, are considered if first-line drugs are ineffective. Medical marijuana is sometimes prescribed as an adjunctive medication. The evidence of effectiveness for the off-label use of these drugs to treat PTSD is limited. The use of benzodiazepines is not recommended for the treatment of PTSD because it is considered ineffective and potentially harmful. Unfortunately, these drugs are frequently prescribed. Antipsychotics, anxiolytics, and antiadrenergic drugs are also prescribed for treatment-resistant PTSD symptoms.

Prazosin, a drug that blocks the noradrenergic stimulation of the alpha$_1$ receptor, has been found to be effective in lessening symptoms associated with PTSD and decreasing nightmares. It is important to monitor for hypotension with this medication.

Medications and psychotherapy are frequently used in combination. This strategy treats both PTSD symptoms and many comorbid conditions that complicate treatment (Reisman, 2016). Refer to Table 10.2 for other useful therapeutic interventions. Refer to Table 10.3 for medications used to treat symptoms of PTSD.

Individuals with mild brain injury plus PTSD report cognitive complaints, such as problems with concentration, attention, and memory. A small study demonstrated that methylphenidate use was associated with significant improvements in PTSD symptoms, depressive symptoms, and postconcussive symptoms in individuals with PTSD, TBI, or

TABLE 10.1 Potential Nursing Diagnoses for Posttraumatic Stress Disorder

Signs and Symptoms	Potential Nursing Diagnoses[a]
Nightmares	*Impaired sleep*
Feeling overwhelmed with small stressors	*Impaired psychological status* *Difficulty coping*
Physical injuries from trauma	*Abuse injury*
Feeling sad, isolating, crying	*Risk for depressed mood* *Risk for loneliness*

[a]The International Classification for Nursing Practice (ICNP) is a product of the International Council of Nurses (ICN). Retrieved from http://www.icn.ch/what-we-do/ICNP-Browser/

TABLE 10.2 Therapeutic Approach

Disorder	Therapeutic Modality
Posttraumatic stress disorder (PTSD)	Cognitive-behavioral therapy (CBT): • Cognitive processing therapy (CPT) • Prolonged exposure (PE) therapy Behavioral therapy: • CPT • PE therapy • Eye movement desensitization and reprocessing (EMDR) Self-help strategy: • **PTSD Coach** smartphone app as a self-management adjunct to psychotherapy

both. Cognitive symptoms also improved (Brown University Psychopharmacology Update, 2016).

Nursing interventions are geared toward helping the patient deal with some of the symptoms associated with an acute exacerbation of the illness.

- If the person experiences **intrusive symptoms** such as **flashbacks and nightmares**, it is important to *stay with the patient* to offer reassurance and emotional safety.

TABLE 10.3 Pharmacology Treatment for Symptoms of Posttraumatic Stress Disorder

First Line	Second Line	Other Drug Categories for Treatment-Resistant Symptoms of PTSD
Antidepressants • Sertraline[a] • Paroxetine[a] • Fluoxetine • Venlafaxine	Antidepressants • Nefazodone • Mirtazapine • Tricyclic antidepressants (imipramine) • Monoamine oxidase inhibitors (phenelzine) • Antiadrenergic: • Prazosin (nightmares)	Antipsychotic drugs Anticonvulsants Antiadrenergic drugs Anxiolytics[b]

Drugs in Clinical Trials for Treatment of PTSD

- Anticonvulsants/antiepileptics (e.g., topiramate)
- Drugs that work on GABA and glutamate
- Cannabis
- Vortioxetine (antidepressant)
- Vilazodone (antidepressant)

GABA, Gamma-aminobutyric acid; *PTSD,* posttraumatic stress disorder.
[a]Approved by the U.S. Food and Drug Administration.
[b]Benzodiazepines are not recommended for long-term use.
Adapted from Reisman, M. (2016). PTSD treatment for veterans: What's working, what's new, and what's next. *Pharmacy and Therapeutics, 41*(10), 623–634.

- Help the person to recognize **avoidance behaviors** and to develop strategies to increase social supports. Psychoeducation can be a useful tool in helping significant others provide support to their loved one.
- **Negative cognitions** that lead to survivor's guilt, depression, and anxiety can increase the risk of suicide, self-harm behaviors, and other types of maladaptive coping. Nurses can provide a therapeutic relationship to share concerns and promote adaptive coping. Safety is a priority.
- **Alterations in arousal** can lead to sleep disturbance, angry outbursts, and reckless behaviors. Providing pharmacological and nonpharmacological interventions to facilitate sleep is necessary. Helping the person find adaptive ways to deal with anger and frustration can decrease destructive behaviors.

Registered nurses (RNs) are in a unique position to help change the lives of people who continue to experience symptoms of psychological trauma. The PTSD Toolkit for Nurses (http://www.nurseptsdtoolkit.org), sponsored by the American Nurses Foundation, was developed to teach nurses how to assess, intervene, and make referrals for veterans struggling with the psychological consequences of stress and trauma (including PTSD). The website also has interactive simulations for nurses to practice these skills (Hanrahan et al., 2016). Many of these skills can also be helpful with nonveterans who experience PTSD symptoms.

Stress Reduction Techniques

Some of the most common techniques that people use to combat stress include the following:

- Elicit the relaxation response using meditation, prayer, mindfulness, and deep breathing.
- Perform physical activity. This deepens breathing, relieves muscle tension, and can elevate levels of the body's endorphins, which induces a sense of well-being. Aerobic exercise for 30 to 60 minutes at least three to four times per week is recommended.
- Seek social support from family and friends. Studies have shown that social interactions provide great buffers against stress and help people cope better with stressful events.

Refer to Box 10.1 for selected stress reduction techniques.

BOX 10.1 Selected Stress Reduction Techniques

Relaxation Techniques

1. These techniques can induce a relaxation state more physiologically refreshing than sleep.
2. They help neutralize stress energy and produce a calming effect.

Reframing

1. Reframing involves changing the way we look at and feel about things.
2. There are many ways to interpret the same reality (e.g., seeing the glass as half full rather than half empty).
3. Reassess the situation. We can learn from most situations by asking some of the following questions:
   - "What positive thing came out of the situation/experience?"
   - "What did you learn in this situation?"
   - "What would you do differently next time?"
4. Considering life from another person's point of view can help dissipate tension and develop empathy. We might even feel some compassion toward the person.
   - "What might be going on with your (spouse, boss, teacher, friend) that would cause him or her to say/do that?"
   - "Is he or she having problems? Feeling insecure? Under pressure?"

Sleep

1. Chronically stressed people are often fatigued.
2. Go to sleep 30 to 60 minutes earlier each night for a few weeks.
3. If still fatigued, try going to bed another 30 minutes earlier.
4. Sleeping later in the morning is not helpful and can disrupt body rhythms.

Exercise (Aerobic)

1. Exercise can dissipate chronic and acute stress.
2. It is recommended for at least 30 minutes, three times a week.

Lower/Eliminate Caffeine Intake

1. Such a simple measure can lead to more energy, fewer muscle aches, and greater relaxation.
2. Wean yourself off coffee, tea, colas, and chocolate drinks.
3. Avoid excessive use of alcohol or other substances as stress relievers.

Stress-Lowering Tips for Life

1. Engage in meaningful, satisfying work.
2. Live with and/or love whom you choose.
3. Associate yourself with gentle people who affirm your personhood.
4. Guard your personal freedom, especially your freedom to:
   - Choose your friends.
   - Live with and/or love whom you choose.
   - Think and believe as you choose.
   - Structure your time as you desire.
   - Set your own life goals.

DISSOCIATIVE DISORDERS

We all dissociate or detach at times, such as when we are daydreaming. We sometimes say we're on *automatic pilot* when we drive home from work but cannot recall the last 15 minutes of the trip. With dissociative *disorders*, people experience significant dysfunction (Black & Andreasen, 2014).

The hallmark of the **dissociative disorders (DDs)** is a disturbance in the normally well-integrated continuum of consciousness, memory, identity, and perception. *Dissociation* is an unconscious defense mechanism to protect the individual against overwhelming anxiety, usually related to past or current trauma. *Symptoms of dissociation* are present in a variety of mental disorders and have been connected to a higher burden of illness and poorer treatment response. *Dissociative symptoms* are strongly associated with borderline personality disorder. *Dissociative disorders* have overlapping features with PTSD. Patients with dissociative disorders have intact reality testing. They do not display delusional thinking or hallucinations.

Prevalence and Comorbidity

It is estimated that 2% of people experience DDs, with women being more likely than men to be diagnosed. Almost half of adults in the United States experience at least one depersonalization/derealization episode in their lives, with only 2% meeting the full criteria for chronic episodes (National Association for Mental Illness [NAMI], 2018). *Dissociative amnesia,* a specific type of dissociative disorder, affects about 1% of men and 2.6% of women in the general population (Cleveland Clinic, 2016). Identification of the *dissociative process* is sometimes overlooked by mental health clinicians who are not trained to recognize these processes.

Comorbid psychiatric disorders include SUDs, depression and anxiety disorders, eating disorders, PTSD, and personality disorders. These individuals have a higher risk for suicidal thoughts and behaviors, self-harm behaviors, significant sleep issues, and problematic work and relationship issues.

Theory

Risk Factors

DDs are thought to be a protective response to past or present trauma. DDs are frequently seen in children exposed to long-term physical, sexual, or emotional abuse. Natural disasters and combat are additional traumas associated with dissociative disorders (NAMI, 2018).

Biological Factors

The precise neurobiological underpinnings of dissociation remain unclear, but there is evidence for a link between dissociative states/traits and altered activity in multiple brain regions. The prefrontal cortex, the part of the brain responsible for rational thought, and the anterior cingulate cortex (ACC), responsible for emotional regulation and cognitive control, become underactivated. The amygdala, responsible for emotional processing and memory, is overactivated, frequently from extreme and repeated trauma (Krause-Utz et al., 2017).

Altered perceptions of self and *fugue* states (loss of orientation to self) occur with neurological diseases such as brain tumors and epilepsy (e.g., complex partial seizure disorder). This suggests a neurological component to the **dissociative disorders**. *Depersonalization* is also experienced by individuals under the influence of psychoactive substances such as alcohol, barbiturates, and hallucinogens.

Genetic Factors

Several studies suggest that **dissociative identity disorder (DID)**, a specific type of DD, is more common among first-degree biological relatives of individuals with the disorder than in the population at large. There is evidence that patients' family histories reveal an increased incidence of dissociative symptoms in siblings and multiple generations (Black & Andreasen, 2014).

Psychosocial Factors

Learning theory may play a role in the continuation of dissociative traits. Depersonalization, derealization, amnesia, and identity confusion can all be thought of as efforts at self-regulation when affect regulation fails. The child experiencing repeated trauma may have unconsciously "learned" that dissociative symptoms were helpful in reducing the overwhelming distress of the trauma experienced. As an adult, the individual may continue to use this same method of dissociation for any distress even though it is no longer adaptive (International Society for the Study of Trauma and Dissociation [ISSTD], 2020).

Cultural Considerations

Certain culturally bound disorders exist in which there may be episodes of trancelike states that demonstrate running or fleeing behaviors that are followed by exhaustion, sleep, and amnesia. These syndromes include *piblokto* among native people of the Arctic, Navajo *frenzy,* witchcraft, and *amok* among western Pacific natives. These episodes must be differentiated from DDs.

Depersonalization/Derealization Disorder

According to the *Diagnostic and Statistical Manual of Mental Disorders*, 5th edition *(DSM-5)*, **depersonalization/derealization disorder** is characterized by recurrent periods of feeling unreal, detached, outside of the body, numb, or dreamlike or experiencing a distorted sense of time or visual perception (APA, 2013). Specifically, *depersonalization* includes experiences of unreality or detachment from one's ***mind, self, or body.*** *Derealization* is experiences of unreality or detachment from *one's* ***surroundings*** (APA, 2013). During the episodes, reality testing remains intact. The symptoms cause significant distress and life impairment and are not related to a medical condition or substance use. Other conditions to be ruled out include schizophrenia and PTSD.

VIGNETTE: A 48-year-old female is admitted to a medical-surgical unit with complaints of a generalized feeling of numbness in her body. During a thorough assessment, she describes an odd perception when she looks in the mirror of not appearing or feeling like herself. "I don't know how to explain it. It just doesn't seem like me." She also reported a detached or floating sensation and is not feeling fully alert. These symptoms began after her son confided that he was HIV positive. Following a complete medical workup to rule out neurological causes, depersonalization in response to her emotional trauma must be considered.

Dissociative Amnesia/Dissociative Amnesia With Fugue

The *DSM-5* describes **dissociative amnesia** as the inability to recall information about the self, usually of a traumatic nature. The memory impairment may be selective for the traumatic event(s) or a particular time period or for one's entire life history (APA, 2013). The symptoms are not a result of drug use or a medical condition, such as head trauma. **Dissociative amnesia with fugue** is associated with amnesia for one's identity or other important autobiographical information. Bewildered wandering or purposeful travel may be part of the clinical picture of a **fugue** state. Black and Andreasen (2014) report that between 5% and 20% of veterans were amnesic for some part of their combat experience.

VIGNETTE: A real-life example of dissociative fugue is the story of Raymond Powers, Jr., a New York attorney who disappeared one day. After his photo was displayed on the television show *America's Most Wanted,* he was recognized by a resident at a homeless shelter in Chicago, where he had been living for 6 months. Even after speaking with his wife by phone, Mr. Powers was unable to remember his children or previous life. Mr. Powers had experienced prolonged and extreme trauma during the Vietnam War. It is believed that the extreme emotional reaction associated with the terrorist attack on the World Trade Center on September 11, 2001, triggered the dissociative fugue episode.

Dissociative Identity Disorder

Dissociative identity disorder (DID) is formerly known as multiple personality disorder and is the most severe of the dissociative disorders. The *DSM-5* criteria include disruption of identity by two or more distinct personality states or **alternate personalities** (sometimes referred to as "**alters**"). The disruption in identity involves loss of the sense of self, accompanied by alterations in affect, behavior, memory, and functioning. Patients "lose time," meaning they do not have a memory of periods of time ranging from minutes to weeks. During the periods of "lost time," an *alter personality* will be in control of the host person. The patient may be unaware of the other personalities before obtaining psychological treatment. The etiology of DID is believed to be severe and repetitive childhood abuse or trauma. Although once considered rare, DID is estimated to exist in 1% of the population, a rate equal to that of schizophrenia. DID is typically caused by trauma occurring at less than 9 years of age (Tracy, 2017). Up to 90% of patients with this disorder are women, which is consistent with higher rates/more severe abuse in females (Black & Andreasen, 2014). Up to 20% of patients admitted for psychiatric or substance use treatment have symptoms consistent with the diagnosis of DID.

Each alter has its own pattern of personality, perception, and memories. Signs of this disorder in adulthood may include finding clothing or other unfamiliar items in your possession, being recognized by unfamiliar persons, different handwriting on documents, and losing periods of time. The change or switch between personalities may be subtle. Borderline personality disorder traits, including self-harm, often co-occur with DID because of their common etiology of childhood trauma. The disorder causes significant distress or impairment in social, occupational, or other important areas of functioning.

It is important to note that there is a portion of the professional psychiatric community that doubts the existence of a separate diagnosis of DID. Even the reported connection between childhood abuse as a cause of DID has been questioned. There is a significant overlapping of symptoms of both borderline personality disorder and a complex presentation of PTSD that can complicate an accurate diagnosis (Tracy, 2015).

VIGNETTE: A 28-year-old woman is being seen for medication management by a psychiatric nurse practitioner (advanced practice registered nurse [APRN]). In the initial psychiatric evaluation, the patient was conservative, well dressed, and articulate. In the third appointment, the patient was wearing a sweatshirt and jeans, used lots of street jargon, and was dismissive and angry. A few appointments later, the patient was almost childlike; wearing a ponytail; and talking in a higher, lisping tone of voice. The APRN began to suspect DID. When questioned, the patient recognized lapses in time, found clothing in her closet that was not her usual style, and noticed different styles of handwriting in personal documents at work. During treatment, the patient revealed three personalities or "alters." The "main" personality was an electrical engineer; a second alter was a teenage male; and the third "alter" was a young girl, who had memories of abuse. The patient had a history of severe sexual abuse beginning at age 2 and continuing until she graduated from high school and moved out of the house. She has never had therapy but had several long periods of depression with two suicide attempts. She initially came for treatment during a depressive episode.

APPLICATION OF THE NURSING PROCESS

ASSESSMENT

The first area of assessment is a **history and physical examination** to rule out physical conditions that cause symptoms that are similar to dissociative symptoms. The examination must rule out conditions such as head injury, brain diseases, temporal lobe epilepsy, extreme sleep deprivation, and drug intoxication or longer-term misuse of psychoactive substances.

A **comprehensive psychiatric assessment** is the next step of the assessment. Patients rarely present for treatment with a chief complaint of dissociation. The clinician must listen for inconsistencies in the patient's history or for symptoms that just don't fit. The following symptoms are suggestive of a dissociative disorder:

- History of abuse, particularly childhood abuse
- Missing blocks of time
- Reported feelings of unreality, being in a dream-like state, or not feeling like self
- Unrecognized handwriting on personal documents
- Finding clothes/items that there is no memory of purchasing
- Friends report the individual acts like a different person sometimes
- Instances of suicidal gestures or self-harm behaviors with no recall of the event
- Clinician-observed switching of alters or distinct personalities

Self-assessment screening tools can be part of a comprehensive assessment. The **Dissociative Experiences Scale II** (Trauma Dissociation, 2018) is a revised version of a screening tool that looks for evidence of both the symptoms of dissociation and dissociative disorders, especially DID (http://traumadissociation.com/des). Those with PTSD also score higher on these tests because of the overlap of symptoms. The Steinberg Depersonalization Test Questionnaire is another tool (http://www.strangerinthemirror.com/questionnaire.html).

Finally, the assessment process looks for evidence of **comorbid conditions and secondary effects** of these conditions. Safety concerns around suicide and self-harm must be immediately addressed. According to the *DSM-5,* more than 70% of patients with dissociative identity disorder have attempted suicide, and self-harm behaviors are common (APA, 2013). Evidence of acute anxiety, panic attacks, flashbacks, and sleep disturbances must also be specifically assessed. Depressive disorders, anxiety disorders, substance use disorders, and personality

TABLE 10.4 Potential Nursing Diagnoses for Dissociative Disorders

Signs and Symptoms	Potential Nursing Diagnoses[a]
Amnesia or fugue related to a traumatic event	*Disturbed personal identity* *Posttrauma response*
Sudden travel from home with an inability to recall previous identity Presence of one or more personalities	*Disturbed personal identity*
Symptoms of depersonalization; feelings of unreality or body image distortions	*Disturbed body image*
Alterations in consciousness, memory, or identity	*Impaired cognition* *Impaired coping process*
Disorganization or dysfunction in usual patterns of behavior (absence from work, withdrawal from relationships, changes in role function)	*Impaired coping process* *Impaired role performance* *Impaired socialization*
Feeling of being out of control related to memory, behaviors, and awareness	*Anxiety* *Powerlessness* *Risk for spiritual distress*
Interrupted family processes related to amnesia or erratic and changing behavior	*Impaired family coping*
Inability to explain actions or behaviors when in an altered state	*Spiritual distress* *Risk for violence* *Altered perception*
Inability to recall (amnesia): Selected event Entire life Own identity Periods of dissociation	*Impaired memory*
Feelings of suicide or self-harm ideation or harm to others in one or more personalities (alters)	*Risk for self destructive behavior* *Risk for suicide* *Risk for self-mutilation* *Risk for violence*

[a]The International Classification for Nursing Practice (ICNP) is a product of the International Council of Nurses (ICN). Retrieved from https://www.icn.ch/what-we-do/projects/ehealth/icnp-browser

disorders are all comorbid conditions that complicate treatment and therefore require careful assessment. The effect of dissociation or alter personalities on the person's role performance and relationships should also be assessed.

DIAGNOSIS

Patients problems and nursing diagnoses for individuals with a diagnosis of a dissociative disorder are suggested in Table 10.4.

OUTCOMES IDENTIFICATION

The general goals are to develop trust, correct faulty perceptions, heal emotional damage resulting from abuse, and encourage the patient to live in the present instead of dissociating (Moorhead et al., 2013). Recovery from DID usual requires long-term therapy to address the abuse and dissolve the amnesic barriers between alter personalities. Integration of identities into a unified, subjective sense of self and development of more adaptive coping strategies are the ultimate goals of treatment.

Indicators that the short-term outcomes are being achieved include the following:

The patient will:

- Refrain from injuring self
- Report a decrease in perceived distress
- Plan coping strategies for stressful situations
- Report comfort with role expectations
- Verbalize a clear sense of personal identity

PLANNING AND IMPLEMENTATION

Nurses usually only encounter a patient with dissociative symptoms when the patient is experiencing a crisis, usually self-harm, suicidal, or homicidal (harm to others) behavior. Care interventions will focus on safety. In the community setting, the patient may initially seek treatment of a comorbid depressive or anxiety disorder. Planning will address the major complaint with appropriate referrals for treatment of the dissociative disorder. Safety, stabilization, and symptom reductions are the first priorities.

Long term, processing of the traumatic experiences and integration of alters is the last part of formal therapy.

Communication Guidelines

Nurses can offer emotional presence during the recall of painful experiences, provide a sense of safety, and encourage an optimal level of functioning. Trust is a central issue in all the dissociative disorders, especially DID, because of the etiology of trauma and abuse. A gentle and supportive approach will help to build therapeutic rapport. Table 10.5 offers examples of interventions for patients with dissociative disorders.

Health Teaching and Health Promotion

Four goals for psychoeducation for patients and families are as follows:

1. Information: learning about the symptoms of the dissociative disorder, causes, and treatment options.
2. Emotional discharge: having opportunities to talk about frustration and an opportunity to exchange ideas with caregivers and peers.
3. Support full participation in therapy, including medication adherence if prescribed.
4. Self-help strategies. Some of the following are strategies suggested on the peer-support website (Mind for Better Health, 2016):
   - Keep a daily journal to increase awareness of feelings and to identify triggers to dissociation.
   - Preplan strategies to interrupt a dissociative episode.
   - Visualization: use your imagination to create internal scenes and environments that help you feel safe.
   - Use mindfulness to help you stay in the present and to decrease dissociation.
   - Grounding techniques can keep you connected to the present to avoid anxiety-provoking intrusive thoughts that can lead to dissociation.
   - Adopt strategies that facilitate sleep, adequate nutrition, and physical activities to decrease stress. Distress leads to increased dissociation.

Milieu Therapy

A safe environment is fundamental for those with a dissociative disorder. High levels of anxiety can lead to increased depersonalization and dissociative episodes. An environment that is quiet, structured, and supportive decreases anxiety.

TABLE 10.5 Interventions for Dissociative Disorders

Intervention	Rationale
1. Provide a safe environment and frequent observation.	1. Safety is a priority.
2. Reassure patient of safety and security by your presence.	2. Dissociative behaviors can be frightening. The presence of a trusted individual provides feelings of security.
3. Orient the patient to current surroundings if necessary (as with dissociative amnesia).	3. Reduces anxiety and helps patient stay in the present.
4. Establish a supportive therapeutic relationship.	4. The nurse–patient relationship is the vehicle for providing support and effective care.
5. Spend time with the patient and allow venting of feelings.	5. To communicate acceptance and concern.
6. Help the patient identify signs and symptoms of anxiety.	6. Awareness of manifestations of anxiety helps the person to recognize signs of escalating anxiety.
7. Help patient recognize the connection between escalating anxiety and dissociative behaviors.	7. Patient may be unaware of the dissociative response to stress.
8. Help the person identify triggers to dissociative behaviors.	8. Allows the person to respond more adaptively to future stressors.
9. Assess the patient's current methods of coping, watching for self-destructive behaviors.	9. Self-injurious behaviors and suicide attempts are maladaptive responses frequently seen in dissociative states.
10. Teach adaptive coping strategies.	10. Developing new coping strategies facilitates healthy coping.
11. Encourage daily journaling.	11. Journaling can help the patient express feelings, develop a sense of self, and lessen the response to triggers.
12. Teach stress reduction techniques.	12. Provides additional methods of anxiety relief.
13. Use grounding techniques (finding or visualizing a safe place, counting, blanket wrapping).	13. Grounding techniques help the person stay in the present, protect against destructive impulses, and increase a sense of security.
14. Involve the person as much as possible in planning own treatment.	14. Increases sense of responsibility and control.
15. Provide support during disclosure of painful experiences.	15. Can be healing while minimizing feelings of isolation.

APPLYING THE ART

A Person With Dissociative Disorder

Scenario

A student nurse attended a coping skills group at a local psychiatric inpatient facility during her psychiatric nursing rotation and noticed a patient staring out the window, seemingly not paying attention.

Therapeutic Goal

By the end of this interaction, the patient will report one concept or coping skill learned during group.

Student–Patient Interaction	Thoughts, Communication Techniques, and Mental Health Nursing Concepts
Student: "Hello. I'm a nursing student. May we sit down and talk for a bit?"	Giving information, general leads, offering self
Patient: "Sure, that's fine."	
Student's feelings: *Relief that patient was willing to talk.*	
Student: "During the group today, I noticed that you were staring out the window and kind of blanking out."	Making observations, seeking information
Patient: "I really wasn't paying attention after the beginning. I wanted to hear what she had to say; I like that group leader, but next thing I know, I was out of it. I don't remember what she was teaching."	
Student's feelings: *Not what I was expecting; I thought she was just ignoring the group.*	
Student: "What was the last thing you remember before feeling out of it?"	Seeking information, placing event in time or sequence; student is noticing a probable dissociative event; patient is bringing up a connection with her mother
Patient: "I was looking at her outfit, the pink flowered shirt and gray skirt ... it looked so much like an outfit my mother had."	
Student's feelings: *I'm really not sure what to say now.*	
Student: "Would that be a good or bad memory related to your mother's outfit?"	Focusing, exploring; student recognizing there may be some trauma or abuse related to patient's mother
Patient: "There weren't too many good memories with my mother."	
Student's feelings: *I don't know if I have the skills to go down this road with her, not sure what all will come up. Will I hurt her by asking questions about sad memories?*	
Student: "Would it be alright if I passed this information on to your therapist? You could process some of the feelings about your mother. The therapist might be able to help you with some techniques to use when you feel triggered and want to blank out mentally."	Formulating a plan of action, suggesting collaboration, offering support; student recognizing some trained professional help is needed to explore childhood issues
Patient: "That would be fine; I appreciate you noticing that I wasn't all there and taking the time to sit and talk with me."	Goal was not met—my patient did not really pay attention in group to report a new skill. But the interaction was still therapeutic and successful.
Student's feelings: *I feel good about this. She appreciated my support, and I can help the treatment team with more information.*	

There are no specific medications for dissociative disorders, but antidepressants or anxiolytic medications are given for comorbid symptoms. Substance use disorders and suicidal and self-harm risk require ongoing assessment.

Evaluation

Treatment is considered successful when outcomes are met. The evaluation looks for achievement of the following:

- Patient safety has been maintained.
- Anxiety has been reduced, and the patient has returned to a functional state.
- Reduction of acute symptoms, including less use of dissociation.

Psychotherapy

Psychotherapy is used to decrease symptom frequency and improve coping strategies for the experience of dissociation. Some of the more common therapies include (NAMI, 2018) the following:

- *Cognitive-behavioral therapy (CBT)* helps change the negative thinking and behavior associated with depression.
- *Dialectical behavioral therapy (DBT)* teaches mood regulation and improved interpersonal relationships and coping skills like mindfulness meditation, regulated breathing, and self-soothing strategies.
- *Eye movement desensitization and reprocessing (EMDR)* is a specialized technique designed to alleviate the distress associated with traumatic memories.
- Individual therapy focuses on working with the client to process traumatic experiences and effectively control the anxiety.
- Group therapy provides a supportive setting in which concerns, problems, fears, and stressors can be discussed. New and functional ways of coping with stressors can be learned.

KEY POINTS TO REMEMBER

- Some stress is useful. *Eustress* is stress that makes us strive to reach our goals, repair important relationships, improve our work, and stimulate creative problem-solving processes.
- Stress is common. When stress is prolonged and increased, it may be experienced more as *distress*. When stress becomes chronic, it can cause physiological harm and emotional difficulties.
- When confronted with a serious stressor, the autonomic nervous system reacts with the fight-or-flight or freeze response. These responses involve a complex network of nerve pathways, brain structures, and glands to help our bodies and minds deal with the stressor.
- The second part of the stress response is activated by the hypothalamus–pituitary–adrenal (HPA) axis.
- Some suggestions for stress reduction are given in Box 10.1.
- Acute stress disorder (ASD) and posttraumatic stress disorder (PTSD) can occur after experiencing or witnessing a severe traumatic event. ASD resolves within 1 month, and PTSD symptoms persist. It is estimated that up to 20% of our combat veterans return with symptoms of PTSD.
- Left untreated, PTSD can lead to serious consequences, including severe depression, alcohol/substance use disorders, and suicide. It leads to social and occupational disruptions for the patient and significant others.
- Evidence-based pharmacological and therapeutic interventions for PTSD have been identified.
- Nurses and other caregivers are at risk for the development of symptoms of compassion fatigue/secondary traumatic stress. Practicing self-care strategies will reduce the risk of developing this disorder.
- Dissociative disorders involve a disruption in consciousness, with a significant impairment in memory, identity, or perceptions of self.
- Patients with dissociative disorders often have a number of comorbid illnesses: depression, anxiety, substance use disorders, and borderline personality disorder.
- Safety is the priority intervention for patients with a diagnosis of dissociative disorders because of the high risk for self-harm and suicidal behaviors.
- Those with dissociative disorders may require long-term treatment.

APPLYING CRITICAL JUDGMENT

1. A friend named Juan arrives to class, breathing hard and looking pale and shaken. He tells you that he just missed getting run over by a car and that his heart keeps pounding. Once Juan becomes calm, how would you explain to Juan his body's physiological response to the fight-or-flight response?
2. Another friend, Teresa, tells you that she failed the midterm exam and cannot stop thinking about her failure. She feels preoccupied and stressed all the time.
   A. If Teresa is experiencing chronic stress, describe what is happening physiologically.
   B. What symptoms might she be at risk of developing?
   C. What suggestions could you offer both Juan and Teresa that might help reduce their stress?
3. After witnessing a brutal murder of four bank guards 3 months ago, Laura continues to have nightmares and jumps at any loud noise. She tells you that she does not sleep well at night and cannot stop thinking about the traumatic event.
   A. If Laura is diagnosed with posttraumatic stress disorder (PTSD), define other signs and symptoms you might notice.
   B. What other areas would you include in a nursing assessment in order to plan effective interventions?
   C. What medication(s) might be prescribed for Laura if she is diagnosed with PTSD?
4. A patient with dissociative identity disorder (DID) has been admitted to the crisis unit for a short-term stay after a suicide threat. On the unit, the patient has repeated the statement that she will kill herself to get rid of "all the others," meaning her alter personalities.
   A. What safety concerns might you have about this patient?
   B. Knowing that she has DID, what types of information should you gather?

CHAPTER REVIEW QUESTIONS

1. A mature, professional couple plans a large wedding in a city that is 100 miles from their home. Which response is most likely to be associated with this experience?
   a. Distress
   b. Eustress
   c. Acute stress
   d. Depersonalization
2. A college student has been experiencing significant stress associated with academic demands. Last month, the student began attending yoga sessions three times a week. Which outcome indicates this activity has been successful?
   a. The student reports improved feelings of well-being.
   b. The student increases the use of caffeine to enhance concentration.
   c. The student reports, "Now I am sleeping about 10 hours every day."
   d. The student says, "I withdrew from two courses to reduce my academic load."
3. An adult required a heart transplant 5 years ago. Multiple medical complications followed, resulting in persistent irritability, depression,

and insomnia. The adult's spouse says, "I've walked on eggshells for 5 years, never knowing when something else will go wrong." What is the nurse's priority intervention regarding the spouse?

a. Explore the spouse's feelings, showing care and compassion.
b. Encourage the spouse to attend a community support group.
c. Teach stress reduction and relaxation techniques to the spouse.
d. Refer the spouse to the primary care provider for health assessment.

4. A veteran of the war in Afghanistan tells the nurse, "Every day, something happens that makes me feel like I'm still there. My family has grown impatient with me. They say it's time for me to move on from that time in my life, but I can't." What is the nurse's first priority?

a. Assess the veteran for suicide risk.
b. Refer the veteran for specialized mental health services.
c. Assess the veteran for evidence of traumatic brain injury.
d. Refer the veteran's family to a posttraumatic stress disorder group.

5. A patient diagnosed with dissociative identity disorder is hospitalized on an acute care psychiatric unit after a suicide attempt. During a team meeting, which staff nurse's comment should prompt the nursing supervisor to intervene?

a. "I have never taken care of a patient diagnosed with this disorder."
b. "I think this patient was misdiagnosed and probably has schizophrenia."
c. "I find myself more fascinated and engaged with this patient than others."
d. "I recently read an autobiographical book about someone with this problem."

REFERENCES

American Bar Organization. (2018). *Compassion fatigue: What is compassion fatigue?* 2018 ABA, Retrieved March 23, 2018 from https://www.americanbar.org/groups/lawyer_assistance/resources/compassion_fatigue.html.

American Psychiatric Association. (2013). *Diagnostic and statistical manual of mental disorders (DSM-5)* (5th ed.). Washington, DC: APA.

American Psychological Association. (2017). *APA stress in America™ survey: US at 'lowest point we can remember;' Future of nation most commonly reported source of stress*, Retrieved from http://www.apa.org/news/press/releases/2017/11/lowest-point.aspx.

Black, D.W., & Andreasen, N.A. (2014). *Introductory textbook of psychology* (6th ed.). Washington, DC: American Psychiatric Publishing.

Brown University Psychopharmacology Update. (2016). Methylphenidate effective on range of symptoms in PTSD. *Brain Injury, 27*(2), 1–7. https://doi.org/10.1002/pu.30115.

Chang, J.-C., et al. (2017). Comorbid diseases as risk factors for incident posttraumatic stress disorder (PTSD) in a large community cohort (KCIS no.PSY4). *Scientific Reports, 7*, 41276. https://doi.org/10.1038/srep41276.

Cleveland Clinic. (2016). *Dissociative amnesia*. Last reviewed May 20, 2016, Retrieved from https://my.clevelandclinic.org/health/diseases/9789-dissociative-amnesia.

Dissociation FAQ Retrieved from http://www.isst-d.org/?contentID=76.

Dissociative Experiences Scale—II. (2018). Traumadissociation.com. Retrieved Apr 16, 2018 from http://traumadissociation.com/des.

Giddens, J. F. (2017). *Concepts for nursing practice* (2nd ed.). St. Louis: Elsevier.

Grieser, Randy (2008–2017) Critical Incident Group Debriefing–Issues and Considerations, Crisis & Trauma Resource Institute Inc. Retrieved March 24, 2018 from: https://blog.ctrinstitute.com/free-resources/critical-incident-group-debriefing-issues-and-considerations/.

Hanrahan, N. P., Judge, K., Olamijulo, G., Seng, L., Lee, M., Herbig Wall, P., et al. (2016). The PTSD Toolkit for Nurses: Assessment, intervention, and referral of veteran. *The Nurse Practitioner, 42*(3), 46–55. https://doi.org/10.1097/01.NPR.0000488717.90314.62.

Harvard Health Publishing. (2016). *Understanding the stress response*. Updated: March 18, 2016. Retrieved March 23, 2018 from https://www.health.harvard.edu/staying-healthy/understanding-the-stress-response.

Hudenko, W. B., Homaifar, B., & Wortzel, H. (2018). *The relationship between PTSD and suicide, PTSD: National Center for PTSD*. Last updated January 29, 2018, Retrieved from: https://www.ptsd.va.gov/professional/co-occurring/ptsd-suicide.asp.

International Society for the Study of Trauma and Dissociation (ISSTD).. (2020). *Dissociation FAQs*. Retrieved from: https://www.isst-d.org/resources/dissociation-faqs/.

Jankowski, K. (2017). *PTSD and physical health PTSD: National Center for PTSD*. updated February 23, 2016, Retrieved from: https://www.ptsd.va.gov/professional/co-occurring/ptsd-physical-health.asp.

Krause-Utz, A., Frost, R., Winter, D., & Elzinga, B. M. (2017). Dissociation and alterations in brain function and structure: Implications for borderline personality disorder. *Current Psychiatry Reports, 19*(1), 6. https://doi.org/10.1007/s11920-017-0757-y.

McLeay., et al. (2017). Physical comorbidities of post-traumatic stress disorder in Australian Vietnam War veterans. *Medical Journal of Australia, 206*(6), 251–257. https://doi.org/10.5694/mja16.00935. Published online: 3 April 2017.

Mind for Better Mental Health. (2016). *Dissociative disorders how can i help myself cope*, Retrieved from: https://www.mind.org.uk/information-support/types-of-mental-health-problems/dissociative-disorders/self-care/#.Wta5AJdG2Uk.

Moorhead, S., Johnson, M., Maas, M.L., & Swanson, E. (2013). *Nursing outcomes classification (NOC)*. (5th ed.). St. Louis: Elsevier.

National Association for Mental Illness (NAMI). (2018). *Dissociative disorders*, Retrieved from: https://www.nami.org/learn-more/mental-health-conditions/dissociative-disorders.

PBS News Hour. (2017). *The stigma that stops veterans from getting help for PTSD*. Mar 29, 2017, Retrieved from: https://www.pbs.org/newshour/show/stigma-stops-veterans-getting-help-ptsd.

Reisman, M. (2016). PTSD treatment for veterans: What's working, what's new, and what's next. *Pharmacy and Therapeutics, 41*(10), 623–634. Retrieved from: https://www.ncbi.nlm.nih.gov/pmc/articles/PMC5047000/.

Scheier, F. R., Vidair, H. B., Vogel, L. R., et al. (2014). Anxiety, obsessive-compulsive, and stress disorders. In Janice, L. Cutler (Ed.), *Psychiatry* (3rd ed.). New York: Oxford University Press.

Tracy, N. (2015). *Dissociative identity disorder controversy: Is DID real?*, HealthyPlace. Retrieved from: https://www.healthyplace.com/abuse/dissociative-identity-disorder/dissociative-identity-disorder-controversy-is-did-real.

Tracy, N. (2017). *Dissociative identity disorder (DID) statistics and facts, HealthyPlace for your mental health*. Last Updated: 23 May 2017, Retrieved from: https://www.healthyplace.com/abuse/dissociative-identity-disorder/dissociative-identity-disorder-did-statistics-and-facts/.

U.S. Department of Health and Human Services Office of Women's Health. (2018). *Alcohol use disorder, substance use disorder, and addiction*. Retrieved from: https://www.womenshealth.gov/mental-health/mental-health-conditions/alcohol-use-disorder-substance-use-disorder-and-addiction/.

U.S. Department of Veterans Affairs. (2016). PTSD: National center for PTSD, how common is PTSD? Updated October 2016, Retrieved from: https://www.ptsd.va.gov/public/PTSD-overview/basics/how-common-is-ptsd.asp.

U.S. Department of Veterans Affairs. (2017). *PTSD: National center for PTSD, treatment of Co-occurring PTSD and substance use disorder in VA*. Update May 2017, Retrieved from: https://www.ptsd.va.gov/professional/co-occurring/ptsd_sud_veterans.asp.

U.S. Department of Veterans Affairs. (2018). *Posttraumatic stress disorder (PTSD)*. Updated, Reviewed Feb 22, 2018, Retrieved from: https://www.research.va.gov/topics/ptsd.cfm.

Wahowiac, L. (2015). *Addressing stigma, disparities in minority mental health: Access to care among barriers*. Retrieved from: http://thenationshealth.aphapublications.org/content/45/1/1.3.full.

Withers, M. (2017). *Trauma-informed care and why it matters*, Retrieved from: https://www.psychologytoday.com/us/blog/modern-day-slavery/201707/trauma-informed-care-and-why-it-matters.

Yurgil, K. A., Barkauskas, D. A., Vasterling, J. J., et al. (2014). Association between traumatic brain injury and risk of posttraumatic stress disorder in active-duty marines. *JAMA Psychiatry, 71*(2), 149–157. https://doi.org/10.1001/jamapsychiatry.2013.3080.

11

Anxiety, Anxiety Disorders, and Obsessive-Compulsive and Related Disorders

Lorraine Chiappetta, Elizabeth M. Varcarolis

http://evolve.elsevier.com/Varcarolis/essentials

OBJECTIVES

1. Differentiate among normal anxiety, acute anxiety, and chronic anxiety.
2. Compare and contrast the four levels of anxiety in relation to perceptual field, ability to learn, and other defining physical and behavioral characteristics.
3. Define at least six defense mechanisms.
4. Rank the defense mechanisms from healthy to maladaptive.
5. Compare predisposing or risk factors associated with the development of anxiety disorders and obsessive-compulsive disorder (OCD).
6. Describe clinical manifestations of each of the most common anxiety disorders.
7. Describe clinical manifestations of OCD.
8. Describe components of interprofessional and intraprofessional practice that facilitate safe and effective care for a person with an anxiety disorder or OCD. **QSEN: Teamwork and Collaboration; Safety**
9. Identify evidence-based practice interventions for individuals with anxiety disorders and OCD. **QSEN: Evidence-Based Practice**
10. Describe realistic outcome criteria for patients with (a) generalized anxiety disorder (GAD), (b) panic disorder (PD), (c) social anxiety disorder, and (d) OCD.
11. Using informatics, compare the advantages and disadvantages of three classes of medications that have demonstrated evidence-based effectiveness in treating anxiety disorders. **QSEN: Informatics**

KEY TERMS AND CONCEPTS

acting-out behaviors, p. 139
acute anxiety, p. 135
agoraphobia, p. 142
altruism, p. 138
anxiety, p. 143
anxiolytic drugs, p. 153
body dysmorphic disorder (BDD), p. 144
chronic anxiety, p. 140
compulsions, p. 144
denial, p. 139
devaluation, p. 139
displacement, p. 138
dissociation, p. 139
fear, p. 135
generalized anxiety disorder (GAD), p. 142
hoarding, p. 145
idealization, p. 139
mild anxiety, p. 135
moderate anxiety, p. 135
noradrenergic drugs, p. 141
normal anxiety, p. 135
obsessions, p. 143
obsessive-compulsive disorder (OCD), p. 143
panic attack, p. 141
panic disorders (PDs), p. 142
panic level of anxiety, p. 135
passive aggression, p. 138
pathological anxiety, p. 135
phobia, p. 142
projection, p. 139
rationalization, p. 138
reaction formation, p. 138
repression, p. 138
selective inattention, p. 135
selective serotonin reuptake inhibitors (SSRIs), p. 141
severe anxiety, p. 135
social anxiety disorder (social phobia) p. 142
somatization, p. 138
specific phobias, p. 142
splitting, p. 139
sublimation, p. 138
suppression, p. 138
undoing, p. 138

CONCEPT: ANXIETY: *Anxiety* is a subjectively distressful experience activated by the perception of threat, which has both a potential psychological and physiological etiology and expression. Anxiety exists along a continuum: mild, moderate, severe, and panic levels of anxiety (Giddens, 2017). Identification of a specific level of anxiety can be used by the nurse as a guide in selecting effective interventions.

INTRODUCTION

An understanding of the symptom of *anxiety* and *defense mechanisms* used to defend against anxiety is basic to the practice of nursing. Anxiety is the most basic of human emotions to which no one is a stranger. Dysfunctional behaviors are often a defense against anxiety. When the behavior is recognized as dysfunctional, interventions to reduce anxiety can be initiated by the nurse. As anxiety decreases, dysfunctional behavior will frequently also decrease.

ANXIETY

Anxiety can be defined as a feeling of apprehension, uneasiness, uncertainty, or dread resulting from a real or perceived threat whose actual source is unknown or unrecognized. According to the *Diagnostic and Statistical Manual of Mental Disorders*, 5th edition *(DSM-5)*, the physiological response of anxiety is more often "associated with muscle tension and vigilance in preparation for future danger with cautious or avoidant behaviors" (American Psychiatric Association [APA], 2013, p. 189). **Fear**, a similar response, is a reaction to a specific danger, and more often the body reacts "with surges of autonomic arousal necessary for fight or flight, thoughts of immediate danger, and escape behaviors" (APA, 2013, p. 189). *Anxiety* can invade the central core of the personality. It may erode the individual's feelings of self-esteem and personal worth.

"Normal" anxiety is an adaptive life force that is necessary for survival. It provides the energy needed to carry out the tasks involved in striving toward goals. *Anxiety* motivates people to make and survive change. It prompts constructive behaviors.

Acute anxiety is precipitated by an imminent real or potential loss or change that threatens an individual's sense of security. It is frequently triggered by an acute stressor. For example, many entertainers experience acute anxiety before performances. Students may experience acute anxiety before an examination. Patients preparing for surgery often experience acute anxiety.

Pathological anxiety differs from normal anxiety in terms of duration, intensity, and disturbance in a person's ability to function. *Pathological* anxiety occurs when (1) the intensity of the emotional response is out of proportion to the threat, (2) the emotional response persists after the threat is resolved, and/or (3) the emotional response becomes generalized to benign situations. Pathological anxiety can lead to the development of anxiety disorders.

A comprehensive understanding of an individual's anxiety responses is necessary to plan and implement effective nursing interventions to help patients. An understanding of one's own anxiety responses is also essential to provide optimal care.

Levels of Anxiety

Levels of anxiety range from mild, to moderate, to severe, to panic. Hildegard Peplau (1968), a nurse theorist, identified four levels of anxiety. These concepts are based on the work of Harry Stack Sullivan (1953), an American psychiatrist and theorist. Assessment of a patient's level of anxiety is necessary to provide the appropriate therapeutic intervention in all health care settings. Although four levels of anxiety have been defined, the boundaries between these levels are not distinct, and the behaviors and characteristics shown by individuals experiencing anxiety often overlap these categories.

Mild Anxiety

Mild anxiety occurs in the normal experience of everyday living. A person's ability to perceive reality is brought into sharp focus. A person sees, hears, and grasps more information, and problem solving becomes more effective. Physical symptoms such as restlessness, mild irritability, or mild tension-relieving behaviors such as nail biting and finger tapping may be present.

Moderate Anxiety

As anxiety escalates, the patient's perceptual field narrows, leading to **selective inattention**. The ability to think clearly is somewhat hampered, but learning and problem solving can still take place. Physical symptoms may include tension, pounding heart, increased pulse and respiration, and other mild somatic symptoms. Voice tremors may be noticed. Mild to **moderate anxiety** levels can be viewed as a signal that something in the person's life needs attention.

Severe Anxiety

The perceptual field of a person experiencing **severe anxiety** is greatly reduced. A person with severe anxiety may become overly focused on one particular detail or may attend to superficial, scattered details. The person may have difficulty noticing events occurring in the environment, even when they are pointed out. Learning and problem solving are significantly affected at this level. Behavior tends to be automatic and aimed at reducing or relieving the anxiety. Often the individual complains of increased severity of somatic symptoms. The most classic experiences are hyperventilation and a sense of dread or impending doom.

Panic Level Anxiety

The **panic level of anxiety** is the most extreme and results in markedly disturbed behavior. An individual is not able to process events in the environment and may lose touch with reality. Confusion, shouting, screaming, or extreme withdrawal may be present. Hallucinations, seeing people or objects that are not present, may be experienced by people at panic levels of anxiety. Erratic, uncoordinated, and impulsive behavior may also be evident. Automatic behaviors are used to reduce and relieve anxiety, although such efforts may be ineffective. Acute panic may lead to exhaustion.

Review the stress response identified in Chapter 10 to help understand how the symptoms of anxiety develop and the relief behaviors we employ to deal with this anxiety. Chapter 10 describes the fight-or-flight response and introduces the "freeze" response. A person may pass out, or individuals may mentally remove themselves from their bodies (dissociate). At times the person may have no (explicit) memory of the feared stressor, as seen with a freeze response. A person is more likely to demonstrate a freeze response in severe and panic levels of anxiety.

Review Table 11.1 to identify the levels of anxiety and review how the level affects (1) perceptual field, (2) ability to concentrate and learn, and (3) physical and other manifestations.

Helpful Interventions

Mild to Moderate Anxiety

A patient experiencing a mild to moderate level of anxiety is still able to solve problems. As anxiety increases, the ability to concentrate decreases. The nurse can help the patient focus and solve problems with the use of specific active listening communication techniques. Restricting topics of communication and introducing irrelevant topics can increase a person's anxiety.

Reducing the patient's level of anxiety and preventing the escalation of anxiety are the goals of these interventions. Remaining calm, recognizing the patient's distress, and being willing to listen are the tasks of the nurse.

TABLE 11.1 Anxiety Levels and Their Characteristics

Mild	Moderate	Severe	Panic
Perceptual Field			
Heightened perceptual field Is alert and can see, hear, and grasp what is happening in the environment Can identify issues that are disturbing and are producing anxiety	Has narrow perceptual field; grasps less of what is occurring Can attend to more *if pointed out by another* (selective inattention)	Has greatly reduced perceptual field Focuses on details or one specific detail Attention scattered May not be able to attend to events in environment *even when pointed out by others* In severe to panic levels of anxiety, the environment is blocked out; it is as if these events were not occurring.	Unable to focus on the environment Experiences the utmost state of terror and emotional paralysis; feels he or she "ceases to exist" In panic, may have hallucinations or delusions that take the place of reality
Ability to Learn			
Able to work effectively toward a goal and examine alternatives	Able to solve problems but not at optimal ability Benefits from guidance of others	Unable to see connections between events or details Has distorted perceptions	May be mute or have extreme psychomotor agitation leading to exhaustion Shows disorganized or irrational reasoning
Mild and moderate levels of anxiety can alert the person that something is wrong and can stimulate appropriate action.		Severe and panic levels prevent problem solving and discovery of effective solutions. Unproductive relief behaviors are implemented, thus perpetuating a vicious cycle.	
Physical or Other Characteristics			
Slight discomfort Restlessness Irritability or impatience Mild tension-relieving behavior: foot or finger tapping, lip chewing, fidgeting	Voice tremors Change in voice pitch Difficulty concentrating Shakiness Repetitive questioning Somatic complaints (urinary frequency and urgency, headache, backache, insomnia) Increased respiration rate Increased pulse rate Increased muscle tension Moderate tension-relieving behavior; pacing, banging hands on table	Feelings of dread Ineffective functioning Confusion Purposeless activity Sense of impending doom More intense somatic complaints (dizziness, nausea, headache, sleeplessness) Hyperventilation Tachycardia Withdrawal Loud and rapid speech Threats and demands	Experience of terror Immobility or severe hyperactivity or flight Dilated pupils Unintelligible communication or inability to speak Severe shakiness Sleeplessness Severe withdrawal Hallucinations or delusions; likely out of touch with reality

Use of the problem-solving method can be a helpful tool for the nurse. This may include:

- Establishing a therapeutic relationship with the patient
- Helping the person to more fully understand the problem using active listening techniques such as broad openings, exploring, reflecting, clarifying, and others
- Assisting the patient to develop self-awareness of verbal and nonverbal relief behaviors
- Assisting the patient to generate possible solutions. Evaluation of effective past coping mechanisms is useful here. Often the nurse can help the patient consider alternatives to problem situations and offer activities that may temporarily relieve feelings of inner tension. The nurse may assist the patient to start to develop new coping strategies.
- Supporting the patient in carrying out the new plan and evaluating the effectiveness of the plan

Table 11.2 identifies interventions useful in assisting people experiencing mild to moderate levels of anxiety.

Severe to Panic Levels of Anxiety

A patient experiencing severe to panic levels of anxiety is unable to solve problems and may have a poor grasp of events occurring in the environment. Unproductive relief behaviors, extreme regression, and aimless behaviors can be behavioral manifestations of a person's intense psychic pain. The nurse must be concerned with the patient's safety and the safety of others. Patients experiencing severe to panic anxiety levels may feel out of control, so they need to know that they are safe from their own impulses. *Staying with the patient* throughout this period is important in helping the patient feel physically and emotionally safe. Physical needs such as food, fluids, and rest must be met to prevent exhaustion and other physical complications.

Anxiety reduction measures may take the form of moving the person to a quiet environment in which there is reduced stimulation. It can also include encouraging gross motor activities, like pacing, to drain some of the tension. The use of medications may be considered. Restraints should only be used to prevent danger and harm and after all less restrictive interventions have failed to decrease anxiety to safer levels.

Although communication may be scattered and disjointed, themes can often be heard that the nurse can address. Feeling understood can decrease the patient's sense of isolation and reduce anxiety. Because of difficulty with concentration, modified communication techniques may be required. *Firm, short, and simple statements* are better understood by the patient. With severe to panic levels of anxiety, the nurse will be more direct since the patient may have a difficult time recognizing what actions need to be taken. *Speaking more slowly, waiting longer for responses, and repeating comments* will facilitate the patient's ability to comprehend.

Recognition and reinforcement of reality may be required when there are distortions. Table 11.3 suggests some basic nursing interventions for patients with severe to panic levels of anxiety.

Numerous studies indicate social support is essential for maintaining physical and psychological health. The protective effects of having

TABLE 11.2 Interventions for Mild to Moderate Levels of Anxiety

Focus of Care: *Anxiety* (moderate) related to situational event or psychological stress, as evidenced by increase in vital signs, moderate discomfort, narrowing of perceptual field, and selective inattention

Intervention	Rationale
1. Identify anxiety. "You look upset."	1. It is important to validate observations with the patient, name the anxiety, and start to work with the patient to lower anxiety.
2. Assess the patient's level of anxiety.	2. Escalation of anxiety to a more disorganizing level is prevented.
3. Use nonverbal language to demonstrate interest (lean forward, maintain eye contact, nod your head).	3. Verbal and nonverbal messages should be consistent. The presence of an interested person provides a stabilizing focus.
4. Encourage the patient to talk about feelings and concerns.	4. When concerns are stated aloud, problems can be discussed, and feelings of isolation decreased.
5. Avoid closing off avenues of communication that are important for the patient. Focus on the patient's concerns.	5. When staff anxiety increases, changing the topic or offering advice is common but leaves the person isolated.
6. Ask questions to clarify what is being said. "I'm not sure what you mean. Give me an example."	6. Increased anxiety results in scattering of thoughts. Clarifying helps the patient identify thoughts and feelings.
7. Help the patient identify thoughts or feelings before the onset of anxiety. "What were you thinking right before you started to feel anxious?"	7. The patient is assisted in identifying thoughts and feelings, and problem solving is facilitated.
8. Encourage problem solving with the patient. The person may need some assistance with this.	8. Encouraging patients to explore alternatives increases sense of control and self-sufficiency while decreasing anxiety.
9. Assist in developing alternative solutions to a problem through role-play or modeling behaviors.	9. The patient is encouraged to try alternative behaviors and solutions to gain confidence and develop alternate skills in dealing with anxiety.
10. Explore behaviors that have worked to relieve anxiety in the past.	10. The patient is encouraged to mobilize successful coping mechanisms and strengths.
11. Provide outlets for dissipating excess energy (walking, exercising).	11. Physical activity can provide relief of built-up tension, increase muscle tone, and increase endorphin levels.

TABLE 11.3 Interventions for Severe to Panic Levels of Anxiety

Focus of Care: *Anxiety* (severe, panic) related to severe threat as evidenced by verbal or physical acting out, extreme immobility, sense of impending doom, inability to differentiate reality, and inability to problem solve

Intervention	Rationale
1. Maintain a calm manner.	1. Anxiety is communicated interpersonally. The quiet calm of the nurse can serve to calm the patient. The presence of anxiety can escalate anxiety in the patient.
2. **Always remain with the person** experiencing an acute severe to panic level of anxiety.	2. Alone with immense anxiety, a person feels abandoned. A caring face may be the patient's only contact with reality when confusion becomes overwhelming.
3. Minimize environmental stimuli. Move to a quieter setting and stay with the patient.	3. Helps minimize distractions and triggers which can further escalate the individual's anxiety.
4. Use clear and simple statements. You may need to repeat statements.	4. A person experiencing a severe to panic level of anxiety has difficulty concentrating and processing information.
5. Use a low-pitched voice; speak slowly.	5. A high-pitched voice can convey anxiety. Low pitch can decrease anxiety.
6. Reinforce reality if distortions occur (seeing objects that are not there or hearing voices when no one is present).	6. Anxiety can be reduced by focusing on and validating what is happening in the environment.
7. Listen for themes in communication.	7. In severe to panic levels of anxiety, verbal communication themes may be the only indication of the patient's thoughts or feelings.
8. Attend to physical and safety needs when necessary (need for warmth, fluids, elimination, pain relief, family contact).	8. High levels of anxiety may obscure the patient's awareness of physical needs.
9. Because safety is an overall goal, physical limits may need to be set. Speak in a firm, authoritative voice: "You may not hit anyone here. If you can't control yourself, we will help you."	9. A person who is out of control is often terrorized. Staff must offer the patient and others protection from destructive and self-destructive impulses.
10. Provide opportunities for gross muscle motor movement and exercise (walk/pace with nurse).	10. Physical activity helps channel and dissipate tension and may temporarily lower anxiety.
11. When a person is constantly moving or pacing, offer high-calorie fluids.	11. Dehydration and exhaustion must be prevented.
12. Assess need for medication.	12. Exhaustion and physical harm to self and others must be prevented.

good social support for those with a mental illness have been well documented. The levels of social support range from formal (a professional) to semiformal (a colleague) to informal (a friend) to close (a partner or relative). Nurses and other health professionals can play an important role by facilitating the development of social supports.

Defense Mechanisms

Unconscious defense mechanisms are used by an individual for anxiety reduction (Shpancer, 2018). Defense mechanisms protect people from painful awareness of feelings and memories that can provoke overwhelming anxiety. Adaptive use of defense mechanisms helps people lower anxiety levels to achieve goals in acceptable ways.

Defense mechanisms operate all the time. When an individual is faced with a situation that triggers high levels of anxiety, that person may become more rigid in the use of these mechanisms and may revert to using less mature defenses. The degree of distortion of reality and disruption in interpersonal relationships and the *frequency, intensity,* and *duration* of use of these defense mechanisms determine if they are adaptive (healthy) or maladaptive (unhealthy).

Sigmund Freud and his daughter Anna outlined most of the defense mechanisms that we recognize today. Five of the most important properties of defense mechanisms are as follows:

1. They are major means of managing unconscious conflict.
2. They are, for the most part, unconscious.
3. They are discrete from one another.
4. They can be seen as part of many psychiatric disorders.
5. They can be both adaptive and pathological.

Healthy Defenses

Altruism. In **altruism**, emotional conflicts and stressors are addressed by meeting the needs of others. Unlike self-sacrificing behavior, in altruism, the person receives gratification either vicariously or from the response of others.

VIGNETTE: Six months after losing her husband in a car accident, Jeanette began to spend 1 day a week doing grief counseling with families who had lost a loved one. She found that she was effective in helping others in their grief, and she obtained a great deal of satisfaction and pleasure from helping others work through their pain.

Sublimation. **Sublimation** is an unconscious process of substituting constructive and socially acceptable activity for strong impulses that are not usually considered acceptable. Often these impulses are sexual or aggressive. A man with strong hostile feelings may choose to become a butcher, or he may participate in rough contact sports.

Humor. Humor makes life easier. An individual may deal with emotional conflicts or stressors by emphasizing the amusing or ironic aspects of the conflict or stressor through *humor*.

VIGNETTE: A man is interviewed for a job by the top executives of a company. He has recently had foot surgery, and on entering the interview room, he stumbles and loses his balance. There is a stunned silence, and then the man states calmly, "I was hoping I could put my best foot forward." With everyone laughing, the interview continues in a relaxed manner.

Suppression. **Suppression** is the *conscious* denial of a disturbing situation or feeling.

VIGNETTE: A student who is studying for the state board examination says, "I can't worry about paying my rent until after my exam tomorrow."

Intermediate Defenses

Repression. **Repression** is the exclusion of unpleasant or unwanted experiences, emotions, or ideas from conscious awareness. Examples include *forgetting* the name of a former boyfriend or girlfriend or *forgetting* an appointment to discuss poor grades. *Repression is considered the cornerstone of the defense mechanisms, and it is the first line of* ***psychological defense against anxiety.***

Displacement. Transfer of emotions associated with a specific person, object, or situation to *another* person, object, or situation that is nonthreatening is called **displacement**. Example: The boss yells at the man, the man yells at his wife, the wife yells at the child, and the child kicks the cat demonstrates the successive use of *displaced* hostility. The use of displacement is common but not always adaptive. Spousal, child, and elder abuse are extreme cases of *displaced* hostility.

Reaction Formation. In **reaction formation**, unacceptable feelings or behaviors are kept out of awareness by developing the opposite behavior or emotion. Example: A person who harbors hostility toward children becomes a Boy Scout leader.

Somatization. **Somatization** occurs when *repressed* anxiety is demonstrated in the form of physical symptoms that have no organic cause. It can be an unconscious way of avoiding a situation that is anxiety provoking or an indirect way to communicate the need for help in a more socially acceptable manner. Example: It is considered "acceptable" to ask for help when you are "physically" sick.

VIGNETTE: A professor develops laryngitis on the day he is scheduled to defend a research proposal to a group of peers.

A woman who does not want to go out with the brother of her boss calls to say, "My back went out," and she cannot make the date.

Undoing. **Undoing** is performing an action to *make up for* a previous behavior. Example: giving a gift to "undo" an argument. A pathological example of undoing is compulsive hand washing. This can be viewed as cleansing oneself of an act or thought perceived as unacceptable.

Rationalization. **Rationalization** consists of justifying illogical or unreasonable ideas, actions, or feelings by developing acceptable explanations for the behavior. Example: "Everybody cheats, so why shouldn't I?" Rationalization is a form of self-deception.

Immature Defenses

Passive Aggression. Passive-aggressive behavior can be seen when an individual deals with emotional conflict or stressors by indirectly and unassertively expressing aggression toward others. The appearance of compliance *masks* covert resistance, resentment, and hostility. In **passive aggression**, the aggression toward others may be expressed through procrastination, failure, inefficiency, or passivity. These types of behaviors occur when the individual feels unable to directly express displeasure or disagreement.

VIGNETTE: A wife is unconsciously annoyed that her husband always works late and "accidentally" burns his dinner.

Acting-Out Behaviors. In acting out, an individual addresses emotional conflicts or stressors by actions rather than by reflections or feelings. A person may lash out in anger verbally or physically to distract the self from threatening thoughts or feelings. Acting out can make a person feel temporarily less helpless or vulnerable. By lashing out at others, an individual can transfer the focus from personal doubts and insecurities to another person or object. **Acting-out behaviors** are a destructive coping style.

> **VIGNETTE:** When Harry was turned down a third time for a promotion, he went to his office and tore apart every patient file in his file cabinet. His initial feelings of worthlessness and lowered self-esteem related to the situation were interpreted by Harry to mean "I am no good." This thinking resulted in Harry quickly transforming these painful feelings into actions of anger and destruction. Temporarily, Harry felt more powerful and less vulnerable.

Dissociation. A disruption in the usually integrated functions of consciousness, memory, identity, or perception of the environment is known as **dissociation**. This defense mechanism is usually only seen with severe stressors.

> **VIGNETTE:** A young mother who saw her son struck by a car was taken to a neighbor's house while the police dealt with the accident. Later she told the policeman, "I really don't remember what happened. The last thing I remember is going out the door to check on Johnny." At that moment, to protect herself from an unbearable situation, she separated the threatening event from awareness until she could begin to deal with her feelings of devastation.

Devaluation. **Devaluation** occurs when emotional conflicts or stressors are handled by attributing negative qualities to self or others. When devaluing another, the individual then appears good by contrast.

> **VIGNETTE:** A woman who is very jealous of a coworker says, "Oh, yes, she won the award. Those awards don't mean anything anyway. I wonder what she had to do to be chosen." In this way, she minimizes the other woman's accomplishments and keeps her own fragile self-esteem intact.

Idealization. In **idealization**, emotional conflicts or stressors are addressed by attributing exaggerated positive qualities to others. Idealization can be an adaptive aspect of the development of the self. Children who grow up with parents they can respect and *idealize* develop healthy standards of conduct and morality.

When people idealize and overvalue a person in a new relationship, disappointment can occur when the object of the idealization turns out to be human. Disappointment leads to lowered self-esteem. Such individuals may then devalue and reject the object of their affection to protect their own self-esteem. If this type of response becomes a pattern, it can lead to interpersonal and occupational problems.

> **VIGNETTE:** Mary met the most "wonderful and perfect" man. No one could tell Mary that Jim was nice but had some quirks, like everyone else. Mary would not listen. When Jim failed to live up to Mary's expectations, she was devastated. Shortly thereafter, she started saying that Jim was, like all men, a brute and that she wanted no more to do with such an insensitive person.

Splitting. **Splitting** is the inability to integrate the positive and negative qualities of oneself or others into a cohesive image. The self or others are either good, loving, worthy, and nurturing or bad, hateful, and worthless. The use of this defense mechanism is prevalent in personality disorders, especially in people who demonstrate borderline personality traits. (See Chapter 13.)

> **VIGNETTE:** Alice viewed her therapist as the most wonderful, loving, and insightful therapist she had ever seen. When her therapist refused to write her a prescription for Valium, Alice shouted at her that she was the "stupidest, most uncaring, and thickheaded person" and demanded another therapist "right away."

Projection. A person unconsciously rejects emotionally unacceptable personal features in one's self and attributes those unacceptable traits to other people, objects, or situations through **projection**. Projection is the hallmark of *blaming*, scapegoating, prejudicial thinking, and stigmatization. People who always feel that others are out to deceive or cheat them may be projecting onto others those characteristics in themselves that they find distasteful and cannot consciously accept. Projection can be associated with paranoia.

Projection can be seen in family, school, business, or political systems. A dysfunctional family system may "scapegoat" (blame) the child for the family problems. The pain and anxiety within the family system are *projected* onto the child: "The problem is Tommy."

Denial. **Denial** involves escaping unpleasant realities by ignoring their existence. Examples: A man believes that physical limitations reflect negatively on his manhood. He then may deny chest pain because it threatens his self-image as a man. A woman whose health has deteriorated because of an alcohol use disorder denies she has a problem with alcohol by saying she can stop drinking whenever she wants. Table 11.4 gives examples of adaptive and maladaptive uses of some common defense mechanisms.

ANXIETY DISORDERS

The symptom of anxiety becomes a problem when it significantly interferes with adaptive behavior, lasts significantly longer than expected, causes physical symptoms, or exceeds a tolerable level. The common element in anxiety disorders is that individuals experience a degree of anxiety that is so uncomfortably high and persistent that it causes dysfunction at work, in social situations, and/or with family functioning.

The diagnosis of anxiety disorders refers to a number of disorders, including panic disorders, phobias, general anxiety disorder, and social anxiety disorder (social phobia), among others.

Prevalence and Comorbidity

Anxiety disorders are the most prevalent lifetime psychiatric disorders leading to stress and impairment worldwide. An estimated 19.1% of U.S. adults had an anxiety disorder in the past year. An estimated 31.1% of U.S. adults experience an anxiety disorder at some time in their lifetimes (National Institute of Mental Health [NIMH], 2017).

Women have a lifetime prevalence rate of approximately 30%, whereas for men, the lifetime rate of anxiety disorders is approximately 19% (Sadock et al., 2015). Anxiety disorders may begin in childhood, adolescence, and early adulthood, with three-fourths of those with an anxiety disorder having a first episode by age 21 or 22 (American Psychological Association, n.d.).

Anxiety disorders are highly treatable, yet only 36.9% of those afflicted receive treatment (American Psychological Association, n.d.). People with an anxiety disorder are three to five times more likely to go

TABLE 11.4 Defense Mechanisms

Defense Mechanism	Adaptive/Within Normal Limits	Maladaptive
Repression	A man forgets his wife's birthday after a marital fight.	A woman is unable to enjoy sex after having pushed out of awareness a traumatic sexual incident from childhood.
Sublimation	A woman who is angry with her boss writes a short story about a heroic woman.	None—the use of sublimation is always constructive.
Regression	A 4-year-old boy with a new baby brother starts sucking his thumb and wanting a bottle.	A person who loses a promotion starts complaining to others, does sloppy work, misses appointments, and arrives late for meetings.
Displacement	A patient criticizes a nurse after his family fails to visit.	A child who is unable to acknowledge fear of his father becomes fearful of animals.
Projection	A man who is unconsciously attracted to other women teases his wife about flirting.	A woman who has repressed an attraction toward other women refuses to socialize. She fears another woman will make homosexual advances toward her.
Compensation	A short man becomes assertive and excels in business.	An individual drinks alcohol when self-esteem is low to diffuse discomfort temporarily.
Reaction formation	A person with a substance use disorder is in recovery. He now constantly preaches about the evils of alcoholic beverages.	A mother who has an unconscious hostility toward her daughter is overprotective to protect daughter from harm, interfering with daughter's normal growth and development.
Denial	A man reacts to news of the death of a loved one by saying, "No, I don't believe you. The doctor said he was fine."	A woman whose husband died 3 years earlier still keeps his clothes in the closet and talks about him in the present tense.
Conversion	A student is unable to take a final examination because of a terrible headache.	A man becomes blind after seeing his wife flirt with other men.
Undoing	After flirting with her male secretary, a woman buys her husband tickets to a show.	A man with rigid and moralistic beliefs and repressed sexuality is driven to wash his hands to gain composure when around attractive women.
Rationalization	An employee says, "I didn't get the raise because the boss doesn't like me."	A father who thinks his son was fathered by another man excuses his malicious treatment of the boy by saying, "He is lazy and disobedient," when that is not the case.
Identification	A 5-year-old girl dresses in her mother's shoes and dress and meets her father at the door.	A young boy thinks a neighborhood pimp with money and drugs is someone to emulate.
Introjection	After his wife's death, the husband has transient complaints of chest pains and difficulty breathing—the symptoms his wife had before she died.	A young child whose parents were overcritical and belittling grows up thinking that she is inferior. She has taken on her parents' evaluation of her as part of her self-image.
Suppression	A businessman who is preparing to make an important speech is told by his wife that she wants a divorce. Although visibly upset, he puts the incident aside until after his speech, when he can give the matter his total concentration.	A woman who feels a lump in her breast shortly before leaving for a 3-week vacation puts the information in the back of her mind until after returning from her vacation.

to a nonpsychiatric doctor and six times more likely to be hospitalized for psychiatric disorders than those who do not suffer from anxiety disorders (Anxiety and Depression Association of America [ADAA], n.d.).

Anxiety disorders frequently *co-occur* with many other psychiatric disorders, including depressive disorders, alcohol/drug use disorders, eating disorders, and bipolar disorders. Major depressive disorder (MDD) occurs in up to half of people with anxiety disorders and leads to greater impairment and poorer response to treatment. Co-occurring substance use disorders have a similar negative effect on overall treatment success.

Other co-occurring conditions have been well documented in the literature. These include cancer, irritable bowel syndrome, kidney and liver dysfunction, reduced immunity, and others. **Chronic anxiety** is thought to be associated with increased risk for cardiovascular morbidity and mortality.

Anxiety can be one of the first symptoms of a medical disorder. Conversely, the symptoms associated with anxiety disorders can mimic symptoms of medical illnesses. It can be challenging to make an accurate differential diagnosis. Patients may visit a variety of medical practitioners seeking an explanation for their symptoms when in fact the basis of their complaints is an anxiety disorder.

Prescription medication can be the source of *new-onset* acute anxiety. These include the following:

- Asthma medicines, such as albuterol, salmeterol, and theophylline
- Blood pressure medicines, such as methyldopa
- Hormones, such as oral contraceptives
- Medicines that contain amphetamines, such as Benzedrine, Dexedrine, and Ritalin
- Steroids, such as cortisone, dexamethasone, and prednisone
- Thyroid medicines
- Other medicines, such as phenytoin, levodopa, quinidine, and some antidepressants

Nonprescription medicines that may cause anxiety include the following:

- Medicines that contain caffeine, such as Anacin, Empirin, Excedrin, No-Doz, and cough medicines
- Decongestants, such as phenylephrine, including Sudafed PE
- Illegal drugs, such as cocaine, crack, or speed (amphetamines)

Theory

Anxiety disorders are most likely caused by a complex interaction of biological, psychological, and environmental factors. Strong evidence suggests that biological factors such as genetic vulnerability may interact with stress or trauma to trigger pathological anxiety. Traumatic life events and psychosocial and sociocultural influences can be significant factors in the etiology of these disorders.

Neurobiology

Although the neurobiology of anxiety and anxiety disorders is very complex, the following discussion identifies some of the major neuroanatomical and neurobiological factors associated with anxiety and anxiety disorders. Refer to Chapter 4 for more information on neurotransmitters and how medications work, and refer to Chapter 10 for more information on the stress response.

The **limbic system**, referred to by some as the "emotional brain," consists of the amygdala, hippocampus, thalamus, hypothalamus, basal ganglia, and cingulate gyrus (Boundless, 2015). All of the components of the limbic system work together to regulate some of the brain's most important processes. The three functions of the limbic system include the following:

- Scanning the environment for threat-relevant cues and assess the magnitude of the threat
- Initiating the body's readiness to respond by eliciting the fight-or-flight (and freeze) response (see Chapter 10)
- Terminating reactivity after external stressors subside and restore the nervous system to a state of homeostasis

The part of the limbic system most associated with anxiety disorders as well as the obsessive-compulsive disorders is the cingulate, where the neural pathways connect to the limbic system and prefrontal lobes. The limbic system is involved in storing memories and creating emotions and is thought to be a major factor in processing anxiety-related information. Some of the other parts of the brain involved in anxiety and anxiety-related disorders are as follows:

- Frontal cortex: cognitive interpretations (potential threat)
- Hypothalamus: activation of the stress response (fight-or-flight and freeze) response (refer to Chapter 10)
- Hippocampus: associated with memory related to fear responses
- Amygdala: fear, especially related to phobic and panic disorders

When an imbalance in certain neurotransmitters in the brain occurs, anxiety is often the result. Based on animal studies and responses to drug treatment, three main neurochemical mediators of anxiety in the central nervous system are implicated in anxiety responses. These are the neurotransmitters serotonin (5-HT), norepinephrine (NE), and γ-aminobutyric acid (GABA) (Sadock et al., 2015).

- Serotonin (5-HT): Because serotonin levels are thought to be decreased in anxiety disorders, it is hypothesized that serotonin dysfunction contributes to anxiety disorders. The **selective serotonin reuptake inhibitors (SSRIs)**, which increase serotonin levels in the brain, are often first-line medications for the treatment of many anxiety disorders.
- Norepinephrine (NE): When a person feels threatened (real or perceived), the level of norepinephrine (adrenaline) increases and can cause hyperarousal and increased anxiety. In some people with anxiety disorders, it is thought that the noradrenergic system is poorly regulated and can cause bursts of activity. **Noradrenergic drugs** such as propranolol, which blocks adrenergic receptor activity, and clonidine, which stimulates α-adrenergic receptors lower anxiety.
- GABA (γ-aminobutyric acid): An inhibitory neurotransmitter in the brain, slows neural transmission, resulting in a calming effect. Benzodiazepine medications facilitate the action of GABA. A number of drugs, including antianxiety agents, sedative-hypnotics, general anesthetics, and anticonvulsant drugs, target the GABA receptor system. It is believed that people with anxiety disorders have diminished benzodiazepine receptor sensitivity. These abnormalities may lead to unregulated anxiety levels.

Other neurotransmitters, like dopamine, hormones, and endorphins, may also be implicated in the development of anxiety.

Genetic Factors

The hypothesis that there are *genetic* components associated with anxiety is substantiated by numerous studies finding that anxiety disorders tend to cluster in families (Sadock et al., 2015). Twin and family studies report that panic disorder has a hereditability of approximately 40%. There is a higher concordance rate (probability) in monozygotic twins as compared with dizygotic twins. It is still uncertain if the genetic influence is specific to panic disorder or to an increased potential to develop general anxiety symptoms. People with a diagnosis of obsessive-compulsive disorder also show a strong genetic predisposition.

Behavioral Theory

Learning theories provide another hypothesis regarding the etiology of anxiety disorders. Behavioral theory conceptualizes anxiety as a *learned response* that can be *unlearned*. Some individuals may *learn* to be anxious from the imitation or *modeling* provided by parents or peers. A mother who is fearful of thunder and lightning may transmit her anxiety to her children, who continue to adopt her behavior into adult life. Behavioral therapies use a variety of techniques to help the individual learn a new way of responding.

Cognitive Theory

Cognitive theorists believe that anxiety disorders are a result of "cognitive distortions" in an individual's thinking and understanding. These cognitive distortions can lead to feelings of acute anxiety. Brain scans taken before and after cognitive therapy treatment support the hypothesis that learning to "reframe" one's thinking can literally change the chemistry and function of the brain. Cognitive-behavioral therapy (CBT) is an evidence-based strategy for both anxiety disorders and many other psychiatric conditions.

Cultural Considerations

Reliable data on the incidence of anxiety disorders among cultures are sparse, but sociocultural variation in symptoms of anxiety disorders has been noted. In some cultures, individuals express anxiety through somatic symptoms, whereas in other cultures, cognitive symptoms predominate. **Panic attacks** in Latin Americans and Northern Europeans often involve sensations of choking, smothering, numbness, or tingling, as well as fear of dying. In other cultural groups, panic attacks involve fear of magic or witchcraft. Social phobias in Japanese and Korean cultures may relate to a belief that the individual's blushing, eye contact, or body odor is offensive to others.

One of the barriers for some cultural groups seeking health care for anxiety disorders is the stigma that various cultures associate with mental disorders in general. For example, African Americans are much less likely to seek mental health services than those from other cultural backgrounds, and Asian Americans are even more reticent to seek help (NIMH, 2015). Interestingly, the incidence of anxiety disorders seems to vary among cultures and countries. Anxiety disorders also vary among immigrants from generation to generation. These findings also generalize to obsessive-compulsive disorder where one must be aware of cultural norms before hastily making a diagnosis such as labeling culturally appropriate ritualistic behavior as a disorder.

Panic Disorders

Panic disorder (PD) consists of recurrent and unexpected, "out of the blue" panic attacks. The *panic attack* is the key feature of panic disorders (PDs). A *panic attack* is the sudden onset of extreme apprehension or fear, usually associated with feelings of impending doom: "I am going to die." Typically, panic attacks occur suddenly, not necessarily in response to an acute stressor. They are extremely intense and can last from 1 to 30 minutes before they subside. Panic attacks can happen at any time during the day or can occur while sleeping at night, causing a person to wake up terrified. The feelings of terror present during a panic attack are so severe that normal function is suspended, the perceptual field is severely limited, and misinterpretation of reality may occur.

People experiencing panic attacks may believe that they are "losing their minds" or are having a "heart attack" because of the uncomfortable physical symptoms that can accompany the panic attack. Physical symptoms experienced may include palpitations, chest pain, diaphoresis, muscle tension, urinary frequency, hyperventilation, breathing difficulties, nausea, feelings of choking, chills, hot flashes, and gastrointestinal symptoms. When a physiologic cause for the symptoms presented is ruled out, the person may need to be referred to a mental health provider to rule out an anxiety disorder. During the intervals between panic attacks, the person may experience low-level constant anxiousness and fear of having another anxiety attack. This is called *anticipatory anxiety*. It is this *anticipatory anxiety* that is an important criterion for this diagnosis of Panic Disorder. Some studies have demonstrated that people who experience panic attacks have an 18% higher rate of suicide attempts as well as a higher rate of completed suicides than the general population (Sadock et al., 2015).

Panic attacks can also be associated with other psychiatric disorders, including the other anxiety disorders. The presence and frequency of panic attacks may predict the level of psychopathology, severity, and outcome of these other disorders. Panic episodes can lead to the development of depressive disorders as well as alcohol or other drug overuse in an attempt to self-medicate.

Preston and Johnson (2015) cite the following pharmacological treatments as efficacious in the treatment of panic disorders:

- Benzodiazepines, such as alprazolam, clonazepam, and lorazepam; usually used for an acute episode and on a ***short-term basis*** only
- Antidepressants such as SSRIs
- Use of cognitive and behavioral therapy either alone or in conjunction with medications to help people learn skills to combat their panic

Phobias

A phobia is a persistent, intense irrational fear of an object, activity, or situation that leads to a *desire* for avoidance, or *actual* avoidance of the object, activity, or situation.

Specific phobias are characterized by the experience of high levels of anxiety or fear in response to *specific* objects, such as dogs, spiders, or heights, or situations, such as closed spaces, tunnels, and bridges. Specific phobias are common and usually do not cause much difficulty because people can contrive ways to avoid the feared object. However, the fear, anxiety, or avoidance in some cases may cause impairment in social, occupational, or other areas of functioning when faced with the feared object or situation.

There is no evidence that specific phobias are related to biological dysfunction. In fact, behavioral therapy seems to be the only effective therapy for specific phobias. Medication is not an effective treatment. According to the *DSM-5*, the prevalence rate for a specific phobia is approximately 7% to 9% over a 12-month period (APA, 2013).

Social anxiety disorders or social phobias are characterized by severe anxiety or fear provoked by exposure to a social situation or a performance situation, resulting in feelings of humiliation or embarrassment. This may include fear of saying something that sounds foolish in public, fear of being unable to answer questions in a classroom, fear of eating in the presence of others, or fear of performing on stage. The intense terror in these situations results from a fear of being evaluated or being rejected by others. Fear of public speaking is the most common social phobia. Many well-known performers suffer from bouts of *performance anxiety* when appearing in front of an audience.

Social anxiety disorders are believed by some to be influenced by psychological factors such as the quality of early attachments, the development of appropriate social skills, inadequate experiences interacting with others, and other negative environmental influences (Sadock et al., 2015). Other theories identify inherited traits, brain structure abnormalities, and learned behaviors as contributing to the etiology of this disorder (Mayo Clinical Staff, 2017).

First-degree relatives of persons with a *social anxiety disorder* are three times more likely to develop this disorder than those in the general population (Sadock et al., 2015). Twin studies suggest a complex genetic transmission of this disorder. There are currently ongoing biological studies to identify specific neurobiological factors associated with anxiety and fear.

The beta blocker propranolol reduces the physiological symptoms of anxiety, although not the cognitive worry symptoms. Propranolol is used effectively by many performers and lecturers before appearing in front of an audience. More pervasive social anxiety may respond to antidepressant therapy, such as SSRIs. CBT interventions, along with social skills training, are helpful for many.

Agoraphobia

Agoraphobia is an intense, excessive anxiety about or fear of being in places or situations where help might not be available, and escape might be either difficult or embarrassing. The feared places or situations are avoided by the individual in an effort to control anxiety. Avoidance behavior is an important part of the diagnosis. The anxiety-producing situations must include at least two of the following to distinguish it from a simple phobia, and the acute anxiety must cause significant distress:

- Using public transportation, such as traveling in a car, bus, or airplane
- Being in open spaces, such as parking lots, marketplaces, or bridges
- Being in enclosed spaces, such as shops, theaters, or cinemas
- Standing in line or being in a crowd
- Being outside of the home alone (APA, 2013)

The avoidance behaviors associated with agoraphobia can be debilitating and life constricting. In its most extreme form, patients may simply refuse to leave their homes, putting great strain on family and friends. Consider the effects on a father whose avoidance renders him unable to leave home and who thus cannot work or participate in his children's school activities. The fears and anxieties may become so intense that the individual may need to rely on others to help meet basic needs and provide everyday services such as shopping, walking the dog, and so on. Complications may ensue when individuals attempt to decrease anxiety through self-medication with alcohol or drugs.

The disorder can be chronic, although it responds well to CBT. Antidepressants, such as SSRIs, help reduce the anxiety and can treat comorbid depression. Panic attacks may precede agoraphobia 30% to 50% of the time (APA, 2013).

Generalized Anxiety Disorder

Generalized anxiety disorder (GAD) is characterized by excessive anxiety and worry about a number of events and activities. People with GAD find it difficult to shake their concerns and report being unable to relax. It is sometimes referred to as the "worry disease" (What if I'm late? … What if I fail? … What if I am fired?). A diagnosis of GAD is made if at least three of the following symptoms are present: restlessness, fatigue, poor concentration, irritability, muscle tension, and sleep disturbance (APA, 2013).

The individual's worry must persist for most days during a 6-month period in order to qualify for *DSM-5* diagnosis. Examples of worries typical in GAD are inadequacy in interpersonal relationships, job responsibilities, finances, and health of family members. These excessive worries can lead to disturbances in relationships and family life, impaired functioning at work, and disturbances in social roles. Sleep disturbance is common because the individual worries about the day's events and real or imagined mistakes, reviews past problems, and anticipates future difficulties during sleep hours. These constant worries leave the limbic system in a perpetual state of alertness. Decision making is difficult because of poor concentration and the dread of making a mistake. Additional somatic symptoms can include sweating, nausea, and diarrhea, chronic muscle tension, fatigue, restlessness, and difficulty concentrating.

GAD results from a combination of genetic, behavioral, developmental, and other factors. The effectiveness of some drug therapies, like buspirone and SSRIs, in reducing the "what if's" and worrying in GAD patients seems to support the biological etiology of the disease (Preston & Johnson, 2015). An overview of medications and therapies for specific anxiety disorders is provided in Table 11.5.

DSM-5 DIAGNOSTIC CRITERIA

Generalized Anxiety Disorder

A. Excessive anxiety and worry (apprehensive expectation), occurring more days than not for at least 6 months, about a number of events or activities (e.g., work or school performance).

B. The individual finds it difficult to control the worry.

C. The anxiety and worry are associated with three (or more) of the following six symptoms (with at least some symptoms having been present for more days than not for the past 6 months):

Note: Only one item is required in children.

a. Restlessness or feeling keyed up or on edge
b. Being easily fatigued
c. Difficulty concentrating or mind going blank
d. Irritability
e. Muscle tension
f. Sleep disturbance (difficulty falling or staying asleep, or restless, unsatisfying sleep)

D. The anxiety, worry, or physical symptoms cause clinically significant distress or impairment in social, occupational, or other important areas of functioning.

E. The disturbance is not attributable to the physiological effects of a substance (e.g., a drug of abuse, a medication) or another medical condition (e.g., hyperthyroidism).

F. The disturbance is not better explained by another mental disorder (e.g., anxiety or worry about having panic attacks in panic disorder, negative evaluation in social anxiety disorder [social phobia], contamination or other obsessions in obsessive-compulsive disorder, separation from attachment figures in separation anxiety disorder, reminders of traumatic events in posttraumatic stress disorder, gaining weight in anorexia nervosa, physical complaints in somatic symptom disorder, perceived appearance flaws in body dysmorphic disorder, having a serious illness in illness anxiety disorder, or the content of delusional beliefs in schizophrenia or delusional disorder).

Other Anxiety Disorders

In the diagnosis of anxiety disorder due to another medical condition, the individual's symptoms of panic attacks and anxiety are a direct physiological result of a medical condition. Examples can include conditions associated with multiple body systems:

- Respiratory
- Cardiovascular
- Endocrine
- Neurological
- Metabolic

To determine whether the anxiety symptoms are caused by a medical condition, a careful and comprehensive assessment of multiple factors is necessary. Evidence must be present in the history, physical examination, and/or laboratory findings to diagnose the medical condition.

When the chronic anxiety is caused by medications or substances, the *DSM-5* diagnosis would be substance/medication-induced anxiety disorder.

Separation anxiety disorder is seen in children and is discussed in Chapter 26. It is important to note, however, that separation anxiety disorder exists in the adult population as well. Children may also demonstrate *selective mutism,* a complex *childhood anxiety disorder* characterized by a child's inability to speak and communicate effectively in select social settings.

OBSESSIVE-COMPULSIVE AND RELATED DISORDERS

Obsessive-compulsive disorder (OCD) is a common, chronic, and long-lasting disorder in which a person has uncontrollable, reoccurring thoughts (obsessions) and behaviors (compulsions) that the person feels the urge to repeat over and over. It affects 1% to 2% of the population. OCD can be extremely disabling and painful.

OCD usually begins during the late teens or early 20s and ranges from mild to severe. There is substantial evidence that OCD has biological origins and is thought by many to be a neurologically based disorder. OCD seems to occur more often in patients with other neurological disorders, such as in Huntington's chorea, epilepsy, Sydenham's chorea, and brain trauma (Black & Andreasen, 2014). OCD frequently co-occurs with Tourette's disorder, a neurological disorder, and these two disorders may be related both in symptom overlap and biological etiology. Other factors that support the neurological etiology of OCD include the following (Black & Andreasen, 2014; Sadock et al., 2015):

- Brain imaging studies show an increase in metabolic activity in patients with OCD, specifically hyperactivity in the prefrontal cortex and dysfunction in the basal ganglia and cingulum.
- There is evidence that OCD has a significant genetic component based on family and twin studies.
- The hypothesis is that dysregulation of serotonin levels is involved in the etiology of OCD. Clinical studies have shown that OCD patients are responsive to SSRIs, whereas other antidepressants are ineffective, with the exception of the tricyclic antidepressant *clomipramine.*

Symptoms of OCD include obsessions and compulsions. **Obsessions** are defined as thoughts, impulses, or images that persist and recur so that they cannot be dismissed from the mind. Obsessions often seem senseless to the individual who experiences them, although they still cause the individual to experience anxiety. Common obsessions include fear of hurting a loved one, fear of contamination, or needing to have things symmetrical or in perfect order.

TABLE 11.5 **Selected Therapies and Interventions for Anxiety and OCD-Related Disorders**

Therapy/Intervention	Characteristics
Cognitive Behavioral Therapy (CBT)	Evidence based Focuses on identifying, challenging, and neutralizing unhelpful thoughts
Acceptance and Commitment Therapy	Moderate evidence Combines behavioral and cognitive behavioral techniques ***Accept*** problematic emotions, then ***commit*** to making changes in behavior
Relaxation Techniques Deep breathing Guided imagery Progressive relaxation Autogenic training Self-hypnosis Meditation Aerobic exercise	Considered adjunct to other forms of therapy Helps people calm emotions and may enhance the effects of therapy
Biofeedback	Uses a device that provides feedback on physiology, measuring things such as blood pressure, muscle tension, and brain wave activity
Mindfulness-Based Stress Reduction (MBSR)	Evidence based Detach from anxious thoughts through awareness, identifying tension, understanding thinking patterns, and learning how to deal with difficult emotions
Aversion Techniques	Undesirable behavior is associated with unpleasant stimulus
Flooding	Prolonged exposure to fear or threat
Systematic Desensitization (sometimes called Exposure Therapy)	Evidence based for phobias Gradually exposes a person to a feared object or situation until free of incapacitating anxiety
Exposure and Response Prevention	Evidence based for phobias, OCD, and anxiety Desensitizes people to their fears by repeatedly facing fears and learning to manage uncomfortable thoughts and emotions

Compulsions are ritualistic behaviors that individuals feel driven to perform in an attempt to reduce anxiety. Common compulsions are repetitive hand washing or checking a door multiple times to make sure it is locked. Compulsions can include mental acts as well, such as counting, praying, or performing a repetitive act that temporarily reduces high levels of anxiety. Anxiety relief is achieved by the compulsive rituals, but because the relief is only temporary, the compulsive act must be repeated many times.

Although obsessions and compulsions can exist independently of each other, they almost always occur together. Behavior associated with OCD exists along a continuum. "Normal" individuals may experience mild symptoms. Nearly everyone has experienced a song playing persistently through the mind, despite attempts to push it away. Many people occasionally have nagging doubts as to whether a door is locked or the stove is turned off. These doubts require the person to go back to check the door or stove. Minor rituals, such as touching a lucky charm, "knocking" on wood, and making the sign of the cross upon hearing disturbing news, are not harmful to the individual.

At the more severe end of the continuum are obsessive-compulsive symptoms that typically center on dirtiness, contamination, and germs and occur with corresponding compulsions, such as cleaning and hand washing. A smaller number focus on safety issues with corresponding repetitive checking rituals. At the most severe levels are persistent thoughts of sexuality, violence, illness, or death. These obsessions or compulsions cause marked distress to the individual. People often feel humiliation and shame regarding these behaviors. The rituals are time-consuming and interfere with normal routine, social activities, and relationships with others. Severe OCD consumes so much of the individual's mental processes and time that the performance of cognitive and behavioral tasks may be impaired. Suicide can be a risk for these individuals, especially in the presence of a co-occurring depression.

BODY DYSMORPHIC DISORDER

Body dysmorphic disorder (BDD) is a highly distressing disorder that ranges along the continuum from distressing to delusional severity. This *DSM-5* diagnosis includes preoccupation with an imagined "defective body part." Patients with BDD usually have a normal appearance, although a small number do show a minor physical defect. The average age of onset is younger than 20 years. The diagnosis can include obsessional thinking, such as thinking "I am ugly or deformed," and compulsive behaviors, such as mirror checking, skin picking, or excessive grooming. There can be an impairment of normal activities related to social, academic, or occupational functioning. The obsessional focus for individuals with BDD frequently center around the face, skin, genitalia, thighs, hips, and hair.

Usually the person feels great shame and hides or withdraws from others. Many will alter their appearance through multiple plastic surgeries in an attempt to fix perceived physical flaws.

The most common co-occurring disorders include major depression, substance use disorder, and social phobia. Individuals with BDD have higher rates of suicidal ideation, suicide attempts, and completed suicides than other individuals. The disorder is often kept secret for many years, and the patient does not typically respond to reassurance. The pharmacological agents of choice for treating people with BDD are SSRI antidepressants and clomipramine, a tricyclic antidepressant. A second-generation antipsychotic added to an SSRI may help in the more severe delusional form of BDD. CBT is another evidence-based treatment strategy.

HOARDING DISORDER

Hoarding disorder is associated with excessive collecting of items that may or may not have value and the persistent difficulty in discarding or parting with these possessions. These individuals often feel shame for their failure to discard excessive amounts of these items. People with hoarding disorder can suffer extreme disruption in daily living and severe distress. Hoarding can be disabling and result in self-imposed social isolation. These individuals may live in unsafe conditions as a result of this behavior. The items hoarded may include garbage and trash, broken objects, old newspapers, books, and old clothing piled indiscriminately in their home. Kitchens may not be usable; beds cannot be slept in; and chairs, couches, and tables may be buried under piles of hoarded items. It has been noted by clinicians that hoarding disorder is associated with the following:

- Increased co-occurring mood or anxiety disorders
- Impairment in the performance of activities of daily living
- Distractibility
- Reduced insight and indecisiveness
- Poor response to standard psychological and pharmacological treatments
- A distinct genetic and neurobiological profile

APPLICATION OF THE NURSING PROCESS

ASSESSMENT

Symptoms of Anxiety

People with anxiety disorders and OCD rarely need hospitalization unless they are suicidal or have compulsions causing injury, such as excessive hand washing. Therefore most patients prone to anxiety are encountered in community settings.

 Assessment Guidelines

There is a critical need to include evidence-based assessment as part of the process of implementing evidence-based practice (EBP) in community settings. There are a number of reliable and valid tools that can be used to identify anxiety and anxiety disorders in adults, adolescents, and children. Three general screening tools for anxiety symptoms that can also be used to monitor symptom change are as follows:

- *The Clinically Useful Anxiety Outcome Scale (CUXOS)*—a 20-question self-report questionnaire that identifies symptoms of anxiety in adult
- *Generalized Anxiety Disorder Screener (GAD-7)*—a seven-question self-report tool for adults
- *Hamilton Rating Scale for Anxiety (HAM-A)*—a 14-question self-report tool for adults and adolescents (Beidas, 2015)

The *Psychiatric-Mental Health Nursing: Scope and Standards of Practice* (American Nurses Association [ANA] et al., 2014) provides guidelines for providing appropriate professional care:

1. Ensure that a complete physical and neurological examination is performed to help determine whether the anxiety is primary or secondary to another psychiatric disorder, a medical condition, or substance use/substance withdrawal issue.
2. Assess potential for self-harm and/or suicide. It is known that people suffering from high levels of intractable anxiety may contemplate, attempt, or complete suicide.
3. Perform a psychosocial assessment. Always ask the person, "What has happened recently that might be increasing your anxiety?" The patient may identify a problem such as stressful marriage, recent loss, stressful job, or school situation that could be addressed through therapy. There may be no identifiable recent event.
4. Assess cultural beliefs and background. Differences in culture can affect how anxiety is manifested.

DIAGNOSES

Nursing diagnoses and the focus of care is based upon the presenting symptoms. Table 11.6 identifies potential nursing diagnoses and patient concerns for the anxious patient. Included are the signs and symptoms that might be found on assessment that support the diagnoses.

OUTCOMES IDENTIFICATION

Table 11.7 identifies short- and long-term outcomes for specific anxiety disorders.

PLANNING AND IMPLEMENTATION

Individuals with anxiety disorders should be encouraged to actively participate in planning care. The Institute of Medicine (IOM, 2001). defines patient-centered care as "care that is respectful of and responsive to individual patient preferences, needs, and values" and that ensures "that patient values guide all clinical decisions." This definition highlights the importance of clinicians and patients working together to produce the best outcomes possible. The QSEN Patient-Centered Care competency addresses these same values. By sharing decision making with the patient, the nurse increases the likelihood of positive outcomes. Shared planning is especially appropriate for a patient with *mild or moderate anxiety*. When experiencing *severe levels of anxiety*, the patient may be unable to fully participate in planning. The nurse may be required to take a more directive role.

Whenever possible, interventions should be based on the *best evidence available*. Overall guidelines for basic nursing interventions are as follows:

1. Use therapeutic communication, milieu therapy, promotion of self-care activities, supportive counseling, health teaching, and health promotion as appropriate.
2. Identify community resources that can offer specialized treatment that is proven to be effective for people with different anxiety disorders.
3. Identify relevant community support groups for patients and significant others.

Communication Guidelines

Communication techniques may need to be modified when working with individuals with high levels of anxiety. The nurse must strive to use clear and concrete communication.

Psychiatric-mental health nurses use therapeutic communication skills to assist patients with anxiety disorders and OCD to reduce anxiety and enhance coping and interpersonal communication skills. The nurse performs assessments and teaching as appropriate.

Health Teaching and Health Promotion

There are four broad goals of health teaching, health promotion, and psychoeducation:

1. Provide information. Teach the patient and family/significant others about anxiety disorders and OCD.
   - Patients may conceal symptoms for years before seeking treatment. More than 50% of people who experience panic attacks seek treatment from a nonpsychiatric practitioner. Helping patients to identify symptoms as potentially being a part of a treatable medical/psychiatric condition is the first step.
   - Teach the patient about signs and symptoms of the disorder and theory regarding causes or risk factors.

TABLE 11.6 Potential Nursing Diagnoses for Patients With Anxiety Disorders and Obsessive-Compulsive Disorders

Signs and Symptoms	Potential Nursing Diagnoses[a]
Acute feelings of anxiety; feelings of acute apprehension, uncertainty, and uneasiness	*Anxiety*
Difficulty concentrating	*Impaired cognition*
Cognitive disorganization associated with exposure to phobic object	*Anxiety* *Impaired concentration*
Concern that a panic attack will occur	*Distress*
Anxiety that interferes with the ability to work, disrupts relationships, and changes the ability to interact with others	*Impaired coping process* *Impaired role performance* *Impaired socialization* *Risk for social isolation*
Avoidance behaviors (phobia, agoraphobia, social phobias)	*Social isolation* *Risk for loneliness* *Impaired socialization* *Impaired role performance* *Withdrawn behaviour*
Presence of obsessive thoughts	*Impaired cognition*
Intrusive thoughts	*Risk for impaired psychological status*
Compulsive behaviors Compulsive hoarding	*Impaired coping process*
Excessive negative thoughts	*Situational low self-esteem* *Chronic low self-esteem* *Risk for depressed mood*
Inordinate time taken for obsession and compulsions	*Impaired role performance* *Impaired coping process*
Inability to go to sleep related to intrusive or ruminative thoughts and excessive worry	*Impaired sleep* *Fatigue*
Feelings of hopelessness, inability to control one's life	*Hopelessness* *Powerlessness* *Chronic low self-esteem* *Situational low self-esteem* *Spiritual distress* *Risk for suicide* *Risk of self-destructive behaviors*
Inability to perform self-care related to rituals	*Self-care deficit*
Skin excoriation related to rituals of excessive washing or excessive picking at the skin	*Impaired skin integrity*
Preoccupation with a perceived body defect (per body dysmorphic disorder)	*Impaired cognition* *Impaired belief* *Disturbed body image* *Impaired socialization*

[a]The International Classification for Nursing Practice (ICNP) is a product of the International Council of Nurses (ICN). Retrieved from http://www.icn.ch/what-we-do/ICNP-Browser/.

- Identify available effective treatments, such as CBT, which gives hope that there can be an improvement in the quality of life for these patients.

TABLE 11.7 Short- and Long-Term Outcomes for Specific Disorders

Anxiety Disorder	Short- or Long-Term Outcomes
Phobia	Patients will: • Develop skills at reframing anxiety-provoking situation (by date). • Work with nurse/clinician to desensitize self to feared object or situation (by date).
Generalized anxiety disorder	Patients will: • State increased ability to make decisions and problem solve. • Demonstrate ability to perform usual tasks even though still moderately anxious (by date). • Demonstrate one cognitive or behavioral coping skill that helps reduce anxious feelings (by date). • Demonstrate one new effective relaxation skill (by date).
Obsessive-compulsive disorder	Patients will: • Reports less time having obsessional thoughts. • Decrease time spent in ritualistic behaviors. • Demonstrate increased amount of time spent with family and friends and on pleasurable activities. • State they have more control over intrusive thoughts and rituals (by date).

- Giving patients information about support groups, useful websites, and the location of nearby clinics is essential.
- Providing written information, such as medication education sheets, is an important part of health teaching and health promotion.
- Discuss the increased risk of developing a comorbid condition, especially substance use disorder and/or clinical depression and suicidality
- Emotional discharge gives an opportunity to exchange ideas about managing the illness and discuss frustrations and concerns.

2. Support treatment adherence through medication teaching.
   - Information on the medications used to target the individual's specific disorder is important to discuss, including the following:
     - The best way to take the medication, such as with food to decrease gastrointestinal (GI) upset
     - Potential side effects and ways to manage these side effects
     - Potential adverse effects that should be reported to the health care provider
     - Reminder to stay on the medications even when symptoms disappear
     - When the patient and the health care provider decide together to stop a medication, it will be done gradually to lessen the chance of relapse.
   - Teach the use of relaxation exercises as adjuncts to medication and therapy.
   - Teach the use of self-help strategies.
3. People with anxiety disorders are usually able to meet their own basic physical needs. Sleep, however, can be a real and serious problem. Patients with anxiety disorders often experience sleep disturbances. Teaching people ways to promote sleep, such as a warm bath, warm milk, or relaxing music, and monitoring sleep through a sleep diary are useful interventions. CBT for insomnia (CBT-I) is an evidence-based treatment for severe insomnia

4. Informatics can be an important part of patient teaching by giving them access to information and continue learning the tools to help them reduce symptoms.
   - There are many smartphone applications (apps) designed to help with relaxation. The research on the effectiveness of apps is limited, but some people may find them useful adjuncts to medication and therapy. The Anxiety and Depression Association of America (ADAA) asked members to rate selected smartphone apps for effectiveness. Some apps with better ratings include AnxietyCoach, Breath 2Relax, Happify, Live OCD Free, MindShift, MoodKit, and Pacifica (see https://adaa.org/finding-help/mobile-apps#).
   - There are additional smartphone apps that also help a person learn to meditate and practice deep-breathing exercises.
   - Many websites also provide strategies to help the person learn to decrease cognitive distortion that may lead to anxiety and to promote relaxation.
   - The ADAA is also an example of an online site that can offer both information and virtual peer support for those struggling with an anxiety disorder or OCD (see https://adaa.org/finding-help/mobile-apps#).

Milieu Therapy

When an inpatient hospital admission is necessary for those with an anxiety disorder, the following features of the therapeutic milieu can be especially helpful to the patient:

- Structure the daily routine to offer physical and emotional safety.
- Provide information about the daily routine to increase predictability, thus reducing anxiety over the unknown.
- Provide daily activities to promote sharing and cooperation.
- Provide therapeutic interactions, including one-on-one nursing care.
- Include the patient in decisions about individualized care.

Teamwork and Collaboration

Psychotherapy

Among the most evidenced-based therapies for the treatment of anxiety disorders is CBT. It can be effective in the treatment of panic disorder, phobias, social anxiety disorder, GAD, and OCD among many other conditions.

CBT examines how negative thoughts or *cognitive distortions* contribute to anxiety and examines how individuals behave and react in situations that trigger anxiety.

The basic premise of CBT is that our thoughts—not external events—affect the way we feel. We may not even be aware of these "automatic" thoughts, just the feeling that results.

For example: There are three people waiting for a bus that is late.

- Person 1, a businessman, becomes upset that he will be late for a very important meeting, "proving" that he is irresponsible.
  - Result: anxiety
- Person 2, a salesperson, becomes upset thinking that this is just the first of many bad things that will happen today.
  - Result: depression
- Person 3, a 15-year-old boy, thinks he will now miss art class.
  - Result: happiness—he doesn't like art class.

CBT teaches patients to challenge the cognitive distortion through "cognitive restructuring":

- Identifying the cognitive distortion
- Challenging the cognitive distortion
- Replacing the cognitive distortion with a more realistic interpretation (Smith et al., 2017).

Acceptance and commitment therapy (ACT) is an action-oriented approach to *psychotherapy* that stems from traditional behavior therapy and CBT. Patients learn to first accept distressing emotions as appropriate to certain situations. With this understanding, patients begin to accept their concerns and commit to making changes in their behavior. There is modest research support for the use of ACT in treating *workplace stress*, test anxiety, *social anxiety disorder, depression, obsessive-compulsive disorder,* and *psychosis* (Hayes, n.d.).

Meditation is a practice that has its roots in Buddhist philosophy. It is used to help the individual enter a state of relaxation or a state of restful alertness. Practices that include meditation with movement, such as yoga and tai chi, can also promote relaxation. **Mindfulness** is a strategy that helps people to become aware of the present moment. Both meditation and mindfulness are practices that may be helpful for anxiety because they enable individuals to reduce worry and be aware without being fearful. Jon Kabat-Zinn combined these two strategies to develop **mindfulness-based stress reduction (MBSR).** The basic premise of this approach is to learn to detach from anxious thoughts. This is achieved by practicing awareness, identifying tension in the body, understanding your thinking patterns, and learning how to deal with difficult emotions. Research supports the efficacy of MBSR in reducing anxiety and increasing a positive sense of self for those with a diagnosis of GAD (Cuncic, 2017). Hoge and colleagues (2016) found a reduction in biological stress-related hormones and a reduction in stress-related inflammation markers in patients with a diagnosis of GAD who completed MBSR training. For a free online MBSR training course modeled on the program founded by Jon Kabat-Zinn, see https://palousemindfulness.com/.

Behavior Therapy and Techniques

There are several forms of behavioral therapy to decrease anxious or avoidant behaviors. Behavioral therapies are based on the premise that all behaviors are learned and that unhealthy behaviors can be "unlearned" or changed. Behavior is "learned" through the environment or through reinforcement (rewards), and punishment. "Faulty learning," called *conditioning,* is the cause of abnormal behavior. The focus of treatment is often on current problems and how to change them. Behavioral therapies are frequently combined with cognitive therapies, such as CBT.

Some formal therapeutic behavioral techniques include the following:

- ***Aversion therapy***—during this therapy, an undesirable behavior is associated with an unpleasant stimulus. For example, drinking alcohol leads to nausea and vomiting because the person was taking a drug that causes vomiting when paired with alcohol. The smell of alcohol produces a memory of vomiting, which stops the desire to drink again. Relapse rates with this technique are high.
- ***Flooding***—uses prolonged exposure to a feared object or situation. The initial fear response is replaced with exhaustion and decreased anxiety levels. This therapy is rarely used but can be effective in very specific cases.
- ***Systematic desensitization***—sometimes called "exposure therapy"; involves gradually exposing a person to a feared object or situation until the person is free of incapacitating anxiety. This therapy is especially helpful with phobias.
- ***Exposure and response prevention (ERP)***—this technique is designed to systematically desensitize people to their fears. By repeatedly facing fears and learning to manage the uncomfortable feelings and thoughts associated with these fears, the patient learns to allow the anxiety to gradually fade. This technique is helpful in dealing with the ritualistic acts that may be part of the diagnosis of OCD.

APPLYING THE ART

A Person With Obsessive-Compulsive Disorder

Scenario

Eight-year-old Tommy Jansen came to see the school nurse I was shadowing for the day. His productive cough and a temperature of 101.2° F prompted the nurse to call his mother. While waiting to see his mother, Tommy looked worried. "Germs make people sick," he said. I nodded. He continued, "How did I get sick when I wash my hands lots of times just like Mommy does?" When Tommy held out his hands, they were red and dry. Tommy took a tissue to cover his cough. "Maybe I got sick because I forgot to use a tissue to hold the doorknob like Mommy does." When Mrs. Jansen arrived, I introduced myself, and we talked privately while Tommy's make-up assignments were being gathered.

Therapeutic Goal

By the end of this interaction, Tommy will acknowledge needing help to manage his anxiety and ritualistic hand washing.

Student–Patient Interaction	Thoughts, Communication Techniques, and Mental Health Nursing Concepts
Mrs. Jansen: "I'm going to get Tommy to his pediatrician this afternoon. He didn't have a fever this morning, although he did act a little grouchy."	Tommy looked relieved to see his mother. I don't observe any signs of abuse or neglect.
Student's feelings: *Poor little guy—I wonder about that.*	
Student: "You're concerned about him." *She nods.* "Mrs. Jansen, Tommy worried that he got sick from germs, despite, as he said, 'washing my hands lots of times like Mommy.'"	He's already a worrier at 8 years old. Sounds like he's afraid that getting sick is his fault.
Student's feelings: *I just met this person yet here I am jumping in, which means I might make a mistake. I guess I'd rather make a mistake by trying to help than by saying nothing. Guess I'm anxious.*	
Mrs. Jansen: *Looking stricken.* "My poor baby! I didn't want my problem to affect him."	I *give information* about Tommy. From looking at Tommy's hands and from what he is saying, this could be a problem. I am concerned that his mother has some obsessive-compulsive traits.
Student: "Your problem?"	I use restatement. Because Mrs. Jansen is able to identify a problem, she may be showing some insight. She also may recognize that she may be "teaching" her child some problematic behaviors
Mrs. Jansen: "Until now I've been convincing myself that I just wanted my house clean."	She was using denial and rationalization.

Student–Patient Interaction	Thoughts, Communication Techniques, and Mental Health Nursing Concepts
Student's feelings: *How could she not see that her behavior represents more than just keeping her house clean?*	
Student: "How do you explain all the hand washing and using tissues to not touch doorknobs?"	
Student's feelings: *I didn't mean to sound like I'm blaming her. This isn't about a logical decision. It's about a disorder.*	Although I asked an *open* question, this came out like I was being critical of her, like I'm *challenging* or even accusing her.
Mrs. Jansen: *Looks down. Silent.*	
Student: "I'm sorry I pushed you for an explanation. This must be so difficult."	I work on restoring trust by attempting to translate into feelings. I hope I did the right thing by saying I'm sorry.
Mrs. Jansen: *Nods, then makes brief eye contact.* "Since Tommy's dad was sent back to Afghanistan as part of the special forces, I worry all the time. I know I sound crazy, but when I try to stop washing my house, my hands, the doorknobs, then I start to become overwhelmed with worry that Tommy's father will be blown up by a suicide bomber."	Worrying "all the time" sounds like generalized anxiety disorder. The obsessive worry that gets relieved by the washing rituals sounds like obsessive-compulsive disorder (OCD). Both disorders cause such distress.
Student's feelings: *I would worry too with my loved one in a war zone. She worries about "sounding crazy." The stigma of mental illness interferes with people feeling okay about seeking treatment. I feel concern toward her.*	
Student: "You feel kind of scared so often and so alone."	I attempt to *translate* into feelings.
Student's feelings: *I want to always show nonjudgmental acceptance. I show empathy when I reflect underlying feelings. I feel sad at all she has to carry. She obviously cares about her son.*	
Mrs. Jansen: *Tears in her eyes.* "While I wash things, my mind rests a minute. Then I look at my bloody raw hands! Now, I've worried Tommy. Poor kid deserves better than me."	Suggests poor self-esteem

Continued

APPLYING THE ART—cont'd

A Person With Obsessive-Compulsive Disorder

Student–Patient Interaction	Thoughts, Communication Techniques, and Mental Health Nursing Concepts
Student: "Mrs. Jansen, sounds like you're feeling really down on yourself."	I assess her *self-esteem.* Low self-esteem, *depressed mood,* and *suicide* ideation go hand in hand. I *validate* to see if I've understood her meaning.
Mrs. Jansen: "Sometimes I feel panicky … like giving up."	
Student: "Like giving up … as in suicide?"	*Asking* about suicide does not plant the idea of suicide.
Student's feelings: *I feel awkward asking about suicide, but I would rather feel funny asking, than overlook a suicide cue.*	
Mrs. Jansen: "No, never. I wouldn't do that to Tommy Jr. The only time I can resist cleaning for a while is when Tommy needs me to help him with something at home or when I watch him play soccer."	She focuses so many of her responses in terms of her son. Mrs. Jansen recognizes that resisting the compulsion is healthy behavior. I *validate* the meaning.
Student's feelings: *I'm so relieved that she answered "no" immediately even if the reason is Tommy rather than herself.*	
Student: "So sometimes you are able to delay the compulsive washing behavior. How do you feel then?"	I *give support* by saying, "you are able to …." I then ask an *open question.*
Student's feelings: *I called the behavior "compulsive." I hope that naming the behavior with the word "compulsive" does not threaten her.*	
Mrs. Jansen: "Proud of myself but also scared for Tom, Sr. You said 'compulsive.' I've heard of that on *Dr. Phil.*"	Mrs. Jansen identified hearing about *OCD* on television. Maybe that helped her readiness to talk about her ritualistic behaviors.
Student: *Nods.* "Obsessive-compulsive disorder responds to medication and therapy. You don't have to do this all by yourself."	I *validate* the meaning and *assess* her feelings. I do a little teaching as I give information that OCD responds to treatment.
Student's feelings: *I feel hopeful that Mrs. Jansen really will seek treatment.*	
Mrs. Jansen: Looking down at her red, raw hands. "I'm ready for Tommy's sake." I watch and wait. "And for myself." As Tommy rejoins us, Mrs. Jansen asks the school nurse for the community mental health number.	

APPLYING EVIDENCE-BASED PRACTICE (EBP)

Problem

A 37-year-old male with a history of anxiety presents to urgent care with hyperventilation and chest pain. The symptoms started in response to an unexpected increase in his job responsibilities to begin on Monday. The patient is a single father and is fearful about not being able to perform these new responsibilities, losing his job, and being unable to support his children. After an examination and electrocardiogram (ECG) are performed, the symptoms are diagnosed as a panic attack. The advanced practice registered nurse (APRN) listens empathetically and then practices a breathing technique with the patient: Breathe in slowly for the count of 4, hold for the count of 4, and breathe out slowly for the count of 8. The APRN modeled the breathing along with the patient for several cycles. The patient expressed surprise at how well the technique worked to settle him down and stop the panic attack.

EBP Assessment

A. **What do you already know from experience?**

- Anxiety can interfere with all areas of life.
- Panic attacks can feel like respiratory distress or even a heart attack, causing fearfulness.
- An acute medical condition must be ruled out first.
- Patients frequently want medication, such as a benzodiazepine, to quickly resolve their symptoms.
- Relaxation and breathing exercises can be very effective if patients are willing to give them a try.

B. **What does the literature say?**

- There is extensive research supporting relaxation and guided imagery, mindfulness, breathing exercises, yoga, massage, exercise, pet therapy, and other alternative therapies in decreasing anxiety.
- Benzodiazepines can be very effective but need to be used with caution.
- Excessive use can also lead to rebound anxiety.
- The use of benzodiazepines and drugs or alcohol can lead to dangerous central nervous system (CNS) depression and increases fall risk.
- The long-term use of benzodiazepines can increase the risk of developing dementia and clinical depression. Long-term use puts the patient at risk for developing tolerance to the effect of the drug and withdrawal when stopped. There is also a risk of developing a substance use disorder.
- It is recommended that these drugs should only be used for short periods of time for acute situations.

C. **What does the patient want?** The patient initially requested a prescription for benzodiazepines and stated that was the only thing that worked for him. By the end of the appointment, he was open to continuing the breathing exercise he had practiced with the APRN as well as following the other recommendations.

Plan

- The patient is referred to a relaxation class at a nearby community mental health clinic.
- The use of relaxation techniques and guided imagery as strategies to decrease anxiety is discussed with the patient.

Continued

APPLYING EVIDENCE-BASED PRACTICE (EBP)—cont'd

- Information on websites and smartphone applications that provide relaxation techniques is provided.
- The patient is encouraged to continue practicing the breathing exercises learned during the appointment.
- A 7-day supply of clonazepam (Klonopin), a long-acting benzodiazepine, was given to help the patient get through his first week of new responsibilities until he could get started with the other recommendations.

QSEN Prelicensure Knowledge, Skills, and Attitudes (KSAs) Addressed

Safety

- APRN ruled out a cardiac etiology or other physiologic causes for the presenting symptoms.
- An anxiolytic, a benzodiazepine, is prescribed for short-term use only.

Patient-Centered Care is given by:

- Providing active listening and mutual goal setting
- Engaging the patient in the practice of a relaxation technique during the visit and evaluating the effectiveness of this intervention for the patient

Informatics is provided by

- Providing information about additional resources to help the patient deal with his increased anxiety

- ***Modeling***—the patient learns new skills by imitating another person, such as a parent or therapist, who performs the behavior to be acquired. It can include "imitating" more adaptive responses to an anxiety-provoking situation.
- ***Thought stopping***—this is a cognitive strategy to get rid of unwanted stressful thoughts. It involves (1) identifying a stressful thought, (2) focusing exclusively on that thought, and then (3) actively interrupting the thought by performing a behavior such as snapping a rubber band on your wrist or saying the word "stop" out loud or in your heard until the thought goes away.

One set of behaviorally based skills is relaxation training. Relaxation techniques have been shown to be effective for a variety of health conditions, including anxiety, stress management, and health maintenance. The goal of each of these techniques is to induce the body's natural relaxation response. To gain the most benefit, these skills must be frequently practiced. Some of the most common types of relaxation techniques are the following:

- **Deep-breathing or breathing exercises**—multiple techniques involve focusing on taking slow, deep, even breaths.
- **Guided imagery**—people are taught to focus on pleasant images to replace negative or stressful feelings. This may be self-directed or led by a practitioner or a recording and can be combined with relaxation breathing.
- **Progressive relaxation**—progressive muscle relaxation involves tightening and relaxing various muscle groups to "teach" the body how to obtain a relaxed state. Progressive relaxation is often combined with guided imagery and breathing exercises.
- **Autogenic training**—the patient is taught to concentrate on the physical sensations of warmth, heaviness, and relaxation in different parts of the body.
- **Self-hypnosis**—people are taught to produce the relaxation response when prompted by a phrase or nonverbal cue (called a "suggestion").
- **Biofeedback-assisted relaxation**—biofeedback equipment measures body functions and give information about them so that the individual can learn to control them. Biofeedback-assisted relaxation uses electronic devices to teach the individual to produce changes in the body that are associated with relaxation, such as reduced muscle tension and relaxed electroencephalogram (EEG) states.

The techniques just mentioned are considered helpful for reducing the symptoms of anxiety, but there is no good evidence that these techniques *alone* are effective in the treatment of anxiety or depressive disorders. These techniques can be important components of other evidence-based behavioral therapies and can be helpful adjuncts (National Center for Complementary and Integrative Health, 2018).

Neurobiology of Anxiety Disorders and the Effects of Anti-Anxiety Medications

An imbalance of certain neurotransmitters are thought to disrupt specific brain regions that contribute to various anxiety disorders.

Frontal cortex: cognitive interpretations (e.g., potential threat)
Hypothalamus: activation of the stress response (fight-or-flight response)
Hippocampus: associated with memory related to fear responses
Amygdala: fear, especially related to phobic and panic disorders

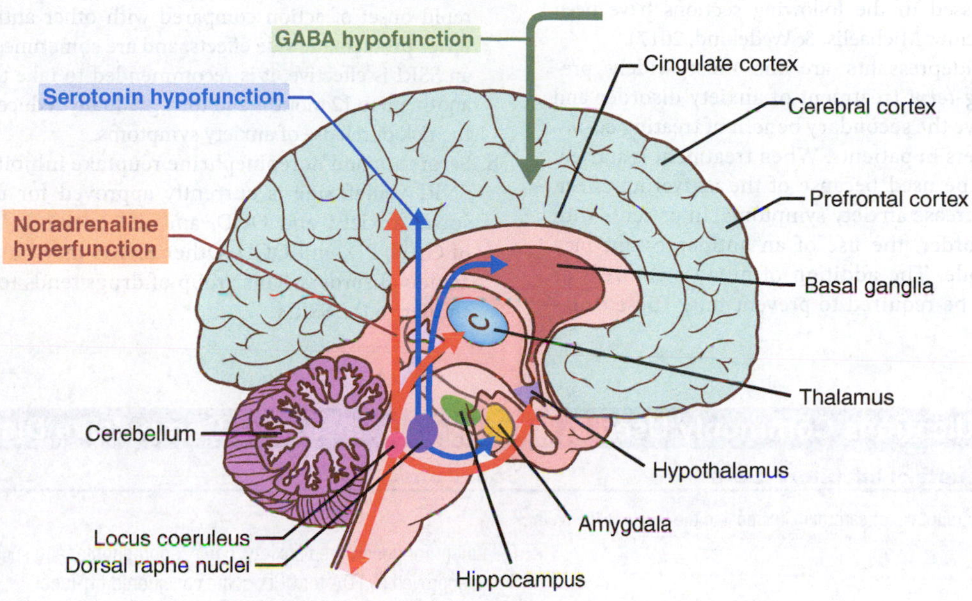

Serotonin: Midbrain, VTA, Cerebral Cortex, and Hypothalamus. Helps regulate mood, sleep, sexual desire, appetite, and inhibits pain. In the anxiety disorders it is believed that there are reduced levels of serotonin transmission and low levels of serotonin are believed to play a role in anxiety disorders as well as depression.

Gamma-aminobutyric acid (GABA): neurotransmitters are widely distributed in the brain. GABA slows neuron activity which plays a role in lowering anxiety and also affects memory. There appears to be strong support that problems with the GABA neurotransmitter system in the brain are related to anxiety disorders.

Norepinephrine (also called Noradrenaline): Midbrain, VTA, Cerebral Cortex, Hypothalamus: plays a role in sensitization, fear conditioning, stress response (increases blood pressure and heart rate). Excessive and unregulated norepinephrine is thought to be related to anxiety disorders.

Antianxiety Agent	How it Works	Examples of Use
SSRIs–first-line treatment	Block reuptake of serotonin-increasing levels in the brain	Paroxetine (Paxil)—helpful in GAD
SNRI–first-line treatment	Blocks both serotonin and norepinephrine in the brain	Venlafaxine (Effexor)—mixed anxiety/depression, anxiety and nerve pain
Noradrenergic drugs	Propranolol—blocks adrenergic receptor activity Clonidine—stimulates-adrenergic receptors	Propranolol—short-term relief of social anxiety and performance anxiety Clonidine—anxiety disorders, panic attacks
Benzodiazepines	Binds to benzodiazepine receptors, facilitates action of GABA, slowing neural transmission thus lowering anxiety	Alprazolam—may be used short-term to treat panic disorder and agoraphobia
Buspirone (BuSpar)	Buspirone functions as a serotonin 5-HT_{1A} receptor partial agonist resulting in anxiolytic and antidepressant effects	Can treat the worry associated with GAD rather than the muscle tension

Pharmacological Therapy

Anxiety disorders are chronic conditions that can be managed and treated. Several classes of medications have been found to be effective in the treatment of anxiety disorders. The combination of psychopharmacology with other therapies, especially CBT, provides the most effective treatment strategy.

The medications discussed in the following sections have been shown to be helpful (Bandelow, Michaelis, & Wedekind, 2017).

Antidepressants. Antidepressants are the most widely prescribed drugs for the *long-term* treatment of anxiety disorder and OCD. Antidepressants have the secondary benefit of treating co-occurring depressive disorders in patients. When treatment is started, low doses of SSRIs must be used because of the activating effect, which can temporarily increase anxiety symptoms. In patients with co-occurring bipolar disorder, the use of an antidepressant may precipitate a manic episode. The addition of mood stabilizers or antipsychotic agents may be required to prevent this. These drugs can increase the risk of suicide. When stopping antidepressants, the drugs must be tapered slowly to prevent a discontinuation syndrome.

The following types of antidepressants are prescribed. Please refer to Table 11.8 for a list of adverse effects.

A. Selective serotonin reuptake inhibitors (SSRIs): First-line treatment for all anxiety disorders, OCD, and BDD. They have a more rapid onset of action compared with other antidepressants, have fewer problematic side effects, and are sometimes more effective. If an SSRI is effective, it is recommended to take the medication for another 6 to 12 months and then gradually reduce the dose to lessen the risk of relapse of anxiety symptoms.
B. Serotonin and norepinephrine reuptake inhibitors (SNRIs). The SNRI venlafaxine is currently approved for use in PD, GAD, social anxiety, and OCD, and duloxetine is approved for use in GAD, PD, and OCD. Other SNRIs may be used off-label for anxiety disorders. This group of drugs tends to have side effects similar to the SSRIs.

TABLE 11.8 Medications Commonly Used in Anxiety and Obsessive-Compulsive Disorder

Selective Serotonin Reuptake Inhibitors (SSRIs)	Comments
Mechanism of Action: Blocks reuptake of serotonin, increasing the levels in the brain	
Citalopram Escitalopram Fluoxetine Fluvoxemine Paroxetine Sertraline	Treatment for generalized anxiety, panic, agoraphobia, and social anxiety Some approved by FDA for OCD; some considered off-label Off-label for body dysmorphic disorder Common side effects: jitteriness, nausea, restlessness, headache, fatigue, changes in appetite, changes in weight, tremor, sweating, QTC prolongation, sexual dysfunction, diarrhea, constipation, hyponatremia, serotonin syndrome
Selective Serotonin Norepinephrine Reuptake Inhibitors (SNRIs)	**Comments**
Mechanism of Action: Blocks reuptake of serotonin and norepinephrine, increasing the levels in the brain	
Duloxetine Venlafaxine	Duloxetine used to treat GAD, PDA, SAD Venlafaxine used to treat GAD Off-label use for OCD Common side effects: jitteriness, nausea, restlessness, headache, fatigue, changes in appetite, changes in weight, tremor, sweating, sexual dysfunction, diarrhea, constipation
Tricyclic Antidepressants (TCAs)	**Comments**
Mechanism of Action: Blocks reuptake of serotonin and norepinephrine, intensifying the effects of the neurotransmitters	
Clomipramine Desipramine Doxepin Imipramine Nortriptyline	Clomipramine used for PDA; FDA approved for OCD This drug category may also be used to treat GAD, PDA, and SAD but not typically prescribed Common side effects: anticholinergic effects, somnolence, dizziness, cardiovascular effects, weight gain, nausea, headaches, sexual dysfunction
Non-Benzodiazapine Anxiolytic	**Comments**
Mechanism of Action: Binds to serotonin and dopamine receptors	
Buspirone	Delayed onset (3 weeks or longer) Reduces symptoms of GAD Less sedating than benzodiazepines No physiological or psychological dependence Common side effects: dizziness, nausea, headache, nervousness, insomnia, light-headedness, excitability

Continued

TABLE 11.8 Medications Commonly Used in Anxiety and Obsessive-Compulsive Disorder—cont'd

Benzodiazepines	Comments
Mechanism of Action: Enhances the action of GABA, slows neuronal transmission	
Alprazolam Oxazepam Triazolam Lorazepam Diazepam Clonazepam Chlordiazepoxide	Depresses neurotransmission in limbic and cortical areas of the brain Useful for short-term anxiety Dependence and tolerance may develop Frequent use linked with rebound anxiety, dementia, increased fall risk, and higher mortality Should not be combined with opioid medications Common side effects: sedation, dizziness, fatigue, impaired driving, impaired cognitive function, CNS depression
Other Medications	**Comments**
Pregabalin	Increases extracellular GABA Used for GAD and SAD Side effects: dizziness, sedation, dry mouth, weight gain, blurred vision, impaired concentration, withdrawal symptoms
Beta Blockers Propranolol Atenolol	Blocks beta-adrenergic receptors Helpful for stage fright or test anxiety Side effects: dizziness, nausea, fatigue, impaired sleep
Quetiapine	Blocks serotonin and dopamine receptors Faster improvements Sometimes used in combination with SSRIs Side effects: sedation, weight gain, cardiac changes, slowed cognition, increased appetite

C. Tricyclic antidepressants (TCAs): Second- or third-line use for the treatment of panic disorder, PTSD, and GAD. Imipramine has shown good efficacy in the treatment of panic disorders. Clomipramine is effective in OCD and PDs with agoraphobia.

D. Monoamine oxidase inhibitors (MAOIs): Examples include phenelzine and tranylcypromine. These drugs are rarely prescribed for the treatment of panic disorder. The use of these drugs is limited due to the dangerous food–drug and drug–drug interactions.

Benzodiazepines. *Benzodiazepines* are **anxiolytic drugs** indicated for *short-term treatment only*. Benzodiazepines are immediately helpful in relieving anxiety but are generally not helpful for the long-term treatment of any of the anxiety disorders. Tolerance to the antianxiety effects of these drugs develops over time, requiring higher and higher dosages to achieve the same calming effect. Sudden stopping of these drugs after long-term use can lead to uncomfortable withdrawal symptoms. There is a risk of developing an addiction when used long term, especially in those with a substance use history. Long-term use is also associated with higher rates of memory and cognitive concerns, including dementia. Benzodiazepine drugs should not be given to women who are pregnant or breast-feeding. In rare instances (up to 5%), benzodiazepines can cause a paradoxical (opposite) agitation in susceptible patients, particularly children and the elderly. *The use of benzodiazepines increases fall risk, increases the risk of the development of dementia, and may lead to increased mortality.* See Box 11.1 for patient teaching related to benzodiazepine use.

Antihistamines. *Antihistamines* such as diphenhydramine or hydroxyzine can provide quick, periodic anxiety relief. They are most effective for short-term use only and are useful for those with a substance use problem because they are not addicting. These drugs can cause acute sedation.

Buspirone. *Buspirone* is a nonaddictive medication used in the management of anxiety disorders and those requiring long-term relief of anxiety disorder symptoms. It is most effective for the treatment of GAD. This drug has a delayed response of 2 to 4 weeks and is not useful for acute episodes of anxiety.

Anticonvulsants. *Anticonvulsants*, such as valproic acid, gabapentin, and pregabalin have shown some usefulness in the treatment of GAD, social anxiety, and panic attacks. These are usually used as adjunct medications. Gabapentin may have some immediate efficacy in the treatment of the symptom of anxiety.

Antipsychotics. Although this class of drugs is not usually used to treat anxiety disorders, *antipsychotics* may be used as calming agents for acute anxiety in certain situations. Quetiapine is not approved by the U.S. Food and Drug Administration but has shown some efficacy for GAD. Refer to Table 11.8.

Complementary and Alternative Medicine

A number of plant-based substances are claimed to relieve anxiety. Unfortunately, available scientific evidence regarding the efficacy of any of these agents in the treatment of anxiety disorders is sparse or of poor quality. The following is a list of some of the more common plant-based substances that have been studied (Bandelow et al., 2017).

- *Kava kava*
  - Inconsistent results on efficacy
  - Significant concerns about the risk of hepatotoxicity
  - Multiple drug–drug interactions; can potentiate the effects of certain medications, such as anticonvulsants, antianxiety agents, diuretics, and many others

BOX 11.1 Patient and Family Medication Teaching: Benzodiazepine Drugs

1. Caution the patient and family:
   - Drug is indicated for short-term use only.
   - Drug may lose its effectiveness over time related to tolerance.
   - Do not increase dose or frequency of use without prior approval of the health care provider.
   - Medications may cause sedation and reduce the ability to handle mechanical equipment and increase fall risk.
   - Avoid alcohol or other central nervous system depressant drugs such as opioid pain medications, because the sedative effect can be compounded and can be fatal.
   - Drug can have an opposite effect in selected individuals—increased anxiety/agitation rather than calming effect—and may cause rebound anxiety.
   - Avoid caffeine because of decreasing the desired effects of the drug.
   - Long-term use can increase mortality and the development of dementia.
   - Avoid for people with a history of substance use disorder; increases risk of developing addiction.
2. Avoid becoming pregnant because these drugs increase the risk of congenital anomalies, especially in the first trimester.
3. Avoid breast-feeding because these drugs are excreted in the milk and would have adverse effects on the infant.
4. Teach the patient the following:
   - Abrupt cessation of benzodiazepine use after 3 to 4 months of daily use may cause withdrawal symptoms such as insomnia, irritability, nervousness, dry mouth, tremors, convulsions, confusion, and even psychosis.
   - Take with meals or snacks to reduce gastrointestinal discomfort.
   - Drug interactions
     - Antacids may delay absorption.
     - Cimetidine interferes with the metabolism of benzodiazepines, causing increased sedation.
     - Central nervous system depressants cause increased sedation.

- *Valerian*
  - Was not effective in placebo-controlled studies of anxious patients
  - May be effective for insomnia
  - May be safe for short-term use; multiple contraindications for use and multiple potential side effects
- *Lavender oil*
  - Shows some effectiveness for GAD and mixed anxiety/depression but more data are needed
- *St John's wort*
  - Is not effective and should not be used with any other antidepressants.

Herbs and dietary supplements are not subject to the same rigorous testing as prescription medications. Also, herbs and dietary supplements are not required to be uniform, and there is no guarantee of bioequivalence of the active compound across preparations. Problems that can occur with the use of psychotropic herbs include toxic side effects and herb–drug interactions.

Self-Care for Nurses

Anxiety is communicated empathetically from person to person. Therefore it is not surprising that being around a person with acute levels of anxiety may cause the nurse to experience intense and uncomfortable emotions. When working with highly anxious patients, students and new clinicians may benefit from the supervision of a more experienced health care professional. Supervision can help nurses identify and intervene when they respond to patient behaviors by becoming negative or demonstrating ineffective interventions. When the nurse feels anger, frustration, or other negative feelings toward the patient, both the nurse and patient may respond with mutual withdrawal.

It is important for caregivers to take time to also care for themselves. Stress management courses, mindfulness, yoga, exercise, creative activities, and humor are all examples of stress reduction techniques to help nurses keep a healthy balance in their personal lives.

EVALUATION

Identified outcomes serve as the basis for evaluation. In general, evaluation of outcomes for patients with anxiety disorders deals with questions such as the following:

- Is there a reduced level of anxiety? Is there a change in intensity?
- Does the patient recognize symptoms as anxiety related? What symptoms does the patient experience when anxiety levels are rising? Does the patient recognize signs of escalating anxiety? Can the patient identify strategies to stop the escalation?
- Are obsessions, compulsions, phobias, worrying, or other symptoms of anxiety disorders present? Quantify the number of increased or decreased symptoms during the day/night/situation.
- List the learned behaviors used by the patient to help manage anxiety.
- Can the patient perform self-care activities or manage health care needs?
- Can the patient maintain satisfying interpersonal relations? How does the patient describe close relationships now as compared with before treatment?
- Can the patient assume usual roles? Are there still areas of role performance that need improvement?
- Is the patient adherent with medication?

KEY POINTS TO REMEMBER

- Anxiety has an unknown or unrecognized source, whereas fear is a reaction to a specific threat.
- Anxiety can be normal, acute, or chronic, as well as adaptive or maladaptive.
- Peplau defined four levels of anxiety. The patient's perceptual field and ability to comprehend and learn are different at each level. There are variable behavioral, cognitive, and physical signs and symptoms of anxiety at each of the different levels (see Table 11.1).
- Effective nursing interventions are different for mild to moderate levels of anxiety and for severe to panic levels of anxiety. Effective nursing approaches are suggested in Tables 11.2 and 11.3.
- Defense mechanisms are used to guard against anxiety. They can be adaptive or maladaptive. Defenses are presented in a hierarchy from healthy to intermediate to immature. Table 11.4 provides examples of adaptive and maladaptive uses of many of the more common defense mechanisms.
- Anxiety disorders are the most common psychiatric disorders in the United States and frequently co-occur with major depression and/or substance use disorders. Obsessive-compulsive disorder (OCD) and body dysmorphic disorder (BDD) also have high rates of co-occurrence with major depressive disorders. All of these disorders increase the risk of suicide.

- Research has identified genetic and biological risk factors in the etiology of anxiety disorders and OCD.
- Patients with anxiety disorders suffer from panic attacks, irrational fears, restlessness, irritability, muscle tension, sleep disturbances, fatigue, and excessive worrying.
- OCD is a chronic disorder in which a person has uncontrollable, reoccurring thoughts (obsessions) and behaviors (compulsions) that the person feels the urge to repeat over and over.
- People with anxiety disorders may consult their primary care providers about multiple somatic complaints without realizing their symptoms may be due to a treatable psychiatric disorder.
- One form of psychotherapy that is effective for treating anxiety disorders, OCD, and milder forms of BDD is cognitive-behavioral therapy (CBT). Psychotherapy can be combined with medication to treat these disorders.
- Nursing interventions include establishing a nurse–patient relationship, providing support counseling, milieu therapy, promotion of self-care activities, psychobiological intervention, and health teaching.

APPLYING CRITICAL JUDGMENT

1. Ms. Smith, a patient with OCD, washes her hands until they are cracked and bleeding. What interventions will you plan to promote healing of her hands?
2. This is Mr. Olivetti's third emergency department visit in a week. He is experiencing severe anxiety accompanied by many physical symptoms. He clings to you, desperately crying, "Help me! Help me! Don't let me die!" Diagnostic tests have ruled out a physical disorder. The patient outcome has been identified as "Patient anxiety level will be reduced to moderate/mild within 1 hour." What are some of the effective interventions you should use?
3. Mrs. Zeamans is a patient with generalized anxiety disorder (GAD). She has a history of substance use disorder and is in recovery. During a clinic visit, she tells you she plans to ask the psychiatrist to prescribe diazepam (Valium) to use when she feels anxious. She asks whether you think this is a good idea. How would you respond? What other kinds of medications might the physician order?

CHAPTER REVIEW QUESTIONS

1. Friends invite an adult diagnosed with type 2 diabetes to go on a mountain hike. The adult replies, "I can't go because I don't have any hiking shoes." Unconsciously, this person is concerned about difficulty with blood glucose management during strenuous activity. Which defense mechanism is evident?
   a. Displacement
   b. Rationalization
   c. Passive aggression
   d. Reaction formation
2. Four adult patients describe frightening events that resulted in panic levels of anxiety/fear. Which patient's report most clearly indicates a reasonable fear response?
   a. "I saw a large spider crawling along my kitchen wall."
   b. "I was at the mall when a gunman began firing an assault weapon."
   c. "I was at home when a storm with heavy thunder and lightning lasted over an hour."
   d. "I was trapped in an elevator that stopped between floors when the power went out."
3. A nursing student arrives late for a clinical experience and is not wearing the correct attire. When the instructor privately criticizes the behavior, the student responds, "I'm always the one who gets caught. You're going to cause me to fail." Select the instructor's best response.
   a. "Other students get caught as well."
   b. "I am not trying to cause you to fail. I am here to help you."
   c. "I am sorry you feel that way. I try to treat all my students equally."
   d. "The requirements for this experience were discussed during our orientation."
4. Select the best example of altruism.
   a. After recovering from a gunshot wound, a police officer attends a local support group.
   b. After recovering from open-heart surgery, an individual plays tennis three times a week.
   c. An individual who received a liver transplant volunteers at a local organ procurement agency.
   d. An individual with a long-standing fear of animals volunteers at a community animal shelter.
5. A disaster relief nurse has just arrived to help efforts after a tornado that destroys a town. Which approach would be most appropriate when talking with survivors?
   a. Provide active listening.
   b. Help the survivors generate possible solutions.
   c. Help the survivors develop self-awareness to understand their stress response.
   d. Offer firm, short, simple statements and instructions.

REFERENCES

American Nurses Association, American Psychiatric Nurses Association, & International Society of Psychiatric-Mental Health Nurses. (2014). *Psychiatric-mental health nursing: Scope and standards of practice*. Silver Springs, MD: Nursesbooks.org.

American Psychiatric Association. (2013). *Diagnostic and statistical manual of mental disorders (DSM-5)* (5th ed.). Washington, DC: APA.

American Psychological Association. (n.d.). *Psychology topics*. Retrieved from: http://www.apa.org/helpcenter/data-behavioral-health.aspx.

Anxiety and Depression Association of America ADAA. (n.d.). Facts and statistics. Retrieved from. https://adaa.org/about-adaa/press-room/facts-statistics.

Bandelow, B., Michaelis, S., & Wedekind, D. (2017). Treatment of anxiety disorders. *Dialogues in Clinical Neuroscience, 19*(2), 93–107.

Beidas, R. S., Stewart, R. E., Walsh, L., Lucas, S., Downey, M. M., Jackson, K., et al. (2015). Free, brief, and validated: Standardized instruments for low-resource mental health settings. *Cognitive and Behavioral Practice, 22*(1), 5–19. https://doi.org/10.1016/j.cbpra.2014.02.002.

Black, D. W., & Andreasen, N. A. (2014). *Introductory textbook of psychology* (6th ed.). Washington, DC: American Psychiatric Publishing.

Boundless. (2015). Retrieved April 5, 2016 from https://www.boundless.com/psychology/textbooks/boundless-psychology-textbook/biological-foundations-of-psychology-3/structure-and-function-of-the-brain-35/the-limbic-system-154-12689/.

Cuncic, A. (2017). The Benefits of Meditation for Generalized Anxiety Disorder Verywell. Updated July 27, 2017. Retrieved from https://www.verywell.com/the-benefits-of-meditation-for-generalized-anxiety-disorder-4143127.

Giddens, J. (2017). *Concepts for nursing practice* (2nd ed.). St. Louis: Elsevier.

Hayes, S. (n.d.). Association for Contextual Behavioral Science, state of the ACT evidence. Retrieved from https://contextualscience.org/state_of_the_act_evidence.

Hoge, E. A., Bui, E., Palitz, S. A., Schwarz, N. R., Owens, M. E., Johnston, J. M., et al. (2016). The effect of mindfulness meditation training on biological acute stress responses in generalized anxiety disorder. *Psychiatry Research*, 2017. pii: S0165- 1781(16)30847-2.https://doi.org/10.1016/j.psychres.2017.01.006.

Institute of Medicine. (2001). Crossing the quality chasm: A new health system for the 21st century. Retrieved from http://www.nationalacademies.org/hmd/~/media/Files/Report%20Files/2001/Crossing-the-Quality-Chasm/Quality%20Chasm%202001%20%20report%20brief.pdf.

Mayo Clinic Staff. (2017). Social Anxiety Disorder (Social Phobia). Mayo Foundation for Medical Education and Research (MFMER). August 29, 2017 Retrieved from: https://www.mayoclinic.org/diseases-conditions/social-anxiety-disorder/symptoms-causes/syc-20353561.

National Center for Complementary and Integrative Health (NCCIH). (2018). *Anxiety at a glance*. Retrieved from https://www.nccih.nih.gov/health/anxiety-at-a-glance.

National Institute of Mental Health. (2015). A New Look at Racial/Ethnic Differences in Mental Health Service Use Among Adults. April 23, 2015 science update. Retrieved from: https://www.nimh.nih.gov/news/science-news/2015/a-new-look-at-racial-ethnic-differences-in-mental-health-service-use-among-adults.shtml.

National Institute of Mental Health. (2017). Any Anxiety Disorder. Retrieved from: https://www.nimh.nih.gov/health/statistics/any-anxiety-disorder.shtml.

Peplau, H. E. (1968). A working definition of anxiety. In S. F. Burd & M. A. Marshall (Eds.), *Some clinical approaches to psychiatric nursing*. New York: Macmillan.

Preston, J., & Johnson, J. (2015). *Clinical psychopharmacology: Made ridiculously simple* (8th ed.). Miami, FL: MedMaster, Inc.

Sadock, B. J., Sadock, V. A., & Ruiz, P. A. (2015). *Kaplan and Sadock's synopsis of psychiatry* (11th ed.). Philadelphia: Wolters/Lippincott Williams & Wilkins.

Shpancer, N. (2018). The wisdom of defense mechanisms managing the internal weather: The concept of psychological defenses. *Psychology Today*. Retrieved from https://www.psychologytoday.com/us/blog/insight-therapy/201802/the-wisdom-defense-mechanisms.

Smith, M. M. A., Segal, R., & Segal, J. (2017). Therapy for Anxiety Disorders. Cognitive Behavioral Therapy. Exposure Therapy, and Other Options HELPGUIDE.ORG. Retrieved from https://www.helpguide.org/articles/anxiety/therapy-for-anxiety-disorders.htm.

Sullivan, H. S. (1953). *The interpersonal theory of psychiatry*. New York: Norton.

12

Somatic Symptom Disorders

Lois Angelo

http://evolve.elsevier.com/Varcarolis/essentials

OBJECTIVES

1. Identify the etiologies and basic symptoms of somatic system disorders.
2. Discuss genetic, cognitive, psychological, interpersonal, and cultural factors influencing the onset and course of somatic symptom disorders.
3. Differentiate the significant differences between somatic symptom disorders and factitious disorder. Explain how this would affect your thought process while giving nursing care.
4. List factors that can make it difficult to identify somatic symptom disorders.
5. Describe the impact of childhood trauma on somatic disorders.
6. Identify the registered nurse (RN) case manager role when working with patients with somatic symptom disorders in both the inpatient and outpatient settings.

KEY TERMS AND CONCEPTS

adverse childhood experiences (ACE), p. 158
assertiveness training, p. 165
case management, p. 165
factitious disorder, p. 161
factitious disorder imposed on another, p. 162
functional neurological disorder (conversion disorder), p. 161
health locus of control, p. 158
holistic approach, p. 158
illness anxiety disorder, p. 160
loneliness, p. 159
malingering, p. 162
Maslow's hierarchy of needs, p. 159
personality types, p. 161
self-compassion, p. 158
somatic symptom disorder, p. 157
somatization, p. 157

CONCEPT: COPING: *Coping* represents continual changes in behavior and cognition in order to modify or adapt the person–environmental relationship to reduce stress (Giddens, 2017). Nurses are in a position to assess, identify, and understand the patient's psychosocial stressors that can contribute to somatic symptom disorders. The nurse attempts to help the patient improve overall functioning through the development of effective coping strategies, such as assertiveness training, problem-solving skills, relaxation techniques, enhancement of social supports, and so on. Nursing interventions should focus initially on establishing rapport with the patient. The therapeutic relationship is vital to treatment success.

INTRODUCTION

Somatic symptom disorders are included in the most controversial and mind-boggling areas of modern psychiatry (Khare & Srivastava, 2016). Somatic symptom disorders, characterized by the presence of one or more physical symptoms, have been around for centuries and have disrupted countless lives. These complex disorders confuse and frustrate patients and health care providers.

SOMATIC SYMPTOM DISORDERS

Patients with somatic symptom disorders often present with numerous symptoms, such as headaches, back pain, persistent lack of sleep, stomach upset, and chronic tiredness (Bhargava, 2016). **Somatization**, defined as a process by which psychological distress is expressed as physical symptoms without a known organic source, causes substantial distress and psychosocial impairment with or without a known general medical disease (Kaviani & Tabrizi, 2016).

The emphasis in the *Diagnostic and Statistical Manual of Mental Disorders,* 5th edition (*DSM-5*; American Psychiatric Association, 2013) is not only on the presence of physical symptoms but also on the way an individual presents and interprets them. It is important to remember that in most somatic symptom disorders, with the exception of factitious disorders, these symptoms are not intentional or under the conscious control of the patient.

Somatic symptom disorders are more prevalent in women than in men, occurring up to 10 times more frequently in women. They are diagnosed most often in children who have experienced a traumatic event (Calahorro, 2017).

Somatization, depression, and anxiety disorders are the most common psychiatric disorders in primary care. It is important for primary care clinicians to be aware of somatic symptoms when they are presented by patients because they may indicate underlying anxiety or depressive disorders (Carlehed, 2016). Somatic disorders impair occupational and social function, resulting in increased work absences, a lower quality of life, and increased health care utilization and costs. The psychological problems are frequently not addressed because the patients are seen by doctors with other areas of medical expertise, which results in increased medical expenses. Complaints by patients suffering from somatic symptoms relate more to the body than to the mind. It is common for medical providers to focus on the physical complaints because they are typically seen as more straightforward to address. This leads to expensive, repetitive medical examinations instead of the provision of psychological care. Meanwhile, many patients "doctor shop," looking for ways to relieve their symptoms. With the stigma associated with mental illness, patients may be hesitant to seek mental health care for their very physical symptoms. Patients with a somatic symptom need to be treated with a mind-body approach (Nakamura et al., 2017).

Physical symptoms may offer a means to indicate distress when patients cannot easily express emotions in words (Greenberg, 2017). Findings suggest that patients low on emotional expressivity may tend to experience and report more bodily pains and complaints than those who are emotionally expressive (Kaviani & Tabrizi, 2016).

This chapter helps prepare nurses to utilize a **holistic approach** for individuals with somatic symptom disorders, emphasizing the multidimensional interplay of biological, psychological, and sociocultural needs. It is also important for nurses who work outside of psychiatric settings to be aware of the influence of the environment, stress, individual lifestyle, support networks, and coping skills of each patient.

Prevalence and Comorbidity

Somatic symptom disorders are pervasive for much of the population, with more than 80% of individuals describing symptoms within the past 7 days (Portrie-Bethke & Hanks, 2017). More than 50% of patients present to outpatient medical clinics with a physical complaint and do not have a diagnosed medical condition (Greenberg, 2017). Because actual diagnosed medical disorders and somatic symptom disorders can exist concurrently, a comprehensive physical and psychosocial examination is imperative. In a recent study of 225 patients, there was a significant correlation of length of sick leave with depression, anxiety, and somatization (Schneider, 2017).

Women have a higher incidence of somatic symptoms, and it is likely due to increased occurrence of abuse in both girls and women and as a result of socialization and social roles. Women may have a greater awareness of somatization in general and are more encouraged to acknowledge distress (Portrie-Bethke & Hanks, 2017).

Theory

Genetic Factors

The genetic basis for somatization is not clear. Some studies indicate a familial pattern for somatization that may be due to genetic or environmental factors, or both. In addition, a genetic influence may represent an inherited predisposition to general distress (Greenberg, 2017).

However, the data do support a genetic theory, in that somatic symptom disorders tend to occur in families, presenting in 10% to 20% of first-degree relatives with somatization disorder (Spratt, 2014). Rates may also be higher in monozygotic twins (Ask et al., 2016). Twin studies looking at the construct of "health anxiety" support somatic symptom disorders as being moderately heritable (Ask et al., 2016).

Psychological Theory

Difficulty with expressing distress verbally is thought to underlie expression through physical symptoms (Spratt, 2014). Positive and negative responses from parents or role models can lead to reinforcement of somatic and illness behaviors (Spratt, 2014). Having a somatic symptom disorder and low **self-compassion** is associated with a number of symptoms and reduced health-related quality of life and is a potential clinically relevant factor that may influence health outcomes (Dewsaran-van der Ven, 2018). Self-compassion is defined as the tendency to be caring, warm, and understanding toward oneself when faced with personal shortcomings, inadequacies, or failures. Although the concept can be found in older Asian Buddhist literature, it is a relatively new topic to the Western world. Self-compassion is viewed as a protective factor that fosters emotional resilience and is particularly relevant to the study of human adaptation to life adversity and stress (Muris & Petrocchi, 2016).

Antecedents of somatization may include living around a family member with an illness; receiving attention for an illness; having an overprotective parenting style; childhood expectations of perfection; or a history of divorce, maltreatment, or trauma (Kurlansik & Maffei, 2016). This may reflect a learned process in which experiencing illness in the environment or the self can lead to a heightened focus on symptoms. In addition, children may not have the ability or training to express distress verbally, which can plant the seeds of somatic behavior. This pattern of focus can carry over into adulthood and be reinforced over time. Before pubescence, the rates of somatizing are equal between boys and girls, with the rate in females being higher after this time (Spratt, 2014). School stressors are a common environmental factor in the development and continuation of these symptoms.

The Self Compassion Scale (SCS) (Box 12.1) is consistent with the definition of self-compassion, a dynamic balance between the compassionate versus uncompassionate ways that individuals emotionally respond to pain and failure with kindness or judgment, cognitively understand their predicament as part of the human experience, and pay attention to suffering in a mindful manner (Neff, 2016). Nurses can use this as a tool for their own self-development, administer it to patients, and use it as a tool for patient education to address areas where the scores are high.

Cognitive Model

Cognitive theorists believe that the somatic disorders are the result of negative, distorted, and catastrophic thoughts and reinforcement of these thoughts. Patients focus on body sensations, misinterpret their meaning, and respond with excessive alarm (Seto & Nakao, 2017).

For the recovery of the patient with a somatic symptom disorder, the management of the concept of **health locus of control** is very important (Box 12.2). Health locus of control is defined as a patient's tendency to think of health-related events as inwardly controlled or controlled by external forces and is found to have a significant relationship with chronic physical and mental illnesses. Health locus of control has a meaningful relationship with health attitudes, behaviors, and outcomes (Bhargava & Pandey, 2016).

Interpersonal Model

Adverse childhood experiences (ACEs) have been shown to contribute to more negative health outcomes in adulthood, including somatic symptoms. Childhood trauma associated with physical or sexual violence is consistently linked with somatization or functional neurological disorders later in life (Greenberg, 2017). Prolonged trauma,

BOX 12.1 Self-Compassion Scale—Short Form

How I Typically Act Toward Myself in Difficult Times

Please read each statement carefully before answering.

To the left of each item, indicate how often you behave in the stated manner, using the following scale:

Almost Never				Almost Always
1	2	3	4	5

1. When I fail at something important to me, I become consumed by feelings of inadequacy. ____
2. I try to be understanding and patient toward those aspects of my personality I don't like. ____
3. When something painful happens, I try to take a balanced view of the situation. ______
4. When I'm feeling down, I tend to feel like most other people are probably happier than I am. _____
5. I try to see my failings as part of the human condition. ______
6. When I'm going through a very hard time, I give myself the caring and tenderness I need.
7. When something upsets me, I try to keep my emotions in balance. ______
8. When I fail at something that's important to me, I tend to feel alone in my failure. ______
9. When I'm feeling down, I tend to obsess and fixate on everything that's wrong. ______
10. When I feel inadequate in some way, I try to remind myself that feelings of inadequacy are shared by most people. ______
11. I'm disapproving and judgmental about my own flaws and inadequacies. ______
12. I'm intolerant and impatient toward those aspects of my personality I don't like. ______

From Raes, F. E., Pommier, K., Neff, D., & Van Gucht, D. (2011). Construction and factorial validation of a short form of the Self-Compassion Scale. *Clinical Psychology and Psychotherapy, 18*, 250–255.

BOX 12.2 Health Locus of Control

Aim of study: To determine the role of health locus of control in patients with somatic disorders.

Internal locus: The belief that an individual is in control of his or her health and can take steps on a personal level to become healthy again.

External locus: The belief that external forces are in control of a patient's health. Patients with an external locus often believe that other people, such as doctors, have control/authority over their health.

Method: Sample consisted of 100 participants from a private clinic. The data were collected using the Patient Health Questionnaire and the Multidimensional Health Locus of Control Scale (Bhargava, 2016). The Multidimensional Health Locus of Control Scale measures four types of beliefs about health locus of control (Gibson, Held, Khawnekar, & Rutherford, 2016):

1. "I am directly responsible for my condition getting better or worse."
2. "Most things that affect my condition happen to me by chance."
3. "Following the doctor's orders to the letter is the best way to keep my condition from getting any worse."
4. "The type of help I receive from other people determines how soon my condition improves."

Individuals with internal health locus of control are more responsible for their health, recovery, and rehabilitation and are more likely to undertake efforts to feel well. An internal locus of control is related to lower severity of symptoms because individuals with an internal locus of control believe that they can control their own destiny. They are likely to be more aware of environmental factors that may influence future behaviors and are more likely to take steps to improve environmental conditions, place greater value on skill or achievement reinforcement, and are resistive to conformity. Patients who believe that they can control their health are more likely to engage in health behavior, which will lead to better health outcomes (Bhargava, 2016).

Conclusion: The higher the internal locus of control, the lower the severity of somatization, which may change patients' perceptions of their own health and affect utilization of the health care system.

especially in childhood, can cause neurobiological changes, such as alterations in the volume and activity levels of major brain structures (Meichenbaum, 2017). Also, children who were victimized by peers show a higher incidence of somatic symptoms (Portrie-Bethke & Hanks, 2017). Childhood adversity is associated with reduced adjustment and social support and increased distress, somatic complaints, and resilience—the ability to recover from setbacks, adapt well to change, and keep going in the face of adversity. Resilient coping is associated with lower distress. Highly resilient subjects show less distress and somatic symptoms despite reported childhood adversities in comparison to those with low resiliency (Beutel et al., 2015).

Loneliness and weak social connections are associated with a reduction in life span similar to that caused by smoking 15 cigarettes a day and even greater than that associated with obesity. High levels of loneliness are associated with exaggerated blood pressure and inflammatory reactivity to acute stress. This, in turn, damages blood vessels and other tissues, increasing the risk of heart disease, diabetes, joint disease, and premature death (Murthy, 2017). There are indications that loneliness may also be related to blunted cardiac, cortisol, and immune responses (Brown & Gallagher, 2017). Because the need for social connections and close, caring relationships is central to human nature, it follows that the failure to fulfill this need is detrimental to mental and physical health. Lonely people have 45% lower odds of survival compared with those who were not lonely (Jaremka & Faqundes, 2013). A lack of social supports can increase the negative impact of stress and lead to an increase in somatic symptoms. Improving social supports is an important part of the treatment plan for someone diagnosed with a somatic symptom disorder. Box 12.3 presents the UCLA Loneliness Scale, the most extensively used scale to assess loneliness.

Cultural Considerations

The tendency to somatize does not vary from culture to culture. One study of somatic symptoms of depressive disorders in 15 primary care centers in 14 countries did not show cultural variability. Although the frequency of somatic disorders is similar across cultures, culture-specific manifestations are often present (Greenberg, 2017). In some cultures, somatic symptoms may be the first indicator of an underlying anxiety or depressive disorder.

Somatic symptoms, such as pain, are frequently seen in immigrant refugees. Somatic symptoms are of considerable concern among traumatized refugees, and different patterns of somatic symptoms are associated with different clusters of posttraumatic stress disorder (PTSD) symptoms. Emphasis should be placed on the importance of screening for PTSD in refugees presenting with pain and somatic symptoms because the somatic complaints may have origins in trauma (Morina et al., 2018).

In contemporary Western culture, there has been unprecedented growth and comfort in the past few decades. Despite an increase in life expectancy, we are seeing that people are sicker but living longer. Core values, such as materialism, consumerism, and individualism, may be damaging to a person's sense of well-being, community, and health, including an increased incidence of somatization. Abraham **Maslow's**

BOX 12.3 Loneliness Scale

The Revised UCLA Loneliness Scale (LS-R) is the most extensively used scale to assess loneliness.

1 = Never, 2 = Rarely, 3 = Sometimes, 4 = Always

1. How often do you feel unhappy doing so many things alone?
2. How often do you feel you have no one to talk to?
3. How often do you feel you cannot tolerate being so alone?
4. How often do you feel as if no one understands you?
5. How often do you find yourself waiting for people to call or write?
6. How often do you feel completely alone?
7. How often do you feel unable to reach out and communicate with those around you?
8. How often do you feel starved for company?
9. How often do you feel it is difficult for you to make friends?
10. How often do you feel shut out and excluded by others?

Scoring

A total score is computed by adding up the response to each question. The average loneliness score on the measure is 20. A score of 25 or higher reflects a high level of loneliness. A score of 30 or higher reflects a very high level of loneliness.

From Ausín, B., Muñoz, M., Martín, T., Pérez-Santos, E., & Ángel Castellanos, M. (2018). Confirmatory factor analysis of the Revised UCLA Loneliness Scale (UCLA LS-R) in individuals over 65. *Journal of Aging and Mental Health, 23*(3), 345–351.

hierarchy of needs indicates that humans shift attention to higher-level needs (social, intellectual, and spiritual) once basic, lower-level needs (food, shelter, clothing) are satisfied. However, Western culture has become fixated on materialism and resists movement to higher-level needs such as love, belonging, and respect for others. Reaching these higher-level needs provides the social inclusion and support that can enhance self-esteem and thus health (Begen & Turner-Cobb, 2015).

Somatic Symptom Disorder

In somatic symptom disorder (formerly known as somatization disorder), medical findings are lacking or less than expected for the magnitude of the complaint. Patient histories may include multiple treatments and surgeries, substance abuse, marital difficulties, suicide attempts, chronic pain, and impaired work and life functioning, including disability and high health care costs. Unfortunately, these individuals frequently refuse psychiatric assistance because they believe their symptoms are medical, even when presented with negative test findings. They tend to not recognize the underlying mental problem and may pressure providers for repeated and unnecessary procedures (Dimsdale, 2015).

Pain response is individual and difficult to measure objectively; however, psychosocial impairments (depression, somatization) are frequently associated with increased pain intensity and disability days (Ahmed, 2017). For example, low back pain is one of the most common musculoskeletal conditions worldwide, with a lifetime prevalence of 84%. In a recent study of college students in the United States, psychological factors such as feeling sad, exhausted, and overwhelmed were directly associated with the prevalence of low back pain. It was determined that there was a relationship between low back pain and depression and somatization. Passive coping, increased depression, and somatization were all associated with greater perceptions of pain (Robertson & Kumbhare, 2017).

Illness Anxiety Disorder

Individuals with illness anxiety disorder (formerly known as hypochondriasis) are preoccupied with having or eventually developing a serious illness. The patient is apprehensive of a particular illness despite

***DSM-5* DIAGNOSTIC CRITERIA**

Somatic Symptom Disorder

A. One or more somatic symptoms that are distressing or result in significant disruption of daily life

B. Excessive thoughts, feelings, or behaviors related to the somatic symptoms or associated health concerns as manifested by at least one of the following:
   1. Disproportionate and persistent thoughts about the seriousness of one's symptoms
   2. Persistently high level of anxiety about health or symptoms
   3. Excessive time and energy devoted to these symptoms or health concerns

C. Although any one somatic symptom may not be continuously present, the state of being symptomatic is persistent (typically more than 6 months).

Specify if:

With predominant pain (previously pain disorder): This specifier is for individuals whose somatic symptoms predominantly involve pain.

Specify if:

Persistent: A persistent course is characterized by severe symptoms, marked impairment, and long duration (more than 6 months).

Specify current severity:

Mild: One of the symptoms specified in Criterion B is fulfilled.

Moderate: Two or more of the symptoms specified in Criterion B are fulfilled.

Severe: Two or more of the symptoms specified in Criterion B are fulfilled, plus there are multiple somatic complaints (or one very severe somatic symptom).

Reprinted with permission from the *Diagnostic and Statistical Manual of Mental Disorders,* Fifth Edition (Copyright © 2013). American Psychiatric Association. All Rights Reserved.

continuous negative medical evaluations and assurances (Khare & Srivastava, 2016).

Individuals with illness anxiety disorder exhibit a high level of anxiety and alarm about their health, lasting at least 6 months, and may either excessively check for problems or avoid medical care. It is important to consider other possible diagnoses, such as anxiety disorders.

The preoccupation with health leads to an encompassing anxiety that severely impairs functioning. These patients are more disturbed by the potential implications of any disorder than with the disorder itself and are alarmed by any new bodily sensations. Patients can misinterpret normal physical sensations, such as sweating, abdominal cramping, or awareness of heartbeat, as indicative of disease (Dimsdale, 2015).

Exposure to media that urge us to use certain health screens or suggest we talk to our doctor about specific medications may also contribute to fears about health. Social media in particular seem to increase fears. For example, following a large-scale trauma or disaster, the use of Twitter and YouTube is significantly associated with higher stress responses (Goodwin, Palgi, & Lavena, 2015). In addition, a recent study found that there are now multiple smartphone apps stating that they can target symptoms of worry and anxiety; however, it is essential that they are consistent with evidence-based interventions (Webb, Rosso, & Rauch, 2017).

Illness anxiety disorder with comorbid depression might be underdiagnosed because some patients do not have depressed mood or loss of interest as the prominent features. It is stressed that a comorbid mood disorder with illness anxiety, especially in middle-aged and elderly patients, could mimic several psychiatric conditions, such as delirium, catatonia, anxiety, and other depressive disorders.

There are a number of case reports of patients with illness anxiety whose condition improved after electroconvulsive therapy (ECT). ECT was found to play a significant role in the modulation of the immunological system. It is believed that the effects of stressors and cytokines may play an important role in the pathophysiology of somatic complaints. Recognizing this in the elderly population would speed up treatment and prevent unnecessary, costly testing and delay. Many practitioners do not consider referral for ECT before multiple medications have been tried, a process that may span many months or even years and leave the patient seriously ill, suffering, and dysfunctional for a prolonged period. ECT has resulted in a fast and complete recovery for people with illness anxiety with comorbid mood disorders (Wong, Pang, & Yiu, 2017).

Functional Neurological Disorder

Functional neurological disorder (FND), also known as **conversion disorder** and historically as "hysteria," involves chronic or brief symptoms of altered voluntary motor or sensory function that cause substantial distress or psychosocial impairment. The diagnosis rests on positive clinical findings that indicate the symptom is incongruent with anatomy, physiology, or known diseases or the symptom is inconsistent at different times (e.g., no ankle dorsiflexion while lying down, but the ability to stand on tiptoes) (Greenberg, 2017). A long-held view of FND is based on psychoanalytic theory. Sigmund Freud proposed that the "unbearable effect" of stressors is "converted" into physical symptoms that provide an escape from an unpleasant conflict—a key feature of the coping mechanism of "repression." He proposed that the physical manifestation reduces the initial stressor by changing the individual's circumstances (e.g., weakness resulting in being unable to return to work where there is workplace bullying). Current studies discuss FND causation as varying from purely biological factors to psychological and traumatic factors such as childhood abuse, child sexual abuse, and family dysfunction, all of which are likely shaped by a combination of genetic programming and environmental factors involving childhood development (Nicholson & Aybek, 2016). A psychiatric comorbidity was present in 73.3% of patients with FND, the most common being depression at 50% and dissociative disorder at 48.3%. Patients with FND tend to be referred to clinics other than psychiatric clinics during the initial stages of the disorder due to barriers to mental health care and concerns about stigma. Because of the very high rate of previous traumatic events in the patient with FND, a comprehensive assessment of trauma history would contribute to the integrative plan of care. Increasing the awareness of society regarding child abuse and neglect may also alleviate the pain experienced by FND trauma survivors (Akyuz & Gokalp, 2017).

VIGNETTE: Jane, age 26, reports physical symptoms such as back pain, nausea, dizziness, poor sleep, and irritable bowel for the past 4 years since she has been working in a very stressful environment. These symptoms appeared episodically at first and slowly became persistent. She changed her primary care provider several times and visited multiple specialists, including a neurologist, an orthopedist, a gastrointestinal specialist, and a rheumatologist. None of the practitioners could explain her symptoms. Most suggested that she should consider seeking a psychiatric consultation. The psychiatric nurse practitioner ordered several medications for mood, sleep, and anxiety. The result was that she just felt more tired and had difficulty going to work each day—until she became aware of a registered nurse (RN) case manager in her primary care provider's office who found Jane to be socially isolated and physically distressed.

Together they developed strategies for Jane to identify ongoing stressors and to slowly become more physically and socially active. Jane joined a gym and initially forced herself to renew old friendships and at least go out to eat with someone once per week. The case manager contacted the psychiatrist, and Jane's medications were slowly reduced to just a mood stabilizer. Jane eventually joined a tennis group and switched jobs, and she states that she is more active and feels much better. Slowly, her physical symptoms decreased, with just periodic episodes of irritable bowel syndrome. Jane maintains her working relationships with her psychiatric nurse practitioner and RN case manager and meets quarterly with both providers.

VIGNETTE: An 18-year-old female was brought to the emergency department during a seizure-like episode. She had been having incidents where she would fall to the ground and exhibit jerky muscle movements, as well as less severe periods of muscle shaking and anxiety. The episodes began after her fiancé broke off their relationship and began dating someone else. The patient's electroencephalogram (EEG) was completely normal, and the episodes had not decreased with the use of the antiseizure medication levetiracetam. Although the patient was still being followed by a neurologist, she was also referred for a psychiatric evaluation and treatment. During the initial assessment, it was discovered that the patient had similar episodes after her parents' divorce while she was in third grade, but they had resolved since then. The patient had never been able to discuss her feelings about the divorce with either parent, but she was allowed to stay home from school and spend more time with them whenever she was ill.

Psychological Factors Affecting Other Medical Conditions

Psychological factors affecting other medical conditions is a disorder that is diagnosed when a general medical condition is adversely affected by psychological or behavioral factors; the factors may precipitate or exacerbate the medical condition, interfere with treatment, or contribute to morbidity and mortality. Conditions that may be affected can involve all physical disorders and diagnoses (Greenberg, 2017). Somatization is strongly associated with anxiety and depression. Depression has a detrimental effect on the cardiovascular system. People suffering from depression are twice as likely as the general population to develop myocardial infarction (MI). A recent study found a positive relationship between negative emotions (anger, hostility, boredom) expressed in Twitter messages and cardiovascular-related death, strengthening the link between negative thinking and cardio-metabolic disorders (Chauvet-Gelinier & Bonin, 2016).

Stress, such as conflicts with family and peers and high workload and job demands; poor supervision; and lack of support are all associated with poor physical and mental health outcomes. Cannon's stress theory explains this response as an imbalance in homeostasis, whereby prolonged exposure to stressors results in a breakdown of the biological system (Khamisa, 2015).

In the history of the concept of stress and somatization, **personality types** were studied. Initially, it was thought that the Type A personality, characterized by a sense of time urgency, high job involvement, strong need for achievement, and competition, was associated with coronary artery disease. However, subsequent studies have focused on hostility and hostile thoughts. Type A personality became more associated with increased survival, especially with coronary heart disease and in diabetes, because Type A individuals are more goal oriented, are often more conscientious, and adhere to healthy lifestyles and thus are associated with better somatic outcomes. Type D personality, as defined by Johan Denollet, associates negative affectivity and social inhibition with coronary heart disease. Type D people experience extreme difficulty in approaching other people and have an avoiding coping style. It is known that a lack of social support/loneliness is associated with cardiovascular disease (Chauvet-Gelinier & Bonin, 2016).

Factitious Disorder Imposed on Self

The essential feature of **factitious disorder** (formerly known as Munchausen syndrome) is intentionally faking symptoms in order to assume the sick role, that is, to be a patient. In addition, there are no obvious external benefits, such as financial gain or avoiding work or criminal prosecution. Patients with factitious disorder tend to have some medical knowledge, and common presentations include wound-healing problems, excoriations, infections, bleeding, hypoglycemia, and gastrointestinal ailments. An extreme presentation occurs in a subgroup of patients who feign disease, move from hospital to hospital, and submit to repeated procedures for an illness they have voluntarily manufactured (Greenberg, 2017).

Malingering is intentionally faking or exaggerating symptoms for an obvious benefit, such as money, housing, medications, avoiding work, or criminal prosecution. Malingering is a behavior and not a psychiatric disorder. Malingering is often used by school-age children to avoid tests/stressful experiences, by "inventing" an ailment, such as "stomach ache" to remain home from school for that day. The motivation for intentionally producing symptoms in malingering is an external incentive, whereas in factitious disorder, the motivation is to assume the role of patient. It is possible to establish feigning only if the patient acknowledges deliberately producing symptoms or if other evidence demonstrates a major inconsistency between reported and observed function (e.g., a patient who reports an inability to walk is subsequently observed playing tennis) (Greenberg, 2017).

The unconscious motivation is thought to be for the purpose of assuming the sick role and receiving nurturance, comfort, and attention, although this is not clear. The cause is unknown, although stress and, often, borderline personality disorder are implicated. The patient is often intelligent, resourceful, and sophisticated regarding medical practices (Dimsdale, 2015). A person may exaggerate, fabricate, simulate, or induce a symptom. For example, a person might inject a caustic substance into the skin to form an abscess, injure himself or herself, use medication inappropriately, falsify lab results or medical reports, or describe suicidal thoughts after the death of a spouse who did not exist. About 1% of hospitalized patients meet the criteria for factitious disorder, although underreporting is likely due to the inherent deception.

Factitious Disorder Imposed on Another

Factitious disorder imposed on another (formerly Munchausen by proxy) has the same criteria as a factitious disorder, except the deliberate fabrication of symptoms or injury is imposed upon another person, often a child or dependent victim. The perpetrator is often a parent or caregiver, and the motivation is to receive attention or nurturing. The diagnosis is given to the perpetrator, not the victim; the victim may be given a diagnosis of abuse. There is a criminal aspect to this disorder because another person is being harmed.

APPLICATION OF THE NURSING PROCESS

Somatic symptoms and actual medical conditions may occur in the same patient at some point. A full assessment cannot be ignored because of a diagnosis of a somatic symptom disorder. The following sections outline several areas that are not normally included in a nursing assessment but are important to assess in a patient with suspected somatic symptom disorders.

ASSESSMENT

Assessment should begin with the collection of data about the nature, location, onset, character, and duration of the symptom(s). Often, patients with functional neurological disorders report having a sudden loss of function of a body part, such as, "I woke up this morning and couldn't move my arm." Patients with any of the somatic symptom disorders may discuss their symptoms in dramatic terms. They may use colorful descriptions, such as, "The pain was searing, like a hot sword drawn across my forehead" or "My symptoms are so rare that none of the doctors can figure it out."

Information should be sought about patients' ability to meet their own basic needs. As with all patients, they should be met where they are and gradually guided toward independence. This process is different for each individual. Anxiety may cause or exacerbate tachypnea and tachycardia. Nutrition, fluid balance, and elimination needs should be evaluated because patients with somatic symptom disorders often complain of gastrointestinal distress, diarrhea, constipation, and anorexia. Sexual desire or performance may be altered by experiences of painful intercourse or pain in another part of the body. Patients should be assessed for a history of childhood trauma because they have an elevated risk of suicidality (Carlier, 2016).

Rest, comfort, recreational activity, and hygiene needs may be altered as a result of problems such as fatigue, weakness, insomnia, muscle tension, and pain. Safety and security needs may be threatened by patient experiences of blindness, deafness, loss of balance and falling, and anesthesia of various parts of the body.

Assessment should also include the dynamics of the family and workplace of the patient. These dynamics can contribute to the development and sustainment of somatic symptoms, which can be seen as expressions of unresolved conflict. Unhealthy or rigid communication patterns also contribute to somatic symptoms (Portrie-Bethke & Hanks, 2017).

Cognitive Style

In general, patients with somatic symptom disorders misinterpret physical stimuli and distort reality regarding their symptoms. For example, sensations a normal individual might interpret as a headache might suggest a brain tumor to a patient with anxiety illness disorder. Exploring the patient's thought processes is enlightening in identifying these distortions.

Ability to Communicate Feelings and Emotional Needs

Patients with somatic symptom disorders have difficulty communicating their emotional needs. As children, their family communication style may have neglected the appropriate expression of anger, depression, fear, and other emotions, and thus they do not recognize feelings or understand how to relate to them. For example, the feeling of anxiety may cause tightness in the stomach, nausea, rapid heartbeat, shortness of breath, dizziness, sweating, and tensing of muscles such as the hands or jaw. If a person is taught to consider the relationship of emotions to physical symptoms, the person will likely identify that he or she is anxious. If this emotional coaching has not occurred, the stage is set to believe only a medical problem could be the cause. Somatization may be a predominant method of expressing feelings in the family, or the child may have received attention for normal symptoms during his or her developmental phase and somatization was thus reinforced. Sometimes there is an obvious connection between symptom and stressor, such as blindness when someone cannot face a situation. More often, the connection is not obvious to the patient or provider.

Dependence on Medication

Individuals experiencing many somatic complaints often become dependent on medication to relieve pain, anxiety, or depression or to induce sleep. Taking anxiolytic agents such as benzodiazepines is common in this population because of high anxiety and concern about symptoms. These medications can become addictive and cause "rebound anxiety" when the dosage wears off, exacerbating the anxiety problem over time.

It is important that the nurse assess the type and amount of medications being used and be alert for a history of numerous prescribers.

Assessment Guidelines

It is always important to ensure that an underlying medical condition has been eliminated from the differential diagnosis, which could be any medical condition, including autoimmune disorders, cardiac disease, and endocrine imbalances. However, as you recall, both a true medical condition and a somatic symptom disorder can co-occur.

Somatic Symptom Disorders

1. Ensure that a thorough physical examination with appropriate medical tests has been completed.
2. Assess for nature, location, onset, characteristics, and duration of the symptom(s).
3. Assess the patient's ability to meet basic needs (level of independence).
4. Assess risks to the safety and security needs of the patient as a result of the symptom(s).
5. Determine whether the symptoms are under the patient's voluntary control.
6. Explore the patient's thought processes and ability to communicate feelings and needs.
7. Determine the type and amount of medication the patient is using.
8. Assess for childhood trauma and risk of suicide.
9. Inquire about previous evaluations/treatments from specialists in any health care area.
10. Explore the patient's interpersonal dynamics/resources, such as network of friends, financial/work stressors, and family dynamics.
11. Assess for the patient's health locus of control and level of self-compassion.

DIAGNOSIS

Patients with somatic symptoms and related disorders present various nursing problems. *Ineffective coping* is frequently diagnosed. Causal statements might include the following:

- Distorted perceptions of body functions and symptoms
- Chronic pain of psychological origin
- Dependence on pain relievers or anxiolytics

Table 12.1 identifies potential nursing diagnoses for patients with somatic symptom disorders.

OUTCOMES IDENTIFICATION

The overall long-term goal in treating individuals with somatic symptom disorders is that people with these disorders will eventually be able to live as normal a life as possible. This includes symptom or pain reduction, improved level of independence, and a better overall quality of life.

The following are examples of potential long-term outcome criteria:

- Patient will identify and articulate feelings such as anger, shame, guilt, and remorse.
- Patient will resume performance of work-role behaviors.
- Patient will identify ineffective coping patterns.
- Patient will make realistic appraisal of strengths and weaknesses.

PLANNING

Because patients are seldom admitted to psychiatric units specifically because of these disorders, long-term interventions usually take place

TABLE 12.1 Potential International Council for Nursing Practice (ICNP) Nursing Diagnoses for Somatic Symptom Disorders[a]

Relationships
1. *Caregiver stress*
2. *Impaired communication*
3. *Lack of knowledge of community services*
4. *Risk for loneliness*
5. *Social isolation*
6. *Impaired socialisation*
Feelings
1. *Anxiety*
2. *Impaired attitude*
3. *Depressed mood*
4. *Despair*
5. *Hopelessness*
6. *Fatigue*
7. *Fear*
8. *Dysfunctional grief*
9. *Helplessness*
10. *Risk for loneliness*
11. *Pain*
12. *Low self-esteem*
13. *Impaired spiritual status/Effective spiritual status*
Coping
1. *Decisional conflict*
2. *Caregiver coping*
3. *Impaired family coping/Effective family coping*
4. *Impaired coping process*
5. *Impaired parenting/Effective parenting*
Perception
1. *Impaired perception*
2. *Powerlessness*
3. *Low self esteem*
Behaviors
1. *Anger control*
2. *Employment problem*
3. *Homebound*
4. *Impaired homemaking*
5. *Housing problem*
6. *Impaired mobility*
7. *Self-care deficit*
8. *Impaired sleep/Adequate sleep*
9. *Withdrawn behavior*
Health Management
1. *Adherence to exercise regimen/Non-adherence to exercise regimen*
2. *Effective gastrointestinal system function/Impaired gastrointestinal system function*
3. *Health-seeking behavior*
4. *Adherence to medication regime/Non-adherence to medication regime*
5. *Impaired nutritional status/Positive nutritional status*
Self-Injurious Behaviors
1. *Drug dependence/Drug abuse*
2. *Risk for suicide*
3. *Self-destructive behaviors*
4. *Suicidal ideation*

[a]The International Classification for Nursing Practice (ICNP) is a product of the International Council of Nurses (ICN). Retrieved from http://www.icn.ch/what-we-do/ICNP-Browser/.

on an outpatient basis. Short-term planning, such as a referral to a psychiatric provider, may be initiated during a medical-surgical admission, which is often of brief duration. Somatic symptom disorders are best treated when a patient has a single, identified care provider who sees the patient on a regular basis.

Nursing interventions should initially focus on establishing rapport with the patient. The therapeutic relationship is vital to treatment success because of the tendency toward defensiveness in these patients. Broaching a nonmedical or psychiatric etiology to the patient's symptoms is threatening. Therapeutic interventions must address helping the patient learn to meet needs without resorting to somatization. The optimal goal is not only to relieve symptoms but also to increase quality of life and independence. Collaboration with family or significant others can be supportive of patient success; however, each situation must be assessed individually because families can also be sources of stress or dysfunction.

IMPLEMENTATION

Innovative, integrated approaches are needed to manage complex patients with overlapping mental health, physical health, and social issues. Fortunately, effective treatment strategies exist that can improve somatic conditions, reinforcing the importance of identifying and engaging affected patients (Pentin, 2016). Establishing trust is essential, and the patient needs to feel respected and understood. One study found that a patient was more likely to report psychological symptoms to a primary care clinician if the patient already had a relationship with that clinician. In taking a history, clinicians should pay attention to how the physical symptoms are related to the patient's emotions and social situation and whether any stressful personal events, such as losses, have occurred. Listening for family, marital, or work conflict is important because conflict is associated with somatic complaints. Clinicians should acknowledge the patient's physical and emotional suffering (Greenberg, 2017).

Communication Guidelines

Generally, for patients with somatic symptom disorders, nursing interventions take place in the outpatient setting. The nurse attempts to help the patient improve overall functioning through the development of effective coping and communication strategies. Through the use of identification and expression of emotions or issues, patients no longer rely only on medical symptoms to unconsciously display their needs. Remember, when patients complain of physical symptoms, take the symptoms seriously. Even if a medical explanation is not found to be understandable, the symptoms are real and distressing to the patient. Table 12.2 lists possible interventions for patients with somatic symptom disorders.

Working with people who have somatic symptom disorders can be frustrating (Box 12.4), and you (and other staff) may find yourself avoiding interaction with them. However, when people feel they are receiving care and attention, the intensity of symptoms tends to diminish. As the symptoms are alleviated and rapport is established, it becomes easier to address emotional issues.

Health Teaching and Health Promotion

When somatization is present, the patient's ability to perform self-care activities may be impaired. In general, nursing interventions involve the use of a straightforward approach to support the highest level of functioning. For example, the patient who demonstrates arm paralysis can be encouraged to eat using the other arm. The patient who is experiencing blindness can be told where foods are located on his or her plate by comparing the plate to a clock face. These strategies are effective in reducing secondary gain.

Assertiveness training is often appropriate to teach a direct means of meeting needs and thereby decreases the need for somatic symptoms. Teaching an exercise regimen, such as doing range-of-motion exercises for 15 to 20 minutes daily, can help the patient feel in control, increase endorphin levels, and help decrease anxiety.

TABLE 12.2 Interventions for Somatic Symptom Disorders

Intervention	Rationale
1. Offer explanations and support during diagnostic testing.	1. Reduces anxiety while ruling out organic illness
2. After physical complaints have been investigated, avoid further reinforcement of the somatic complaints.	2. Directs focus away from physical symptoms
3. Spend time with the patient at times other than when he or she is expressing a physical complaint (e.g., when talking about a pet or TV program), and give the "reward" of extra attention during those times.	3. Rewards non–illness-related behaviors and encourages repetition of desired behavior
4. Observe and record frequency and intensity of somatic symptoms.	4. Establishes a baseline and later enables evaluation of effectiveness of interventions
5. Do not imply that symptoms are not real.	5. Acknowledges that psychogenic symptoms are real to the patient
6. Shift focus from somatic complaints to feelings or to neutral topics.	6. Conveys interest in patient as a person rather than patient's symptoms; reduces need to gain attention via symptoms
7. Assess secondary gains that physical illness provides for patient, such as attention, lack of work responsibility, or guilt of a spouse causing them to stay rather than leave the patient.	7. Allows these needs to be met in healthier ways and thus minimizes secondary gains
8. Use straightforward approach to patient exhibiting resistance or covert anger.	8. Avoids power struggles, demonstrates acceptance of anger, and permits discussion of angry feelings
9. Have patient direct all requests to a designated nurse or clinician.	9. Reduces manipulation
10. Show concern for patient but avoid fostering dependency needs.	10. Shows respect for patient's feelings while minimizing secondary gains from illness; encourages progress toward independence
11. Reinforce patient's strengths and problem-solving abilities.	11. Contributes to positive self-esteem; helps patient realize that needs can be met without resorting to somatic symptoms
12. Teach assertive communication skills and techniques.	12. Provides patient with a positive way of identifying feelings and meeting emotional needs; reduces feelings of helplessness and need for manipulation
13. Teach patient stress reduction techniques, such as meditation, relaxation, and mild physical exercise.	13. Provides alternate coping strategies; reduces need for medication

BOX 12.4 Working With Patients Displaying Somatic Symptoms

Managing somatic symptom disorders is a common problem for medical students and results in anxiety, frustration, anger, and challenging situations. The current biomedical model of medical education continues to produce clinicians who rely solely on biomedical decision making with a reticence to address psychological issues. This results in inappropriate referrals and suboptimal patient care, and it affects students emotionally.

The following are several comments from medical students regarding working with patients displaying somatic symptoms:

- "I could find myself getting really agitated with him and getting cross as well. I've got lots of other things to do. I don't have time for this."
- "It's very satisfying when you have worked with patients like this. No one has really bothered to work with them before—to gradually get people off being so focused on that particular symptom is really satisfying because you think 'I've seen them change.'"
- "It's a way of ending the consultation—to send her for blood work or a chest x-ray."
- "Really trying to pay attention to the psychological side of things early on—ask them about what else is going on in their lives."
- "It's actually quite therapeutic for her just to come in and complain."

Communication skills teaching was described as being particularly useful for the students. Researchers have proposed a curriculum that focuses on psychosocial assessment. Teaching techniques such as cognitive-behavioral therapy to medical staff and nurse practitioners has shown some positive impact on patient management of somatic symptom disorders (Howman, 2016).

Assertiveness Training

"**Assertiveness training** is a form of behavior therapy designed to help people stand up for themselves—to empower themselves, in more contemporary terms. Assertiveness is a response that seeks to maintain an appropriate balance between passivity and aggression. Assertive responses promote fairness and equality in human interactions, based on a positive sense of respect for self and others" (*Encyclopedia of Mental Disorders*, 2019).

Assertiveness training uses "I" statements to help defuse a combative/aggressive response. Instead of saying *"You always say you're going to study, and you don't study—you'll never amount to anything,"* for example, a less accusatory approach using "I" statements could decrease the aggressive tone and help the listener feel less defensive ("When you … I feel …"). For example, *"When you don't study, I feel so upset and frustrated because I want you to get the skills that will make you successful in life."*

Case Management

Case management can help limit health care costs by meeting with patients regularly and helping the patient identify when a medical visit is necessary. Case managers may recommend more frequent visits to primary care for simple check-in appointments and discourage unnecessary visits to urgent care or emergency rooms for somatic symptoms. The patient who establishes a relationship with the case manager often feels less anxiety because he or she has an advocate and feels someone is managing and aware of his or her care. Nurse case managers play a key role in managing patients' conditions and enhancing clinical and self-management skills, particularly with patients with somatic symptoms, targeting their psychosocial as well as physical needs. Case managers can also help gather medical records because multiple specialists are often involved, and they can coordinate care with these providers. In one study, case managers had their own offices inside the primary care practice to meet with patients. The case managers did an initial assessment, checking patients' perspectives, personal resources, and motivation for change. In cooperation with patients, they developed specific objectives to be achieved toward their health care goals. Together, they decided on a hierarchy of goals, from smaller to larger ones, and strategies to meet these goals. Strategies included developing a trusting relationship; identifying continuing, persistent stressors; identifying resources and activating physical and social networks; providing psycho-educational counseling; checking the availability of treatment options in the patients' local vicinity; assessing patients' economic resources; comparing costs of treatments; calculating patients' time to access services; coordinating care with patients' other providers, and enhancing patients' self-care (Zimmerman & Puschmann, 2016).

Psychotherapy

Cognitive and behavioral approaches can be effective in helping patients to cope with their symptoms, express underlying emotions, and develop alternative strategies for expression of feelings (Webb et al., 2017). Trauma-focused psychotherapy is recommended for patients with a history of childhood trauma (Carlier, 2016). Behavior modification can provide incentives, motivation, and rewards to help patients control their symptoms. Family and group therapy can increase awareness of communication patterns and help patients gain strategies to improve social skills (Koelen et al., 2014). Nurses may be involved with teaching patients alternative coping skills as well, such as relaxation and breathing techniques, or cognitive restructuring to aid in controlling anxiety and reframing faulty thinking.

Family/relationship therapy can also be beneficial. It is important to explore the patient's emotional connections with family, friends, and coworkers and identify strengths and wellness behaviors, encouraging traditional and alternative therapies that can help to alleviate anxiety/depression and, often, physical symptoms as well (Portrie-Bethke & Hanks, 2017).

Group cognitive-behavioral therapy (CBT) provides communication and interaction among the group members as a vehicle of change. Group models offer positive peer modeling opportunities, reinforcement, and most importantly, social support (Khare & Srivastava, 2017). Over the past two decades, Internet-based cognitive-behavioral therapy (iCBT) programs have proliferated. A growing body of research supports the efficacy of iCBT for depression and other psychiatric conditions, and these programs may help address barriers that hinder access to effective treatment (Webb et al., 2017).

Pharmacological Therapies

Currently, there are no medications specified for somatic symptom disorders. Psychopharmacology treatment is focused on comorbid depression or anxiety. A selective serotonin reuptake inhibitor (SSRI), such as citalopram, may be used to help alleviate symptoms of anxiety and depression and reduce pain. In contrast, benzodiazepines are becoming less frequently used due to the potential for abuse and rebound symptoms.

Nursing responsibilities include administering these medications and providing patient teaching.

EVALUATION

Evaluation of progress toward therapeutic goals is a straightforward process when measurable behavioral outcomes have been written clearly and realistically in the care plan. Even partially met goals are considered a success because of the considerable resistance to change in this population. Remission of symptoms is a process over time, and patients are likely to report the continuing presence of somatic symptoms, although they report less intensity and focus on the symptoms.

APPLYING EVIDENCE-BASED PRACTICE (EBP)

Problem

A 30-year-old woman has been referred for a psychiatric evaluation by her primary care provider (PCP). She brings pillows for joint support and asks that the lights be turned down during appointments. The first two sessions have been spent talking about her numerous medical conditions, and she has shared a three-ring binder of medical records with the psychiatric nurse practitioner. Her complaints include back, neck, and knee pain as well as migraine headaches. Her records indicate mild osteoarthritis that is inconsistent with the level of pain and inability to work that she reports. She has had second and third opinions with similar findings. She has an appointment with a neurologist because she is concerned her headaches may be indicative of a tumor. Her husband and friends avoid her, stating they are tired of hearing about her medical problems all the time.

EBP Assessment

A. **What do you already know from experience?** This patient seems significantly more concerned about her conditions in comparison to the average person. Mild osteoarthritis is unlikely to present with a severe level of pain or result in the inability to work. Similar patients have tended to be defensive when possible psychiatric aspects to their problems have been broached.

B. **What does the literature say?** People with somatic symptom disorder often present with several medical issues. Symptoms are often exaggerated in comparison to the medical findings. Patients with this disorder focus on medical problems to a degree that creates high anxiety and interferes with life functioning. Several providers may have been consulted, and patients are frequently unaware of the psychological aspects of their condition. Antidepressants, anxiolytics, cognitive-behavioral therapy, and hypnotherapy have been shown to be helpful.

C. **What does the patient want?** This client is seeking help with a disability claim that had been denied. She requests assistance with anxiety related to the denied claim. She is interested in the nurse practitioner's opinion of her medical records and the quality of care she has received.

Plan

Although this patient does not see the connection between her psychological stressors and her medical problems, treating her anxiety is a good place to start. She has requested help with this, so she should be cooperative, and the treatment of anxiety will likely improve her physical symptoms as well. As therapeutic rapport is established, the connection between psychological and physical symptoms can be gently discussed. A selective serotonin reuptake inhibitor (SSRI) antidepressant such as sertraline will be prescribed, and a referral will be given for counseling to help with anxiety and relationships.

QSEN Prelicensure Knowledge, Skills, and Attitudes (KSAs) Addressed

Teamwork and Collaboration by referring the patient for therapy, reviewing medical records, and making contact with other providers

Evidence-Based Care by utilizing what the literature says about best practice, past experience, and patient desires in the plan of care

KEY POINTS TO REMEMBER

- Somatic symptom disorders are characterized by the presence of multiple, real physical symptoms for which there is most often no evidence of medical illness.
- There is strong evidence that psychological/interpersonal/cognitive conditions may precipitate and often increase the severity of physical symptoms. Patients with somatic symptom disorders often have a number of comorbid psychiatric illnesses, primarily depression and anxiety. A suicide assessment should be performed with any psychiatric patient. Patients with somatic symptom disorders may be especially prone to self-harm behaviors.
- The nursing assessment is important to identify a history of adverse childhood events and symptoms of depression and anxiety and to clarify the history, interpersonal dynamics, current stressors, and course of past symptoms. The nurse case manager is in a key position to assist other health care personnel to take an integrated, holistic approach toward patients in both inpatient and outpatient settings.
- Integrated holistic interventions, particularly in primary care offices, target both the psychological and medical problems. This increases adherence to the care regimen, promotes healing, minimizes health care costs, and maximizes quality of life.

APPLYING CRITICAL JUDGMENT

1. A patient with suspected somatic symptom disorder has been admitted to the medical-surgical unit after an episode of chest pain. While on the unit, she frequently complains of palpitations, asks the nurse to check her vital signs, and begs staff to stay with her. She does not believe that her electrocardiogram was normal and repeatedly asks for it to be interpreted again. Some nurses retake her pulse and blood pressure measurements when she asks. Others evade her requests. Most staff try to avoid spending time with her. Consider why staff members tend to avoid her.
   - **A.** What could you do, as a nursing team, to improve care and support one another with this difficult patient? Think about both communication and structured interventions.

CHAPTER REVIEW QUESTIONS

1. A patient at a general medical clinic tells the nurse, "I have so many ailments that I need to see six different doctors. None of them has discovered what is really wrong with me." Which comment should the nurse offer next?
   - **a.** "Let's review all the medications you currently take."
   - **b.** "Tell me about allergic reactions you've had to medication."
   - **c.** "Selecting one primary care provider would be better for you."
   - **d.** "I'm not sure I understand how you can afford these expenses."
2. A nurse in an outpatient medical clinic talks to a patient with a long history of malingering and doctor-shopping. The patient continues to express complaints of multiple problems. Select the nurse's best comment to the patient.
   - **a.** "The treatment team believes you would benefit more from seeing a mental health professional."
   - **b.** "The treatment team discussed your case and wants to begin a special case management program for you."
   - **c.** "Because you take a number of medications, it would be safer to have them all filled at the same pharmacy."
   - **d.** "Diagnostic testing has shown no medical problems, and you are using more than your fair share of health care services."
3. A patient in the emergency department was seen for the third time in a month with complaints of tremors and paresthesia in the lower extremities. Neurological functional disorder was diagnosed. While preparing for discharge, the patient says, "Now I'm having chest pain, but it's probably nothing." How should the nurse respond?
   - **a.** Assess the patient's most current laboratory values.
   - **b.** Interrupt the discharge and arrange additional medical evaluation of the patient.

c. Remind the patient, "The diagnostic tests showed you did not have a medical problem."
d. Tell the patient, "Being in the emergency department for a long time can be very distressing."

4. A patient has been identified as having a somatoform disorder. Which of the following should the nurse do when interacting with the patient?
a. Ignore feelings to avoid promoting progression of symptoms.
b. Redirect conversation away from feelings but show interest toward the patient.
c. Encourage the use of benzodiazepines on a consistent basis to reduce anxiety.
d. Suggest the patient direct all questions to the nurse and not the medical provider.

5. Which disorder would the nurse suspect when a person takes their child from doctor to doctor and from hospital to hospital with a variety of intentionally induced symptoms?
a. Illness anxiety disorder
b. Functional neurological disorder
c. Factitious disorder imposed by another
d. Rumination disorder

REFERENCES

Ahmed, H. (2017). Psychosocial symptoms as Predictors for persistent pain in Temporomandibular disorder University of Washington Libraries.

Akyuz, F., & Gokalp, P. (2017). Conversion disorder comorbidity and childhood trauma. *Archives of Neuropsychiatry, 54*(1), 15–20.

American Psychiatric Association. (2013). *Diagnostic and statistical manual of mental disorders (DSM-5)* (5th ed.). Washington, DC: APA.

Ask, H., Waaktaar, T., Seglem, K. B., & Torgersen, S. (2016). Common etiological sources of anxiety, depression, and somatic complaints in adolescents: A multiple rater twin study. *Journal of Abnormal Childhood Psychology* (44), 101–114.

Begen, F., & Turner-Cobb, J. M. (2015). Benefits of Belonging: Experimental manipulations of social inclusion to enhance psychological and physiological health parameters. *Psychology and Health, 30*(5), 568–582.

Beutel, M., Tibubos A. N., Klein, E. M., et al. (2015). [period] Childhood adversities and distress - The role of resilience in a representative sample. https://doi.org/10.1371/journal.pone.0173826.

Bhargava, T., & Pandey, R. (2016). Effect of Health locus of control on patient with somatization. *International journal of Indian Psychology, 4*(1).

Brown, E., & Gallagher, S. (2017). Loneliness and acute stress reactivity: A systematic review of psychophysiological studies. *Psychophysiology*.

Calahorro, C. M. (2017). Gynecological Symptoms in somatization disorder. *European Psychiatry, 41*, S406–S407.

Carlehed, G. (2016). *Somatic symptoms of depression and anxiety: A population based study.* Umea University, Student thesis.

Carlier, I. (2016). Characteristics of suicidal outpatients with mood, anxiety and somatic disorders: The role of childhood abuse and neglect. *International Journal of Social Psychiatry*.

Chauvet-Gelinier, J. C., Bonin, B. (2016). Stress, anxiety and depression in heart disease patients: A major challenge in cardiac rehabilitation. ScienceDirect.com, 1-11.

Dewsaran-van der Ven, C., van Broeckhuysen-Kloth, S., Thorsell, S., Scholten, R., De Gucht, V., & Geenen, R. (2018). Self-compassion in somatoform disorder. *Psychiatry Research, 262*, 34–39. https://doi.org/10.1016/j.psychres.2017.12.013

Dimsdale, J. E. (2015). Somatic symptom disorder. *Merck manual professional version.* Retrieved from www.merckmanuals.com/professional/psychiatric-disorders/somatic-symptom-and-related-disorders/somatic-symptom-disorder.

Encyclopedia of Mental Disorders. (2019). *Assertiveness training.* Retrieved from http://www.minddisorders.com/A-Br/Assertiveness-training.html#ixzz3yHMZ9Tle.

Gibson, E. L., Held, I., Khawnekar, D., & Rutherford, P. (2016). Differences in knowledge, stress, sensation seeking and locus of control linked to dietary adherence in hemodialysis patients. *Frontiers in Psychology, 7*, 1864.

Giddens, J. F. (2017). *Concepts for nursing practice* (2nd ed.). St. Louis: Elsevier.

Goodwin, R., Palgi, Y., & Lavena, O. (2015). Association between media use, acute stress disorder and psychological distress. *Psychotherapy and Psychosomatics, 84*, 253–254.

Greenberg, D. (2017). *Somatization: Epidemiology, pathogenesis, clinical features, medical evaluation, and diagnosis.* Wolters Kluwer.

Howman, M. (2016). Kate Walters, "You kind of want to fix it don't you?" Exploring general practice trainees's experience of managing patients with medically unexplained symptoms. *BMC Medical Education, 16*, 27.

Jaremka, L., & Faqundes, C. (2013). Loneliness promotes inflammation during acute stress. *Psychol Research, 24*(7).

Kaviani, H., & Tabrizi, M. (2016). Emotional expressivity and somatization symptoms in clinical depressed patients. *Clinical Depression, 2*(113).

Khamisa, N. (2015). Work Related Stress, burnout, job satisfaction and general health of nurses. *International Journal of Environmental Research and Public Health, 12*(1), 652–666.

Khare, S., & Srivastava, M. N. (2017). Validity of current treatment Protocols to Overcome hypochondriasis. *Journal of Clinical and Diagnostic Research, 11*(1), VE01–VE04. https://doi.org/10.7860/JCDR/2017/22509.9262.

Koelen, J. A., Houtveen, J. H., Abbass, A., Luyten, P., Eurelings-Bontekoe, E. H. (2014). Effectiveness of psychotherapy for severe somatoform disorder: Meta-analysis. *British Journal of Psychiatry*, doi: 10.1192/bjp.bp.112.12.121830.

Kurlansik, S. L., & Maffei, M. S. (2016). Somatic symptom disorder. American Family Physician, 93(1), 49–54. Retrieved from https://www.aafp.org/afp/2016/0101/p49.html.

Meichenbaum, D. (2017). *Evolution of cognitive behavioral therapy.* New York: Routledge.

Morina, N., Kuenburg, A., Schnyder, U., Bryant, R. A., Nickerson, A., & Schick, M. (2018). The association of Post-traumatic and Postmigration stress with pain and other somatic symptoms: An Explorative Analysis in Traumatized Refugees and Asylum Seekers. *Pain Medicine, 19*(1), 50–59.

Muris, P., & Petrocchi, N. (2016). Protection or Vulnerability? A Meta-analysis of the Relations between the positive and negative components of self-compassion and psychopathology. *Clinical Psychology & Psychotherapy, 24*(2), 373–383.

Murhy, V. (2017). Connecting at work. *Harvard Business Review*, Retrieved from https://hsc.unm.edu/school-of-medicine/education/assets/doc/wellness/murthy-loneliness.PDF.

Nakamura, Y., Takeuchi, T., Hashimoto, K., & Hashizume, M. (2017). Clinical features of outpatients with somatization symptoms treated at a Japanese psychosomatic medicine clinic. *BioPsychoSocial Medicine, 11*, 16.

Neff, K. (2016). The self-compassion scale is a valid and theoretically coherent measure of self compassion . Mindfullness, 7(1) DOI: 10.1007/s12671-015-0479-3.

Nicholson, T. R., & Aybek, S. (2016). Life events and escape in conversion disorder. *Psychological Medicine, 46*, 2617–2626.

Pentin, P. (2016). Somatoform disorders and related Syndromes. *Family Medicine*, 449–458.

Portrie-Bethke, T., & Hanks, B. (2017). *Systemic ecology in understanding somatic symptom and related disorders, DSM-5 and Family Systems edited by Jessica Russo.* Springer Publishing.

Robertson, D., & Kumbhare, D. (2017). Associations between low back pain and depression and somatization in a Canadian emerging adult population. *Journal of the Canadian Chiropractic Association, 61*(2), 96–105.

Schneider, A, Hilbert, S., Hamann, J., Skadsem, S., Glaser, J., Löwe, B., Bühner, M. (2017). The implications of psychological symptoms for length of sick leave: Burnout, depression, and anxiety as Predictors in a primary care setting. *School Deutsches Ärzteblatt International, 114*(17), 291–297.

Seto, H., & Nakao, M. (2017). Relationships between catastrophic thought, bodily sensations and physical symptoms. *BioPsychoSocial Medicine Japanese*, 201711:28. https://doi.org/10.1186/s13030-017-0110-z.

Spratt, E. G. (2014). Somatoform disorder. *Medscape.* Retrieved from http://emedicine.medscape.com/article/918628-overview.

Webb, C. A., Rosso, I. M., & Rauch, S. L. (2017). Internet-based cognitive-behavioral therapy for depression: Current progress and future Directions. *Harvard Review of Psychiatry, 25*(3), 114–122.

Wong, M. M. C., Pang, P. F., & Yiu, M. G. C. (2017). Hypochondriacal delusion in an elderly man with good response to electroconvulsive therapy but complicated with febrile reaction. *Archives of Depression and Anxiety, 3*(2), 038–041. https://doi.org/10.17352/2455-5460.000021.

Zimmerman, T., & Puschmann, E. (2016). Collaborative nurse-led self-management support for primary care patients with anxiety, depressive or somatic symptoms. *International Journal of Nursing Studies, 63*, 101–111.

13

Personality Disorders

Lorraine Chiappetta, Elizabeth M. Varcarolis

http://evolve.elsevier.com/Varcarolis/essentials

OBJECTIVES

1. Compare predisposing factors associated with the development of personality disorders.
2. Summarize four characteristics shared by people with personality disorders.
3. Compare and contrast the signs and symptoms associated with the different personality disorders.
4. Describe at least four co-occurring conditions that are often present in individuals with a personality disorder.
5. Define the defense mechanisms associated with personality disorders.
6. Identify evidence-based practice interventions for individuals with a personality disorder. **QSEN: Evidence-Based Practice**
7. Apply communication strategies that facilitate patient-centered care for the individual with a personality disorder. **QSEN: Patient-Centered Care**
8. Describe components of interprofessional and intraprofessional teamwork and collaboration that facilitate safe and effective care for individuals with personality disorders. **QSEN: Teamwork and Collaboration; Safety**
9. Identify those individuals with personality disorders who have the highest potential for safety risk (suicide, self-harm, and harm to others).
10. Discuss intervention strategies to lessen the manipulative and impulsive behaviors frequently seen with patients with personality disorders.
11. Identify caregiver responses that can interfere with the effective treatment of the individual with a personality disorder.

KEY TERMS AND CONCEPTS

CONCEPT: SELF-MANAGEMENT: *Self-management* is the ability of individuals to engage in the daily tasks required to maintain health and well-being. A strong patient–nurse relationship serves as the vehicle through which optimal self-management occurs (Giddens, 2017). Individuals with personality disorders display significant challenges in *self-management,* often having difficulty regulating painful emotions in ways that are healthy (Halter, 2018).

INTRODUCTION

Personality refers to individual differences in characteristic patterns of thinking, feeling, and behaving (Cherry, 2018). Personality *traits* are characteristics that all people bring to social relationships, including shyness, seductiveness, rigidity, suspiciousness, or passive-aggressive traits. In ordinary/nonpathological states, personality traits are flexible and adaptive. When these individuals experience stressors, the defenses against anxiety that are used tend to be more mature and functional.

PERSONALITY DISORDERS

Personality disorders (PDs) are defined as an enduring pattern of inner experience and behavior that deviates from the individual's culture (American Psychiatric Association [APA], 2013). In people with PDs, personality traits tend to be inflexible and unpredictable, and coping strategies tend to be more primitive and immature (Blaise et al., 2016). PDs range from mild to moderate to severe based on disturbances in functionality. Most people with PDs demonstrate maladaptive patterns in cognition, affectivity (emotional responses), interpersonal functioning, and impulse control that lead to distress or impairment in functioning (APA, 2013). People with a diagnosis of *PD* are frequently unaware that their own personality traits are causing problems, and they often blame others for their difficulties or even deny they have a problem.

Maladaptive patterns of behavior, lack of insight about how these patterns of behavior contribute to distress, and the tendency to blame others combine to make caring for individuals with a PD very challenging for the health care professional. Nurses will encounter patients with problematic personality traits and PDs in every health care setting. This chapter will help the nurse understand those with a PD and provide strategies to work with common problematic behaviors.

Prevalence and Comorbidity

The National Institute of Mental Health (NIMH, 2017) reported the following:

- The past-year prevalence of any PD was 9.1%, and that for borderline PD was 1.4%.
- Sex and race were not found to be associated with the prevalence of PDs.
- Of people with past-year PDs, 84.5% also had one or more other mental disorder(s).
- Comorbidity was highest with borderline PD.
- Of those with any PD, 39% reported receiving mental health treatment in the past 12 months, as did 42.4% of those with borderline PD.

PDs often co-occur with other PDs, with other mental disorders (substance use disorder, somatic symptom disorders, eating disorders, posttraumatic stress disorder, depression, anxiety disorders), or with general medical conditions. In fact, comorbidity seems to be the rule and not the exception. Comorbidity frequently leads to a poorer treatment outcome.

The lack of insight ("there is nothing wrong with me") associated with most individuals with a diagnosis of PD usually means that they do not enter treatment for their PD alone. Most often, the presenting set of symptoms is about the person experiencing some type of psychological crisis. Therefore a complete psychosocial assessment must always include formal or informal screening for PDs.

Depression is more common in the background of patients with borderline PDs; antisocial disorders have a high rate of concordance with alcohol/substance use disorders (Sadock, Sadock, & Ruiz, 2015).

Theory

There is no single cause for the development of PDs. The etiology of these disorders includes genetic, biological, developmental, and environmental factors. The different types of PDs may have individualized etiological factors.

Genetic Factors

Current research supports a more dominant role of genetics. In a study of identical and fraternal twins who were raised apart, identical twins were found to have more similar personality traits than fraternal twins (Sadock et al., 2015).

There seems to be good evidence for the heritability of paranoid PD, schizoid PD, and schizotypal PD. There is a possible genetic link with paranoid PD and schizophrenia and schizotypal PD and schizophrenia. There is strong support for a genetic contribution to antisocial PD and modest evidence of heritability for obsessive-compulsive PD (Bienenfeld, 2016). Some identical twin studies of borderline PD have shown that 42% to 69% of the variance in borderline PD is caused by genetics (Salters-Pedneault, 2020). There is less evidence for the heritability of the other PDs.

As with many psychiatric disorders, most likely a genetic/biological predisposition combined with environmental factors leads to the development of PDs.

Neurobiological Factors

In patients with a PD, abnormalities have been observed in the frontal, temporal, and parietal lobes of the brain. These abnormalities may be caused by perinatal injury, encephalitis, trauma, or genetics. The exact relationship of these abnormalities (whether it is a cause or an effect) to PDs is not clear, however (Bienenfeld, 2016).

Disturbances in the levels of the neurotransmitter serotonin (5-hydroxytryptamine, 5-HT) have been linked with irritability, impulsivity, and hypersensitivity. Affective instability is thought to be a result of excessive limbic reactivity in GABAergic/glutamatergic/cholinergic circuits. These symptoms of irritability, impulsivity, hypersensitivity, and affective instability are prominent symptoms of borderline PD. This suggests that dysregulation of serotonin and the GABAergic circuits are associated with borderline PD (Bienenfeld, 2016). Individuals who have a specific variation of the serotonin gene may be more likely to develop borderline PD (Salters-Pedneault, 2020). Lower serotonin neurotransmission may also be associated with antisocial PD (Black & Andreasen, 2014).

In people with *borderline PD*, abnormalities in the size of the hippocampus, the size and functioning of the amygdala, and the functioning of the frontal lobes have been found. These areas of the brain are associated with regulating emotions and integrating thoughts with emotions (Dryden-Edwards, 2016). Individuals with antisocial PD have demonstrated altered metabolism in the prefrontal regions of the brain and reduced autonomic activity. This may underlie the low arousal, poor fear conditioning, and decision-making deficits described in those with an antisocial PD (Bienenfeld, 2016).

Psychological Influences

Childhood trauma is a significant risk factor for the development of any PD in general and for borderline and antisocial PDs in particular (Black & Andreasen, 2014). Physical and sexual abuse, early separation from caregivers, emotional or physical neglect, and parental insensitivity are distressing childhood experiences that are frequently, *but not always,* seen in those who develop borderline PD (Salters-Pedneault, 2020). Linehan (1993), a theorist, further defines *parental insensitivity* as creating an "invalidating experience" in which a child's emotional responses are consistently invalidated or punished or where there is a caregiver overreaction.

Individuals diagnosed with *antisocial PD* often have a history that includes excessively harsh or erratic discipline, inadequate parental supervision, parent(s) with a substance use disorder, and parents who are criminals or display antisocial behaviors themselves. Those with this diagnosis are more likely to have a history of child abuse (Black, 2017).

Cultural Considerations

When making a psychiatric diagnosis, it is important to be aware of cultural implications and what is considered normal in a particular culture. It is especially true when a clinician is making a diagnosis of PD. Research findings about race, ethnicity, and PDs are conflicting. It is generally believed that PDs exist across all races, ethnic groups, and socioeconomic groups. It has also been noted that the presentation of any one of the PDs may be different in different ethnic or racial groups.

Clinical Picture

Individuals with PDs often use coping strategies or "defense mechanisms" that allow them to deny responsibility for their feelings and actions. One defense mechanism is called splitting. It is defined as the division or polarization of beliefs, actions, objects, or persons into *good and bad*. It is sometimes known as "black and white" thinking and is commonly seen in borderline and other PDs.

Another defense mechanism is called *projective identification*. Projection is the unconscious act of attributing a (usually difficult) thought or belief inside ourselves to someone else. (Example: I hate my boss but accuse my boss of hating me. In reality, my boss may actually like me.) Projective identification builds upon projection and occurs within a relationship. The "someone else" starts to unconsciously adopt the "difficult thought" being "projected." (Example: My boss starts to dislike me.) For example, if someone believes that he or she is being persecuted, the person may alter his or her behavior in such a way as to look suspicious in the presence of others. Others' suspicious looks would only act to further strengthen the person's belief that he or she is being persecuted. This defense mechanism is evidenced in paranoid PDs and other PDs.

Most symptoms of PDs begin in early adulthood and present in a variety of contexts (APA, 2013). Over time, the most dramatic symptoms associated with many of the PDs decrease in intensity, with less intensive symptoms shown in those who are middle-age and older.

The PDs can be grouped into three "clusters" based on similarities in the clinical picture. Although these classifications are useful in research and education (refer to the following table), clinically, a person may have more than one PD from more than one cluster.

SYMPTOMS SEEN IN PERSONALITY DISORDERS

Cluster A	Cluster B	Cluster C
Odd or eccentric behavior	Dramatic, emotional behavior	Anxious, fearful behavior
Suspicious	Attention-seeking behavior	Tense
Cold	Labile	Overcontrolled
Withdrawn	Shallow	Depressed
Irrational	Increased rates of substance use and suicide	

Cluster A Disorders

Individuals with Cluster A disorders, described as **odd or eccentric**, demonstrate behaviors sometimes seen in schizophrenia. They come into the health care system either because of a co-occurring disorder, acute distress, or a brief psychotic episode.

Cluster A disorders include schizotypal PD, schizoid PD, and paranoid PD.

Schizotypal Personality Disorder

Individuals with schizotypal personality disorder show a pattern of social and interpersonal deficits marked by a reduced capacity for close relationships. There are cognitive and perceptual distortions, peculiar behavior, and **odd speech** (APA, 2013). These individuals avoid interpersonal relationships and may be indifferent to the reactions of others.

People with this diagnosis most closely resemble people with the diagnosis of schizophrenia and are perceived by others as having strikingly **odd thinking and beliefs**. These individuals demonstrate **magical thinking** *and rituals*, **ideas of reference** (believing innocuous events have strong personal significance), and **unusual perceptual experiences** that are *not* consistent with cultural norms. The person may have an **inappropriate affect** and an **odd, eccentric, or peculiar appearance.** Their **speech is peculiar** in phrasing and syntax and may have meaning only to them. Reactions of confusion by others to their illogical speech may cause these individuals to become **suspicious of others and eventually to develop paranoid thinking**. Their eccentric and *unkempt appearances, strange behaviors, and nonadherence to social conventions* make it difficult for them to have give-and-take conversations.

Because of these odd styles of behavior and inattention to social conventions, they **lack friends.** People with this disorder may be genuinely unhappy about their lack of relationships and their **social anxiety.** Under increased stress, these individuals may exhibit psychotic symptoms (APA, 2013; Sadock et al., 2015).

Up to 10% of people with schizotypal PD complete suicide. Some individuals with this disorder later develop schizophrenia (Sadock et al., 2015).

(**Bolded words** are part of the *Diagnostic and Statistical Manual of Mental Disorders*, 5th edition [DSM-5; APA, 2013] diagnostic symptoms for schizotypal PD.)

VIGNETTE: Ms. Sands is a 36-year-old female who lives alone. She describes herself as a "writer" and lives on Social Security benefits. She only goes to a nearby grocery store at night because, she says, "their magic does not work at night." She dresses in several layers of multicolored and mismatched clothes, even in warmer weather. She wears a turban on her head to "keep them from seeing my thoughts." Each night, she tells the grocer in a flat and formal manner that she is going to be a famous director and star. She knows this because "it hasn't snowed yet, and that means the coast is clear."

Paranoid Personality Disorder

People with paranoid personality disorder (PPD) exhibit traits that are characterized by **pervasive,** persistent, and inappropriate **suspiciousness and distrust of others** (APA, 2013). Individuals with **PPD** are no strangers to the health care system. Nurses may consider this diagnosis when patients present with *hostile, irritable, angry* mood and affect. These individuals frequently **suspect that others are exploiting or deceiving them**. There is a **reluctance to confide in others for fear the information will be used against them.** This person **reads hidden meanings into benign remarks** and **perceives attacks that are not apparent to others.** There is an **inability to forgive perceived insults.** They are **suspicious** and believe that others are lying, cheating, **exploiting**, or **trying to harm** them in some way. There can be **recurrent suspicion without justification about the infidelity of a spouse or partner.** These individuals lack warmth, pay close attention to power and rank, and express disdain for those who are weak, sickly, and impaired. Although they may appear businesslike and efficient, they often generate fear and conflict in others through their hostile, stubborn, and sarcastic expressions (APA, 2013; Sadock et al., 2015). Even when others are loyal, they can become preoccupied **with unjustifiable doubts about the trustworthiness of others.** It has been said that individuals with paranoid personality traits "lack the milk of human kindness."

(**Bolded words** are part of the *DSM-5* diagnostic symptoms for the diagnosis of paranoid PD.)

VIGNETTE: Mr. Cole, a 58-year-old man, comes into the emergency department (ED) with chest pains. He refuses to give background information "because the information could be used against me." He is demeaning to the nurse, saying, in a loud and angry voice, "Get someone in here who knows something. I know when I am being treated unfairly." When the nurse turns her back to Mr. Cole to speak to the physician, Mr. Cole shouts, "What lies is she telling you about me? Do either one of you know what you are doing? Are you both in this together?"

Schizoid Personality Disorder

People with schizoid personality disorder are characterized by an **inability to establish relationships with others and a restricted range of emotions in interpersonal settings** (APA, 2013). They are seen by others as eccentric, isolated, or lonely and **take pleasure in few things.** They may exist on the periphery of society, content to avoid even the most superficial relationships. Their affect is usually flat, which projects **emotional coldness.** They appear **indifferent to praise or criticism** by others. They tend to **choose solitary activities, lack friends,** and **have little desire for close relationships,** including **sexual experiences with another.** Although they invest little interest or energy in human relationships, they may invest enormous energy in nonhuman interests such as mathematics and astronomy. Typically loners, they spend much time daydreaming and are often very attached to animals. There is some evidence that people with schizoid personality traits may later develop schizophrenia or a delusional disorder. Although aloof, some individuals with schizoid traits have conceived, developed, and given our world genuinely original and creative ideas.

(**Bolded words** are part of the *DSM-5* diagnostic symptoms for the diagnosis of schizoid PD.)

VIGNETTE: Mr. Ortiz, a 38-year-old unmarried bookkeeper, was assaulted on his way home from work. A bystander called 911, and Mr. Ortiz was taken to the emergency department in an unconscious state. Once awake, he answers questions in a monotonal voice and avoids making eye contact. He often looks away and does not respond at all. He is adherent and remains a passive recipient of his treatment. Mr. Ortiz rejects all nursing interventions aimed at increasing socialization.

Cluster B Personality Disorders

Cluster B disorders appear to share emotional reactivity, such as dramatic, erratic, flamboyant behavior; poor impulse control; and an unclear sense of identity (APA, 2013). There seems to be a great deal of overlap among these disorders with other mental health disorders, including substance use, depression, and eating disorders. **Manipulation** is a common behavioral mechanism among people with these disorders. Their behaviors can be challenging no matter what part of the health care system is caring for their needs.

These disorders include antisocial, borderline, histrionic, and narcissistic PDs.

Antisocial Personality Disorder

Antisocial PD is characterized by a persistent disregard for and violation of the rights of others, with a lack of remorse for actions or hurting others (APA, 2013).

People with antisocial personality disorder have a sense of **entitlement**, which means they believe they have the right to take what they want, treat others unfairly, destroy the property of others, and even hurt others if it is in their best interest. They do not adhere to traditional values or standards of morality as boundaries for their actions. There is little restraint on their behavior, and they feel little sense of responsibility for their actions. People who have **antisocial PD lack regard for the law and the rights of others** and may engage in **criminal behaviors.** There is frequently a history of persistent **lying, deception, and conning of others for profit or pleasure.**

These patients may be charming, engaging, and uncanny in their ability to find just the right angle to lure a person into their intrigue with the intent to exploit them for money, favors, or more sadistic purposes. Behavior can be described as manipulative and **irresponsible.** Promiscuity, **reckless disregard for the safety of others, physical aggressiveness, failure to honor work or financial commitments,** and drunk driving are common events in their lives. They are frequently **impulsive and fail to plan ahead.** They may have a history of **irritability and aggression** that includes partner abuse, child abuse, anger in response to minor slights, and vindictive behavior toward others that can result in physical or emotional pain. People with **antisocial PD** often become bored and engage in risky and dangerous sports or other activities, sometimes claiming they participate in such behaviors just to "feel alive." This diagnosis can only be made in people 18 years of age or older. Often there is evidence of a psychiatric history of a *conduct disorder* (fire setting, cruelty to animals, stealing) with onset before the age of 15 years (APA, 2013).

These individuals account for a disproportionate number of **criminal arrests,** including violent offenses (Verona & Patrick, 2015). This diagnosis is more common in males. The challenge for treatment in this population is that these individuals have difficulty learning from mistakes and are unresponsive to punishment. (See the *DSM-5* Antisocial Personality Disorder box.)

(**Bolded words** are part of the *DSM-5* diagnostic symptoms for the diagnosis of antisocial PD.)

DSM-5 DIAGNOSTIC CRITERIA

Antisocial Personality Disorder

A. A pervasive pattern of disregard for and violation of the rights of others, occurring since age 15 years, as indicated by three (or more) of the following:
   1. Failure to conform to social norms with respect to lawful behaviors, as indicated by repeatedly performing acts that are grounds for arrest.
   2. Deceitfulness, as indicated by repeated lying, use of aliases, or conning others for personal profit or pleasure.
   3. Impulsivity or failure to plan ahead.
   4. Irritability and aggressiveness, as indicated by repeated physical fights or assaults.
   5. Reckless disregard for safety of self or others.
   6. Consistent irresponsibility, as indicated by repeated failure to sustain consistent work behavior or honor financial obligations.
   7. Lack of remorse, as indicated by being indifferent to or rationalizing having hurt, mistreated, or stolen from another.

B. The individual is at least age 18 years.

C. There is evidence of conduct disorder with onset before age 15 years.

D. The occurrence of antisocial behavior is not exclusively during the course of schizophrenia or bipolar disorder.

VIGNETTE: Mr. Jones has been extorting money from lonely widows by charming them, "helping them with their finances," promising to marry them, and then taking off with their money. When in court, he laughed when he was asked if he felt guilty for taking the life savings of these elderly, lonely widows and stated, "Hey, I gave them what they wanted." Fingerprints revealed that his name was really Oliver Torres, with a long list of aliases, as well as a history of family violence and burglary. He had abandoned his wife and three children 8 years previously.

Borderline Personality Disorder

The symptoms of borderline personality disorder (BPD) can be summarized as experiencing ongoing patterns of *difficulty with self-regulation*, an inability to soothe oneself in times of stress. Characteristic symptoms include trouble with **instability in mood,** thinking, behavior, and personal relationships; an **unstable self-image;** and **marked impulsivity.** Individuals with BPD traits develop maladaptive behaviors that can be difficult for friends and families to understand, often resulting in chaotic relationships.

The individual with *BPD* traits tends to have a **pattern of unstable and intense relationships** that are characterized by **alternating between idealization** ("you are the best") **and devaluation** ("you are the worst") of the person who is part of the interpersonal relationship. Because of the **identity disturbance (unstable sense of self)** sometimes associated with this diagnosis, the individual with BPD traits sometimes "takes on" the behaviors and values of the *idealized* person. Those with BPD traits desperately seek relationships to avoid feelings of abandonment and **chronic feelings of emptiness.** Characteristic behaviors of those with borderline personality traits include **frantic efforts to avoid real or imagined abandonment,** like begging, clinging, or excessive jealousy. Because these behaviors can be experienced by others as being excessively *needy* and problematic, significant others frequently respond with physical or emotional distance. This further reinforces the fear of abandonment. There can be an extreme sensitivity to perceived rejection. The previously *idealized* person can quickly be *devalued* if it is perceived that this need for overinvolvement is not being met. A previously *idealized* person is viewed as either perfect or horrible, nothing in between. This is an example of the defense mechanism of *splitting.*

Individuals with BPD traits tend to have extreme emotional sensitivity. Some describe it as feeling as if there were an exposed nerve ending. Small things can trigger intense reactions. **Inappropriate, intense anger or difficulty controlling anger** can occur. In the context of relationships, these angry outbursts can be very disturbing to significant others. Once upset, the individual with BPD traits may have a hard time calming down. **Recurrent suicidal behavior, gestures, or threats of self-mutilating behavior** can occur in response to stress and perceived rejection. **Potentially damaging impulsive behaviors, such as excessive spending and risky sex, and eating disorders** tend to go along with this **affective instability.** These mood swings can be intense but tend to pass rather quickly (unlike the mood swings of bipolar disorder). Under extreme levels of **stress,** the individual with BPD traits can become **paranoid** or experience **dissociation** (feeling foggy, spaced out, or outside one's body).

BPD is a disorder of emotion regulation affecting up to 5% of the population and 20% of individuals on behavioral health units (National Education Alliance for Borderline Personality Disorder, 2018). Up until a few decades ago, those diagnosed with the disorder were thought to be untreatable. Despite this shift, individuals living with BPD continue to face stigma.

Feelings of depression and anxiety are common. Complaints of feeling "empty" contribute to chronic feelings of suicidality. Self-mutilation can be a maladaptive attempt to deal with either extreme levels of anxiety (as a release) or an attempt to deal with the emptiness (to feel something). The frequent use of splitting not only strains personal relationships but also creates turmoil in health care settings. The individual may attempt to *split* staff and other patients into "good" or "bad," making consistency of care difficult. The *emotional dysregulation* and *unstable interpersonal relationships* demonstrated as part of this disorder can create many problems in a therapeutic milieu.

It is useful to remember that the same symptoms that can cause chaotic relationships and personal distress can have positive aspects. Positive feelings are also stronger for those with a BPD trait. On good days, these individuals can be passionate and fiercely loyal as friends. They frequently sense the emotions of others instinctively and can be extremely empathetic.

(**Bolded words** are part of the *DSM-5* diagnostic symptoms for the diagnosis of BPD.)

VIGNETTE: Mrs. Kit is twice divorced and has been hospitalized several times for suicidal ideation. She also engages in self-injury by cutting her inner thighs and arms with a razor when anxious or experiencing feelings of abandonment. She has arrived for today's therapy session. Mrs. Kit's nurse therapist is leaving for a 2-week vacation and has been preparing Mrs. Kit for the separation for more than 2 months. The therapist has given Mrs. Kit the name and phone number of another therapist to call and see while she is away. Mrs. Kit arrives at the office with fresh razor marks on her arms and tells the nurse that she is quitting therapy because the nurse really does not like her anyway and she might as well kill herself. "Go, have a good time; I might not be here when you get back," she says. Mrs. Kit then storms out of the office and refuses to answer her phone all day.

DSM-5 DIAGNOSTIC CRITERIA

Borderline Personality Disorder

A pervasive pattern of instability of interpersonal relationships, self-image, and affect and marked impulsivity, beginning by early adulthood and present in a variety of contexts, as indicated by five (or more) of the following:

1. Frantic efforts to avoid real or imagined abandonment. (**Note:** Do not include suicidal or self-mutilating behavior covered in Criterion 5.)
2. A pattern of unstable and intense interpersonal relationships characterized by alternating between extremes of idealization and devaluation.
3. Identity disturbances: markedly and persistently unstable self-image or sense of self.
4. Impulsivity in at least two areas that are potentially self-damaging (e.g., overspending money, sex, substance abuse, reckless driving, binge eating). (**Note:** Do not include suicidal or self-mutilating behavior covered in Criterion 5.)
5. Recurrent suicidal behavior, gestures, or threats, or self-mutilating behavior.
6. Affective instability due to a marked reactivity of mood (e.g., intense episodic dysphoria, irritability, or anxiety usually lasting a few hours and only rarely more than a few days).
7. Chronic feelings of emptiness.
8. Inappropriate, intense anger or difficulty controlling anger (e.g., frequent displays of temper, constant anger, recurrent physical fights).
9. Transient, stress-related paranoid ideations or severe dissociative symptoms.

Narcissistic Personality Disorder

Narcissistic personality disorder (NPD) is a maladaptive response characterized by a person's *grandiose* sense of self-importance. There can be a preoccupation with fantasies of unlimited success. People with this disorder consider themselves special and expect special treatment. Their demeanor may be arrogant and haughty, and their sense of entitlement is striking. These individuals require excessive admiration. They lack empathy for the needs or feelings of others and exploit others to meet their own needs. Their relationships are shallow and superficial and based on what the other person can do for them. If they are at fault in some way, they always blame others for the problems they themselves have caused. Patients with *NPD* are often envious of the successes or possessions of others or believe others are envious of them.

Of individuals with *NPD*, 50% to 75% are male. Because of their fragile self-esteem, they are prone to depression, interpersonal difficulties, occupational problems, and feelings of rejection (Sadock et al., 2015). Comorbid conditions associated with this disorder are mood disorders, eating disorders, substance-related disorders and other PDs, including *antisocial PD*. Patients with *NPD* can be abusive and prone to impulsive and reckless behaviors (Mayo Clinic, 2020).

(**Bolded words** are part of the *DSM-5* diagnostic symptoms for the diagnosis of NPD.)

VIGNETTE: Mr. Chad is the vice president of a successful business. He is very arrogant and always reminds people of what he has done for the company and where it would be without him. As an aside, he will say that it is he who really runs the company, and it is he who should be the president. When employees disagree with him or have a different or novel way to implement change or progress, he listens to their ideas and plans and later takes credit for the good ideas. He is known to lose his temper on the slightest provocation, such as having to wait for someone to start a meeting. On the other hand, he is usually late for meetings and appointments and feels others should wait for him. His need for admiration is insatiable, and he is preoccupied with fantasies of unlimited success, power, brilliance, and ideal love.

Histrionic Personality Disorder

The essential feature of *histrionic PD* is a pattern of **excessive emotionality and attention seeking.** People with *histrionic PDs manipulate* others through self-dramatization, theatricality, and exaggerated expression of emotion. Their style of speech may be excessively impressionistic and lacking in detail. The excessive displays of emotions are an attempt to be and remain the **center of attention,** so they can get the love and admiration that they require. They may *act out* with displays of temper, tears, and accusations when they are not getting the attention or praise they believe they deserve. Interactions are often characterized by inappropriate and sexually seductive or provocative behavior to draw others into a relationship or work project. They may **use** physical appearance to draw attention **to themselves.** There can be **sudden emotional shifts and emotional lability** (rapid change in mood). When a relationship is initiated with someone with histrionic PD traits, it can appear that relationships are more intimate than they actually are. In reality, relationships tend to be superficial and shallow. In general, relationships do not last long because of the **constant need for attention** and insensitivity to the needs of others. These individuals tend to be highly suggestible.

Histrionic PD is more prevalent in females than males. There is usually a lack of insight about their role in the failure of relationships. They may seek treatment for depression or another comorbid condition.

(**Bolded words** are part of the *DSM-5* diagnostic symptoms for the diagnosis of histrionic PD.)

VIGNETTE: Ms. Miller, a 45-year-old woman, meets her therapist, Dr. Jim, for the first time. She is dressed in a tight top and short skirt and wearing a lot of makeup. She becomes flirtatious and tells Dr. Jim that she wants extra time today because her story is so long, and she is most likely more interesting than his other patients. Her speech is flamboyant and dramatic but lacking in substance and facts. When the therapist reiterates the terms of the contract and reminds Ms. Miller that they have 20 minutes remaining in today's session to discuss her issues, she becomes angry and insulting and tells Dr. Jim he had better admit her to the hospital immediately or she will commit suicide.

Cluster C Personality Disorders

The main characteristics of Cluster C disorders are *anxiety and fearfulness*. Individuals with avoidant PD deal with acute anxiety in social situations through social inhibitions. Those with dependent PD feel acute anxiety around the need to be taken care of. With obsessive-compulsive PD, anxiety is managed by behaviors that attempt to maintain control.

Avoidant Personality Disorder

People with avoidant personality disorder have high levels of anxiety and outward signs of fear with feelings of low self-worth. They are **hypersensitive to criticism or rejection;** therefore they tend to **avoid situations that require socialization.** Even though they have a strong desire for affection and for relationships, they are fearful of rejection, disappointment, criticism, or ridicule. They can spend most of their time in self-imposed social isolation and experience depression and anxiety. They may view themselves as **socially inept, personally unappealing, or inferior to others** and consequently have very low self-esteem. They are **reluctant to take personal risks for fear of embarrassment.** The **feelings of inadequacy** lead to **inhibition in new interpersonal relationships** and interpersonal intimacy. These individuals are frequently described as "shy," "timid," and "isolated." The problems associated with this disorder are impairments in both social and occupational functioning. Virtually all people with **avoidant PDs** have social phobias.

(**Bolded words** are part of the *DSM-5* diagnostic symptoms for the diagnosis of avoidant PD.)

VIGNETTE: Keith is a 32-year-old computer programmer. He is excessively shy and rarely speaks with his coworkers other than perfunctory "hellos." He has never had a relationship with a woman and tries to avoid situations in which he will be alone with any of the female employees. Sometimes the group goes out after work for a drink, and when Keith is asked, he becomes very anxious and makes excuses for why he must decline. His sense of loneliness has become intolerable, and he finally seeks psychotherapy for depression, not knowing where else to turn.

Obsessive-Compulsive Personality Disorder

People with obsessive-compulsive personality disorder (OCPD) are preoccupied with orderliness and mental and interpersonal control at the expense of openness or efficiency. The disorder is marked by a pervasive pattern of perfection and inflexibility.

These individuals are cautious and consider all choices in a methodical and inflexible manner. They are **preoccupied with rules and details** and follow them rigidly, believing there is only one way to do things correctly. They have great difficulty incorporating new ideas or viewpoints (**rigid perfectionism). Perfectionism** can sometimes **interfere with task completion because strict standards are not met**. They may be **reluctant to delegate tasks.** They are high achievers and do well in the sciences and intellectually demanding fields that require attention to detail. These individuals may obtain their sense of self-worth from work and productivity. Their **devotion to work may exclude pleasurable activities and friendships.**

They often have a very formal demeanor, lack a sense of humor, and have limited interpersonal skills. Behaviors are described as **rigid and stubborn,** especially in **matters of morality, ethics, or values.** They are uncomfortable with their feelings and relationships. They can experience distress in situations they cannot **control** or in which events are unpredictable. Even though they may have deep and genuine affection for others, their intimacy in *relationships is superficial* and rigidly controlled. People with OCPD are **financially extremely stingy,** and it is **difficult for them to part with personal objects even if they are broken or worthless.** Unlike people with *obsessive-compulsive disorder (OCD)* (refer to Chapter 11), people with this disorder do not display unwanted obsessions or compulsive ritualistic behavior. People with OCPD may come into therapy because their rigidity and need for control are causing problems in their interpersonal or work relationships. Interestingly, many people with OCPD may initially come across as high functioning.

(**Bolded words** are part of the *DSM-5* diagnostic symptoms for the diagnosis of OCPD.)

VIGNETTE: Mike is a 45-year-old middle manager for a microchip company. He works late and sometimes on the weekends, avoiding social and recreational activities. He has a need to get everything done to perfection, which has pushed back the deadline on many projects. He has experienced some heartburn now for a month, and his wife has been insisting he see a physician. He tells her he will go when this project is finished but hates to "waste" his money on physicians. In the physician's office, he says he does not have time to take a treadmill test. When the physician tells Mike that he cannot make a diagnosis until he gets all the test results, Mike becomes very anxious.

Dependent Personality Disorder

Those with dependent personality disorder are inhibited and fearful or reluctant to express disagreement for fear of rejection and loss of support. Unlike a person with a borderline PD, they do not respond with anger to rejection but, rather, withdraw or become passive.

People with dependent PD traits are fearful that they are incapable of surviving if left alone and have an **excessive need to be taken care of.** They solicit caretaking by **clinging and being excessively submissive.** By early adulthood, these individuals **have difficulty making everyday decisions without excessive advice** and have **difficulty initiating projects because of a lack of self-confidence**. They **need others to take responsibility for most major areas of their lives.** Their intense fear of separation and being alone is so great that they tolerate poor, even abusive treatment in order to stay in a relationship. They are **fearful and reluctant to express disagreement for fear of loss of support and may go to great lengths to obtain nurturance and support**. Once a relationship ends, there is an urgent need to get into another related to extreme feelings of helplessness when alone. They are **unrealistically preoccupied with fears of being left alone to take care of themselves.** The individuals may ruminate about abandonment even when it is not threatened. Their high levels of anxiety intensify their **inability to complete anything on their own.**

People with dependent PD are at greater risk for anxiety and mood disorders, and this disorder often co-occurs with borderline, avoidant, and histrionic PDs. This condition can sometimes be seen in individuals who have a general medical condition or disability that requires them to be dependent on others.

(**Bolded words** are part of the *DSM-5* diagnostic symptoms for the diagnosis of dependent PD.)

VIGNETTE: Mr. Martin, 49 years old, has lived with his mother since high school. His mother cooks, cleans, and shops for him. He works as a shipping dock clerk and has had the job for 30 years. He even has to ask his mother's advice on what to wear each day for work. He has become extremely anxious and fearful because his mother has been scheduled for surgery and will be away from the home for 5 days. He is terrified that he cannot cope without her to care for him.

Passive-Aggressive Traits

Although not a *DSM-5* PD diagnosis, passive-aggressive personality traits are disruptive to interpersonal relationships. It is helpful for nurses and others to be aware of these traits because working with people who have passive-aggressive traits can be very confusing and disruptive to others.

Passive-aggressive personality traits can be hard to spot even when you're feeling the psychological consequences. Characteristic of these traits is the tendency to engage in *indirect expression of hostility through acts* such as subtle insults, sullen behavior, stubbornness, or a deliberate failure to accomplish required tasks. The work of those with these traits is often characterized by *procrastination and intentional inefficiency*. There may a sullenness to the person's behavior and an inability to compromise due to stubbornness. People with passive-aggressive behavioral traits are more likely to *express their negative/hostile feelings indirectly,* such as being chronically late or "forgetting" to do something. Although they may openly agree to another's demands or requests, they rarely complete those demands or requests. In fact, the actions of people with passive-aggressive personality traits are usually the opposite of their promises. Therefore a person with passive-aggressive traits often *disrupts or sabotages* other people's projects or plans. Working with people who have passive-aggressive personality traits is usually very difficult.

VIGNETTE: A nursing instructor is perceived by her coworkers to be constantly complaining and avoiding responsibility in any way. The instructor was put in charge of one of the committees involved with an upcoming accreditation visit. As the months before the accreditation visit passed, it became more noticeable that this instructor had canceled many of the meetings for her committee, missed deadlines, and failed to complete her committee work. In fact, the day the draft was to be compiled, she called in sick. When one of the committee members suggested that the accreditation material was in her office, it was discovered that absolutely nothing had been done on the report. When this individual realized that others had been in her office, she became furious that anyone should invade her privacy. She then took the next 2 weeks off from work due to "illness," essentially jeopardizing the project.

APPLICATION OF THE NURSING PROCESS

ASSESSMENT

Primitive Defenses

People with PDs often attempt to modulate painful feelings by using less mature (primitive) defense mechanisms, like splitting, dissociation, and projection in a rigid fashion. (See Chapter 11 for definitions of healthy and immature or primitive defenses.) The symptoms associated with PDs can significantly interfere with the provision of appropriate health care interventions. Frequently labeled as "difficult patients," these individuals may require a different approach to care.

Assessment Tools

Several structured interview tools are used to diagnose PDs. These tools are not used in all clinical settings because they require lengthy interviews and evaluation.

Taking a full medical history can help determine if the problem is psychiatric, medical, or both. Always start with the assumption that you must first rule out medical illness as the cause of symptoms. Important issues in assessment for PDs include the following: a history of suicidal thoughts, self-harm behavior, aggressive ideation or actions, past and current use of medicines, substance use disorders, ability to handle money, and a history of legal problems. Other important areas that should be investigated include current or past physical, sexual, or emotional abuse. Finally, it is helpful to understand the acute stressful event (precipitant) to the current crisis state.

Assessment Guidelines

1. Assess for past and current suicidal, self-harm, or homicidal thoughts. If these are present, the patient will need immediate attention. Safety is a priority.
2. Determine whether the patient has a medical disorder or another psychiatric disorder that may be responsible for the symptoms (especially a substance use disorder).
3. Determine if there is a comorbid psychiatric or medical diagnosis.
4. View the assessment of personality functioning from within the person's ethnic, cultural, and social background.
5. Determine whether the patient experienced a recent acute stressor or important loss. Problematic behaviors associated with PDs are often exacerbated after the loss of a significant supporting person or as the result of a disruptive social situation.
6. Be aware of the strong negative emotions these patients may evoke in you as the caregiver.

DIAGNOSIS

The focus of treatment for the patient with a PD is usually centered around acute symptoms secondary to the PD. People with a diagnosis of BPD or antisocial PD are the most challenging to work with and are most likely to be seen in any treatment setting. The behaviors central to these disorders often cause the most disruption in psychiatric and medical-surgical settings. Safety is always the priority, so the risk for self-injury, suicide, and harm to others is usually addressed first. Emotions such as anxiety, rage, and depression and behaviors such as withdrawal, paranoia, and manipulation are among the most frequent symptoms that health care workers need to address. See Table 13.1 for common potential patient problems/concerns.

OUTCOMES IDENTIFICATION

Brief, focused hospitalization with predetermined goals for discharge is the most therapeutic use of inpatient admissions. Much of the therapeutic work occurs in outpatient settings.

General *short-term* goal setting for all the PDs centers around the following:

1. Crisis stabilization, which includes safety—resolution of acute ideation and behaviors related to suicide, self-harm, and harm to others
2. Engagement in the therapeutic treatment/therapy—recognizing need for help
3. Symptom control:
   a. Modifying dysfunctional thoughts, emotions, and behaviors that are causing interpersonal and personal distress

Long-term goal setting is based on the perspective that personality change involves one learned skill at a time. There is an expectation that long-term change takes time and repetition. Long-term outcome criteria might include the following:

1. Minimizing self-destructive or aggressive behaviors
2. Reducing the effect of manipulating behaviors
3. Linking consequences to functional as well as dysfunctional behaviors
4. Initiating functional alternatives to prevent a crisis
5. Practicing ongoing management of anger, anxiety, shame, and happiness
6. Creating a lifestyle that prevents regression

PLANNING AND IMPLEMENTATION

Planning must incorporate helping staff to acknowledge and cope with the disruptive behaviors associated with PDs. Staff should be taught specialized techniques to prevent acute disruptions in the health care setting through instruction and ongoing supervision.

It is often difficult to create a therapeutic relationship with individuals with PDs because of symptoms like suspiciousness, aloofness, and hostility. The guarded and secretive style of many of these patients tends to produce an atmosphere of combativeness. It can help when the nurse understands that these "attacks" may be a consequence of the patient feeling threatened. The more intense the complaints, the greater the perceived fear of potential harm or loss.

When the patient:

1. Acts in a suspicious manner:
   - Institute behaviors to help the person feel safe emotionally. Explain reasons for actions in a *matter-of-fact manner.*
2. Lacks the ability to trust:
   - Give the patient a sense of control over what is happening by *giving the patient choices* when possible (e.g., appointment in the morning or afternoon) to facilitate adherence to treatment.
3. Is hypersensitive to criticism yet has no strong sense of autonomy:
   - Teach/model new interpersonal skills by *building on existing skills.*
4. Falsely attributes malevolent intentions to the nurse or others:
   - Discuss these cognitive distortions and present facts in a matter-of-fact manner.
5. Insults or threatens the nurse or caregiver:
   - Ignore insults or sarcasm, but set limits on abusive language or threats of violence while continuing to provide care.
6. Reports feeling hurt or rejected by others:
   - *Allow the person to discuss* the situation. *Listen* to understand the situation and offer *empathy. Acknowledge the distress.* Help *educate the person* regarding how people, systems, families, and relationships work.

Ritter and Platt (2016) identified five common characteristics of evidence-based treatment for people with a diagnosis of PD:

- Provide patients with a structured approach to problem solving.
- Encourage patients to practice self-control.
- Help patients connect feelings to events and actions.
- Be active and responsive so that the person feels validated.
- Discuss countertransference issues (negative feelings toward the patient by staff) with staff members.

TABLE 13.1 Potential Nursing Diagnoses for People With Personality Disorders

Signs and Symptoms	Potential Nursing Diagnoses[a]
Psychological crisis symptoms: • High levels of anxiety • Labile and unstable mood	*Impaired coping process* *Anxiety* *Labile moods*
Dissociation in borderline personality disorder associated with acute anxiety	*Disturbed personal identity*
Anger outbursts	*Labile moods* *Anger* *Risk for violence* *Impaired coping process* *Impaired impulse control*
Aggressive behavior	*Aggressive behavior*
Violence (physical and sexual abuse toward others)	*Risk for violence (specify type)*
Withdrawal	*Withdrawn behavior* *Social isolation* *Impaired socialization*
Paranoia	*Fear* *Risk for confusion*
Chronic depression	*Risk for depressed mood* • *Hopelessness* • *Helplessness* • *Risk for suicide* • *Risk for self-mutilation* • *Chronic low self-esteem* • *Risk for spiritual distress* • *Low self-efficacy*
Difficulty with decision making	*Decisional conflict*
Difficulty in relationships, manipulation, and clinging behavior	*Impaired coping process* *Impaired socialization* *Impaired role performance* *Risk for loneliness* *Low self-efficacy*
Interpersonal problems with family	*Impaired family coping* *Impaired role performance* *Impaired socialization*
Failure to keep medical appointments, late arrival for appointments, failure to follow treatment or medication regimen	*Denial* *Non-adherence to therapeutic regime* *Impaired health-seeking behavior*

[a]The International Classification for Nursing Practice (ICNP) is a product of the International Council of Nurses (ICN). Retrieved from http://www.icn.ch/what-we-do/ICNP-Browser/.

Communication Guidelines

People with PDs may be excessively dependent, demanding, manipulative, or stubborn, or they may self-destructively refuse treatment. Nurses greatly enhance their ability to be therapeutic when they combine limit setting, trustworthiness, manipulation management, and authenticity with their own natural style.

- For Cluster A PDs:
  - *Develop a trusting relationship* by being genuine, respectful, and punctual and doing what you say you will do.
  - *Use a business-like approach* that is not overly warm to reduce suspiciousness.
  - *Acknowledge* patient concerns and perceptions of circumstances without debate or agreement; avoid confrontation.
  - *Respect the patient's need for interpersonal distance* by maintaining a professional demeanor without withdrawing from the patient.
- For Cluster B PDs:
  - *Develop a trusting relationship* by demonstrating respect and positive regard, expressing empathy, and following through on promises.
  - *Avoid the use of "why" questions* to decrease defensiveness.
  - *Maintain interpersonal professional boundaries*; do not "punish" or reject the person for maladaptive behaviors (e.g., angry outbursts), and gently resist the patient's attempt to establish an overly familiar relationship.
  - *Give the patient an opportunity to describe current stressors* that lead to the suicidal or self-harm behaviors to help identify triggers.
  - Support the patient to *talk* to staff to discuss sad and angry feelings or when thinking of hurting himself or herself, instead of acting on impulses.
  - Assign only one or two staff members to the patient to *minimize splitting behaviors.*
  - *Implement a clear and structured plan of care* that is closely followed by the patient and all members of the treatment team.
  - Consider the use of a *behavioral contract* to concretely spell out acceptable behaviors and support personal safety.
  - *Set limits on manipulative behavior in a calm, nonaccusatory manner.* Use objective and specific language to describe the problematic behavior, and discuss the more adaptive behaviors that can be substituted.
- For Cluster C PDs:
  - *Develop a trusting relationship* by providing empathy for the person's distress.
  - *Avoid unnecessary power struggles,* especially with the person with OCPD.
  - *Encourage the patient to assume responsibility* for thoughts and behaviors without blame or shame.
  - *Initiate collaborative problem solving* to facilitate anxiety reduction and improved coping.

Refer to Table 13.2 for interventions for manipulative behaviors and to Table 13.3 for interventions for impulsive behaviors.

Milieu Therapy

Individuals with PDs may be treated within a therapeutic milieu to promote safety. Short-term hospitalization occurs when an individual is assessed to be suicidal or self-harms or is a harm to others. Patients with a diagnosis of BPD requiring hospital admission for attempted suicide have an increased risk of adverse outcomes and require careful clinical monitoring. Hospitalization is of unproven value for long-term suicide prevention among patients with BPD because those with this disorder may be chronically suicidal. A combination of brief, intensive, emergency-type treatment that connects to a comprehensive outpatient program may be a cost-effective alternative to inpatient hospitalization.

The primary therapeutic goal of milieu therapy is *affect management* in a group context. Community meetings, problem-solving

TABLE 13.2 **Interventions for Manipulation**

Intervention	Rationale
1. Assess your own reactions toward patient. If you feel angry, discuss with peers ways to reframe your thinking to defray feelings of anger.	1. Anger is a natural response to being manipulated. It is also a block to effective nurse–patient interaction.
2. Assess patient's interactions for a short period before labeling as manipulative.	2. A patient might respond to one particular, high-stress situation with maladaptive behaviors but use appropriate behaviors in other situations.
3. Set limits on any manipulative behaviors, such as: • Arguing or begging • Flattery or seductiveness • Instilling guilt, clinging • Constantly seeking attention • Pitting one person, staff, group against another • Frequently disregarding the rules • Constant engagement in power struggles • Angry, demanding behaviors	3. From the beginning, limits need to be clear. It will be necessary to refer to these limits frequently because it is to be expected that the patient will test these limits repeatedly.
4. Intervene in manipulative behavior. • Set limits in a calm and nonpunitive way. • Be consistent: All limits adhered to by *all* staff involved. • Behaviors should be documented objectively (give concrete descriptions of time, dates, circumstances). • Provide clear boundaries and consequences. • Enforce the consequences.	4. Patients will test limits, and once they understand that the limits are solid, this understanding can motivate them to work on other ways to meet their needs. It is hoped that this will be done with the nurse clinician by following problem-solving alternative behaviors and learning new effective communication skills.
5. Be vigilant; **avoid:** • Discussing yourself or other staff members with the patient • Promising to keep a secret for the patient • Accepting gifts from the patient • Doing special favors for the patient	5. Patients can use this kind of information to manipulate you and/or split staff. Decline all invitations in a firm, but straightforward manner—for example: • "I am here to focus on you." • "I cannot keep secrets from other staff. I will share it with the treatment team so that everyone is available to support you." • "I cannot accept gifts, but I am wondering what this means to you." • "You are to return to the unit by 4 PM on Sunday, period."

TABLE 13.3 **Interventions for Impulsive Behaviors**

Intervention	Rationale
1. Discuss previous impulsive acts.	1. Helps to identify previous triggers impulsive action.
2. Identify the thoughts and feelings preceding the impulsive acts.	2. Helps link pattern of thoughts or events that trigger impulsive action.
3. Explore effects of such acts on self and others.	3. Helps patients evaluate the results of their behaviors on self and others—may motivate change.
4. Discuss potential alternative behaviors to impulsive acts.	4. Once cues are recognized, planning alternatives to impulsive actions is possible.
5. Teach or refer patient to appropriate place to learn needed coping skills (anger management, assertive skills).	5. Special skills training can potentiate positive change in behaviors.

groups, coping skills groups, and socializing groups are all areas in which patients can interact with peers, consider relationship problems, delegate and take responsibility for certain tasks, discuss goals, collectively deal with problems that arise in the milieu, and learn problem-solving skills. Milieu therapy provides a safe environment for the person to practice communicating needs more clearly instead of acting them out in a socially unacceptable manner.

It is essential for the *entire treatment team* to act in a *consistent and congruent* manner. This starts by maintaining effective communication and collaboration with the entire treatment team. A *concise, structured, and written plan of care* that concretely describes clear boundaries can facilitate this process. *Mutual goal setting* with the patient and treatment team in the form of a *behavioral contract* is another strategy to consider. Limit setting in a calm and respectful manner can help to avoid escalation of angry outbursts.

A small study from the United Kingdom indicated that an intervention called democratic therapeutic communities (DTC) was more effective than "treatment as usual" in improving outcomes in PD. DTC is a form of psychosocial treatment based on a collaborative and deinstitutionalized approach to staff–patient interaction that emphasizes empowerment, personal responsibility, shared decision making, and participation in communal activity (Pearce et al., 2017).

Psychotherapy

Cognitive-behavioral therapy and *interpersonal therapy* have demonstrated some effectiveness with many of the PDs. Some specialized therapies were originally developed for the treatment of borderline PDs and are now sometimes used to treat other disorders.

Dialectical Behavior Therapy

Dialectical behavior therapy (DBT) is an *evidence-based* type of cognitive-behavioral therapy originally developed by Marsha Linehan (1993). It helps change the self-destructive behaviors associated with the diagnosis of BPD. The therapy addresses strategies for the extreme mood swings, the tendency to see the world in black and white, and the nonstop crises that are part of BPD. It includes individual sessions that emphasize problem solving within the context of a supportive therapeutic relationship, plus groups sessions where participants learn adaptive behavioral skills. There are four core concepts:

1. Mindfulness—living in the moment
2. Interpersonal effectiveness—skills that maximize the chance of achieving a goal without damaging a relationship or one's self-respect
3. Distress tolerance—learning to bear emotional pain skillfully by accepting self and the current situation
4. Emotional regulation—recognizing and coping with negative emotions in a healthy manner

Specially trained therapists, such as advanced practice nurses, provide this therapy. Between sessions, participants are given "homework" to practice these skills. Another strategy to reinforce these adaptive skills is the use of smartphone applications (apps). Some recommended apps are:

- DBT Diary Card and Skills Coach—*provides coaching to help an individual use DBT skills*
- DBT Trivia & Quiz—*provides a fun way to become familiar with DBT concepts*
- Buddhify—described as *modern mindfulness* on the go (VonBank, 2015)

Other evidence-based strategies for BPD include the following (Choi-Kain et al., 2017):

- *Systems training for emotional predictability and problem solving (STEPPS)*: A modification of DBT in which educational training in a group setting focuses on emotional and behavioral skills.
- *Mentalization-based treatment (MBT):* Mentalization is the capacity to understand behavior and feelings and how they are associated with specific mental states in ourselves and others. This therapy focuses on learning these skills in a supportive therapy relationship.
- *Schema-focused therapy (SFT)*: Connects maladaptive *adult* behavior to distortions emerging from *childhood* experiences. The therapy attempts to "re-parent" the adult.
- *Transference-focused psychotherapy (TFP)*: Emotions that develop within the interpersonal relationship with the therapist are identified and compared to responses in other situations. More adaptive coping mechanisms are then taught and practiced.

Pharmacological Therapy

Medication is considered adjunctive therapy used to treat symptoms associated with a PD or for comorbid disorders that complicate treatment. Generally, benzodiazepines for anxiety are not appropriate because of the potential for misuse leading to addiction and the possibility of overdose.

Because there is an increased risk for suicidal gestures and self-harm, medications with low toxicity are appropriate for patients with BPD. Because patients with a diagnosis of BPD may become psychotic under stress, a second-generation atypical antipsychotic can be helpful to control high levels of anxiety. Depression is highly comorbid in these patients; therefore the selective serotonin reuptake inhibitors (SSRIs) and venlafaxine are good choices because they are the least toxic in overdose. The SSRIs can also help patients with a diagnosis of BPD who have co-occurring panic attacks. Carbamazepine (anticonvulsant) to help target impulsivity, uncontrolled behaviors, and self-harm has been useful. Other mood stabilizers can be helpful for mood dysregulation and impulsivity. Lithium, anticonvulsants, or SSRIs may be helpful to minimize the aggression seen with antisocial PD and other PDs.

People with Cluster A traits, especially schizotypal PD, may be helped by low-dose antipsychotic medications, which help ameliorate anxiety and the psychosis-like features associated with this disorder. OCPD is often helped with clomipramine (a tricyclic antidepressant) and SSRIs to ameliorate ruminative thinking and comorbid depression.

Self-Care for Nurses

Finding an approach for helping patients with PDs who have overwhelming needs can be daunting. The intense feelings evoked in the nurse/clinician often mirror the feelings being experienced by the patient. Health care workers may feel confused, helpless, angry, and frustrated. These patients are often hostile, calling the nurse inadequate or incompetent; many are abusive of authority and are often successful in using splitting behaviors with the staff—praising or disparaging the nurse to peers in such a way that peers begin

APPLYING THE ART

A Person With Borderline Personality Disorder

Scenario: Maria is an 18-year-old female who has already met with me three times on the young adult unit. She always wore long sleeves even though the unit was warm. The last time we met, Maria shared her poetry, which expressed themes of loneliness amid the beauty of nature. Each time she seemed glad to see me while simultaneously disparaging the evening shift staff.

Therapeutic Goal: By the end of this interaction, Maria will choose to express her feelings using a nondestructive form of communication rather than through self-mutilating behavior.

Student–Patient Interaction	Thoughts, Communication Techniques, and Mental Health Nursing Concepts
Maria: "I wondered if you'd actually come back."	According to her chart, she has many reasons to mistrust, starting with her dad, who sexually abused her. She started self-mutilating in middle school when her parents divorced.

APPLYING THE ART—cont'd

A Person With Borderline Personality Disorder

Student–Patient Interaction	Thoughts, Communication Techniques, and Mental Health Nursing Concepts
Student: "Hi, Maria. I came back as I said I would, but next Tuesday is my last day here." ***Student's feelings:*** *Sometimes I feel guilty to enter my patients' lives only to leave again. I don't want to be one more person to let her down.*	I *give information* reminding Maria of our *original nurse–patient contract.* Maria reacts with surprise but avoids any discussion about *termination* of the *nurse–patient relationship.*
Maria: *Avoids eye contact.* "Read this." *Hands me her poem.* ***Student's feelings:*** *I feel okay about her bossiness. I recognize that I'm in charge of my own boundaries. Actually, I'm relieved that Maria and I get along. She gets in so much trouble with the staff. I've seen the staff get frustrated with Maria.*	Maria says, "Read this" almost as a command. The abuse in her childhood left her feeling powerless. She needs to feel in charge of something.
Student: "Your poem describes the mother as 'daisy.' 'Daisy deigning to decorate my life.'" *Maria nods.* "The 'my life' person might feel lonely with such a powerful mother who drops by to decorate only." *We make eye contact.* "Is this about you, Maria?"	I reflect on feeling "lonely" and seek to clarify that the poem actually refers to Maria and her mother.
Maria: "She loves me, she loves me not." ***Student's feelings:*** *I'm beginning to feel a little lost in the poetry. I need to pay better attention in my English classes!*	Through the poem, Maria uses *symbolism* to safely express her thoughts and sad feelings. Is this also an example of black-and-white thinking?
Student: "At first I didn't catch the meaning of 'daisy' in your poems. 'She loves me, she loves me not.' You're sharing about your mother." ***Student's feelings:*** *I feel so sad that she's so young yet still must battle this mental torment that so disrupts her life and her happiness. She shows so much talent in her writings.*	
Maria: "She says I can't come back to live with her! She's such a ____!"	Maria shows anger in her swearing. Fear and loss fuel her anger. Her mood changes so fast! *Emotional lability,* that's the term.
Student: "You feel abandoned. Maybe thrown away like the daisy petals." ***Student's feelings:*** *I know from her history the chaos evident in her family. I also recognize that Maria pulls people close and then pushes them away. Still, I can't imagine not being able to turn to my family. I feel lonely at the thought.*	I use *reflection,* remembering that patients with *borderline personality disorder* vacillate between feeling *engulfed* by the person they move close to and needing to push that person away to *individuate* self again. Unfortunately, they often *devalue* the other person, get rejected, and then experience *abandonment depression* until once again they move too close.
Maria: "I don't feel anything. Just numb. I have to go to the bathroom."	Maria says she is numb, not *depressed.* The numbness *isolates* her feelings from awareness.
Student: "Okay." When Maria leaves, I tell my instructor and the nurse what just happened. The nurse immediately goes to find Maria. ***Student's feelings:*** *I feel upset with myself for not immediately understanding that after this exchange, Maria might cut herself!*	I probably should have gone with her or asked if she felt like cutting when she said she felt numb. Self-mutilation breaks through the numbness that has its roots in Maria's past. As a child, Maria had to *dissociate* to survive the sexual abuse.
Maria: *Standing in front of me.* "You told on me!" *Raises voice but sits down two chairs away.* ***Student's feelings:*** *I feel uncomfortable being yelled at, and my anxiety level begins to elevate some.*	I understand her behavior; it will just take me a while to not take a patient's behavior so personally and look beyond the behavior to the patient's reason for the behavior.
Student: "Maria, I told the nurse that you felt upset about your mom and maybe about my leaving. I was concerned that you would be okay." ***Student's feelings:*** *I feel anxious, but I know that in reporting, I did the right thing. I want Maria to know I am concerned for her safety.* **Maria:** "I don't want to talk to you anymore." ***Student's feelings:*** *I feel sad as Maria rejects me. I know this isn't really about me, but still, I feel sad.*	When Maria confronts me, I *give truthful information.* When we *contracted,* I said I would need to share important information with the *treatment team.*
Student: *Quietly.* "You're really upset at me and at your mother, yet you were still able to stop yourself from cutting." ***Student's feelings:*** *I feel good that so far I'm able to contain my feelings in light of her angry and rejecting behavior toward me. I do know she needs me to stay calm and not be pushed away no matter how hard she tries.*	I *reflect* feelings and make an observation and give *support* by identifying her nondestructive choice and that she has some control over not cutting herself.
Maria: "I'm so ____ at you. A fine nurse you'll be!" *Storms away.*	With the sarcasm, Maria *devalues* me. I remember devaluing as the other pole to *idealizing* others, also part of the disorder. Nevertheless, using words to express her anger shows some progress. She uses *withdrawal* in leaving me. The closeness threatens her safety by encroaching on her *ego boundaries.* Maria's deeper loss, which pertains to her mother, gets *displaced* into the anger at me.

Continued

APPLYING THE ART—cont'd

A Person With Borderline Personality Disorder

Student–Patient Interaction	Thoughts, Communication Techniques, and Mental Health Nursing Concepts
Student: *I stay seated about 5 minutes. I notice Maria glancing over at me a few times before she leaves for lunch.* ***Student's feelings:*** *Maria acts so very angry at me. I feel my heart rate pick up (guess it makes me anxious). Okay, I'll take some mindful breaths. It's hard to wait here but I want Maria to know she's worth waiting for.*	Because I promised Maria that the 45 minutes we contracted was for her, I will make myself available to her for the contracted period of time.
Student: *I leave to debrief with my clinical group.* ***Student's feelings:*** *I hope Maria will let me talk to her later today or at least on the last day I come.*	Maria's self-esteem and even her sense of identity are fragile. She restores some kind of control or power by leaving me before I terminate with her.

APPLYING EVIDENCE-BASED PRACTICE (EBP)

Problem

A 40-year-old female presents to the mental health clinic with a history of extreme mood swings and irritability. She is unable to keep a job or a relationship because of her frequent outbursts. She feels people are always abandoning her. She has a history of hitting herself on the head and legs, as well as pulling out pieces of hair, to relieve emotional pain. She is diagnosed with borderline personality disorder (BPD) in addition to her other issues.

EBP Assessment

A. **What do you already know from experience?** People with BPD can be difficult to treat because of feeling abandoned and having difficulty with emotional regulation. They tend to have tumultuous relationships and demonstrate self-harm behaviors. They often have co-occurring diagnoses such as mood disorders or substance use disorders. The psychiatric history often reveals a history of abuse or disrupted relationships with their caregivers in childhood.

B. **What does the literature say?** There is no medication to specifically treat a personality disorder, but selective serotonin reuptake inhibitor (SSRI) antidepressants or mood stabilizers may be used for relief of symptoms that coexist. The dysfunctional behaviors displayed helped the patient survive a chaotic childhood but create difficulties in adult life. Dialectical behavior therapy (DBT) has been shown to be the most effective treatment for BPD. DBT is a form of cognitive-behavioral therapy (CBT) that incorporates the acceptance of uncomfortable thoughts or feelings and the development of coping skills and mindfulness practices.

C. **What does the patient want?** This patient states she wants to feel better, but she has been resistant to medications or therapy, attending appointments but not following through with the recommendations. This response is common in patients with personality disorders because change can feel scary. Often, it will take a major loss or threat of a loss (e.g., loss of a relationship or job) for the patient to accept the need to change.

Plan

The psychiatrist has remained supportive throughout the fluctuations in patient mood and anger during appointments. Medications have been introduced slowly and in very small dosages because of resistance. The patient is in DBT but feels the exercises assigned by the therapist are "really stupid." She has been encouraged to do them anyway. The patient is ashamed of her mental illness and does not want to pass on her behaviors to her children. This has been used therapeutically as an incentive to accept growth and change.

QSEN Prelicensure Knowledge, Skills, and Attitudes (KSAs) Addressed

Informatics was used by the psychiatrist to provide quality online information for the patient because the patient had been relying on inappropriate and inaccurate sources

Teamwork and Collaboration occurred through frequent communication between the psychiatrist and DBT therapist and the development of a consistent treatment plan

to react negatively toward one another. Usually this is the patient's attempt to defend against feelings of frustration and powerlessness. When staff are split, the result is often substantial conflict within the treatment team. In fact, staff conflict that centers around the care of a specific patient can be seen as a *warning flag* that the patient has a PD.

Untrained and unsupported staff may easily regress or become vengeful in response to a patient's sense of entitlement, manipulation, dependency, ingratitude, impulsivity, and rage. *Frequent communication among staff and continuous availability of supervision and support are vital when the behaviors of these patients start to affect the confidence, feelings, behaviors, and effectiveness of staff members.*

Nurses and other health care workers should practice self-health management. This includes acknowledging and accepting their own emotional responses and attempting to ensure personal well-being.

EVALUATION

Evaluating treatment effectiveness in this patient population is difficult. Health care providers may never know the real results of their interventions, particularly in acute care settings. Even in long-term

Neurobiology of Borderline Personality Disorder/Emotional Deregulation (EDR)

Borderline Personality Disorder (BPD) is actually a serious and disabling brain disease marked by impulsivity and dysregulation.

Serotonin: altered functioning of serotonin in the brain has been linked to depression, aggression and difficulty in controlling destructive urges. The serotonin transporter gene 5-HTT is thought to have shorter alleles in BPD which have been associated with lower levels of serotonin and greater impulsive aggression.

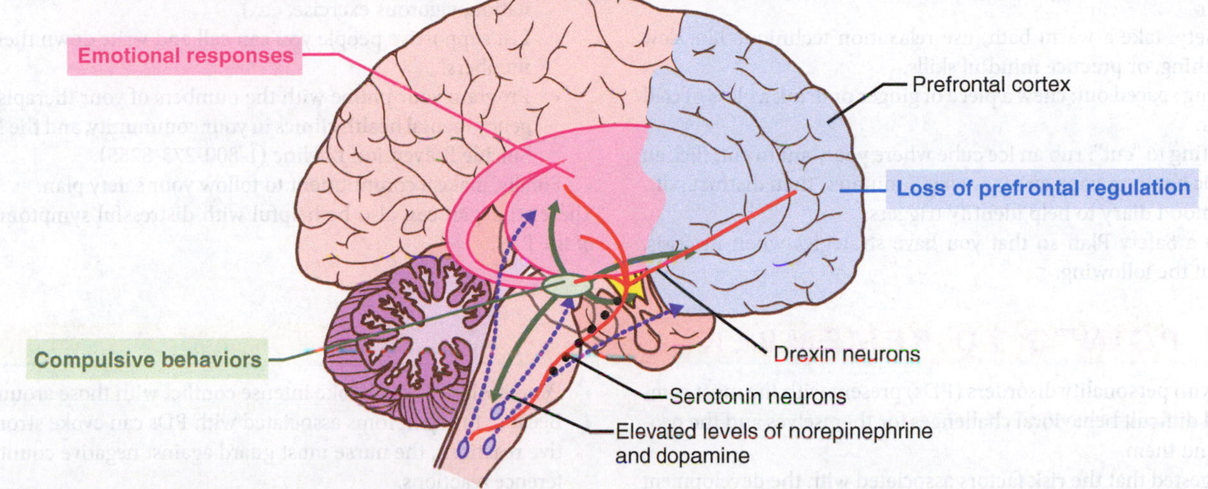

Emotional Dysregulation and the Brain

Emotional dysregulation: emotional responses that are poorly modulated (e.g., angry outbursts, rage, marked fluctuation of mood, self-harm that can shift within seconds, minutes, or hours).

Brain Imaging (fMRI) Supports:

Prefrontal cortex: in times of stress, this part of the brain helps us regulate emotions, restrain from inappropriate actions, helps with reality testing, and guides attention and thought. In people with BPD this part of the brain *doesn't respond*; instead there is an extreme perception and intensity of negative emotions.

Limbic system/ amygdala: in BPD, parts of the emotional center of the brain are overstimulated and take longer to return to normal. Also, it is believed that **certain neurotransmitters** that act as constraints in normal circumstances under-function in BPD, thus leaving a person in a prolonged state of the fight/flight response.

Medications/Therapy to Help Individuals Regulate Their Emotions

Method	What's Involved	What It Does
Dialectic behavioral therapy (DBT)	Mindfulness, deep breathing, relaxation techniques	Helps brain switch from sympathetic nervous system (arousal) to the parasympathetic (relaxation mode)
Medications	SSRIs, anticonvulsants, second-generation antipsychotics, lithium	Helps dampen angry, impulsive, labile behavior

Dialectical Living. Emotion Dysregulation. http://www. dialecticalliving.ca/emotion-regulation-disorder-dpd/
Neural correlates of negative emotionality in borderline personality disorder: an activation-likelihood-estimation meta-analysis (2013) Ruocco, A. C., Amirthavasagam, S., Choi-Kain ,L. W., & McMain, S. S. Biological Psychiatry, 73(2)
Nauert, R. (2015). Brain scans clarify borderline personality disorder. Psych Central. Retrieved October 21, 2015, from http://psychcentral.com/news/2009/09/04/brain-scans-clarify-borderline-personality-disorder/8184.html

outpatient treatment, many patients find the relationship too intimate an experience to remain long enough for successful treatment. However, some motivated patients may be able to learn to change their behavior, especially if positive experiences are repeated. Each therapeutic episode offers an opportunity for patients to observe themselves interacting with caregivers who consistently try to teach positive coping skills. Perhaps effectiveness can be measured by how successfully the nurse is able to be genuine with the patient, maintain a helpful posture, offer substantial instruction, and still care for the patient. Specific short-term outcomes may be accomplished, and the patient can be given the message of hope that quality of life can always be improved.

There are several self-help strategies that are especially useful for symptoms associated with BPD. Because of the impulsivity and emotional dysregulation associated with this disorder, it is important to develop strategies to minimize suicidal and self-harm behaviors. Patient teaching might include the following self-help strategies:

- Take care of your physical health:
  - Get enough sleep.
  - Eat regular, high-quality meals (less "junk" food).
  - Get regular exercise.
  - Spend time in nature if possible.
  - Avoid drugs and alcohol.

- Develop strategies to "get through" distressful feelings:
  - Anger/frustration: rip up newspaper, engage in vigorous exercise, or listen to loud music.
  - Depression: wrap yourself in a blanket, cuddle a pet or stuffed animal, or write out negative thoughts and then tear up the paper.
  - Anxiety: take a warm bath, use relaxation technique like slow breathing, or practice mindful skills.
  - Feeling spaced out: chew a piece of ginger or drink a glass of cold water.
  - Wanting to "cut": rub an ice cube where you want to cut; flick an elastic band on your wrist; or wait 5 minutes, then distract self.
- Keep a mood diary to help identify triggers.
- Develop a Safety Plan so that you have strategies when in crisis. Write out the following:
  - Identify risk behaviors (thoughts of suicide).
  - Identify triggers so that you can avoid them.
  - Identify five self-soothing techniques for when you can't avoid the trigger.
  - Make a list of coping techniques that work for you (music, meditation, vigorous exercise, etc.).
  - List supportive people you can call and write down their phone numbers.
  - Program your phone with the numbers of your therapist, emergency mental health clinics in your community, and the National Suicide Prevention Lifeline (1-800-273-8255).
- Finally, make a commitment to follow your safety plan.

These strategies can also be helpful with distressful symptoms of any of the PDs.

KEY POINTS TO REMEMBER

- People with personality disorders (PDs) present with the most complex and difficult behavioral challenges for themselves and the people around them.
- It is suggested that the risk factors associated with the development of PDs are genetics, biochemical and neurobiological changes, and environmental factors.
- People with these disorders respond to stress with more primitive defenses and less adaptive defense mechanisms.
- People with PD have inflexible and maladaptive ways of handling stress. These disorders can lead to dysfunction in work and intimate relationships.
- People with PD can experience great distress and have difficulty managing impulses.
- PDs often co-occur with other mental health disorders, including depression, substance use disorders, somatization, eating disorders, posttraumatic stress disorder, anxiety disorders, other PDs, and general medical conditions.
- People with PD can evoke intense conflict with those around them.
- Because the symptoms associated with PDs can evoke strong negative reactions, the nurse must guard against negative countertransference reactions.
- Safety is a first priority. Assessment of past and present suicide/homicide/self-mutilation ideation is essential. The presence of co-occurring disorders is also a vital part of the initial assessment interview.
- Communication guidelines for manipulative and impulsive behaviors are outlined.
- Medication is used for symptom relief for those with PD or a co-occurring condition.
- There are a variety of therapies available for the treatment of PDs. Therapies based on cognitive-behavioral therapy (CBT) seem to be the most effective. Dialectical behavior therapy (DBT), a specialized type of CBT, has been shown to be especially effective in people with borderline PD. These therapies are generally long term.

APPLYING CRITICAL JUDGMENT

1. Ms. Pemrose is brought to the emergency department (ED) after slashing her wrist with a razor. Her past history reveals a previous drug overdose and a history of addiction. During a previous ED admission, she was described as sarcastic, belittling, and aggressive to those who tried to care for her. She has a history of difficulty with interpersonal relationships at her job. Upon initial examination, Ms. Pemrose initially presented as polite and cooperative, telling the nurse, "You are the best nurse I've ever seen. I truly want to change." When the nurse refused to support her request for diazepam (Valium) and Oxycodone for "pain," she became upset, yelling, "You are a stupid excuse for a nurse. I want a physician immediately." Ms. Pemrose has been diagnosed with borderline personality disorder (BPD).
   A. What defense mechanism is Ms. Pemrose using?
   B. How could the nurse set limits while still demonstrating empathy and concern?
   C. What might you expect to find in Ms. Pemrose's psychosocial history, including behavioral issues, family history, and potential comorbidities?
   D. What is the priority safety concern when planning care for this patient?
   E. Describe one evidence-based treatment regimen that has shown effectiveness with people with a diagnosis of BPD.
   F. When Ms. Pemrose becomes manipulative, identify specific steps that can help minimize the negative effects of manipulation.
   G. Identify nursing interventions that might help when working with someone like Ms. Pemrose who exhibits impulsive behavior.

CHAPTER REVIEW QUESTIONS

1. A person shoplifts merchandise from a community cancer thrift shop. When confronted, the person replies, "All this stuff was donated, so I can take it." This comment suggests features of which personality disorder?
   a. Antisocial
   b. Histrionic
   c. Borderline
   d. Schizotypal
2. After a power outage, a facility must serve a dinner of sandwiches and fruit to patients. Which comment is most likely from a patient diagnosed with a narcissistic personality disorder?
   a. "These sandwiches are probably contaminated with bacteria."
   b "I suppose it's the best we can hope for under these circumstances."
   c. "You should have ordered a to-go meal from a local restaurant for me."

CHAPTER REVIEW QUESTIONS—CONT'D

d. "I would rather wait to eat until the dietary department can prepare a meal."

3. A nurse plans care for a patient diagnosed with borderline personality disorder. Which patient problem is most likely to apply to this patient?
   a. Ineffective relationships related to frequent splitting
   b. Social isolation related to fear of embarrassment or rejection
   c. Ineffective impulse control related to violence as evidenced by cruelty to animals
   d. Disturbed thought processes related to recurrent suspiciousness of people and situations
4. The nurse assesses a new patient suspected of having a schizotypal personality disorder. Which assessment question is this patient most likely to answer affirmatively?
   a. "Do some types of situations frighten you?"
   b. "Do you often have episodes of prolonged crying?"
   c. "Has anyone in your family ever been diagnosed with a mental illness?"
   d. "Is it ever very important for you to do everything correctly?"
5. A mental health nurse assesses a patient diagnosed with an antisocial personality disorder. Which comorbid problem is most important for the nurse to include in the assessment?
   a. Generalized anxiety
   b. Alcohol or substance use disorder
   c. Compulsions and phobias
   d. Dysfunctional sleep patterns

REFERENCES

American Psychiatric Association. (2013). *Diagnostic and statistical manual of mental disorders (DSM-5)* (5th ed.). Washington, DC: American Psychiatric Publishing.

Bienenfeld, D. (2016, February 15). Personality disorders. *Medscape.* Retrieved from https://emedicine.medscape.com/article/294307-overview#a4.

Black, D. (2017). Antisocial personality disorder causes. *Psychiatry Central.* Retrieved on April 17, 2018, from https://psychcentral.com/disorders/antisocial-personality-disorder/causes/.

Black, D. W., & Andreasen, N. C. (2014). Personality disorders. In *Introductory textbook of psychiatry*. Washington, DC: American Psychiatric Publishing.

Blaise, M. A., Smallwood, P., Groves, J. E., et al. (2016). Personality and personality disorders. In Stern, T., et al. (Eds.), *Massachusetts General Hospital comprehensive clinical psychiatry*. Philadelphia: Saunders/Elsevier.

Cherry, K. (2018). *Personality Psychology,* Verywellmind. Retrieved from https://www.verywellmind.com/personality-psychology-4157179.

Choi-Kain, L. W., Finch, E. F., Masland, S. R., Jenkins, J. A., & Unruh, B. T. (2017). What works in the treatment of borderline personality disorder. *Current Behavioral Neuroscience Reports, 4*(1), 21–30. https://doi.org/10.1007/s40473-017-0103-z.

Dryden-Edwards, R. (2016). *Borderline personality disorder.* Retrieved January 20, 2016, from http://www.medicine.com/borderline_personality_disorder/page9htm#how_can_ borderline_personality_disorder_be_prevented.

Giddens, J. (2017). *Concepts for nursing practice* (2nd ed.). St. Louis: Elsevier.

Halter, M. (2018). *Varcarolis' Foundations of psychiatric-mental health nursing* (8th ed.). St. Louis: Elsevier.

Linehan, M. M. (1993). *Understanding borderline personality disorder: A dialectical approach.* New York: Guilford.

Mayo Clinic. (2020). Narcissistic personality disorder. Retrieved from https://www.mayoclinic.org/diseases-conditions/narcissistic-personality-disorder/symptoms-causes/syc-20366662.

National Education Alliance for Borderline Personality Disorder. (2018). *Overview of BPD.* Retrieved from https://www.borderlinepersonalitydisorder.com/what-is-bpd/bpd-overview/.

National Institute of Mental Health (NIMH). (2017). *Personality disorders.* Retrieved from https://www.nimh.nih.gov/health/statistics/personality-disorders.shtml.

Pearce, S., et al. (2017). Democratic therapeutic community treatment for personality disorder: Randomised controlled trial. *The British Journal of Psychiatry, 210*(2), 149–156. https://doi.org/10.1192/bjp.bp.116.184366.

Ritter, S., & Platt, L. M. (2016). What's new in treating in patients with personality disorders? Dialectical behavior therapy and old-fashioned, good communication. *Journal of Psychosocial Nursing, 54*(1), 38–45.

Sadock, B. J., Sadock, V. A., & Ruiz, P. (2015). *Kaplan & Sadock's synopsis of psychiatry: Behavioral sciences/clinical psychiatry* (11th ed.). Philadelphia: Wolters Kluwer.

Salters-Pedneault, K. (2020). *Genetic causes of borderline personality disorder.* Retrieved from https://www.verywellmind.com/genetic-causes-of-borderline-personality-disorder-425157.

Verona, E., & Patrick, C. J. (2015). *Psychobiological aspects of antisocial personality disorder, psychopathy, and violence.* Retrieved November 2, 2016, from http://www.psychiatrictimes.com/special-reports/psychobiological-aspects-antisocial-personality-disorder-psychopathy-and-violence#sthash.oHFdg1Du.dpuf.

VonBank, B. (2015). *3 apps worth Downloading to practice your DBT skills, IntinpschPsych woman.* Retrieved from http://intrinpsychwoman.com/2015/10/3-apps-worth-downloading-to-practice-your-dbt-skills/.

14

Eating Disorders

Lorraine Chiappetta[a]

http://evolve.elsevier.com/Varcarolis/essentials

OBJECTIVES

1. Compare predisposing factors associated with the development of eating disorders.
2. Differentiate between the signs and symptoms of anorexia nervosa and bulimia nervosa.
3. Identify priority assessments for individuals with an eating disorder to facilitate safe and effective care. **QSEN: Safety**
4. Apply behavioral and communication strategies that facilitate patient-centered care for the individual with an eating disorder. **QSEN: Patient-Centered Care**
5. Identify evidence-based practice interventions for both the acute phase and the long-term phase of anorexia nervosa and bulimia nervosa. **QSEN: Evidence-Based Practice**
6. Describe components of interprofessional and intraprofessional teamwork and collaboration to effectively treat eating disorders. **QSEN: Teamwork and Collaboration**
7. Use informatics to compare the advantages and disadvantages of treatment strategies used to treat eating disorders. **QSEN: Informatics**

KEY TERMS AND CONCEPTS

anorexia nervosa, p. 184
binge-eating disorder, p. 184
bulimia nervosa, p. 184
cachectic, p. 187
cognitive distortions, p. 190
eating disorder, p. 184
harm-reduction approach, p. 192
ideal body weight, p. 189
lanugo, p. 187
purging, p. 188
refeeding syndrome, p. 189

CONCEPT: NUTRITION: *Nutrition* encompasses the process by which food and nutrients affect growth and development, cellular function and repair, health promotion, and disease prevention. It can be viewed on a continuum from optimal to suboptimal (Giddens, 2017). People with *eating disorders* experience severe disruptions in normal eating patterns and a disturbance in the perception of body shape and weight. They are among the most lethal of all psychiatric diseases (Halter, 2018).

INTRODUCTION

For most people, eating provides nourishment for the body as well as the soul. Families and friends gather around the table to break bread as they celebrate, mourn, laugh, cry, and share. However, for some individuals, eating is not a pleasant experience. For those with an **eating disorder**, there are severe disruptions in normal eating patterns, high levels of anxiety around eating, and a significant disturbance in the perception of body shape and weight.

EATING DISORDERS

The *Diagnostic and Statistical Manual of Mental Disorders,* 5th edition (*DSM-5;* American Psychiatric Association [APA], 2013) groups psychiatric disorders associated with eating under "Feeding and Eating Disorders." The eating disorders included in this chapter are anorexia nervosa, bulimia nervosa, and binge-eating disorders. Individuals with **anorexia nervosa (AN)** have intense irrational beliefs about their shape and weight. They engage in self-starvation, express intense fear of gaining weight, and have a disturbance in self-evaluation of weight and its importance (APA, 2013). There are two subtypes of AN: one in which the individual restricts intake of food and one in which the individual restricts foods but also has periods of binge eating and purging.

Individuals with **bulimia nervosa (BN)** engage in repeated episodes of binge eating (consuming large amounts of calories) followed by inappropriate *compensatory* behaviors such as self-induced vomiting; misuse of laxatives, diuretics, other medications; or excessive exercise.

Binge-eating disorder (BED) is diagnosed when individuals engage in repeated episodes of binge eating followed by significant distress. These individuals do not regularly use the compensatory behaviors seen in patients with bulimia nervosa, and obesity often results. There are several other less common eating disorders described in the *DSM-5* (APA, 2013).

The *DSM-5* (APA, 2013) describes the specific criteria required for a formal diagnosis of an eating disorder. It is important to note that

[a]The authors acknowledge Kathleen Ibrahim for prior contributions to this chapter.

individuals may experience periods of *disordered eating behavior* prior to demonstrating the full criteria for these diagnoses.

The most effective treatments involve an interdisciplinary team approach that enlists the expertise of various health care professionals, including primary care providers, medical specialists, advanced practice psychiatric nurses, psychologists, psychiatrists, and nutritionists. Family psychoeducation and participation in treatment can be an important component of effective treatment.

Prevalence

Prevalence rates of the different eating disorders are as follows (Franco et al., 2017):

Anorexia nervosa (AN):

- Lifetime prevalence: 0.6%; three times higher in females compared with males

Bulimia nervosa (BN):

- Overall prevalence in the past year: 0.3%; five times higher in females compared with males
- BN is more common than AN and has a better prognosis.
- Lifetime prevalence is 1.0%.

Binge-eating disorders (BED):

- Overall prevalence in the past year: 1.2%; twice as many females as males
- Of those with the disorder, 18.5% had severe impairment.
- Lifetime prevalence is 2.8%.

Prevalence of eating disorders in adolescents (ages 13 to 18):

- The lifetime prevalence of eating disorders is 2.7%.
- The prevalence of *subthreshold* eating disorders is up to 11%.
- Eating disorders are more than twice as prevalent among females than males (National Institute of Mental Health [NIMH], 2017).
- Eating disorders are the third most common chronic illness among adolescents.

It is challenging to get accurate statistics on the incidence of eating disorders, particularly "subthreshold" disordered eating that does not meet the full diagnostic criteria. The following are additional observations about those who struggle with eating issues:

- Eating disorders affect up to 30 million Americans.
- One in five women struggles with an eating disorder or disordered eating.
- Middle-aged women are the fastest-growing segment of the population being diagnosed with eating disorders.
- Bullying about body size and appearance is the most common form of bullying in schools.
- Of 10-year-old children, 81% are afraid of "being fat."
- Up to 60% of girls between the ages of 6 and 12 are concerned about their weight (Smolak, 2011).
- At least 10% to 15% of those with AN and BN are male.
- Of American adults, 61% are either overweight or obese (Mirasol, n.d.).

The most common age of onset for eating disorders is during adolescence, although eating disorders can occur in patients of any age, gender, race, or ethnicity. The risk is highest for young men and women between 13 and 17 years of age (National Institute for Health and Care Excellence [NICE], 2017). The onset of BEDs is most common in the mid-20s (Franco et al., 2017).

Comorbidity

Eating disorders usually present with other comorbid psychiatric illnesses. More than 50% of people with anorexia have a concurrent psychiatric disorder, and almost 95% of people with bulimia have a concurrent psychiatric disorder (Sadock, Sadock, & Ruiz, 2015). Most eating disorders have the highest comorbidity with an anxiety disorder. Additional comorbid conditions include major depressive disorder or dysthymia (50% to 75%), sexual abuse history (20% to 50%), obsessive-compulsive disorder, substance use disorders, and bipolar disorder. There is a higher incidence of substance use disorders with bulimia nervosa (Franco et al., 2017). Eating disorders are also associated with a high risk for suicide and self-harm.

There are multiple medical complications related to weight loss, purging/vomiting, laxative misuse, and appetite suppressant abuse that can significantly compromise every organ system of the body. AN can cause muscle wasting, heart and brain damage, and multiorgan failure (Weir, 2016). In fact, AN has been reported to have one of the highest mortality rates of any psychiatric disorder (Hamilton, Cullar, & Elenback, 2015). Untreated BN can lead to serious gastrointestinal problems, electrolyte imbalance, and cardiovascular disease. BEDs may have additional medical comorbidities associated with the obesity that occurs. Without treatment, up to 20% of people with a serious eating disorder die, usually as a result of cardiovascular complications or suicide.

Adolescent girls with type 1 diabetes are twice as likely to have disordered eating behavior than their nondiabetic counterparts and may omit insulin as a weight-reduction strategy (**Blazek, 2015**). There is a lack of solid research on effective strategies to reach this population. Pregnancy also presents additional challenges for treating females with eating disorders.

Course and Prognosis

Generally, about a third of patients with an eating disorder recover fully, a third retain subthreshold symptoms, and a third maintain a chronic eating disorder (Franco et al., 2017).

Long-term follow-up shows recovery rates ranging from 44% to 76%, with prolonged recovery time (57 to 59 months) for AN. There is a better overall prognosis for BN. Short-term success is 50% to 70%, with a relapse rate of 30% to 50% after 6 months for those with BN (Franco et al., 2017).

Theory

The etiology of eating disorders is complex. It appears that a biological vulnerability or predisposition may be activated by genetic, psychosocial, and cultural factors. The exact etiology remains unknown.

Neurobiological and Neuroendocrine Models

A faulty reward-processing system seems to be an important feature of these diseases. It is thought that those with AN have difficulty benefitting from a "reward," like the pleasant sensation of eating. Those with AN may also be oversensitive to punishment (Weir, 2016). Dopamine activity, an important component of the reward system, appears to be altered in both bulimia and anorexia. People with AN often report that sitting down to a meal makes them feel worried. This may be related to the release of the neurotransmitter dopamine in the dorsal striatum that triggers anxiety rather than the pleasure that many of us feel when preparing to eat. Those with BN may have a weaker-than-normal response to the dopamine-related reward circuitry. Experiencing less pleasure when eating "usual" amounts of food may explain the desire to binge eat. Structural and functional areas of the brain associated with the reward system also appear to be altered in individuals with an eating disorder. These areas include the orbitofrontal cortex, which signals us to stop eating; the right insula, involved in the ability to sense one's own bodily signals; and a subregion of the insula associated with an anxious temperament. Malnutrition causes significant brain changes, making it challenging to figure out if these observed brain changes are *the cause* or *the consequence* of an eating disorder.

Serotonin is a neurotransmitter involved with well-being, anxiety, and appetite. Norepinephrine is a stress hormone. In addition to dopamine, there appear to be abnormal levels of these and other neurotransmitters in people with an eating disorder (Gleissner, 2017).

Recent research addresses the overlap between uncontrolled compulsive eating and compulsive drug seeking in drug addiction. Reduction in ventral striatal dopamine is found in both of these groups. Lower frequency of dopamine D_2 receptors was associated with higher body mass index. Obese persons might eat to temporarily increase activity in these reward circuits (Franco et al., 2017).

Genetic Factors

First-degree female relatives and monozygotic twin offspring of people with AN have higher rates of AN and BN. Children of persons with AN have a lifetime risk that is tenfold that of the general population (5%). Families of patients with BN have higher rates of substance use disorders, particularly alcoholism, affective disorders, and obesity (Franco et al., 2017).

Finally, a large-scale, international whole-genome analysis found evidence that *AN* is associated with genetic anomalies on chromosome 12 (Duncan et al., 2017).

Psychological and Psychosocial Models

Sociocultural and psychological factors have long been implicated in the etiology of eating disorders. External factors such as cultural pressure, parental attitudes, and stressful or traumatic life events have all been implicated. Environmental factors that may increase one's risk of developing an eating disorder include the following:

- Dysfunctional family and interpersonal relationships: Families with adolescents diagnosed with AN tend to report interpersonal boundary problems in which there may be *separation and individuation* developmental issues. This developmental issue is based on the idea that a child must learn to achieve a separateness from the primary caregiver and develop a sense of being a separate individual so that the child will be able to achieve autonomy, independence, and identity as an adult. Dysfunctional families may demonstrate a poor tolerance of conflicts and low levels of satisfaction in the family. Parents of adolescents diagnosed with BN described their families as more chaotic. Families of female adolescents with BED showed significantly low emotional and affective involvement (Cerniglia et al., 2017).
- Trauma: The types of child maltreatment most closely associated with any eating disorders are sexual abuse and physical neglect among men and sexual abuse and emotional abuse among women (Affi et al., 2017).
- Participation in career or sports in which being thin is promoted/required.
- Cultural/peer pressure to be thin: When assessing the adolescent, inquire about bullying and teasing about weight and body issues because this is a common stressor for this population (NICE, 2017).
- Stressful life transitions: Although environment can certainly play a role, as we learn more about the brain, it becomes more evident that faulty neurobiology may be the most significant etiologic factor. It has been noted that people who later develop AN and BN demonstrated anxious, obsessive, perfectionistic, and achievement-oriented traits *before* the onset of the eating disorder (Weir, 2016).
- Comorbid anxiety disorder (Ekern, 2017).

Cultural Considerations

Eating disorders are more common in industrialized societies where there is an abundance of food and being thin is considered attractive. In the United States, eating disorders are common in young Latin American, Native American, and African American women, but the rates are still lower than in Caucasian women. African American women are more likely to develop bulimia and more likely to purge. First-generation daughters of Asian immigrants are at higher risk than U.S. females of the same age. This appears to be related to cultural expectations (Franco et al., 2017). Female athletes involved in running, gymnastics, or ballet and male bodybuilders or wrestlers are at increased risk (Franco et al., 2017).

Clinical Picture

AN and BN present two different clinical pictures:

- Box 14.1 identifies the signs and symptoms of these disorders.
- Box 14.2 identifies a number of complications that can occur in individuals with eating disorders.
- Box 14.3 identifies when an individual should be hospitalized.

Eating disorders are often characterized by denial, rationalization, minimization, or concealment of the disordered behaviors from others. This may be related to stigma and shame (Marcon et al., 2017). Fundamental to the care of individuals with eating disorders is the establishment and maintenance of a therapeutic relationship. This may take time. In addition, information and interventions must be tailored to the person's age and level of development (NICE, 2017).

APPLICATION OF THE NURSING PROCESS

ASSESSMENT: ANOREXIA NERVOSA

Formal assessment tools can be used to help identify those at risk for developing AN and other eating disorders. The **SCOFF questionnaire** is an example of a standardized, validated screening tool available to primary care providers to assess for eating disorders (Schreiner, 2015). Answering yes to two or more questions may indicate an eating disorder:

- <u>S</u>ick: Do you make yourself sick or vomit after a meal because you feel uncomfortably full?
- <u>C</u>ontrol: Do you fear loss of control over how much you eat?

BOX 14.1 Possible Signs and Symptoms of Anorexia Nervosa and Bulimia Nervosa

Anorexia Nervosa

- Terror of gaining weight
- Preoccupation with thoughts of food
- View of self as fat even when emaciated
- Peculiar handling of food:
  - Cutting food into small bits
  - Pushing pieces of food around plate
- Possible development of rigorous exercise regimen
- Possible self-induced vomiting; use of laxatives and diuretics
- Cognitive distortions: individual judges own self-worth by weight
- Controls eating to feel powerful to overcome feelings of helplessness

Bulimia Nervosa

- Binge-eating behaviors
- Binging may occur after attempts to fast to prevent weight gain
- Compensatory behavior, often self-induced vomiting (or laxative or diuretic use) after bingeing
- History of anorexia nervosa in one-fourth to one-third of individuals
- Depressive signs and symptoms
- Problems with:
  - Interpersonal relationships
  - Self-concept
  - Impulsive behaviors; reports feeling "out of control" at times
- Increased levels of anxiety and compulsivity
- Possible comorbid substance use disorder
- Bingeing may be motivated by feelings of emptiness or attempts to feel less depressed

BOX 14.2 Some Medical Complications of Anorexia Nervosa and Bulimia Nervosa

Anorexia Nervosa

- Bradycardia
- Hypotension
- Orthostatic changes in pulse rate or blood pressure
- Cardiac murmur—one-third with mitral valve prolapse
- Sudden cardiac arrest caused by profound electrolyte disturbances
- Prolonged QT interval on electrocardiogram
- Acrocyanosis (bluish color of hands and feet caused by slow circulation)
- Leukopenia
- Lymphocytosis
- Carotenemia (elevated carotene levels in blood), which produces skin with a yellow pallor
- Hypokalemic alkalosis (with self-induced vomiting or use of laxatives and diuretics)
- Elevated serum bicarbonate levels, hypochloremia, and hypokalemia
- Electrolyte imbalances, which lead to fatigue, weakness, and lethargy
- Osteoporosis, indicated by low bone density
- Fatty degeneration of the liver, indicated by elevation of serum enzyme levels
- Elevated cholesterol levels
- Amenorrhea
- Abnormal thyroid functioning
- Hematuria
- Proteinuria

Bulimia Nervosa

- Cardiomyopathy (rare occurrence due to diminished protein synthesis, malnutrition)
- Cardiac dysrhythmias
- Sinus bradycardia
- Sudden cardiac arrest as a result of profound electrolyte disturbances
- Orthostatic changes in pulse rate or blood pressure
- Cardiac murmur; mitral valve prolapse
- Electrolyte imbalances
- Elevated serum bicarbonate levels (although they can be low, which indicates metabolic acidosis)
- Hypochloremia
- Hypokalemia
- Dehydration, which results in volume depletion, leading to stimulation of aldosterone production, which in turn stimulates further potassium excretion from kidneys; thus there can be an indirect renal loss of potassium as well as a direct loss through self-induced vomiting
- Severe attrition and erosion of teeth, producing irritating sensitivity and exposing the pulp of the teeth
- Loss of the dental arch
- Diminished chewing ability
- Parotid gland enlargement associated with elevated serum amylase levels
- Esophageal tears caused by self-induced vomiting
- Severe abdominal pain indicative of gastric dilation
- Russell's sign (callus on knuckles from self-induced vomiting)

- One stone: Has the patient lost 14 lb in a 3-month period? (A stone is a unit of weight in Great Britain equivalent to 14 lb.)
- Fat: Do you believe you are fat even when others tell you that you are too thin?
- Food: Does food dominate your life?

Diagnostic symptoms for AN include *dangerously low body-weight* measurements relative to the age and gender of the patient, *intense fear of gaining weight,* and *disturbances in how one's body weight is experienced.* Body mass index (BMI) is a specific measurement used to identify the severity of AN. An ideal BMI is thought to be between 19 and 25 kg/m^2. See the *DSM-5* Diagnostic Criteria for Anorexia Nervosa box for specific BMI ranges. Pediatric growth tables can also be used for children. Other symptoms associated with low body weight that can suggest a problem include rapid weight loss, dieting or restrictive eating practices, or family reports of changes in eating behaviors. Physical signs associated with low body weight suggestive of AN may include the following:

- Malnutrition, including poor circulation, dizziness, palpitations, fainting, or pallor
- Menstrual or other endocrine disturbances
- Unexplained gastrointestinal symptoms (NICE, 2017)
- **Cachectic** appearance (severely underweight with muscle wasting)
- **Lanugo** (a growth of fine, downy hair on the face and back)

A comprehensive psychosocial assessment can be used to identify some of the other prominent symptoms associated with AN. Areas of assessment include the following:

- The person's perception of the problem
- Eating habits, especially ritualistic eating patterns
- History of dieting or restrictive eating
- Methods used to achieve weight control (restricting, purging, exercising)
  - Exercise might include long periods (hours) of daily excessive exercise, further compromising physiologic safety.
- Value attached to a specific shape and weight
- Comorbid mental health issues, including depression, anxiety, and obsessive-compulsive traits
- Alcohol or substance misuse
- Self-harm and suicidal ideation
- Interpersonal and social functioning (e.g., Does the person participate in high-risk activities associated with eating disorders, like modeling or professional sports?)
- Avoidance of social functions and interpersonal withdrawal

Unlike the *symptom* of anorexia in which the person may not experience hunger, the person with AN frequently feels great hunger and makes attempts to gain control over this sensation. Over time, the

BOX 14.3 Criteria for Hospital Admission of Individuals With Eating Disorders

Physical Criteria

- Weight loss of more than 30% over 6 months
- Rapid decline in weight
- Inability to gain weight with outpatient treatment
- Severe hypothermia caused by loss of subcutaneous tissue or dehydration (body temperature lower than 36° C or 96.8° F)
- Heart rate less than 40 beats per minute
- Systolic blood pressure less than 70 mm Hg
- Hypokalemia (less than 3 mEq/L) or other electrolyte disturbances not corrected by oral supplementation
- Electrocardiographic changes (especially dysrhythmias)

Psychiatric Criteria

- Suicidal or self-mutilating behaviors
- Uncontrollable use of laxatives, emetics, diuretics, or street drugs
- Failure to adhere to treatment contract
- Severe depression
- Psychosis
- Family crisis

individual may lose the ability to experience feelings of hunger in the context of lower caloric intake.

Individuals with the binge/purge type of AN may have additional physiologic concerns:

- Prominent parotid glands because of hyperstimulation from repeated vomiting
- Atypical dental erosion and caries related to vomiting
- Severe electrolyte imbalance because of **purging** or misuse of laxatives or diuretics

Assessment Guidelines

Anorexia Nervosa

1. Safety is the priority concern:
   a. Determine if medical or psychiatric condition warrants hospitalization (see Box 14.3).
   b. Determine if there are additional medical complications.
   c. Determine if there are additional psychiatric comorbidities, especially suicidal ideation and risk for self-harm.
2. Assess the patient's level of insight about the disordered eating and feelings regarding weight.
3. Assess the patient's and family's understanding about the disease, the therapeutic goals, and the treatment plan.

VIGNETTE: Tina, a 16-year-old girl who is at 60% of her ideal body weight, is cachectic on admission to an inpatient psychiatric unit. She has lanugo over most of her body and prominent parotid glands. She is hypotensive (86/50 mm Hg) and dehydrated. In addition, she has a low serum potassium level and dysrhythmias. A decision is made to transfer her to the intensive care unit until she is medically stabilized. As an intravenous (IV) catheter is inserted, her severe fear of gaining weight is underscored when she cries, "There's not going to be sugar in the IV, is there?" The nurse responds, "I hear how frightened you are. We are helping you to get past this physiological crisis."

DIAGNOSIS

Priority patient problems and nursing diagnoses tend to be focused on the physiologic consequences of malnutrition, vomiting, and dehydration. These conditions can affect all body systems. *Impaired nutritional status* and *Risk for injury* related to cardiac output, electrolyte imbalances, and imbalanced fluid volume and other body system problems may be relevant International Classification for Nursing Practice (ICNP) nursing diagnoses. Psychologically focused patient problems include *Disturbed body image, Negative self-image, Low self-esteem,* and *Difficulty coping.* Acute levels of *Anxiety* are frequently seen during the treatment of these disorders. There is an increased risk for maladaptive coping behaviors such as self-harm (*Risk for self-mutilation*) and suicide (*Risk for suicide*). *Impaired health-seeking behavior* and *Non-adherence* are nursing diagnoses that may also be associated with this disorder. *Impaired family coping* is frequently seen with eating disorders.

OUTCOMES IDENTIFICATION

Outcomes need to be measurable and include a time frame. Common outcome criteria for patients with anorexia nervosa include the following:

The patient will:

- Refrain from suicidal behaviors or self-harm.
- Normalize eating patterns by eating 75% of three meals per day plus two snacks.
- Achieve 85% to 90% of ideal body weight.
- Be free of physical complications.
- Demonstrate improved self-acceptance, as evidenced by verbal and behavioral data.
- Address maladaptive beliefs, thoughts, and activities related to the eating disorder.
- Participate in treatment of associated psychiatric symptoms (mood dysregulation and mood intolerance, poor self-esteem).
- Demonstrate at least one new adaptive coping behavior.
- Participate in long-term treatment to prevent relapse.

DSM-5 DIAGNOSTIC CRITERIA

Anorexia Nervosa

A. Restrictions of energy intake relative to requirements, leading to a significantly low body weight in the context of age, sex, developmental trajectory, and physical health. Significantly low weight is defined as a weight that is less than minimally normal or, for children and adolescents, less than that minimally expected.

B. Intense fear of gaining weight or becoming fat, or persistent behavior that interferes with weight gain, even though at a significantly low weight.

C. Disturbance in the way in which one's body weight or shape is experienced, undue influence of body weight or shape on self-evaluation, or persistent lack of recognition of the seriousness of the current low body weight.

Coding note: The ICD-9-CM code for anorexia nervosa is 307.1, which is assigned regardless of the subtype. The ICD-10-CM code depends on the subtype (see below).

Specify whether:

(F50.01) Restricting type: During the last 3 months, the individual has not engaged in recurrent episodes of binge eating or purging behavior (i.e., self-induced vomiting or the misuse of laxatives, diuretics, or enemas). This subtype describes presentations in which weight loss is accomplished primarily through dieting, fasting, and/or excessive exercise.

(F50.02) Binge-eating/purging type: During the last 3 months, the individual has engaged in recurrent episodes of binge eating or purging behavior (i.e., self-induced vomiting or the misuse of laxatives, diuretics, or enemas).

Specify if:

In partial remission: After full criteria for anorexia nervosa were previously met. Criterion A (low body weight) has not been met for a sustained period, but either Criterion B (intense fear of gaining weight or becoming fat or behavior that interferes with weight gain) or Criterion C (disturbances in self-perception of weight and shape) is still met.

In full remission: After full criteria for anorexia nervosa were previously met, none of the criteria have been met for a sustained period of time.

Specify current severity:

The minimum level of severity is based, for adults, on current body mass index (BMI) (see below) or, for children and adolescents, on BMI percentile. The ranges below are derived from World Health Organization categories for thinness in adults; for children and adolescents, corresponding BMI percentiles should be used. The level of severity may be increased to reflect clinical symptoms, the degree of functional disability, and the need for supervision.

Mild: BMI ≥ 17 kg/m^2
Moderate: BMI 16 to 16.99 kg/m^2
Severe: BMI 15 to 15.99 kg/m^2
Extreme: BMI <15 kg/m^2

PLANNING

Planning is affected by the acuity of the patient's situation. Immediate physiologic stabilization, usually on a medical unit, is required for extreme electrolyte imbalance or for weight that is less than 70% to 75% of **ideal body weight** or for slowed or unstable vital signs. Refeeding, nutritional plans, and weight restoration are crucial parts of the medical stabilization process. A potentially deadly complication of the refeeding process is the development of **refeeding syndrome**. This can occur when starved patients begin to eat and metabolize calories. The body shifts from a catabolic state (a state of breaking down tissues for nutrients) to an anabolic state (a state of rebuilding tissues/growth), causing a shift in fluids and electrolytes. Associated complications of this shift can include heart failure, arrhythmias, respiratory failure, muscle breakdown, and death. Close monitoring while calorie intake is gradually increased tends to prevent the development of *refeeding syndrome* (Ekern, 2018).

Once a patient is medically stable, acute cognitive symptoms, reduced ability to concentrate, rigidity of thinking, and problems processing information tend to improve. Other symptoms of the disease can now be addressed through psychotherapy, nutrition education, continued medical monitoring, and sometimes medications. The specific treatments are individualized for each person (Mayo Clinic Staff, 2017).

Continued longer-term outpatient treatment includes individual, group, and family therapy as well as psychopharmacological therapy during different phases of the illness.

The following are the focus of care for all eating disorders:

1. Stabilize acute medical symptoms.
2. Restore the patient's nutritional state.
   a. For AN, this means restoring weight to within a normal range.
   b. For BN, this means ensuring a balanced metabolic state.
3. Modify the patient's distorted eating behaviors.
4. Help change distorted and erroneous beliefs about weight and body image.

IMPLEMENTATION

See Table 14.1 for specific interventions regarding AN.

Acute Care

Following physiologic stability, the patient is usually transferred to a behavioral health unit or a specialized unit for those with eating disorders. An interdisciplinary treatment approach is used that incorporates nutritional, medical, and psychosocial components.

Weight monitoring, monitoring eating patterns, and weight restoration are part of intervention strategies that can be implemented using a behavioral approach. Nursing interventions may include the following:

- Weigh the patient regularly or daily at the same time of day (before breakfast), in the same attire (e.g., a hospital gown), after voiding. Care must be given to prevent water loading by the patient or other measures to "cheat" during a weigh-in.
  - Rationale: Weight restoration is an objective measure of meeting treatment goals.
- Observe or sit with the patient while eating.
  - Rationale: To prevent hoarding or inappropriate disposing of food.
- The choice of foods will be made in consultation with a nutritionist.
  - Rationale: To prevent odd/unhealthy eating behaviors.
- The patient is given a limited time to complete a meal (e.g., 30 minutes).
  - Rationale: To model "normal" eating and prevent procrastination as a way to not eat.

TABLE 14.1 Interventions for Anorexia Nervosa

Intervention	Rationale
1. Acknowledge the emotional and physical difficulty the patient is experiencing.	1. A first priority is to establish a therapeutic alliance.
2. Assess for suicidal thoughts/self-injurious behaviors.	2. The potential for a psychiatric crisis is always present.
3. Monitor physiological parameters (vital signs, electrolytes) as needed.	3. The life-threatening effects of weight restriction and/or purging need to be monitored.
4. Weigh patient wearing only bra and panties/underwear on a routine basis (same time of day after voiding and before drinking/eating). Some protocols include weighing with the patient's back to the scale.	4. The weigh-in process is a high-anxiety time. In the weight-gain phase, the patient is expected to gain ½ to ¾ lb at specified weigh-in intervals according to a set unit protocol. The underweight patient might try to manipulate the weight by drinking fluids or placing heavy objects in clothing before being weighed. Discussion of weight gain (or loss) may be postponed for the primary therapist.
5. Monitor patient during and after meals to prevent throwing away food and/or purging.	5. The compelling force of the illness makes it difficult to stop certain behaviors.
6. Recognize the patient's distorted image/overvalued ideas of body shape and size without minimizing or challenging the patient's perceptions.	6. A straightforward statement that the nurse's perceptions are different will help to avoid a power struggle. Arguments and power struggles intensify the patient's need to control.
7. Educate the patient about the ill effects of low weight and resultant impaired health.	7. The treatment goal of gaining weight is what the patient most resists. Focus on the benefits of improved health and increased energy at a more normalized weight.
8. Work with patients to identify strengths.	8. When patients are feeling overwhelmed, they no longer view their lives objectively.

- Continue supervision of the patient after eating (1 to 3 hours).
  - Rationale: To prevent vomiting after the meal.
- Some programs base unit privileges on weight gain. Privileges, such as attending an occupational activity or being able to leave the room, are withdrawn if weight is not gained.
  - Rationale: Behavioral approach to reward treatment adherence.
- Tube feedings and liquid supplements are sometimes given if weight is lost or a prescribed percentage of food (e.g., 75%) is not consumed at each meal. These should be administered in a matter-of-fact manner.
  - Rationale: Physiologic safety.
- Excessive exercise and use of laxatives or diuretics should be avoided because these are used to rid the body of calories.
  - Rationale: To prevent expending calories in unhealthy ways.

Communication Guidelines

Nurses on a behavioral health inpatient unit may function as both a primary nurse and a group leader. Interventions include milieu therapy, teaching, and counseling. The development of a therapeutic relationship is very important in keeping patients safe. As individuals start to gain weight, they can experience increased impulses to self-harm or act on suicidal feelings. Safety is always a priority.

A key research finding on *AN* and the nurse–patient relationship showed that patient motivation to adhere to treatment was likely to increase when the nursing approach was *person centered* and when nurses' attitudes were characterized by presence, genuine commitment, and motivation (Salzmann-Erikson & Dahlén, 2017). The effective nurse can be viewed as a companion in the recovery process of the patient (Table 14.2).

Milieu Therapy

Inpatient units designed to treat individuals with an eating disorder include a combination of therapeutic modalities provided by an interdisciplinary team. The milieu of an eating disorder unit is purposefully organized to assist the patient in establishing more adaptive behavioral patterns, including normalization of eating.

Psychotherapy

The following therapies have demonstrated effectiveness in treating eating disorders and are geared toward recovery:

- **Cognitive-behavioral therapy** is used to diminish distortions in the patient's thinking that result in problematic attitudes and eating-disordered behaviors. Box 14.4 identifies some common types of cognitive distortions characteristic of people with eating disorders.
- **Enhanced CBT (CBT-E)** is a structured, time-limited treatment specifically for eating disorders. The primary focus is to establish a regular pattern of stable, flexible eating and to address factors that reinforce the eating problem (NICE, 2017).
- **Dialectical behavioral therapy** is a form of CBT adapted to address emotional dysregulation. It has demonstrated effectiveness with adults with BN and BED, but there is less evidence for effectiveness with AN.

TABLE 14.2 Four Broad Goals of Health Teaching and Psychoeducation

1. **Information:**
   a. Teach patient and family/significant others about the etiological factors associated with eating disorders, including neurobiological risks factors. Avoid blame.
   b. Explain the biological, psychosocial, and cognitive changes associated with these diseases/disorders.
   c. Nutrition education:
      1. Explain the risk of malnutrition.
      2. Describe healthy eating and healthy body weight.
   d. Be aware that the family members/significant others may also experience severe distress.
      1. Assess the emotional impact that the eating disorder has on significant others.
      2. Education should include practical support and emergency plans if the person with an eating disorder develops a medical or psychiatric crisis. (NICE, 2017)
2. **Emotional discharge:** Give opportunities to exchange ideas about managing the illness and to discuss frustrations and concerns.
3. **Support treatment adherence:**
   a. Because most eating disorders begin in adolescence, family involvement in treatment is essential.
   b. Psychotherapy is the cornerstone of treatment for all the eating disorders.
   c. Pharmacology can play a secondary role in treatment, especially with bulimia nervosa and binge-eating disorders.
   d. Develop a relapse prevention plan that includes emergency contacts.
4. **Teach the use of self-help strategies:**
   a. Help individuals differentiate healthy support groups and websites/apps from destructive ones.
   b. Support self-efficacy (one's belief in one's ability to succeed or accomplish a task).
   c. Facilitate learning more constructive coping skills, improving social skills, and developing problem-solving and decision-making skills.

APPLYING THE ART

A Person With an Eating Disorder: Anorexia

Scenario

I met 15-year-old Stacie on the eating disorders unit. A "straight A" student, Stacie was 5 feet 7 inches tall and weighed 90 pounds. Her mother was a physician and her father a college professor. Her older brother was the quarterback of his college team. We set up the contract that morning, and she had just finished the post-lunch focus group.

Therapeutic Goal

By the end of this interaction, Stacie will express at least one painful feeling directly instead of acting out with self-destructive behavior.

Student–Patient Interaction	Thoughts, Communication Techniques, and Mental Health Nursing Concepts
Stacie: "They think we're all going to go and vomit after lunch, so they keep us talking. Like that's going to help."	I should *clarify indefinite pronouns.* She used "they" a lot, but I am guessing she means the staff. Her feelings take precedence right now.
Student's feelings: *I am feeling a bit overwhelmed. Where to start! She looks like a skeleton, and here I am always struggling with my own weight.*	
Student: "You sound pretty frustrated."	*Reflection* rarely fails to continue the interaction. I am aware of my own potential for *countertransference* in this situation.
Student's feelings: *Her thinness scares me.*	

APPLYING THE ART—cont'd

A Person With an Eating Disorder: Anorexia

Student–Patient Interaction	Thoughts, Communication Techniques, and Mental Health Nursing Concepts
Stacie: "I am! Sometimes I feel like a piece of taffy being pushed and pulled and stretched by everyone else." ***Student's feelings:*** *I'm feeling some anxiety about being able to figure this out. She shares how controlled she feels by making an analogy to candy. Is her whole life about food?*	Control sounds like a key issue. She is revisiting *autonomy versus shame and doubt*. I remember that adolescents re-encounter all of Erikson's earlier stages as part of *identity versus role confusion*.
Student: "Pushed and pulled?"	*Restatement* and *encouraging her to elaborate*. I hope this shows Stacie I am really listening by using her exact words.
Stacie: "Try being in that family of mine! You can't stay unless you're at the top of your game." ***Student's feelings:*** *I am feeling drawn into her story. How overwhelming for her.*	I wonder which carries the most emotional impact for her: achievement or staying in the family.
Student: "You feel a lot of pressure to excel … at everything?" ***Student's feelings:*** *I feel uncertain here. I probably should have focused first on the family part. Hope we can get back to her family stuff, too.*	I *restate* again.
Stacie: "My mom would say, 'Honey, just be yourself,' but she'd really mean, 'as long as you get straight A's and make the family proud, like your brother does!'" ***Student's feelings:*** *I kind of feel intimidated by her straight A's. She accomplishes more than I do in my own studies. Why can't that be enough? I feel sad that she never feels good enough.*	Could this be a cognitive distortion?
Student: "Somehow you never quite feel good enough." *Concerned look, leaning toward her.*	I reflect her feelings. I hope to convey *empathy* with my nonverbal behavior.
Stacie: "That's it, exactly." *Eyes fill with tears. I pause to let her cry.* ***Student's feelings:*** *I want to comfort her, but I stop myself because the tears are healthy. She actually lets herself feel frustration and now sadness.*	When a person is crying, feelings are very close to the surface. Saying comforting things might help her push her feelings down. Expressing emotions directly is much healthier for her than using food to *displace* feelings.
Stacie: *Crying.* "I can't tell you how long it's been since I actually cried." ***Student's feelings:*** *I'm glad she could unbottle some of her feelings and that she felt safe to do so with me.*	
Student: "Maybe crying is not such a bad thing?"	I ask an *indirect question*. Maybe she will see that she can let out some of her painful feelings and that it is okay.
Stacie: "It's not done in my family." ***Student's feelings:*** *Seems like she never lets go of the pressures she feels from her family. In some ways, I understand that, with the way my family keeps me plugging through nursing; I feel like I'd really let them down if I failed.*	The family theme pervades her thoughts.
Student: "I wonder if a person can stay in the family yet still feel and do things a little differently than everyone else?" ***Student's feelings:*** *I feel like Stacie really made some progress and we can build a foundation for the next time we talk. I feel more hopeful for her.*	Again, an *indirect question* asks Stacie to ponder without feeling interrogated. The work of *identity versus role confusion* means separating and *individuating* oneself as distinct from one's family.
Stacie: "Maybe. I never thought of it that way." *Takes the tissue I offer, looking thoughtful.*	I'll report this to my instructor and chart about her being able to cry.

- **Interpersonal psychotherapy (ITP)** is an evidence-based therapy that focuses on resolving interpersonal stressors that may trigger feelings of loss, bodily changes, interpersonal disputes, and/or isolation.
- **Maudsley anorexia nervosa treatment for adults (MANTRA)** covers nutrition, symptom management, and behavior change. Motivation and encouraging the person to work collaboratively with the practitioner are emphasized (NICE, 2017).
- **Specialist supportive clinical management (SSCM)** therapy focuses on education and support while allowing the person to decide what else should be included as part of the therapy.
- **Maudsley/family-based therapy (FBT)** has consistently been shown to be the best treatment for children and adolescents with AN, and it demonstrates good effectiveness for children and adolescents with BN. This therapy is time efficient (once-per-week meetings), cost-effective, and delivered in a "real-life" setting (home) (Gerson, 2016).
- **Group therapy** offers support to patients who feel isolated while offering a place to explore the various issues and concerns inherent in eating disorders.
- Other useful therapies following weight stabilization include motivational therapy, and psychodynamic therapy (Bernstein & Pataki, 2016). All are delivered in a variety of settings. The goals of treatment remain the same: maintaining weight, normalization of eating habits, and initiation of the treatment of the psychological, interpersonal, and social issues that perpetuate the disease. The approach to diagnosis and treatment must always be culturally informed.

BOX 14.4 Cognitive Distortions Related to Eating Disorders

Overgeneralization: A single event affects unrelated situations.
- "He didn't ask me out. It must be because I'm fat."
- "I was happy when I wore a size 6. I must get back to that weight."

All-or-nothing thinking: Reasoning is absolute and extreme, in mutually exclusive terms of black or white, good or bad.
- "If I have one Popsicle, I must eat five."
- "If I allow myself to gain weight, I'll blow up like a balloon."

Catastrophizing: The consequences of an event are magnified.
- "If I gain weight, my weekend will be ruined."
- "When people say I look better, I know they think I'm fat."

Personalization: Events are overinterpreted as having personal significance.
- "I know everybody is watching me eat."
- "People won't like me unless I'm thin."

Emotional reasoning: Subjective emotions determine reality.
- "I know I'm fat because I feel fat."
- "When I'm thin, I feel powerful."

Adapted from Bowers, W. A. (2001). Principles for applying cognitive-behavioral therapy to anorexia nervosa. *Psychiatric Clinics of North America, 24*(2), 293–303.

Families often report feeling powerless in the face of some of the mystifying behaviors associated with eating disorders. Patients can sometimes express that they want their families to care about them but are unable to recognize expressions of care. Families sometimes experience the tension of saying or doing the wrong thing and then feeling responsible if a setback occurs. Psychiatric nurse clinicians have an important role in assisting families and significant others in developing strategies for improved communication and searching for ways to be comfortably supportive to the patient.

Pharmacological Treatment

Fluoxetine, a selective serotonin reuptake inhibitor (SSRI), is sometimes prescribed for AN when weight has been stabilized to treat depression and obsessive-compulsive symptoms. There is little evidence that it treats symptoms of AN directly but helps more with associated symptoms or comorbid mental health issues. SSRIs increase the risk of suicide. Olanzapine, an atypical antipsychotic, has been found to be helpful with weight gain and to change obsessive thinking. There are safety concerns with this class of drugs related to cardiac complications in this population (Bernstein, 2020).

Long-Term Treatment

AN can be a chronic illness that waxes and wanes. Recovery is evaluated as a stage in the process rather than a fixed event. Factors that influence the stage of recovery include the percentage of ideal body weight that has been achieved, the extent to which self-worth is defined by shape and weight, and the amount of disruption existing in the patient's personal life. The patient may require long-term treatment.

As part of discharge planning, the nurse needs to explore the patient's participation in social media, which can both support and interfere with recovery. Websites like e-Ana and e-Mia perpetuate the myth that excessive thinness and disordered eating can be a lifestyle choice. These websites describe, endorse, and motivate users to continue their efforts with eating-disordered behaviors. Despite the destructive aspects of these sites, those who use the sites report that the forums provide a sense of community and belonging (Mariani, 2016). The challenge for those who treat individuals with eating disorders is to help them find a supportive community that promotes healthy alternatives to disordered eating.

Websites such as those sponsored by the National Eating Disorder Association may support patients in healthy ways. Smartphone applications (apps) can also be part of recovery. The most effective ones are those that contain a feature allowing for self-monitoring of food intake without calorie counting and include fields to log behaviors, thoughts, and feelings. Apps that incorporate healthy coping strategies can be especially useful. The use of apps may contribute to recovery, especially if used in conjunction with a treatment provider (Fairburn & Rothwell, 2015).

In chronic AN, a **harm-reduction approach** is sometimes an option (Bernstein & Pataki, 2016). In this treatment approach, the goal is to improve quality of life and minimize harm through symptom management, skill development, and an understanding of the benefits and risks of symptoms (Gerson, 2017).

EVALUATION

Evaluation is ongoing, and short-term and intermediate goals are revised as necessary to achieve the treatment outcomes established. The long-term outcome for AN is less favorable than that for BN.

APPLICATION OF THE NURSING PROCESS

ASSESSMENT: BULIMIA NERVOSA

People with BN may not initially appear to be physically or emotionally ill. They are often at or slightly above ideal body weight. However, as the nurse makes further observations, physical and emotional problems become apparent. The patient may demonstrate enlargement of the parotid glands and dental erosion and caries associated with induced vomiting, plus skin problems and problems associated with dehydration. These individuals tend to display the same acute desire to be thin and are overly concerned with weight and appearance. Symptoms of anxiety and depression are quite common. The history may reveal difficulties with impulsivity as well as compulsivity. Family relationships demonstrate varying levels of dysfunction.

Refer to Box 14.1 for a listing of the characteristics of BN and AN.

Assessment Guidelines

Bulimia Nervosa

1. Medical stabilization is the first priority.
2. A thorough physical examination is essential. Pertinent laboratory testing includes the following:
   - Electrolyte levels
   - Glucose level
   - Thyroid function tests
   - Complete blood count
   - Electrocardiogram (ECG)
3. Psychiatric evaluation is advised because of the high frequency of coexisting psychiatric disorders that accompany BN.
4. Risk assessment is essential because this disorder increases the risk for suicide and self-harm.

5. In addition to assessing for the use of diuretics, vomiting, or laxatives, ask patients if they are taking any diet pills, amphetamines, energy pills, or diet teas that claim to be all-natural.

VIGNETTE: I was a three-sport athlete throughout high school and then played volleyball in college. How did the bingeing and purging start? How did it happen to me? I began to consume thousands of calories at my parents' house and secretly go to the bathroom and purge, and then start all over again. By the time I went to college, I would go to several fast-food restaurants and order cheeseburgers, fries, tacos, and milkshakes. I would consume them all by the time I got home and then induce vomiting the minute I walked through the door. As time went by, the cycles became worse. I despised what I was doing and what it was doing to me. I had broken blood vessels in my face, causing my eyes to swell. My shame made me deceive everyone. I hated it so much that each time I binged and purged, I swore to myself that it would never happen again.

DIAGNOSIS

Priority patient problems and nursing diagnoses for this disorder continue to be focused on the physiologic consequences of malnutrition, vomiting, and dehydration. Many of the diagnoses associated with AN also apply to BN. All body systems are potentially affected. *Impaired nutritional status* and *Risk for injury* related to cardiac output, electrolyte imbalances, and imbalanced fluid volume and other body system problems may be relevant nursing diagnoses. Psychologically focused patient problems include *Disturbed body image*, *Negative self-image*, *Low self-esteem*, and *Difficulty coping*. *Low volition* or *Low self-control* may be associated with the binge–purge behaviors. Acute levels of *Anxiety* are frequently seen during the treatment of these disorders. There is an increased risk for maladaptive coping behaviors, such as self-harm (*Risk for self-mutilation*) and suicide (*Risk for suicide*). *Impaired health-seeking behavior* and *Non-adherence* are nursing diagnoses that may also be associated with this disorder. *Impaired family coping* is frequently seen with eating disorders.

OUTCOMES IDENTIFICATION

Measurable outcome criteria for patients with bulimia nervosa include the following:

The patient will:

- Obtain and maintain normal electrolyte balance and stable vital signs.
- Refrain from binge–purge behaviors.
- Be free of self-harm behaviors and suicidal ideation/behaviors.
- Demonstrate at least two new skills for managing stress/anxiety/shame in a non–food-related way.
- No longer demonstrate high levels of anxiety related to fear of gaining weight.
- Demonstrate improved self-esteem by naming two personal strengths.
- Verbalize a desire to participate in ongoing treatment.

PLANNING

The criteria for inpatient admission of a patient with BN are presented in Box 14.3. As with AN, the patient with bulimia may be treated for life-threatening complications, such as gastric rupture (rare), electrolyte imbalance, and cardiac dysrhythmias, in an acute care unit of a hospital. If the patient is admitted to a general inpatient psychiatric unit because of acute suicidal risk, it is usually short term. Planning will include appropriate referrals for continuing outpatient treatment.

DSM-5 DIAGNOSTIC CRITERIA

Bulimia Nervosa

A. Recurrent episodes of binge eating. An episode of binge eating is characterized by both of the following:
   1. Eating, in a discrete period of time (e.g., within any 2-hour period), an amount of food that is definitely larger than what most individuals would eat in a similar period of time under similar circumstances.
   2. A sense of lack of control over eating during the episode (e.g., feeling that one cannot stop eating or control what or how much one is eating).

B. Recurrent inappropriate compensatory behavior in order to prevent weight gain, such as self-induced vomiting; misuse of laxatives, diuretics, or other medications; fasting; or excessive exercise.

C. The binge eating and inappropriate compensatory behaviors both occur, on average, at least once a week for 3 months.

D. Self-evaluation is unduly influenced by body shape and weight.

E. The disturbance does not occur exclusively during episodes of anorexia nervosa.

Specify if:

In partial remission: After full criteria for bulimia nervosa were previously met, some, but not all, of the criteria have been met for a sustained period of time.

In full remission: After full criteria for bulimia nervosa were previously met, none of the criteria have been met for a sustained period of time.

Specify current severity:

The minimum level of severity is based on the frequency of inappropriate compensatory behaviors (see below). The level of severity may be increased to reflect other symptoms and the degree of functional disability.

Mild: An average of 1 to 3 episodes of inappropriate compensatory behaviors per week.

Moderate: An average of 4 to 7 episodes of inappropriate compensatory behaviors per week.

Severe: An average of 8 to 13 episodes of inappropriate compensatory behaviors per week.

Extreme: An average of 14 or more episodes of inappropriate compensatory behaviors per week.

IMPLEMENTATION

See Table 14.3 for intervention guidelines for a patient with bulimia nervosa.

Acute Care

A patient who is medically compromised as a result of BN is referred to an inpatient unit for comprehensive treatment of the illness. Weight monitoring, monitoring of eating patterns, and interruption of the binge–purge cycle are also implemented using a behavioral approach.

- Weigh the patient regularly or daily at the same time of day, in the same attire.
- Observe or sit with the patient while eating to prevent binging.
- Continue supervision of the patient (1 to 3 hours) to prevent vomiting after the meal.

- The patient is frequently observed for any other type of compensatory behavior designed to eliminate calories, such as excessive exercise.

Therapy is begun to examine the underlying conflicts and distorted perceptions of body shape and weight that sustain the illness. Treatment of comorbid disorders, such as major depression and substance use disorders, is also undertaken. In most cases of substance use disorders, the treatment of the eating disorder must occur after the substance use disorder is stabilized.

Communication Guidelines

Compared with the food-restricting patients, the patient with BN may have an easier time establishing a therapeutic alliance with the nurse because the patient also desires to stop the bingeing–purging behavior. The therapeutic alliance allows the nurse, along with other members of the interdisciplinary team, to provide counseling that gives useful feedback regarding the distorted beliefs held by the patient. See Box 14.4 for a list of common cognitive distortions.

In working with a patient who has *bulimia nervosa*, the nurse needs to be aware that the patient is sensitive to the perceptions of others. The patient may feel significant shame and a loss of control. In building a therapeutic alliance, the nurse needs to empathize with feelings of low self-esteem, worthlessness, and dysphoria (sadness or unease). An accepting, nonjudgmental approach, along with a comprehensive understanding of the subjective experience of the patient, will help to build trust.

TABLE 14.3 Interventions for Bulimia Nervosa

Intervention	Rationale
1. Assess mood and presence of suicidal thoughts/ behaviors and self-harm.	1. Emotional dysregulation is at the core of bulimic behaviors, and there is always the risk for self-destructive behaviors.
2. Monitor physiological parameters (vital signs, electrolyte) as needed.	2. The life-threatening effect of weight restriction and/or purging needs to be monitored.
3. Monitor the patient's weight as needed.	3. The weigh-in intervals are determined by the unit protocol for the patient with bulimia depending on the percentage above or below ideal body weight.
4. Explore dysfunctional thoughts that maintain the binge–purge cycle.	4. Nonjudgmental reframing can balance and combat distorted thinking and challenge automatic behaviors.
5. Educate the patient that fasting can lead to continuation of bingeing and the binge–purge cycle, emphasizing its self-perpetuating nature.	5. The binge–purge cycle is maintained by the pattern of restricting, hunger, and bingeing and purging accompanied by feelings of shame, then repetition of the cycle.
6. Monitor the patient during and after meals to prevent throwing away food and/or purging.	6. A straightforward statement that the nurse's perceptions are different will help avoid a power struggle. Arguments and power struggles intensify the patient's need to control.
7. Acknowledge the patient's overvalued ideas of body shape and size without minimizing or challenging the patient's perceptions.	7. Cognitive-behavioral approaches can be very effective in helping the patient identify irrational beliefs about self and body image.
8. Encourage the patient to keep a journal of thoughts and feelings.	8. A journal can provide information to identify irrational thinking and identify triggers that induce disordered eating behaviors. Reframing distorted beliefs and thinking can lead to healthier behaviors.

Milieu Therapy

The primary goals of a highly structured milieu of an inpatient unit are interrupting the binge–purge cycle and helping to normalize eating patterns. The interdisciplinary team uses a comprehensive approach that includes therapy, education, and support to address the emotional and behavioral problems that arise when the patient is no longer binge eating or purging.

Health Teaching and Health Promotion

Health teaching focuses not only on the eating disorder but also on the importance of meal planning, the use of relaxation techniques, maintenance of a healthy diet and exercise, implementation of coping skills, and knowledge of the physical and emotional effects of bingeing and purging as well as the effects of cognitive distortions.

Upon discharge from the hospital, the individual may be referred to an intensive outpatient program, where he or she will continue to receive support and therapy for 3 or more hours a day, at least 3 days a week. Long-term and intensive care can help solidify the goals that have been achieved, address the attitudes and perceptions that maintain the eating disorder, and deal with the underlying psychological issues that attend the illness. The patient and family can benefit from connecting with support networks that address eating disorders, such as the National Eating Disorders Association (NEDA; http://www.nationaleatingdisorders.org).

Psychotherapy

Most therapies listed for the treatment of AN are also effective in treating BN.

Pharmacological Treatment

Fluoxetine (Prozac) is approved by the U.S. Food and Drug Administration (FDA) for the treatment of BN. Binge-eating and purging behaviors are noted to be significantly decreased with this medication. As an SSRI, fluoxetine has an increased risk of suicide. Other antidepressants may also be helpful. Mood-stabilizing drugs like topiramate may help people with BN to suppress the urge to binge and reduce the preoccupation with eating and weight. Medication use in conjunction with therapy tends to be the most successful strategy (Randhawa, 2016).

EVALUATION

Evaluation is ongoing, and short-term and intermediate goals are revised as necessary to achieve the treatment outcomes established. The goals provide a daily guide for evaluating success and must be continually reevaluated for their appropriateness.

SELF-CARE FOR NURSES

Nurses caring for patients with AN may find it difficult to appreciate the seriousness of this illness. A lack of knowledge about the neurobiological components of these diseases can lead to the belief that weight restriction, bingeing, and purging are self-imposed lifestyle choices. Common behaviors associated with eating disorders, such as rigidity of thinking, perfectionism, obsessive thoughts, and compulsive actions relating to food, can pose challenges to the nurse.

The nurse must take care not to cross the line toward authoritarianism in an effort to be helpful. The patient's *terror* at gaining weight can be difficult to understand. Empathy, compassion, and respect are important here. The primary goal of treatment—weight gain—is the very outcome the client fears most. Frequent acknowledgment of the difficulty of the situation for the patient will help during times of extreme resistance. If countertransference/personal feelings are not recognized and examined, withdrawal may result in an effort to avoid feelings of frustration. Being supervised by a competent, supportive, more experienced clinician and sharing with peers help minimize feelings of frustration and can contribute to therapeutic growth.

BINGE-EATING DISORDER

BED was first formally recognized as a specific disorder in the *DSM-5* (APA, 2013). *Binge-eating disorder* is a variant of compulsive overeating. Although controversy exists over whether this proposed diagnosis constitutes a separate eating disorder, 20% to 30% of obese individuals seeking treatment report binge eating. These individuals report recurrent episodes of eating a large amount of food in a short period of time and usually feel guilty or shameful after bingeing. The pattern is similar to BN, but with BED, there are no compensatory mechanisms used (e.g., self-induced vomiting or inappropriate use of diuretics/laxatives). The *DSM-5* makes a distinction between BED and obesity, stating that most obese individuals do not engage in recurrent binge-eating behaviors. The *DSM-5* does not include obesity as a mental disorder. BED usually exists with co-occurring psychiatric disorders such as bipolar disorder, depressive disorder, anxiety disorder, and to a lesser extent, substance use disorders (APA, 2013).

Overeating is sometimes seen as a symptom of depression (atypical depression). Those who binge eat report a history of major depression significantly more often than those who do not binge eat. For those with a formal disorder, the binge-eating behavior is described as soothing and helps to regulate their moods. Although a period of dieting is almost always the behavior observed just before binge eating in BN, in approximately 50% of a sample of obese binge eaters, no attempt to restrict dietary intake occurred before bingeing (APA, 2013). A range of interdisciplinary intervention strategies can be implemented to treat BED. Specialized cognitive behavior therapies offered individually or in a group setting, such as CBT-ED, have shown some effectiveness in changing problematic behaviors that perpetuate the disease. Guided self-help programs with supportive counseling have also demonstrated some effectiveness in modifying behaviors. Because psychological treatments do not have a significant impact on weight loss, obesity management interventions must be included. Treatment of co-occurring psychiatric disorders is also recommended (NICE, 2017). Table 14.4 list some specific recommended treatment strategies.

TABLE 14.4 Interventions for Binge-Eating Disorder

Intervention	Rationale
1. Assess mood, psychosocial factors, and risk factors such as suicide and self-harm ideation.	1. Psychological distress frequently operates as a trigger, and dysphoria is common.
2. Along with the interdisciplinary team, determine treatment objectives.	2. The treatment focus may be primarily to interrupt binge eating with or without weight loss.
3. Provide nutritional counseling.	3. Approximately one-third of binge eaters are obese and are at risk for cardiovascular complications, including diabetes mellitus type 2. In some patients, a weight-control program may trigger a resurgence of binge eating.
4. Provide psychosocial treatment.	4. Binge eating is associated with significant mood disturbance and psychosocial stress. There is evidence-based support for cognitive-behavioral therapy.

Medication should not be offered as the sole treatment for BED. SSRIs may help reduce the symptoms of binge eating and can improve mood in patients who have BED who are also struggling with depression or anxiety. Fluoxetine is FDA approved for this disorder. Lisdexamfetamine (Vyvanse), a stimulant used to treat attention-deficit/hyperactivity disorder (ADHD), is FDA approved for moderate to severe BED in adults. Antiepileptic drugs, such as topiramate (Topamax), are used to treat the obsessive and compulsive behaviors associated with this disorder (Bernstein, 2019). The drug dasotraline, a dopamine and norepinephrine reuptake inhibitor, is showing promise for the treatment of BED (APA, 2017).

APPLYING EVIDENCE-BASED PRACTICE (EBP)

Problem

A 47-year-old male is on a surgical unit after having bariatric surgery to promote weight loss. The registered nurse (RN) brings him his first meal tray, which consists of 15 mL of clear liquid. The patient appears shocked and raises his voice in frustration, stating, "This is not what I expected—get me some food!" The nurse sits down to talk with the patient and discovers he had been binge eating large amounts up until the day before the surgery and had not attended nutrition classes or counseling to prepare for the significant lifestyle changes post-surgery.

EBP Assessment

A. What do you already know from experience?

Patients can be psychologically unprepared and have a lack of education regarding the changes that can occur after bariatric surgery.

Binge eating can be the result of a learned habit, metabolic or medical issues, or a response to past trauma or stress.

Changing eating patterns can be difficult.

Obese individuals experience prejudice and stigma.

B. What does the literature say?

Protocol dictates that patients be referred for a psychiatric evaluation prior to surgery. Individuals should be encouraged to attempt losing weight through dietary and other lifestyle changes prior to surgery.

Obesity has a variety of contributing factors besides binge eating. Severely obese individuals may not be able to lose weight in any other manner besides surgery.

Most patients maintain most of their weight loss after bariatric surgery, contrary to popular belief.

C. What does the patient want?

The patient wants to feel better but is very uncomfortable without eating his usual amounts.

He wants to lose weight and be healthier but is distressed at this time.

He is demanding food, which would result in surgical complications.

Plan

The RN reports the patient's response to the surgeon. The nurse sits down with the patient to provide support and patient education. A nursing staff member is enlisted to stay with the patient at all times for support during the initial stages of adjustment. Social services is notified to provide therapeutic support. The dietician begins to work with the patient to provide the education he did not obtain prior to surgery. The RN administers a prn sedative as needed.

QSEN Prelicensure Knowledge, Skills, and Attitudes (KSAs) Addressed

Safety was maintained by staying with the patient while distraught; surgical complications were prevented

Teamwork and Collaboration were displayed by involving the RN, surgeon, social services, dietician, and the patient in the treatment plans

KEY POINTS TO REMEMBER

- A number of theoretical models help explain the risk factors associated with the development of eating disorders.
- Neurobiological theories identify an association between eating disorders, depression, and neuroendocrine abnormalities.
- Genetic theories suggest vulnerabilities that may predispose people toward eating disorders.
- Psychological theories explore issues of control in anorexia and affective instability and poor impulse control in bulimia, but these are not considered causes of eating disorders.
- Sociocultural factors that may affect etiology look at our present societal ideal of being thin.
- Families can serve as important allies in treatment.
- *Anorexia nervosa (AN)* is a potentially life-threatening eating disorder that includes severe levels of being underweight; low blood pressure, pulse rate, and temperature measurements; dehydration; electrolyte imbalances; and cardiac dysrhythmias. *AN* may be treated in an inpatient treatment setting, and treatment includes weight restoration, milieu therapy, psychotherapy, development of self-care skills, and psychobiological interventions.
- Eating disorders are most commonly diagnosed in adolescents but are also being diagnosed in people 35 years of age and older.
- Long-term treatment of eating disorders is provided on an outpatient basis and aims to help patients maintain a healthy weight. Treatment modalities include individual therapy, family therapy, group therapy, psychopharmacology, and nutrition counseling.
- Individuals with *bulimia nervosa (BN)* are typically within the normal weight range, but some may be slightly below or above ideal body weight.
- Assessment of a patient with BN may show enlargement of the parotid glands, dental erosion, and other symptoms associated with induced vomiting.
- Acute care may be necessary when life-threatening complications are present, such as gastric rupture (rare), electrolyte imbalance, and cardiac dysrhythmias.
- The primary goal of intervention for a patient with BN is to interrupt the binge–purge cycle and correct disordered eating patterns. Issues of body image distortion are also addressed.
- Psychotherapy and self-care skills training are used to facilitate treatment.
- Long-term treatment focuses on therapy aimed at addressing any coexisting depression, substance use disorders, and/or personality disorders that are causing the patient distress and interfering with quality of life. Self-worth and interpersonal functioning eventually become issues that must be addressed in therapy for long-term remission.
- There are a variety of subthreshold problematic eating patterns that do not meet the full criteria as set forth in the *DSM-5*. These can cause physiologic problems and patient distress and may require interventions.
- Those with a *binge-eating disorder (BED)* demonstrate binge eating without compensatory purging behavior. This frequently results in obesity. Major depressive disorder symptoms are frequently seen in this population.
- Effective treatment for those with BED includes psychological therapies to reduce the disordered eating patterns and improve mood dysregulation. Additional weight management strategies must also be applied to reduce obesity and the secondary problems associated with obesity.

APPLYING CRITICAL JUDGMENT

1. A 19-year-old model has experienced a rapid decrease in weight over the past 4 months, after his agent told him he would need to lose weight or lose a coveted account. The model is 6 ft 2 in tall and weighs 132 lb, down from his usual 176 lb. He is brought to the emergency department with a pulse rate of 40 beats per minute and dysrhythmias. His laboratory workup reveals hypokalemia. He has become extremely depressed, saying, "I'm too fat … I won't take anything to eat. If I gain weight, my life will be ruined. There is nothing to live for if I can't model." His parents are startled and confused and feel powerless to help him. "I tell him he needs to eat or he will die. I tell him he is a skeleton, but he refuses to listen to me. I don't know what to do," his mother says.
   - **A.** Which physical and psychiatric criteria suggest that he should be immediately hospitalized? What other physical signs and symptoms may be found on assessment?
   - **B.** What are some of the questions you would eventually ask when evaluating his biopsychosocial functioning?
   - **C.** What are your feelings toward someone with anorexia? Is there a distinction between your thoughts and feelings toward women with anorexia nervosa and toward men with anorexia nervosa?
   - **D.** What are some things you could do for his parents in terms of offering them information, support, and referrals? Identify specific referrals.
   - **E.** Explain the types of interventions or restrictions that may be used while he is hospitalized (weighing, observation after eating or visits, exercise, therapy, self-care).
   - **F.** What are some of the cognitive distortions that would be a target for therapy?
   - **G.** Identify at least five criteria that would indicate there is improvement.
2. You and your close friend have been together since nursing school, and you are now working on the same surgical unit. Your friend told you that in the past, she has made several suicide attempts. Today you accidentally come upon her bingeing while off the unit, and she looks embarrassed and uncomfortable when she sees you. Several times, you notice that she spends time in the bathroom, and you hear sounds of retching. In response to your concern, she admits that she has been bingeing–purging for several years, but now these symptoms are getting out of control, and she feels profoundly depressed.
   - **A.** Although she does not show any physical signs of bulimia nervosa, what would you look for when assessing an individual with bulimia?
   - **B.** What types of emergencies could result from bingeing and purging?
   - **C.** What would be the most useful type of psychotherapy, and what issues would need to be addressed?
   - **D.** What types of new skills does a person with bulimia nervosa need to learn to lessen the compulsion to binge and purge?
   - **E.** What would be some signs that she is recovering?

CHAPTER REVIEW QUESTIONS

1. The school nurse assesses four adolescents who appear to have a healthy weight. Which comment would lead the nurse to explore further for an eating disorder?
   - **a.** "I usually try to exercise 30 minutes a day."
   - **b.** "I know everything in my life will be better once I lose 15 more pounds."
   - **c.** "I forgot my lunch today, so I will only be eating an apple."
   - **d.** "I know I shouldn't eat potato chips, but I just love them."
2. A nurse assesses four adolescents diagnosed with various eating disorders. Which comment would the nurse expect from the adolescent diagnosed with anorexia nervosa?
   - **a.** "I look good because whenever I overeat, I purge myself."
   - **b.** "I love sweets. I make myself throw up so I can eat more."
   - **c.** "I've lost 60 pounds, but I'm still a size 2. I want to be a size 0."
   - **d.** "I've hidden my eating disorder from everyone, even my parents."
3. While weighing patients on an eating disorders unit, the nurse overhears a psychiatric technician say, "I wish I had an eating disorder; maybe I'd lose a little weight." What is the nurse's best action?
   - **a.** Report the clinical observation to the nursing supervisor.
   - **b.** Ask the psychiatric technician, "What did you mean by that comment?"
   - **c.** Privately discuss the importance of sensitivity with the psychiatric technician.
   - **d.** Immediately interrupt the interaction between the patient and the psychiatric technician.
4. Shortly after hospitalization, an adolescent diagnosed with anorexia nervosa says to the nurse, "Being fat is the worst thing in the world. I hope it never happens to me." Which response by the nurse is appropriate?
   - **a.** "You need to gain weight to become healthier."
   - **b.** "Your world would not change if you gained a few pounds."
   - **c.** "Tell me how your world would be different if you were fat."
   - **d.** "Your attractiveness is not defined by a number on the scale."
5. A patient is hospitalized with a diagnosis of anorexia nervosa. The nurse reviews the patient's laboratory results, as follows:
   Sodium 143 mEq/L
   Potassium 3.1 mEq/L
   Chloride 102 mEq/L
   Magnesium 2.2 mEq/L
   Calcium 8.4 mg/dL
   Phosphate 3.0 mg/dL
   The nurse should take which action next?
   - **a.** Measure the patient's body temperature.
   - **b.** Inspect the patient's skin and sclera for jaundice.
   - **c.** Assess the patient's mucous membranes for erosion.
   - **d.** Auscultate the patient's heart rate, rhythm, and sounds.

REFERENCES

Afifi, T. O., Sareen, J., Fortier, J., Taillieu, T., Turner, S., Cheung, K., et al. (2017). Child maltreatment and eating disorders among men and women in adulthood: Results from a nationally representative United States sample. *The International Journal of Eating Disorders*, *50*(11), 1281–1296. https://doi.org/10.1002/eat.22783.

American Psychiatric Association (APA). (2013). *Diagnostic and statistical manual of mental disorders (DSM-5)* (5th ed.). Arlington, VA: APA.

American Psychiatric Association (APA). (2017). *Dasotraline for the treatment of moderate to severe binge eating disorder in adults: Results from a randomized, double-blind, placebo-controlled study*. Abstract presented at the American Psychiatric Association Annual Meeting; May 23, 2017; San Diego, CA. Retrieved from https://www.psychcongress.com/article/dasotraline-shows-positive-results-binge-eating-study.

Bernstein, B. (2020). Anorexia nervosa medication. Retrieved from https://emedicine.medscape.com/article/2221362-treatment#d9.

Bernstein, B. (2019). Binge eating disorder (BED) treatment & management. Retrieved from https://emedicine.medscape.com/article/912187-medication.

Bernstein, B. E., & Pataki, C. (2016). Anorexia nervosa treatment and management. http://emedicine.medscape.com/article/912187-treatment.

Blazek, N. (2015). Recognizing disordered eating in teen girls with type 1 diabetes. Clinical Advisor, May 18, 2015, Retrieved from: https://www.clinicaladvisor.com/napnap-2015-meeting-coverage/teens-eating-disorders-type-1-diabetes/article/403374/.

Cerniglia, L., Cimino, S., Tafà, M., Marzilli, E., Ballarotto, G., & Bracaglia, F. (2017). Family profiles in eating disorders: Family functioning and psychopathology. *Psychology Research and Behavior Management*, *10*, 305–312. https://doi.org/10.2147/PRBM.S145463.

Duncan, C. M., et al. (2017). Significant locus and metabolic genetic correlations revealed in genome-wide association study of anorexia nervosa. *American Journal of Psychiatry*, 1. https://doi.org/10.1176/appi.ajp.2017.16121402.appi.ajp.2017.

Ekern, J. (2017). Eating disorders: Causes, symptoms, signs & treatment help, eating disorder information help & resources, updated May 1, 2017 Retrieved from https://www.eatingdisorderhope.com/information/eating-disorder.

Ekern, M.S. (2018). Original author, Mascolo, M, Refeeding Patients with Anorexia Nervosa: What Does Research Show? https://www.eatingdisorderhope.com/information/anorexia/refeeding-patients-with-anorexia-nervosa-what-does-research-show.

Fairburn, C. G., & Rothwell, E. R. (2015). Apps and eating disorders: A systematic clinical appraisal. *International Journal of Eating Disorders*, *48*(7), 1038–1046.

Franco, K. N., Sieke, E. H., Dickstein, L., & Falcone, T. (2017). Eating disorders. Cleveland Clinic Center For Continuing Education. Retrieved from http://www.clevelandclinicmeded.com/medicalpubs/diseasemanagement/psychiatry-psychology/eating-disorders/.

Gerson, M. (2016). Best Practices: The Evidence-Base for Eating Disorder Treatment, Columbus Park, Eating Disorder Experts. Retrieved from: https://columbuspark.com/2016/09/19/best-practices-the-evidence-base-for-eating-disorder-treatment/.

Gerson, M. (2017). Specialist supportive clinical management treatment. Project Heal. Retrieved from http://theprojectheal.org/specialist-supportive-clinical-management-treatment/.

Giddens, J. F. (2017). *Concepts for nursing practice* (2nd ed.). St. Louis: Elsevier.

Gleissner, G. (2017). Can the Brain Fuel an Eating Disorder? Eating Disorder Recovery Specialists, March 6, 2017, Retrieved from http://eatingdisorderspecialists.com/can-brain-fuel-eating-disorder/.

Halter, M. J. (2018). *Varcarolis' foundations of psychiatric-mental health nursing: A clinical approach* (8th ed.). St. Louis: Elsevier.

Hamilton, G., Cullar, L., & Elenback, R. (2015). Eating disorder hope: Anorexia nervosa – highest mortality rate of any mental disorder: Why? Retrieved from http://www.eatingdisorderhope.com/information/anorexia/anorexia-nervosa-highest-mortality-rate-of-any-mental-disorder-why.

Marcon, T. D., Girz, L., Stillar, A., Tessier, C., & Lafrance, A. (2017). Parental involvement and child and adolescent eating disorders: Perspectives from residents in psychiatry, pediatrics, and family medicine. *Journal of the Canadian Academy of Child and Adolescent Psychiatry*, *26*(2), 78–85. https://www.ncbi.nlm.nih.gov/pmc/articles/PMC5510936/.

Mariani, M. (2016). How pro-anorexia websites exacerbate the eating disorder epidemic. Newsweek. Retrieved from http://www.newsweek.com/2016/07/01/pro-ana-websites-anorexia-nervosa-473433.html.

Mayo Clinic Staff. (2017). Eating disorder treatment: Know your options. July 14, 2017. Retrieved from https://www.mayoclinic.org/diseases-conditions/eating-disorders/in-depth/eating-disorder-treatment/art-20046234.

Mirasol. (n.d.). Eating Disorder Statistics. Retrieved from https://www.mirasol.net/learning-center/eating-disorder-statistics.php.

National Institute for Health and Care Excellence (NICE). (2017). Eating disorders: Recognition and treatment [NG69]. Retrieved from https://www.nice.org.uk/guidance/ng69.

National Institute of Mental Health (NIMH). (2017). Eating Disorders. Retrieved from: https://www.nimh.nih.gov/health/statistics/eating-disorders.shtml.

Randhawa, G. (2016). Bulimia Nervosa, Medscape. Retrieved from: https://emedicine.medscape.com/article/286485-overview#a1.

Sadock, B. J., Sadock, V. A., & Ruiz, P. (2015). *Kaplan and Sadock's synopsis of psychiatry* (11th ed.). Philadelphia: Wolters Kluwer/Lippincott Williams & Wilkins.

Salzmann-Erikson, M., & Dahlén, J. (2017). Nurses' establishment of health promoting relationships: A descriptive synthesis of anorexia nervosa research. *Journal of Child and Family Studies*, *26*(1), 1–13. https://doi.org/10.1007/s10826-016-0534-2 https://www.ncbi.nlm.nih.gov/pmc/articles/PMC5219017/.

Schreiner, J. (2015). Eating disorder screening: Implementation of the SCOFF questionnaire. Presented at AANP 2015. June 9–14, 2015, LA.

Smolak, L. (2011). Body image development in childhood. In T. Cash, & L. Smolak (Eds.). *Body image: A handbook of science, practice and prevention*. (2nd ed.). New York: Guilford.

Weir, K. (2016). New insights on eating disorders. *American Psychiatric Association, Monitor on Psychology*, 47(4). http://www.apa.org/monitor/2016/04/eating-disorders.aspx.

15

Mood Disorders: Depression

Lorraine Chiappetta, Elizabeth M. Varcarolis

http://evolve.elsevier.com/Varcarolis/essentials

OBJECTIVES

1. Compare predisposing factors associated with the development of depressive disorders.
2. Summarize the stress-diathesis model of depression and the other biological models of depression.
3. Differentiate between major depressive disorder (MDD) and persistent depressive disorder (dysthymia) (PDD).
4. Identify assessment findings for the individual experiencing clinical depression in each of the following areas: (a) mood and affect, (b) thought content and processes, (c) physical signs and symptoms, and (d) characteristic communication styles.
5. Identify evidence-based practice interventions for individuals with a depressive disorder. **QSEN: Evidence-Based Practice (EBP)**
6. Apply communication strategies that facilitate patient-centered care for the individual with a depressive disorder. **QSEN: Patient-Centered Care**
7. Describe components of interprofessional and intraprofessional teamwork and collaboration that facilitate safe and effective care for a person with a depressive disorder. **QSEN: Teamwork and Collaboration; Safety**
8. Applying evidence-based practice, identify clinical indications for the use of electroconvulsive therapy (ECT). **QSEN: Evidence-Based Practice**
9. Using informatics, compare the advantages and disadvantages of both the selective serotonin reuptake inhibitors (SSRIs) and the tricyclic antidepressants (TCAs). **QSEN: Informatics**
10. Identify two atypical antidepressants, and explain the unique advantages of each.
11. Explain the mechanism of action and special precautions when a monoamine oxidase inhibitor (MAOI) antidepressant is prescribed.

KEY TERMS AND CONCEPTS

anergia, p. 201
anhedonia, p. 201
atypical antidepressants, p. 216
automatic negative thoughts, p. 202
deep brain stimulation, p. 222
dual-action reuptake inhibitor, p. 216
electroconvulsive therapy (ECT), p. 221
hypersomnia, p. 208
learned helplessness, p. 203
light therapy, p. 222
major depressive disorder (MDD), p. 200
mood, p. 199
persistent depressive disorder (dysthymia) (PDD), p. 200
psychomotor agitation, p. 208
psychomotor retardation, p. 208
reframing, p. 203
S-adenosylmethionine (SAMe), p. 222
selective serotonin reuptake inhibitor (SSRI), p. 215
serotonin and norepinephrine reuptake inhibitors (SNRIs), p. 216
St. John's wort, p. 222
transcranial magnetic stimulation (TMS), p. 222
tricyclic antidepressants (TCAs), p. 216
unipolar depression, p. 200
vagus nerve stimulation (VNS), p. 221
vegetative signs of depression, p. 208

CONCEPT: MOOD AND AFFECT: Mood is defined as the way a person feels, and *affect* is defined as the observable response to a person's behavior. Mood and affect are on a continuum from depressed to normal to elevated. Nurses must be able to recognize the different affective states that affect a person's functional status (Giddens, 2017). Depressive disorders lead to painful levels of low self-esteem that can erode a person's quality of life and contribute to hopelessness and helplessness. There are many therapies available to decrease depression and increase quality of life.

INTRODUCTION

We all have low moods, feel sad, and have "blue" days. According to Sadock, Sadock, and Ruiz (2015), though, people with formal mood disorders describe a distinct quality to their depressive state. It is difficult to convey the profound anguish that is experienced by an individual suffering a severe depressive episode unless we ourselves have had a similar experience.

MOOD DISORDERS

The term *depression* is an umbrella term for a variety of disorders that range from mildly to moderately to severely disabling. Depression is a syndrome rather than a disease. "While a disease is a specific condition characterized by a common underlying cause and consistent physical traits, a syndrome is a collection of signs and symptoms known to frequently appear together, but without a single known cause" (Chen, 2015). Clinical depressive syndromes can cause severe impairment in psychosocial functioning and lead to increased mortality. Depressive disorders represent a group of syndromes that often share some common symptoms but may have different etiologies, courses, and treatments. Treatments for depression do work, but finding the right combination of interventions may take time.

Major depressive disorder (MDD) is a medical illness that affects how you feel, think, and behave, causing persistent feelings of sadness and loss of interest in previously enjoyed activities. MDD represents the classic condition in this group of disorders. The second most common presentation of depressive symptoms is the diagnosis of **persistent depressive disorder (dysthymia) (PPD)**. When a person experiences depression without ever experiencing an excessively elevated mood or mania, it is also sometimes labeled **unipolar depression**.

Prevalence

The World Health Organization (WHO, 2017) identified depression as the leading cause of disability worldwide.

- The lifetime prevalence of MDD is 28.2%.
- The 12-month prevalence of MDD is approximately 6.7 % (National Institute of Mental Health [NIMH], 2017).

The incidence of depression appears to be increasing in all age groups worldwide. Women are 70% more likely than men to experience depression during the course of their lifetimes and are more likely to seek help for depression. Men are more likely to self-medicate depressive symptoms with alcohol/substances (Lliades, 2015).

PDD is a more chronic presentation of a set of depressive symptoms.

- The lifetime prevalence rate of PDD with persistent major depressive episode (MDE) is 15.2%.
- The lifetime prevalence rate is 3.3% for PDD with pure dysthymia, a milder but more chronic form of depression.
- The lifetime prevalence rate is 9.1% for other specified depressive disorders (OSDDs), or disorders that do not fully meet the criteria for a major depressive episode (Vandeleur et al., 2017).

Comorbidity

Depressive symptoms frequently accompany many other psychiatric disorders. This comorbidity complicates the treatment of both disorders. Comorbidity has been shown to result in a higher rate of suicide, greater severity of depression, and greater impairment in social and occupational functioning. People with a diagnosis of anxiety disorders, posttraumatic stress disorder (PTSD), schizophrenia, substance use disorders, eating disorders, obsessive-compulsive disorders, and schizoaffective disorder commonly present with depression (American Psychiatric Association [APA], 2013). People with a diagnosis of personality disorders, particularly borderline personality disorder, also frequently experience clinical depression.

Individuals with chronic medical problems are at a higher risk of developing depression compared with those in the general population. These chronic illnesses may include cancers, stroke, chronic pain, or heart disease (Mayo Clinic Staff, 2017). Neuroendocrine diseases also increase the risk of developing clinical depression.

The prevalence of depression ranges from 5% to 60%, with a median of 33%, among all hospitalized patients. Depression in hospitalized individuals has been associated with poorer functional outcomes, worse physical health, and increased returns to the hospital after discharge (IsHak et al., 2017). Early recognition and referral for the treatment of comorbid depressive symptoms are priorities for all nurses.

Medications such as heart and high blood pressure medications, steroids, birth control pills, sleeping pills, and antibiotics/antivirals are some of the more common classes of medication that can induce depression in susceptible individuals (Harvard Health Publishing, 2017).

Chronic pain may also play a role in the etiology of depressive symptoms. Chronic pain and depression are closely correlated from the perspectives of both the brain regions affected and the functioning of the neurological system. Chronic pain may lead to clinical depression. Clinical depression can make chronic pain worse. Common brain changes affect the occurrence and development of these two disorders (Jiyao et al., 2017).

Symptoms of depression occur during bereavement and are expected as part of the normal process of mourning. The symptoms of MDD must be differentiated from "usual" symptoms associated with bereavement

Children and Adolescents

The incidence of severe depression in youth increased from 5.9% in 2012 to 8.2% in 2015 (Mental Health America, 2018). Children as young as 3 years of age have been diagnosed with MDD, with an incidence of 2.5% for those under the age of 12. Depression in children and adolescents may present differently. Children may initially present with symptoms such as irritability, physical complaints, decline in school performance, or social withdrawal. After puberty, girls are twice as likely to develop depression. Children with depressive symptoms may start using drugs and alcohol at an earlier age (WebMD Medical Reference, 2016). Early intervention for depressive symptoms may prevent the development of comorbid conditions.

For youth (age 12 to 17), the incidence of having at least one **MDE** in the past year is 11.93% (Nguyen et al., 2017). Adolescents may mask depression through sulking, being negative or grouchy, getting into trouble at school, feeling misunderstood, withdrawing from others, or running away from the home (*Psychology Today*, 2017). Major depression among adolescents is often associated with substance use disorders, behavior problems, and other mental illnesses. This can obscure accurate diagnosis and lower levels of treatment response. The prevalence rate of depression in individuals 18 to 29 years old is three times higher than in individuals 60 years old or older (APA, 2013).

After recovery from an acute depressive episode, 30% to 70% of children tend to relapse. In adolescents, 20% to 50% may relapse (Bonin, 2016).

Older Adults

Clinical depression occurs in 7% of the general older population, with significant disability for those affected (WHO, 2017). Estimates of incidence in the older adult are as follows:

- In older people living in the community, the incidence ranges from less than 1% to about 5%.
- In those requiring home health care, the incidence is 13.5%.
- In older hospital patients, the incidence is 11.5% (Centers for Disease Control and Prevention [CDC], 2017).
- Of all older adults, 10% to 15% have clinically significant depressive symptoms even in the absence of an MDD.

There are factors that increase the risk of the development of depression in older adults. As a group, these individuals may be more likely to have chronic medical conditions or to be taking medications that contribute to the development of depressive symptoms. This disorder frequently goes unrecognized and undiagnosed. Older adults are less likely to recognize symptoms of treatable depression, assuming that symptoms are an inevitable part of aging. They are also less likely to seek help from a mental health professional (National Institute of Health, National Institute of Aging, 2017). Suicide rates are high for this age group (Kok & Reynolds, 2017).

Two key symptoms that distinguish late-life depressive disorders in older adults are (1) complaints of sadness are less prominent, and (2) there is excessive concern with physical health compared with those who are younger. Sometimes older adults who are depressed complain of feeling tired, have trouble sleeping, or seem grumpy and irritable. Confusion or attention problems caused by depression can sometimes look like Alzheimer's disease or other brain disorders. The *Geriatric Depression Scale* is considered a best-practice assessment tool in the nursing care of older adults. More consistent use of this tool could facilitate the WHO goal of providing integrated mental health care for the elderly in community-based settings. Refer to Chapter 28 for more on depression in the older adult.

Theory

Predisposing Factors

Depression is a complex disease with many possible causes. It is believed that the causes of this disorder are a combination of genetic vulnerability, biochemical and physical changes in the brain, environmental stressors, traumatic events, and other physiologic and psychological factors.

There are common risk factors for the development of this serious psychiatric illness (Box 15.1).

Genetic Factors

Twin studies support the idea that genetic factors play a role in the development of depressive disorders. If one monozygotic (twins sharing the same genetic constitution) twin is affected by unipolar depression, the second has a 50% chance of also being affected. The percentage for dizygotic twins (different genetic constitution) is 20%. These statistics imply that although there may be a genetic link, other factors must also be involved in the etiology of this disease.

Adoptive studies also support a genetic contribution to the development of depression. The risk for the development of depression in children born to a parent or parents with a depressive illness is the same when these children are adopted by a family that does not have a psychiatric history of depression

Family studies further support the idea of inherited traits as being a causative factor for this disorder. Individuals who have a first-degree family member with depression are two to four times more likely to become depressed (APA, 2013; NIMH, 2015). Increased heritability is associated with an earlier age of onset, a greater rate of comorbidity (especially alcohol use disorders and psychosis), and an increased risk of recurrent illness. However, genetic factors must interact with environmental and neurobiological preconditions for depression to develop. Some theories of causation identify temperament or *how* you respond to environmental stressors as being a significant risk factor. This idea combines the interaction of an inherited trait, like temperament, with outside influences, like environmental stressors, as being important contributors to the development of these illnesses.

Biochemical Factors

One theory states that depression is thought to involve changes in receptor–neurotransmitter relationships in the following areas of the brain:

1. Limbic system (emotional alterations)
2. Hypothalamus (mood regulation)
3. Prefrontal cortex (decreased mood, problems concentrating)
4. Hippocampus (memory impairments; feelings of worthlessness, hopelessness, and guilt)
5. Amygdala (anxiety and reduced motivation)

It is believed that many neurotransmitters are involved in the appearance of depressive symptoms, including the monoamines: serotonin, norepinephrine, and dopamine. Changes in the availability of these monoamines in the brain seem to be important in the development of clinical depression.

- Serotonin, 5-hydroxytryptamine (5-HT), is an important regulator of sleep, appetite, and libido. A serotonin-circuit dysfunction can result in poor impulse control, low sex drive, decreased appetite, disturbed regulation of body temperature, and irritability.
- Decreased levels of norepinephrine (NE) in the medial forebrain bundle (MFB) may account for the symptoms of **anergia** (reduction in or lack of energy), **anhedonia** (an inability to find meaning or pleasure in existence), decreased concentration, and diminished libido.
- Dopamine (DA) neurons in the mesolimbic system are thought to play a role in the reward and incentive behavior processes, emotional expression, and learning processes that are disrupted in depression. This is particularly true in melancholic depression.

BOX 15.1 Primary Risk Factors for Depression

- History of prior episodes of depression
- Family history of depressive disorder, especially in first-degree relatives
- History of suicide attempts or family history of suicide
- Member of the lesbian, gay, bisexual, transgender, queer or questioning (LGBTQ) community
- Female gender
- Age 40 years or younger
- Postpartum period
- Chronic medical illness
- Absence of social support
- Negative, stressful life events, particularly early trauma
- Active alcohol or substance use disorder
- History of sexual abuse

Further research has identified other neurotransmitters, such as glutamate, gamma-aminobutyric acid (GABA), and acetylcholine, as playing a role in the etiology of depression (Harvard Health Publishing, 2017).

One type of dysfunction of these neurotransmitters appears to be abnormalities in the number of *receptor sites,* which increase or decrease the activity of these neurotransmitters. Medication that helps regulate specific neurotransmitters and the various subtypes of these neurotransmitters has proven effective in the treatment of depressive symptoms in many patients. The relationship among the monoamines—serotonin, norepinephrine, and dopamine—with other transmitters, like glutamate, acetylcholine, and GABA, need further assessment and study. Fig. 15.1 shows a positron emission tomography (PET) scan of the brain of a woman with depression before and after taking medication.

Bio-/Psychosocial Theories

The Stress-Diathesis Model of Depression. The stress-diathesis model of depression is a bio-/psychosocial theory that explains depression from an environmental, interpersonal, and life-events perspective combined with biological vulnerability or predisposition (diathesis). Psychosocial stressors and interpersonal events can trigger certain neurophysiological and neurochemical changes in the brain. For example, early life trauma can result in long-term hyperactivity of the corticotropin-releasing factor (CRF) and norepinephrine systems of the central nervous system (CNS). This can induce neurotoxic effects in the hippocampus that can lead to neuronal loss. Norepinephrine, serotonin, and acetylcholine play a role in stress regulation and can become overtaxed through stressful events. Neurotransmitter depletion may occur and cause permanent neuronal damage, leaving the person vulnerable to depression later in life (Sadock et al., 2015). Stressful events can cause brain changes that can lead to depression in a vulnerable brain.

Cognitive Theory. Aaron T. Beck, one of the early proponents of cognitive therapy, applied cognitive-behavioral theory to the treatment of depression. Beck proposed that people acquire a psychological predisposition to depression through early life experiences. These experiences contribute to negative, illogical, and irrational thought processes that may remain dormant until they are activated during times of stress (Beck & Rush, 1995). The central concept of cognitive behavioral therapy is as follows: What you think = What you feel (and do).

Beck found that people with depression process information in negative and distorted ways, even in the midst of positive factors that affect the person's life. See Box 15.2 for a list of common cognitive distortions. Beck believed that three automatic negative thoughts or cognitive distortions—called Beck's cognitive triad—are responsible for the development of depression:

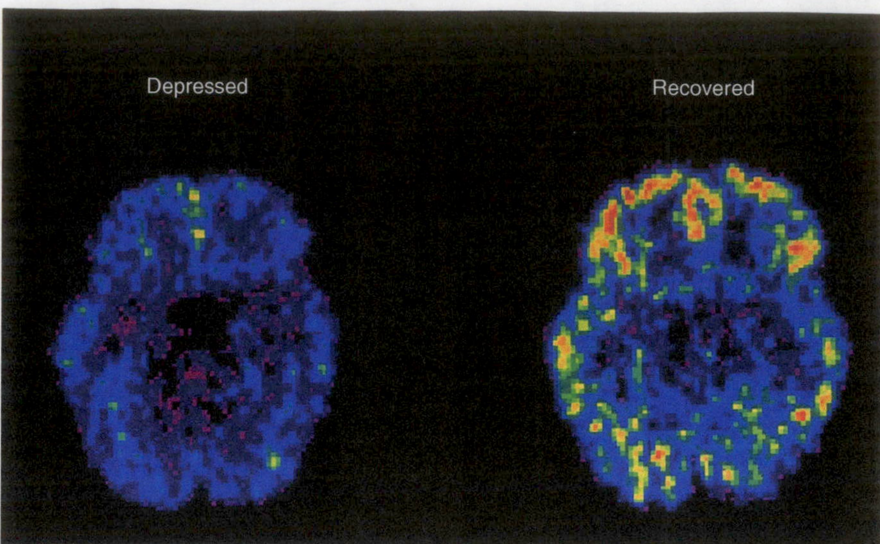

Fig. 15.1 Positron emission tomography (PET) scans of a 45-year-old woman with recurrent depression. The scan on the left was taken when the patient was not taking medication and was very depressed. The scan on the right was taken several months later when the patient was well, after she had been treated with medication for her depression. Note that her entire brain, particularly the left prefrontal cortex, is more active when she is well. (Courtesy Mark George, MD, Biological Psychiatry Branch, National Institute of Mental Health, Bethesda, MD.)

BOX 15.2 Common Cognitive Distortions

Filtering	Taking negative details and magnifying them while filtering out all positive aspects of a situation.
Polarized thinking (or "black-and-white" thinking)	Things are either "black or white." We have to be perfect or we're a failure—there is no middle ground or shades of gray.
Overgeneralization	Coming to a general conclusion based on a single incident or a single piece of evidence. If something bad happens only once, we expect it to happen over and over again.
Jumping to conclusions	Without individuals saying so, we think we know what they are feeling and why they act the way they do.
Catastrophizing	We expect disaster to strike, no matter what. We exaggerate the importance of insignificant events.
Personalization	A distorted belief that everything others do or say is somehow about us.
Control fallacies	We see ourselves as helpless, a victim of fate, having no control, or we assume total responsibility for the pain and happiness of everyone around us (overcontrol).
Fallacy of fairness	We feel resentful because we think we know what is fair, but other people won't agree with us.
Blaming	We hold other people responsible for our feelings and behaviors. Nobody can "make" us feel any particular way—only we have control over our own emotions and emotional reactions.
Shoulds	We have a list of ironclad rules about how we and others should and must behave.
Emotional reasoning	We believe that what we feel must be true automatically. "I feel it; therefore it must be true."
Global labeling	We generalize one or two qualities into a negative global judgment. For example, "I'm a loser" verses "In one situation, I failed."
Always being right	I have to prove my opinions and actions are correct. Being wrong is unthinkable.

Adapted from Grohol, J. (2017). *15 common cognitive distortions*. Retrieved from https://psychcentral.com/lib/15-common-cognitive-distortions/; and American Academy of Family Physicians. (2017). *Postpartum depression. Retrieved from https://familydoctor.org/condition/postpartum-depression/?adfree=true*

1. *A negative, self-deprecating view of self*: "I really never do anything well; everyone else seems smarter."
2. *A pessimistic view of the world*: "Once you're down, you can't get up. Look around—poverty, homelessness, sickness, war, and despair are every place you look."
3. *The belief that negative reinforcement (or no validation for the self) will continue*: "It doesn't matter what you do; nothing ever gets better. I'll be in this stupid job for the rest of mylife."

The phrase **automatic negative thoughts** refers to anxiety-provoking thoughts that are automatically triggered in a person by a particular situation. These automatic thoughts can be unfavorable and may not be recognized by the person.

The cognitive model states that the way individuals understand a situation is more closely connected to their reaction than to the situation itself. The goal of cognitive-behavioral therapy (CBT) is to change the way a patient thinks to help relieve the reaction or the depressive symptoms that are experienced. This is accomplished by assisting the patient in the following:

1. Identifying and "testing" negative or distorted cognitions or viewpoints
2. Developing alternative thinking patterns by challenging the cognitive distortions
3. Rehearsing new cognitive and behavioral responses

CBT has identified a list of common automatic negative thoughts frequently seen in depressed patients. For example, John reports the following:

- When John was walking in the hall, he said "Hi" to his supervisor.
- John's supervisor failed to also say hello.
- John responds to these events by feeling demoralized and disrespected and becomes sad.

This is an example of one type of cognitive distortion: John personalized the situation. The tools of CBT would help John to "challenge" the thinking errors (cognitive distortion):

Therapist: "In this instance, the supervisor's behavior may have nothing to do with you, John. The supervisor may have just been preoccupied and didn't hear the greeting."

The goal is to change the reaction to the situation to improve mood by (1) identifying the cognitive distortion and then (2) challenging the cognitive distortion by **reframing** or identifying alternative ways of viewing the situation.

Cognitive-behavioral therapy for insomnia (CBT-I) is a promising treatment for insomnia, a frequent comorbid condition of depression. There is some evidence that insomnia improvement as a result of CBT-I may lead to an improvement in depressive symptoms (Cunningham & Shapiro, 2018).

Based on a CBT-based skill-building approach, a program entitled Creating Opportunities for Personal Empowerment (COPE) has been shown to be effective in reducing depressive and anxiety symptoms in children and adolescents. It is an evidence-based strategy that helps this population to reduce negative thoughts, increase healthy behaviors, and improve communication and problem-solving skills (Lusk, 2017).

Learned Helplessness. **Learned helplessness** is a theory of causation proposed by Martin Seligman (1973). He stated that although anxiety is the initial response to a stressful situation, anxiety is replaced by depression if the person feels no control over the outcome of that situation. People who believe that an undesired event is their fault and/or that nothing can be done to change it are prone to depression. The theory of learned helplessness has been used to explain the development of depression in certain social groups, such as older adults, people living in impoverished areas, and women.

Cultural Considerations

Depressive disorders among diverse cultures may show substantial differences in symptom presentation. In many countries, depressive disorders remain unrecognized because somatic symptoms often are the presenting complaint (APA, 2013).

The 12-month prevalence rate for an MDE in 2015 according to race was as follows:

- 7.5% for Caucasians
- 4.9% for African Americans
- 4.8% for Hispanics
- 4.1% for Asians
- 5.2% for Native Hawaiian/other Pacific Islander
- 8.9% for American Indians/Alaska Natives

For those who identify with more than one race, the prevalence rate is 12.2 % (NIMH, 2017).

It can be hard to evaluate these kinds of statistics because members from minority groups often have presenting symptoms that may differ from those of Caucasians. Minorities may not seek health care and may not have the finances to afford health care.

Individuals who are lesbian, gay, bisexual, or transgender or those having variations in the development of genital organs that aren't clearly male or female (intersex) demonstrate significantly increased rates of depression if there is a nonsupportive psychosocial environment (Mayo Foundation for Medical Education and Research [MFMER], n.d.).

Nurses are in an ideal position to facilitate early recognition of clinical depression in all populations so that appropriate referrals can be made. Knowing who is at highest risk can facilitate this early recognition and lessen the negative consequences.

Clinical Picture

Major Depressive Disorder (Single Episode or Recurrent)

People with MDD can experience substantial emotional pain and suffering, as well as psychological, social, and occupational disability. The individual may not be unable to function "normally."

Symptoms of an episode of MDD may sometimes lessen or even resolve within 3 months for 20% of individuals and within 1 year for 80% of individuals even without treatment. When there is one reoccurrence of symptoms, there is an increased risk for multiple future reoccurrences. When reoccurrence episodes do occur, they are usually longer and more severe (Fava, Ostergaard, & Cassano, 2016). Comorbidity with medical illnesses or other psychiatric disorders increases morbidity and mortality.

All forms of depression share common symptoms, which can make it difficult to make a correct diagnosis. Use the mnemonic SIG E CAPS to help recognize the symptoms associated with clinical depression:

- **S**leep disturbance (too much sleep or insomnia) and **S**ad mood
- **I**nterest diminished in pleasurable activities
- **G**uilt feeling; feelings of worthlessness
- **E**nergy decreased or fatigue and (self)-**E**steem loss
- **C**oncentration diminished and indecisiveness
- **A**ppetite changes (decreased or increased) with weight changes
- **P**sychomotor retardation (slowing) or agitation
- **S**uicidal thoughts and behaviors and thoughts of death

The current level of severity of the episode (mild, moderate, or severe) is added to the diagnosis. A more detailed explanation of some of these symptoms is found under Assessment.

A number of additional specifiers are used to more clearly identify severity or further descriptions of MDD, including MDD with anxious distress, with psychotic features, with peripartum onset or with seasonal pattern, and others. See the *DSM-5* Diagnostic Criteria box for specific symptoms.

Persistent Depressive Disorder

PDD is a disorder characterized by depressive symptoms that have been present for at least 2 years. Because PDD is more chronic in nature, the disorder can be hard to distinguish from the person's *apparent* "usual pattern of functioning": "I've always been this way. It's just the way I *am*." Although people with PDD suffer from social and occupational distress, it is usually not severe enough to warrant hospitalization unless the individual becomes suicidal. The age of onset is usually adolescence, although it can occur in adulthood after severe stress. PDD is present longer and presents with less severe symptoms compared with an episode of MDD. Additional symptoms seen in individuals diagnosed with PDD may include the following:

- Daytime fatigue
- Can function at work and in social situations but not at an optimal level
- Chronic low-level depressed/irritable mood

DSM-5 DIAGNOSTIC CRITERIA

Major Depressive Disorder

A. Five (or more) of the following symptoms have been present during the same 2-week period and represent a change from previous functioning; at least one of the symptoms is either (1) depressed mood or (2) loss of interest or pleasure.

Note: Do not include symptoms that are clearly attributable to another medical condition.

1. Depressed mood most of the day, nearly every day, as indicated by either subjective report (e.g., feels sad, empty, hopeless) or observation made by others (e.g., appears tearful). (**Note:** In children and adolescents, can be irritable mood.)
2. Markedly diminished interest or pleasure in all, or almost all, activities most of the day, nearly every day (as indicated by either subjective account or observation).
3. Significant weight loss when not dieting or weight gain (e.g., a change of more than 5% of body weight in a month) or decrease or increase in appetite nearly every day. (**Note:** In children, consider failure to make expected weight gain.)
4. Insomnia or hypersomnia nearly every day.
5. Psychomotor agitation or retardation nearly every day (observable by others, not merely subjective feelings of restlessness or being slowed down).
6. Fatigue or loss of energy nearly every day.
7. Feelings of worthlessness or excessive or inappropriate guilt (which may be delusional) nearly every day (not merely self-reproach or guilt about being sick).
8. Diminished ability to think or concentrate, or indecisiveness, nearly every day (either by subjective account or as observed by others).
9. Recurrent thoughts of death (not just fear of dying), recurrent suicidal ideation without a specific plan, or a suicide attempt or a specific plan for committing suicide.

B. The symptoms cause clinically significant distress or impairment in social, occupational, or other important areas of functioning.

C. The episode is not attributable to the physiological effects of a substance or to another medical condition.

Note: Criteria A through C represent a major depressive episode.

Note: Responses to a significant loss (e.g., bereavement, financial ruin, losses from a natural disaster, a serious medical illness or disability) may include the feelings of intense sadness, rumination about the loss, insomnia, poor appetite, and weight loss noted by Criterion A, which may resemble a depressive episode. Although such symptoms may be understandable or considered appropriate to the loss, the presence of a major depressive episode in addition to the normal response to a significant loss should also be carefully considered. This decision inevitably requires the exercise of clinical judgment based on the individual's history and the cultural norms for the expression of distress in the context of loss.

D. The occurrence of the major depressive episode is not better explained by schizoaffective disorder, schizophrenia, schizophreniform disorder, delusional disorder, or other specific and unspecified schizophrenia spectrum and other psychotic disorders.

E. There has never been a manic episode or a hypomanic episode.

Note: This exclusion does not apply if all the manic-like or hypomanic-like episodes are substance-induced or are attributable to the physiological effects of another medical condition.

VIGNETTE: Sally is a bright, successful 34-year-old businesswoman. Over the past few weeks, she has become more withdrawn. Her life has become empty of meaning. She has difficulty getting out of bed in the mornings but finds it hard to sleep more than 3 to 4 hours a night. She is constantly exhausted.

Sally finds it impossible to concentrate at work and has called in sick the past 2 days. She feels unable to find the energy to dress, bathe, groom, or even eat. She has not eaten for 3 days except for some water, a few glasses of milk, and a few crackers. She has lost considerable weight.

When her best friend calls to find out why she has not shown up for work, Sally tells her, "I don't know. I just can't concentrate; I can't focus on anything. Nothing seems to be worth doing. I feel so heavy and empty inside. I don't see things getting any better." When her friend tries to coax her out of her mood, Sally snaps at her and tells her to mind her own business and leave her alone. Later, Sally is filled with remorse, telling herself she is a horrible person and does not deserve her friend's concern and loyalty. She wonders what it would be like if she no longer had to deal with all this pain. She is not sure if she can take this much longer.

- Eating too much or too little
- Difficulty with sleeping: usually difficulty getting to sleep and, once asleep, excessive sleeping (hypersomnia)
- Loss of energy, fatigue, and chronic tiredness even for simple tasks
- Decreased capacity to experience pleasure, enthusiasm, or motivation
- Irritability
- Negative, pessimistic thinking
- Low self-esteem (Preston & Johnson, 2015)

There are several other types of depressive disorders per the *DSM-5* (APA, 2013).

Disruptive mood dysregulation disorder is a relatively new diagnosis that is seen in children and features a chronic, severe, persistent irritability with outbursts larger than would be expected for the child's age or the situation. *Premenstrual dysphoric disorder* occurs when depressive symptoms are present in the week before the onset of menses and gradually improve and remit after the onset of menses. *Depressive disorder due to another medical condition* occurs when a pathophysiological consequence of a medical condition is causing or contributing to depressive symptoms. *Substance/medication-induced depressive disorder* occurs during or soon after exposure to a substance or medication. A diagnosis of *other specified or unspecified depressive disorder* is used when someone does not meet the full criteria for one of the other depressive disorders but symptoms are severe enough to cause impairment.

Refer to the Assessment section for a more thorough discussion of the signs and symptoms of depression.

VIGNETTE: Sam had another bad week at work. He cannot seem to perform the way he thinks he should. He never gets things right. Although his work seems acceptable to others, he constantly puts himself down. He wanted to take a class to improve his computer skills but cannot seem to find the energy or the time. His weekends are filled with "hanging around" his apartment. "Nothing much going on … there is never much going on. Life is dull; has it ever been otherwise?" His brother is always telling him that he has a face as long as a football field. "What's the matter with you, bro? You're good looking, smart. Go find a girl and have some fun in life. Why can't you just enjoy anything?" Sam just sighs. Who would be interested in him? He gets a cold beer from the fridge and continues watching reruns on TV.

APPLICATION OF THE NURSING PROCESS

ASSESSMENT

The first challenge in the assessment of clinical depression is recognition of the symptoms of the disorder. Depression in older adults can be missed. Depression in children and adolescents may remain undiagnosed when attention is focused on behavioral problems only. Racial and economic disparities in health care can lead to underdiagnosis and undertreatment of African Americans, Hispanics, and other minorities. Undiagnosed and untreated depression is associated with more severe disability and more long-term complications.

Although symptoms of depression are prevalent among primary care patients, few patients discuss these symptoms directly with their primary care clinicians. Instead, two-thirds of primary care patients with depression present with somatic symptoms (headache, back problems, or chronic pain), making detection of depression more difficult (Williams & Nieuwsma, 2018). The U.S. Preventive Services Task Force (USPSTF, 2016) recommends regular screening for depression in the general adult population, including pregnant and postpartum women. Postpartum depression can impair the bonding and attachment between mother and baby. Screening should be implemented, with adequate systems in place to ensure accurate diagnosis, effective treatment, and appropriate follow-up.

Assessment Tools

Numerous standardized screening tools can help the clinician assess the type of depression a person may be experiencing. Reliable and valid screening tools include the Beck Depression Inventory, the Hamilton Depression Scale, the Geriatric Depression Scale, and Zung's Self-Rating Depression Scale. The Patient Health Questionnaire (PHQ-9) is an easy-to-complete, nine-question instrument given to patients in a primary care setting to screen for the presence and severity of depression. Refer to Fig. 15.2 for a list of signs and symptoms associated with the diagnosis of depression.

The Edinburgh Postnatal Depression Scale (EPDS) is an effective screening tool for the identification of depression in pregnant and postpartum women (O'Connor et al., 2016). A systematic review of the literature shows evidence suggesting that programs that screen pregnant and postpartum women reduced the prevalence of depression and increased remission and treatment response. Screening is a recommended standard of practice for this population (O'Connor et al., 2016).

Suicide and Homicide Potential (QSEN: Safety)

A patient who appears depressed should always be evaluated for suicidal and homicidal ideation. Suicide is the 10th-leading cause of death for all age groups. Related statistics are as follows:

- Of all completed suicides, 78% are male, which is four times the rate for females.
- Suicide is:
  - The third-leading cause of death among people ages 10 to 14
  - The second-leading cause of death for people ages 15 to 34
  - The fifth-leading cause of death for people ages 45 to 54
  - The eighth-leading cause of death for people ages 55 to 64
  - The 17th-leading cause of death among persons ages 65 years and older
- Middle-aged adults account for the largest proportion of suicides.
- Ethnicity:
  - American Indian/Alaska Natives have the highest rates of suicide.
  - White/non-Hispanics have the second-highest rates (CDC, 2015).

Assessment Guidelines

Suicide Assessment

Evaluation for suicidal potential might include the following statements or questions:

- "You have said you are depressed. Tell me what that is like for you." (exploring)
- "When you feel depressed, what thoughts go through your mind?" (clarifying)
- Have you ever thought about taking your own life in the past? (suicidal ideation assessment—past)
- Are you thinking about killing yourself now? (suicidal ideation assessment—present)
- Assess for evidence of suicidal planning: evidence of a plan and the means to carry out the plan
  - When you think about killing yourself, do you have a way you would do this?
  - Do you have a plan? Do you have the means to carry out your plan?
- Is there anything that would prevent you from carrying out your plan? (protective factors)
- Have you ever attempted to kill yourself in the past? (assessing history of past attempts)

Homicide Assessment

A similar assessment is needed for ideation (thoughts) related to harm to others (homicidal ideation). Evaluation for homicide potential might include the following statements or questions:

- (Normalize) When someone feels as upset as you do, they may have thoughts about hurting the person who has upset or hurt them. What thoughts have you had like this? (homicidal ideation)
- If you decided to try to hurt ________, how would you do it? Tell me about the plans you've made. (planning [means])
- You mentioned that if you were to hurt ________, you'd probably do it by (describe method). How easy would it be for you to do this? (access to means)
- (Normalize) People often have very mixed feelings about harming other people. What are some reasons that would stop you or prevent you from trying to hurt ________? What is it that most holds you back from actually doing this? (protective factors)
- What have been your past experiences related to hurting people who have hurt you? (history of past attempt)

Depression

1. Always evaluate the patient's risk of suicide or harm to others. **(QSEN: Safety)** Overt hostility is highly correlated with suicide (see Chapter 23).
2. A thorough medical and neurological examination helps determine if the depression is primary or secondary to another disorder. Depression can be secondary to a host of medical or other psychiatric disorders, as well as medications or other substances. Evaluate the following:
   - Has the patient used or is the patient currently using drugs or alcohol?
   - Are there co-occurring/comorbid medical conditions?
   - Is there a history of a co-occurring psychiatric disorder (e.g., eating disorder, borderline personality disorder, anxiety disorder)?
   - Is there evidence of psychosis? This may require additional interventions and safety measures.
3. Assess for a history of depression. If the patient has a history of previous episodes of depression, determine therapies used previously that were effective. Some of the following questions can be asked:
   - "Have you ever gone through or felt anything like this before?"
   - "What seemed to help you at that time?"

The Hamilton Rating Scale for Depression

Patient's Name ______________________ Date of Assessment ____________

To rate the severity of depression in patients who are already diagnosed as depressed, administer this questionnaire. The higher the score, the more severe the depression.
For each item, write the correct number on the line next to the item. (Only one response per item)

1. DEPRESSED MOOD (Sadness, hopeless, helpless, worthless)
______ 0 = Absent
1 = These feeling states indicated only on questioning
2 = These feeling states spontaneously reported verbally
3 = Communicates feeling states non-verbally—i.e., through facial expression, posture, voice, and tendency to weep
4 = Patient reports VIRTUALLY ONLY these feeling states in his spontaneous verbal and non-verbal communication

2. FEELINGS OF GUILT
______ 0 = Absent
1 = Self reproach, feels he has let people down
2 = Ideas of guilt or rumination over past errors or sinful deeds
3 = Present illness is a punishment. Delusions of guilt
4 = Hears accusatory or denunciatory voices and/or experiences threatening visual hallucinations

3. SUICIDE
______ 0 = Absent
1 = Feels life is not worth living
2 = Wishes he were dead or any thoughts of possible death to self
3 = Suicidal ideal or gesture
4 = Attempts at suicide (any serious attempt rates 4)

4. INSOMNIA EARLY
______ 0 = No difficulty falling asleep
1 = Complains of occasional difficulty falling asleep—i.e., more than 1/2 hour
2 = Complains of nightly difficulty falling asleep

5. INSOMNIA MIDDLE
______ 0 = No difficulty
1 = Patient complains of being restless and disturbed during the night
2 = Waking during the night—any getting out of bed rates 2 (except for purposes of voiding)

6. INSOMNIA LATE
______ 0 = No difficulty
1 = Waking in early hours of the morning but goes back to sleep
2 = Unable to fall asleep again if he gets out of bed

7. WORK AND ACTIVITIES
______ 0 = No difficulty
1 = Thoughts and feelings of incapacity, fatigue or weakness related to activities; work or hobbies
2 = Loss of interest in activity; hobbies or work—either directly reported by patient, or indirect in listlessness, indecision and vacillation (feels he has to push self to work or activities)
3 = Decrease in actual time spent in activities or decrease in productivity
4 = Stopped working because of present illness

8. RETARDATION: PSYCHOMOTOR (Slowness of thought and speech; impaired ability to concentrate; decreased motor activity)
______ 0 = Normal speech and thought
1 = Slight retardation at interview
2 = Obvious retardation at interview
3 = Interview difficult
4 = Complete stupor

9. AGITATION
______ 0 = None
1 = Fidgetiness
2 = Playing with hands, hair, etc.
3 = Moving about, can't sit still
4 = Hand wringing, nail biting, hair-pulling, biting of lips

10. ANXIETY (PSYCHOLOGICAL)
______ 0 = No difficulty
1 = Subjective tension and irritability
2 = Worrying about minor matters
3 = Apprehensive attitude apparent in face or speech
4 = Fears expressed without questioning

Fig. 15.2 The Hamilton Rating Scale for Depression. (From Hamilton, M. [1960]. A rating scale for depression. *Journal of Neurology, Neurosurgery and Psychiatry, 23*, 56–62.)

11. ANXIETY SOMATIC: Physiological concomitants of anxiety (i.e., effects of autonomic overactivity, "butterflies," indigestion, stomach cramps, belching, diarrhea, palpitations, hyperventilation, paresthesia, sweating, flushing, tremor, headache, urinary frequency). Avoid asking about possible medication side effects (i.e., dry mouth, constipation).
_____ 0 = No difficulty
1 = Subjective tension and irritability
2 = Worrying about minor matters
3 = Apprehensive attitude apparent in face or speech
4 = Fears expressed without questioning

12. SOMATIC SYMPTOMS (GASTROINTESTINAL)
_____ 0 = None
1 = Loss of appetite but eating without encouragement from others. Food intake about normal
2 = Difficulty eating without urging from others. Marked reduction of appetite and food intake

13. SOMATIC SYMPTOMS GENERAL
_____ 0 = None
1 = Heaviness in limbs, back or head. Backaches, headache, muscle aches. Loss of energy and fatigability
2 = Any clear-cut symptom rates 2

14. GENITAL SYMPTOMS (Symptoms such as: loss of libido; impaired sexual performance; menstrual disturbances)
_____ 0 = Absent
1 = Mild
2 = Severe

15. HYPOCHONDRIASIS
_____ 0 = Not present
1 = Self-absorption (bodily)
2 = Preoccupation with health
3 = Frequent complaints, requests for help, etc.
4 = Hypochondriacal delusions

16. LOSS OF WEIGHT
A. When rating by history:
_____ 0 = No weight loss
1 = Probably weight loss associated with present illness
2 = Definite (according to patient) weight loss
3 = Not assessed

17. INSIGHT
_____ 0 = Acknowledges being depressed and ill
1 = Acknowledges illness but attributes cause to bad food, climate, overwork, virus, need for rest, etc.
2 = Denies being ill at all

18. DIURNAL VARIATION
A. Note whether symptoms are worse in morning or evening. If NO diurnal variation, mark none
_____ 0 = No variation
1 = Worse in A.M.
2 = Worse in P.M.

19. DEPERSONALIZATION AND DEREALIZATION (Such as: Feelings of unreality; Nihilistic ideas)
_____ 0 = Absent
1 = Mild
2 = Moderate
3 = Severe
4 = Incapacitating

20. PARANOID SYMPTOMS
_____ 0 = None
1 = Suspicious
2 = Ideas of reference
3 = Delusions of reference and persecution

21. OBSESSIONAL AND COMPULSIVE SYMPTOMS
_____ 0 = Absent
1 = Mild
2 = Severe

Total score: _____

Fig. 15.2 cont'd

4. Assess support systems, including family and significant others. Determine if there is a need for information and referrals.
   - "With whom do you live?"
   - "Whom do you trust?"
   - "To whom do you talk when you are upset?"
5. Assess for any events that might have "triggered" a depressive episode.
   - "Has anything happened recently to upset you?"
   - "Have you had any major changes in your life?"
   - "Have you had any recent losses: job, divorce, loss of partner, child moving away, deaths?"
6. Complete a psychosocial assessment that includes cultural beliefs and spiritual practices related to mental health and treatment. Determine if the depression is affecting the patient's beliefs and practice.
   - "How do you view depression?"
   - "Have you tried taking any over-the-counter remedies such as (herbs) to help with your depression?"
   - "Do you find solace in spiritual activities or a place of worship?"

Refer to Chapter 23 for more on suicide assessment, prevention, and intervention and to Chapter 24 for more on homicide assessment.

Detailed Assessment

Mood and Affect

Anxiety is a common symptom associated with depression. It is seen in about 60% to 90% of depressed patients. Some additional feelings that accompany a depressed mood are as follows:

- Feelings of worthlessness range from feeling inadequate to having an unrealistic evaluation of self-worth. These feelings reflect low self-esteem. Statements such as "I am no good; I'll never amount to anything" are common. Themes of one's inadequacy and incompetence are repeated relentlessly.
- Guilt is commonly seen with depression. A person may ruminate over present or past failings. Extreme guilt can assume psychotic proportions: "I have committed terrible sins." "I have caused terrible pain and destruction to everyone I have ever known, and now I'm paying for it."
- Helplessness is evidenced by believing that "everything," even usual tasks, is too difficult to accomplish. During a depressed period, people believe that things will never change. This can lead some to consider suicide as a way to escape the constant mental pain.
- Hopelessness is one of the core characteristics of depression and suicide. Hopelessness results in negative expectations for the future and a sense of loss of control over future outcomes.
- Anger and irritability are natural outcomes of profound feelings of helplessness. Anger in depression is often expressed inappropriately through destruction of property, hurtful verbal attacks, or physical aggression toward others. Anger may also be directed toward the self in the form of suicidal or self-destructive behaviors, such as alcohol or drug misuse, overeating, and smoking. These behaviors often contribute to feelings of low self-esteem and worthlessness.
- Affect: The patient may not make eye contact, may speak in a monotone voice, may show little or no facial expression (flat affect), and may answer with only yes-or-no responses. Frequent sighing is common. The range of facial expressions may be decreased.

Physical Changes—Clinical Symptoms

A person who is depressed sees the world through gray-colored glasses. Posture is poor, and the patient may look older than the stated age. Facial expressions convey sadness and dejection, and the patient may have frequent bouts of weeping. Conversely, patients may say that they are unable to cry.

Nearly 97% of people with depression have *anergia* (lack of energy). Feelings of fatigue can result in slowed movements, called **psychomotor retardation**. The continuum in psychomotor retardation may range from slowed and difficult movements to complete inactivity and incontinence. At other times, the nurse may note **psychomotor agitation**. Patients may pace, bite their nails, smoke, tap their fingers, or engage in some other tension-relieving activity. At these times, patients report feeling fidgety and unable to relax.

Grooming, dress, and personal hygiene are markedly neglected. People who usually take pride in their appearance and dress may be poorly groomed and allow themselves to look shabby and unkempt.

Vegetative signs of depression include somatic changes and alterations in those activities necessary to support physical life and growth, such as eating, sleeping, elimination, and sex. About 60% to 70% of people who experience a *major depressive episode* report having decreased appetite. Overeating occurs more often in PDD.

Changes in sleep patterns are a classic sign of depression. Often, people have early insomnia, difficulty falling asleep, or middle insomnia, waking at 3 or 4 AM and staying awake. Sometimes sleep problems consist of sleeping only for short periods. The light sleep of a depressed person tends to prolong the agony of depression. Sleep can be increased (**hypersomnia**) and provides an escape from painful feelings. This is more common in younger depressed individuals or those with depression as part of a bipolar disorder. Sleep that does occur is usually described as not being restful or refreshing.

Changes in bowel habits are common. Constipation is seen most frequently in patients with psychomotor retardation. Diarrhea occurs less frequently, often in conjunction with psychomotor agitation. Interest in sex declines (loss of libido) for men and women during depression. Some men experience impotence. These sexual problems can further complicate marital relationships.

Approximately 50% to 75% of people suffering from depression complain of pain with or without reporting psychological symptoms. People who suffer from chronic pain need careful assessment to differentiate for depression as a primary disease or as a comorbid condition.

Cognition and Thought Content

When people are depressed, their thinking is slowed. Memory and ability to concentrate may be affected. Depressed people may dwell on (rumination) and exaggerate their perceived faults and failures and are unable to focus on their strengths and successes.

When depressed, a person's ability to solve problems and think clearly is negatively affected. Judgment may be poor, and indecisiveness is common.

Evidence of delusional thinking may be seen in a person with MDD with psychotic features. This diagnosis is a severe form of this mood disorder that is characterized by delusions and/or hallucinations.

Example: "I am a terrible person, so God put snakes in my stomach and told me not to eat." This would be an example of a mood-congruent delusion (I am a bad person; therefore I am being punished).

DIAGNOSIS

Depressed individuals have a variety of needs that will guide the focus of care. The following are the most common patient problems and associated nursing diagnoses that are the focus of acute care:

- Risk of harm: Is the patient suicidal, homicidal, or at risk for self-harm?
- Mood regulation/stability: Feelings of hopelessness, helplessness, and worthlessness all increase the risk of harm to self or others.
- Withdrawn behavior leads to social isolation and impaired socialization.
- Lack of motivation and impaired volition lead to self-care deficits or problems with bathing, grooming, and other activities of daily living (ADLs).

TABLE 15.1 Potential Nursing Diagnoses for Depression

Signs and Symptoms	Potential Nursing Diagnoses[a]
Previous suicidal attempts Putting affairs in order Giving away prized possessions Suicidal ideation Overt or covert statements regarding killing self	*Attempted suicide* *Risk for self-destructive behavior* *Risk for suicide* *Risk for self-mutilation*
Feelings of helplessness, hopelessness, worthlessness, and powerlessness	*Despair* *Hopelessness* *Helplessness*
Vegetative signs of depression; changes in • Grooming and hygiene • Sleeping • Eating • Elimination • Sexual patterns	*Self care deficit* *Impaired sleep* *Impaired nutritional status* *Constipation* *Impaired sexual functioning*
Sad mood	*Depressed mood*
Withdrawn behavior, becoming isolative	*Impaired socialization* *Risk for loneliness* *Withdrawn behavior*
Difficulty with simple tasks, inability to function at previous level, verbalizations of inability to cope	*Impaired coping process* *Impaired cognition* *Impaired role performance*
Noncommunicativeness; speech that is only in monosyllables	*Impaired verbal communication*
Difficulty making decisions, poor concentration, poor problem solving, poor cognitive functioning, ruminations	*Decisional conflict* *Impaired thought process*
Feelings of inability to make positive change in one's life or have a sense of control over one's destiny	*Powerlessness* *Impaired coping process* *Low self-efficacy*
Questioning meaning of life and own existence, inability to participate in usual religious practices, conflict over spiritual beliefs, anger toward spiritual deity or religious representatives	*Spiritual distress*
Feelings of worthlessness, poor self-image, negative sense of self, self-negating verbalizations, feeling of being a failure, expressions of shame or guilt, hypersensitivity to slights or criticism	*Chronic low self-esteem* *Situational low self-esteem* *Shame*

[a]The International Classification for Nursing Practice (ICNP) is a product of the International Council of Nurses (ICN). Retrieved from http://www.icn.ch/what-we-do/ICNP-Browser/.

- Loss of appetite can lead to weight loss or impaired nutritional intake and lack of appetite.
- Disturbances of sleep and fatigue can lead to impaired sleep.
- Impairment in self-esteem can reduce quality of life and lead to feelings of depression, anxiety, and shame.

Table 15.1 identifies signs and symptoms commonly experienced in depression and offers possible nursing diagnoses.

OUTCOMES IDENTIFICATION

Outcomes should include goals for safety. Even if the patient is not having current self-destructive thoughts, one goal should be the development of a safety plan:

- Identifying symptoms associated with beginning a relapse
- Reminders of healthy coping
- Listing who can be contacted if the patient starts to feel suicidal

Goals for the outcomes of vegetative or physical signs of depression are also formulated; examples may include the following:

- Evidence of weight gain
- Return to normal bowel activity
- Sleep of 6 to 8 hours per night
- Reports of restful sleep
- Return of sexual desire

PLANNING

The planning of care for patients with depression is geared toward the particular symptoms the person is exhibiting. The increased risk for suicide, self-harm, or harm to others is ongoing during the care of the depressed person. (**QSEN: Patient-Centered Care**) Safety is always the highest priority. Safe administration of medications is included in this phase. Recognizing and helping the patient tolerate side effects increases medication adherence. Facilitating a supportive nurse-patient relationship is an ongoing intervention.

Planning must take into account the presence of vegetative signs of depression as well as changes in concentration, activity level, social interaction, or personal appearance.

IMPLEMENTATION

Communication Guidelines

A person who is depressed may speak slowly and take longer to comprehend and respond. The lack of an immediate response by the patient does not mean that the person has not heard or chooses not to reply. The patient may need a little more time to compose a reply.

In extreme cases, some depressed patients are so withdrawn that they are unwilling or unable to speak. Nurses may feel uncomfortable with silence and not being able to "do anything" to effect immediate change. The intervention of "offering self" by sitting with a patient in silence may be a valuable intervention. It is important to be aware that this time spent together can be meaningful to the depressed person, especially if the nurse has a genuine interest in the depressed individual.

VIGNETTE: Doris, a senior nursing student, was assigned to a woman with a diagnosis of depression. On admission, she admitted to having suicidal ideation and describes herself as being withdrawn. The instructor notices that Doris spends a lot of time talking with other students and their patients and little time with her own patient. While talking to her nursing instructor, Doris acknowledges feeling threatened and useless and says that she wants a patient who will interact with her. After reviewing the symptoms of depression and clarifying the needs of depressed individuals with her instructor, Doris turns her attention back to her patient. She spends short time periods sitting in silence, making observations, and offering to walk with her patient up and down the halls. Upon leaving for the day, the patient tells Doris, "Thanks for spending time with me; it helped me focus on other things."

It is difficult to say when a withdrawn or depressed person will be able to respond. However, certain techniques are known to be useful in guiding effective nursing interventions. Some communication interventions to use with a severely withdrawn patient are listed in Table 15.2. Additional communication interventions to use when caring for depressed patients are offered in Table 15.3.

Facilitating the development of a nurse–patient relationship may require brief, frequent contact with the patient. Once the patient feels comfortable with the one-to-one relationship, encourage participation in milieu group activities. A therapeutic milieu that provides a structure of group and other activities alternating with periods for rest can be helpful to the individual with depression. Accompanying the patient to the group activities may be required initially. Give positive reinforcement for increased participation in activities and interactions with peers on the unit.

Health Teaching and Health Promotion

There are four broad goals of health teaching and psychoeducation:

1. Information:
   a. Teach patient and family/significant others that depression is a medical illness over which the patient has no voluntary control.
   b. Explain the biological, psychosocial, and cognitive changes associated with a depressive disorder.
   c. Explain the overt and covert signs of suicidal ideation, and know precautionary measures to take if the warning signs of suicidal thinking or planning occur (see Chapter 23).
   d. Emotional discharge gives an opportunity to exchange ideas about managing the illness and to discuss frustrations and concerns.
2. Support treatment adherence through medication teaching:
   a. Review the patient's medications and adverse reactions. Give information about ways to lessen side effects to increase medication adherence.
   b. Written information is helpful to reinforce understanding. Repeating the information taught back to the nurse confirms comprehension. Be aware of the patient's cultural background and ability to understand and/or read English.
   c. Remind patients and families that medications take several weeks to become effective. This can be discouraging for those struggling with the symptoms of depression.
   d. Reinforce the need to stay on medications even after symptoms have been relieved.
   e. Reinforce the role of psychotherapy and other treatments in helping a person with a depressive disorder.

TABLE 15.2 Interventions for Severely Withdrawn Individuals: Communication

Intervention	Rationale
1. When a patient is mute, use the technique of *making observations:* "There are many new pictures on the wall" or "You are wearing your new shoes."	1. When a patient is not ready to talk, direct questions can raise the patient's anxiety level and frustrate the nurse. Pointing to commonalities in the environment addresses the "here and now" and reinforces reality.
2. Use simple, concrete words.	2. Slowed thinking and difficulty concentrating impair comprehension.
3. Allow time for the patient to respond.	3. Slowed thinking necessitates time to formulate a response.
4. Listen for covert messages and ask about suicide plans: "Have you had thoughts of killing or harming yourself or others in any way?"	4. People often experience relief and decrease in feelings of isolation when they share thoughts of suicide, self-harm, or harm to others.
5. Avoid false reassurances such as, "Things will look up" or "Everyone gets down once in a while."	5. These tend to minimize the patient's feelings and can increase feelings of guilt and worthlessness because the patient cannot "look up" or "snap out of it."

TABLE 15.3 Interventions for Depression: Communication

Intervention	Rationale
1. Help the patient question underlying assumptions and beliefs and consider alternate explanations to problems.	1. Reconstructing a healthier and more hopeful attitude about the future can alter depressed mood.
2. Work with the patient to identify cognitive distortions that encourage negative self-appraisal. For example: a. Overgeneralizations b. Self-blame c. Mind reading d. Discounting of positive attributes	2. Cognitive distortions reinforce a negative, inaccurate perception of self and world. a. The patient takes one fact or event and makes a general rule out of it ("He always …"; "I never …"). b. The patient consistently blames self for everything perceived as negative. c. The patient assumes others do not like him or her, and so forth, without any real evidence that assumptions are correct. d. The patient focuses on the negative.
3. Encourage activities that can raise self-esteem. Identify need for (a) problem-solving skills, (b) coping skills, and (c) assertiveness skills.	3. Many depressed people feel unable to problem-solve and use adaptive coping skills. Increasing social, family, and job skills can change negative self-assessment.
4. Discuss physical activities the patient enjoys, such as running. Explain that initially 10 to 15 minutes a day 3 or 4 times a week has short-term benefits.	4. Exercise can help reduce tension, alleviate depression and anxiety, improve self-concept, and shift the neurochemical balance.
5. Encourage the formation of supportive relationships through support groups, therapy, and peer support.	5. Such relationships reduce social isolation and enable the patient to work on personal goals and relationship needs among people who share similar experiences.
6. Provide information and referrals for spiritual/religious information.	6. Spiritual and existential issues may be heightened during depressive episodes—many people find strength and comfort in spirituality or religion.

f. Develop a relapse prevention plan that includes emergency contacts in case the person starts to have suicidal thoughts and feelings.
g. Whenever possible, psychoeducation should begin early and be carried out with the patient and the patient's significant others. Including significant others in counseling facilitates the following:
   - Increased understanding and acceptance of the depressed family member
   - Increased understanding of symptoms that signal a relapse
3. Teach the use of self-help strategies. It is believed that there are interactions between diet, sleep, and exercise and major depression.
   a. Maintain a healthy diet. A healthful dietary pattern is associated with a decreased risk of depression (Li et al., 2017).
   b. Promote good sleep hygiene. There is evidence that sleep problems are both symptoms of and causal factor in the occurrence of depression (Freedman et al., 2017).
   c. Maintain a regular exercise regime. Although the exact neurobiological mechanism is not fully understood, regular exercise does have an antidepressant effect (Schuch et al., 2016).
4. Informatics: The Internet offers multiple self-help websites, such as the following:
   a. **MoodGYM**— https://moodgym.com.au/: Information, quizzes, games, and skills training to help prevent depression (You do need to register for this site, but it is free.)
   b. **Blue Pages**—https://bluepages.anu.edu.au/: Evidence-based self-help website. At 6 weeks, reductions in symptoms of depression were greater in both the Blue Pages and MoodGYM groups compared with a control group.
   c. **Living Life to the Full** —https://llttf.com/: Free online life skills course for people feeling distressed. Helps you understand why you feel as you do and make changes in your thinking, activities, sleep, and relationships.
   d. University of Michigan Depression Center, Depression Tool Kit—https://www.depressioncenter.org/depression-tool-kit: Useful information about self-help strategies to treat depression.

Some effective interventions targeting the physical needs of the depressed patient are listed in Table 15.4.

TABLE 15.4 Interventions Targeting the Physical Needs of the Depressed Patient

Intervention	Rationale
Nutrition: Anorexia	
1. Offer small, high-calorie, and high-protein food and drinks frequently throughout the day and evening.	1. Low weight and poor nutrition render the patient susceptible to illness and contribute to feelings of fatigue. Small, frequent snacks are more easily tolerated than large plates of food when the patient is anorectic.
2. Offer fluids frequently throughout the day and evening.	2. Fluids prevent dehydration and can minimize constipation.
3. When possible, encourage family or friends to remain with the patient during meals.	3. This strategy reinforces the idea that someone cares, can raise the patient's self-esteem, and can serve as an incentive to eat.
4. Ask the patient which foods or drinks are preferred. Offer choices. Involve the dietician.	4. The patient is more likely to eat the foods provided.
5. Weigh the patient weekly and observe the patient's eating patterns.	5. Monitoring the patient's status gives the information needed for revision of the intervention.
Sleep: Insomnia	
1. Provide periods of rest after activities.	1. Fatigue can intensify feelings of depression.
2. Encourage the patient to get up and dress and to stay out of bed during the day.	2. Minimizing sleep during the day increases the likelihood of sleep at night.
3. Encourage the use of relaxation measures in the evening (warm bath, warm milk, progressive muscle relaxation techniques).	3. These measures induce relaxation and sleep.
4. Reduce environmental and physical stimulants in the evening—provide decaffeinated coffee, soft lights, soft music, quiet activities.	4. Decreasing caffeine and environmental stimulation increases the possibility of sleep. Playing relaxing music can help the patient sleep.
Self-Care Deficits	
1. Encourage the use of toothbrush, washcloth, soap, makeup, shaving equipment, and so forth.	1. Being clean and well-groomed can temporarily increase self-esteem.
2. When appropriate, give step-by-step reminders such as, "Wash the right side of your face, now the left."	2. Slowed thinking and difficulty concentrating make organizing simple tasks difficult.
Elimination: Constipation	
1. Specifically monitor bowel movements.	1. Many depressed patients are constipated. If the condition is not checked, fecal impaction can occur.
2. Offer foods high in fiber and provide periods of exercise.	2. Roughage and exercise stimulate peristalsis and help with the evacuation of fecal material.
3. Encourage the intake of fluids.	3. Fluids help prevent constipation.
4. Evaluate the need for laxatives and enemas.	4. These measures prevent fecal impaction.

APPLYING THE ART

A Person With Depression

Scenario

I met Nadia, a 39-year-old mother of three, in the mental health clinic where I was doing my psychiatric rotation. Her main complaint was severe fatigue, anhedonia, and inertia. She states she no longer has the energy to care for her children or her marriage, saying, "I am not fit to be a mother or wife."

Therapeutic Goal

By the conclusion of this interaction, Nadia will state that she understands that depression is a treatable disorder and that it is her symptoms that are causing her despondent behavior.

Student–Patient Interaction	Thoughts, Communication Techniques, and Mental Health Nursing Concepts
Nadia: *Speaking slowly, eyes downcast.* "I couldn't face all those people."	
Student: "You're looking down like you are sad." *No response from Nadia.* "I wonder what facing the group means to you."	Depression slows everything: thoughts, feelings, and responses to others. I *make an observation* and *attempt to translate into feelings,* then shift to an *indirect question.* Because depression hinders Nadia's processing of information, I need to slow my pace. Allow more silence.
Student's feelings: *I should have stayed with "sad." I aimed for her feelings, then did not wait for her to share any feelings.*	
Nadia: *Slowly shakes her head back and forth. Silent for 3 minutes. No eye contact.*	
Student: *With a concerned look.* "You shake your head as if you are saying no."	I use *silence* along with attending behavior. I *make an observation* and then use *restatement.*
Student's feelings: *I know it's the right thing to do, but waiting during the silence makes me so anxious. I need to stay mindfully alert and attentive. I can endure the silence for Nadia's sake.*	
Nadia: "Everybody in the group makes progress. I just keep sinking deeper."	
Student: "Sinking deeper?"	Nadia has just started taking antidepressant medication. Most affect *serotonin or norepinephrine neurotransmitter levels,* but therapeutic effectiveness takes 2 to 3 weeks. I use *restatement* to encourage Nadia to say more.
Nadia: "Into depression. I can't pull it together even though I know my kids need me." *Makes eye contact.*	Depression erodes self-esteem, and low self-esteem, in turn, exacerbates depression.
Student's feelings: *I know from experience that it's hard to pull anything together when you feel depressed.*	
Student: "You care about your children." *She nods.* "Sounds like you find it difficult at this time to care about yourself very much."	I *attempt to translate into feelings* adding "at this time" to imply a temporary state.
Student's feelings: *I've noticed that sometimes, like Nadia, nurses find it easier to care for others than take care of self, even basic self-care or prevention measures.*	
Nadia: *Sustaining eye contact.* "I can't do anything right. I have nothing to show for my life."	
Student: "Think about what you've accomplished! You have your children, your marriage, your teaching career." *Nadia shrugs, eyes downcast.*	I inadvertently minimized her feelings by giving *approval* and *advice,* which is *nontherapeutic.* Even though all the things I pointed out may be valid, none of it rings true for Nadia right now.
Student's feelings: *She has so much going for her. Why can't she see that?*	One step that helps with depression would be for Nadia to problem-solve and work through any cognitive distortions ("I can't do anything right"). *Cognitive-behavioral therapy,* like antidepressant medication, takes time, but depression is a treatable disorder. *My response causes Nadia to pull away by withdrawing eye contact. When I deliver positives about Nadia before she feels more positive about herself, I discount her experience, which interferes with trust.* *I need to remember that support and nonjudgmental acceptance provide the foundation for the nurse–patient relationship.*
Student: *After waiting for 2 minutes.* "Nadia, I am here to be with you right where you are at this moment. No pressure."	I offer self and acceptance.
Nadia: *Looking up.* "Thank you. You don't know how much that means. I do want to get better and not feel like depression consumes who I am."	
Student: *Nods.* "You want to get better. You were able to take the first courageous step. In deciding to get admitted, you acknowledge that your symptoms are a problem, and they are the symptoms of depression, a disorder."	I *give support.* Separating oneself as distinct from the disorder of depression restores some sense of control to Nadia.
Student's feelings: *Nadia feels swallowed up (consumed) by the depression. I want her to know that depression need not be her life.*	
Nadia: "Oh, I never thought of it that way … as a first step, not a sign of failure. My symptoms are from the depression."	
Student's feelings: *As a nurse, my belief in Nadia's ability to battle the depression offers hope.*	
Student: *Nods.* "A treatable disorder." *I continue to sit with Nadia in silence for a short while.*	At some level, Nadia acknowledges a self not fully consumed by depression.
Nadia: "Yes, depression is a disorder, not all that I am."	Hope will grow as Nadia begins to take charge of her disorder through active investment in treatment.

Neurobiology of Depression and the Effect of Antidepressants

Imbalance of certain neurotransmitters (serotonin and norepinephrine) thought to contribute to depression in certain parts of the brain.

Prefrontal cortex (PFC): regulates role in executive functions and emotional control and memory.

Limbic system: (amygdala, hypothalamus, hippocampus) regulates activities such as emotions, physical and sexual drives, and the stress response (as well as processing, learning, and memory).

Anterior cingulate cortex (ACC): decreases motivation and ability to stay focused on a task, and disrupts ability to manage appropriate emotional reactions

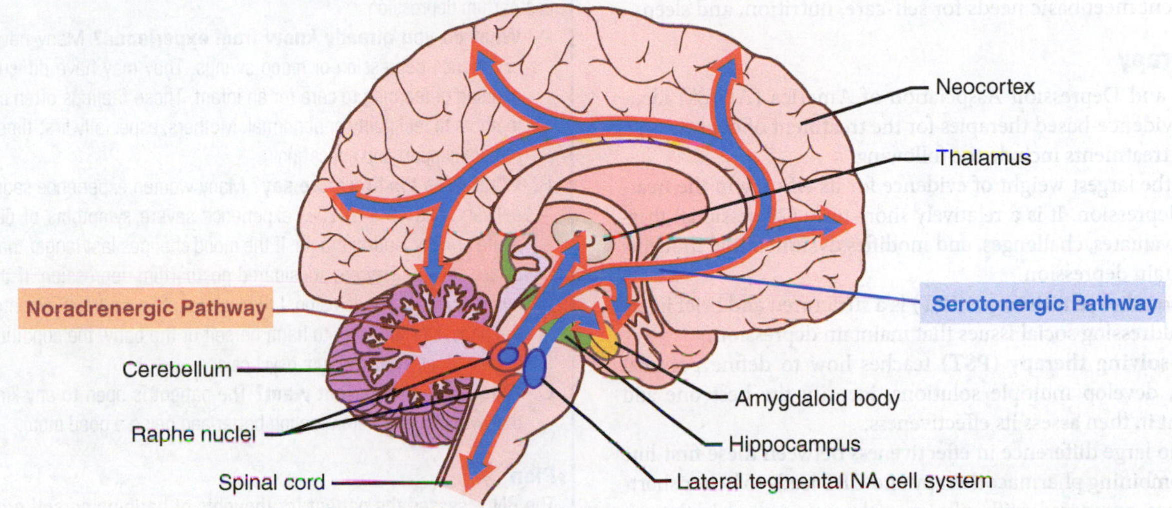

Various Parts of the Brain Along the Noradrenergic Pathway

The axons of these neurons project upward through the forebrain to the cerebral cortex, the limbic system, the thalamus, and the hippocampus.

Noradrenaline and the Noradrenergic System (NE): plays a major role in mood and emotional behavior as well as energy, drive, anxiety, focus, and metabolism.

Various Parts of the Brain Along the Serotonergic Pathway

The axons of serotonergic neurons originate in the raphe nuclei of the brainstem and project to the cerebral cortex, the limbic system, cerebellum, and spinal cord.

Serotonin and the Serotonergic System (5-HT): involved in the regulation of pain, depression, pleasure, anxiety, panic arousal, and sleep cycle, carbohydrate craving, PMS.

Medications for Depression

Medications for depression include the selective serotonin reuptake inhibitors (**SSRIs**), serotonin/norepinephrine reuptake inhibitors (**SNRIs**), noradrenergic and specific serotonergic antidepressants (**NaSSAs**), tricyclic antidepressants (**TCAs**), monoamine oxidase inhibitors (**MAOIs**), and atypical antidepressants.

They all work equally as well and are chosen by their safety profile and side effects.* All have a delayed response, a discontinuation syndrome, Black Box Warning-suicide.

Patient's Problem*	Side Effect Profile*	Example of Drug*
Fatigue	Stimulates the CNS	Fluoxetine (SSRI)
Insomnia	Substantial sedation	Mirtazapine (NaSSAs)
Sexual dysfunction	Enhances libido	Bupropion (atypical)
Chronic pain	Relieves pain	TCAs or duloxetine (SNRI)

*Adapted from page 341 *Lehne's Pharmacology for Nursing Care*, 9th edition (2016) by Jacqueline Burchum DNSc APRN BC (Authors), Laura Rosenthal DNP ACNP (Author)

Milieu Therapy

When a person is acutely and severely depressed, the structure of the hospital setting may be necessary. The depressed person may need support so that he or she does not act on suicidal thoughts. A therapeutic milieu provides a physically safe environment. In addition, the presence of nursing staff provides a psychologically safe environment by offering consistent emotional support. Hospitals have protocols for suicidal observation and protection that can be implemented when the person is experiencing suicidal thinking. Nursing staff also help the patient meet basic needs for self-care, nutrition, and sleep.

Psychotherapy

The Anxiety and Depression Association of America (ADAA) identified some evidence-based therapies for the treatment of depression.

First-line treatments include the following:

- **CBT** has the largest weight of evidence for its efficacy in the treatment of depression. It is a relatively short-term (20 sessions) therapy that evaluates, challenges, and modifies dysfunctional thoughts that maintain depression.
- **Interpersonal psychotherapy** (**IPT**) is a structured and brief intervention addressing social issues that maintain depression.
- **Problem-solving therapy** (**PST**) teaches how to define personal problems, develop multiple solutions, identify the best one and implement it, then assess its effectiveness.

There is no large difference in effectiveness between these first-line therapies. Combining pharmacotherapy and CBT leads to better short-term outcomes compared with pharmacotherapy or psychotherapy treatment alone (MDD Clinical Practice Review Task Force, 2016).

CBT-I is an evidenced-based therapy to deal with the symptoms of insomnia, a common and troublesome symptom seen in depression (Cunningham & Shapiro, 2018).

Second-line treatments include the following:

- **Social skills training (SST):** Behavioral treatment that teaches skills and behaviors that help build and maintain social relationships; often also includes assertiveness training.
- **Behavioral activation (BA):** Involves activity scheduling and increasing pleasant activities or positive interactions between a person and the environment.
- **Psychodynamic therapy (PT):** Aims to increase understanding, awareness, and insight about repetitive conflicts (intrapsychic and intrapersonal).

The evidence for the effectiveness of these treatments is small to moderate (MDD Clinical Practice Review Task Force, 2016).

Imaging studies have been used to attempt to predict which patients will respond to which specific therapies. This opens up another area for researchers to explore to provide individualized, patient-centered care (Crowther et al., 2015; Derewicz, 2015).

Mindfulness-Based Cognitive Therapy

There are increasing numbers of studies looking at the use of **mindfulness-based cognitive therapy (MBCT)** and its effectiveness in treating people who are experiencing a relapse/reoccurrence of MDD (MacKenzie & Kocovski, 2016). MBCT is a combination of CBT and mindfulness-based stress reduction (MBSR) techniques. MBSR was developed by Kabat-Zinn at the University of Massachusetts in the early 1970s (Dickson, 2020). Mindfulness is a meditation technique that has been used successfully in patients coping with a variety of medical or mental health disorders.

Group Therapy

Group therapy is another type of treatment for depression. Support groups and group therapy offer patients an opportunity to share common feelings and concerns as well as provide patients with the opportunity to reach out and support others. Belonging to a group can help decrease feelings of isolation, hopelessness, helplessness, and alienation. It can also increase the number of people who can receive treatment at a decreased cost per individual.

Medication groups for patients and families focus on understanding the medications used for treatment. They provide strategies to use these medications properly and to lessen distressing side effects. Treatment adherence is facilitated by identifying outside influences that may be interfering with staying on prescribed medication.

APPLYING EVIDENCE-BASED PRACTICE (EBP)

Problem

A registered nurse (RN) visits a new mother for a home visit to provide lactation and infant care support and education. This is the 19-year-old mother's first child. When the RN enters the home, she finds the curtains drawn, and the new mother appears exhausted and unkempt. She begins crying while talking to the nurse and expresses feelings of guilt that she does not feel closer to her baby or happy and excited. The RN suspects that the new mother has postpartum depression.

A. **What do you already know from experience?** Many new mothers experience depression or mood swings. They may have difficulties with bonding or learning to care for an infant. These feelings often cause new mothers to feel guilty or abnormal. Mothers, especially first-time mothers, require support and education.

B. **What does the literature say?** Many women experience sadness after delivery, and 10% to 20% experience severe symptoms of depression, acute anxiety, and/or mania. If the mood changes last longer than 10 days or are severe, they are considered postpartum depression. If the mother has hallucinations, delusional thinking (e.g., "everything is contaminating the baby"), or thoughts to harm herself or the baby, the condition may be more serious—postpartum psychosis.

C. **What does the patient want?** The patient is open to any kind of help that would assist her in feeling better and being a good mom.

Plan

The RN assessed the patient for thoughts of harming herself or the baby. The mother denied having such thoughts either now or in the past. The RN referred the mother for a psychiatric evaluation to see if therapy or medications would be appropriate. She helped the mother think of supportive friends and relatives who could help her with the baby and allow her to get regular sleep. The RN provided lactation assistance and education because the mother was struggling to nurse her baby. The RN and patient agreed to a weekly visit until she is feeling better, and the client was provided with resources to call in a crisis.

QSEN Prelicensure Knowledge, Skills, and Attitudes (KSAs) Addressed

Safety was addressed through evaluation of suicidal or homicidal thoughts and the provision of psychiatric resources.

Patient-Centered Care was provided by identifying what the mother wants, addressing the patient's pain and suffering, and empowering the patient.

Pharmacological Therapies

Antidepressant Medication Therapy

Approximately 40% to 60% of people taking an antidepressant notice an improvement in their symptoms. Unfortunately, 23% of those taking an antidepressant relapse within 1 to 2 years. Antidepressants work best for moderate to severe depression and are less effective for mild depression. There is evidence that the combination of nonpharmacological therapies and pharmacotherapy may be the most effective strategy for the treatment of depressive disorders and may reduce the risk of recurrence or relapse of MDD and PDD. It is believed that the core symptoms of depression improve with antidepressant therapy, and quality-of-life measures improve with certain psychotherapies.

Antidepressant target symptoms include the following:

- Sleep disturbance
- Appetite disturbance (decreased or increased)
- Fatigue
- Decreased sex drive
- Psychomotor retardation or agitation
- Diurnal variations in mood (feeling sluggish and tired in the morning and enervated at night)
- Impaired concentration or forgetfulness
- Anhedonia (loss of ability to experience joy or pleasure in living)

One significant drawback to the use of antidepressant medication is that improvement in mood may take 1 to 3 weeks or longer. If a patient is acutely suicidal, this may be too long to wait. At these times, other options may be indicated.

Although there are many antidepressants available, there is no clear-cut way to determine if any specific drug will be effective for an individual patient. This trial-and-error approach can significantly prolong the suffering of the depressed patient. Currently, research is attempting to decipher which particular biomarkers will predict an individualized response to a particular antidepressant (Solis, 2016).

Safety

There is the possibility that children, adolescents, and young adults taking antidepressants, particularly **selective serotonin reuptake inhibitors (SSRIs)**, may experience both suicidal ideation and aggressive behaviors as side effects. There is a **Black Box warning** associated with **all** antidepressants for the increased risk of suicide in children and adolescents, but no formal mention of aggressive behavior. A recent analysis of the most commonly prescribed antidepressants revealed that these drugs could double the risk of suicide and aggressive behavior in those under 18 years old (Knapton, 2016).

As with all medications, the use of antidepressants in the elderly must take into consideration the side-effect profile and the risk of drug–drug interactions. Doses must be adjusted. Due to slowed renal function associated with aging, the risk of hyponatremia is higher when using SSRIs and some of the newer antidepressants. Some antidepressants with long half-lives should be avoided in this population because of generalized slow drug metabolism. The accepted practice for older adults is always, "Start low, go slow."

Taking any medications during pregnancy is of concern. For SSRIs, there is a concern that inhibiting serotonin during critical fetal development may result in birth defects (Davenport, 2016). There may also be a slightly higher risk of the development of autism in the children of women that have used antidepressants during pregnancy (Schendel, 2017). The risks associated with the illness of depression must always be weighed against the risk of the side effects of the treatment.

Another area of concern is the increased risk of cerebral microbleeds in those age 45 or older who take these drugs (Melville, 2016).

Classes of Antidepressants

Although all antidepressants work equally well, they certainly do not all work well for all individuals. Because the complex interplay of neurotransmitters responsible for depression is unique for different individuals, a variety of antidepressants or a combination of antidepressants may need to be tried before the most effective regimen is found. Each antidepressant has adverse effects as well as cost, safety, and maintenance considerations. The following are some of the primary and secondary considerations when choosing a specific antidepressant:

- Primary considerations
  - Previous response to antidepressants
  - Ease of administration
  - Safety and medical comorbidities (diabetes, cardiac disease)
  - Associated symptoms of psychiatric comorbidity (obsessive-compulsive disorder [OCD], PTSD, bipolar disorder, anxiety disorder, energy level)
- Secondary considerations
  - Neurotransmitter specificity
  - Family history of response
  - Cost

Neurotransmitters and receptor sites in the brain are the targets of pharmacological intervention (Table 15.5). While reading the following section and using Table 15.5 as a guide, see if you can identify potential side effects caused by the blockage of the given neurotransmitter.

Studies that compare the efficacy of more recent SSRIs and newer dual-action antidepressants to the tricyclic antidepressants (TCAs) generally fail to find support for one group over the other. The difference lies

TABLE 15.5 Potential Effects of Receptor Blockade of Various Medications for Depression

Receptor Blocked		Potential Effects
NE	Norepinephrine	Decreased depression Tremors Tachycardia Erectile and/or ejaculatory dysfunction
α_1	Specific receptor for epinephrine	Antipsychotic effect Postural hypotension Dizziness Reflux tachycardia Ejaculatory dysfunction and/or impotence Memory dysfunction
α_2	Specific receptor for norepinephrine	Priapism
5-HT	Serotonin	Decreased depression Antianxiety effects Gastrointestinal disturbance Sexual dysfunction
5-HT_2	Serotonin	Decreased depression Decreased suicidal behavior Antipsychotic effects Hypotension Ejaculatory dysfunction Weight gain and carbohydrate craving
DA	Dopamine reuptake blocked	Decreased psychosis Psychomotor agitation Parkinsonian effect
Ach	Acetylcholine	Anticholinergic effects
H_1	Histamine	Sedation Weight gain Cognitive impairment

in the quality and quantity of adverse effects, complications, and patient compliance. Basic antidepressant classes include the following:

- First-line agents
  - SSRIs
  - Dual-action antidepressants (serotonin norepinephrine reuptake inhibitors [SNRIs], norepinephrine–dopamine reuptake inhibitors [NDRIs] and others)
  - Atypical antidepressants
- Second-line agents
  - Cyclic antidepressants (TCAs)
  - Monoamine oxidase inhibitors (MAOIs)

All subclasses of antidepressants share the following special considerations:

- They can precipitate a manic episode in a patient with bipolar disorder (BD). This can be prevented by administering a mood stabilizer, such as lithium, concurrently.
- They may precipitate a psychotic episode in a person with schizophrenia (rare).
- They have a delayed onset of effectiveness of several weeks.
- They must be discontinued slowly to prevent a *discontinuation syndrome.*
  - Symptoms may include anxiety, insomnia or vivid dreams, headaches, dizziness, tiredness, irritability, flu-like symptoms, including achy muscles and chills, nausea electric shock sensations, and return of depression symptoms.
- They have a Black Box warning for an increased risk of suicide.

Selective Serotonin Reuptake Inhibitors

SSRIs selectively block the neuronal uptake of serotonin (5-HT, 5-HT_1 receptors), leaving more serotonin available at the synaptic site. (See Chapter 4 for detailed information on the mechanism of action of SSRIs.)

SSRIs have a lower incidence of *anticholinergic side effects* (dry mouth, blurred vision, urinary retention), less cardiotoxicity, and faster onset of action than some other categories of antidepressants. SSRIs, SNRIs, and some of the newer antidepressants are considered first-line drugs of choice for the treatment of depression because they are better tolerated, with better medication adherence. The SSRIs seem to be effective in depression with anxiety features as well as in depression with psychomotor agitation. SSRIs are also safer in the event a patient attempts to overdose and may be preferred if suicidal ideation is a concern.

Indications. In addition to their use in treating depressive disorders, the SSRIs have been prescribed with success to treat some anxiety disorders, such as panic disorder, PTSD, and obsessive-compulsive spectrum disorders (refer to Chapter 11). Fluoxetine (Prozac) has been found to be effective in treating some women who suffer from premenstrual dysphoric disorder and bulimia nervosa.

Vortioxetine (Trintellix), a novel antidepressant, may effectively treat the symptoms of both depression and cognitive dysfunction in adults with MDD. This appears to be the only antidepressant that also improves cognition. The mechanism of action is similar to SSRIs, but it also acts as a 5-HT (serotonin) agonist, antagonist, and transport inhibitor. The most commonly reported negative side effects of vortioxetine are headache and nausea (Connolly & Thase, 2016).

Common Adverse Reactions. Agents that selectively enhance synaptic serotonin within the CNS may induce agitation, anxiety, sleep disturbance, tremor, sexual dysfunction (primarily anorgasmia in women), or tension headaches. The effect of SSRIs on sexual performance may be the most significant undesirable outcome reported by patients. These include loss of sexual desire and delayed or absent orgasm.

Autonomic reactions such as dry mouth, sweating, weight change, mild nausea, and loose bowel movements also may be experienced with the SSRIs. SSRIs show an increased risk of bleeding. See Table 15.6 for a general side-effect profile of the SSRIs.

Potential Toxic Effects. One rare and life-threatening event associated with the SSRIs is **serotonin syndrome.** This is thought to be related to overaction of the central serotonin receptors, caused by either too high a dose or by interaction with other drugs.

Use the S*H*I*V*E*R*S memory tool to help you recognize the symptoms of **serotonin syndrome:**

- **S**hivering
- **H**yperreflexia and myoclonus; muscular rigidity only in more severe cases
- **I**ncreased temperature, usually only in severe cases; likely caused by muscular hypertonicity
- **V**ital sign instability, presenting as tachycardia, tachypnea, and/or labile blood pressure
- **E**ncephalopathy—mental status changes such as agitation, delirium, and confusion
- **R**estlessness and incoordination—common because of excess serotonin activity
- **S**weating (diaphoresis)—an autonomic response to excessive serotonin stimulation

Severe manifestation can induce hyperpyrexia (excessively high fever), cardiovascular shock, or death.

The risk of this syndrome seems to be the greatest when an SSRI is administered in combination with a second serotonin-enhancing agent, such as a monoamine oxidase inhibitor (MAOI), another category of antidepressants, and/or over-the-counter cold medications. When switching between antidepressants, there needs to be a 2- to 5-week "washout" period of the SSRI or other antidepressants before starting an MAOI.

Box 15.3 gives emergency treatment guidelines for serotonin syndrome. Box 15.4 is a useful tool for patient and family teaching about SSRIs.

Serotonin–Norepinephrine Reuptake Inhibitors and Norepinephrine–Dopamine Reuptake Inhibitors

SNRI and NDRI antidepressants are referred to as dual-action reuptake inhibitors. Table 15.6 introduces dual-action reuptake inhibitors and identifies their strengths and side-effect profiles.

Atypical Antidepressants

Atypical antidepressants don't fit neatly into any of the other antidepressant categories. They include trazodone, mirtazapine, vilazodone, bupropion, and others. These drugs have different mechanisms of action and may be effective when the side effects of other antidepressants are problematic. (see Table 15.6).

Tricyclic Antidepressants

The tricyclic antidepressants (TCAs) increase levels of norepinephrine and serotonin and block the action of acetylcholine. Scientists believe that depression is relieved by restoring the balance of these neurotransmitters in the brain (Katz, 2016).

Patients must take therapeutic doses of TCAs for 4 to 8 weeks before full effectiveness is reached. Relief of some symptoms, such as insomnia and anorexia, may be noted sooner. A person who has shown a positive response to TCA therapy would probably be maintained on that medication for 6 to 12 months to prevent an early relapse.

A patient who is lethargic and fatigued may have the best results with a more stimulating TCA, such as desipramine (Norpramin) or protriptyline (Vivactil). If a more sedating effect is needed for agitation or restlessness, drugs such as amitriptyline (Elavil) and doxepin (Sinequan) may be more appropriate choices.

TABLE 15.6 Characteristics of Antidepressants

Special Considerations: All Antidepressants

- Black Box warning: Antidepressants increase the risk of suicidal thinking and behavior (suicidality) in children, adolescents, and young adults
- Increased risk of activation of mania/hypomania in susceptible individuals
- Delayed clinical response (most take 4–8 weeks for full effect)
- Remain on medication even when symptoms resolve
- Drugs must be tapered when discontinued to prevent a discontinuation syndrome

Subclass	Commonly Used Drugs	Potential Side Effects	Special Considerations/ Toxic Side Effects
Selective serotonin reuptake inhibitors (SSRIs)	Citalopram Escitalopram[a,b] Fluoxetine[b] Fluvoxamine[b] Paroxetine Sertraline[a,b]	Headaches Gastrointestinal disturbance Insomnia, fatigue Initial anxiety Sexual problems: reduces sexual drive; problems having and enjoying sex Agitation, feeling jittery and nervous Increased bleeding risk Can also treat anxiety disorders	Risk of **serotonin syndrome:** **S**hivering **H**yperreflexia **I**ncreased temperature **V**ital sign changes **E**ncephalopathy **R**estlessness **S**weating Hyponatremia Increased bleeding tendencies Avoid alcohol and herbal medications
Selective serotonin–norepinephrine reuptake inhibitor (SNRI) (Dual-action reuptake Inhibitors)	Venlafaxine Desvenlafaxine Duloxetine[b] Levomilnacipran	Initial increases in anxiety Insomnia Restlessness Sedation Possible sexual dysfunction Headaches Nausea Insomnia Dry mouth Elevated blood pressure (rare) Can also treat anxiety disorders	Risk of serotonin syndrome Hyponatremia Avoid alcohol and herbal medications
Atypical antidepressants	Nefazodone (serotonin antagonist and reuptake inhibitor [SARI])	Some formulations taken off the market due to acute liver failure	
	Mirtazapine (noradrenergic antagonist-specific serotonin antagonist [NaSSA])	Sedation Changes to appetite (less or increased) May help with insomnia and anxiety symptoms No sexual dysfunction or weight gain	Avoid alcohol
	Trazodone (serotonin antagonist and reuptake inhibitor [SARI])	Sedation Nausea Priapism (rare) May help with insomnia and anxiety symptoms	Avoid alcohol
	Bupropion (norepinephrine–dopamine reuptake inhibitor [NDRI])	Headache Agitation Insomnia Loss of appetite and weight loss Sweating No sexual side effects	Avoid alcohol and herbal medications
	Vilazodone (serotonin partial agonist–reuptake inhibitor [SPARI])	Fewer sexual side effects Less weight gain Gastrointestinal problems Helps reduce anxiety	Serotonin syndrome Caution taking vilazodone with foods/herbal product with antiplatelet/anticoagulant properties
	Vortioxetine (serotonin modulator and simulator [SMS])	Low risk of sexual side effects Weight gain Sedation May improve cognitive functioning in adults	Serotonin syndrome Increased risk of abnormal bleeding Hyponatremia

Continued

TABLE 15.6 **Characteristics of Antidepressants—cont'd**

Subclass	Commonly Used Drugs	Potential Side Effects	Special Considerations/ Toxic Side Effects
Tricyclic antidepressants (TCAs)	Imipramine[b] Amitriptyline Doxepin Desipramine Nortriptyline Clomipramine[b] Maprotiline Protriptyline Trimipramine Amoxapine	Weight gain Sedation Nausea Anticholinergic symptoms: dry mouth, blurred vision, urinary retention, constipation, tachycardia Orthostatic hypotension	Cardiotoxic side effects Avoid alcohol and herbal medications
Monoamine oxidase inhibitors (MAOIs)	Isocarboxazid Phenelzine Tranylcypromine Selegiline (comes in transdermal patch form for treatment of depression)	Weight gain Fatigue and sedation Sexual dysfunction Hypotension Muscle cramps Urinary hesitancy and constipation	Multiple **food–drug** and **drug–drug** interactions, causing **serotonin syndrome** and/or **hypertensive crisis:** • Severe increase in blood pressure • Tachycardia and shortness of breath • Chest pain • Severe headache • Nausea and vomiting • Sweating and severe anxiety • Nosebleeds NEVER to be taken with another antidepressant

[a]Indicates highest rates of continued medication compliance.
[b]Approved by the U.S. Food and Drug Administration (FDA) for use in children age 8 and older for the treatment of psychiatric disorders.
Santarsieri, D., & Schwartz, T. L. (2015). Antidepressant efficacy and side-effect burden: A quick guide for clinicians. *Drugs in Context, 4,* 212290. http://doi.org/10.7573/dic.212290

BOX 15.3 **Emergency Measures for Serotonin Syndrome**

1. Discontinue offending agent(s); call health care practitioner *immediately.*
2. Initiate symptomatic treatment per orders:
   - **Muscle relaxants.** Benzodiazepines can help control agitation, seizures, and muscle stiffness; (and /or) dantrolene for muscle relaxation.
   - **Serotonin-production blocking agents,** such as cyproheptadine, can help by blocking serotonin production.
   - **Oxygen and intravenous (IV) fluids.** O_2 helps maintain normal oxygen blood levels, and IV fluids treat dehydration and fever.
   - **Drugs that control heart rate and blood pressure.** These may include the following:
     - Esmolol (Brevibloc) or nitroprusside (Nitropress), to reduce increased heart rate or high blood pressure
     - Phenylephrine (Neo-Synephrine) or epinephrine (Adrenalin, EpiPen) for hypotension
   - Cooling blankets for high fever
   - Use of a breathing tube and machine and medication to paralyze muscles

TCAs have been used to treat nocturnal enuresis and as an adjunctive medication for chronic pain.

Common Adverse Reactions. The anticholinergic side effects of TCAs include dry mouth, blurred vision, tachycardia, constipation, urinary retention, esophageal reflux, photophobia, and sexual dysfunction. These adverse effects are usually not serious and are often transitory. Measures such as sips of water and sugarless gum or lozenges can help with dry mouth. Increasing fluid intake and diet changes to increase fiber can lessen constipation. Acute urinary retention and severe constipation warrant immediate medical attention. Have the patient void before taking the next dose of medication to lessen the potential effects of urinary hesitancy or retention.

The α-adrenergic blockade effects of TCAs can produce postural orthostatic hypotension and tachycardia. Postural hypotension can lead to dizziness and increase the risk of falls. Reminding patients to change positions slowly is helpful.

The histamine effect of TCAs causes sedation and weight gain. Administering the total daily dose of the TCA at night is beneficial for two reasons. First, the sedative effects aid sleep, and second, the minor side effects occur during sleep, which increases adherence with drug therapy. Table 15.6 reviews the side effects of commonly prescribed TCAs.

Potential Toxic Effects. The most serious side effects of the TCAs are cardiovascular in nature, including dysrhythmias, tachycardia, myocardial infarction, and heart block. Because the cardiac side effects are so serious, TCA use is considered a risk in patients with cardiac disease and in older adults. Patients should have a thorough cardiac workup before beginning TCA therapy. TCAs have a very high potential for lethality with overdose. These drugs can lower the seizure threshold and should be used with caution in people with pre-existing seizure disorders.

Drug–Drug Interactions. Individuals taking TCAs can have adverse reactions to numerous other medications. Common medications that should be avoided while taking TCAs are listed in Box 15.5. A patient who is taking any of these medications with a TCA should have a medical clearance beforehand because some of the reactions can be fatal.

Contraindications. Individuals who have recently had a myocardial infarction or other cardiovascular problems and those with narrow-angle glaucoma, benign prostatic hypertrophy, or a

BOX 15.4 Patient and Family Teaching About Selective Serotonin Reuptake Inhibitors (SSRIs)

- SSRIs may cause sexual dysfunction (impotence; difficulty achieving orgasm, especially in women) or lack of sex drive. Inform the health care provider. This can be treated.
- SSRIs may cause insomnia, anxiety, and nervousness. Some people also experience headache, fatigue, nausea, diarrhea, dry mouth, dizziness, or tremor. Symptoms tend to subside within a few weeks. Inform nurse or physician if they persist.
- SSRIs may cause a serious interaction with other medications and make other medications less effective. Be sure the physician knows all other medications the patient is taking. SSRIs should not be taken within 14 days of the last dose of a monoamine oxidase inhibitor (MAOI).
- No over-the-counter drugs should be taken, especially cold medications and herbal supplements, without first notifying the physician.
- Because of the potential for drowsiness and dizziness, do not drive or operate machinery until these side effects are ruled out.
- Alcohol should be avoided. People report increased effects of alcohol while taking an SSRI. Alcohol is also a central nervous system (CNS) depressant that may work against the desired effect of the SSRI.
- Liver and renal function tests should be performed, and blood counts checked periodically.
- Medication should not be discontinued abruptly to prevent a *discontinuation syndrome*: dizziness, nausea, diarrhea, muscle jerkiness, tremors, and rebound depression. If side effects from the SSRIs become bothersome, the patient should ask the health care professional about changing to a different drug. The drug will be slowly tapered before starting a new antidepressant.
- SSRIs should be used with caution in the elderly and in pregnant women. The benefits versus the risk must be considered in this population.
- Any of the following symptoms should be reported to a physician immediately:
  - Increase in depression or suicidal thoughts
  - Rash or hives
  - Rapid heartbeat
  - Sore throat
  - Difficulty urinating
  - Fever, malaise
  - Anorexia and weight loss
  - Unusual bleeding
  - Initiation of hyperactive behavior
  - Severe headache

BOX 15.5 Drugs to Be Used With Caution in Patients Taking a Tricyclic Antidepressant

- Phenothiazines ("conventional" antipsychotic)
- Barbiturates
- Monoamine oxidase inhibitors (risk for serotonin syndrome)
- Disulfiram (Antabuse)
- Oral contraceptives (or other estrogen preparations) (may decrease effectiveness)
- Anticoagulants
- Some antihypertensives (clonidine, guanethidine, reserpine)
- Benzodiazepines
- Alcohol
- Nicotine (may lower drug serum levels)
- St. John's wort
- Antihistamines (additive anticholinergic and sedative effects)

BOX 15.6 Patient and Family Teaching About Tricyclic Antidepressants

- Improvement in mood may take from 7 to 28 days after initiation of treatment. Families should be encouraged to reinforce this frequently. People with depression may have trouble remembering and respond to ongoing reassurance.
- Provide reassurance that drowsiness, dizziness, and hypotension usually subside after the first few weeks.
- Use caution when working around machines, driving cars, and crossing streets because of possible altered reflexes, drowsiness, or dizziness.
- Change position slowly to prevent dizziness upon standing.
- Dry mouth can be treated with sips of water, sugarless gum, and lozenges.
- Voiding before taking the medication can lessen urinary retention.
- Eat foods high in fiber and stay hydrated to decrease constipation.
- Alcohol can block the effects of antidepressants and increases sedative effects. Refrain from drinking alcohol.
- Take the full dose at bedtime to reduce sedation during the day.
- If bedtime dose or the once-a-day dose is missed, the next dose should be taken within 3 hours; otherwise, the patient should wait until the usual medication time the next day. Do not double the dose.
- Suddenly stopping TCAs can cause a discontinuation syndrome: nausea, altered heartbeat, nightmares, and cold sweats in 2 to 4 days. They are tapered slowly when discontinued.
- If suicidal ideation is present, have a family member limit access to medication. TCAs can be fatal in overdose.

history of seizures should not be treated with TCAs. Pregnant women should avoid the use of TCAs, except with extreme caution and careful monitoring.

Areas for the nurse to discuss when teaching patients and their families about TCA therapy are presented in Box 15.6.

Monoamine Oxidase Inhibitors (MAOIs)

MAOIs are antidepressant medications for patients who have not responded to other antidepressant medications and for atypical depression clinical presentation (see Table 15.6).

MAOIs can be useful in treating other disorders, such as panic disorder, social phobia, generalized anxiety disorder, obsessive-compulsive disorder, PTSD, bulimia, and refractory anxiety states. It is believed that MAOIs prevent the breakdown of norepinephrine, serotonin, and dopamine, which increases the levels of these amines in the brain, resulting in an elevated mood. (See Chapter 4 for detailed information on the mechanism of action of MAOIs.) Common adverse reactions and potential toxic effects of MAOIs are outlined in Table 15.6.

The MAOIs inhibit the breakdown of dietary tyramine in the liver. Increased levels of tyramine can lead to high blood pressure, hypertensive crisis, and potentially a cerebrovascular accident (stroke) and death. A hypertensive crisis is considered a medical emergency. Treatment consists of administering drugs to lower hypertension as quickly as possible.

Beginning clinical symptoms of a hypertensive crisis include the following:

- Severe headache or blurry vision
- Increasing chest pain and tachycardia
- Increasing shortness of breath
- Diaphoresis and anxiety
- Mental status changes; confusion
- Nausea and vomiting

TABLE 15.7 Foods That Can Interact With Monoamine Oxidase Inhibitors

Foods That Can Be Used in Small Amounts		
Chocolate	Contains phenylethylamine, large amounts can cause a reaction	
Ginseng	Headache, tremulousness, and mania-like reactions have occurred	
Caffeinated beverages	Caffeine is a weak pressor agent; large amounts may cause a reaction	
Category	**Unsafe Foods (High Tyramine Content)**	**Safe Foods (Little or No Tyramine) (Fresh Foods)**
Vegetables	Avocados, especially if overripe; fermented bean curd; fermented soybean; soybean paste; broad beans (fava bean pods); sauerkraut	Most fresh vegetables
Fruits	Figs, especially if overripe; bananas in large amounts (banana peel is extremely high in tyramine)	Most fresh fruits
Meats	Meats that are fermented, smoked, cured, or otherwise aged; spoiled meats; liver, unless very fresh	Meats that are known to be fresh (exercise caution in restaurants; meats may not be fresh)
Sausages	Fermented varieties: bologna, pepperoni, salami, air-dried sausages, others	Nonfermented varieties
Fish	Pickled herring and smoked salmon; lungfish roe, sliced schmaltz herring in oil, salmon mousse; dried, pickled, or cured fish; fish that is fermented, smoked, or otherwise aged; spoiled fish	Fish that is known to be fresh; vacuum-packed fish, if eaten promptly or refrigerated only briefly after opening
Milk, milk products	Practically all cheeses, especially hard cheeses	Milk, yogurt, cottage cheese, cream cheese
Foods with yeast	Yeast extract (e.g., Marmite, Bovril)	Baked goods that contain yeast
Beer, wine	Some imported beers, tap (draft) beers, some wines, Chianti	Major domestic brands of beer; most white wines
Other foods	Protein dietary supplements; soups (may contain protein extract); shrimp paste; soy sauce	

From Burchum, J., & Rosenthal, J. (2015). *Lehne's pharmacology for nursing care* (9th ed.). St. Louis: Elsevier.

Therefore people taking MAOIs must restrict their intake of tyramine so that their blood pressure does not rise to dangerous levels. See Table 15.7 for a list of foods that are high in tyramine and need to be avoided.

See Table 15.6 for an overview of MAOIs in current use. These are all given in an oral form. In 2006 the U.S. Food and Drug Administration (FDA) approved an MAOI that is delivered through a transcutaneous skin patch called the selegiline transdermal system (STS). Because of the unique delivery system, the liver and gastrointestinal (GI) system can function to break down dietary tyramine while still increasing the availability of neurotransmitters in the brain that help alleviate depression. STS does **not** require a tyramine-restricted diet at the 6-mg dosage over 4 hours. At higher doses (9 or 12 mg), dietary restrictions must be observed.

Box 15.7 can be used as an MAOI teaching guide and lists common adverse effects of MAOIs.

MAOIs also have multiple drug–drug interactions that can cause life-threatening adverse reactions. MAOIs should never be taken with another antidepressant. Patients should be advised to check with a physician when taking any additional medication or over-the-counter supplement.

Contraindications. The use of MAOIs may be contraindicated when one of the following is present:

- Cerebrovascular disease
- Hypertension and congestive heart failure
- Liver disease
- Consumption of foods containing tyramine, tryptophan, and dopamine (see Table 15.7)
- Use of multiple medications
- Recurrent or severe headaches
- Surgery in the previous 10 to 14 days
- Age younger than 16 years

Decisions about which specific drug to prescribe for any individual takes into account the specific symptoms displayed, the side-effect

BOX 15.7 Patient and Family Teaching About Monoamine Oxidase Inhibitors

- Review and provide a list of foods that must be avoided to prevent a serious adverse reaction.
- Give the patient a wallet card describing the monoamine oxidase inhibitor (MAOI) regimen.
- **Common side effects include** sedation, weakness, fatigue, weight gain, sexual dysfunction, muscle cramps, and cardiac rhythm problems.
- **Hypotension** is the most critical side effect, especially in the elderly (increased fall risk).
- Tell the patient to go to the **emergency department immediately** if a severe headache, chest pain, and severe nausea and vomiting develop from a drug–drug or food–drug reaction. These symptoms may indicate a medical emergency: hypertensive crisis.
- Monitor the patient's blood pressure for both hypotensive and hypertensive effects.
- Instruct the patient that dietary and drug restrictions should be maintained for 14 days after discontinuing MAOIs.
- Patients should be advised to tell their health care professional that they are taking an MAOI before starting any other over-the-counter or prescription medication.

profile, and comorbidities. Some subclasses of antidepressants and even specific drugs within a subclass work better for specific sets of symptoms.

Antipsychotics and Other Drugs

The FDA has approved aripiprazole and quetiapine slow-release tablets as an adjunctive treatment for depressive disorders and has approved the combination of olanzapine and fluoxetine for treatment-resistant depression. Other antipsychotics are used off-label to augment the effect of antidepressants for treatment-resistant depression. When these drugs are used, the patient must be monitored for the serious side effects associated with this class of drugs.

- Augmenting the treatment of depressive symptoms with the addition of lithium is another option for some individuals (Khouzam, 2016).
- There continue to be many new drugs in development for the treatment of depression. Many of these drugs have novel mechanisms of action. Some examples include the following:
  - ALKS 5461 (buprenorphine and samidorphan): a partial opioid agonist plus an opioid antagonist that rebalance brain function in patients with treatment-resistant depression
  - CERC-301: a selective *N*-methyl-D-aspartate (NMDA) receptor antagonist being developed as an adjunctive treatment for MDD
  - Amitifadine: inhibits serotonin, norepinephrine, and dopamine uptake

Ketamine (Ketalar), an anesthetic drug, and ketamine-like NMDA antagonists hold promise as a treatment for depression. These drugs also act on opioid receptors, which can impact pain and depression and neurotransmitters like glutamate. Studies indicate that ketamine can dramatically improve mood with just one dose and can be effective for treatment-resistant depression. The fact that they are quick acting makes these drugs especially useful for acutely suicidal patients. Ketamine is usually administered intravenously, and an intranasal formulation has recently become available. For most patients, the initial effect of the drug on depression fades within 1 to 3 days. Repeated treatment over months or even years may be required. The usual side effects include increased blood pressure and heart rate and a feeling of dissociation. These symptoms tend to resolve within hours. Some studies indicate that regular use of ketamine leads to memory and thinking issues. Currently, there are not enough comprehensive studies on the long-term effects of repeated use of these drugs to verify safety. This treatment is not widely available at this time but remains a promising treatment option (Watson, 2017).

Brain Stimulation Therapies

Electroconvulsive Therapy

Electroconvulsive therapy (ECT) is a procedure, done under general anesthesia, in which small electric currents are passed through the brain, intentionally triggering a brief seizure. *ECT* seems to cause changes in brain chemistry that can quickly reverse the symptoms of certain mental illnesses (Mayo Clinic Staff, 2018).

ECT remains one of the most effective treatments for treatment-resistant depression and major depression with psychotic symptoms and for the treatment of patients with life-threatening psychiatric conditions such as self-harm and acute mania. Clinical depression is considered treatment resistant when two or more pharmacological interventions fail. Treatment-resistant depression accounts for 20% to 30% of depressed individuals. ECT may also be used when the side effects of antidepressants are too uncomfortable or have been ineffective.

Although stigmatized for many years, ECT is safe and effective and can achieve a 70% to 90% remission rate in depressed patients within 1 to 2 weeks. The following list describes when ECT may be indicated:

- There is a need for a rapid, definitive response when a patient is suicidal or homicidal.
- The patient exhibits extreme agitation or psychomotor retardation and stupor.
- The patient has severe mania.
- The patient develops a life-threatening illness because of refusal of foods and fluids.
- The patient has a history of poor drug response, a history of good ECT response, or both.
- Standard medical treatment has no effect.

ECT is not necessarily effective in patients with chronic depression, atypical depression, personality disorders, drug dependence, or depression secondary to situational or social difficulties. The usual course of ECT for a depressed patient is 2 or 3 treatments per week for a total of 6 to 12 treatments.

Procedure. The procedure is explained to the patient, and informed consent is obtained. A short-acting general anesthetic (e.g., methohexital sodium) is used to allow the patient to be asleep during the short procedure. A neuromuscular blocking agent (e.g., succinylcholine chloride) is used to lessen the potential side effects of the induced seizure that is part of the procedure. An anticholinergic agent (e.g., glycopyrrolate) may also be used to lessen secretions and modulate the vagal response to the procedure. The patient is carefully monitored throughout the short procedure through the use of electroencephalogram (EEG) and electrocardiogram (ECG) monitoring.

Potential Adverse Reactions. Upon awakening from ECT, the patient may be confused and disoriented. The nurse may need to reorient the patient frequently during the postprocedure recovery period. Patients may complain of headache, muscle soreness, and nausea. These generally resolve quickly. Many patients state that they have short-term memory deficits for the first few hours to weeks after treatment. Memory deficits usually resolve. ECT is not a permanent cure for depression. Treatment following ECT usually includes resuming psychiatric medications and therapy for residual symptoms and to lessen the incidence of relapse. Maintenance ECT (once a week to once a month) may also help to decrease relapse rates for patients with recurrent depression. This procedure can be performed both inpatient and outpatient.

Although there are many treatment options available, some individuals continue to struggle with symptoms despite treatment. New methods are needed to help this group of individuals obtain relief from this debilitating illness (Mayo Clinic Staff, 2018).

Vagus Nerve Stimulation

Vagus nerve stimulation (VNS) is an FDA-approved adjunctive, long-term treatment for patients with treatment-resistant depression. The exact mechanism of action of VNS is not totally understood. VNS does affect blood flow to specific parts of the brain and affects neurotransmitters, including serotonin and norepinephrine, which are implicated in depression. A recent 5-year study confirmed the efficacy of this procedure for treatment-resistive depression (Aaronson et al., 2017). VNS involves surgically implanting a device called a pulse generator (similar to a pacemaker) into the upper left chest. The pulse generator is connected by a wire to the left vagus nerve. When the generator is stimulated, electrical impulses are transmitted to areas of the brain that affect mood, resulting in an improvement of depressive symptoms. Because the vagus nerve affects many functions of the brain, VNS is being studied for other conditions, such as anxiety disorders, Alzheimer's disease, migraines, and chronic pain/fibromyalgia.

Transcranial Magnetic Stimulation

Transcranial magnetic stimulation (TMS) applies the principles of noninvasive electromagnetism to deliver an electrical field to the cerebral cortices. Unlike in ECT, the waves do not result in generalized seizure activity. An electromagnetic coil is placed against the scalp near the forehead. The electromagnet painlessly delivers a magnetic pulse that stimulates nerve cells in the region of the brain involved in mood control and depression. It requires a series of 30- to 60-minute treatment sessions to be effective. Generally, sessions are carried out daily, five times a week, for 4 to 6 weeks. Symptoms relief may take a few weeks of treatment (Mayo Clinic Staff, 2018).

TMS it is considered safer than ECT and has minimal side effects, such as headache, scalp discomfort, or lightheadedness, that tend to resolve quickly. This treatment is considered effective for medication-resistant depression and some anxiety disorders (Rodriguez, 2016).

Deep Brain Stimulation

Deep brain stimulation (DBS), used in the treatment of Parkinson's patients and for chronic pain, is being used experimentally in patients with severe, treatment-resistant depression or OCD (NIMH, 2016). Electrodes must be surgically implanted into several areas of the brain affected by depression. An insulated wire is connected to an impulse generator, which is connected to a battery-powered device that generates stimulation to specific areas of the brain. The procedure carries the risk of brain hemorrhage and stroke, infection, disorientation and mood changes, movement disorders, lightheadedness, and trouble sleeping (NIMH, 2016). The efficacy of this treatment for depression has not been determined.

Complementary and Integrative Therapies

Light therapy is one method to treat seasonal affective disorder or the *DSM-5* diagnosis of major depressive disorder with seasonal pattern. Full-spectrum wavelength light is the specific type of light used. People with seasonal affective disorder often live in climates in which there are marked seasonal differences in the amount of daylight. Light therapy also may be useful as an adjunct to medications in treating chronic MDD or PDD with seasonal exacerbations. Light therapy is thought to be effective because of the influence of light on melatonin. Melatonin is secreted by the pineal gland and is necessary for maintaining and shifting biological rhythms. Exposure to light suppresses the nocturnal secretion of melatonin, which seems to have a therapeutic effect on people with seasonal affective disorder. Light therapy also appears to increase the availability of serotonin. Treatments consist of exposure to light balanced to replicate the effects of sunlight for 30 to 60 minutes a day.

Like all treatments, there are potential side effects. For those with bipolar depression, light therapy may trigger a manic episode or irritability. Other potential side effects are headache, nausea, and eyestrain. It is best to use this treatment after discussion with a mental health professional.

St. John's Wort

St. John's wort *(Hypericum perforatum)* is an over-the-counter whole-plant product with antidepressant properties that is not FDA approved. There are conflicting reports of the efficacy of this remedy. In one comprehensive study, the efficacy was generally comparable to low-dose TCAs and less so to SSRIs for mild depression and not effective for MDD. The herb is contraindicated for children and for women who are pregnant (WebMD Medical Reference, 2018). St. John's wort poses multiple harmful drug–drug interactions that can result in significant toxic effects on the liver. This plant is not regulated by the FDA, so there is no guarantee as to the amount of St. John's wort contained in over-the-counter preparations.

S-Adenosylmethionine

A study of **S-adenosylmethionine (SAMe)**, an over-the-counter dietary supplement, found it to be effective as an adjunct treatment in people with MDD who are resistant to other treatment. Multiple studies support the idea that SAMe is both safe and effective when used alone or as an add-on treatment for MDD (Sharma & Mischoulon, 2017). It is generally well tolerated.

Peer Support

We all experience positive results when talking to good friends regarding a problem or situation that is causing us difficulty. Studies indicate that peer support and support groups are important in helping people with depression. Support groups can decrease feelings of isolation, provide a buffer against stressful events, increase health information, and offer role models.

Self-Care for Nurses

People who are depressed often reject the presence of, friendship with, or interactions with others. Over time, family, friends, and health care workers can experience feelings of frustration, hopelessness, ineffectiveness, and annoyance. They may withdraw their concern and presence from the depressed individual. When working with depressed patients, nurses can experience the following:

- **Unrealistic expectations of self.** Setting unrealistic goals for the treatment of depressed individuals may result in the nurse feeling anxious, hurt, angry, and helpless or incompetent when the goals are not met. Identifying realistic expectations is one way to decrease feelings of helplessness and can increase the nurse's self-esteem and therapeutic potential.
- **Becoming depressed yourself.** It is common to experience feelings of hopelessness or depression when around a person who is depressed. This can occur subconsciously when we overidentify with the depressed individual and can result in withdrawal from the patient. The ability to recognize the true source of our own feelings is important. Consultation with a more experienced nurse/clinician can be helpful in dealing with any feelings that interfere with providing optimal care.

The Future of Treatment

There is a great need for earlier detection and intervention, achievement of remission, prevention of progression, and integration of neuroscience and behavioral science in the treatment of depression. High-risk ages and groups are in need of screening to facilitate early intervention. These include the following:

- Individuals in late adolescence and early adulthood (usual age of onset)
- Women in their reproductive years
- Adults and older adults with medical problems
- People with a family history of depression

There is also a need for education, particularly about the connection between physical symptoms and depression.

Future research may result in better genetic screening tools and a better understanding of the pharmacogenetics of depression treatment. The use of neuroimaging may soon become a common diagnostic tool.

EVALUATION

Short-term indicators and outcome criteria are continually evaluated. The nurse evaluates whether the patient still has suicidal or self-harm thoughts. Measurable outcome indicators include the ability to state alternatives to suicidal impulses in the future and to be able to explore thoughts and feelings that precede suicidal impulses. Outcomes relating to thought content and processes, self-esteem, and social interactions are frequently formulated because these areas are often problematic in people who are depressed.

Physical needs also warrant specific attention. Has there been an improvement in appetite, bowel functioning, and sleep? Is the person able to complete ADLs independently?

If the indicators have not been met, an analysis of the data, patient treatment goals, and planned nursing interventions is made. The patient's clinical picture and priority needs should be reassessed and the care plan reformulated when necessary.

KEY POINTS TO REMEMBER

- Depression is a very common psychiatric syndrome.
- There are a number of different presentations of depressive illnesses. Two primary depressive disorders are major depressive disorder (MDD) and persistent depressive disorder (dysthymia) (PDD).
- The symptoms in MDD are usually severe enough to interfere with a person's social or occupational functioning. Symptoms can include a sad mood, an inability to experience pleasure (anhedonia), significant weight loss, insomnia or hypersomnia, extreme fatigue (anergia), psychomotor agitation or retardation, diminished ability to think or concentrate, feelings of worthlessness, and suicidal ideation or recurrent thoughts of death.
- A person with MDD may or may not have psychotic symptoms.
- In PDD, the symptoms last for at least 2 years and can be mild to moderate. Usually, a person's social or occupational functioning is not as significantly impaired, although this illness can cause significant distress. The symptoms of PDD may appear to be the person's "usual" pattern of functioning.
- The most accepted theory of causation of depression is the biopsychosocial theory. A genetic predisposition combined with environmental stressors leads to brain changes that result in clinical depression. Cognitive theory, learned helplessness theory, and stressful life events help explain triggers to depression and the maintenance of depressive thoughts and feelings.
- Nursing assessment includes the evaluation of mood and affect; thought processes and thought content, especially suicidal thoughts or thoughts to harm others; physical symptoms and behavior; and communication changes. The nurse also needs to be aware of atypical symptoms associated with depression.
- The focus of care must include multiple areas:
  - Safety issues, including the risk of suicide, self-harm, and harm to others.
  - Mood states that may contribute to risk are an important focus of care. Look for feelings of hopelessness, helplessness, and worthlessness.
  - Psychosocial issues, such as problems with low self-esteem, issues with social interaction, and spiritual distress
  - Physical problems, such as decreased appetite, constipation, and sleep disturbances
  - Ability to complete ADLs independently
  - Coping and role performance
- Nursing interventions with patients who are depressed include the following:
  - Using specific principles of communication
  - Administering or participating in psychopharmacological therapy
  - Maintaining a therapeutic environment
  - Providing patient and family education
- There are several subclasses of antidepressants available to treat depressive disorders. Each subclass has different mechanisms of action, usual side effects, and toxic effects that influence the effectiveness of these drugs and how well they are tolerated by individual patients.
- Short-term psychotherapies that are effective in the treatment of depression include cognitive-behavioral therapy (CBT), interpersonal psychotherapy (IPT), and some forms of group therapy.
- Brain stimulation techniques include electroconvulsive therapy (ECT), transcranial magnetic stimulation (TMS), and vagus nerve stimulation (VNS). Each can be effective for treatment-resistant depression. Light therapy can be effective for seasonal affective disorder.
- Evaluation is ongoing throughout the nursing process. Patients' outcomes are compared with the stated outcome criteria and short-term and intermediate treatment goals. The plan of care is revised when desired outcomes are not being met.

APPLYING CRITICAL JUDGMENT

1. You notice that your patient, Mr. Plotsky, avoids eye contact, slouches in his seat, and displays a sad affect. Mr. Plotsky's psychiatry history reveals numerous bouts of major depression. He states, "This will be my last depression. I will never go through this again."
   A. What is your priority concern? What are the appropriate questions to ask Mr. Plotsky at this time?
   B. Give an example of the kinds of signs and symptoms you might find when you assess a patient with depression. What are expected behaviors, thought processes, activities of daily living, and ability to function at work and at home?
   C. Mr. Plotsky asks what causes depression. In simple terms, how might you respond?
   D. Mr. Plotsky asks you about the herb St. John's wort. What is some information he should have about its effectiveness, drug-drug interactions, and safety concerns?
   E. What are some of the brain stimulation treatment option for a patient who does not respond to drug therapy?
   F. Mr. Plotsky tells you that he has never tried therapy. What information could you give him about various therapeutic modalities that have proven effective?
2. When you are teaching Ms. Mac about the selective serotonin reuptake inhibitor (SSRI) sertraline, she asks you, "What makes this such a good drug?"
   A. What are some of the positive attributes of SSRIs? What are the side effects and toxic effects of the SSRIs?
   B. Devise a teaching plan for Ms. Mac.

CHAPTER REVIEW QUESTIONS

1. A 28-year-old second-grade teacher is diagnosed with major depressive disorder. She grew up in Texas but moved to Alaska 10 years ago to separate from an abusive mother. Her father died by suicide when she was 12 years old. Which combination of factors in this scenario best demonstrates the stress-diathesis model?
   a. Cold climate coupled with history of abuse
   b. Current age of 28 coupled with family history of depression
   c. Family history of mental illness coupled with history of abuse
   d. Female gender coupled with the stressful profession of teaching
2. A patient tells the nurse, "No matter what I do, I feel like there's always a dark cloud following me." Select the nurse's initial action.
   a. Assess the patient's current sleep and eating patterns.
   b. Explain to the patient, "Everyone feels down from time to time."
   c. Suggest alternative activities for times when the patient feels depressed.
   d. Say to the patient, "Tell me more about what you mean by 'a dark cloud.'"
3. A patient experiencing depression says to the nurse, "My health care provider said I need 'talk' therapy, but I think I need a prescription for an antidepressant medication. What should I do?" Select the nurse's best response.
   a. "Which antidepressant medication do you think would be helpful?"
   b. "There are different types of talk therapy. Most patients find it beneficial."
   c. "Let's consider some ways to address your concerns with your health care provider."
   d. "Are you willing to give 'talk therapy' a try before starting an antidepressant medication?"
4. The nurse cares for a hospitalized adolescent diagnosed with major depressive disorder. The health care provider prescribes a low-dose antidepressant. In consideration of published warnings about the use of antidepressant medications in younger patients, which action(s) should the nurse employ? (Select all that apply.)
   a. Notify the facility's patient advocate about the new prescription.
   b. Teach the adolescent about Black Box warnings associated with antidepressant medications.
   c. Monitor the adolescent closely for evidence of adverse effects, particularly suicidal thinking or behavior.
   d. Remind the health care provider about warnings associated with the use of antidepressants in children and adolescents.
5. Over the past 2 months a patient made eight suicide attempts, with increasing lethality. The health care provider informs the patient and family that electroconvulsive therapy (ECT) is needed. The family whispers to the nurse, "Isn't this a dangerous treatment?" How should the nurse reply?
   a. "Our facility has an excellent record of safety associated with use of electroconvulsive therapy."
   b. "Your family member will eventually be successful with suicide if aggressive measures are not promptly taken."
   c. "Yes, there are hazards with electroconvulsive therapy. You should discuss these concerns with the health care provider."
   d. "Electroconvulsive therapy is very effective when urgent help is needed. Your family member was carefully evaluated for possible risks."

REFERENCES

Aaronson, S. C., et al. (2017). A 5-Year observational study of patients with treatment-resistant depression treated with vagus nerve stimulation or treatment as usual: Comparison of response, remission, and suicidality. *American Journal of Psychiatry 2017, 174*(7), 640–648. https://doi.org/10.1176/appi.ajp.2017.16010034.

American Psychiatric Association (APA). (2013). *Diagnostic and statistical manual of mental disorders (DSM-5)* (5th ed.). Washington, DC: APA.

Beck, A. T., & Rush, A. J. (1995). Cognitive therapy. In H. I. Kaplan, & B. J. Sadock (Eds.), *Comprehensive textbook of psychiatry* (6th ed.) (Vol. 2) (pp. 1847–1856). Baltimore: Williams & Wilkins.

Bonin, L. (2016). *Patient education: Depression in children and adolescents (Beyond the Basics)*. UpToDate, Inc., Topic 4867 Version 21.0, Retrieved from https://www.uptodate.com/contents/depression-in-children-and-adolescents-beyond-the-basics.

Centers for Disease Control and Prevention (CDC). (2015). Suicide facts at a glance 2015 national center for injury prevention and control, Division of

Violence Prevention. Retrieved from https://www.cdc.gov/violenceprevention/pdf/suicide-datasheet-a.pdf.

Centers for Disease Control and Prevention (CDC). (2017). Depression is not a normal part of growing older. Division of Population Health, National Center for Chronic Disease Prevention and Health Promotion, Retrieved from https://www.cdc.gov/aging/mentalhealth/depression.htm.

Chen, J. (2015). *Why depression needs a new definition.* Retrieved January 22, 2016, from http://www.theatlantic.com/health/archive/2015/08/why-depression-needs-a-new-definition/399–9021.

Connolly, K. R., & Thase, M. E. (2016). Vortioxetine: A new treatment for major depressive disorder. *Expert Opinions in Pharmacotherapy*, *17*(3), 421–431. https://doi.org/10.1517/14656566.2016.1133588.

Crowther, A. (2015). Resting-state connectivity predictors of response to psychotherapy in major depressive disorder. *Neuropsychopharmacology.* https://doi.org/10.1038/npp.2015.12.

Cunningham, J. E. A., & Shapiro, C. M. (2018). Cognitive Behavioural Therapy for Insomnia (CBT-I) to treat depression: A systematic review. *Journal of Psychosomatic Research*, *106*, 1–12. https://doi.org/10.1016/j.jpsychores.2017.12.012.

Davenport, L. (2016). *Widely prescribed antidepressant linked to birth defects.* Retrieved January 23, 2016, from http://www.medscape.com/viewarticle/857244.

Derewicz, M. (2015). *Brain scans predict effectiveness of talk therapy to treat depression.* Retrieved September 15, 2015, from http://news.unchealthcare.org./2015/january/brain-scans-predict-effectiveness-of-talk-therapy-to-treat-depression.

Dickson, E. (2020). *A message from Dr. Eric Dickson.* Retrieved from https://www.umassmemorialhealthcare.org/umass-memorial-center-mindfulness.

Fava, M., Ostergaard, S. D., & Cassano, P. (2016). Mood disorders: Depressive disorders (major depressive disorders). In T. A. Stern, M. Fava, T. E. Wilens, et al. (Eds.), *Massachusetts General Hospital comprehensive clinical psychiatry* (2nd ed.). China: Elsevier, Inc.

Freedman, D., et al. (2017). The effects of improving sleep on mental health (OASIS): A randomised controlled trial with mediation analysis, *The Lancet. Psychiatry*, *4*(10), 749–758. https://doi.org/10.1016/S2215-0366(17)30328-0.

Giddens, J. (2017). *Concepts for nursing practice* (2nd ed.). St. Louis: Elsevier.

Harvard Health Publishing. (2017). What causes depression?. Retrieved from https://www.health.harvard.edu/mind-and-mood/what-causes-depression.

IsHak, W., et al. (2017). Screening for depression in hospitalized medical patients. *Journal of Hospital Medicine*, *12*(2), 118–125. Retrieved from https://www.journalofhospitalmedicine.com/jhospmed/article/130454/hospital-medicine/screening-depression-hospitalized-medical-patients.

Katz, M. (2016). Tricyclic antidepressants (TCAs) drugs FAQ. Retrieved from https://www.rxlist.com/tricyclic_antidepressants_tcas/drugs-condition.htm.

Khouzam, H. R. (2016). Second-generation antipsychotics for treatment-resistant major depressive disorder in primary care. *Consultant*, *56*(3), 217–220. Retrieved from https://www.consultant360.com/articles/second-generation-antipsychotics-treatment-resistant-major-depressive-disorder-primary-care.

Knapton, S. (2016). *Antidepressants can raise the risk of suicide, biggest ever review finds.* Retrieved from http://www.telegraph.co.uk/science/2016/03/14/antidepressants-can-raise-the-risk-of-suicide-biggest-ever-revie/.

Kok, R. M., & Reynolds, C. F. (2017). Management of depression in older adults: A review. *Journal of the American Medical Association*, *317*(20), 2114–2122. https://doi.org/10.1001/jama.2017.5706.

Li, Ye, et al. (2017). Dietary patterns and depression risk: A meta-analysis. *Psychiatry Research*, *253*, 373–382. https://doi.org/10.1016/j.psychres.2017.04.020.

Lliades, C. (2015). *Stats and facts about depression in America. Everyday health.* Retrieved June 18, 2015, from www.everydayhealth.com/health-report/major-depression/depression-statistics.aspx.

Lusk, P. (2017). *APNA 30th Annual Conference, October 19-22, 2016, Hartford, Connecticut.* Paper presented at the Journal of the American Psychiatric Nurses Association.

MacKenzie, M. B., & Kocovski, N. L. (2016). Mindfulness-based cognitive therapy for depression: Trends and developments. *Psychology Research and Behavior Management*, *9*, 125–132. https://doi.org/10.2147/PRBM.S63949.

Mayo Clinic Staff. (2018). *Electroconvulsive Therapy.* Retrieved March 2018, https://www.mayoclinic.org/tests-procedures/electroconvulsive-therapy/about/pac-20393894.

Mayo Foundation for Medical Education and Research (MFMER) (n.d). (2017). *Mayo Clinic, depression (major depressive disorder).* Retrieved from https://www.mayoclinic.org/diseases-conditions/depression/symptoms-causes/syc-20356007.

MDD Clinical Practice Review Task Force. (2016). Clinical practice review for major depressive disorder, Anxiety and Depression Association of America, February 2, 2016, Retrieved from https://adaa.org/resources-professionals/practice-guidelines-mdd.

Melville, N. A. (2016). *Antidepressant use linked to increase brain bl eed risk.* Retrieved January 22, 2016, from https://www.medscape.com/viewarticle/857102.

Mental Health America. (2018). The state of mental health in America. Retrieved from http://www.mentalhealthamerica.net/issues/state-mental-health-america.

National Institute of Health, National Institute of Aging. (2017). Depression and older adults, content reviewed. Retrieved from https://www.nia.nih.gov/health/depression-and-older-adult.

National Institute of Mental Health (NIMH). (2015). *Depression in children and adolescents fact sheet.* Retrieved June 18, 2015, from www.nimh.nih.gov.

National Institute of Mental Health (NIMH). (2016). Brain stimulation therapies. Retrieved March 25, 2018, https://www.nimh.nih.gov/health/topics/brain-stimulation-therapies/brain-stimulation-therapies.shtml.

National Institute of Mental Health (NIMH). (2017). Major depression. Retrieved from https://www.nimh.nih.gov/health/statistics/prevalence/major-depression-among-adults.shtml.

Nguyen, Theresa, et al. (2017). State of mental health in America. Retrieved from http://www.mentalhealthamerica.net/issues/state-mental-health-america#Key.

O'Connor, E., Rossom, R. C., Henninger, M., et al. (2016). *Screening for depression in adults: An updated systematic evidence review for the U.S. preventive services task force.* Rockville, MD: Agency for Healthcare Research and Quality. (Evidence Syntheses, No. 128.) Retrieved from https://www.ncbi.nlm.nih.gov/books/NBK349027/.

Preston, J., & Johnson, J. (2015). *Clinical psychopharmacology made ridiculously simple* (8th ed.). Miami: MedMaster.

Psychology Today. (2017). Depressive disorders (Children and Adolescents). Retrieved from https://www.psychologytoday.com/conditions/depressive-disorders-children-and-adolescents.

Rodriguez, T. (2016). *Transcranial magnetic stimulation effective for major depressive disorder.* Retrieved March 2018 from http://www.psychiatryadvisor.com/apa-2016-coverage/transcranial-magnetic-stimulation-effective-treatment-for-mdd-and-gad/article/497801/.

Sadock, B. J., Sadock, V. A., & Ruiz, P. (2015). *Kaplan & Sadock's synopsis of psychiatry: Behavioral sciences/clinical psychiatry* (11th ed.). Philadelphia: Lippincott Williams & Wilkins.

Schendel, D. (2017). Prenatal antidepressant use and risk of autism. *British Medical Journal*, *358*. https://doi.org/10.1136/bmj.j3388.

Schuch, F. B., Deslandes, A. C., Stubbs, B., Gosmann, N. P., Silva, C. T., & Fleck, M. P. (2016). Neurobiological effects of exercise on major depressive disorder: A systematic review. *Neuroscience & Biobehavioral Reviews*, *61*, 1–11. https://doi.org/10.1016/j.neubiorev.2015.11.012. Epub 2015 Dec 2.

Seligman, M. E. (1973). Fall into hopelessness. *Psychology Today*, *7*, 43.

Sharma, A., & Mischoulon, D. (2017). Expert's corner: When should SAMe be considered for major depression? *Psychiatric News.* Retrieved from https://psychnews.psychiatryonline.org/doi/full/10.1176/appi.pn.2017.pp7b3.

Sheng, J., Liu., S, Wang, Y, Cui., R., & Zhang., X. (2017). The link between depression and chronic pain: Neural mechanisms in the brain. *Neural Plasticity*, *10, 9724371*. https://doi.org/10.1155/2017/9724371.

Solis, Michele (2016). Personalised treatment for depression on the horizon: predicting response to antidepressants. *Pharmaceutical Journal*, Retrieved from https://www.pharmaceutical-journal.com/news-and-analysis/features/personalised-treatment-for-depression-on-the-horizon-predicting-response-to-antidepressants/20201782.article.

U.S. Preventive Services Task Force (USPSTF). (2016). Depression in adults: Screening, recommendation summary. Retrieved from https://www.uspreventiveservicestaskforce.org/Page/Document/UpdateSummaryFinal/depression-in-adults-screening1.

Vandeleur, C. L. et al. (2017). Prevalence and correlates of DSM-5 major depressive and related disorders in the community, *Psychiatry Research*, *250*, 50–58. Retrieved from http://www.psy-journal.com/article/S0165-1781(16)31416-0/abstract.

Watson, S. (2017). Ketamine and depression: FAQ. WebMD Health News. Retrieved from https://www.webmd.com/mental-health/news/20170706/ketamine-and-depression-faq.

WebMD Medical Reference. (2016). *Children and depression*. Retrieved from https://www.webmd.com/depression/guide/depression-children#1.

WebMD Medical Reference. (2018). St. John's Wort for Treating Depression. Retrieved from https://www.webmd.com/depression/guide/st-johns-wort#1.

Williams, J., & Nieuwsma, J. (2018). Screening for depression in adults. UpToDate. Retrieved from https://www.uptodate.com/contents/screening-for-depression-in-adults.

World Health Organization (WHO). (2017). Depression fact sheet. Retrieved from http://www.who.int/mediacentre/factsheets/fs369/en/.

16

Bipolar Spectrum Disorders

Lorraine Chiappetta, Elizabeth M. Varcarolis

http://evolve.elsevier.com/Varcarolis/essentials

OBJECTIVES

1. Compare predisposing factors associated with the development of bipolar spectrum disorders.
2. Identify the different clinical manifestations of the bipolar spectrum disorders, including hypomania, mania, and delirious mania.
3. Discuss the behaviors, speech patterns, thought processes, and thought content of a person diagnosed with bipolar spectrum disorders.
4. Describe evidence-based practice interventions for bipolar spectrum disorders. **QSEN: Evidence-Based Practice**
5. Contrast physical, safety, personal, and legal considerations when providing safe and effective care to a patient in an acute phase of mania. **QSEN: Safety**
6. Discuss patient-centered communication strategies that are effective with patients in an acute manic state. **QSEN: Patient-Centered Care**
7. Describe components of interprofessional and intraprofessional teamwork and collaboration that facilitate safe and effective care for a person in the acute phase of mania. **QSEN: Teamwork and Collaboration; Safety**
8. Describe components of a safe milieu for a hospitalized patient in an acute manic state.
9. Compare and contrast treatment for a person in the acute manic phase and maintenance phase of bipolar I disorder.
10. Using informatics, identify expected side effects of lithium therapy. **QSEN: Informatics**
11. Distinguish between the signs and symptoms and of early and severe lithium toxicity and associated nursing interventions.
12. Using informatics, describe the use of antiepileptic drugs (AEDs) as mood stabilizers in the treatment of bipolar disorders. **QSEN: Informatics**
13. Using informatics, identify which antipsychotic medications are used in the treatment of bipolar disorders. **QSEN: Informatics**
14. Develop a patient-centered teaching plan for a person diagnosed with bipolar disorder. **QSEN: Patient-Centered Care**

KEY TERMS AND CONCEPTS

acute phase, p. 236
antiepileptic drugs (AEDs), p. 240
bipolar I disorder, p. 228
bipolar II disorder, p. 228
clang associations, p. 234
continuation phase, p. 235
cyclothymic disorder, p. 229
electroconvulsive therapy (ECT), p. 242
finger foods, p. 238
flight of ideas, p. 234
hypomania, p. 228
lithium, p. 237
maintenance phase, p. 235
mania, p. 228
mixed episode, p. 228
pressured speech, p. 234
psychoeducation, p. 242
rapid cycling, p. 228
seclusion protocol, p. 237

CONCEPT: ADHERENCE: *Adherence* is a self-initiated action taken to promote wellness, recovery, and rehabilitation. Adherence to prescribed therapy is a key component of care in mental health settings. One in four patients experiencing psychosis demonstrates nonadherence. Estimates of medication nonadherence for patients with mental illness are 24% to 90%. Some suggest patients are more likely to adhere when the treatment recommended fits with their expectations (Giddens, 2017). It is important not to reject, blame, or shame the patient when nonadherence occurs. Instead, label it simply an issue for continuing focus and accept that achieving adherence often requires numerous attempts.

INTRODUCTION

Bipolar disorders, previously known as manic-depressive illness, are a group of brain diseases characterized by unusual shifts in mood, energy, and activity levels leading to difficulties in carrying out day-to-day tasks (National Institute of Mental Health [NIMH], 2016). These can include recurring depression and/or recurrent elevated, expansive, and irritable moods (mania) alternating with periods of normalcy. The term *bipolar spectrum disorders* (BSDs) refers to conditions that include bipolar disorder and other types of mental conditions that can involve depression or mood swings (WebMD Medical Reference, 2017).

BSDs are labeled as bipolar and related disorders in the *Diagnostic and Statistical Manual of Mental Disorders,* 5th edition (*DSM-5*; American Psychiatric Association [APA], 2013). The labels can be used interchangeably. These disorders are chronic, recurrent, and life-threatening illnesses that require lifetime monitoring. They can lead to significant morbidity and disability. According to Brooks (2015), bipolar disorders are increasingly being diagnosed at younger ages. BSDs can be difficult to accurately diagnose. Some individuals live 8 to 10 years with symptoms before obtaining a diagnosis and proper treatment.

BSDs are currently conceptualized as a bridge between depressive disorders and schizophrenia spectrum disorders in terms of symptomatology, family history, and genetics (APA, 2013). They include a range of symptoms on a continuum. At one end is **mania**, which constitutes an exaggerated, elevated, expansive, or irritable mood, accompanied by a persistent increase in activity and/or energy. This end of the spectrum can also include hypomania, a lower intensity of mania (APA, 2013). On the other end is depressive symptoms. Persons with this disorder may experience an acute episode of mania or hypomania or an acute episode of depression at any one time. A person can also experience a **mixed episode** in which there are concurrent symptoms of both depression and mania. Periods of normal functioning may alternate with these acute episodes of illness. Slightly less than half of individuals with BSDs regain full occupational, interpersonal, and/or social functioning even during remission.

BIPOLAR SPECTRUM DISORDERS

The following list includes the most common presentations of the disorder (APA, 2013):

- **Bipolar I disorder** is characterized by at least one episode of "persistent or elevated, expansive or irritable mood" (mania), accompanied by changes in activity and energy. The diagnosis frequently includes a major depressive episode as part of a person's psychiatric *history.* (Refer to Chapter 15 on depressive disorders.) There is marked impairment in social and occupational functioning. Psychosis may accompany the manic episode or the depressive episode, and hospitalization may be warranted.
- The criteria for **bipolar II disorder** include at least one period of **hypomania** alternating with one or more periods of depression. Those with a bipolar II disorder never experience a full manic episode. Typically, an individual seeks treatment during a depressive episode. The brief periods of hypomania may be missed. "*A decreased need for sleep and a lot of daytime fatigue are the red flags for hypomania*" (Preston & Johnson, 2015, p. 21). Those with bipolar II disorder tend to have more severe depressive symptoms and spend more time in a depressive state.

As described in the *DSM-5* (APA, 2013), when determining a diagnosis of bipolar and related disorders, it is useful to identify the following:

- Current episode (manic, hypomanic, or depressed)
- Severity (mild, moderate, or severe)
- With psychosis (if this is present)
- Whether the episode is active or in partial or full remission

Additional *specifiers* are added to identify important sets of symptoms that may accompany the disorder. These include the following:

- With anxious distress—those with significant anxiety symptoms.
- With mixed features—presence of depressive symptoms with hypomanic or manic symptoms. The essential symptoms for the specifier "with mixed features" include the following:
  - Significant suicide risk
  - Marked irritability
  - Pessimism and unrelenting worry and despair
  - Decreased need for sleep (Preston & Johnson, 2015)
- With **rapid cycling**—four or more mood episodes in a 12-month period. Rapid cycling usually indicates less global functioning and greater resistance to conventional somatic treatments.
- With melancholic features—a depressive episode with a significant inability to feel pleasure.
- With atypical features—symptoms of the depressive episode are not the usual symptoms of depression.
- With peripartum onset—mood symptoms begin during or in the months after pregnancy.
- With seasonal pattern—when depressive symptoms occur during certain seasons.
- With psychotic features—symptoms of psychosis (hallucinations, delusions, paranoia) occur during a mood episode; the psychosis may be mood congruent, meaning the content of the psychosis goes with the current mood or mood incongruent, when the content doesn't go with the current mood.
- With catatonic features—extremes of physical activity and speech. (APA, 2013)

The distinction between bipolar I and bipolar II diagnoses in conjunction with the identification of specifiers is crucial. Each of these different presentations dictates the most appropriate medical interventions. This is particularly true of the mixed-features and rapid-cycling specifiers (Preston & Johnson, 2015).

Manic Episode

Symptoms associated with mania are as follows (Box 16.1):

- Feelings of euphoria and elation or irritability and anger
- Impulsive, high-risk behavior, including grand shopping sprees, drug and alcohol misuse, and sexual promiscuity
- Increased activity and aggressive behavior
- Increased energy and rapid speech
- Fleeting, often grandiose ideas
- Decreased sleep (typically the individual doesn't feel tired after as few as 3 hours of sleep)
- Decreased appetite
- Difficulty concentrating; disorganized thoughts
- Inflated self-esteem
- Delusions and hallucinations (in severe cases) (Tartakovsky, 2017)

(Please refer to the *DSM-5* [APA, 2013] diagnostic criteria for more details.)

Hypomanic Episode

Hypomania is a less severe and less intense form of mania and must last at least 4 days. The hypomanic episode must include a noticeable change in functioning that is uncharacteristic of the individual. Occupational and social functioning are less impaired. Psychotic symptoms are not present (APA, 2013). Refer to Table 16.1 for the differences between hypomania and mania.

BOX 16.1 Memory Tool for Symptoms of Mania

- **D**istractibility
- **I**mpulsivity
- **G**randiosity
- **F**light of ideas/racing thoughts
- **A**ctivity/energy increase
- **S**leep needs diminish
- **T**alkative

TABLE 16.1 Mania on a Continuum

Hypomania	Acute Mania
Communication	
1. Talks and jokes incessantly, is the "life of the party," and gets irritated when not center of attention 2. Treats everyone with familiarity and confidentiality; often borders on crude 3. Talk is often sexual—can reach obscene, inappropriate propositions to total strangers 4. Talk is tangential; jumps from one topic to the next; *pressure of speech* (rapid talking, loud, and can be difficult to interrupt)	1. May change suddenly from laughing to anger or depression; *mood is labile* 2. Becomes inappropriately demanding of people's attention, and intrusive nature repels others 3. Speech may be marked by profanities and crude sexual remarks to everyone (nursing staff in particular). 4. Speech marked by *flight of ideas,* in which thoughts race and fly from topic to topic; may have *clang associations.*
Affect and Thinking	
1. Persistently elevated, expansive, or irritable mood 2. Full of pep and good humor, feelings of euphoria and sociability; may show inappropriate intimacy with strangers 3. Feels boundless self-confidence and enthusiasm. Has elaborate grandiose schemes for becoming rich and famous. Initially, schemes may seem plausible. 4. Judgment often poor. Gets involved with schemes in which job, marriage, or financial status may be destroyed. 5. May write large quantities of letters to rich and famous people regarding schemes 6. Decreased attention span to internal and external cues 7. Limited insight	1. Abnormally persistently elevated, expansive, or irritable mood 2. Good humor gives way to increased irritability and hostility and short-lived period of rage, especially when controls are set on behavior. May have quick shifts of mood from anger to submissive. 3. Grandiose delusions—may come to believe they are famous or especially gifted without any basis in fact 4. Judgment is extremely poor. 5. Decreased attention span and distractibility are intensified. 6. Lack of insight about illness or consequences of behavior
Physical Behavior	
1. Overactive, distractible, buoyant, and busily occupied with grandiose plans (not delusions); goes from one action to the next 2. Increased sexual appetite; sexually irresponsible and indiscreet. Unplanned pregnancies and sexually transmitted diseases. Sex used for escape, not for relating to another human being. 3. May have a voracious appetite, eat on the run, or gobble food during brief periods 4. May go without sleeping; unaware of fatigue; may be able to take short naps 5. Financially extravagant, goes on buying sprees, gives money and gifts away freely, can easily go into debt	1. Extremely restless, disorganized, and chaotic. Physical behavior may be difficult to control. May have outbursts, such as throwing things or becoming briefly assaultive when crossed. 2. No time to eat—too distracted and disorganized 3. No time for sleep—psychomotor activity too high; if unchecked, can lead to exhaustion and death 4. Same as in hypomania but in the extreme
Delirious Mania	
1. Most severe form of mania; less common 2. Acute onset and rapid progression 3. Consists of symptoms of both delirium and mania 4. Severe clouding of consciousness, disorientation, fluctuating sensorium, psychosis, catatonia, and manic symptoms (excitement, grandiosity, insomnia, etc.)	

Depressive Episode

Symptoms associated with depression are as follows:

- Feelings of hopelessness and sadness
- Inability to sleep or sleeping too much
- Loss of interest in formerly enjoyable activities; loss of energy
- Changes in appetite and weight
- Feelings of worthlessness and inappropriate guilt
- Inability to concentrate or make a decision
- Thoughts of death and suicide (Tartakovsky, 2017)

(Please refer to the *DSM-5* [APA, 2013] diagnostic criteria for more details.)

Cyclothymic Disorder

Cyclothymic disorder presents with hypomanic episodes alternating with persistent depressive episodes (dysthymia) for at least 2 years' duration, or 1 year in children. Individuals with cyclothymia tend to have irritable hypomanic episodes (APA, 2013).

There are significant differences between unipolar and bipolar depression. **Unipolar depression** is (see Chapter 15) characterized by a history of one or more major depressive episodes with no history of manic or hypomanic symptoms. **Bipolar depression** is best understood as the presence of symptoms of a major depressive disorder in a person with a history of mania or hypomania. Distinguishing *bipolar disorder (BP)* from *unipolar depression* has important relevance for prognosis and treatment.

Patients with **bipolar depression** are less likely to be female and to report symptoms of diminished interest. There is an increased risk of an earlier initial onset, with more total episodes over time. Disturbances in sleep include hypersomnia, excessive tiredness, and difficult morning waking. Changes in appetite occur, such as binge eating and cravings for carbohydrates. These may alternate with periods of loss of appetite. Bipolar depression is more often marked by psychomotor retardation (a slowing down of motor activity). There is a higher risk of substance use disorders and suicide as compared to unipolar depression. Labile emotions (frequently changing emotional states), including more irritability, are frequently present. Psychosis may be

DSM-5 DIAGNOSTIC CRITERIA

Bipolar I Disorder

For a diagnosis of bipolar I disorder, it is necessary to meet the following criteria for a manic episode. The manic episode may have been preceded by and may be followed by hypomanic or major depressive episodes.

Manic Episode

A. A distinct period of abnormally and persistently elevated, expansive, or irritable mood and abnormally and persistently increased goal-directed activity or energy, lasting at least 1 week and present most of the day, nearly every day (or any duration if hospitalization is necessary).

B. During the period of mood disturbance and increased energy or activity, three (or more) of the following symptoms (four if the mood is only irritable) are present to a significant degree and represent a noticeable change from usual behavior:
  1. Inflated self-esteem or grandiosity.
  2. Decreased need for sleep (e.g., feels rested after only 3 hours of sleep).
  3. More talkative than usual or pressure to keep talking.
  4. Flight of ideas or subjective experience that thoughts are racing.
  5. Distractibility (i.e., attention too easily drawn to unimportant or irrelevant external stimuli), as reported or observed.
  6. Increase in goal-directed activity (either socially, at work or school, or sexually) or psychomotor agitation (i.e., purposeless non-goal-directed activity).
  7. Excessive involvement in activities that have a high potential for painful consequences (e.g., engaging in unrestrained buying sprees, sexual indiscretions, or foolish business investments).

C. The mood disturbance is sufficiently severe to cause marked impairment in social or occupational functioning or to necessitate hospitalization to prevent harm to self or others, or there are psychotic features.

D. The episode is not attributable to the physiological effects of a substance (e.g., a drug of abuse, a medication, other treatment) or to another medical condition.

Note: A full manic episode that emerges during antidepressant treatment (e.g., medication, electroconvulsive therapy) but persists at a fully syndromal level beyond the physiological effect of that treatment is sufficient evidence for a manic episode and, therefore, a bipolar I diagnosis.

Note: Criteria A through D constitute a manic episode. At least one lifetime manic episode is required for the diagnosis of bipolar I disorder.

Hypomanic Episode

A. A distinct period of abnormally and persistently elevated, expansive, or irritable mood and abnormally and persistently increased activity or energy, lasting at least 4 consecutive days and present most of the day, nearly every day.

B. During the period of mood disturbance and increased energy and activity, three (or more) of the following symptoms (four if the mood is only irritable) have persisted, represent a noticeable change from usual behavior, and have been present to a significant degree:
  1. Inflated self-esteem or grandiosity.
  2. Decreased need for sleep (e.g., feels rested after only 3 hours of sleep).
  3. More talkative than usual or pressure to keep talking.
  4. Flight of ideas or subjective experience that thoughts are racing.
  5. Distractibility (i.e., attention to easily drawn to unimportant or irrelevant external stimuli), as reported or observed.
  6. Increase in goal-directed activity (either socially, at work or school, or sexually) or psychomotor agitation.
  7. Excessive involvement in activities that have a high potential for painful consequences (e.g., engaging in unrestrained buying sprees, sexual indiscretions, or foolish business investments).

C. The episode is associated with the unequivocal change in functioning that is uncharacteristic of the individual when not symptomatic.

D. The disturbance in mood and the change in functioning are observable by others.

E. The episode is not severe enough to cause marked impairment in social or occupational functioning or to necessitate hospitalization. If there are psychotic features, the episode is, by definition, manic.

F. The episode is not attributable to the physiological effects of a substance (e.g., a drug of abuse, a medication, other treatment).

Note: A full hypomanic episode that emerges during antidepressant treatment (e.g., medication, electroconvulsive therapy) but persists at a fully syndromal level beyond the physiological effect of that treatment is sufficient evidence for a hypomanic episode diagnosis. However, caution is indicated so that one or two symptoms (particularly increased irritability, edginess, or agitation following antidepressant use) are not taken as sufficient for diagnosis of a hypomanic episode, nor necessarily indicative of a bipolar diathesis.

Note: Criteria A through F constitute a hypomanic episode. Hypomanic episodes are common in bipolar I disorder but are not required for the diagnosis of bipolar I disorder.

Major Depressive Episode

A. Five (or more) of the following symptoms have been present during the same 2-week period and represent a change from previous functioning; at least one of the symptoms is either (1) depressed mood or (2) loss of interest or pleasure.

Note: Do not include symptoms that are clearly attributable to another medical condition.
  1. Depressed mood most of the day, nearly every day, as indicated by either subjective report (e.g., feels sad, empty, or hopeless) or observation made by others (e.g., appears tearful). (**Note:** In children and adolescents, can be irritable moods.)
  2. Markedly diminished interest or pleasure in all, or almost all, activities most of the day, nearly every day (as indicated by either subjective account or observation).
  3. Significant weight loss when not dieting or weight gain (e.g., a change of more than 5% of body weight in a month) or decrease or increase in appetite nearly every day. (**Note:** In children, consider failure to make expected weight gain.)
  4. Insomnia or hypersomnia nearly every day.
  5. Psychomotor agitation or retardation nearly every day (observable by others; not merely subjective feelings of restlessness or being slowed down).
  6. Fatigue or loss of energy nearly every day.
  7. Feelings of worthlessness or excessive or inappropriate guilt (which may be delusional) nearly every day (not merely self-reproach or guilt about being sick).
  8. Diminished ability to think or concentrate, or indecisiveness, nearly every day (either by subjective account or as observed by others).
  9. Recurrent thoughts of death (not just fear of dying), recurrent suicidal ideation without a specific plan, or a suicide attempt or a specific plan for committing suicide.

B. The symptoms cause clinically significant distress or impairment in social, occupational, or other important areas of functioning.

C. The episode is not attributable to the physiological effects of a substance or another medical condition.

Note: Criteria A through C constitute a major depressive episode. Major depressive episodes are common in bipolar I disorder but are not required for the diagnosis of bipolar I disorder.

DSM-5 DIAGNOSTIC CRITERIA—cont'd

Bipolar I Disorder

Note: Responses to a significant loss (e.g., bereavement, financial ruin, losses from a natural disaster, a serious medical illness or disability) may include the feelings of intense sadness, rumination about the loss, insomnia, poor appetite, and weight loss noted in Criterion A, which may resemble a depressive episode. Although such symptoms may be understandable or considered appropriate to the loss, the presence of a major depressive episode in addition to the normal response to a significant loss should also be carefully considered. This decision inevitably requires the exercise of clinical judgment based on the individual's history and the cultural norms for the expression of distress in the context of loss.

Bipolar I Disorder

A. Criteria have been met for at least one manic episode (Criteria A through D under "Manic episode" above).

B. The occurrence of the manic and major depressive episode(s) is not better explained by schizoaffective disorder, schizophrenia, schizophreniform disorder, delusional disorder, or other specified or unspecified schizophrenia spectrum and other psychotic disorder.

part of the clinical picture. Cognitive symptoms that affect memory, judgment, comprehension, and the ability to concentrate may be seen. There is much more variability of symptoms with bipolar depression.

Prevalence and Comorbidity

The lifetime prevalence of bipolar disorders varies around the world, but in the United States, it is estimated to be 4.4% (NIMH, 2017). Onset of bipolar disorders occurs throughout the life span and can occur as late as 60 or 70 years. The average age of onset is 18 years (APA, 2013). One-third of the initial symptoms of BSD occurs before the age of 13, and another third occurs between the ages of 13 and 18. Early onset leads to greater comorbidity and functional impairment (Perlis & Ostacher, 2015). For bipolar I, the male-to-female ratio is approximately 1:1, and for bipolar II, it is 1:2. The initial presentation of this disorder for men is usually mania; for females, it is depression.

Cyclothymia usually begins in adolescence or early adulthood and has a lifetime prevalence of 0.4% to 1%. There is a 15% to 50% risk that an individual with cyclothymia will subsequently develop bipolar I or bipolar II disorder (APA, 2013).

Comorbidity with other mental disorders is quite high with both bipolar I and bipolar II disorders. The most common co-occurring disorders are anxiety disorders. Impulse control disorders, attention-deficit/hyperactivity disorder (ADHD), and substance use disorders (SUDs) occur in over half of those with a diagnosis of bipolar disorder. Persons with a diagnosis of bipolar disorder and co-occurring substance use problems seem to experience more rapid cycling and more mixed or dysphoric mania (anger and irritability), and they report more hospitalizations. Co-occurring substance use and anxiety disorders worsen the prognosis and greatly increase the risk of suicide.

Between 25% and 50% of people with a diagnosis of BSD attempt suicide, with completed suicides seen in 15% to 20% (Perlis & Ostacher, 2015). BSDs account for one-quarter of all completed suicides in those with any mental disorder (APA, 2013).

The BSDs also have a high rate of *medical* comorbidity, especially cardiovascular and metabolic diseases, endocrine disorders, type 2 diabetes, and obesity.

Some medical conditions are associated with *manic-like symptoms.* These include central nervous system (CNS) tumors or trauma, hyperthyroidism, seizure disorders, and some infectious diseases, such as human immunodeficiency virus (HIV). Some drugs, such as amphetamines, may mimic manic symptoms. The use of antidepressants during a mixed or depressive phase of the illness without a mood stabilizer can trigger a manic episode in susceptible individuals.

Life Span: Children and Adolescents

Over 60% of adults with bipolar spectrum disorders have an age of onset during childhood or adolescence. Diagnosing bipolar spectrum disorders in childhood and adolescence can be complicated by both developmental and illness features. Pediatric bipolar disorder is characterized by significant mood disturbances, including elated or irritable mood, cycling mood episodes, rage, grandiosity or inflated self-esteem, hypersexual behavior, decreased need for sleep, and poor insight. There is an overlapping of some symptoms of disruptive mood dysregulation disorder, making a definitive diagnosis difficult. Comorbid ADHD is present in 50% to 70% of children with bipolar disorder, which further complicates the clinical picture (APNA, 2015).

Theory

The cause of BSDs involves a complex interaction of environmental, genetic, and neurochemical factors that is poorly understood.

Genetic Factors

Twin, family, and adoption studies provide evidence that bipolar disorders have a strong genetic component. However, the inheritance of bipolar disorders is an expression of multiple genes. First-degree relatives of a person with a bipolar disorder are 7 to 10 times more likely to develop bipolar disorder compared with the general population (Perlis & Ostacher, 2015). A child with two parents with bipolar disorder has up to a 50% chance of developing the disorder. Siblings of persons with the disorder have a 10% to 25% chance, and identical twins have up to an 80% chance of developing the illness (Perlis & Ostacher, 2015; WebMD Medical Reference, 2017).

Epidemiologists are attempting to predict the development of bipolar disorder for "at-risk" children of people with a bipolar disorder diagnosis. Earlier age of onset of the disorder in the parent increases the risk of the child developing the disorder. The strongest predictor of later development of bipolar disorder is when the child displays premorbid symptoms of anxiety/depression, affective lability, and low-level manic symptoms prior to the first episode. Having multiple risk factors can lead to a 49% chance of developing bipolar disorders (NIMH, 2016).

Researchers are finding evidence that there is a genetic overlap on specific chromosomes among five different major mental illnesses that share the same common inherited genetic variations. The genetic connection is strongest between schizophrenia and bipolar disorder; more moderate between bipolar disorder, depression, and ADHD; and to a lesser extent between schizophrenia and autism.

These shared genetic roots may provide new insight into both the cause of these chronic disabling disorders and our understanding of each of these diagnostic entities (Perlis & Ostacher, 2015).

Neurobiological Factors

Experts believe bipolar disorder is partly caused by an underlying problem with specific brain circuits and brain neurotransmitter dysfunction. The neurotransmitters dopamine, norepinephrine, glutamate, serotonin, and gamma-aminobutyric acid (GABA) have all been implicated.

Disruption of neural circuits that communicate using dopamine may be implicated in the psychosis associated with mania. It is hypothesized that higher levels of dopamine, norepinephrine, and glutamate result in manic phases, and lower levels of dopamine and norepinephrine lead to bipolar depression. Serotonin can be too low in a depression phase or can cause aggression and poor impulse control in the manic phase. The action of GABA is significantly blunted in the brains of those with bipolar disorder. The release of melatonin is altered in patients with bipolar disorder, which may contribute to poor sleep (Lingohr-Smith, 2017).

Neuroendocrine Factors. The hypothalamic–pituitary–adrenal (HPA) axis modulates the stress response and is involved in maintaining homeostasis. It is suggested that bipolar disorder is associated with abnormalities of stress-related molecular pathways of the HPA axis in several brain areas that are triggered by acute environmental stress. The disease is associated with higher levels of adrenocorticotropic hormone (ADH) and cortisol, but not corticotropin-releasing *hormone* (*CRH*) (Belvederi et al., 2016).

Hormones may play a role in the development of the severity of symptoms of bipolar disorder in women. Women with mood disorders can experience more severe symptoms of premenstrual syndrome. Late-onset bipolar disorder has been associated with menopause. Women with a bipolar diagnosis are seven times more likely to have an exacerbation of their illness during and after pregnancy (WebMD Medical Reference, 2016).

Inflammatory factors interact with the HPA axis; the autonomic nervous system; and key neurotransmitters like glutamate, serotonin, and dopamine. Recent studies in patients with bipolar disorder have confirmed the presence of a chronic inflammatory state in this disorder (Muneer, 2016).

Neuroanatomical Factors. *The pathophysiology of bipolar disorder suggests that both neurodevelopmental and neurodegenerative processes contribute to the disease* (Fears et al., 2015). Magnetic resonance imaging (MRI) studies comparing patients with bipolar disorder to controls demonstrate subtle deficits in gray-matter volume, especially in brain regions underpinning mood regulation. There is also white-matter disorganization in tracts connecting various brain regions (McDonald, 2015).

The reduced hippocampal volume and the dysfunction in the prefrontal cortex and limbic system observed in patients with bipolar disorder emphasize the importance of these brain regions in the development of the disease. A reduced volume of the amygdala and striatal regions leads to problems with cognition and processing of emotional stimuli. Dysfunctions in neural growth, which result in loss of synaptic function, are also indicated in both schizophrenia and bipolar disorders. Preston and Johnson (2015) concluded there are both structural and functional abnormalities at multiple levels of the CNS. Whether these neuroanatomical differences cause the illness or are part of the progression of the illness is still not fully understood (APNA, 2015).

Environmental and Psychological Influences

According to the behavioral approach system (BAS) dysregulation model, individuals with bipolar disorder experience extreme fluctuations in the activation and deactivation of the BAS, a reward system in the brain. Excessive activation of the BAS leads to hyperresponsiveness to certain environmental stimuli, resulting in manic symptoms. Depressive symptoms result from deactivation of the BAS. This is an integrated model for understanding the psychosocial and biological etiologic factors of bipolar disorder (Dempsey, Gooding, & Jones, 2017).

Social rhythm theory states that disruptions of our circadian rhythms and sleep deprivation may provoke or exacerbate the symptoms commonly associated with bipolar disorder (Grohol, 2016). Some have theorized that disruption in *social zeitgebers* or social demands/tasks that set the *biological clock* can lead to instability in circadian rhythms. These environmental disruptions can trigger bipolar episodes (Boland et al., 2016). Severe social rhythm disruptions, such as returning from an international trip, are associated with the onset of mania. Psychosocial therapies have been developed that emphasize the importance of maintaining circadian rhythms and routines in a patient's life, including eating, sleeping, and other daily activities (Grohol, 2016).

Although stress is not a cause of bipolar disorders, stressful life events can trigger symptoms of an acute episode. Family conflict and altered sleep patterns were the most commonly reported stressful life events associated with the initial episodes of the illness (Subramanian et al., 2017).

Some key findings of a comprehensive long-term study of those with bipolar disorder include the following (McInnis et al., 2017):

- Migraine headaches are three and a half times more common with this illness.
- Eating disorders, anxiety disorders, substance-related and addictive problems, and metabolic syndrome are also common.
- There is a higher incidence of childhood trauma.
- Poor sleep is associated with the severity of depressive and manic symptoms.
- Two genes, *CACNA1* and *ANK3,* increase susceptibility to developing bipolar disorder.
- A wide range of cognitive abilities, including memory, executive functioning, and motor skills, were found to be poorer in those patients with a diagnosis of bipolar disorder.
- Key features of speech patterns were found to be predictive of mood states; this finding may lead to an earlier intervention to prevent relapse.
- Neurons derived from the cells of patients with bipolar disorder were found to be more excitable than comparisons.

Cultural Considerations

Bipolar disorders can be difficult to diagnose because many of the symptoms overlap with those of other mental illnesses. The psychotic symptoms of a manic episode can look like symptoms of schizophrenia. The lack of emotional regulation of borderline personality disorder can look like symptoms of bipolar disorder. Both anxiety disorders and bipolar disorders share the symptoms of agitation, anxiety, and irritability. In addition, a person who meets the criteria for bipolar disorder may have a comorbid condition that makes it difficult to differentiate symptoms. Cocaine and amphetamine misuse can mimic mania, for example. About 40% of patients with bipolar disorder are initially diagnosed with major (or unipolar) depression, which does not involve mood swings or mania (Thomas, 2016). Cultural differences and beliefs can vastly influence which symptoms are displayed when acutely ill. Clinicians who are not familiar with the culture of a patient may miss important cues and misinterpret what is being reported. For example, African Americans presenting with psychotic symptoms are more likely to be diagnosed as having schizophrenia.

More careful assessments of a person's past behaviors/symptoms and obtaining a collateral history from significant others may help with a more accurate diagnosis.

Clinical Picture

Mania may begin gradually over the course of a few weeks, but it more typically has an abrupt onset. With effective treatment, the prognosis of any single manic episode is good. Unfortunately, reoccurrence is likely. A manic episode may last for a few days to months and may be followed by a depressive episode that may occur suddenly. During this time, there may be remorse for inappropriate behavior displayed during a manic episode. This can lead to an increased risk for suicide. Suicide can occur in both the manic and depressive phases of the bipolar disorder and is more likely in the depressed phase.

APPLICATION OF THE NURSING PROCESS

ASSESSMENT

Fig. 16.1 presents the Mood Disorder Questionnaire (MDQ). Although this is an older screening tool, the overall diagnostic accuracy of the MDQ is still valid (Wang et al., 2015). This is *not* a diagnostic test; rather, it is a helpful screening device for assessment purposes.

The euphoric mood or manic state associated with a bipolar illness is unstable and *labile* (continually fluctuating). It can include variable states of hypomania, depression, irritability, and euphoria. During euphoria, patients may state they are experiencing "an intense feeling of well-being," or are "cheerful in a beautiful world," or are becoming "one with God." This mood may change to irritation and quick anger when the elated person is thwarted. The irritability and belligerence may be short-lived or may become the prominent feature of a person's manic episode. When the person is elated, the overly joyous mood may seem out of proportion to what is occurring in the person's environment, and a cheerful mood may be inappropriate to the circumstances.

People in a manic state may laugh, joke, and talk in a continuous stream, with uninhibited familiarity. During mania, people demonstrate boundless enthusiasm, treat everyone with confident friendliness, and incorporate everyone into their plans and activities. "They know no strangers." Energy and self-confidence seem boundless.

As the clinical course progresses, sociability and euphoria are replaced by a stage of hostility, irritability, and paranoia. The following vignette is how one patient describes this experience (Jamison, 1995, p. 67).

Mood Disorder Questionnaire

Instructions: Please answer each question as best you can.

1. Has there ever been a period of time when you were not your usual self and...	Yes	No
you felt so good or so hyper that other people thought you were not your normal self or you were so hyper that you got into trouble?	☐	☐
you were so irritable that you shouted at people or started fights or arguments?	☐	☐
you felt much more self-confident than usual?	☐	☐
you got much less sleep than usual and found you didn't really miss it?	☐	☐
you were much more talkative or spoke much faster than usual?	☐	☐
thoughts raced through your head or you couldn't slow down your mind?	☐	☐
you were so easily distracted by things around you that you had trouble concentrating or staying on track?	☐	☐
you had much more energy than usual?	☐	☐
you were much more active or did many more things than usual?	☐	☐
you were much more social or outgoing than usual; for example, you telephoned friends in the middle of the night?	☐	☐
you were much more interested in sex than usual?	☐	☐
you did things that were unusual for you or that other people might have thought were excessive, foolish, or risky?	☐	☐
spending money got you or your family into trouble?	☐	☐

2. If you answered "Yes" to more than one of the above, have several of these ever happened during the same period of time?

3. How much of a problem did any of these cause you—like being unable to work; having family, money, or legal troubles; or getting into arguments or fights? Please select one response only.

☐ No problem ☐ Minor problem ☐ Moderate problem ☐ Serious problem

4. Have any of your blood relatives (children, siblings, parents, grandparents, aunts, uncles) had manic-depressive illness or bipolar disorder? ☐ ☐

5. Has a health care professional ever told you that you have manic-depressive illness or bipolar disorder? ☐ ☐

Criteria for Results: Answering "Yes" to 7 or more of the events in question 1, answering "Yes" to question 2, and answering "Moderate problem" or "Serious problem" to question 3 are considered a positive screen result for bipolar disorder.

Fig. 16.1 The Mood Disorder Questionnaire. (From Hirschfeld, R. M. A., et al. [2000]. Development and validation of a screening instrument for bipolar spectrum disorder: The Mood Disorder Questionnaire. *American Journal of Psychiatry, 157*[11], 1873-1875. Copyright © 2004 Eli Lilly and Company.)

VIGNETTE: At first when I'm high, it's tremendous ... ideas are fast, like shooting stars you follow until brighter ones appear. All shyness disappears; the right words and gestures are suddenly there. Uninteresting people and things become intensely interesting. Sensuality is pervasive; the desire to seduce and be seduced is irresistible. Your marrow is infused with unbelievable feelings of ease, power, well-being, omnipotence, euphoria ... you can do anything. But somewhere this changes.

The fast ideas become too fast and there are far too many. Overwhelming confusion replaces clarity. You stop keeping up with it—memory goes. Infectious humor ceases to amuse—your friends become frightened ... everything now is against the grain. You are irritable, angry, frightened, uncontrollable, and trapped in the blackest caves of the mind—caves you never knew were there. It will never end. Madness carves its own reality.

Behavior

Mania

When in full-blown *mania,* a person may constantly switch from one activity to another, one place to another, and one project to another. Projects may be started, but few are completed. Hyperactivity may range from mild to frenetic, wild activity. Individuals can become involved in pleasurable activities that can have painful consequences. For example, spending large sums of money on frivolous items, giving money away indiscriminately, or making foolish business investments can leave a family penniless. Sexual indiscretion can dissolve relationships and ruin marriages.

During mania, individuals can be manipulative, profane, fault finding, and adept at exploiting others' vulnerabilities. They push the limits of acceptable behavior. These behaviors often alienate family, friends, employers, health care providers, and others.

All persons experiencing mania sleep less, and some people may not sleep for several days in a row. The person can become too distracted or busy to eat. **This nonstop physical activity and the lack of sleep and food can lead to physical exhaustion and even death if not treated and therefore constitutes an emergency.** Modes of dress may be described as outlandish, bizarre, colorful, and noticeably inappropriate. Makeup may be garish or overdone. During mania, people are highly distractible, with a poor ability to concentrate. Judgment is poor and impulsive, and as a result, marriages and divorces may occur.

People often emerge from a manic state startled and confused by the shambles of their lives. The following description conveys one patient's experience (Jamison, 1995, p. 68).

VIGNETTE: Now there are only others' recollections of your behavior—your bizarre, frenetic, aimless behavior. At least mania has the grace to dim memories of itself now [that] it's over, but is it? Incredible feelings to sort through. Who is being too polite? Who knows what? What did I do? Why? And most hauntingly, will it, when will it, happen again? Medication to take, resist, resent, forget ... but always to take. Credit cards revoked ... explanations at work ... bad checks and apologies overdue ... memory flashes of vague men (what did I do?) ... friendships gone, a marriage ruined.

Hypomania

During *hypomania,* individuals show signs and symptoms similar to mania, just not as extreme. When in a hypomanic state, the person may experience voracious appetites for food as well as for indiscriminate sex. There is still a felt need for less sleep, but short naps are possible.

Delirious Mania

Delirious mania is a rare disorder characterized by the rapid onset of delirium, plus mania, and may include psychosis. Hyperactive catatonia is often a prominent feature of the syndrome. It can be life threatening if not recognized and treated. Treatment usually includes high doses of a benzodiazepine, like lorazepam, and/or electroconvulsive therapy (ECT).

Refer to Table 16.1 for the characteristics of a person experiencing states of mania.

Thought Content and Thought Processes

Approximately 50% of patients have psychotic symptoms during a manic episode (Black & Andreasen, 2014). Thought content can include delusions or hallucinations. A manic individual may think they have special powers or abilities. They may have altered sensory perception and believe they are hearing messages from God. They may become paranoid or believe things such as the government having the ability to read their mind, or they may fear they are being controlled by alien technology. They may worry that people are out to get them. Thought content is often sexually explicit and can range from mildly inappropriate to vulgar.

The individual's thought process is revealed by his or her speech. Pressured speech and flight of ideas are common when a patient is having a manic episode. **Pressured speech** is often loud and difficult to interrupt. **Flight of ideas** is a nearly continuous flow of speech with abrupt changes in topics. Speech is rapid, verbose, and circumstantial. When severe, speech may be disorganized and difficult to follow. With increasing mania, speech becomes more disorganized and may include **clang associations**, the stringing together of words because of the rhyming sounds without regard to meaning:

"Cinema I and II, last row. Row, row, row your boat. Don't be a cutthroat. Cut your throat. Get your goat. Go out and vote. And so I wrote."

Grandiosity or grandiose thinking is also often present during a manic episode. Persons with grandiosity may believe they are exceptional artists or brilliant business leaders when their skills may be mediocre. They may also overinflate their accomplishments.

Cognitive Function

The onset of bipolar disorder is often preceded by comparatively high cognitive function. In fact, bipolar illness is often associated with creativity and high achievement (Black & Andreasen, 2014). Unfortunately, one-third of patients with a diagnosis of bipolar disorder display significant and persistent cognitive difficulties. These include problems with verbal memory, sustained attention, and occasionally executive functioning as the disease progresses. These deficits often persist, even in periods of remission. Cognitive impairment appears to be a core feature of bipolar disorder and a contributing factor to poor psychosocial outcomes.

Despite the recognition of the importance of treating cognitive symptoms, there is no strong evidence that medications or therapies can effectively treat these symptoms.

Potential prevention strategies to decrease cognitive dysfunction include the following:

- Prevent multiple episodes with effective pharmacotherapy and implementation of psychoeducation programs.
- Treat subclinical depressive symptoms.
- Control comorbidity (mental and psychiatric).
- Implement cognitive or functional remediation.
- Promote healthy habits.
- Promote aerobic physical exercise (Solé et al., 2017).

Assessment Guidelines

1. Assess physiological safety. **(QSEN: Safety)**
    - **Need for hospitalization** to physically stabilize the individual
    - **Medical examination** to determine if manic symptoms are one of the following:

- Primary: bipolar disorder or cyclothymia
- Secondary to a co-occurring condition or use of a drug or substance or toxin exposure
- Part of a different medical condition, such as a brain disease; certain infections, including HIV; and endocrine disorders
- **Dehydration:** A person in acute mania may become severely dehydrated, as evidenced by poor skin turgor, dark and scant urinary output, and poor skin integrity.
- **Cardiac status**: Severe exhaustion and dehydration can lead to cardiac collapse.
- **Poor sleep** and constant activity lead to physiological exhaustion.

2. Other areas of safety. **(QSEN: Safety)**
   - Assess whether the patient is a danger to self:
     - Not sleeping (as described previously)
     - Not eating (The patient may hoard food while not eating.)
     - Poor impulse control that may result in harm to self or others
     - Poor judgment
     - Inappropriate sexual activity
     - Uncontrolled spending (Protect the patient in mania from bankruptcy.)
3. When the patient is clinically stable, assess the patient's and family's understanding of bipolar disorder, including knowledge of medications and knowledge of support groups and organizations that provide information.

DIAGNOSIS

The focus of nursing care is related to the symptoms displayed by the patient. Nursing diagnoses vary for a patient with a bipolar disorder. Priority diagnoses may include the following:

Acute phase:

- Safety risks: self
  - *Impaired sleep*—lack of sleep leading to exhaustion and cardiac collapse
  - Manic state: *Impaired neurological status*; *Impaired psychomotor activity*
  - *Impaired cognition:* poor judgment—may accidentally hurt self
- Self-care deficits
  - *Impaired fluid intake*—with potential for dehydration
  - *Deficient food intake*
- Safety risk toward others
  - *Impaired impulse control*
  - *Impaired interactive behavior*
  - *Anger control*—impaired related to interpersonal intrusiveness and aggressive behavior toward others
- Lack of insight
  - *Nonadherence to medication regime*—refusal to take prescribed meds

Impaired mood regulation and *labile emotional control* are additional patient problems encountered during a manic episode.

Refer to Table 16.2 for a list of potential patient problems for those with bipolar disorders.

OUTCOMES IDENTIFICATION

Phase I (Acute Mania)

The overall goal during the acute manic phase is to **prevent injury** and **maintain safety. (QSEN: Safety)** Both physiological and behavioral issues are stated in measurable terms within realistic time frames. For example, the patient will:

- Be well hydrated within 24 hours, as evidenced by good skin turgor with urinary output and concentration within normal limits.
- Maintain stable cardiac status, as evidenced by stable vital signs.
- Maintain tissue integrity, as evidenced by the absence of infection or absence of untreated cuts or abrasions.
- Get sufficient sleep and rest, as evidenced by 4 to 6 hours of sleep at night and 10-minute rest periods every hour.
- Demonstrate self-control with the aid of staff presence or medication, as evidenced by the absence of harm to others.
- Make no attempt at self-harm with the aid of staff presence or medication, as demonstrated during regular, formal, eyes-on safety checks throughout the period of acute mania.

Phase II and Phase III (Continuation and Maintenance)

The overall outcome of phase II, the **continuation phase**, and phase III, the **maintenance phase**, is to continue the resolution of problematic symptoms, prevent relapse, and limit the severity and duration of future episodes. Strategies to accomplish this goal are as follows:

1. Patient and family will attend psychoeducational classes that include the following:
   - Knowledge of disease process
   - Knowledge of medication, including side effects and toxic effects

TABLE 16.2 Potential Nursing Diagnoses for Bipolar Disorders

Signs and Symptoms	Potential Nursing Diagnoses[a]
Lack of rest and sleep	*Impaired sleep*
Excessive motor activity	*Hyperactivity*
Poor nutritional intake (food and fluids)	*Impaired nutritional status* *Impaired fluid volume*
Poor judgment	*Impaired cognition*
Impulsivity	*Impaired psychological status* *Risk for injury*
Loud, profane, hostile, combative, aggressive, demanding behaviors	*(Risk for) Self-destructive behaviors* *(Risk for) Aggressive behavior*
Inability to control behavior	*(Risk for) Emotional problem: anger*
Provocative behaviors	*Impaired psychological status*
Property destruction or lashing out at others in a rage reaction	*(Risk for) Difficulty with coping*
Intrusive behaviors	*Impaired interactive behaviors*
Grandiosity; grandiose delusions	*Impaired cognition*
Giving away valuables, neglecting family, making impulsive major life changes (divorce, career changes)	*Impaired role performance* *Caregiver stress* *Impaired family coping*
Continuous pressured speech jumping from topic to topic *(flights of ideas)*	*Impaired verbal communication*
Labile mood	*Labile moods*
Failure to eat, groom, bathe, dress self because too distracted, agitated, and disorganized	*Self-care deficit (specify bathing/hygiene, dressing/grooming)*

[a]The International Classification for Nursing Practice (ICNP) is a product of the International Council of Nurses (ICN). Retrieved from http://www.icn.ch/what-we-do/ICNP-Browser/.

- Recognition of the importance of medication and treatment adherence
- Consequences of substance use as a significant risk factor for future relapse
- Recognition of other risk factors for relapse and early signs and symptoms of relapse

2. Support groups
   - Bipolar disorder or recovery support groups
   - Substance use support groups (if applicable)
3. Therapies: psychoeducational groups, cognitive-behavioral therapy (CBT), interpersonal social rhythm therapy (IPSRT), and family-focused therapy (FFT) are all evidence-based treatment modalities. **(QSEN: Evidence-Based Practice)**
4. Communication and problem-solving skills training

PLANNING

The planning of care for an individual with bipolar disorder usually is targeted toward the specific phase of the illness, the severity of the symptoms, and co-occurring issues identified in the assessment.

Phase I (Acute Mania)

During the acute phase, planning focuses on the physiological stability of the patient while maintaining **safety.** Hospitalization is usually the safest option for a patient with acute manic symptoms. Nursing care is often geared toward the following:

1. Decreasing excessive physical activity
2. Maintaining adequate food and fluid intake
3. Ensuring at least 4 to 6 hours of sleep per night
4. Alleviating any bowel or bladder problems
5. Intervening to ensure self-care needs are met
6. Providing careful medication management

Some patients may require close observation, seclusion, or electroconvulsive therapy (ECT) for severe symptoms.

Phase II and Phase III (Continuation and Maintenance)

Planning focuses on maintaining adherence with the medication regimen and preventing relapse. Interventions are planned in accordance with the assessment data. Areas to consider are as follows (Fuentes, Rizo-Mendez, & Jarne-Esparcia, 2016):

1. The patient's interpersonal skills, including communication skills and problem solving
2. The patient's stress-reduction skills
3. Cognitive functioning—poor neuropsychological functioning is associated with lower medication adherence for people with a diagnosis of bipolar disorder.
4. Employment status and any legal issues
5. Substance-related problems
6. Social support systems
7. Individualized relapse prevention plan **(QSEN: Patient-Centered Care)**

Residual problems resulting from reckless, violent, withdrawn, or bizarre behavior that may have occurred during a manic episode can now be addressed. These can often leave lives shattered and family and friends hurt and distant. For many patients, psychotherapy is needed to address these issues.

IMPLEMENTATION

Phase I (Acute Mania)

Hospitalization provides **safety** for a patient in acute mania by imposing external controls on destructive behaviors and providing medical stabilization.

Communication

Communicating with a patient who is acutely manic can be challenging, but specific and effective approaches are available (Table 16.3). The goal is to first engage the agitated individual, establish a collaborative relationship, and then verbally de-escalate or help the person return to a less agitated state (Spencer & Johnson, 2016).

Safety is a priority during the acute phase. Setting limits in a *firm, nonthreatening, and neutral* manner prevents further escalation of mania and provides safe boundaries for the patient and others. *Early intervention* in escalating behavior helps the patient stay in better control and leads to better outcomes. Attempts should be made to avoid a power struggle with the patient by setting limits on behavior only when it is necessary for safety reasons (Table 16.4).

Milieu Therapy

While hospitalized, the ideal therapeutic milieu for persons who are hyperactive and easily distracted is an atmosphere with *decreased stimulation*. There should be space for solitary or noncompetitive activities, such as writing, drawing, or pacing/walking. The staff members need to maintain close observation and intervene to protect the patient from potentially embarrassing behaviors on the unit. Interactions with others on the unit must also be observed. The intrusive behaviors of the person in a manic state may lead to confrontation by other patients in the therapeutic community. A patient should be assigned a private room when possible and encouraged to return to the room when showing beginning signs of agitation. When a patient's activity begins to escalate, the staff members need to employ additional interventions. Spencer and Johnson (2016) summarized verbal de-escalation techniques as strategies for dealing with agitated or aggressive behaviors. Refer to Chapter 24 for effective verbal de-escalation techniques. Immediate administration of a sedating medication, like antipsychotics or benzodiazepines to decrease anxiety, is also a useful option. When verbal de-escalation techniques do not work, seclusion may be necessary to prevent harm to self or others.

Seclusion

When a patient is dangerously out of control, and *all other approaches have been unsuccessful,* seclusion or restraints may be indicated. Seclusion is defined as the involuntary, solitary confinement of an individual (Substance Abuse and Mental Health Services Administration [SAMHSA], 2015). Restraint refers to any method, device, or equipment that immobilizes or reduces an individual's ability to freely move the arms, legs, body, or head (SAMHSA, 2015). A chemical restraint is sedating a person to control or overpower by giving medication that is not a standard treatment or dosage for the condition (World Health Organization [WHO], 2017). Giving medication to decrease anxiety is acceptable. Chemical restraints should only be used in extreme situations when people pose a threat to themselves or others.

Seclusion may provide comfort and relief to a patient who can no longer control his or her own behavior by:

- Reducing overwhelming environmental stimuli
- Protecting a patient from injuring self, others, or staff
- Preventing the destruction of personal property or the property of others

Seclusion may be warranted when documented data reflect the following points:

- There is a substantial risk of harm to others or self.
- The patient is unable to control his or her actions.
- Problematic behavior continues or escalates despite other measures.
- *Less restrictive measures* have failed.

TABLE 16.3 Interventions for Acute Mania: Communication

Intervention	Rationale
1. Use firm and calm approach: "John, come with me. Eat this sandwich."	1. External structure and control are provided for patient who is out of control. Feelings of security can result: "Someone is in control."
2. Use short and concise explanations or statements.	2. Short attention span limits comprehension to small bits of information.
3. Remain neutral; avoid power struggles and value judgments.	3. Patient can use inconsistencies and value judgments as justification for arguing and escalating mania.
4. Be consistent in approach and expectations.	4. Consistent limits and expectations minimize potential for patient's manipulation of staff.
5. Have frequent staff meetings to plan consistent approaches and to set agreed-on limits.	5. Consistency of all staff is needed to maintain controls and minimize manipulation by patient.
6. With other staff, decide on limits and tell patient in simple, concrete terms with consequences; for example, "John, do not yell at or hit Peter. If you cannot control yourself, we will help you" or "The seclusion room will help you feel less out of control and prevent harm to yourself and others."	6. Clear expectations help patient experience outside controls as well as understand reasons for medication, seclusion, or restraints (if unable to control behaviors).
7. Continue to use active listening to hear and act on legitimate complaints.	7. Underlying feelings of helplessness are reduced, and acting-out behaviors are minimized.
8. Firmly redirect energy into more appropriate and constructive channels. Use distraction techniques as a tool to de-escalate.	8. Distraction is the nurse's most effective tool during the patient's manic phase.

Staff members need to be well prepared and knowledgeable about unit protocol regarding seclusion.

The use of seclusion or restraints is associated with complex therapeutic, ethical, and legal issues. Most state laws prohibit the use of unnecessary physical restraint or isolation. There is an attempt by health professionals to completely eliminate the use of seclusion and/or restraints (WHO, 2017). Most hospitals have well-defined protocols for the use of seclusion/restraints. **Seclusion protocol** usually includes documentation of attempts to use the *least restrictive interventions* and usually requires an order from a physician. Refer to Chapter 24 for more on seclusion and restraints and accepted protocols and to Chapter 6 for more on legal parameters.

Pharmacological Therapies

Mood stabilization is the primary goal of pharmacological treatment. This starts with treatment of the type of acute episode the person is experiencing—mania, hypomania, or depression. The continued goal of pharmacological therapy is to reduce the risk and incidence of relapse. Medications may need to be continued indefinitely. The specific mood stabilizer prescribed considers individual patient factors. Factors to consider include tolerability, the occurrence of rapid cycling, family history, comorbid conditions (e.g., substance use disorders and suicidality), and how well the drug is tolerated.

Mood Stabilizers

Lithium. **Lithium** is the first-line treatment used for bipolar disorder. Multiple studies have demonstrated effectiveness in the treatment of acute mania, acute bipolar depression, and the prevention of manic and depressive episodes. Less effective when used alone for the treatment of depression, lithium is the most effective *added* agent in treatment-resistant depression. It has significant anti-suicidal effects. The neuroprotective effects of lithium have also been demonstrated. Starting lithium early in the course of the disorder reduces the rates of treatment nonresponse (Zivanovic, 2017).

The exact mechanism of how lithium normalizes the effects of bipolar disorder remains unknown but appears to be related to changes in the brain. It is also known that lithium modulates neurotransmitters, particularly dopamine, glutamate, and GABA neurotransmission. Lithium also acts at the intracellular level, including inhibiting intracellular proteins, stabilizing calcium channels, and decreasing neuronal activity (Guzman, 2017b).

Adverse Effects. Lithium tends to require 3 to 6 weeks to show a full therapeutic response and needs monitoring of serum levels due to the narrow range from therapeutic to toxic levels. Therapeutic serum levels in treating acute mania are 0.5 to 1.2 mEq/L, maintenance serum levels are 0.6 to1.0 mEq/L, and toxic concentrations are greater than 1.5 mEq/L (Stahl, 2017). Serum lithium levels are drawn at a trough level (10 to 12 hours after the last dose). Older adults may have good symptom control with lower serum levels of the drug.

Cases of severe lithium toxicity with levels of 2 mEq/L or greater constitute a life-threatening emergency. Symptoms include the following:

- Neurologic: coarse tremor, slurred speech, ataxia, seizures, stupor, coma
- Gastrointestinal (GI): severe nausea, vomiting, and diarrhea
- Cardiac: hypotension, bradycardia, electrocardiogram (ECG) abnormalities
- Renal: renal failure

In such cases, gastric lavage and treatment that facilitates more rapid lithium excretion are used. Hemodialysis may be used in extreme cases. Refer to Table 16.5 for side effects, signs of lithium toxicity, and interventions.

Because fluid and electrolyte balance can affect serum lithium levels, the lithium level must be monitored more frequently if the patient experiences any condition that causes fluid and electrolyte imbalances. This might include excessive sweating, dehydration or excessive hydration, and high sodium intake. Patients living in hot, dry areas need to be especially careful to avoid dehydration because this can quickly cause the serum lithium to increase to toxic levels.

Non–dose-related side effects that people find particularly bothersome are as follows:

- Essential fine-motor tremors
- Alterations in taste
- Slowed cognition
- Delayed sexual response
- Weight gain

TABLE 16.4 Interventions for Acute Mania: Safety and Physical Needs

Intervention	Rationale
Structure in a Safe Milieu	
1. Maintain low level of stimuli in patient's environment: away from bright lights, loud noises, and people.	1. Decreases escalating anxiety.
2. Provide structured, noncompetitive or solitary activities with nurse or aide.	2. Structure provides security and focus.
3. Redirect agitated behavior through physical exercise such as walking.	3. Physical exercise can decrease tension and provide focus.
4. Use antipsychotics, sedative drugs, and seclusion to minimize physical harm when clinically indicated.	4. Exhaustion and death can result from dehydration, lack of sleep, and constant physical activity.
5. Observe for signs of lithium toxicity.	5. There is a small margin of safety between therapeutic and toxic doses.
6. Protect patient from giving away money and possessions. Hold valuables in hospital safe until rational judgment returns.	6. Patient's "generosity" is in fact a symptom of the disease and can lead to catastrophic financial ruin for patient and family.
7. Protect patient from inappropriate behavior, such as sexual acting out.	7. There may be shame and embarrassment about this behavior when no longer in a manic state.
Nutrition	
1. Monitor intake, output, and vital signs.	1. Adequate fluid and caloric intakes are ensured; development of dehydration and cardiac collapse is minimized.
2. Offer frequent high-calorie protein drinks and milkshakes and **finger foods** such as sandwiches and fruit.	2. Constant fluid and calorie replacement are needed. Patient may be too active to sit at meals. Finger foods allow "eating on the run."
3. Frequently remind patient to eat. "Tom, finish your milkshake." "Sally, eat this banana."	3. During mania, the patient is unaware of bodily needs and is easily distracted. Needs supervision to eat.
Sleep/Rest	
1. Encourage frequent rest periods during the day.	1. Lack of sleep can lead to exhaustion and death.
2. Keep patient in areas of low stimulation.	2. Relaxation is promoted, and manic behavior is minimized.
3. At night, provide warm baths, soothing music, and medication when indicated. Avoid giving patient caffeine.	3. Promotes relaxation, rest, and sleep.
Hygiene	
1. Supervise choice of clothes; minimize flamboyant and bizarre clothing, such as unmatched colors or sexually provocative clothing.	1. The potential is decreased for ridicule, which can lower self-esteem and increase the need for manic defense. The patient is helped to maintain dignity.
2. Give simple, step-by-step reminders for hygiene and dress. "Here is your razor. Shave the left side … now the right side. Here is your toothbrush. Put the toothpaste on the brush."	2. Distractibility and poor concentration are countered through simple, concrete instructions.
Elimination	
1. Monitor bowel habits; offer fluids and foods that are high in fiber. Evaluate need for laxative. Encourage patient to go to the bathroom.	1. Fecal impaction resulting from dehydration and decreased peristalsis is prevented.

APPLYING THE ART

A Person With Bipolar Disorder

Scenario

I approached Gloria, a 33-year-old woman who had seemed edgy and distracted when we talked earlier. She had been admitted to the hospital for the third time after becoming angry and threatening suicide over losing a job she loved. She is on suicide precautions.

Therapeutic Goal

By the end of this session, Gloria will show an increased ability to problem solve, as evidenced by the insight that stopping medication exacerbates the disorder.

Student–Patient Interaction	Thoughts, Communication Techniques, and Mental Health Nursing Concepts
Student: *Smiling.* "Hi, Gloria. Would you talk some more about your feelings when you heard you were going to be fired from your job?"	I know that "could" or "would" acts like an *indirect question* rather than a *direct question,* meaning I will get more than a yes or no answer.
Gloria: "Get the ________ away from me! I'm sick of you people asking about that ________ job." *Clenching fists, practically yelling.*	
Student's feelings: *I forgot to tune in to Gloria as a person before I jumped in with questions. She's loud, but I'm okay. Her fear and loss fuel all that anger. Okay, self, mindfully breathe.*	I forgot to *assess* first! I must remember that she is afraid and *displacing* her frustration onto me. Each time she gets admitted means starting over. If only she had kept taking her Depakote and Abilify.

APPLYING THE ART—cont'd

A Person With Bipolar Disorder

Student–Patient Interaction	Thoughts, Communication Techniques, and Mental Health Nursing Concepts
Student: *Quiet and concerned.* "Gloria, I'm ________, your nursing student. You've been through such a rough time. You feel upset about the job and anyone who asks you about it."	Using *reflection* makes sense because I hope that reflecting the feelings lets my *empathy* get through to her.
Student's feelings: *I can do this. I'll step back a little, slow things down, and keep telling myself that her anger is not really about me. I care about Gloria, so I'm not going to be pushed away that easily.*	
Student's feelings: *I'm struggling with anxiety, too.*	I remember now. Anxiety is communicated interpersonally.
Gloria: "I need to walk." *Starts pacing quickly down the hall.*	Gloria is using walking as a healthy relief behavior for her anxiety.
Student's feelings: *I hope she'll let me walk with her. Walking will help my anxiety, too!*	
Student: "Good idea. Let's walk together. Tell me what's happening inside." *We quickly walk down the hall.*	I am offering myself by walking with her. Using an indirect question often helps the patient talk without feeling interrogated.
Student's feelings: *As she responds while we walk, I'm feeling calmer, too.*	
Gloria: "I feel like, why even try anymore? While I worked at the pet store, I felt like my life meant something. Then I go and stop taking my medicine. It's just so expensive. I'm such a loser." *Eyes fill with tears.*	
Student's feelings: *I feel so sad for her. She struggles so hard and then seems to give in by quitting her medication. Sometimes I feel like a loser. Sometimes I feel like nursing school pressures me too much, especially when I bomb a test. I need to put my own "failure worries" on hold to handle later and refocus to fully tune in to Gloria.*	
Student: "Sounds like right now, you're blaming yourself for what you've lost." *I pause, handing her a tissue.* "Gloria, I care about what happens to you. When you say, 'why even try,' what do you mean …?"	By saying "right now," I plant the idea that she may not always choose to see herself as a failure. I must stay alert for countertransference. Using Gloria's name and reminding her who I am factoring in that she is probably experiencing moderate anxiety, so her *perceptual field* of what she is able to take in decreases. I need to assess even a *covert reference* to *suicide,* especially with Gloria's history.
Gloria: "Don't worry. I don't want to kill myself anymore. But I just keep screwing up! I even let my animals down." *Glancing at me.*	When Gloria tells me not to worry, she may be using *projection,* in that she may still have some latent concern about her suicide potential. She is still on *15-minute checks,* which continues to be necessary, and I will report and chart about all this.
Student's feelings: *I wish she could see the survivor I see when I'm with her. I'm relieved Gloria recognizes she wants to live now. I have so much hope inside for her.*	
Student: "Talk some more about your animals."	By using a focusing approach, I remind her of what she values. She may also remember what she was able to do well, which may help her self-esteem. She said, "my animals," so I deliberately restated, "your animals" because they are so important to her.
Gloria: "I loved caring for all of the animals, but especially the puppies. One little beagle had such sad eyes, I took him home. That's when I got in trouble. I know I wouldn't have done that if I'd kept taking my meds."	Was Gloria using identification? The beagle's "sad" eyes may have resonated with Gloria's own sadness.
Student: "So you recognize a link between stopping your meds and doing some things you wouldn't usually do when you take charge of your bipolar disorder by staying on your meds?"	I am using the behavior modification technique of positive reinforcement by attending to Gloria's insight when she connects her impulsive behavior with stopping her psychotropics. I am also empowering her by deliberately associating taking her medications with taking charge of her disorder.
Student's feelings: *I feel kind of proud of myself for knowing to praise her about the meds.*	
Gloria: "I still get mad too easily, but I'm starting to think more clearly since my Abilify's been upped. I've been wondering if my boss would give me a second chance. I did well with the animals. My boss said so before I got sick again. My case manager made sure the beagle pup got back okay."	Gloria is actually able to problem solve now, so that means her anxiety has decreased to mild.
Student: "I hear you reminding yourself that your skills in pet care endure even through this bout in the hospital."	I think the animals provide some of Gloria's love and belonging needs, which precede self-esteem needs. I validate with Gloria about her pet care skills.
Gloria: "I really love those animals. I'm going to run this idea past the nurse and work out when and how to phrase things to call my boss."	The treatment team will be doing discharge planning.
Student's feelings: *She's taking charge of this. Wow! I feel honored that Gloria trusted me. I'm beginning to trust myself some, too.*	
Student: "You are able to find a goal to work toward, maybe even begin to believe in yourself a little."	I give Gloria support by naming her mentally healthy verbalizations as a goal. I am careful to add qualifiers—"maybe," "begin to," and "a little"—to insert the idea about believing in herself without overwhelming her.
Gloria: *Nods.*	

TABLE 16.5 Lithium Side Effects and Signs of Lithium Toxicity

Level	Signs	Interventions
Expected Side Effects		
<0.4 to 1 mEq/L (therapeutic level)	Fine hand tremor, polyuria, and mild thirst Mild nausea and general discomfort Weight gain sedation Acne Cognitive problems Hair loss	Symptoms may persist throughout therapy. These symptoms may subside. Give with food to decrease nausea. Weight gain may be helped with diet, exercise, and nutritional management.
Early Signs of Toxicity		
<1.5 mEq/L	Increased nausea, vomiting, diarrhea, thirst, polyuria, slurred speech, muscle weakness	Hold medication. Measure blood lithium levels. Re-evaluate dosage.
Advanced Signs of Toxicity		
1.5 to 2 mEq/L	Coarse hand tremor, persistent gastrointestinal upset, mental confusion, muscle hyperirritability, electroencephalographic (EEG) changes, incoordination	Hold medication, obtain blood level, re-evaluate dose, and treat more serious symptoms.
Severe Toxicity		
2 to 2.5 mEq/L	Ataxia, serious EEG changes, blurred vision, clonic movements, large output of dilute urine, tinnitus, blurred vision, seizures, stupor, severe hypotension, coma; death is usually secondary to pulmonary complications	No known antidote for lithium poisoning. Stop drug and facilitate excretion: • If alert, give emetic. • Gastric lavage • Treatment with urea, mannitol, and aminophylline to hasten excretion
>2.5 mEq/L	Symptoms may progress rapidly; coma, cardiac dysrhythmia, peripheral circulatory collapse, proteinuria, oliguria, and death	In addition to the previously listed interventions, hemodialysis may be used in severe cases.

Data from Burchum, J., & Rosenthal, L. (2016). *Lehne's pharmacology for nursing care* (9th ed.). St. Louis: Elsevier.

Lithium can cause mild GI distress, which can be lessened by giving with food. Other adverse reactions include frequent urination, thirst, sedation or lethargy, impaired coordination, hair loss, and acne.

Longer-term side effects that require regular laboratory monitoring include the following:

- Medication-induced hypothyroidism and goiter
- Medication-induced kidney dysfunction (nephrogenic diabetes insipidus)

Lithium used alone is only effective with one-third to one-half of those with a bipolar disorder. In addition, some individuals have difficulty tolerating the side effects of this drug.

During the maintenance phase of the illness, the provision of patient and family education becomes essential for the safe use of this medication and to support medication adherence. Box 16.2 outlines patient and family teaching. Medication education should include:

1. The purpose of lithium therapy
2. Adverse effects and ways to minimize these
3. Drug–drug interactions, including avoiding nonsteroidal antiinflammatory drugs (NSAIDs), diuretics, and others
4. Risk for fetal harm
5. Toxic effects and long-term complications and when to notify the health care provider
6. The need to maintain adequate fluid intake and consistent dietary sodium
7. Conditions that can increase the risk of toxicity, such as excessive sweating and dehydration, excessive diarrhea, or vomiting
8. The need to stay on the medication even when acute symptoms have improved
9. How medication adherence prevents relapse

Anticonvulsant Drugs. Anticonvulsant drugs or **antiepileptic drugs (AEDs)** are another major class of medications used to treat bipolar disorders. Some specific AEDs are used either alone or in combination with lithium. Some have been shown to be more effective for certain specifiers of bipolar disorder compared with lithium. Specific AEDs are approved by the U.S. Food and Drug Administration (FDA) for the treatment of bipolar disorder, and others are used off-label. All AEDs can increase the risk for suicide and have a potential for serious adverse effects. All AEDs must be tapered slowly when discontinuing the drug to prevent an acute relapse of symptoms. Patients who do not respond well to lithium may show symptom reduction when treated with antiepileptic drugs.

Valproic Acid. Valproic acid is considered a first-line treatment for bipolar mania or hypomania or mixed states. The two common derivatives of the drug are divalproex and several different forms of valproate. These drugs are useful in treating those who do not respond to lithium, who are in acute mania, who experience rapid cycles, or who are in a dysphoric mania. These drugs are also helpful in preventing manic episodes and depressive episodes but are less effective than lithium. They affect glutamate and GABA, which appears to contribute to the mood-regulating effects.

Valproate is effective in treating bipolar disorders with multiple comorbid conditions, including alcohol use disorder, mental retardation, anxiety and panic attacks, posttraumatic stress disorder, marked sleep disturbances, explosive dyscontrol and aggression, and comorbid migraine (Shah, Grover, & Rao, 2017).

Common side effects of valproate are GI pain, tremor, sedation, hair loss, and weight gain. It is important to obtain a full blood count panel, monitor liver function, and measure serum amylase and lipase due to the risk of blood dyscrasias, hepatotoxicity, and pancreatitis. Valproate use may lead to birth defects and developmental delays in children exposed in utero and is contraindicated in women of childbearing age. There are multiple drug–drug interactions that must be considered when taking this drug. Therapeutic blood levels are monitored and collected 12 hours after the last dose. Ataxia, confusion, somnolence, and coma are signs of toxicity (Goodwin et al., 2016). Monitoring for weight gain, glucose dysregulation, and increased lipids is recommended with long-term use.

Carbamazepine. Some patients with treatment-resistant bipolar disorder improve after taking carbamazepine and lithium concurrently or carbamazepine and an antipsychotic concurrently. Carbamazepine seems to work better in patients with rapid cycling, mixed states, and acute mania. It is helpful in preventing relapse of manic symptoms.

Blood levels of carbamazepine should be monitored at least weekly for the first 8 weeks of treatment because the drug can increase the levels of liver enzymes that accelerate the metabolism of the drug. Serious side effects include hepatic disease, blood dyscrasias, risk of fluid overload and hyponatremia, and life-threatening dermatological reactions. It should not be used in pregnancy and can decrease the effectiveness of birth control pills. Common dose-related adverse reactions include fatigue; nausea; and neurological symptoms such as diplopia, blurred vision, and ataxia as beginning signs of toxicity.

Lamotrigine. Lamotrigine is a first-line treatment for bipolar depression and is approved for acute and maintenance therapy. It is generally well tolerated, but there are two concerns with this agent. One is a rare but serious dermatological reaction: a potentially life-threatening rash called Stevens–Johnson syndrome. Patients should be instructed to seek immediate medical attention if a rash appears, although in most cases rashes are benign. Aseptic meningitis is another rare but serious side effect of lamotrigine. Symptoms include fever, chills, photophobia, painful headache and stomachache, and stiff neck. Lamotrigine can lower the effectiveness of oral contraceptives, and oral contraceptives can lower the effectiveness of lamotrigine.

Other Anticonvulsant Drugs. Other antiepileptic drugs may be used in the treatment of refractory bipolar disorder, but there is a lack of evidence-based studies to support their use in most cases. Topiramate has shown evidence of being helpful in treating mania

BOX 16.2 Patient and Family Teaching About Lithium Therapy

Education should include the following:

- Lithium works to stabilize your mood and reduces extremes in behavior. It also helps prevent relapse. Continue taking the drug even when your current symptoms are no longer present.
- Lithium blood levels must be monitored very closely because the difference between the correct amount and taking too much is small.
- **Kidney function** should be assessed before treatment and then yearly (creatinine, blood urea nitrogen [BUN], and glomerular filtration rate [GFR]).
- Thyroid-stimulating hormone (TSH) should be measured to determine thyroid dysfunction (goiter) before treatment and then yearly.
- Lithium is not addictive.
- Eat a normal diet with consistent salt and fluid intake (8 to 12 glasses per day). Do not change the amount of salt in your diet unless recommended by your **health care professional (HCP)**.
- **Stop taking lithium and call your HCP** if you have excessive diarrhea, vomiting, or sweating (excessive exercise, hot weather, fever). These symptoms can lead to dehydration. Dehydration can lead to lithium toxicity.
- Take lithium with meals to prevent gastrointestinal (GI) irritation.
- Tell your **HCP** your entire medical history, including all prescribed medications.
- Do not take diuretics (water pills) while you are taking lithium.
- Do not take any over-the-counter medicines, especially nonsteroidal antiinflammatory drugs (NSAIDs) and antacids, without first checking with your physician.
- If you plan to become pregnant, consult with your **HCP first.** This drug is not recommended during the first trimester. Breastfeeding while on this drug is not recommended.
- Consult your **HCP** or nutritionist if you change your diet significantly.
- Keep a list of side effects and toxic effects handy (see Table 16.5), along with the name and number of a contact person.
- If lithium is to be discontinued, the dosage will be tapered gradually to minimize the risk of relapse.
- Always feel free to ask your **HCP** any questions about your illness or your medication.

APPLYING EVIDENCE-BASED PRACTICE (EBP)

Problem

A 63-year-old female is brought to the emergency department (ED) by ambulance. She is combative, hitting and grabbing at anyone within arm's length. She speaks rapidly in a loud voice. She demonstrates flight of ideas: "People are trying to kill me, and I don't know where my cat Bubbles is. Look how nice my hair looks; don't touch it. I will not take that medication … those people are laughing at me."

There are self-inflicted scratches on her face and arms. The emergency medical technician (EMT) reports that the patient has not been taking her Depakote for 2 weeks because she ran out of medication and did not have transportation to the clinic.

EBP Assessment

1. **What do you already know from experience?**
   a. Patient has a diagnosis of bipolar disorder and has been in the ED before.
   b. Patients in a manic state are often hyperverbal and combative and do not eat, drink, or sleep enough. They can hallucinate or be delusional. Moods may be elevated, angry and irritable, or rapidly shifting. They may lash out at staff, family, or themselves.
2. **What does the literature say?**
   a. Guidelines recommend eliminating the use of seclusion and restraint in the treatment of people with mental and/or substance use disorders.
   b. Currently, these methods are viewed as traumatizing practices.
   c. Studies have shown that the use of seclusion and restraint can result in psychological harm, physical injuries, and death.
   d. Best practice now dictates the use of alternative methods, such as one-to-one staff, de-escalation techniques, walking, relaxation techniques, voluntary time out, as-needed (PRN) medications, and moving others away from the patient for safety.

Continued

APPLYING EVIDENCE-BASED PRACTICE (EBP)—cont'd

e. Seclusion and restraint are limited to situations of imminent danger to self or others, usually must have a physician order, and have clear time and safety guidelines.

3. **What does the patient want?**
    a. The patient is unable to clearly articulate her needs.
    b. She is fearful.
    c. She has been acting as a danger to herself and others, requiring intervention.

Plan

1. The ED supervisor assigned a registered nurse (RN) who was known to this patient from a prior visit.
2. The supervisor assisted until the patient was calm and safe.
3. Orders were obtained for Depakote, a mood stabilizer, and a PRN benzodiazepine, a sedative drug.
4. The patient was allowed adequate time to voluntarily take the medication.
5. Staff slowly paced with patient, decreased stimulation by lowering lighting, and gently held her hand to prevent lashing out.
6. Patient did agree to take the medication.
7. Small bites of food and sips of fluid were frequently offered.
8. Staff stayed with patient during this period of acute anxiety until calmer.
9. Seclusion and restraints were avoided by the use of alternative methods of de-escalation.
10. Psychiatry was called for a consult to determine further care.

QSEN Prelicensure Knowledge, Skills, and Attitudes (KSAs) Addressed

Safety was maintained by having two staff with the patient, assigning an RN with a good rapport, and avoiding the use of restraints.

Evidence-Based Practice was implemented by using de-escalation communication techniques. Least restrictive, alternative methods were used instead of seclusion or restraint.

Patient-Centered Care was provided by allowing time for the patient to participate in the treatment decision to help herself by taking the medication.

and does not appear to cause weight gain. Oxcarbazepine, a structural variant of carbamazepine, has the advantage of being better tolerated and has a more favorable drug interaction profile than other anticonvulsants. See Table 16.6 for commonly prescribed AEDs and their adverse reactions.

Anxiolytics

Clonazepam and Lorazepam. Clonazepam and lorazepam are considered adjunctive agents in the treatment of acute mania. These drugs can be helpful in managing the psychomotor agitation seen in acute mania and are typically given for a short period. Lorazepam has a beneficial role in catatonia. Both drugs should be avoided in patients with a history of substance use disorders.

Selective serotonin reuptake inhibitors (SSRIs) such as fluoxetine, sertraline, and others can trigger manic episodes and should be used with extreme caution and in combination with another mood stabilizing medication.

Second-Generation Antipsychotics. Atypical antipsychotics have demonstrated significant mood-stabilizing properties, as follows:

- First-line management of **acute mania:**
    - Olanzapine, quetiapine, aripiprazole, risperidone, paliperidone, ziprasidone, and asenapine
- First-line treatment of **bipolar depression:**
    - Quetiapine monotherapy
    - Olanzapine and fluoxetine combination in the management of bipolar depression
    - Lurasidone for an acute episode of bipolar depression
- Prevention of relapse of **mania** and **depression:**
    - Olanzapine and quetiapine monotherapy
    - Olanzapine and quetiapine as adjunctive medications to lithium or valproate

There is evidence to suggest that when lithium or valproate is combined with antipsychotics in the management of acute mania, the efficacy is higher, and the onset of action is faster than that reported for a single agent (Shah et al., 2017). Long-acting, injectable forms of antipsychotic medications can prevent relapse when adherence is questionable (Goodwin et al., 2016).

Electroconvulsive Therapy

Electroconvulsive therapy (ECT) is used for treatment-resistant bipolar disorder and for severe symptoms of the illness. Possible indications for the use of ECT include the following:

- Catatonic symptoms
- Treatment-resistant manic and depressed symptoms
- Need for rapid control of symptoms
- Severe suicidal behavior, agitation, or violent behavior
- Severe depression or mania during pregnancy (Shah et al., 2017) See Chapter 23.

Phase II and Phase III (Continuation and Maintenance)

The outcome for the continuation/maintenance phase is to prevent relapse. Medication adherence during this phase is perhaps the most important treatment outcome. Follow-up care is frequently handled through a community mental health center. In an outpatient setting, case managers evaluate appropriate follow-up care for patients and their families.

Health Teaching and Health Promotion

During the acute phase of the illness, the patient may not be receptive to health teaching. Significant others and family may benefit from information about the symptoms and progression of the illness and treatment strategies and goals. Opportunities to allow the family to share fears and concerns should be provided.

Once the symptoms of the acute illness have stabilized, the patient is more likely to benefit from education. Health teaching and health promotion can be facilitated through the use of psychoeducation.

The general aim of **psychoeducation** is to help the patient and family gain an understanding of the illness. This includes an understanding of the disease process, treatment options, and medication education. It also must include the importance of treatment adherence and relapse prevention, lifestyle regularity, and stress management strategies. Psychoeducation provides opportunities for both the patient and caregivers

TABLE 16.6 Mood Stabilizers and Other Drugs Used to Treat Bipolar Disorders

Antiepileptic Drug (AED) Therapy	Indications and Major Adverse Effects
FDA Approved for Bipolar Disorder	
Carbamazepine (Therapeutic serum level 4-12)	Indication: Manic episodes, mixed episodes; less effective for bipolar depression Usually added to another medication for bipolar disorder Increased risk for birth defects Weight gain Blood dyscrasias: Agranulocytosis, aplastic anemia, thrombocytopenia Skin rashes, hives, Stevens-Johnson syndrome, toxic epidermal necrolysis (TEN) Hyponatremia Jaundice **Symptoms of Toxicity:** Mild to moderate: Ataxia, nystagmus, dyskinesia, dystonia Severe: Seizures, respiratory depression, coma, tachycardia
Valproic acid, valproate, divalproex (Therapeutic serum level 85-125)	Indication: First-line treatment for manic episodes, mixed episodes, and rapid cycling Especially helpful for patients with comorbidities, including alcohol use disorders, anxiety, PTSD, and sleep disorders Can be used in combination with lithium Birth defects, especially neural tube defects May increase risk for polycystic ovarian syndrome Hepatitis Pancreatitis Thrombocytopenia Encephalopathy (related to high ammonia level) Weight gain and metabolic issues **Symptoms of Toxicity**: Ataxia, confusion, coma, dizziness, hallucinations, irritability, somnolence
Lamotrigine	Indication: Bipolar depression, long-term maintenance; less effective for mania Concurrent use with valproic acid can increase blood level and side effects Risk of birth defects although often the preferred medication for bipolar disorder during pregnancy May be lowered by birth control; dose of lamotrigine may need to be increased if birth control is started Weight gain Stevens-Johnson syndrome or TEN Aseptic meningitis: Headache, fever, nausea, stiff neck, confusion
Off-label Use: Not FDA Approved for Bipolar Disorder	
Topiramate	Indication: Treatment-resistant mania, bipolar depression, mixed states; less useful for mania Slight risk of birth defects Weight loss Impaired concentration, cognitive dulling/slowing Fatigue Visual disturbances: Blurring, double vision, eye pain (report immediately)
Oxcarbazepine	Indication: Mania, mixed states, hypomania, rapid cycling, relapse prevention Hyponatremia Increased risk of fetal harm May reduce effectiveness of birth control

to vent feelings and share concerns. Refer to Box 16.3 for more detailed guidelines.

Knowledge of community supports and self-help groups also facilitates health promotion.

Psychosocial Interventions

Pharmacotherapy and continuous psychosocial support are essential in the treatment of bipolar spectrum disorders. There is good evidence that early, high-quality intervention can change the trajectory and course of illness for the better. Early pharmacological and nonpharmacological interventions at the first episode have been shown to reverse cognitive deficits and preserve gray-matter volume, especially in those who remain episode-free (Berk et al., 2017). A large multicenter study showed increased rates of recovery from an acute episode using CBT, IPSRT, and FFT (Perlis & Ostacher, 2015).

Common treatment elements for these therapies are as follows:

- Psychoeducation (see Box 16.3).
- Communication and problem-solving training
- Strategies for early detection and intervention for relapse

These interventions can reduce the risk of relapse, improve functioning, and facilitate treatment adherence.

In the following vignette, one patient describes her feelings about drug therapy and psychotherapy (Jamison, 1995).

VIGNETTE: I cannot imagine leading a normal life without lithium. From starting and stopping of it, I now know it is an essential part of my sanity. Lithium prevents my seductive but disastrous highs, diminishes my depressions, clears out the weaving of my disordered thinking, slows me, gentles me out, keeps me in my relationships, in my career, out of a hospital, and in psychotherapy. It keeps me alive, too.

But psychotherapy heals, it makes some sense of the confusion, it reins in the terrifying thoughts and feelings, it brings back hope and the possibility of learning from it all. Pills cannot, do not, ease one back into reality. They bring you back headlong, careening, and faster than can be endured at times. Psychotherapy is a sanctuary, it is a battleground, and it is where I have come to believe that someday I may be able to contend with all of this. No pill can help me deal with the problem of not wanting to take pills, but no amount of therapy alone can prevent my manias and depressions. I need both.

Cognitive-Behavioral Therapy

Cognitive-behavioral therapy (CBT) teaches a person how to recognize, challenge, and change flawed or distorted thoughts that lead to problematic mood states. It also helps the individual identify and correct troublesome behavior patterns. Developed by Aaron Beck, this therapy was originally used to treat depressive and anxiety disorders. For bipolar disorder, the focus is on managing symptoms, avoiding triggers for relapse, and problem solving (Jones et al., 2015).

The focus of *recovery-oriented* CBT for bipolar disorder includes the following:

- Accepting your diagnosis
- Monitoring your mood
- Undergoing cognitive restructuring: correcting flawed thought patterns by learning how to become more aware of the role thoughts play in determining your mood
- Practicing problem-solving skills
- Enhancing social skills
- Stabilizing personal routine: maintaining a regular and predictable rhythm each day, with consistent sleep and mealtimes (Lingohr-Smith, 2017)

CBT has been shown to be effective in decreasing affective symptoms, increasing social functioning, reducing the rate of relapse, and reducing the number of hospital admissions.

Interpersonal and Social Rhythm Therapy

Interpersonal and social rhythm therapy (IPSRT) is based on the idea that problems in interpersonal relationships and disruptions in daily routines can contribute to the recurrence of manic and depressive episodes in an individual with a bipolar disorder. IPSRT has been found effective in shortening a depressive episode in patients with bipolar I. There is some evidence that those receiving this intervention had better vocational functioning in the maintenance phase of the illness. The therapy may lengthen periods of mood stability (Grohol, 2016).

Family-Focused Education/Therapy

Behavioral family management, family therapy, and psychoeducation help to improve family functioning and lead to lower rates of rehospitalization.

BOX 16.3 Psychoeducation for Patients With Bipolar Disorder and Their Families

Four Broad Goals for Psychoeducation

1. Information: learn about symptoms, causes, and treatment of the illness.
   a. Bipolar disorder has a chronic, cyclic, and episodic course.
   b. These are long-term illnesses requiring ongoing treatment.
2. Emotional discharge: gives an opportunity to exchange ideas about managing the illness and to discuss frustrations and concerns.
   a. Increases acceptance of the illness
3. Support medication and other treatment adherence.
   a. Mood-stabilizing medication must be taken even when not experiencing symptoms.
   b. Tell your health care worker about troubling side effects. Most side effects can be managed. Do not just stop taking medication.
   c. Medications to treat bipolar disorders usually require regular blood work to monitor for toxic adverse effects. Know the beginning signs of toxicity and what to do if they occur.
   d. Develop a relapse prevention plan.
      (1) It can feel like signs and symptoms of relapse come "out of the blue." Learn your specific early warning signs.
      (2) Tracking your mood over time may give clues to when you are most at risk for relapse. Keep a mood diary (smartphone apps can help with this).
      (3) Family members and others can be helpful in recognizing the beginning symptoms of relapse.
      (4) Emergency contact numbers should be readily available.
   e. Group and individual psychotherapy.
      (1) Supports increased insight and acceptance of illness
      (2) Decreases self-stigma
      (3) Helps to develop skills in relapse prevention
      (4) Provides social support
      (5) Helps improve coping skills in interpersonal relations
      (6) Improves treatment and medication adherence
4. Use self-help strategies.
   a. Maintain good sleep hygiene. Lack of sleep can be a beginning symptom of a manic episode relapse.
   b. Re-establish sleep and wake rhythms and other daily routines.
   c. Avoid alcohol and drugs; they can precipitate a relapse. Caffeine and over-the-counter drugs should be used with caution because they can interfere with medications.
   d. Re-engage with social, familial, and occupational roles.
   e. Learn ways to manage stress.
      (1) Psychosocial and environmental stressors are frequently the precipitant of an acute episode.

Health care workers need to remember the following:

1. Lack of insight is a significant problem, especially during acute mania. Minimization and denial are common defenses that require empathy, active listening, and gradual introduction of facts when partnering with the patient.
2. Anger and abusive remarks are symptoms of the acute illness and are not personal.

Data from Australian Institute of Psychological Counsellors. (2014). *Psychoeducation: Definition, goals and methods.* Retrieved from http://www.aipc.net.au/ articles/psychoeducation-definition-goals-and-methods/; and Guzman, F. (2017). *Bipolar disorder treatment guidelines: A 2018 Update, 2017 psychopharmacology institute, Last update Dec 24, 2017.* Retrieved from: https://psychopharmacologyinstitute.com/guidelines/bipolar-disorder-guidelines/?utm_source=email&utm_medium=emailARCkit&utm_campaign=Email-Bipolar-Guidelines&convertkit_id=lchiappetta@wccnet.edu&ck_subscriber_id=158592472.

Family-focused therapy (FFT), a specific type of family therapy, involves psychoeducation and teaches communication and problem-solving skills to patients and caregivers. There is evidence that this therapy leads to improvements in the quality of family relationships and physical well-being (O'Donnell et al., 2017). FFT works to restore a healthy and supportive home environment. Educating family members about the disease and how to cope with its symptoms is a major component of treatment.

Informatics

Despite the evidence for the need to provide both pharmacological and psychological treatment to improve the outcome and quality of life for people with bipolar disorders, such specialized treatment is not always available. Technology may provide solutions. For example, telepsychiatry can involve providing a range of services from a distance. It can include psychiatric evaluations, therapy (individual therapy, group therapy, family therapy), patient education, and medication management through the use of technology tools like videoconferencing.

Smartphone applications (apps) are another potentially effective use of technology. Apps can provide everything from medication and meditation reminders to mood-tracking strategies. Unfortunately, there remains a significant absence of reliable data about the effectiveness of specific apps (Nicholas et al., 2015). Smartphone apps seem to work best when used in conjunction with formal therapy.

An app called Predicting Individual Outcomes for Rapid Intervention (PRIORI) is part of a long-term study by the University of Michigan. It allows speech features to be recorded and analyzed securely, making it possible to detect changes in mood. Eventually, it will include a feedback loop to the patient and the treatment team and even a chosen family member (University of Michigan, 2014).

Support Groups

Patients with bipolar disorder and their significant others can benefit from support groups. Examples include the Depression and Bipolar Support Alliance (DBSA), the National Alliance on Mental Illness (NAMI), and the National Depressive Manic-Depressive Association (NDMDA).

Self-Care for Nurses

During the acute manic phase, a patient can elicit numerous intense, unpleasant, and negative emotions in health care professionals. During mania, the patient lacks internal controls and resists being controlled. The patient may use humor, manipulation, or demanding behavior to prevent or minimize the staff's ability to set limits or control dangerous behaviors. The patient might get involved in power plays with the staff, such as by pointing out faults or oversights and drawing negative attention to one or more staff members. Manic behavior that goes unchecked can escalate further.

Clear and consistent limit setting is required to keep the patient, the staff, and the therapeutic milieu safe. **Teamwork and collaboration** are essential to achieving this **consistency. (QSEN: Teamwork and Collaboration)** All health care workers need to communicate with one another and reestablish limit setting in clear terms. *Behavioral contracts* that concretely describe acceptable and unacceptable behaviors can be a useful tool when the patient is less acutely ill.

Patients with bipolar disorders are often ambivalent about treatment. They may minimize the destructive consequences of their behaviors or deny the seriousness of the disease. Some are reluctant to relinquish the increased energy, euphoria, and heightened sense of self-esteem of hypomania. Unfortunately, nonadherence to the regimen of mood-stabilizing medication is a major cause of relapse. Establishing a therapeutic alliance with the individual who has a bipolar disorder is crucial.

EVALUATION

Evaluation is used to determine whether the goals of nursing interventions have been met. The nurse evaluates short- and longer-term goals. Some examples of outcome indicators include the following:

1. Stable vital signs?
2. Is the patient well hydrated?
3. Does the person sleep at least 4 or 5 hours per night?
4. Is self-control maintained?
5. Do the patient and family have a clear understanding of the patient's disease?
6. Do the patient and family know which community agencies may help them?

If the goals of treatment are not achieved, it is important to consider how to modify care.

Longer-term goals include adherence to the medication regimen; resumption of functioning in the community; achievement of stability in family, work, and social relationships and in mood; and improved coping skills for reducing stress.

KEY POINTS TO REMEMBER

- There is strong support that biological factors play a role in the etiology of bipolar disorders.
  - Strong genetic correlates have been shown.
  - Imbalance in neurotransmitters has been associated with symptoms of bipolar disorders.
  - Neuroendocrine and neuroanatomical changes are associated with a diagnosis of bipolar disorder.
- Bipolar disorders often remain unrecognized. Early detection and intervention can help promote more positive long-term outcomes and diminish co-occurring substance use disorders, suicide, and declines in social and personal relationships.
- The nurse assesses the patient's mood, behavior, thought processes, and thought content and is alert to cognitive dysfunction.
- During the acute phase of mania, physical needs often take priority. Deficient fluid volume, imbalanced nutrition, elimination disturbances, and disturbed sleep pattern must be addressed.
- The use of consistent limit-setting strategies using a neutral tone is most effective when a patient displays intrusive interpersonal behaviors. Early intervention in impulsive and aggressive behaviors helps maintain safety.
- Support groups, psychoeducation, and guidance for the family can greatly affect the patient's adherence to the medication and treatment regimen.
- Nursing care involves identifying the specific needs of the patient and family during acute episodes and during the continuation/maintenance phases of the disease.
- Pharmacological treatments for bipolar disorders include the following:
  - Lithium is the first-line treatment used to treat and prevent both mania and depression. The narrow therapeutic index requires thorough patient and family teaching and regular follow-up.
  - Antiepileptic drugs such as carbamazepine, lamotrigine, and valproic acid are useful, especially in treating people who do not respond well to lithium therapy.
  - Atypical antipsychotic drugs are used for both sedation and mood stabilization. Some atypical antipsychotics can be used

KEY POINTS TO REMEMBER—Cont'd

as both a first-line treatment and an adjunctive treatment for patients who do not respond well to lithium treatment.

- For some patients, electroconvulsive therapy (ECT) may be the most appropriate medical treatment for acute illness.
- There are therapies that can enhance well-being and improve the quality of family relationships when used with medications.
- Evaluation includes examining the effectiveness of the nursing interventions and making changes to the treatment regimen as needed. Evaluation is an ongoing process and is part of each of the other steps in the nursing process.

APPLYING CRITICAL JUDGMENT

1. A patient is taken into the emergency department after threatening in a loud voice to "Blow up the world to save the poor, and many more, where's the door? No more, no more. Let me loose." He had attacked a bartender who would not give him any more to drink. He has not eaten or slept for more than 1 week and only takes sips of fluids when offered. He talks nonstop and moves constantly, flailing his arms and bumping into objects as he walks rapidly.
   A. Identify the patient's immediate needs. Describe the interventions you would plan for his physiological safety, including milieu management.
   B. Discuss the most appropriate communication techniques for the patient. Give examples of what you would say and how you would say it.
   C. What medications would most likely be given immediately? Long term?
   D. Write a medication psychoeducation plan for the patient and his family.
   E. Describe at least four evidence-based therapeutic modalities for a patient with a diagnosis of bipolar disorder.
   F. What symptoms would help you evaluate if a patient with a diagnosis of bipolar disorder was currently in a hypomania or mania state?
   G. Name the most important interventions you would institute for each of the clinical presentations listed in the previous question.

CHAPTER REVIEW QUESTIONS

1. A patient has a long history of bipolar disorder with frequent episodes of mania secondary to stopping prescribed medications. The patient says, "I will use my whole check next month to buy lottery tickets. Winning will solve my money problems." Select the nurse's best action.
   a. Educate the patient about the low odds of winning the lottery.
   b. Present reality by saying to the patient, "That is not a good use of your money."
   c. Confer with the treatment team about appointing a legal guardian for the patient.
   d. Tell the patient, "If you buy lottery tickets, your money will run out before the end of the month."
2. Which comment by a patient diagnosed with bipolar disorder best indicates the patient is experiencing mania?
   a. "I have been sleeping about 6 hours each night."
   b. "Yesterday I made 487 posts on my social network page."
   c. "I am having dreams about my father's death 8 years ago."
   d. "My appetite is so robust that I've gained 4 pounds in the past 2 weeks."
3. A community mental health nurse counsels a group of patients about the upcoming flu season. What instruction does the nurse provide for patients who are prescribed lithium?
   a. "Call the clinic if you have nausea, vomiting, and/or diarrhea or are unable to stay well hydrated."
   b. "Remember that lithium reduces your immunity, so you are more vulnerable to catching the flu."
   c. "The flu is contagious. Isolate yourself if you get the flu so that you avoid exposing others to it."
   d. "Because you take lithium, you may have flu symptoms that are not typically experienced by others."
4. A patient was diagnosed with bipolar disorder many years ago. The patient tells the nurse, "When I have a manic episode, there's always a feeling of gloom behind it, and I know I will soon be totally depressed." What is the nurse's best response?
   a. "Most patients diagnosed with bipolar disorder report the same types of feelings."
   b. "Feelings of gloom associated with depression result from serotonin dysregulation."
   c. "If you take your medication as it is prescribed, you will not have those experiences."
   d. "Your comment indicates you have an understanding of and insight about your disorder."
5. A patient diagnosed with bipolar disorder lives in the community and is showing early signs of mania. The patient says, "I need to go visit my daughter, but she lives across the country. I put some requests on the Internet to get a ride. I'm sure someone will take me." What is the nurse's most therapeutic response?
   a. "I'm concerned about your safety when meeting or riding with strangers."
   b. "Have you asked friends and family to donate money for your airfare?"
   c. "You are not likely to get a ride. Let's consider some other strategies."
   d. "Have you asked your daughter if she wants you to come for a visit?"

REFERENCES

American Psychiatric Association. (2013). *Diagnostic and statistical manual of mental disorders (DSM-5)* (5th ed.). Washington, DC: Author.

APNA e-Series. (2015). *Issue 1 bipolar spectrum disorders: Assessment, diagnosis, and epidemiology using a recovery Paradigm.*

Australian Institute of Psychological Counsellors. (2014). *Psychoeducation: Definition, goals and methods.* Retrieved from: https://www.aipc.net.au/articles/psychoeducation-definition-goals-and-methods/.

Belvederi Murri, M., Prestia, D., Mondelli, V., Pariante, C., Patti, S., Olivieri, B., et al. (2016). The HPA axis in bipolar disorder: Systematic review and meta-analysis. *Psychoneuroendocrinology, 63*, 327–342. https://doi.org/10.1016/j.psyneuen.2015.10.014.

Berk, M., Post, R., Ratheesh, A., Gliddon, E., Singh, A., Vieta, E., et al. (2017). Staging in bipolar disorder: From theoretical framework to clinical utility. *World Psychiatry, 16*(3), 236–244. https://doi.org/10.1002/wps.20441.

Black, D. W., & Andreasen, N. C. (2014). *Introductory textbook of psychiatry* (6th ed.). Washington, DC: American Psychiatric Publishing.

Boland, E. M., Strange, J. P., Labelle, D. R., Shapero, B. G., Weiss, R. B., Abramson, L. Y., et al. (2016). Affective disruption from social rhythm and Behavioral Approach System (BAS) Sensitivities: A test of the integration of the social zeitgeber and BAS Theories of bipolar disorder. *Clinical Psychological Science, 4*(3), 418–432. https://doi.org/10.1177/2167702615603368.

Brooks, M. (2015). *Bipolar disorder recognized earlier, mortality remains high.* Medscape. Retrieved from: www.medscape.com/viewarticle/8454150.

Dempsey, R. C., Gooding, P. A., & Jones, H. (2017). A prospective study of bipolar disorder vulnerability in relation to behavioural activation, behavioural inhibition and dysregulation of the Behavioural Activation System. *European Psychiatry, 44*, 24–29. https://doi.org/10.1016/j.eurpsy.2017.03.005.

Fears, S. C., et al. (2015). Brain structure–function associations in multi-generational families genetically enriched for bipolar disorder. *Brain, 138*(Pt 7), 2087–2102. https://doi.org/10.1093/brain/awv106. Epub 2015 May 5.

Fuentes, I., Rizo-Mendez, A., & Jarne-Esparcia, A. (2016). Low compliance to pharmacological treatment is linked to cognitive impairment in euthymic phase of bipolar disorder. *Journal of Affective Disorders, 195*, 215–220. https://doi.org/10.1016/j.jad.2016.02.005.

Giddens, J. (2017). *Concepts of nursing practice.* St. Louis: Elsevier.

Goodwin, G. M., Haddad, P. M., Ferrier, I. N., et al. (2016). Evidence-based guidelines for treating bipolar disorder: Revised third edition Recommendations from the British Association for Psychopharmacology. *Journal of Psychopharmacology (Oxford, England), 30*(6), 495–553. https://doi.org/10.1177/0269881116636545.

Grohol, J. (2016). *Interpersonal and social rhythm therapy.* Psych Central. Retrieved from https://psychcentral.com/lib/interpersonal-and-social-rhythm-therapy/.

Guzman, F. (2017a). Bipolar disorder treatment guidelines: A 2018 Update, 2017 Psychopharmacology Institute. Retrieved from: https://psychopharmacologyinstitute.com/guidelines/bipolar-disorder-guidelines/?utm_source=email&utm_medium=emailARCkit&utm_campaign=Email-Bipolar-Guidelines&convertkit_id=lchiappetta@wccnet.edu&ck_subscriber_id=158592472

Guzman, F. (2017b). Lithium's mechanism of action: An Illustrated review, Psychopharmacology Institute. Retrieved from: https://psychopharmacologyinstitute.com/mood-stabilizers/mechanism-action-lithium-illustrated-review/

Jamison, K. R. (1995). *An unquiet mind.* New York: Knopf.

Jones, S. H., Smith, G., Mulligan, L. D., et al. (2015). Recovery-focused cognitive–behavioural therapy for recent-onset bipolar disorder: Randomised controlled pilot trial. *The British Journal of Psychiatry, 206*(1), 58–66. https://doi.org/10.1192/bjp.bp.113.141259.

Lingohr-Smith, M. (2017). What Chemicals Are Involved with Bipolar Disorder? Livestrong.com. Retrieved from: https://www.livestrong.com/article/234421-what-chemicals-are-involved-with-bipolar-disorder/.

McDonald, C. (2015). Brain structural effects of Psychopharmacological treatment in bipolar disorder. *Current Neuropharmacology*. Retrieved from https://doi.org/10.2174/1570159X13666150403231654.

McInnis, M., et al. (2017). Cohort profile: The Heinz C. Prechter Longitudinal study of bipolar disorder. *International Journal of Epidemiology*. Retrieved from https://doi.org/10.1093/ije/dyx229.

Muneer, A., et al. (2016). Bipolar disorder: Role of inflammation and the development of disease biomarkers. *Psychiatry Investigation. 13*(1), 18–33. https://doi.org/10.4306/pi.2016.13.1.18.

National Institute for Health and Care Excellence (NICE) (2016). NICE Guidance: Clinical guideline [CG185], Bipolar disorder: Assessment and management. Retrieved from: https://www.nice.org.uk/guidance/cg185/chapter/1-Recommendations#how-to-use-medication.

National Institute of Mental Health (NIMH). (2016, February 26). *Symptoms Outdo diagnoses in predicting bipolar disorder in at-risk Youth.* Science Update. https://www.nimh.nih.gov/news/science-news/2016/symptoms-outdo-diagnoses-in-predicting-bipolar-disorder-in-at-risk-youth.shtml.

National Institute of Mental Health (NIMH). (2017). Bipolar Disorder. Retrieved from: https://www.nimh.nih.gov/health/statistics//bipolar-disorder.shtml.

Nicholas, J., Larsen, M.E, Proudfoot, J., Christensen H. (2015). Mobile apps for bipolar disorder: A systematic review of features and content quality. *Journal of Medical Internet Research, 17*(8):e198. URL: http://www.jmir.org/2015/8/e198, DOI: 10.2196/jmir.4581, PMID: 26283290 PMCID: 4642376

O'Donnell, L. A., Axelson, D. A., Kowatch, R. A., Schneck, C. D., Sugar, C. A., & Miklowitz, D. J. (2017). Enhancing quality of life among adolescents with bipolar disorder: A randomized trial of two psychosocial interventions. *Journal of Affective Disorders*. https://doi.org/10.1016/j.jad.2017.04.039.

Perlis, R. H., & Ostacher, M. (2015). Bipolar disorder. In T. A. Stern, M. Fava, T. E. Wilens, & J. F. Rosenbaum (Eds.), *Massachusetts General Hospital comprehensive clinical psychiatry* (2nd ed.). St. Louis: Elsevier.

Preston, J., & Johnson, J. (2015). *Clinical psychopharmacology made ridiculously simple* (8th ed.). Miami: MedMasters.

Shah, N., Grover, S., & Rao, G. P. (2017). Clinical practice guidelines for management of bipolar disorder. *Indian Journal of Psychiatry, 59*(Suppl. 1), S51–S66. Retrieved from https://doi.org/10.4103/0019-5545.196974.

Solé, B., Jiménez, E., Torrent, C., Reinares, M., Bonnin, C., del, M., et al. (2017). Cognitive impairment in bipolar disorder: Treatment and prevention strategies. *International Journal of Neuropsychopharmacology, 20*(8), 670–680. Retrieved from https://doi.org/10.1093/ijnp/pyx032.

Spencer, S., & Johnson, P. (2016). De-escalation techniques for managing aggression (Protocol). *Cochrane Database of Systematic Reviews, 2016*(1), CD012034. Retrieved from https://doi.org/10.1002/14651858.CD012034.

Stahl, S. M. (2019). *Stahl's essential psychopharmacology. Prescriber's guide* (6th ed.). Cambridge: Cambridge University Press.

Subramanian, K., Sarkar, S., Kattimani, S., Philip Rajkumar, R., & Penchilaiya, V. (2017). Role of stressful life events and kindling in bipolar disorder: Converging evidence from a mania-predominant illness course. *Psychiatry Reviews, 258*, 434–437. Retrieved from https://doi.org/10.1016/j.psychres.2017.08.073.

Substance Abuse and Mental Health Services Administration. (2015). *Alternatives to seclusion and restraint.* Retrieved from https://www.samhsa.gov/trauma-violence/seclusion.

Tartakovsky, M. (2017). Bipolar disorder fact Sheet. Psych Central. Retrieved from https://psychcentral.com/disorders/bipolar/bipolar-disorder-fact-sheet/.

Thomas, J. (2016). *The challenge of accurately diagnosing bipolar disorder, health Newsletter*. Retrieved from: http://www.health.com/health/condition-article/0,,20275016,00.html.

University of Michigan. (2014). *Listening to bipolar disorder: Smartphone app detects mood swings via voice analysis.* Retrieved from: http://www.eecs.umich.edu/eecs/about/articles/2014/app_for_mood_swings.html.

Wang, H. R., Woo, Y. S., Ahn, H. S., Ahn, I. M., Kim, H. J., & Bahk, W.-M. (2015). The Validity of the mood disorder Questionnaire for screening bipolar disorder: A meta-analysis. *Depression and Anxiety, 32*, 527–538. Retrieved from https://doi.org/10.1002/da.22374.

WebMD Medical Reference. (2016). *Women with bipolar disorder. Reviewed by Joseph Goldberg*. Retrieved from: https://www.webmd.com/bipolar-disorder/guide/bipolar-disorder-women#1.

WebMD Medical Reference. (2017). *What is bipolar disorder? Reviewed by Smitha Bhandari*. Retrieved from: https://www.webmd.com/bipolar-disorder/guide/bipolar-spectrum-categories#1.

World Health Organization (WHO). (2017). *Strategies to end the use of seclusion, restraint and other coercive practices*. Retrieved from: http://apps.who.int/iris/handle/10665/254809.

Zivanovic, O. (2017). Lithium: A classic drug—frequently discussed, but, sadly, seldom prescribed! *Australian and New Zealand Journal of Psychiatry, 51*(9), 886–896. Retrieved from http://journals.sagepub.com/doi/pdf/10.1177/0004867417695889.

17

Schizophrenia Spectrum Disorders and Other Psychotic Disorders

Lorraine Chiappetta, Elizabeth M. Varcarolis

http://evolve.elsevier.com/Varcarolis/essentials

OBJECTIVES

1. Compare predisposing factors associated with the development of schizophrenia.
2. Use evidence-based data to explain the physiological factors that support the premise that schizophrenia is a disease of the brain. **QSEN: Evidence-Based Practice**
3. Compare and contrast the positive and negative symptoms of schizophrenia and how these symptoms affect quality of life and progression of the disease.
4. Explain how cognitive/neurocognitive symptoms and mood symptoms of schizophrenia affect both the prognosis of the disease and a person's quality of life.
5. Name and describe at least four other primary psychotic disorders.
6. Describe components of interprofessional and intraprofessional teamwork and collaboration that facilitate safe and effective care for a person with a schizophrenic disorder during the different phases of the illness. **QSEN: Teamwork and Collaboration; Safety**
7. Discuss principles of effective communication when caring for a person who is experiencing symptoms of psychotic, including (a) hallucinating, (b) experiencing paranoid ideation, or (c) experiencing delusional thinking. **QSEN: Patient-Centered Care**
8. Compare and contrast the similarities and differences between the properties of first-generation antipsychotics (typical/conventional) and those of second-generation (atypical) antipsychotic drugs.
9. Discuss evidence-based psychosocial therapies for patients with schizophrenia and their families. **QSEN: Evidence-Based Practice**
10. Using informatics, identify available web-based and other resources to support appropriate patient and family care for those with a psychotic disorder. **QSEN: Informatics**

KEY TERMS AND CONCEPTS

acute dystonia, p. 272
affect, p. 256
akathisia, p. 272
associative looseness, p. 255
catatonia p. 255
circumstantial (circumstantiality), p. 255
clang association, p. 255
cognitive/neurocognitive symptoms, p. 251
concrete thinking, p. 255
delusions, p. 254
dysphoria, p. 257
echolalia, p. 255
echopraxia, p. 255
extrapyramidal symptoms (EPSs), p. 270
first-generation antipsychotics (FGAs)/typical/conventional antipsychotics, p. 270
hallucinations, p. 255
ideas of reference (delusions of reference), p. 254
illusions, p. 255
negative symptoms, p. 251
neologisms, p. 255
neurogenesis, p. 252
neuroleptic malignant syndrome (NMS), p. 272
neuroleptics, p. 270
paranoia, p. 257
positive symptoms, p. 251
projection, p. 257
pseudoparkinsonism, p. 272
psychotic, p. 250
recovery model of mental illness, p. 268
second-generation antipsychotics (SGAs)/atypical antipsychotics, p. 270
stereotyped behaviors, p. 257
tangential (tangentiality), p. 255
tardive dyskinesia (TD), p. 271
thought broadcasting, p. 254
thought insertion, p. 254
thought withdrawal, p. 254
waxy flexibility, p. 257
word salad, p. 255

CONCEPT: PSYCHOSIS: *Psychosis* is a syndrome of neurocognitive symptoms that impairs cognitive capacity, leading to deficits in perception, functioning, and social relatedness. Society's relative lack of understanding of psychosis leads to stigma and has allowed social injustice to flourish.

Primary psychosis is associated with discrete psychiatric disorders, like schizophrenia spectrum disorders, whereas secondary psychosis is part of other organic disorders, like substance intoxication and dementia. Primary and secondary forms of psychosis are not mutually exclusive; not only do they coexist, but in some instances, they potentiate the other (Giddens, 2017).

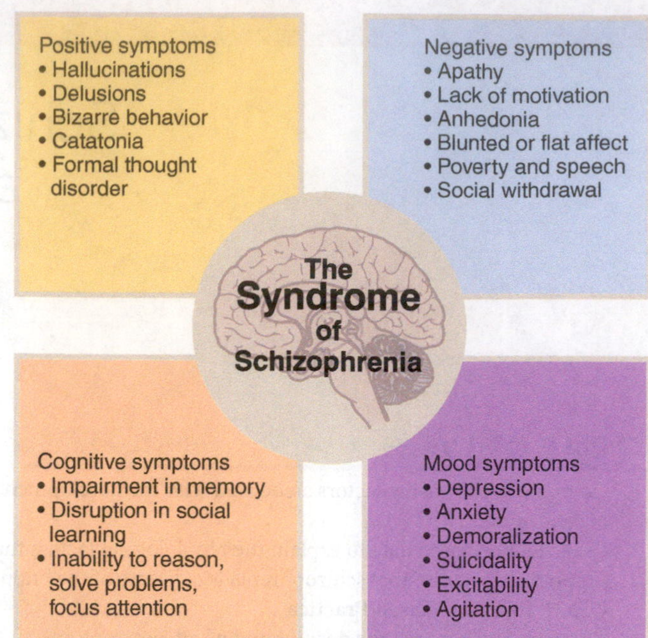

Fig. 17.1 Treatment-relevant dimensions of schizophrenia.

INTRODUCTION

Schizophrenia is a devastating brain disease that is typically diagnosed in late adolescence or early adulthood. It is best understood as being part of a spectrum or continuum of a broad range of disorders, rather than one homogenous disease (American Psychiatric Association [APA], 2013). *Schizophrenia spectrum disorders* are some of the more disabling types of mental illnesses. They are usually chronic and affect how a person thinks, feels, and behaves.

SCHIZOPHRENIA

Schizophrenia is considered a *primary* psychotic disorder. The word *psychosis* is used to describe a set of symptoms that affects the mind when there has been some loss of contact with reality (National Institute of Mental Health [NIMH], 2016). Psychotic disorders can lead to abnormalities in five different symptomatic domains: delusions, hallucinations, disorganized thoughts, disorganized or abnormal motor behavior, and "negative symptoms" (APA, 2013). *Secondary* psychotic symptoms can also be observed with other diseases that affect the neurological system.

Although every person must be approached as a unique individual, there is a set of common symptoms associated with the *primary psychotic disorder* of schizophrenia. These symptoms are described in detail in this chapter and summarized in Fig. 17.1. Other primary psychotic disorders are identified in Box 17.1.

Prevalence

The lifetime prevalence of schizophrenia is said to be approximately 1% worldwide, with no differences related to race, social status, culture, gender, or environment (Sadock, Sadock, & Ruiz, 2015). With an early age of onset, there is more evidence of structural brain abnormalities, more prominent *negative* and disabling symptoms, and a poorer prognosis. Males tend to have an earlier age of onset (18 to 25 years). Individuals with a later onset (25 to 35 years) are more likely to be female, have less evidence of structural brain abnormalities, and have better long-term outcomes. Childhood-onset schizophrenia is rare.

An abrupt onset of symptoms with good premorbid functioning usually has a better prognosis, with a greater chance of remission or complete recovery. A slow, insidious onset over a period of 2 or 3 years tends to have a poorer prognosis. A childhood history of withdrawn, reclusive, eccentric, and tense behavior is an unfavorable diagnostic sign that usually indicates a more disabling form of the disease in adulthood.

Comorbidity

Knowledge of the most common comorbid conditions associated with schizophrenia helps the nurse to complete a more comprehensive assessment to prevent the incidence and complications associated with these conditions.

Substance use disorders occur in more than 50% of individuals with schizophrenia (Sadock et al., 2015). Of those with a diagnosis of schizophrenia, 50% also have a tobacco use disorder (APA, 2013). Epidemiological observations have demonstrated a strong association between cannabis use and the risk of developing a psychotic disorder, including schizophrenia (Vaucher et al., 2017). Risk factors associated with the development of schizophrenia also increase the risk of using/misusing cannabis. This suggests some type of genetic link between the two disorders (Gage et al., 2017). Comorbid substance use disorders can lead to significant morbidity and mortality.

Those with a diagnosis of schizophrenia have an increased risk for additional psychiatric disorders. Co-occurring depressive symptoms/disorders are frequently observed in schizophrenia, with suicide as the leading cause of premature death in this population. Approximately 20% of those with a diagnosis of schizophrenia *attempt* suicide during their lifetime, and 6% to 10% *complete* a suicide (APA, 2013). It has been shown that a higher IQ and shorter illness length are factors that increase the risk of *completed* suicides in this population. Psychosocial factors that include a history of depression, a history of problematic drug use, and a positive family psychiatric history were significant predictors of suicide attempts (Cassidy et al., 2017). The rates of co-occurring anxiety disorders, obsessive-compulsive disorder, and panic attacks are also significantly higher in this population compared with the general population. Individuals diagnosed with schizotypal and paranoid personality disorders may later progress to full-blown schizophrenia (APA, 2013).

Adults with schizophrenia are more than 3.5 times more likely to die from premature death due to nonpsychiatric illnesses. This is related to the increased incidence of cardiovascular disease, respiratory disease, influenza, and pneumonia and diseases associated with alcohol/drug use disorders (Olfson et al., 2015). *Metabolic syndrome* is another leading cause of morbidity and mortality in patients with schizophrenia, with a prevalence rate twice that of nonpsychiatric populations. Metabolic syndrome is usually associated with the antipsychotic medications used to treat schizophrenia. Signs and symptoms of *metabolic syndrome* include dyslipidemia, hypertension, obesity, and type 2 diabetes, leading to increased risk of cardiovascular disease and premature death (Rawat et al., 2017).

BOX 17.1 Other Psychotic Disorders

Disorder	Course	Description
Schizophreniform disorder	Symptoms must last at least 1 month but not more than 6 months	*Essential features* are identical to those of schizophrenia but of *shorter duration*
Brief psychotic disorder	Usually no longer than a month; person returns to premorbid functioning; usually precipitated by extreme stress	A sudden onset of psychotic symptoms
Schizoaffective disorder	Better prognosis than schizophrenia but significantly worse than a mood disorder	Symptom of a mood disorder: major depressive, manic, or mixed episode, concurrent with symptoms that meet the criteria for schizophrenia Common psychotic disorder
Schizotypal personality disorder (refer to Chapter 13)	May progress to developing schizophrenia	Personality disorder considered part of the schizophrenia spectrum disorders *(DSM-5)*; shares common genetics and neuropsychiatric characteristics
Delusional disorder	Ranges from remission without relapse to chronic waxing and waning; symptoms must last at least 1 month	Involves nonbizarre delusions such as being followed, infected, loved at a distance, or deceived by a spouse; having some great or unrecognized insight; ability to function is not markedly impaired and behavior is not obviously odd or bizarre. Delusions of persecution are the most common.
Substance-/medication-induced psychotic disorder	Psychosis *usually* resolves	Caused by ingestion of or withdrawal from a substance

DSM-5, Diagnostic and Statistical Manual of Mental Disorders.

The incidence of human immunodeficiency virus (HIV) and acquired immune deficiency syndrome (AIDS) in those with a diagnosis of schizophrenia is 1.5 times more likely compared with the general population (Blank, 2016). The diagnosis of schizophrenia has also been associated with increased incidences of incarceration, homelessness, and being the victim of violence.

Course and Prognosis

The clinical course of schizophrenia frequently includes recurrent, acute exacerbations of psychosis with periods of full or partial remission of symptoms. Newer public health initiatives can potentially have a positive impact on the course and long-term outcome of this illness.

Primary and secondary intervention strategies include targeting people at "high risk" for developing schizophrenia, intervening in the prodromal (early or pre-illness) phase of schizophrenia, and reducing the "duration of untreated psychosis" (DUP) during a psychotic episode (Fusar-Poli, McGorry, & Kane, 2017). In general, the earlier someone with schizophrenia is diagnosed and stabilized on an appropriate treatment regimen, the better the chance of recovery (Fusar-Poli et al., 2017). Preventing relapse is important because with every relapse into psychosis, there is an increase in residual dysfunction and deterioration (Sadock et al., 2015).

The following are the phases of the disease:

- Prodromal phase: includes signs and symptoms that precede the acute, fully manifested signs and symptoms of disease. Prodromal symptoms occur in up to 80% to 90% of people with schizophrenia before the emergence of frank psychosis (acute phase). Early prodromal symptoms include social withdrawal and deterioration in functioning, depressive mood, perceptual disturbances, magical thinking, and peculiar behavior. Changes in self-care, sleeping or eating patterns, and school or work performance may also be evidenced. Prodromal symptoms can appear a month to a year before the first psychotic "break" (episode).

    Health care workers can play a role in primary and secondary prevention through early recognition of prodromal symptoms of schizophrenia and facilitating early treatment to prevent full-blown psychotic symptoms.

- Acute phase: Period of "florid" or severe and well-developed symptoms grouped into four categories: (1) **positive symptoms** (hallucinations, delusions), (2) **negative symptoms** (apathy, withdrawal, lack of motivation); (3) **cognitive/neurocognitive symptoms** (problematic ability to understand and make decisions, attention problems, and problems with "working memory") and (4) *mood symptoms* (depression and anxiety). (See Dimensions of Schizophrenia in the next section.)
- Stabilization phase: Period in which acute symptoms, particularly the "positive symptoms," decrease in severity.
- Maintenance phase: Period in which symptoms are in remission, although there might be milder persistent symptoms (residual symptoms).

Although schizophrenia is a chronic illness, the level of disability associated with this illness is on a continuum. The National Alliance on Mental Illness (NAMI, n.d.) estimates that many people with a diagnosis of schizophrenia can recover significantly if they get treatment. The *DSM-5* states that 20% of diagnosed individuals demonstrate a favorable outcome. Some have recovered completely (APA, 2013). However, 20% of patients diagnosed with schizophrenia will relapse within a year after successful treatment of an acute episode, even when taking medications as prescribed. As with other chronic illnesses, some patients do extremely well in managing their illness, whereas others continue to be symptomatic and need ongoing support and assistance. As treatment options continue to improve, the prognosis for those diagnosed with schizophrenia also tends to improve. *The generalist nurse can play a significant role in early case findings by having knowledge of the typical age of onset of this disorder and an understanding of the early symptoms of the disease.*

Theory

Risk Factors

Determining the causes of schizophrenia is a complicated matter. This disease is a "no-fault" biological illness. Schizophrenia most likely occurs as a result of a combination of inherited genetic factors and nongenetic factors that impact the brain. Alterations in brain structure, disruptions in the brain's neurotransmitter system, and alterations to neural circuits caused by these genetic and nongenetic factors are all implicated in the etiology of schizophrenia.

Neurochemical Contributing Factors

For many years the *dopamine hypothesis* was the most widely accepted explanation for the biochemical pathophysiology in schizophrenia. It concluded there was hyperactivity of the neurotransmitter dopamine in the limbic regions of the brain. The *revised dopamine hypothesis* proposes *hyperactive* dopamine transmission in the mesolimbic areas and *hypoactive* dopamine transmission in the prefrontal cortex in patients with schizophrenia. In addition, there is evidence of dopamine dysregulation in multiple other areas of the brain in schizophrenia (Brisch et al., 2014).

Abnormal levels of the neurotransmitter serotonin might also play a role in causing some of the negative and mood symptoms associated with schizophrenia. The *NMDA receptors hypofunction hypothesis* suggests that *N*-methyl-D-aspartate (NMDA), an amino acid similar to glutamate, is implicated in the psychotic, negative, and cognitive symptoms associated with schizophrenia (Black & Andreasen, 2014). The *glutamate hypothesis* suggests that excess or insufficient glutamate activity may cause some symptoms of schizophrenia partly through the interaction of glutamate with other neurotransmitters, such as dopamine and gamma-aminobutyric acid (GABA) (Patel et al., 2014). Many of these theories are based on the study of the mechanism of action of drugs that mimic symptoms of schizophrenia, such as amphetamines and hallucinogens. Researchers also formed hypotheses about the pathophysiology of schizophrenia based on an understanding of the mechanism of action of the medications (antipsychotics) used to treat this disorder.

Genetic Factors

Numerous studies suggest schizophrenia has a strong genetic component. Having one parent with schizophrenia leads to a 5% to 6% chance of developing the disease, whereas having two parents with schizophrenia leads to a 46% likelihood of developing schizophrenia (Black & Andreasen, 2014). The lifetime risk for developing schizophrenia is 10% for siblings, up to 14% for fraternal (dizygotic) twins, and up to 50% for identical (monozygotic) twins (Dein, 2017). For identical twins reared apart, the concordance rate (incidence of developing the illness) for schizophrenia is similar.

Schizophrenia is not a "one gene, one illness" disease. Researchers have identified a group of eight genetically different types of schizophrenias. They found evidence that there are different networks of 42 genes that work together to produce specific symptom profiles, including positive symptoms, cognitive symptoms, and thought disorganization symptoms, associated with the illness (Nauert, 2015).

Recent research has focused on a gene called *C-4* that is responsible for a neurodevelopmental process called *synaptic pruning. Synaptic pruning* is described as the cutting back of weak or redundant connections between neurons in the area of the brain associated with thinking and planning skills. This normal developmental process occurs naturally in the teen years. The current hypothesis is that this gene causes excessive or inappropriate "pruning" of neural connections, resulting in some of the problematic cognitive symptoms seen in schizophrenia (Chavan, 2016; Rettner, 2016).

Neuroanatomical Factors

Schizophrenia is sometimes viewed as having a neurodegenerative component that occurs after the onset of the disease. Brain imaging techniques show tissue volume decreases in both gray and white matter, especially in the frontal lobes of the brain (Weinmann, Aderhold, & Haegele, 2015), and decreases in cortical gray matter. Other structural brain abnormalities observed include decreased brain volume, larger lateral and third ventricles, atrophy in the frontal lobe, and more cerebrospinal fluid (Black & Andreasen, 2014). Positron emission tomography (PET) scans show a lower rate of blood flow and glucose metabolism in the frontal lobes of the cerebral cortex of those diagnosed with schizophrenia. Neural circuitry (how neurons interact with each other) is thought to be faulty in schizophrenia, especially between the prefrontal cortex (PFC) and other brain areas like the thalamus (Cold Spring Harbor Laboratory, 2015). These neuroanatomical abnormalities may account for the cognitive dysfunctions (planning, memory, decision making, and attention) associated with schizophrenia. Although these studies are of interest for research, they presently have limited clinical relevance (Gerstein & Shlamovitz, 2015).

Nongenetic Risk Factors

The *neurodevelopmental vulnerability model* is one of the widely accepted hypotheses of the etiology of schizophrenia. **Neurogenesis** refers to the process by which neurons or nerve cells are generated and develop within the brain. This process is most active during prenatal development, when a baby's brain is being formed. Neurogenesis is altered in schizophrenia through both genetic and nongenetic factors (Nour & Howes, 2015).

Prenatal risk factors that may impact this neurogenesis and increase the risk for development of schizophrenia include viral infection (e.g., influenza, toxoplasmosis, and genital/reproductive infection), poor maternal nutrition or starvation, and exposure to toxins. Perinatal complications and birth injuries, including lack of oxygen during birth, are also significant risk factors. Closed head injuries that occur after birth increase the risk for the development of this disease later in life. Advanced paternal age (over 45 years) may also be a risk factor for adult schizophrenia (Fond et al., 2017).

Another theory suggests that the immune response may play a role in the etiology of schizophrenia. The illness may be triggered by environmental risk factors like infections or significant stress that activate the immune response. Further research in this area is needed (Pouget et al., 2016).

Several studies indicate a higher potential of developing psychosis in first- and second-generation immigrants (Tarricone et al., 2015). This higher risk is also associated with refugees (Dapunt, Kluge, & Heinz, 2017). Living in an urban environment is associated with an increased prevalence of specific mental health disorders, particularly schizophrenia, and may be related to the increased exposure to social stressors (Howes et al., 2017).

In addition to cannabis, the drugs methamphetamine and lysergic acid diethylamide (LSD) may increase the risk of developing schizophrenia in vulnerable individuals. This is especially true of those younger than age 21, in whom the brain is still developing.

Finally, social, psychological, and physical stressors may precipitate the illness in vulnerable individuals. Although stress is not considered a direct cause of schizophrenia, it may play a role in the severity and course of the disease.

Many questions remain regarding how these risk factors interact and contribute to the cause and progression of schizophrenia.

Cultural Considerations

Although the developmental pattern of schizophrenia is fairly consistent across cultures, studies find that some symptoms of schizophrenia can be interpreted differently in industrialized nations compared with developing countries. Anthropologists have noted that hallucinations associated with serious psychotic disorders are shaped by local cultural expectations and meaning. Rural Africans are more likely to hallucinate about ancestor worship; Christians are more likely to experience hallucinations about Christ, Mary, and Satan. Patients in the United States are more likely to use diagnostic labels and to report hearing auditory hallucinations of violent commands. Those in India and Ghana are more likely to report rich relationships with their hallucinations or voices (Luhrmann et al., 2015).

Even within the United States, types of hallucinations have differed over time. In East Texas, the command hallucinations of the 1930s were primarily benign and religious ("live right"; "lean on the Lord"), but those of the 1980s were negative and highly destructive ("kill yourself"; "kill your mother") (Dein, 2017).

Cultures differ in their attributions of the source of mental illness. Is the cause of symptoms attributed to religious, spiritual, or supernatural beliefs, or is there a biomedical explanation for symptoms? Understanding how an individual and family understands the cause of serious mental illness has implications for treatment and may affect medication adherence and treatment outcomes. For example, one consumer-driven movement, the Hearing Voices Network, introduces the idea that it may be possible to improve a person's relationships with the voices by teaching the person to respect the voices and to build relationships with them, to reduce their caustic or destructive qualities (HVN, 2020; Luhrmann et al., 2015) (**QSEN: Patient-Centered Care**).

It is currently unclear how cultural factors interact with biological factors in the causation and presentation of schizophrenia. Cultural factors might act as stressors that build on a biological vulnerability to stress (Dein, 2017).

Psychosis can be seen in the more severe forms of several psychiatric disorders, such as bipolar disorder, psychotic depression, and postpartum psychosis.

Secondary Causes

Secondary causes of psychosis include brain tumors or cysts, dementias, late-stage neurological diseases like Parkinson's disease and Huntington's chorea, HIV/AIDS, and infections of the brain. Secondary psychosis can also be part of the clinical picture of neurological diseases like stroke and some forms of epilepsy.

Finally, drugs associated with misuse and addiction, some prescription medications, and environmental toxins can precipitate secondary psychosis.

Clinical Picture

The signs and symptoms of schizophrenia are numerous. Not all symptoms apply to all individuals with the diagnosis. Symptoms are discussed in more detail under the assessment section Application of the Nursing Process in this chapter. Fig. 17.1 list many of the more common symptoms displayed. The *Diagnostic and Statistical Manual of Mental Disorders*, 5th edition (*DSM-5*; APA, 2013) diagnostic criteria for schizophrenia are also listed in this chapter.

Schizophrenia and Other Psychotic Disorders

People with schizophrenia may have multiple disturbing and disabling symptoms that necessitate a multifaceted approach to care and treatment.

Table 17.4 later in the chapter lists some common patient-centered concerns and nursing diagnoses that are the focus of care by the nurse.

BOX 17.2 Positive Symptoms of Schizophrenia

Hallucinations

See Table 17.2, Summary of Hallucinations and Other Perceptual Distortions

Delusions

See Table 17.1, Summary of Delusions

Types of Formal Thought Disorder and Disorganized Speech

- Derailment or loose associations (phrases that are not logically connected)
- Tangentiality (replies are off topic)
- Incoherence (lack of logical thoughts/speech)
- Circumstantiality (speech includes too many irrelevant details)
- Pressure of speech (increased rate of speech that is difficult to interrupt)
- Distractible speech (trouble staying on topic)
- Clang associations (word choice is governed by the sound of the words rather than meaning)

Types of Grossly Disorganized Behavior

- Repetitive, stereotyped behavior
- Bizarre mannerisms
- Odd clothing and appearance
- Agitated or aggressive behavior
- Catatonia

Dimensions of Schizophrenia

The major symptoms of schizophrenia can be grouped into positive, negative, cognitive, and mood. Fig. 17.1 presents an overview of these major symptom groups. A more detailed explanation of these symptoms and the ways in which they can affect an individual's ability to work, have satisfying relationships, and take care of self is as follows:

1. *Positive* symptoms are "add-on" symptoms, sometimes called "florid" symptoms. Some common "positive" symptoms seen in schizophrenia include hallucinations, delusions, bizarre behavior, and paranoia (Box 17.2).
2. *Negative* symptoms are "deficit" symptoms, which include thoughts and behaviors that the individual no longer demonstrates. They can include apathy, lack of motivation, and anhedonia (inability to experience pleasure). These symptoms are harder to treat. They affect a person's quality of life and ability to experience life-fulfilling activities (see Box 17.2).
3. *Cognitive* symptoms are perhaps the most debilitating symptoms. These include impairment in memory, disruption in social learning, and a decreased ability to reason and solve problems or focus attention. The greater the degree of *negative and cognitive* symptoms, the more likely it is that the person will have difficulty functioning on a job, engaging in social activities, and caring for self adequately and safely.
4. *Mood* symptoms include depression, anxiety, dysphoria, and suicidality (Freudenreich, Brown, & Holt, 2016).

Positive Symptoms. Positive symptoms are usually associated with an acute onset of the illness, normal premorbid functioning, and less brain pathology. These symptoms are more likely to lessen in response to antipsychotic medications. The positive symptoms appear early in the acute phase of the illness and often precipitate hospitalization. The positive symptoms presented here represent alterations in thinking, speech, perception, and behavior.

Alterations in Thinking

Delusions. Delusions are defined as *false fixed beliefs* that cannot be corrected by reasoning. A person experiencing delusions is convinced that what is believed to be real is real. Delusions are a type of "thought content" problem. Approximately 75% of people with schizophrenia experience delusions at some time during their illness.

Delusional thinking frequently involves the following themes:

1. Delusions of reference or "ideas of reference": the person believes a neutral event has a special and personal meaning.
   Example: A person drives by a billboard and starts to believe the message on the billboard was a private and personal message.
2. Paranoid or delusion of persecution: a belief that "others" are out to harm that person. Paranoid delusions put the patient at risk for harm to self and others. **(QSEN: Safety)**
   Example: "I know my enemies were actively trying to interfere with my activities, were trying to harm me, and even kill me."
3. Grandiosity: an unrealistic sense of superiority.
   Example: "I felt that I had the power to determine the weather, which responded to my inner moods."
4. Somatic: a belief about the meaning of a physical sensation.
   Example: "Snakes are eating out my stomach."
5. Jealousy: a feeling of envy over someone else's achievements or advantages or unfounded suspicion that someone is unfaithful.
   Example: "My spouse is always cheating on me."
6. Control: belief that one's body or mind is controlled by an outside force or agency.
   Example: "There's a man from darkness who controls my thoughts with electrical waves."

Table 17.1 provides definitions and examples of some of these common types of delusions. Delusions can also involve unique religious ideas. A person's thinking often reflects underlying feelings of great fear, anxiety, and isolation.

Other common delusions observed in schizophrenia include the following:

- Thought broadcasting: belief that one's thoughts can be heard by others. This type of delusion can make the assessment of a patient's thinking more challenging for the nurse.
  Example: A woman refuses to explain her problem, saying, "I know you know what I'm thinking. Everybody hears what I'm thinking."
- Thought insertion: belief that thoughts of others are being inserted into one's mind.
  Example: "They make me think bad thoughts."
- Thought withdrawal: belief that thoughts have been removed from one's mind by an outside agency. People experiencing thought withdrawal may experience other irregularities in speech and thinking, such as thought blocking.
  Example: "The devil takes my thoughts away and leaves me empty."

TABLE 17.1 Summary of Delusions

Type of Delusion (positive symptom)	Definition (a delusion is a false belief held and maintained as true, even with evidence to the contrary[a])	Example
Ideas of reference	Misconstruing trivial events and remarks and giving them personal significance	When Maria saw the doctor and nurse talking together, she believed they were plotting against her. When she heard on the radio that a hurricane was coming, she believed this was really a message that harm was going to befall her.
Persecution	The false belief that one is being singled out for harm by others; this belief often takes the form of people in power conspiring against the person or following the person, or being persecuted by friends or colleagues	Sam believed that the Secret Service was planning to kill him. He believed that the Secret Service was poisoning his food. Therefore he would only eat food that he was certain was safe.
Grandeur	The false belief that one is a very powerful and important person, having special abilities, or possessing great wealth or beauty	Sally believed that she was Mary Magdalene and that Jesus controlled her thoughts and was telling her how to save the world.
Somatic delusions	The false belief that the body is changing in an unusual way (e.g., rotting inside, heart is no longer beating)	David told the doctor that his brain was rotting away.
Jealousy	The false belief that one's mate is unfaithful; may have so-called proof	Harry accused his girlfriend of going out with other men, even though this was not the case. His "proof" was that she came home from work late twice that week. He persisted in his belief, even when the girlfriend's boss explained that everyone had worked late.
Erotomania	The false belief that another person, usually a stranger or high-class or famous person, is in love with him or her	Samantha is firmly convinced that Johnny Depp, the famous movie star, is madly in love with her. She imagines that callers who claim to have the wrong number are really Johnny. She sends him love letters and flowers through his agent. She repeatedly tries to get his home address.
Nihilistic	Exaggerated belief in the futility of everything; may deny his or her own existence and believe that he or she is literally dead	Jason is becoming more preoccupied with the belief that the world will end soon. He questions his own existence, sometimes wondering if he is already dead.
Bizarre delusions	Clearly implausible and incomprehensible false beliefs that do not derive from ordinary experiences	Phoebe is obsessed with the idea that aliens are taking over her mind and are replacing parts of her brain with parts of an alien brain.

[a]This does not include unusual beliefs maintained by one's culture or subculture.

- Thought blocking: a person's speech is suddenly interrupted by silences that may last a few seconds to a minute or longer. The person may be unaware of the stopping of speech or may report that "Someone took the thought out of my head."

Concrete Thinking. Concrete thinking refers to an overemphasis on specific details and a literal interpretation of ideas. It is contrasted with abstract thinking. The answer is literal; the ability to use abstract reasoning is lessened or absent.

Example: During an assessment, the nurse might ask a patient, "What brought you to the hospital? A concrete response might be "a cab" rather than explaining the reason for seeking medical or psychiatric assistance.

Example: When asked to give the meaning of the proverb "People in glass houses shouldn't throw stones," the person with concrete thinking might answer, "Don't throw stones or the windows will break."

Alterations in Thought Process (as Evidenced in Alterations in Speech). Disorganized or alterations in speech typically arise from *alterations in thought processes* or how thoughts are connected. Associations are the threads that tie one thought to another and one concept to another. In schizophrenia, these threads are missing, and connections are interrupted.

Associative Looseness. In associative looseness (or looseness of associations), thinking becomes haphazard, illogical, and confused. There are illogical shifts between topics. Zelda Fitzgerald wrote to her husband, the writer F. Scott Fitzgerald, an account of going mad:

> *Then the world became embryonic in Africa—and there was no need for communication ... I have been living in vaporous places peopled with one-dimensional figures and tremulous buildings until I can no longer tell an optical illusion from a reality ... head and ears incessantly throb, and roads disappear.*
>
> (Vidal, 1982, p. 82)

Circumstantiality. Circumstantiality is using excessive detail that distracts from the central idea of a conversation. The patient has difficulty separating relevant and irrelevant information when describing an event. The speaker does eventually complete the thought.

Example: "You asked about my knee brace. I was riding my bike to go get a pack of gum from the store and while I was riding my bike, there was a car that started to turn in front of me. The driver almost hit me. I didn't end up getting the gum I went for. I was going to get spearmint gum. It's my favorite flavor. I try to keep a pack with me in case I meet that special person. I almost got hit but I didn't fall to the ground. The guy in the car pulled over to help me. I think it scared him more than he scared me. But when he turned in front of me, I put my leg down to stop quickly and I twisted my knee. I went to urgent care and they said I sprained it and told me to wear the knee brace for a month."

Tangentiality. Tangential speech is when the train of thought of a speaker wanders off in another direction, never returning to the initial topic.

Example: "I went downtown last night. Nighttime is the best time of day. Daybreak brings sunshine."

Neologisms. Neologisms are "made-up" words that have special meaning for the person.

Example: "I was going to tell him the *mannerologies* of his hospitality just won't do." "I want all the *vetchkisses* to leave the room and let me be."

Use of neologisms in children and creative writers is considered imaginative, constructive, and adaptive. In people with a diagnosis of schizophrenia, neologisms represent a disruption in *thought and speech.*

Word Salad. Word salad represents further deterioration of the ability to connect thoughts in a coherent fashion. It is a term used to identify a jumble of words that is meaningless to the listener and perhaps to the speaker as well. It may include a string of *neologisms.*

Example: "I sang out for my mother ... for this to hell I went. How long is road? These little said three hills hop aboard, share the appetite of the Christmas mice spread ... within three round moons the devil will be washed away."

Echolalia. Echolalia is the pathological repeating of another's words by imitation. Echolalia is the counterpart of echopraxia, defined as mimicking the movements of another. Both are often seen in people with catatonia.

Clang Association. Clang association is the meaningless rhyming of words, often in a forceful manner. The rhyming is often more important than the context of the word. This disruptive speech pattern may be associated with schizophrenia; bipolar disorder during a manic phase; or a cognitive disorder, such as Alzheimer's disease or HIV-related dementia.

Example: "On the track ... have a Big Mac ... or get the sack."

Alterations in Perception

Hallucinations. Hallucinations can be defined as sensory perceptions for which no external stimulus exists. When they occur, "they are vivid and clear, with the full force and impact of normal perceptions, and not under voluntary control" (APA, 2013, p. 87). Table 17.2 provides a description and examples of common types of hallucinations.

It is estimated that up to 90% of people with schizophrenia experience hallucinations at some time during their illness. Auditory hallucinations are the most common and may or may not go away with treatment. During acute illness, these hallucinations tend to be negative or derogatory voices that can make the individual feel awful. Such hallucinations contribute to the poor self-esteem associated with the diagnosis of schizophrenia. Auditory hallucinations may consist of one or more voices speaking directly to the person or commenting on the person's behavior. A person may believe that the voices are from God, the devil, deceased relatives, or strangers. Auditory hallucinations may also take the form of sounds like buzzing, scratching, banging, or indistinct whispering. Visual hallucinations occur less frequently in people with schizophrenia.

Command hallucinations refer to hearing a voice that "commands" the person to do something, such as hurt self or others. Command hallucinations may signal a ***psychiatric emergency*** because patients describe feeling compelled to respond to the command. Command hallucinations are often terrifying for the individual. Command hallucinations put the patient at higher risk for self- or other-directed harm through behavioral acting out.

Example: A patient might report that "the voices" are saying "jump out the window" or "take a knife and kill your child."

Patients may be unwilling to admit to hallucinations. The nurse should be alert to behavioral signs that may indicate an auditory hallucination, such as turning or tilting the head, as if the person is listening to someone or appearing to be carrying on a conversation with someone. Frequent blinking of the eyes, movement of the eyes as if tracking a moving object, and grimacing or responding verbally to "unseen others" may be an indicator of visual hallucinations. This patient behavior is described as "responding to internal stimuli."

Illusions. Illusions are another type of perceptual abnormality. They are misinterpretations of real experiences.

Example: A man sees a coat hanging in a closet but misinterprets what is seen; he believes he sees a bear.

Personal Boundary Difficulties. People with schizophrenia often lack a sense of where their bodies end in relation to where others' bodies begin. Patients might say that they are merging with others or are part of inanimate objects. For example:

- Depersonalization: a nonspecific feeling of having lost one's identity; the self is different or unreal. People may be concerned that

TABLE 17.2 Summary of Hallucinations and Other Perceptual Distortions

Type of Hallucination (Positive Symptom)	Definition (A hallucination is a false sensory perception for which no external stimulus exists)	Example
Auditory (most common type of hallucination in schizophrenia)	Hearing voices or sounds that do not exist in the environment but are thought to be projections of inner thoughts or feelings	Anna reports hearing numerous voices talking about how worthless she is.
Visual	Seeing a person, object, or animal that does not exist in the environment	Charles, who is experiencing alcohol withdrawal delirium, reports seeing hungry rats hovering around him.
Olfactory (most common in temporal lobe epilepsy)	Smelling odors that are not present in the environment	Theresa smells her insides rotting.
Gustatory (rare; may be part of persecutory delusion)	Tasting sensations that have no stimulus in reality	Sam will not eat his food because he tastes the poison the FBI is putting in his food.
Tactile (common in amphetamine/cocaine/alcohol withdrawal)	Feeling strange sensations where no external objects stimulate such feelings; common in delirium tremens	Judy, who is a heavy cocaine user, screams that bugs are crawling under her skin.
Type of Altered Perception		
Illusion	Misperceptions or misinterpretations of a real object or experience	A man sees his coat hanging on a coat rack and believes it to be a bear about to attack him.
Depersonalization	Feeling disconnected or detached from one's body and thoughts	"I feel like I am observing myself from outside my body" or "I am not connected to my arm."
Derealization	*Alteration* in the *perception* or experience of the external world so that it seems unreal.	Sights and sounds may be described as muted, strange, or unreal.

body parts do not belong to them, or they may have an acute sensation that the body has drastically changed.

Example: A woman may see her fingers as snakes or her arms as rotting wood.

Example: A man may look in a mirror and state that his face is that of an animal.

- Derealization is the false perception that the environment has changed.

  Example: The person expresses that everything seems bigger or smaller, or familiar surroundings have become strange and unfamiliar.

The use of touch should be limited to medically necessary procedures during the acute phase of this illness. It can be experienced as an aggressive act by the patient. If it is required, explain what you are doing first and move slowly.

Alterations in Behavior (Grossly Disorganized or Catatonic). Bizarre behavior may take the form of a stilted, rigid demeanor and eccentric dress, grooming, and rituals.

When patients with schizophrenia are acutely ill, impulse control may be impaired. Frequently, the lack of impulse control is expressed in socially inappropriate and agitated behaviors such as grabbing another's cigarette or throwing food on the floor or through regressed behaviors like soiling oneself.

Negative Symptoms. Negative symptoms are associated with a history of dysfunctional premorbid symptoms and a more insidious onset of the disease. They are also associated with more brain pathology and are less responsive to antipsychotic medication. The presence of negative symptoms contributes to the person's poor social functioning and social withdrawal. It can affect the individual's ability to follow through with adequate hygiene and grooming and maintain a job or productive activity. Some of these negative symptoms are outlined in Table 17.3.

Affect is the observable behavior that expresses a person's emotions. In people with a diagnosis of schizophrenia, affect may be altered. Some examples commonly seen in schizophrenia are as follows:

- Flat affect—immobile facial expression or a blank look
- Blunted affect—minimal range of emotional response
- Inappropriate affect—an emotional response to a situation that is not congruent with the tone of the situation

TABLE 17.3 Negative Symptoms Observed in Schizophrenia

Phenomenon	Explanation
Affective blunting[a] (diminished emotional expression)	Severe reduction in the expression of emotions on the face, lack of eye contact, bland intonation of speech, etc.; often referred to as *flat affect* when no facial or other expressions of emotion are present
Anergia	Lack of energy: passivity, lack of persistence at work or school
Anhedonia	Inability to experience any pleasure in activities that usually produce pleasurable feelings; result of profound emotional barrenness
Avolition[a]	Lack of motivation: inability to initiate tasks, such as social contacts, grooming, and other aspects of activities of daily living
Poverty of content of speech	Speech that is adequate in amount but conveys little information because of vagueness, empty repetitions, or use of stereotypes or obscure phrases
Poverty of speech	Restriction in the amount of speech: answers range from brief to monosyllabic, one-word answers

[a]Avolition and affective blunting are the most prominent negative symptoms observed in schizophrenia (APA, 2013).

Example: A young man breaks into laughter when told that his father has died.

- Bizarre affect—can include grimacing, giggling, and mumbling to oneself. This is especially prominent in the disorganized form of schizophrenia.

Neurocognitive/Cognitive Symptoms. Cognitive symptoms represent a third dimension of symptoms associated with schizophrenia. Problematic cognitive symptoms affect 40% to 60% of people with a diagnosis of schizophrenia. These symptoms can sometimes be subtle but can significantly affect a patient's ability to hold a job, initiate or maintain a social support system, or live independently. Cognitive dysfunction negatively affects a person's ability to manage his or her own health care and participate fully in relapse-prevention programs, which impacts long-term recovery. The presence of good verbal memory is one cognitive indicator that is predictive of a better long-term prognosis. The cognitive dysfunctions are as follows:

- Poor "executive functioning" (the ability to absorb and interpret information and make decisions based on that information)
- Inability to sustain attention
- Problems with "working memory" (the ability to keep recently learned information in mind and use it right away) (WebMD, 2019)

Impairment of insight is considered a hallmark of schizophrenia (Joseph, Narayanaswamy, & Venkatasubramanian, 2015). It is associated with both cognitive and negative symptoms of the disease. The term *insight* refers to (1) the ability to recognize that one has a psychiatric illness, (2) the ability to label unusual psychological experiences as pathological, and (3) the ability to adhere to the advised treatment regimen.

Mood Symptoms. A fourth dimension involves variations in mood, such as anxiety, depression, suicidality, and **dysphoria** (a state of feeling emotionally unwell). A phenomenon known as post-psychotic depressive disorder occurs in up to 25% of people after an acute psychotic episode and increases the risk of suicide. Comorbid depression increases the likelihood of suicide, substance misuse, and impaired functioning.

Specifier: Catatonia. The *DSM-5* (APA, 2013) uses the term *specifier* to further describe the nature or course of a person's disorder. For the diagnosis of schizophrenia, one specifier listed is catatonia, in which a particular set of behavioral symptoms is present and may predominate. The essential feature of catatonia is extreme and abnormal motor behavior, either extreme motor agitation or extreme psychomotor retardation, which is a slowing-down of thought and a reduction of physical movements that can lead to total psychomotor immobility or stupor.

During the very *withdrawn phase,* the person may not move or eat, thus becoming vulnerable to pressure ulcers, contractures, malnutrition, and circulatory issues. Patients may exhibit the following:

- **Stereotyped behaviors** are motor patterns that originally had meaning to the person (sweeping the floor or washing windows) but are now mechanical and lack purpose.
- *Automatic obedience* is the performance of all simple commands in a robot-like fashion.
- *Bizarre posturing* is the voluntary assumption and maintenance of inappropriate or bizarre posture or bodily position.
- **Waxy flexibility** is the excessive maintenance of posture. Patients can hold unusual postures for long periods, potentially causing physiological problems related to immobility, such as circulatory problems.
- *Negativism* is equivalent to behavioral resistance. In active negativism, the patient does the opposite of what one is told to do. When a person does not perform activities that are normal expectations, such as getting out of bed, dressing, and eating, the behavior is termed *passive negativism.*
- *Stupor* refers to a state in which the catatonic patient is motionless for long periods and may even appear to be in a coma.

Problematic speech patterns may include echolalia (repeating/mimicking of another's speech). Echopraxia (mimicking another's movement) may be present. Although individuals may be mute during these episodes of catatonia, they can be acutely aware of activities that occur around them.

During *extreme motor activity,* the patient may run about ceaselessly and without purpose, leading to exhaustion, cardiac difficulties, or physical collapse.

The onset of catatonia is usually abrupt, and the prognosis is favorable. Fortunately, with the advances in pharmacotherapy and improved individual management, severe catatonic symptoms are rarely seen today. Catatonia can also occur in the context of other disorders, including brain damage, neurodevelopmental disorders, and extreme manic or depressed phases of bipolar disorder.

VIGNETTE: Mary has been motionless and has not spoken for days. When her husband raises her arm to dress her and take her to the hospital, her arm stays raised in the air until he lowers it (waxy flexibility). When she starts to move, she does everything she is told to do (get up, sit down) and only moves on command (automatic obedience). When he speaks to her, she repeats everything he says—for example, "Mary, drink this water." "Mary, drink this water" (echolalia).

The mental health clinician may clarify the diagnostic picture by adding additional information. The addition might "specify if" (1) this is a first episode or multiple episodes, an acute episode, or an episode in partial remission; (2) if these symptoms include catatonia; and (3) the current severity.

Other Clinical Presentations. Individuals who have a schizophrenia spectrum disorder have different neuroanatomical findings, distinct courses of disease development, individual responses to treatment, and different prognoses. Although not all patients will meet all *DSM-5* (APA, 2013) criteria for schizophrenia spectrum disorders, it is helpful to be aware of possible prominent presentations of the spectrum of illness.

The following presentations provide the reader with a clinical picture of some of the specialized presentations of this illness.

Paranoia. Any intense and strongly defended irrational suspicion can be regarded as **paranoia**. Paranoid ideas cannot be corrected by experiences and cannot be modified by facts or reality. **Projection** is the most common defense mechanism used by people who are paranoid. For example, when paranoid individuals experience *unconscious* feelings of being self-critical, they *consciously* experience others as being harshly critical toward them. When they feel angry, they experience others as being unjustly angry at them, as if to say, "I'm not angry—you are!"

People who are paranoid are unable to trust the actions of those around them, so they are usually guarded, tense, and reserved. Although patients may keep themselves aloof from interpersonal contacts, impairment in actual functioning in other areas may be minimal. To ensure interpersonal distance, they may adopt a superior, hostile, or sarcastic attitude. With

DSM-5 DIAGNOSTIC CRITERIA

Schizophrenia

A. Two (or more) of the following, each present for a significant portion of time during a 1-month period (or less if successfully treated). At least one of these must be (1), (2), or (3):
   1. Delusions.
   2. Hallucinations.
   3. Disorganized speech (e.g., frequent derailment or incoherence).
   4. Grossly disorganized or catatonic behavior.
   5. Negative symptoms (i.e., diminished emotional expression or avolition).

B. For a significant portion of the time since the onset of the disturbance, level of functioning in one or more major areas, such as work, interpersonal relations, or self-care, is markedly below the level achieved prior to the onset (or when the onset is in childhood or adolescence, there is failure to achieve expected level of interpersonal, academic, or occupational functioning).

C. Continuous signs of the disturbance persist for at least 6 months. This 6-month period must include at least 1 month of symptoms (or less if successfully treated) that meet Criterion A (i.e., active-phase symptoms) and may include periods of prodromal or residual symptoms. During these prodromal or residual periods, the signs of the disturbance may be manifested by only negative symptoms or by two or more symptoms listed in Criterion A present in an attenuated form (e.g., odd beliefs, unusual perceptual experiences).

D. Schizoaffective disorder and depressive or bipolar disorder with psychotic features have been ruled out because either (1) no major depressive or manic episodes have occurred concurrently with the active-phase symptoms, or (2) if mood episodes have occurred during active-phase symptoms, they have been present for a minority of the total duration of the active and residual periods of the illness.

E. The disturbance is not attributable to the physiological effects of a substance (e.g., a drug of abuse, a medication) or another medical condition.

F. If there is a history of autism spectrum disorder or a communication disorder of childhood onset, the additional diagnosis of schizophrenia is made only if prominent delusions or hallucinations, in addition to the other required symptoms of schizophrenia, are also present for at least 1 month (or less if successfully treated).

Specify if:

The following course specifiers are only to be used after a 1-year duration of the disorder and if they are not in contradiction to the diagnostic course criteria:

First episode, currently in acute episode: First manifestation of the disorder meeting the defining diagnostic symptom and time criteria. An acute episode is a time period in which the symptom criteria are fulfilled.

First episode, currently partial remission: Partial remission is a period of time during which an improvement after a previous episode is maintained and in which the defining criteria of the disorder are only partially fulfilled.

First episode, currently in full remission: Full remission is a period of time after a previous episode during which no disorder-specific symptoms are present.

Multiple episodes, currently in acute episode: Multiple episodes may be determined after a minimum of two episodes (i.e., after a first episode, a remission and a minimum of one relapse).

Multiple episodes, currently in partial remission

Multiple episodes, currently in full remission

Continuous: Symptoms fulfilling the diagnostic symptom criteria of the disorder are remaining for the majority of the illness course, with subthreshold symptom periods being very brief relative to the overall course.

Unspecified

Specify if:

With catatonia (refer to the criteria for catatonia associated with another mental disorder for definition).

Coding note: Use additional code 293.89 (F06.1), catatonia associated with schizophrenia, to indicate the presence of the comorbid catatonia.

Specify current severity:

Severity is rated by a quantitative assessment of the primary symptoms of psychosis, including delusions, hallucinations, disorganized speech, abnormal psychomotor behavior, and negative symptoms. Each of these symptoms may be rated for its current severity (most severe in the last 7 days) on a 5-point scale ranging from 0 (not present) to 4 (present and severe). (See Clinical-Rated Dimensions of Psychosis Symptom Severity in the chapter "Assessment Measure.")

Note: Diagnosis of schizophrenia can be made without using this severity specifier.

paranoid delusions, an individual misinterprets the messages of others or gives private meaning to the communications of others (ideas of reference).

Example: A patient might see his wife talking to a man at a checkout counter at a supermarket and believe they are lovers and plotting to get rid of him.

Minor oversights are often interpreted as personal rejections. It can be intimidating to be in the presence of an extremely paranoid individual.

People with a prominent paranoid presentation of symptoms usually have a later age of onset of the disease (late 20s to 30s). There tends to be less cognitive dysfunction, and these individuals often have a better response to medications. The result is that with treatment, these individuals can work and tend to experience improved long-term outcomes. Work that involves solitary pursuits and projects where a person's paranoia is less likely to be stimulated seem to lead to more occupational success.

The website Schizophrenia.com is an online resource offering support and education for patients and family members dealing with schizophrenia. This resource identified some helpful guidelines to use when working with an individual who shows paranoid behavior (Schizophrenia.com, 2004):

1. Speak indirectly. Avoid speaking directly about the person. Substitute pronouns such as *he* or *she* for the words *I* and *you*. The purpose is to direct paranoid symptoms toward external and more general "real-world" issues.
2. Identify with, rather than fight, the patient. The goal is to help the patient feel understood by empathizing with the feelings and attitudes without supporting the delusional thinking. Meet frustration with understanding. ("I can see how frustrating that must have been.") A paranoid individual is not thinking rationally, and any attempt on your part to explain "why" will be met with resistance.
3. Share mistrust. Rather than trying to persuade a person to be more trusting, it is better to align with the need to feel guarded or suspicious. No attempt should be made to correct or contradict the patient or to present reality. The assumption behind this technique is that in the midst of a paranoid state, the patient is overburdened and overwhelmed by a mixture of real-life stresses and distress from psychotic symptoms. Without supporting the delusion, you should

attempt to find certain believable or credible aspects of the paranoid belief system. This allows you to agree with the patient on something. For example, rather than confront a patient's own behavior that led to a police arrest, the clinician might agree that some police are not trustworthy.

See Table 17.7 later in the chapter for other interventions for paranoid individuals.

VIGNETTE: Sam stares at the nurse as she explains how to replace a bandage after minor surgery on his face. He frequently looks at the door and places himself near it. His general demeanor is condescending, and he becomes sarcastic when the nurse drops a bandage, asking, "Are you the best they could give me?" When the nurse answers the phone, he says, "So they got to you, too. You are all plotting against me" (ideas of reference). He starts to mutter to himself and looks to his side as if he is talking to someone (auditory hallucinations).

Disorganized. People who display disorganized components of schizophrenia represent the most regressed and socially impaired of all individuals with schizophrenia. These individuals are often homeless, which makes them easy targets for maltreatment. A person who presents with these symptoms of schizophrenia may have marked looseness of associations, grossly inappropriate affect, bizarre mannerisms, and incoherent speech. They may display extreme social withdrawal and severe cognitive impairment. Although delusions and hallucinations are present, they are fragmentary and poorly organized. Behavior may be considered odd, and giggling or grimacing in response to internal stimuli is common.

Often, individuals with these symptoms have an earlier age of onset (early to middle teens), with symptoms that develop insidiously (slowly). Disorganized symptoms are associated with poor premorbid functioning, a significant positive family history, and a poor prognosis. To be able to live in the community, these patients may require a structured and well-supervised setting to maintain safety. Families living with someone who is this vulnerable and disorganized need significant community support, respite care, and even day hospital affiliations. People with schizophrenia with profound disorganization are discussed further in Chapter 27.

VIGNETTE: Pete pushes his grocery cart loaded with rags, bottles, bags, and such down the street. He appears disheveled, dressed in a dirty plaid shirt, a dirty baseball hat, and ragged jeans. He is giggling and laughing to himself. Once in a while he shouts out something, "Alms for the poor me ... howdy to you all. ... Where is it? Where is it?" (looseness of associations). He goes from garbage can to garbage can rummaging for food. He often sleeps under a bridge, with a cardboard box as protection, and when the weather becomes too hot or too cold, he sometimes seeks help at a nearby shelter.

Schizoaffective Disorder

Schizoaffective disorder is a mental disorder characterized by psychotic symptoms similar to schizophrenia with concurrent symptoms of a mood disorder. The diagnosis is made when the person has features of both schizophrenia plus a mood component of either bipolar disorder (mania) or major depression but does not strictly meet diagnostic criteria for either alone (APA, 2013). Interventions include treating both the symptoms of psychosis while also treating the symptoms of the specific mood disorder.

APPLICATION OF THE NURSING PROCESS

ASSESSMENT

Assessment Guidelines

Schizophrenia and Other Psychotic Disorders

1. Rule out medical or substance-induced psychosis through a formal medical workup.
2. Assess for command hallucinations (voices telling the person to harm self or another). If present, ask the patient:
   - Do you plan to follow the command?
   - Do you feel able to resist the command?
   - Do you believe the voices are real?
   - Do you recognize the voices?
3. Review the patient's belief system. Is it fragmented? Is it poorly or well organized? Is it systematized? Is the system of beliefs unsupported by reality (delusion)? Determine if:
   - The patient admits to/understands the presence of an illness (insight).
   - Delusions focus on someone trying to harm the patient.
   - The patient is planning to retaliate against a person or organization in response to the delusion.
   - Safety precautions need to be taken.
4. Assess for co-occurring conditions, including the following:
   - Depression
   - Suicidality (past and present)
     - Perform a current suicide assessment.
   - Anxiety disorder
   - Alcohol and other substance use/substance use disorder
   - History of violence (past and present)
     - Perform a current violence assessment.
5. Inventory the patient's medications and assess whether the patient is adhering to the medication regimen.
   - If the person is nonadherent with medications, ask what makes it difficult to follow this medication regimen (fear of side effects, forgetting, lack of money).
   - Record reasons for nonadherence and what will be done to help the person to become more adherent (social services for monetary reasons, recovery group, medication group, etc.).
6. Determine the family's response to increased symptoms.
   - Are they overprotective, hostile, suspicious, or overwhelmed?
7. Assess the way the patient and family members relate.
8. Review the support system. Families can play a significant role in facilitating recovery.
   - Is the family well informed about the disease?
   - Does the family understand the need for medication adherence?
   - Is the family familiar with support groups available in the community for both the family and the patient?
   - Are they aware of locations where respite and family support may be offered?
   - Have family members received or been referred for psychoeducation?

DIAGNOSIS

People with a diagnosis of schizophrenia may have multiple disturbing and disabling symptoms that necessitate a multifaceted approach to care and treatment for both the individual and family. Table 17.4 lists potential nursing diagnoses associated with these symptoms.

TABLE 17.4 Potential Nursing Diagnoses for Schizophrenia

Symptoms	Potential Nursing Diagnoses[a]
Hallucinations	
Hears voices that others do not	*Altered perception* *Fear*
Hears voices telling person to hurt self or others *(command hallucinations)*	*Altered perception* *Risk for:* *Self-mutilation* *Suicide*
Delusions	
Ideas of reference Persecutory Grandeur Somatic Jealousy Erotomania Nihilistic Bizarre	*Distorted thinking process* *Impaired cognition* *Fear* *Anxiety* *Difficulty coping* *Risk for:* *Self-mutilation* *Suicide*
Communication Difficulties	
Looseness of associations: Phrases that do not appear to be logically connected to each other *Clang association:* Uses words that rhyme in a nonsensical fashion *Echolalia:* Repeats words that are heard *Mutism:* Does not speak *Circumstantiality:* Delays getting to the point of communication because of unnecessary and tedious details	*Impaired verbal communication*
Negative Symptoms	
Uncommunicative, withdrawn, makes no eye contact Preoccupied with own thoughts	*Impaired socialization* *Social isolation*
Is stigmatized for diagnosis of schizophrenia Talks about self as "bad" or "no good" Feelings of anxiety and depression	*Situational low self-esteem* *Chronic low self-esteem* *Risk for self-mutilation* *Risk for suicide* *Hopelessness* *Powerlessness* *Anxiety*
Shows lack of energy (anergia) Shows lack of motivation (avolition), unable to initiate tasks (social contact, grooming, and other aspects of daily living)	*Difficulty coping* *Self-care deficit* *Impaired adjustment* *Impaired role performance* *Social isolation*
Lack of insight	*Denial* *Difficulty coping*
Other	
Families and significant others become confused or overwhelmed Have lack of knowledge about disease or treatment Feel powerless in ability to help patient at home May not be able to care for patient in home setting	*Caregiver stress* *Impaired family coping* *Lack of knowledge* *Impaired homemaking*
Patient and family may have difficulty accessing community supports	*Impaired family processes* *Social isolation*
Nonadherence to Medication and Treatment	
Lack of insight Patient stops taking medication Patient stops going to therapy groups Lack of knowledge of relapse-prevention strategies	*Denial* *Impaired health-seeking behavior* *Non-adherence to:* *Medication regime* *Therapeutic regime* *Impaired health maintenance* *Lack of knowledge (specify) of disease:* *Medication regime* *Treatment regime*

[a]The International Classification for Nursing Practice (ICNP) is a product of the International Council of Nurses (ICN). Retrieved from http://www.icn.ch/what-we-do/ICNP-Browser/.

OUTCOMES IDENTIFICATION

Phase I (Acute)

During the acute phase of the illness, the overall goal is *patient safety and medical stabilization.* Therefore if the patient is at risk for harm to self or others, initial outcome criteria should address safety issues: **(QSEN: Safety)**

- Patient consistently refrains from inflicting injury to self (self-harm or suicide) or others.
- Patient consistently refrains from acting on delusions or hallucinations.

Medication adherence is a vital outcome for all phases of recovery. Ideally, outcomes should focus on enhancing the patient's strengths and minimizing the patient's deficits.

Phase II (Stabilization) and Phase III (Maintenance)

Outcome criteria during the stabilization and maintenance phases focus on helping patients adhere to medication regimens, understand their disease, and participate in psychoeducational activities with their families:

- Improvement in functioning through participation in social, vocational, or self-care skills training and involvement in social groups.
- Anxiety control and relapse prevention to reduce the patient's vulnerability to psychosis

The Wellness Recovery Action Plan, or WRAP, is an example of a formalized program for recovery that can be implemented during the stabilization and maintenance phases. It centers on instilling hope for recovery, taking personal responsibility for recovery, being informed about ways to stay well, self-advocacy, and support to get help to facilitate recovery. WRAP has been studied extensively and is listed in the Substance Abuse and Mental Health Services Administration (SAMHSA) National Registry of Evidence-Based Programs and Practices (SAMHSA, 2017a). **(QSEN: Evidence-Based Practice)**

PLANNING

Phase I (Acute)

During the acute phase of schizophrenia, brief hospitalization is frequently indicated if the patient is considered a danger to self or others, refuses to eat or drink, or is too disorganized to provide self-care. Another indication for hospitalization is the need for specific observation, neurological workup, or other medically related tests or treatments for co-occurring disorders. The planning process continues to focus on the best strategies to ensure patient safety and provide symptom stabilization.

At this time, the treatment team starts to identify aftercare needs for follow-up and support, as well as the appropriate referrals that will benefit the patient and family. Discharge planning considers both external factors, such as the patient's living arrangement, economic resources, social supports, and family relationships, and internal factors, especially the patient's vulnerability to stress. Once a person develops schizophrenia, the individual can become acutely sensitive to environmental and psychosocial stressors. This acquired acute sensitivity can strongly affect recovery and relapse. Because relapse can be devastating to long-term functioning, vigorous efforts must be instituted to connect the patient (and family) with community agencies that provide social supports and programs designed to help the patient remain well (see Chapter 5).

Phase II (Stabilization) and Phase III (Maintenance)

Planning during the stabilization and maintenance phases of treatment focuses on strategies to provide patient and family education and skills training (psychosocial education), including the following:

- Identifying the social, interpersonal, coping, and vocational skills needed
- Teaching relapse-prevention strategies
- Determining how and where these needs can best be met within the community

IMPLEMENTATION

Phase I (Acute)

Interventions geared toward the acute phase of schizophrenia can be found in Table 17.5. During this phase, the clinical focus is on crisis intervention, acute symptom stabilization, medication adherence, and safety. **(QSEN: Safety)** Inpatient hospitalization is used in the short term for acute crisis situations. Alternatives to inpatient hospitalization can sometimes be used. These include partial hospitalization, halfway houses, and day treatment programs, as described later in this chapter.

Phase II (Stabilization) and Phase III (Maintenance)

Once the acute symptoms are somewhat stabilized, follow-up treatment occurs in the community, where appropriate treatment can be carried out during the maintenance and stabilization phases. Effective long-term care of an individual with schizophrenia relies on a three-pronged approach: medications, nursing interventions, and community support. Patient and family psychoeducation (Box 17.3), as well as community support, are key components of effective treatment. Health promotion and health maintenance interventions support optimal wellness in the community (see the section Health Teaching and Health Promotion).

Peer-support services can help a person feel more connected to the community. Frequently associated with community mental health services, *peer-support specialists* offer support, strength, and hope to a person struggling with mental illness. These are trained individuals who also have a diagnosis of schizophrenia or other mental disorder (SAMHSA, 2017b).

Communication Guidelines

Therapeutic strategies for communicating with patients with schizophrenia focus on lowering anxiety, decreasing defensive patterns, encouraging participation in therapeutic and social events, raising feelings of self-worth, and increasing medication adherence. Familiarity with the specialized communication principles used for dealing with phenomena such as hallucinations, delusions, paranoia, and looseness of associations is helpful for establishing rapport and being effective.

When a person is responding to internal stimuli, it can be helpful to adjust how you communicate:

- Wait longer for the person to think about or *process* your questions and then respond, especially during the acute phase.
- Repeat questions or gently redirect the person when necessary.
- Use shorter phrases and concrete language to facilitate more effective communication.

Helpful Interventions

Hallucinations

With auditory hallucinations, the nurse should initially try to understand what the voices are saying or telling the person to do. Suicidal or homicidal (harm to others) messages require the nurse to initiate safety measures. Can the person recognize the identity of the voice? Is the voice supportive, or is it threatening in some way? Can the

TABLE 17.5 **Treatment Focus at Different Phases of Schizophrenia**

PHASE I		PHASE II	PHASE III
Acute	**Subacute or Convalescent**	**Stabilization Phase**	**Maintenance Phase Health Promotion**
Clinical Focus			
Crisis intervention Safety Acute symptom stabilization	Ability to take care of basic needs Social supports Living arrangements Economic resources	Understanding and acceptance of illness Developing strategy to manage illness	Achieving optimal wellness Lessening residual or secondary disability
Intervention			
Acute psychopharmacological treatment Psychiatric, medical, and neurological evaluation Therapeutic milieu Supportive and directive care Give support and involve family in treatment decisions	Psychosocial evaluation Linkage with community supports Social services Human services Community mental health treatment agencies Psychoeducational interventions with patient and families	Support and teaching Medication teaching and side effect management Illness management Relapse prevention: Direct assistance with situational problems Identification of prodromal and acute symptoms and signs of relapse Continued psychoeducational work with families as needed	Continued support and teaching Cognitive and social skills enhancement Medication maintenance Vocational rehabilitation Continued psychoeducational intervention with families as needed Involvement with recovery groups and strategies
Professional Teamwork and Collaboration			
Community crisis intervention Inpatient treatment team Internist, neurologist, and other specialists Crisis residential alternative to hospitalization	Social work department Health and human services Partial hospitalization programs and community mental health services	Community mental health support staff Case management Assertive community treatment programs Family support groups Individual and group therapists Self-help groups for patient and families (e.g., National Alliance on Mental Illness [NAMI])	Therapists Community mental health support staff Social, vocational, and self-care providers Clubhouse model of psychosocial rehabilitation Self-help groups for patient and families

Adapted from Gabbard, G. O. (2001). *Treatments of psychiatric disorders* (3rd ed.). Washington, DC: American Psychiatric Publishing.

person resist the urge to act upon what the "voices" are telling the person to do?

Hallucinations are real to the person who is experiencing them and are frightening to the individual. Nurses should approach individuals who are hallucinating in a nonthreatening and nonjudgmental manner. Empathize with the feelings underneath the hallucination. Lowering the patient's anxiety may lower the distress associated with the hallucination. Decreasing environmental stimulation may also decrease anxiety.

During the acute phase of the illness, the nurse should maintain eye contact, call the patient by name, and speak simply.

Patient: "I hear my mother's voice saying terrible things about me. She says I am a horrible person and she wishes I had never been born."

Nurse: "That must be very upsetting [empathy], Tom. Are you feeling upset?" (helps the person identify the feeling) Nurse waits for a response.

Patient: "Yes, yes … she makes me feel bad."

Nurse: "Tell your voice to go away. (asks the person to turn away from the voices). (The nurse then suggests a reality-based activity.) "I hear you are very good at card games. Let's go over to the table and play a game of cards."

Here, the nurse uses empathy, tries to identify the feelings the patient is experiencing (clarifies), asks the person to turn away from the voices, distracts attention, and focuses on a reality-based activity. Table 17.6 lists interventions for hallucinations.

The patient can also be advised to listen to music through earphones; sing softly to self; or engage in nonstressful, reality-based activities, like playing a game, as ways to distract self from "the voices."

Delusions

Delusions reflect a distortion in thought content. When the nurse attempts to see the world as it appears through the eyes of the patient, it is easier to understand the patient's delusional experience and provide supportive care.

Patient: "I see now … you are an ISIS fighter in disguise who wants to drain my brain … you all want me destroyed."

Nurse: "I don't want to hurt you, Tom. [addresses the implied feeling] I am your nurse for the day. [reality-based information] Thinking that others want to destroy you must be very frightening." (empathy)

BOX 17.3 Psychoeducational Strategies for the Patient and Family

Four Broad Goals for Psychoeducation

1. Information:
   a. Learn about symptoms, causes, course of disease, and treatment options.
   b. Acknowledge and lessen the role of stigma as a barrier to seeking treatment and to recovery.
   c. Discuss ways to manage symptoms associated with the illness.
   d. Minimize comorbid conditions like substance use disorders, depression, and metabolic syndrome.
   e. Attend psychoeducational groups and support groups (see list at the end of this box).
      - National Alliance on Mental Illness (NAMI) for education and support
      - National Institute of Mental Health (NIMH) for current information about the illness and treatment
2. Emotional discharge—provides an opportunity to talk about frustrations and exchange ideas with others
   a. Teach families how to provide a healing environment.
   Encourage families to:
      - Understand symptoms as part of the disease; do not take personally.
      - Support realistic and attainable goals; recovery can be a slow process.
      - Offer praise and offer hope frequently.
      - Provide a calm atmosphere with low stimulation.
      - Support acceptance, belonging, and encouragement of their loved one.
3. Support medication and treatment adherence.
   a. Adherence to treatment
      - People cope best when given individualized treatment that works for them; psychoeducation may help.
      - Troubling medication side effects (sexual problems, weight gain, "feeling funny") should be reported rather than just stopping medications. Most side effects can be treated or lessened.
      - Foster recovery through cognitive and social skills enhancement.
   b. Develop a relapse-prevention plan.
      - Know the early warning signs of relapse (social withdrawal, increased or decreased sleep, increased bizarre or magical thinking).
      - Know whom to call and where to go when early signs of relapse appear.
      - Relapse is part of the illness, not a sign of failure.
      - Maintain hope. This is a long-term illness that can be managed.
4. Use self-help strategies.
   a. Participate in family, group, and individual education/therapy.
   b. Learn new behaviors and cognitive coping skills to help handle intrafamily stress and interpersonal, social, and vocational difficulties.
   c. Everyone needs a place to address their fears and losses and learn new ways of coping.
   d. Avoid alcohol and drugs; they can act on the brain and can precipitate a relapse.
   e. Keep in touch with supportive people.
   f. Keep healthy—stay in balance.
      - Self-care deficits can lead to high rates of medical comorbidity.
      - Maintain a regular sleep pattern.
      - Maintain self-care (diet, hygiene).
   g. Keep active (hobbies, friends, groups, sports, job, special interests).
   h. Learn ways to reduce stress.
   i. Identify web-based and community resources for patient and family support. **(QSEN: Informatics)**

Some examples:

- **NAMI and NIMH,** as previously noted
- **Clubhouse model** of psychiatric rehabilitation (https://www.nami.org/Learn-More/Treatment/Psychosocial-Treatments): Offers people living with mental illness opportunities for friendship, productive activity, and supported employment activities to facilitate recovery and full participation as valued and respected members of society.
- **Mental Health America** (http://www.mentalhealthamerica.net/who-we-are): Community-based nonprofit dedicated to addressing the needs of those living with mental illness and to promoting the overall mental health of all Americans.
- **MentalHelp.net** (https://www.mentalhelp.net/about/): Provides online mental health and wellness education.
- **Schizopherenia.com** (http://schizophrenia.com/): Provides in-depth information about treatment and recovery and online support groups.
- **Schizophrenia and Related Disorders Alliance of America** (SARDAA), Health Storylines (https://sardaa.org/schizophrenia-app/): A web-based tool and app to help document self-care activities and symptoms experienced for better care coordination and communication with health care provider.
- **Janssen Canada** (https://www.schizophrenia24x7.com/): A sponsored website that provides updated information and tools and support for both caregivers and patients.

Adapted from Australian Institute of Psychological Counsellors. (2014). *Psychoeducation: Definition, goals and methods.* Retrieved from https://www.aipc.net.au/articles/psychoeducation-definition-goals-and-methods

In this example, the nurse clarifies the reality of the patient's experience and empathizes with the patient's apparent experience and feelings of fear. The nurse avoids being drawn into the conversation regarding the content of the delusion but attempts to identify the feelings that the patient is experiencing. Talking about the person's feelings is helpful; talking about delusional material is not.

It is rarely useful to argue or try to "reason" with the patient regarding the content of the delusion. Doing so can intensify the patient's irrational beliefs. However, it is helpful for the nurse to clarify misinterpretations of the environment.

Patient: "I see the doctor is here, and he is part of this plan to destroy me."

Nurse: "It is true the doctor wants to see you, but he wants to talk to you about your treatment and find out if the medication is helping you. Would you feel more comfortable talking to him in his office without people around?"

Interacting with the patient about concrete realities in the environment helps minimize the time available for the patient to focus on delusional thoughts. Performance of specific manual tasks within the scope of the patient's abilities is also useful in distracting the patient from delusional thinking. The more time the patient spends engaged in reality-based activities or with people, the more opportunity the patient has to become comfortable with reality. Table 17.7 lists interventions for a patient experiencing delusions.

Paranoia

A paranoid individual may make offensive yet accurate criticisms of the nurse or the unit policies. It is important that the staff not

TABLE 17.6 Interventions for Hallucinations

Intervention	Rationale
1. Watch patients for cues that they may be hallucinating (eyes darting to one side, muttering, or staring sideways; changes in facial expressions).	1. Patients are usually experiencing high levels of anxiety at this time. Early intervention may help interrupt the hallucinatory process and lessen the patient's anxiety and potential for harm.
2. Ask patients directly if they are hallucinating. "Are you hearing voices?" "What are you hearing the voices say to you?"	2. Asking about auditory hallucinations and their content assesses for psychosis and any safety concerns.
3. If voices are telling patients to harm self or others (command hallucinations): a. If in the community: Notify appropriate authority (police, physician, administrator according to agency protocols). There may be a "duty to warn"; evaluate need for hospitalization. b. If inpatient: Place patient on close observation.	3. People often obey hallucinatory commands to harm self or others. Early assessment and intervention could save lives.
4. Document what patients say, if they are a threat to self or others, and who was notified and when.	4. If the patient threatens self or others, documentation shows that correct legal protocols were followed. Otherwise, nurses, physicians, and institutions can be held legally responsible.
5. Accept the fact that the voices are real to patients, but explain that you do not hear the voices. Refer to the voices as "your voices" or "the voices that you hear."	5. Validating that your reality does not include voices may help patients cast doubt on their voices.
6. Present a calm demeanor and stay with patients while they are hallucinating. At times, you can tell patients to tell the "voices they hear" to go away.	6. When patients feel comfortable with a nurse, they can sometimes learn to push the voices aside when given repeated instruction.
7. Maintain a calm milieu free of overstimulating activities.	7. A stimulating environment may increase anxiety, which can make hallucinations more prominent.
8. Keep patients focused on simple, basic, reality-based topics and activities. Help patients focus on one idea at a time.	8. Hallucinating patients are confused; this intervention helps patients focus on people and what is real. A concrete task may act as a distraction from the hallucination.
9. Help patients identify times and situations when hallucinations are the most prevalent and intense.	9. Helps nurse and patients identify situations and times that are the most threatening and find ways to mitigate perceived threats.
10. Assess for signs of increased anxiety, fear, or agitation and intervene as soon as possible.	10. The earlier intervention takes place, the easier it is to calm patients and prevent harm. Help the patient make the connection between increased anxiety and increased hallucinations.

react to these criticisms with anxiety or rejection of the patient. Staff conferences, nursing peer groups, and clinical supervision are effective ways of looking beyond the behaviors to the motivations of the patient. Staff treatment team meetings can provide opportunities to develop ways to reduce the patient's anxiety and increase staff effectiveness.

It is important to approach a patient who is paranoid in a nonjudgmental, respectful manner and use clear and simple language. This helps minimize the opportunity for the patient to misconstrue the meaning of a message. A matter-of-fact or business-like approach allows for the interpersonal distance the patient initially requires and may decrease suspiciousness. Be honest and consistent with the patient regarding expectations when enforcing rules. Explaining to the patient what you are going to do prepares the patient and minimizes the opportunity for misinterpreting your intent as hostile or aggressive. Avoid laughing, whispering, or talking quietly when the patient cannot hear what is being said. Suspicious patients may automatically think that they are the target of the interaction and interpret it in a negative manner (ideas of reference). Refer to Table 17.7.

Paranoid patients may perceive the hospital environment with suspicion. This can affect the patient's ability to meet basic needs, including sleeping and eating. Please review the information included under Milieu Therapy for strategies to help patients feel safe.

Associative Looseness

The symptom of associative looseness often mirrors the patient's autistic thoughts (retreating into an inner fantasy world) and reflects the person's poorly organized thinking. An increase in this type of communication often indicates that the patient is feeling increased anxiety. The patient's ramblings may confuse and frustrate the nurse. The following communication guidelines are useful with a patient whose speech is confused and disorganized:

- Do not pretend that you understand the patient's communications when you are confused by words or meanings.
- Tell the patient that you are having difficulty understanding.
- Verbalize the implied. For example, "You seem to be upset about the food on your tray."
- Place the difficulty in understanding on yourself, not on the patient. For example, say, "I am having trouble following what you are saying," not "You are not making any sense."
- Look for recurring topics and themes in the patient's communications. For example, "You've mentioned trouble with your brother several times. Tell me about your brother."

TABLE 17.7 Interventions for Delusions

Intervention	Rationale
1. Assess if external controls are needed: if the patient is agitated and believes someone is going to inflict harm, the patient may harm someone else to survive; use safety measures.	1. Beliefs are real for the patient, and delusional thinking might dictate a need for self-defense. Evaluate the least restrictive alternatives (confer with others if helpful).
2. Be aware that the patient's delusions represent the way that person is experiencing reality.	2. Identifying the patient's experience helps the nurse to understand the patient's feelings.
3. Identify feelings:	3. The nurse can focus on feelings, not delusional content.
a. If the patient believes there is an attempt to "get" the patient, then the patient is experiencing *fear.*	a. "If you believe the CIA is out to kill you, you must feel frightened; are you feeling frightened?" "This is a safe place."
b. If the belief is that someone is controlling the patient's thoughts, then the patient is experiencing *helplessness.*	b. "If you believe your thoughts are being controlled, are you feeling helpless?" "What would help you feel more comfortable?"
4. Engage the individual in yoga, exercise, walking, etc.	4. Shift the focus from the delusions and engage the patient in reality-based activities.
5. Do not argue with the patient's beliefs or try to correct false beliefs with logic or facts.	5. Arguing will only increase the patient's defensive position, thereby reinforcing false beliefs.
6. Do not touch the patient; use gestures very carefully, particularly if the patient is paranoid.	6. Give a delusional patient a lot of personal space. Touching may be misconstrued as an aggressive or sexual gesture.
Paranoid Individual	
1. Place yourself beside the patient, not face to face.	1. A face-to-face position can be interpreted by a paranoid individual as confrontational (either standing or sitting).
2. Avoid direct eye contact.	2. This can be construed as confrontational or threatening.
3. Use a matter-of-fact or business-like approach.	3. A warm interpersonal approach may be misconstrued.
4. A paranoid patient might not eat or drink, thinking the food is poisoned. Offer food and fluids in closed containers, such as a carton of milk, a carton of yogurt, unpeeled fruit, or a hardboiled egg.	4. Food that has not "been tampered with" is "safe" to eat, and some nutritional intake is possible.
5. After understanding the patient's underlying feelings (fear, helplessness), engage the patient in reality-based activities, such as cards or crafts.	5. When the patient is focused on reality-based activities, feelings associated with delusions are momentarily lessened.
6. If the patient is paranoid, intellectual functioning is often higher, and the patient may respond better to more intellectually taxing, noncompetitive activities.	6. The more a person is focused on reality, the greater the delusions can be minimized during that time.
7. Observe for events that trigger delusions.	7. Observe for events that make the patient anxious and fearful. Problem-solve ways to mitigate the effect of these situations or events.
8. If anxiety escalates and the patient loses control, use least restrictive interventions (one-to-one therapy, prn [as needed] medications, last-resort seclusion). Always follow unit protocol and provide detailed documentation.	8. A calm, nonthreatening presence during high levels of anxiety usually helps lower anxiety levels.

- Emphasize what is going on in the patient's immediate environment (here and now), and involve the patient in simple reality-based activities. These measures can help the patient to focus thoughts.
- Tell the patient what you do understand, and reinforce clear communication and accurate expression of needs, feelings, and thoughts.

Health Teaching and Health Promotion

Psychoeducation is an indispensable intervention to facilitate optimal wellness in the person with a schizophrenic spectrum disorder. Ideally, it should include the patient and family. Providing practical education can increase a person's ability to manage symptoms of the disease, instill hope, promote wellness, and increase a person's self-esteem. Education for families must start by helping families to understand the illness and giving strategies to support appropriate treatment. Psychoeducation must also include information that helps to support the recovery of the person and gives opportunities for success. Effective family education leads to better outcomes for the individual struggling with symptoms associated with schizophrenia. See Box 17.3 for additional psychoeducational strategies for the patient and family.

When people lack understanding of the disease and its symptoms, they may misinterpret a patient's apathy and lack of drive as laziness. This erroneous assumption can foster hostility in family members, caregivers, or others in the community. Further teaching about the negative and positive symptoms of schizophrenia can reduce these tensions.

It is vital that nurses, physicians, and social workers be aware of the community support resources and make this information available to patients and their families. Examples of such resources include community mental health services, home health services, work support programs, day hospitals, social skills training and support groups, family educational skills groups, and respite care.

Milieu Therapy

Although hospital stays are usually short, effective hospital care involves more than protection from family, social, or work environments that are stressful or disruptive. Many patients need the structure provided by hospitalization. In fact, patients in the acute phase of schizophrenia improve more on a unit with a structured milieu than on an open unit that allows greater freedom. Nursing staff provide 24-hour care during a hospitalization and are responsible for facilitating therapeutic milieu therapy.

A milieu (hospital environment) that is not understimulating or overstimulating will help the person feel less anxious. Patients with

APPLYING THE ART

A Person With Schizophrenia

Scenario

I noticed Aaron standing barefooted in the hallway with both shoes in his outstretched hand. He almost looked like a statue with his blank, unaware demeanor. He deliberately picked up each foot and then slowly rubbed the ball of each foot against the carpet.

Therapeutic Goal

By the end of the present encounter, Aaron will demonstrate increased comfort with the student nurse, as evidenced by voluntarily walking together in the hallways of the psychiatric unit.

Student–Patient Interaction	Thoughts, Communication Techniques, and Mental Health Nursing Concepts
Student: "Aaron, I am _____, one of the nursing students. Aaron, I'm standing next to you, on your right side."	With *schizophrenia*, it is important to say his name and say my own name to make clear our separateness.
Student's feelings: *I'm kind of nervous. How scary and lonely his world must be.*	
Aaron: *Quietly murmuring.* "Don't know left, right, right, correct. I can't quite gather first one, last one. Can't last long … long … long lost soul. Soul train."	He may have an *ego-boundary* disturbance. He also holds his shoes far away from his body. What are the clues inside his *loose associations?* He looks stuck just standing there, yet he holds his shoes like he is *ambivalent* about going somewhere.
Student's feelings: *I wonder why he rubs each foot against the floor like he really needs to feel where the floor is.*	
Student's feelings: *That part, "long lost soul," makes me feel sad. I felt lost when I first arrived here at school, without a single friend. When I let myself know what I'm feeling, memories of the losses in my childhood begin to stir.*	I need to focus on Aaron and deal with potential *countertransference* later. His most intense words are "long lost soul." That phrase is near the end of his rambling associations. He may remember the last words he spoke at some level. I will *restate* and then use *reflection* of feelings.
Student: "Long lost soul. You're feeling kind of lost right now. It's hard to decide what to do next."	Maybe he wants to get away on his own "soul train." Is he an *elopement* risk? Probably not. He is too confused right now to plan anything, although he may follow easily. I'll give some structure to meet *safety needs.* I will use the techniques of expressing empathy and verbalizing the implied.
Student: "Aaron, it's _____. Come with me and we'll figure out how to help you." *I touch his arm to direct him toward the day area.*	
Aaron: *Abruptly tilts his head toward opposite wall. He begins mumbling like he's responding to an unseen other.*	The touch violated his precarious *ego boundary.* He's *hallucinating*—my touch must have increased his anxiety. I need to speak in short sentences with many pauses to slow this down.
Student's feelings: *I'm so upset with myself. I acted without thinking about how threatening my touch would be without asking first. I so want to help him, and now I've scared him. I want to say, "I'm sorry," but that's my need. I'll tell him later when he's able to process information. Okay, keep focused. He needs to feel safe more than anything.*	
Student: "Aaron, I'm here. I'll stay with you."	I *offer self.*
Aaron: *Mumbles.* "The mistop … don't … can't …." *Looks panicked.*	He is approaching *panic-level* anxiety. "Mistop." What is that? Is it a *neologism?*
Student: "Aaron, talk to me. What are the voices saying?"	
Student's feelings: *My first job is to stay calm myself. He looks terrified. I need to let him know he's safe. I am okay. Even if I don't say everything right, I do care.*	
Aaron: *Shakes his head.* "Soul train, blame, shame, going to the end of the line … supine … surprise … demise."	He is making *clang associations.* I hear covert references that may be to suicide. I will *restate* and then ask a *direct question* to assess suicide potential.
Student: "The end of the line; demise. Aaron, are the voices telling you to hurt yourself or someone else?"	He probably cannot *reality test* enough to tell me whether the voices tell him to kill himself. I must report this now, but I also do not want to leave him alone if there is the slightest potential for suicide. He needs *close, constant observation.*
Student's feelings: *Overwhelmed, I can't do this alone. Maybe medication will help. I hope at some level he will feel safer.*	
Aaron: *Mumbles.*	Before he did not come with me. Now he is walking beside me. He feels more comfortable with me now.
Student: *Without crowding him, I position myself so that he can see my face. Quiet and concerned.* "Let's go together to talk to the nurse." *Aaron slowly walks with me.*	

paranoid ideation (ideas) may be suspicious of food served and be afraid to sleep. Serving sealed food (like a yogurt container) and providing explanations of safety measures on the unit ("We make rounds every half hour throughout the night to make sure everyone is safe") may lessen suspiciousness. A therapeutic milieu provides emotional and physical safety, useful activities, resources for resolving conflicts, and opportunities for learning social and vocational skills. **(QSEN: Safety)**

An individual with schizophrenia or other related psychotic disorders, especially in the acute phase, is at higher risk for harm to self or others, often in response to hallucinations (voices telling them others are out to harm or kill them or telling them to jump out a window) or delusions (believing that another is out to harm or kill them). During this time, measures need to be taken to protect the patient and others. If verbal de-escalation efforts and sedative medications (antipsychotic medication and/or benzodiazepines) fail to lessen the patient's anxiety/aggression, physical restraints and seclusion may be used as a very last resort (see Chapters 6, 15, and 23).

With the shifting of care for the seriously mentally ill from inpatient to community-based treatment centers, the need for transitional care is heightened, and the role of the nurse in providing a therapeutic milieu is broadened. Alternatives to hospitalization include residential crisis services, partial hospitalization, day treatment services, and halfway houses.

- Crisis residential services: Patients receive short-term, consumer-centered treatment in a supportive, home-like environment in the community for adults who are experiencing an acute psychiatric crisis but may not require inpatient hospitalization.
- Partial hospitalization/day treatment programs: Patients attend a structured program during the day and return to a halfway house or their own home in the evening. These are sometimes used to help the patient transition more smoothly from inpatient hospitalization to home.
- Halfway houses: Patients live in the community with a group of other patients, sharing expenses and responsibilities. Staff members are present in the house 24 hours a day, 7 days a week.

Some of these programs may include group therapy, supervised activities, individual counseling, or specialized training and rehabilitation (see Chapter 5).

Psychotherapy and Psychoeducation

Program of Assertive Community Treatment

The Program of Assertive Community Treatment (PACT) or Assertive Community Treatment (ACT) is designed for the most marginally adjusted and poorly functioning patients. The aim of treatment is to prevent relapse, maximize social and vocational functioning, and keep the individual in the community. PACT/ACT is a team approach and provides *expanded case management* available around the clock. It emphasizes the patient's strengths in adapting to the community, provides support and assertive outreach, and involves almost all aspects of the patient's life (food, shelter, schooling, grooming, budgeting, and transportation). PACT/ACT outpatient programs may provide mobile crisis intervention, supportive cognitive and behavioral therapy, and substance use treatment, to name a few. These programs have been shown to reduce hospital admissions and improve quality of life for many of these patients (Black & Andreasen, 2014). Medication adherence is emphasized.

Family Psychoeducation/Therapy

Most evidence-based approaches emphasize the value of family participation in treatment. Families with members who are struggling with schizophrenia often endure considerable hardships while coping with the psychotic and residual symptoms of the illness. Often these families become isolated from their relatives and communities. Families are perhaps the most consistent factor in patients' lives. More than half of patients discharged from a psychiatric facility return to their family of origin. The following example shows how a family came to distinguish between "Martha's problem" and "the problem caused by schizophrenia."

VIGNETTE: It was a good idea, us all meeting in the comfort of our own home to discuss my sister's illness. We were all able to say how it felt, and for the first time I realized that I knew very little about what she was suffering from or how much—the word *schizophrenia* meant nothing to me before but it's much clearer now. I used to think she was just being lazy until she told me in the meeting what it was really like.

Family psychoeducation seeks to engage family members as partners, complementing interventions by clinicians by teaching specialized interactions and coping skills that counter the neurologic deficits inherent in those with psychotic disorders. Psychoeducation can be provided in single-family and multi-family groups. For multi-family groups, practitioners invite five to six patients and their families to participate in a weekly psychoeducation group for at least 6 months.

The original goal was to help the family modify the family's (emotional) living environment. The level of "expressed emotion" (EE) (overinvolvement, yelling, shouting, fighting, or critical comments) by caregivers is correlated with relapse rates. Low-EE skills are taught to family members as a strategy to reduce relapse. This intervention was also found to improve caregivers' positive well-being and reduce the burden of care. When this intervention was used in first-episode and prodromal symptoms of psychosis, it led to a substantial return of functioning for the individual and avoidance of psychosis altogether (McFarlane, 2016).

Cognitive-Behavioral Therapy

Recovery-oriented cognitive therapy (CT-R), a form of cognitive-behavioral therapy, appears to be highly successful in the treatment of individuals with chronic schizophrenia who have difficulty integrating into the community. The therapy targets the distress and disturbance that are often a consequence of the experience of psychotic symptoms by correcting self-defeating beliefs (Moran, 2014).

Cognitive Remediation

Cognitive remediation/cognitive enhancement is an intervention that uses specific learning activities to improve cognitive skill. It is aimed at improving attention, memory, language, and/or executive functions. It seems to be most effective in the early course of schizophrenia and for people at risk for the development of psychosis (Cella et al., 2017).

Social Skills Training

Poor social and interpersonal skills can prevent people from interacting effectively with other people in the community. Social skills training (SST) involves training to improve social interactions, social cognition (accurately perceiving and understanding social interactions), self-management and illness management skills, community participation, and workplace skills.

There is evidence that social skills training can improve social interactions. There is also some benefit in terms of improved community functioning, improvement in negative symptoms, and improved emotion perception (understanding other people's mental states). Relapse rates were reduced, and quality-of-life indicators showed improvement (Almerie et al., 2015).

The Recovery Model and Recovery-Oriented Care

The recovery model of mental illness moves beyond just symptom management. Interventions are geared toward the patient's strengths, highest level of functioning, and quality of life (Jacob, 2015). **(QSEN: Evidence-Based Practice)** The recovery model is based on a program used by SAMHSA. It defines recovery as *a process of change* through which individuals improve their health and wellness, live self-directed lives, and strive to reach their full potential (SAMHSA, 2017b). This model is based on the knowledge and belief that anyone can recover and/or manage their condition successfully. The four dimensions that support recovery are as follows:

1. Health: overcoming or managing your disease
2. Home: having a stable place to live
3. Purpose: having meaningful daily activities and the resources to participate in society
4. Community: having supportive relationships and hope

The recovery model fosters hope, rebuilds self-image, helps people to cope with life's challenges, and helps to give individuals some control over their illness. The individual is a partner in planning individualized goals and formulating a treatment plan (Jacob, 2015; SAMHSA, 2017b). **(QSEN: Patient-Centered Care; Evidence-Based Practice)**

See Chapters 5 and 19 for more on the recovery model.

Recovery After an Initial Schizophrenia Episode (RAISE) Project. In 2008, the National Institute of Mental Health (NIMH) launched a large-scale research initiative called the *Recovery After an Initial Schizophrenia Episode (RAISE)* Project. It was designed to study the best ways to intervene after a person begins to experience psychotic symptoms to prevent long-term disability. This approach combines medication, psychosocial therapies, case management, family involvement, and supported education and employment services to develop a personal treatment plan for people with first-episode psychosis. The study found that participants in the treatment stayed in treatment longer. They reported a greater improvement in their symptoms, with improved interpersonal relationships and quality of life. The current challenge is to help more communities implement this evidence-based care (Kane et al., 2015). **(QSEN: Evidence-Based Practice)**

Pharmacological, Biological, and Integrative Therapies

Drugs used to treat psychotic disorders are called antipsychotic medications. This class of medication may alleviate many of the symptoms of schizophrenia but cannot cure the underlying psychotic processes. When patients stop taking their medications, psychotic symptoms usually return. With each relapse following medication discontinuation, it can take longer to achieve remission after restarting medications. This leads to the possibility that the patient will eventually become unresponsive to treatment.

APPLYING EVIDENCE-BASED PRACTICE (EBP)

Problem

A 52-year-old male with a diagnosis of paranoid schizophrenia has been a patient at a community mental health clinic for about 10 years. Due to the scarcity of psychiatric professionals in this rural area, he sees his psychiatric nurse practitioner (NP) via telemedicine. He has a history of being nonadherent with his appointments and medications, and as a result, his symptoms have escalated. During the worst periods, the patient does not eat, drink, or sleep adequately; has vivid and terrifying hallucinations of bloody people and demons; and becomes very paranoid. He isolates himself in his home much of the time, and when he does come to town, he appears disheveled and rants and raves loudly, which scares others. He has been arrested on several occasions because of his behaviors.

EBP Assessment

A. **What do you already know from experience?**

1. This patient has a pattern of missing appointments and medications.
2. This patient has complained frequently about the telemedicine appointments.
3. The patient says he doesn't like talking to a machine, and at times feels he is being recorded and his thoughts are being broadcast through the computer to the government.

B. **What does the literature say?**

1. Telemedicine is a cost-effective option in many settings.
2. In general, patient perceptions of the usefulness of telemedicine vary.
3. Nonadherence is an issue in up to 72% of patients with schizophrenia.
4. Patients who adhere to their treatment plan have much better outcomes.
5. The relationship between the health care professional, other staff, and the patient is an important component of adherence to treatment.

C. **What does the patient want?**

1. The patient does not like the telemedicine appointments.
2. When taking his medications and thinking more clearly, he recognizes the need for treatment.
3. During an acute psychotic episode, he becomes extremely paranoid, and it is difficult to reason with him.

Plan

Due to the long-standing problems with this patient, the clinic devised an individualized plan of care. The patient was assigned a local peer-support person who visits him several times a week. Transportation was provided to a city about 75 miles away so that the patient can meet with his psychiatric NP face to face, accompanied by his peer-support person for support.

Result

The patient became more adherent as he developed relationships with his caregivers. His symptoms were monitored more closely, and his paranoia decreased. He eventually accepted telemedicine appointments part of the time.

QSEN Prelicensure Knowledge, Skills, and Attitudes (KSAs) Addressed

Informatics was used to provide health care through telemedicine to the majority of patients in this rural setting.

Patient-Centered Care incorporated the patient's preferences in the treatment plan.

Teamwork and Collaboration was incorporated as the clinic worked with the psychiatric NP and peer-support person to providew individualized care.

Neurobiology of Schizophrenia and the Effects of Antipsychotics

The antipsychotics affect a number of neurotransmitters including dopamine, noradrenaline/norepinephrine, serotonin, and GABA Excess of serotonin may contribute to both the positive and negative symptoms of schizophrenia. GABA regulates dopamine activity and in some people with schizophrenia, there is a loss of GABAergic neurons in the hippocampus, potentially causing hyperactivity of dopamine. However, since dopamine is the most studied and most prominent of the neurotransmitters (D1, D2, D3, D4, and D5) in schizophrenia, the role of dopamine is presented here.

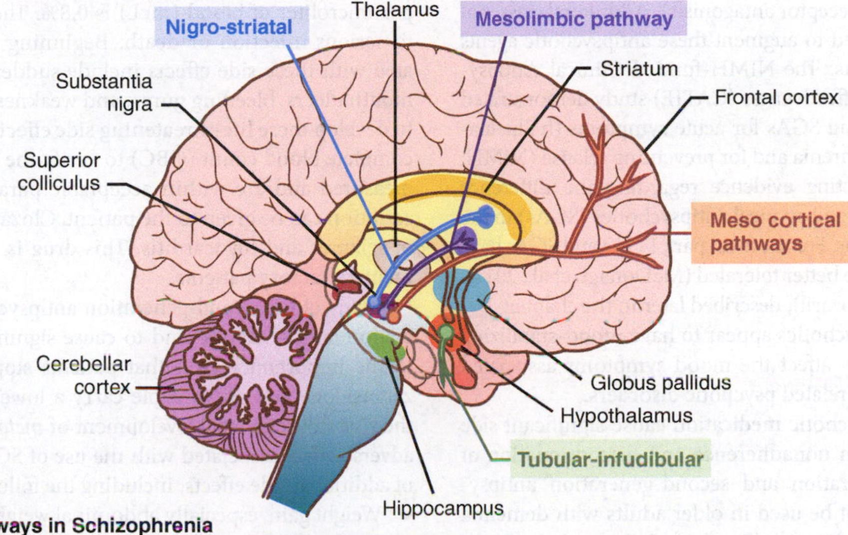

Dopamine Pathways in Schizophrenia

Mesolimbic pathway: reward motivation, emotions and positive symptoms of schizophrenia.

Meso cortical pathways: relevant to cognitive function and executive function and negative symptoms of schizophrenia

Nigro-striatal: normally responsible for purposeful movement.

Tubuler-infundibular: normally responsible for regulation of prolactin.

First-generation antipsychotic (FGA) drugs are potent antagonists/blockers of D2.

Second-generation antipsychotics (SGA) have less affinity for D2 receptors, and tend to bind with D3 and D4 receptors. Since the expression of D3 and D4 is limited to the neurons of the limbic system and cerebral cortex, the action of these drugs is limited to areas involved in the pathology of schizophrenia. Second-generation drugs also inhibit the serotonin (5-HT) receptors. Since serotonin inhibits the release of dopamine, the dopaminergic transmission is affected.

The potential serious effects of the SGAs (metabolic effects: weight gain, diabetes, and dyslipidemia) come from the blockade of noradrenaline/norepinephrine (alpha-1), histamine, and acetylcholine.

Dopamine Pathways and Antipsychotic Responses

Dopamine Pathway	Abnormality in Schizophrenia	Responses to Antipsychotic Drugs
Mesolimbic pathway connects the VTA to the nucleus accumbens Associated with reward, motivation, and emotion	Hyperactive in schizophrenia Associated with positive symptoms (hallucinations, delusions, disorganized thought)	**FGA**—D2 blockage results in reduction in positive symptoms **SGA**—D3 and D4 antagonism results in reduction of positive symptoms
Mesocortical pathway made up of dopaminergic neurons that project from the ventral tegmental area to the prefrontal cortex Relevant to cognition, executive function, emotions, and affect	Hypofunction in schizophrenia results in cognitive impairment and negative symptoms (apathy, anhedonia, lack of motivation)	**FGA**—D2 blockage may result in a worsening of these symptoms **SGA**—Since there are more serotonin (5-HT) receptors than D2 receptors in this area, blockage of 5-HT is more profound. Blockage of 5-HT may help improve negative symptoms
Tuberoinfundibular pathway consists of dopaminergic projections from the hypothalamus to the pituitary gland Inhibits prolactin release	Unaffected	**FGA** (to a less degree SGA)—Blockade of D2 receptors increases prolactin levels resulting in hyperprolactinemia and lactation
Nigrostriatal pathway-substantial nigra to basal ganglia Responsible for purposeful movement	Unaffected	**FGA** (to a lesser degree SGA)—Long-term blockade of D2 receptors can cause upregulation (increase response to a stimulus) to those receptors, which may lead to extrapyramidal side effects (e.g., tardive dyskinesia [TD]).

There are two basic groups of antipsychotic drugs. One group includes the **first-generation antipsychotics (FGAs) or conventional or typical antipsychotics**. These drugs are also called **neuroleptics** and are also known as dopamine antagonists (D2 receptor antagonists). Another group is called **second-generation antipsychotics (SGAs) or atypical antipsychotics**. These are sometimes called serotonin–dopamine antagonists (5-HT2A and 5-HT2C receptor antagonists). Additional classes of medication are sometimes used to augment these antipsychotic agents for treatment-resistant patients. The NIMH-funded Clinical Antipsychotic Trials of Intervention Effectiveness (CATIE) study demonstrated equal effectiveness of FGAs and SGAs for acute symptoms (hallucinations and delusion) of schizophrenia and for preventing relapse (NIMH, 2005). There is some conflicting evidence regarding the difference between conventional (FGAs) and atypical antipsychotics (SGAs) in the treatment of negative symptoms. For the most part, FGAs and SGAs have equal efficacy, but the SGAs are better tolerated (McDonagh et al., 2017). The exception is clozapine (Clozaril), described later in the chapter.

The newer atypical antipsychotics appear to have mood-stabilizing properties that may positively affect the mood symptoms associated with schizophrenia and other related psychotic disorders.

Both subclasses of antipsychotic medication cause significant side effects, which is one factor in nonadherence and discontinuation of medications. Both first-generation and second-generation antipsychotic medications should not be used in older adults with dementia because they double the mortality risk (Burchum & Rosenthal, 2016).

Antipsychotic medications can be given using multiple routes of administration. Individual medications may or may not be available in these multiple routes of administration.

1. Oral form (tablet or liquid) that is swallowed—most common
2. Oral disintegrating tablets that dissolve on the tongue—when the nurse suspects a patient may be "cheeking" meds (not taking/swallowing the medication given)
3. Short-acting intramuscular (IM)—when the sedative effects are needed quickly in an acute situation
4. A long-acting IM form, sometimes called "depot" (effect lasts 1 to 4 weeks)—for people who are nonadherent or are forgetful about taking daily medications
5. A longer-acting IM form (3-month length of effectiveness)—only INVEGA TRINZA currently fits this category (Janssen Pharmaceuticals, 2020)
6. Intravenous (IV) for an extremely fast-acting response—rarely used

Various new routes of drug administration are in development. These include a long-acting transdermal patch that eliminates the need to take a daily pill, long-acting IM injections that have an immediate antipsychotic effect, a drug implant that is effective for 6 months, and the use of a digital tracking system that transmits information about medication adherence.

Antipsychotic medications are central nervous system (CNS) depressants, so the initial response is sedation. Individuals may notice some positive effects of antipsychotic medication within 1 to 2 days. It may take 2 to 4 weeks for more noticeable improvement and several months for full antipsychotic effects (Burchum & Rosenthal, 2016). Most individuals with schizophrenia respond at least partially to antipsychotic drug therapy. However, without drug treatment, up to 70% to 80% of individuals will relapse within a year.

Second-Generation Antipsychotics/Atypical Agents

SGAs/atypical agents (except for clozapine) are usually chosen as first-line antipsychotics and are the treatment of choice for patients experiencing their first episode of schizophrenia.

The second-generation antipsychotics first emerged in the early 1990s with clozapine (Clozaril). It was one of the first antipsychotics to treat the negative symptoms of schizophrenia. Unfortunately, the incidence of neutropenia (neutrophil count [ANC] less than 1500/mc) among clozapine-treated patients is 2%, and the incidence of agranulocytosis (white blood cell count [WBC] below 3500 WBCs per microliter of blood (mcL) is 0.8%. These abnormalities can lead to serious infection or death. Beginning clinical symptoms associated with these side effects include sudden fever, chills, sore throat, mouth ulcers, bleeding gums, and weakness. Because of the potential to develop these life-threatening side effects, prescribers must order a complete blood count (CBC) to verify the WBC and ANC have been measured and are within acceptable parameters before a new prescription can be given to the patient. Clozapine also increases the risk of seizures and myocarditis. This drug is only used today for treatment-refractory patients.

Many older second-generation antipsychotics and some first-generation antipsychotics tend to cause significant weight gain, and this is one important reason that patients stop taking their medication. Ziprasidone and aripiprazole carry a lower risk for weight gain, but the risk still remains. Development of *metabolic syndrome* is a serious adverse effect associated with the use of SGAs and includes a cascade of additional side effects, including the following:

- Weight gain, especially abdominal weight gain
- Insulin resistance/glucose dysregulation, which increases the risk of developing type 2 diabetes
- Hypercholesterolemia and dyslipidemia, which increase the risk of developing cardiovascular disease/stroke
- Hypertension, which increases the risk of stroke
- Diminished self-esteem related to weight, which leads to problems in adherence to the medication regimen

There have been some cases in which the first indication of *metabolic syndrome* was discovered when the patient developed diabetic coma.

Many SGAs or atypical second-generation antipsychotics have fewer **extrapyramidal symptoms (EPSs)** and fewer *anticholinergic side effects* at lower dosages. *EPSs and anticholinergic symptoms* are described in detail later in the chapter. Other side effects observed with this class of medication are sedation; orthostatic hypotension; lowered seizure threshold; hormonal dysregulation, such as increased prolactin levels; and cardiac dysrhythmias, including prolonged QTc intervals. Sexual dysfunction is also included in this list. Some SGAs have a warning associated with increased suicidal ideation (Table 17.8).

First-Generation Antipsychotics/Conventional Drugs

The first-generation antipsychotics/conventional or typical drugs (FGAs) are generally used less frequently. In the CATIE study, the use of FGAs tended to lead to high discontinuation rates due to multiple side effects (National Institute of Mental Health [NIMH], 2005).

The FGAs block a variety of receptors within and outside the CNS, including dopamine (D1 and D2 receptors), acetylcholine, histamine, and norepinephrine, serotonin, and GABA (Halter, 2018). Refer to Table 17.10 later in the chapter for adverse effects related to the receptor blockage caused by antipsychotics. Blockage of D2 receptor sites in the motor areas of the brain is responsible for some of the most troubling side effects of the FGAs, namely, the *EPSs* described in the following section. Other adverse reactions include *anticholinergic effects* (described later in the chapter).

TABLE 17.8 Second-Generation Antipsychotics (SGAs): General Side-Effect Profile

SGAs have the potential for exhibiting multiple side effects, as listed here. Specific drugs in this category have higher or lower incidences of each of these side effects.

Side Effects

Anticholinergic
- Urinary retention, constipation
- Dry mouth, blurry vision, tachycardia

Cardiovascular events
- QTc interval prolongation and sudden death
- Myocarditis and cardiomyopathy
- Orthostatic hypotension

Extrapyramidal side effects (EPSs)
- Dystonias
- Akathisia
- Parkinsonian symptoms
- Tardive dyskinesia (TD)

Metabolic syndrome
- Central or abdominal obesity
- ↑ Triglycerides
- ↑ High-density lipoprotein (HDL) cholesterol
- ↑ Blood pressure
- ↑ Fasting blood glucose

Seizures

Sedation/somnolence

Blood dyscrasias such as agranulocytosis

↑ Prolactin elevation
- Gynecomastia, galactorrhea, menstrual problems

Sexual problems

Nausea and vomiting

↑ Suicide risk

Contraindicated use in elderly with dementia
- Cardiovascular or infection complications

Neuroleptic malignant syndrome (NMS)

Common SGAs

Clozapine (Clozaril)
Amisulpride (Solian)
Aripiprazole (Abilify)
Asenapine (Saphris)
Iloperidone (Fanapt)
Lurasidone (Latuda)
Olanzapine (Zyprexa) (short- and long-acting forms)
Paliperidone (Invega) (long- and very-long-acting forms)
Quetiapine (Seroquel)
Risperidone (Risperdal) (short- and long-acting forms)
Sertindole (Serdolect)
Ziprasidone (Geodon)
Brexpiprazole (Rexulti)
Cariprazine (Vraylar)

When the FGAs are used, the specific drug is often chosen for its side-effect profile. For example, chlorpromazine (Thorazine), a low-potency FGA, is the most sedating agent and has fewer EPSs than do other antipsychotic agents, but it causes hypotension in large dosages. Haloperidol (Haldol), a high-potency FGA, is the least sedating and is often used in larger doses to reduce assaultive behavior, but it has a high incidence of EPSs. Haloperidol is effective in treating aggressive behaviors because it controls problematic symptoms with a low incidence of hypotension. People who are functioning at work or at home may prefer less sedating drugs; patients who are agitated or excitable may do better with a more sedating medication (Table 17.9).

TABLE 17.9 First-Generation Antipsychotics (FGAs): General Side-Effect Profile

FGAs have the potential for exhibiting multiple side effects, as listed here. Specific drugs in this category have higher or lower incidences of each of these side effects.

Side Effects

Anticholinergic
- Urinary retention, constipation
- Dry mouth, blurry vision, tachycardia

Cardiovascular events
- QTc interval prolongation and sudden death
- Myocarditis and cardiomyopathy
- Orthostatic hypotension

Extrapyramidal side effects (EPSs)
- Dystonias
- Akathisia
- Parkinsonian symptoms
- Tardive dyskinesia (TD)

Weight gain

Drug-induced liver disease

Cataracts

Photophobia

Seizures

Sedation/somnolence

Blood dyscrasias such as agranulocytosis

↑ Prolactin elevation
- Gynecomastia, galactorrhea, menstrual problems

Sexual problems

Nausea and vomiting

Contraindicated use in elderly with dementia
- Cardiovascular or infection complications

Neuroleptic malignant syndrome (NMS)

Hypersensitivity: skin rash

Common FGA Agents

Haloperidol (Haldol)
Trifluoperazine (Stelazine)
Fluphenazine
Loxapine (Loxitane)
Perphenazine
Chlorpromazine (Thorazine)
Thioridazine (Mellaril)

Extrapyramidal Symptoms. *EPS* are motor symptoms associated with the use of antipsychotic drugs. **Tardive dyskinesia (TD)** is an EPS that usually appears after prolonged treatment. *TD* consists of involuntary tonic muscular spasms of the face and jaw. *TD* is most frequently seen in older women and older patients and varies from mild to moderate. It can be disfiguring or incapacitating.

Early symptoms of *TD* are fasciculations (very tiny involuntary motor movements) of the tongue or constant lip smacking. These early oral movements can develop into uncontrollable biting, chewing, or sucking motions and lateral movements of the jaw. If these beginning symptoms are identified early, *TD* disappears when the antipsychotic medication is discontinued. In other cases, symptoms are not reversible and may progress. In 2017, the U.S. Food and Drug Administration (FDA) approved the first drug to be used for the treatment of *TD*, valbenazine (Ingrezza). It is considered standard practice to regularly monitor all persons on long-term use of antipsychotic medication for movement disorders. The *Abnormal Involuntary Movement Scale (AIMS)* is one instrument used in the early detection of *TD*; it also provides a method for ongoing surveillance of *TD* and other movement disorders. The *AIMS test* can be obtained online or via mobile devices (Psychiatric Times Supplement, 2013).

TD is less likely to occur with SGAs, but monitoring for symptoms is still required.

In addition to *TD*, three of the more common *EPSs* are the following:

- **Acute dystonia**: severe spasms of the muscles of the tongue, head, and neck; fixed upward deviation of the eyes; and severe back spasms that arch the trunk forward and thrust the head and lower limbs backward
- **Akathisia**: internal restlessness and external restless pacing or fidgeting; sometimes mistaken for psychotic agitation or comorbid anxiety
- **Pseudoparkinsonism**: stiffening of muscular activity in the face, body, arms, and legs; salivation; shuffling gait; tremor; bradykinesia

These symptoms are quite uncomfortable and need to be recognized and treated quickly. Treatment usually consists of lowering the dosage of the antipsychotic medication or prescribing additional medications, such as the following:

- Trihexyphenidyl (Artane)—anticholinergic/antiparkinsonian drug; PO (by mouth) form only
- Benztropine mesylate (Cogentin)—anticholinergic/antiparkinsonian drug; PO, IM, intravenous (IV)
- Diphenhydramine hydrochloride (Benadryl)—antihistamine; PO, IM, IV
- Biperiden (Akineton) and amantadine hydrochloride (Symmetrel)—antiparkinsonian drugs; PO only
- Benzodiazepines such as lorazepam—for acute treatment only

Treatment with anticholinergic drugs is not completely benign because of the potential to develop additional side effects associated with these drugs.

Anticholinergic side effects are seen with the use of anticholinergic medications and are also part of the side-effect profile of antipsychotic agents (FGAs and some SGAs). Anticholinergic side effects include blurry vision, dry mouth, constipation, urinary hesitancy/retention, sexual dysfunction, and tachycardia.

Concurrent use of these two classes of drugs, antipsychotics and anticholinergics, can result in an anticholinergic delirium with symptoms of agitation, pressured, incoherent speech, and visual and/or auditory hallucinations.

Neuroleptic malignant syndrome (NMS) is characterized by greatly increased muscle rigidity (with elevation in creatine phosphokinase [CPK]); elevated temperature; altered level of consciousness; and autonomic dysfunction, including labile (changeable) hypertension, tachycardia, tachypnea, diaphoresis, and drooling. Treatment consists of early detection and stopping the medication. The patient should be taught to call the health care provider immediately if these symptoms appear. Medical treatment consists of reduction of temperature, monitoring of fluid balance, and monitoring for complications. Mild cases of NMS are treated with bromocriptine (Parlodel), a dopamine receptor agonist. More severe cases are treated with intravenous dantrolene (Dantrium), a muscle relaxant, and even with electroconvulsive therapy in some cases. See Table 17.10 for the side effects, onset, and nursing measures for *EPS* and *NMS*. NMS is estimated to occur in about 0.2% to 1% of patients who have taken antipsychotic agents. It is believed that the acute reduction in brain dopamine activity plays a role in the development of NMS. It is fatal in about 10% of cases. It usually occurs early during therapy but has been reported in people after 20 years of treatment.

Agranulocytosis is also a rare but serious side effect of the FGAs.

Drug-induced liver problems are another a rare side effect of FGAs. Symptoms may include intense itchiness, dark urine, light-colored feces, and yellowing of the skin or whites of the eyes. Nurses need to be aware of the prodromal signs and symptoms of these rare but life-threatening side effects. Patients and families should be taught to recognize these symptoms and report them to the psychiatric provider immediately.

Many side effects often appear early in therapy and can be minimized with treatment. Patients should be taught to report side effects rather than stopping the medication. Some side effects can be managed with simple remedies, like modifying the diet to decrease constipation, for example. Some patients develop tolerance over time to some side effects. For all antipsychotics, the patient should be cautioned not to stop the drug abruptly. This can result in a discontinuation syndrome (nausea, vomiting, headache, tremulousness, and insomnia)

Pharmacogenetics describes the use of genetic factors to predict an individual's response to a drug, in terms of both efficacy and side effects. Genetic variations may account for differences in the efficacy of antipsychotics and the development of side effects. For example, the drug olanzapine caused greater weight gain in African American patients with schizophrenia than in Caucasian patients (Kishi et al., 2017). There is a continued effort to implement pharmacogenetics in the development of new treatments for psychiatric diseases.

Analysts have identified five unmet needs in the pharmacological treatment of schizophrenia. They include the need to develop the following:

- Drugs that address cognition deficits
- Drugs that treat negative symptoms (e.g., lethargy, apathy, and social withdrawal)
- Drugs that provide improved options for treatment-resistant patients
- Drugs with enhanced safety profiles and fewer side effects
- Drugs that increase adherence (Fellner, 2017)

The focus of current drug development attempts to address these unmet needs. Newer drug treatments target different mechanisms of action, including drugs that affect different neurotransmitters, drugs that affect the immune response, and other mechanisms.

A Caveat: How Antipsychotics Cause Brain Damage. The progressive changes in brain volume seen in schizophrenia are thought to be due principally to the disease process. There is recent concern, though, that antipsychotics may be contributing to brain damage and may contribute to the severity of the cognitive symptoms seen in individuals with schizophrenia. The use of antipsychotic medication may lead to decreased neural connections in the prefrontal region and the loss of white- and gray-matter volume (Vita, De Peri, & Deste, 2015).

It is recommended that antipsychotics are used only when necessary, and it is important to prescribe the minimal effective dose to lessen the potential of the development of these serious secondary effects.

Adjuncts to Antipsychotic Drug Therapy

Antidepressants. Antidepressants are added to antipsychotics when symptoms meeting the criteria for major depressive disorder cause severe distress or are disabling. In fact, a study by Tiihonen and colleagues (2016) found that the use of antidepressants was associated with markedly decreased suicidal deaths. Antidepressants are often used to target negative symptoms.

Benzodiazepines. Although benzodiazepines have been used in the past as an adjunct to antipsychotics, a new study demonstrated that benzodiazepine use was associated with a marked increase in morbidity (Tiihonen et al., 2016). Benzodiazepines can be most useful during an acute episode of the illness to help reduce

TABLE 17.10 Nursing Measures for Medication Side Effects: Extrapyramidal Symptoms and Neuroleptic Malignant Syndrome

	EXTRAPYRAMIDAL SYMPTOMS (EPS)	
Side Effect	**Onset**	**Nursing Measure**
1. **Pseudoparkinsonism:** masklike facies, stiff and stooped posture, shuffling gait, drooling, tremor, "pill-rolling" phenomenon	5 hours to 30 days	1. Alert medical staff. Administer: • Anticholinergic agent: trihexyphenidyl (Artane) or benztropine (Cogentin) or • Dopamine agonist: amantadine (Symmetrel)
2. **Acute dystonic reactions:** acute spasms of tongue, face, neck, and back (tongue and jaw first) • **Opisthotonos:** tetanic heightening of entire body, head and belly up • **Oculogyric crisis:** eyes locked upward	A few hours to 5 days	2. Administer diphenhydramine hydrochloride (Benadryl) IM/IV or benztropine IM/IV. Relief occurs in minutes. Prevent further dystonia with any anticholinergic agent. Experience is very frightening. **Take patient to quiet area** and stay until relief of symptoms.
3. **Akathisia:** distressing motor inner-driven restlessness (e.g., tapping foot incessantly, rocking forward and backward in chair, shifting weight from side to side)	2 hours to 60 days	3. Reduce dosage, switch to a low-potency antipsychotic, or trial an atypical antipsychotic. Treat with anticholinergic, benzodiazepine, or beta blockers. Is sometimes mistaken for psychotic agitation

4. **Tardive dyskinesia (TD):**
• **Facial:** protruding and rolling tongue, blowing, smacking, licking, spastic facial distortion
• **Limbs:**
  • Choreic: rapid, purposeless, and irregular movements
  • Athetoid: slow, complex, and serpentine movements
• **Trunk:** neck and shoulder movements, dramatic hip jerks and rocking, twisting pelvic thrusts
	Months to years	4. Treatment
		a. Stopping drug and switching to newer antipsychotic agent may help for beginning symptoms. Discontinuing drug does not always relieve symptoms.
		b. Occurs in 15% to 20% of patients taking these drugs for more than 2 years.
		c. Eating difficulties; malnutrition can occur because of tongue and mouth involvement.
		d. Most disabling symptom.
		e. Use Abnormal Involuntary Movement Scale (AIMS) to help detect TD in early stages.
		f. Ingrezza (valbenazine)—first FDA-approved (2017) drug to treat adults with TD; side effects: sleepiness, QT prolongation

	NEUROLEPTIC MALIGNANT SYNDROME (NMS) (SOMEWHAT RARE, POTENTIALLY FATAL)	
Symptoms Memory Tool F * E * V *E * R	**Course of Illness and Risk Factors**	**Treatment**

Fever (Hyperpyrexia: >103°F or above 38°C)
Elevated CPK/WBC
Vital sign instability (autonomic instability)
• Fluctuating BP, pallor, tachycardia
• Excessive sweating, salivation, tremors, incontinence
Encephalopathy
• Confusion, agitation, altered level of consciousness
(Muscle) **R**igidity
	Course of illness:
	• Can occur in first 1–4 wk of drug therapy; may occur at any time during treatment
	• Rapid progression over 2–3 days after initial symptoms
	• Mortality 5%–11%
	Risk factors:
	• Use of more than one psychotropic medication
	• Higher in those under age 40 and male
	• Presence of a mood disorder (40%)
	• Higher dosage, rapid titration, use of long-acting (depot) drugs
		• Stop drug immediately.
		• Early recognition increases chance for full recovery.
		• Aggressive treatment of symptoms, including:
		  • Antipyretics to treat hyperpyrexia
		  • Dantrolene to reduce muscle spasms/rigidity
		  • IV fluids for dehydration
		• Treat complications of multiple body systems

BP, Blood pressure; *CPK*, creatinine phosphokinase; *FDA*, U.S. Food and Drug Administration; *IM*, intramuscular; *IV*, intravenous; *WBC*, white blood cell.

panic levels of anxiety and aggressiveness. The long-term use of benzodiazepines is linked with dementia and cognitive decline.

Self-Care for Nurses

A person who is psychotic is intensely anxious, lonely, dependent, and distrustful. Health care professionals may respond with similar emotions. An individual who is extremely paranoid and hostile can be frightening and challenging even to experienced staff. Deciphering incomprehensible language (looseness of associations) and working with a person who is hallucinating or who has strong delusional systems (paranoid) can lead to high levels of anxiety in the nurse. Nurses who are new to the psychiatric setting, especially the student nurse, may adopt defensive behaviors such as denial or withdrawal and avoidance. These are responses that can interfere with providing optimal care. Supervision and support from more experienced nurses and staff should always be available in these situations. The student's part in the supervisory process is a willingness to discuss and identify personal feelings and behavioral responses to clinical situations. This is often accomplished in group supervision or through peer-group supervision.

There are technical platforms like virtual reality and YouTube videos that simulate the experience of psychosis. These can be used by health care providers and family members to help caregivers develop an empathetic understanding of some of the acute symptoms associated with schizophrenia. YouTube testimonials by those with a diagnosis of schizophrenia can also further an empathetic understanding of the disease.

EVALUATION

Evaluation is always an important step in the planning of care and is especially important for people who have chronic psychotic disorders. Realistic outcomes that are mutually agreed upon by the nurse and the patient tend to be more successful. It is critical for staff to remember that change is a process that occurs over time. For a person diagnosed with schizophrenia, the period may be prolonged.

It is important to schedule regular evaluations for chronically ill patients so that new data can be considered and the patient's problems can be reassessed. Areas to consider include the following:

1. Have distressing symptoms lessened? If not, why not?
2. Are the patient's strengths and interests used to achieve the outcomes?
3. Is the patient taking medications as prescribed?
4. If not, what is contributing to the nonadherence?
5. Are family members involved? Do they understand the patient's disease and treatment issues to help them be more supportive?
6. Are the patient and family aware of relapse issues (prodromal symptoms of relapse, need for medication adherence)?
7. Are the patient and family working with effective community supports and treatments?

Active staff involvement and interest in the patient's progress communicate concern and help to prevent feelings of helplessness and burnout. Input from the patient can offer valuable information about possible causes of the failure to achieve a desired behavior or situation.

KEY POINTS TO REMEMBER

- Schizophrenia is a devastating brain disease. It is not one disorder but a group of disorders that appear on a spectrum along with other psychotic disorders. The psychotic symptoms found in schizophrenia are more pronounced and disruptive than are the symptoms found in some other psychotic disorders.
- Neurochemical, genetic, and neuroanatomical findings help explain the symptoms of schizophrenia. At present, no one theory accounts for all phenomena found in schizophrenic disorders.
- The nursing assessment is used to identify the presence of symptoms associated with the four specific dimensions of schizophrenia. These include positive, negative, cognitive, and mood symptoms.
- The positive symptoms are more florid (hallucinations, delusions, looseness of associations) and tend to lessen with antipsychotic drug therapy. Assessment of these symptoms takes priority during acute illness to maintain safe and effective care. **QSEN: Safety**
- The negative symptoms (poor social adjustment, lack of motivation, withdrawal) are more debilitating and do not respond as well to antipsychotic drug therapy.
- Cognitive impairment is perhaps one of the most serious groups of symptoms in the schizophrenia spectrum disorders. Careful assessment and interventions must be implemented to increase the person's quality of life and ability to function in the community.
- Co-occurring illnesses need to be identified and treated to lower the potential for suicide, substance use disorders, and further mortality and morbidity.
- Patient problems, nursing diagnoses, and the focus of care can be determined based on the recognition of thoughts, feelings, and behaviors associated with schizophrenia spectrum disorders. Additional areas of intervention are family focused (see Table 17.4).
- Planning of outcomes starts by identifying the phase of schizophrenia and assessing the patient's individual needs based on functional ability. It involves identifying individualized short-term and intermediate goals. **QSEN: Patient-Centered Care**
- Specific specialized communication strategies are necessary when dealing with a patient who is experiencing hallucinations, delusions, or paranoia. **QSEN: Patient-Centered Care**
- Patient and family health teaching and family psychoeducation are essential aspects of care. Other strategies include milieu management, psychotherapy, and pharmacological therapies. **QSEN: Teamwork and Collaboration**
- The recovery model emphasizes hope and a strong belief that it is possible for people with mental illness to regain a meaningful life. It focuses on the person and self-management, rather than just alleviating symptoms. **QSEN: Patient-Centered Care**
- The nurse must understand the properties, adverse effects, and toxic effects of the typical and atypical antipsychotic medications and other medications used to treat schizophrenia. **QSEN: Evidence-Based Practice**
- Psychoeducation and health teaching for the patient and family should include information about the illness; medication education, including the importance of medication adherence; identification of wellness strategies; and development of a relapse-prevention plan.
- Psychoeducation must also include knowledge of web-based and community supports for patients and families. Reliable web-based sources of current, evidence-based information about the course and treatment of these illnesses should be explored with patients and families to facilitate recovery. **QSEN: Informatics**

APPLYING CRITICAL JUDGMENT

1. Differentiate between the short-term and long-term needs of people with a diagnosis of schizophrenia. Identify the basic focus and interventions for the different phases of the illness.
2. Read the following case study and collaborate with a peer to answer the questions that follow.

Jamie, a 29-year-old woman, is being discharged in 2 days from the hospital after her first psychotic break. She is extremely paranoid. Jamie is recently divorced and has been working as a legal secretary. Recently, her work became erratic, and her suspicious behavior prompted a hospital admission. Jamie will be discharged to her mother's care until she is able to resume working. Jamie's mother is overwhelmed and asks the nurse how she is going to cope. "Jamie has become so distant, and she always takes things the wrong way. I can hardly say anything to her without her misconstruing everything. She is very mad at me because I called 911. I had her admitted after she told me she was going to get justice back in the world by blowing up evil forces that have been haunting her life. She then proceeded to try to run over her ex-husband, thinking he was the devil. She told me there is nothing wrong with her, and I am concerned she won't take her medication once she is discharged. What am I going to do?"

A. What are some of the priority concerns that should be addressed prior to discharge?
B. How would you explain to Jamie's mother some of the symptoms that Jamie is experiencing? What suggestions do you have to address the mother's immediate concerns?
C. What strategies might help to facilitate better medication adherence after discharge for this patient?
D. Identify and describe three community resources that could be supportive for this patient and family.
E. How would you describe the prognosis for Jamie? Support your hypothesis.
F. Discuss how you think the recovery model might help Jamie with some of her problems once she becomes less psychotic and paranoid.

3. Visit the National Alliance on Mental Illness (NAMI) website (http://www.NAMI.org) and identify a local chapter of the organization. List places in your community that are available to help people with severe mental illnesses (e.g., day treatment centers, respite centers, clubhouse model, group homes). **QSEN: Informatics**
4. Read about the Substance Abuse and Mental Health Services Administration (SAMHSA) recovery model at https://www.samhsa.gov/treatment/mental-health-disorders/schizophrenia#recovery-social-support-services. **(QSEN: Informatics)** Do you believe that the components of the recovery model can be applied to people with a psychotic disorder?

CHAPTER REVIEW QUESTIONS

1. A patient smiles broadly at the nurse and says, "Look at my clean teeth. I brushed them with scouring powder because the label said, 'It brightens and whitens everything.'" Which term should the nurse include when documenting this encounter?
   a. Circumstantiality
   b. Concrete thinking
   c. Poverty of speech
   d. Associative looseness
2. A patient diagnosed with schizophrenia says, "I hear the voices every day. They always say bad things about me." Which action by the nurse has the highest priority?
   a. Assess the patient for suicidal thinking and plans.
   b. Review the patient's medication regimen and adherence.
   c. Educate the patient about symptoms associated with schizophrenia.
   d. Suggest distracters for the patient to use when auditory hallucinations occur.
3. Three days after beginning a new regime of haloperidol (Haldol), the nurse observes that a hospitalized patient is drooling, has stiff and extended extremities, and has skin that is damp and hot to the touch. The patient has difficulty responding verbally to the nurse. What is the nurse's correct analysis and action in this situation?
   a. A seizure is occurring; place the patient in a lateral recumbent position and monitor.
   b. Serotonin syndrome has developed; place an intravenous line and rapidly infuse D5½ normal saline (NS).
   c. Neuroleptic malignant syndrome has developed; prepare the patient for immediate transfer to a medical unit.
   d. An acute dystonic reaction is occurring; promptly administer an intramuscular injection of diphenhydramine (Benadryl).
4. A patient diagnosed with schizophrenia complains to the nurse about persistent feelings of restlessness and says, "I feel like I need to move all the time." What is the nurse's next action?
   a. Add an activity group to the patient's plan of care.
   b. Assess the patient for other extrapyramidal symptoms.
   c. Perform a full mental status evaluation of the patient.
   d. Educate the patient about the psychomotor agitation associated with schizophrenia.
5. A nurse begins a therapeutic relationship with a patient diagnosed with schizophrenia. The patient has severe paranoia. Which comment by the nurse is most appropriate?
   a. "Let's begin by talking about the goals you have for yourself."
   b. "I understand that you have problems with fear and suspiciousness of others."
   c. "As you get to know me better, I hope you will feel comfortable talking to me."
   d. "I am part of your treatment team. Our goal is to help stabilize your symptoms."

REFERENCES

Almerie, M., Okba, A., Marhi, M., Jawoosh, M., Alsabbagh, M., Matar, H. E., et al. (2015). Social skills programmes for schizophrenia. *Cochrane Database of Systematic Reviews 2015*, 6, CD009006. https://doi.org/10.1002/14651858.CD009006.pub2.

American Psychiatric Association (APA). (2013). *Diagnostic and statistical manual of mental disorders (DSM-5)* (5th ed.). Washington, DC: APA.

Australian Institute of Psychological Counsellors. (2014). *2014 Mental Health Academy, psychoeducation: Definition, goals and methods*, Retrieved from: https://www.aipc.net.au/articles/psychoeducation-definition-goals-and-methods/.

Black, D. W., & Andreasen, N. C. (2014). *Introductory textbook of psychiatry* (6th ed.). Washington, DC: American Psychiatric Publishing.

Blank, M. (2016). An overview of the interface between HIV/AIDS infection and mental illness. *Psychiatric Times*. Retrieved from: https://www.scribd.com/document/346141466/Psychiatric-Times-Mental-Health-and-HIVAIDS-2017-01-03-1-pdf.

Brisch, R., Saniotis, A., Wolf, R., Bielau, H., Bernstein, H.-G., Steiner, J., et al. (2014). The role of dopamine in schizophrenia from a neurobiological and evolutionary perspective: Old fashioned, but still in vogue. *Frontiers in Psychiatry*, 5, 47. https://doi.org/10.3389/fpsyt.2014.00047.

Burchum, J., & Rosenthal, L. (2016). *Lehne's pharmacology for nursing care* (9th ed.). St. Louis: Elsevier.

Cassidy, R. M., Yang, F., Kapczinski, F., & Passos, I. C. (2017). Risk factors for suicidality in patients with schizophrenia: A systematic review, meta-analysis, and meta-regression of 96 studies. *Schizophrenia Bulletin, September 23*, 2017. https://doi.org/10.1093/schbul/sbx131.

Cella, M., Preti, A., Edward, C., Dow, T., & Wykes, T. (2017). Cognitive remediation for negative symptoms of schizophrenia: A network meta-analysis. *Clinical Psychology Review, 52*, 43–51.

Chavan, P. (2016). Harvard & MIT scientists identify C4-A, the gene that causes schizophrenia. Retrieved from http://www.thehealthsite.com/Harvard-MIT-scientists-identity-c-4-a-the-gene-that-courses-schizophrenia-poO116/.

Cold Spring Harbor Laboratory. (2015). Discovery of communication link between brain areas implicated in schizophrenia. *ScienceDaily*. Retrieved from www.sciencedaily.com/releases/2015/04/150407210901.htm.

Dapunt, J., Kluge, U., & Heinz, A. (2017). Risk of psychosis in refugees: A literature review. *Translational Psychiatry, 7*(6), e1149. https://doi.org/10.1038/tp.2017.119.

Dein, S. (2017). Recent work on culture and schizophrenia: Epidemiological and anthropological approaches. *Global Journal of Archaeology & Anthropology, 1*(3), 555562.

Fellner, C. (2017). New schizophrenia treatments address unmet clinical needs. *Pipeline Plus, 42*(2), 130–134.

Fond, G., et al. (2017). Advanced paternal age is associated with earlier schizophrenia onset in offspring. Results from the national multicentric FACE-SZ cohort. *Psychiatry Research, 254*, 218–223. https://doi.org/10.1016/j.psychres.2017.04.002.

Freudenreich, O., Brown, H. E., & Holt, D. J. (2016). Psychosis and schizophrenia. In T. A. Stern, M. Fava, T. E. Wilens, & J. F. Rosenbaum (Eds.), *Massachusetts General Hospital comprehensive clinical psychiatry* (2nd ed.). St Louis, MO: Elsevier.

Fusar-Poli, P., McGorry, P. D., & Kane, J. M. (2017). Improving outcomes of first-episode psychosis: An overview. *World Psychiatry, 16*, 251–265. https://doi.org/10.1002/wps.20446.

Gage, S. H., et al. (2017). Assessing causality in associations between cannabis use and schizophrenia risk: A two-sample mendelian randomization study. *Psychological Medicine, 47*, 971–980. https://doi.org/10.1017/S0033291716003172.

Gerstein, P. S., & Shlamovitz, G. Z. (2015). Emergent treatment of schizophrenia. Retrieved from http://e medicine.medscape.com/article/805988-overview#a4.

Giddens, J. (2017). *Concepts for nursing practice*. St. Louis: Elsevier.

Halter, M. (2018). *Varcarolis' foundations of psychiatric-mental health nursing* (8th ed.). St. Louis: Elsevier.

Hearing Voices Network (HVN). (2020). HVN: A positive approach to voices and visions. Retrieved from: http://www.hearing-voices.org/about-us/hvn-values/.

Howes, O. D., McCutcheon, R., Owen, M. J., & Murray, R. (2017). The role of genes, stress and dopamine in the development of schizophrenia. *Biological Psychiatry, 81*(1), 9–20. https://doi.org/10.1016/j.biopsych.2016.07.014.

Jacob, K. S. (2015). Recovery model of mental illness: A complementary approach to psychiatric care. *Indian Journal of Psychological Medicine, 37*(2), 117–119. https://doi.org/10.4103/0253-7176.155605.

Janssen Pharmaceuticals. (2020). Invega Trinza. Retrieved from: https://www.invegatrinzahcp.com/administration/injection-video.

Joseph, B., Narayanaswamy, J. C., & Venkatasubramanian, G. (2015). Insight in schizophrenia: Relationship to positive, negative and neurocognitive dimensions. *Indian Journal of Psychological Medicine, 37*(1), 5–11. https://doi.org/10.4103/0253-7176.150797.

Kane J. M., Schooler, N. R., Marcy, P., et al. (2015). The RAISE early treatment program for first-episode psychosis: Background, rationale, and study design. *J Clin Psychiatry, 76*, 240–246.

Kishi, T., Ikuta, T., Matsunaga, S., Matsuda, Y., Oya, K., & Iwata, N. (2017). Comparative efficacy and safety of antipsychotics in the treatment of schizophrenia: A network meta-analysis in a Japanese population. *Neuropsychiatric Disease and Treatment, 13*, 1281–1302. https://doi.org/10.2147/NDT.S134340.

Luhrmann, T. M., Padmavati, R., Tharoor, H., & Osei, A. (2015). Differences in voice-hearing experiences of people with psychosis in the USA, India and Ghana: Interview-based study. *The British Journal of Psychiatry, 206*(1), 41–44.

McDonagh, M. S., Dana, T., Selph, S., et al. (2017). *Treatments for schizophrenia in adults: A systematic review [Internet]*. Rockville, MD: Agency for Healthcare Research and Quality (US). (Comparative Effectiveness Reviews, No. 198.) Evidence Summary. Retrieved from: https://www.ncbi.nlm.nih.gov/books/NBK487620/.

McFarlane, W. R. (2016). Family interventions for schizophrenia and the psychoses: A review. *Family Process, 55*(3), 460–482. https://doi.org/10.1111/famp.12235.

Moran, M. (2014). CBT addresses most-debilitating symptoms in chronic schizophrenia. *Psychiatric News*. Retrieved from http://psychnews.psychiatryonline.org/doi/full/10.1176%2Fappi.pn.2014.1b10.

National Alliance on Mental Illness NAMI. (n.d.). Psychosocial treatments. Retrieved from: https://www.nami.org/Learn-More/Treatment/Psychosocial-Treatments.

National Institute of Mental Health. (2005). Questions and answers about the NIMH Clinical Antipsychotic Trials of Intervention Effectiveness Study (CATIE)—phase 1 results. Retrieved from https://www.nimh.nih.gov/funding/clinical-research/practical/catie/phase1results.shtml.

National Institute of Mental Health. (2016). Fact sheet: First episode psychosis. NIH Publication No. OM 16-4306. Retrieved from: https://www.nimh.nih.gov/health/publications/raise-fact-sheet-first-episode-psychosis/index.shtml.

Nauert, R. (2015). *Eight different types of schizophrenia*. Retrieved from http://psychcentral.com/news/2015/eight-different-types-of-schizophrenia/80805.html.

Nour, M., & Howes, O. (2015). Interpreting the neurodevelopmental hypothesis of schizophrenia in the context of normal brain development and ageing. *Proceedings of the National Academy of Sciences, 112*(21), E2745.

Olfson, M., Gerhard, T., Huang, C., Crystal, S., & Stroup, T. (2015). Premature mortality among adults with schizophrenia in the United States. *JAMA Psychiatry, 72*(12), 1172–1181. https://doi.org/10.1001/jamapsychiatry.2015.1737.

Patel, K. R., Cherian, J., Gohil, K., & Atkinson, D. (2014). Schizophrenia: Overview and treatment options. *Pharmacy and Therapeutics, 39*(9), 638–645.

Pouget, J. G., Gonçalves, V. F., Schizophrenia Working Group of the Psychiatric Genomics Consortium, et al. (2016). Genome-wide association studies suggest limited immune gene enrichment in schizophrenia compared to 5 autoimmune diseases. *Schizophrenia Bulletin, 42*(5), 1176–1184. http://doi.org/10.1093/schbul/sbw059.

Psychiatric Times Supplement. (2013). Tardive dyskinesia a review: AIMS abnormal involuntary movement scale. *Psychiatric Times Supplement*. Retrieved from: http://www.psychiatrictimes.com/clinical-scales-movement-disorders/clinical-scales-movement-disorders/aims-abnormal-involuntary-movement-scale.

Rawat, V. S., et al. (2017). Prevalence and predictors of metabolic syndrome in patients with schizophrenia and healthy controls: A study in rural South Indian population, *Schizophrenia Research, 181–190*. Retrieved from: https://doi.org/10.1016/j.schres.2017.04.039. 2017.

Rettner, R. (2016). Schizophrenia gene discovery sheds light on possible cause; improper "pruning" of neural connections could lead to the development of mental illness. *Scientific American*. Retrieved February 1 from *www.scientificamerican.com/article schizophrenia-gene-discovery-sheds-light-on-possible-causes/*.

Sadock, B. J., Sadock, V. A., & Ruiz, P. (2015). *Kaplan & Sadock's synopsis of psychiatry* (11th ed.). Philadelphia: Wolters Kluwer/Lippincott Williams & Wilkins.

Schizophrenia.com. (2004). *How to manage 5 common symptoms of schizophrenia*. http://www.schizophrenia.com/family/mansymptoms.htm.

Substance Abuse and Mental Health Services Administration (SAMHSA). (2017a). *National registry of evidence-based programs and practices. Wellness Recovery Action Plan (WRAP)*. Retrieved from https://nrepp.samhsa.gov/ProgramProfile.aspx?id=1231.

Substance Abuse and Mental Health Services Administration (SAMHSA). (2017b). *Recovery and recovery support*. Retrieved from: https://www.samhsa.gov/recovery.

Tarricone, S., Tosato, P., Clanconi4, M., Braca, A., Fiorillo, L., & Valmaggia, C. M. (2015). Migration history, minorities status and risk of psychosis: An epidemiological explanation and a psychopathological insight. *Journal of Psychopathology, 21*, 424–430.

Tiihonen, J., Mittendorfer-Rutz, E., Torniainen, M., & Alexanderson, K. (2016). *American Journal of Psychiatry, 173*(6), 600–606. https://doi.org/10.1176/appi.ajp.2015.15050618. Epub 2015 Dec 7.

Vaucher, J., et al. (2017). Cannabis use and risk of schizophrenia: A Mendelian randomization study. *Molecular Psychiatry 23*, 1–6. Retrieved from: https://www.nature.com/articles/mp2016252.

Vidal, G. (1982). *The second American revolution and other essays (1976–1982)*. New York: Random House.

Vita, A., De Peri, L., & Deste, G. (2015). *The effect of antipsychotic treatment on cortical gray matter changes in schizophrenia: Does the class matter? A meta-analysis and meta-regression of longitudinal magnetic resonance imaging studies.* Retrieved from https://www.ncbi.nlm.nih.gov/pubmed/25802081.

WebMD. (2019). *Schizophrenia symptoms.* Retrieved from https://www.webmd.com/schizophrenia/cognitive-symptoms-schizophrenia.

Weinmann, S., Aderhold, V., & Haegele, C. (2015). *Brain atrophy and antipsychotic medication—a systematic review.* Retrieved from http://www.europsy-journal.com/article/S0924-9338(15)30055-9/abstract?cc=y=.

18

Neurocognitive Disorders

Lorraine Chiappetta, Elizabeth M. Varcarolis

http://evolve.elsevier.com/Varcarolis/essentials

OBJECTIVES

1. Describe the signs and symptoms associated with delirium.
2. Discuss the safety needs of a patient with delirium and nursing interventions to facilitate safe and effective care for these individuals. **QSEN: Safety**
3. Identify nursing interventions used to provide patient-centered care for an individual experiencing delirium. **QSEN: Patient-Centered Care**
4. Describe the *Diagnostic and Statistical Manual of Mental Disorders,* 5th edition *(DSM-5)* criteria and other signs and symptoms associated with Alzheimer's disease (AD).
5. Identify evidence-based practice interventions when caring for a patient with AD.
6. Describe essential teaching for family members caring for someone with AD.
7. Describe components of interprofessional and intraprofessional teamwork and collaboration that facilitate the short-term and long-term treatment of individuals with delirium and AD. **QSEN: Teamwork and Collaboration**
8. Using informatics, identify pharmacological interventions and individual and family community supports for a person with AD. **QSEN: Informatics**

KEY TERMS AND CONCEPTS

agnosia, p. 290
agraphia, p. 288
Alzheimer's disease (AD), p. 284
aphasia, p. 290
apraxia, p. 290
cognition, p. 278
confabulation, p. 290
delirium, p. 279
dementia, p. 284
hallucinations, p. 281
hypermetamorphosis, p. 288
hyperorality, p. 288
hypervigilance, p. 281
illusions, p. 281
major neurocognitive disorder, p. 278
mild cognitive impairment (MCI), p. 284
mild neurocognitive disorders, p. 278
perseveration, p. 290
pseudodementia, p. 289
sundown syndrome, p. 279
tau protein, p. 286

CONCEPT: COGNITION: *Cognition* is defined as the mental action or process of acquiring knowledge and understanding through thought, experience, and the senses. It is a comprehensive term used to refer to all the processes involved in human thought (Giddens, 2017). Cognition has a distinctive personalized impact on the individual's physical, psychological, social, and spiritual life. The ability to remember the connections between related actions and how to initiate them depends on cognitive processing and has a direct relationship with activities of daily living (Halter, 2018).

INTRODUCTION

Neurocognitive disorders (NCDs) affect the structural or functional areas of the brain and cause disturbances in normal **cognition** (thinking). The criteria for the various NCDs are based on defined cognitive domains. These include:

- Complex attention
- Executive functioning: planning, decision making, working memory, responding, and mental flexibility
- Learning and memory
- Language usage
- Perceptual-motor abilities
- Social cognition: recognition of emotions (American Psychiatric Association [APA], 2013)

This chapter discusses three main categories of the neurocognitive/cognitive disorders: (1) *delirium,* (2) *mild neurocognitive disorder,* and (3) *major neurocognitive disorder*. Alzheimer's disease will be used as an example (exemplar) of a *major neurocognitive disorder.*

Delirium is a transient cognitive disorder caused by an underlying physiological disturbance and is separate from the other two broad categories known as **mild neurocognitive disorders** and **major neurocognitive disorders**. All neurocognitive disorders affect the individual's ability to function intellectually, emotionally, socially, and occupationally. With a *mild neurocognitive disorder,* the person can still function but at a lower level. With a *major neurocognitive disorder*, almost all aspects of brain function are affected. As the disease progresses, it leaves a shell of a once vital, functioning human being whose personality, life memories, and abilities are gone forever.

Refer to Table 18.1 for subtypes of the neurological disorders based on etiology.

DELIRIUM

Delirium is always *secondary to another condition*. Medical conditions, substance use (intoxication and withdrawal), and medication or toxin exposure are possible causes of delirium. If the underlying physiological disturbances that caused the delirium are corrected in a timely manner, complete recovery occurs. If the underlying etiologies of delirium are not addressed, dementia and even death may follow.

Delirium is one of the most commonly encountered medical conditions seen in medical practice, with the elderly being at greatest risk. Unfortunately, it is often overlooked or misdiagnosed. From 15% to 53% of postsurgical older adults develop delirium, and 70% to 87% of those who are in intensive care and up to 60% of nursing home residents also experience delirium (APA, 2013). Delirium is associated with increased mortality, falls, functional decline, cognitive decline, and significant additional health care costs. Nurses are in an ideal position to prevent, identify, and manage delirium (Table 18.2). Table 18.3 offers some guidelines for distinguishing among delirium, depression, and dementia.

Box 18.1 lists many of the common causes of delirium.

The detailed features of delirium are as follows:

- Disturbance in *attention and awareness*, with reduced ability to direct, focus, sustain, and shift focus. There can be a reduced orientation to the environment. Sometimes the person becomes withdrawn, with little or no response to the environment.
- Disturbance in *cognition* or thinking skills: This includes memory deficit, particularly for recent events. The person can become disoriented to person or place and time. Language deficits, such as rambling speech, difficulty speaking or understanding speech, and difficulty writing or reading, also occur. There can be perceptual distortion, including hallucinations (seeing things that don't exist) and illusions (misinterpreting things that are seen) and reduced visuospatial ability.
- Specific criteria for the diagnosis are that the symptoms *develop rapidly* over hours to days and *fluctuate in severity during the course of the day*. **Sundown syndrome**, in which symptoms and problem behaviors become more pronounced in the evening and at night, is an example of fluctuating symptoms that may occur in both delirium and dementia.
- There must be evidence that the disturbance develops as a *direct physiological consequence of another medical condition* (APA, 2013).

Behavioral symptoms can include restlessness; agitation and combativeness; disturbed sleep, including reversal of night–day/sleep–wake cycles; withdrawal; and slowed speech. Emotional responses can be rapidly changing, with an unpredictable mood/affect. These emotional responses include being irritable and angry, euphoric, depressed, anxious, apathetic, and paranoid.

There are three different types of delirium:

- **Hyperactive**: restlessness, pacing, and agitation, with rapid mood swings and sometimes hallucinations
- **Hypoactive**: reduced motor activity, sluggishness, drowsiness or seeming dazed; least recognized presentation
- **Mixed**: includes both hypoactive and hyperactive symptoms, switching from one type to another (Mayo Clinic, 2018)

TABLE 18.1 Subtypes of Neurocognitive Disorders

• Alzheimer's disease	• Substance/medication use
• Frontotemporal dementia	• HIV infection
• Vascular disease	• Prion disease
• Traumatic brain injury	• Parkinson's disease
• Lewy body disease	• Huntington's disease
	• Another medical condition/multiple etiologies

APPLICATION OF THE NURSING PROCESS: DELIRIUM

ASSESSMENT

Assessment starts by *screening patients for risk factors* and implementing *prevention and early intervention strategies. Ongoing assessment and recognition* of delirium symptoms should continue as needed (American Nurses Association [ANA], 2016a). There are a number of validated screening tools that can be used to identify delirium. The **Confusion Assessment Method (CAM)** is one tool frequently used. The CAM short form (SF) and 3D-CAM are shortened versions of

TABLE 18.2 Interventions for Problematic Behaviors

Anger and Aggression

- Try to determine cause (pain or a triggering event).
- Focus on feelings.
- Speak in a soft, reassuring, and calm tone.
- Limit distractions.
- Use music or other relaxing activities.
- Ensure safety; if the person remains aggressive, call 911 or other help.

Anxiety and Agitation

- Listen to the person's frustration and provide reassurance.
- Modify the environment (decrease noise, maintain routine, introduce new environments slowly).
- Break down complex tasks into small steps.
- Find outlets for energy (a walk or a car ride).

Forgetfulness

- Respond with simple, brief explanations.
- It can be frustrating to repeat things over and over; remain calm.
- Use labels on objects when appropriate.
- Show photos as reminders.
- Use memory aids, such as calendars, notes, and clocks.

Suspiciousness

- Don't take personally.
- Don't argue.
- Offer a simple explanation.
- Use distraction; switch focus.

TABLE 18.3 Comparison of Delirium, Dementia, and Depression

	Delirium	Dementia	Depression
Onset	Sudden, over hours to days	Slowly, over months to years	May have been gradual with exacerbation during crisis or stress
Cause or contributing factors	Hypoglycemia, fever, and dehydration, hypotension; infection, other conditions that disrupt the body's homeostasis; adverse drug reaction; head injury; change in environment (e.g., hospitalization); pain; emotional stress; B_{12} and folate deficiencies	Alzheimer's disease, vascular disease, human immunodeficiency virus infection, neurological disease, chronic alcoholism, head trauma, B_{12} and folate deficiencies	Lifelong history, losses, loneliness, crises, declining health, medical conditions
Cognition	Impaired memory, judgment, calculations, and attention span; can fluctuate throughout the day	Impaired memory, judgment, calculations, attention span, and abstract thinking; agnosia	Difficulty concentrating, forgetfulness, inattention
Level of consciousness	Altered	Not altered	Not altered
Activity level	Can be increased or reduced; restlessness; behaviors may worsen in evening (sundown syndrome); sleep–wake cycle may be reversed	Not altered; behaviors may worsen in evening (sundown syndrome)	Usually decreased; lethargy, fatigue, and lack of motivation; may sleep poorly and awaken in early morning
Emotional state	Rapid swings; can be fearful, anxious, suspicious, and aggressive and have hallucinations and/or delusions	Flat affect, suspiciousness, catastrophic reactions, anxiety, anger, aggressiveness	Extreme sadness, apathy, irritability, anxiety, paranoid ideation
Speech and language	Rapid, inappropriate, incoherent, rambling	Incoherent, slow (sometimes due to effort to find the right word), inappropriate, rambling, repetitious	Slow, flat, low
Prognosis	Reversible with proper and timely treatment	Not reversible; progressive	Reversible with proper and timely treatment

BOX 18.1 Common Causes of Delirium

Postoperative States
- Surgery and other invasive procedures
- Anesthesia medications and pain medications used

Drug Intoxications and Withdrawals
- Alcohol, anxiolytics, opioids, and central nervous system (CNS) stimulants (cocaine, crack cocaine, and others)
- Alcohol withdrawal (delirium tremens) is a medical emergency (see Chapter 19).

Infections
- Systemic: pneumonia, typhoid fever, malaria, urinary tract infection, and septicemia
- Intracranial: meningitis and encephalitis

Metabolic Disorders
- Dehydration
- Hypoxia (pulmonary disease, heart disease, and anemia)
- Hypoglycemia
- Sodium, potassium, calcium, magnesium, and acid–base imbalances
- Hepatic encephalopathy or uremic encephalopathy
- Thiamine (vitamin B_1) deficiency (Wernicke's encephalopathy)
- Endocrine disorders (thyroid and parathyroid)
- Hypothermia or hyperthermia
  - Elevated temperature is most common cause in children
- Diabetic acidosis
- Vitamin B_{12} and folate deficiencies

Drugs
- Digitalis, steroids, lithium, levodopa, anticholinergics, benzodiazepines, CNS depressants, tricyclic antidepressants
- Anticholinergic delirium from the use of multiple drugs with anticholinergic side effects
- Please refer to the American Geriatrics Society 2015 updated Beers Criteria for potentially inappropriate medication use in older adults.

Neurological Diseases (CNS Pathology)
- Seizures
- Head trauma
- Hypertensive encephalopathy
- Dementia (secondary delirium especially during a hospitalization)

Tumor
- Primary cerebral

Other
- Relocation or other sudden changes
- Sensory deprivation or overload
- Sleep deprivation
- Immobilization
- Pain
- Of people with a terminal illness, 75% to 85% develop delirium near death.

the assessment. Forms are available at http://www.hospitalelderlife-program.org/delirium-instruments/confusion-assessment-method-long-cam. The particular tool used is dependent on the treatment team's needs and goals and the population being assessed (Bull, 2015).

Use the following memory tool (MINDSPACES) to screen for risk factors associated with delirium (see Box 18.1 for additional specific causes):

M—Medications: polypharmacy, multiple classes of medications, medication weaning/withdrawal (refer to "Beers Criteria" for drugs to avoid[a])
I—Infection and advanced illness
N—Number of co-occurring conditions/comorbidities (hypertension, heart failure, chronic obstructive pulmonary disease [COPD], obstructive sleep apnea [OSA])
D—Disorders of substance or alcohol use (including withdrawal)
S—Surgery and/or invasive procedures (including anesthesia medications)
P—Pain (uncontrolled), perfusion problems
A—Age: young children and older adults are most at risk but may occur at any age
C—Cognitive impairment and/or dementia
E—Emotional or mental illness (depression, anxiety)
S—Sleep disturbances and altered patterns of sleep (ANA, 2016b)

Cognitive and Perceptual Disturbances

It may be difficult to engage *delirious* individuals in conversation because they are easily distracted due to significant attention deficits and because their memory is impaired. In mild delirium, memory deficits may only be seen on careful questioning. In more severe delirium, memory problems usually take the form of obvious difficulty in processing and remembering recent events. A mother might ask when her son is coming to visit, even though her son left a half hour earlier. Perceptual misinterpretations of reality are common and may take the form of illusions or hallucinations.

Illusions are errors in the accurate perception of sensory stimuli. A person may mistake the folds in bedclothes for white rats or the cord of a window blind for a snake. The stimulus is a real object in the environment; however, it is misinterpreted and often becomes the object of the patient's projected fear. *Illusions,* unlike delusions or hallucinations, *can be explained and clarified for the individual.*

Hallucinations are false sensory stimuli (see Chapter 17 for guidelines for dealing with hallucinations). *Visual* hallucinations are common in delirium. *Tactile* hallucinations may also be present. Individuals with delirium may become terrified when they "see" giant spiders crawling over the bedclothes or "feel" bugs crawling on their bodies. Auditory hallucinations occur more often in other psychiatric disorders, such as schizophrenia.

The *delirious* individual generally has an awareness that something is very wrong. This person may state, "My thoughts are all jumbled." When perceptual disturbances are present, the emotional response is frequently fear and anxiety. Nurses should be alert for and intervene with *verbal and psychomotor signs of agitation.*

Physical Needs

Physical Safety

A person with *delirium* may become disoriented and try to "go home." Alternatively, persons may think they *are* home and may jump out of a window in an attempt to get away from "invaders." Wandering, pulling out intravenous lines and Foley catheters, and falling out of bed are common dangers that require preventative nursing interventions. Persons with *delirium* may immediately "forget" instructions to call for the nurse before getting out of bed, increasing fall risks.

An individual experiencing *delirium* has difficulty processing stimuli in the environment. This confusion magnifies the inability to recognize what is real. The physical environment should be made as simple and as clear as possible. Objects such as clocks and calendars can maximize orientation to time. Eyeglasses, hearing aids, and adequate lighting without glare can maximize the person's ability to more accurately interpret the environment. The nurse should interact with the patient whenever the patient is awake. Short periods of social interaction help reduce anxiety and misperceptions.

Biophysical Safety

Elevations in autonomic responses, such as tachycardia, sweating, flushed face, dilated pupils, and elevated blood pressure, are often present in the context of delirium. *These changes must be monitored and documented carefully and may require immediate medical attention.*

Changes in the sleep–wake cycle can occur, with complete reversal of the night–day/sleep–wake cycle. The patient's level of consciousness may range from lethargy to stupor or from semi-coma to hypervigilance. In **hypervigilance**, patients are extraordinarily alert, and their eyes constantly scan the room; they may have difficulty falling asleep or may be actively disoriented and agitated throughout the night.

Moods and Behaviors. The *delirious* individual's behavior and mood may change dramatically within a short period. Moods may fluctuate from fear, anger, and anxiety to euphoria, depression, and apathy. These labile moods (quickly changing) are often accompanied by behaviors associated with feeling states. A person may strike out from fear or anger or may cry, call for help, curse, moan, and tear off clothing and then, within a minute, become apathetic or laugh uncontrollably. Behavior and emotions are erratic and fluctuating.

Assessment Guidelines

Delirium

All patients must be assessed upon admission, during every shift, and with any change in the clinical picture.

1. **Patient safety**: Prevent physical injuries and self-harm as a result of confusion, aggression, or electrolyte and fluid imbalance.
   a. Assess vital signs, including pulse oximetry, level of consciousness, and neurological signs.
   b. Assess the potential for injury, especially fall risk, the potential for wandering, and so forth.
2. History and information gathering from family and significant others
   a. Obtain baseline behaviors/cognitive ability.
   b. Assess for past confusional states that increase risk: prior dementia diagnosis; previous delirium associated with past substance use/withdrawal.
   c. Identify any electroencephalographic, neuroimaging, or laboratory abnormalities documented in the patient's record.
3. Physical examination and a comprehensive nursing assessment to aid in identifying the cause
   a. Identify other physiological conditions that increase risk, such as infection, dyspnea, edema, and the presence of jaundice.
   b. Perform an assessment of cognitive functioning using a validated instrument.
      - The Confusion Assessment Method (CAM), Mini-Mental Status Examination, the Visual Analog Scale for Confusion, and the digit span test are examples.

[a]Starting in 1991, Dr. Mark Beers and colleagues developed a list of drugs, called the **"Beers Criteria,"** that have a high potential to cause delirium and other harm in patients age 65 or older. The current edition of this list also provides alternative drugs to use (American Geriatrics Society, 2015).

c. Assess for abnormal diagnostic findings:
   - Serum chemistries (electrolytes, blood urea nitrogen [BUN], creatinine, BUN/creatinine ratio, liver and thyroid, ammonia, lactic acid)
   - Urinalysis (UA), complete blood count (CBC), arterial blood gases (ABGs), cultures, drug levels (digoxin, phenytoin), and chest x-ray

d. Assess patient's ability to take care of own basic needs, especially fluid and food intake and elimination.

e. Assess sleep history and sleep–wake cycle.

4. Assess the need for interventions to optimize comfort and orientation.

a. Assess the need for comfort measures, including pain control, feeling chilled, and positioning.

b. Assess ways to increase the patient's orientation (glasses, hearing aids, clocks, calendars, pictures from home, raising head of bed to increase reality-based environment). Orientation and level of consciousness may fluctuate throughout the day, requiring ongoing assessment (ANA, 2016c).

DIAGNOSIS

Safety needs play a substantial role in nursing care, so *Risk for injury* is always the greatest consideration.

Physiologic symptoms fall within the general category of *Impaired body process* and *Impaired physiological status.* An elevated temperature is diagnosed as *Impaired thermoregulation.* The symptoms of dehydration and decreased fluid intake, decreased urinary output, decreased skin turgor, and dry skin or mucous membranes can be conceptualized as *(Risk for) Impaired fluid intake, Impaired fluid volume,* and *Electrolyte imbalance.* Other physiologically based diagnoses include *Impaired gas exchange, Impaired nutritional status, Impaired sleep,* and *Impaired self toileting.*

The memory difficulties, confusion, and other cognitive problems lend themselves to a general nursing diagnosis of *Impaired cognition* with more specific diagnoses of *Delirium, Acute confusion, Disorientation,* and *Impaired memory.* Perception disturbances can be diagnosed as *Impaired perceptions,* with a specific focus of *Hallucination* and/or *Illusions.*

Sustaining communication with a delirious patient is difficult. *Impaired communication* related to cerebral hypoxia or decreased cerebral blood flow, as evidenced by confusion or clouding of consciousness, may be diagnosed.

Self-care deficit, Negative mood status, Fear, Anxiety, and *Impaired socialization,* are also potential diagnoses. Table 18.4 identifies nursing diagnoses for a confused patient.

OUTCOME IDENTIFICATION

The predominant goal is a return to the premorbid level of functioning. Appropriate outcomes involve safety:

- Patient will remain safe and free from injury while in the hospital.
- Patient will demonstrate increased periods of being oriented to person, place, and time.
- Patient will remain free from falls and injury while confused.
- Patient's tubes (nasogastric, intravenous, oxygen) will remain in place.

PLANNING AND IMPLEMENTATION

Immediate medical intervention to determine the underlying cause of the *delirium* to prevent permanent damage is the priority. In very specific and infrequent situations, low doses of antipsychotics or antianxiety agents may be helpful in controlling behavioral symptoms.

A patient in acute *delirium* should never be left alone. In the past, friends or family would often sit with the patient, and this can be encouraged. It is not, however, appropriate for family members to be given the responsibility of keeping the patient safe. Even when family members are visiting, **safety** remains the responsibility of the staff. Acute care facilities utilize "sitters," who are trained to work with patients who are confused. Refer to Table 18.5 for guidelines for caring for a patient with delirium and to Table 18.2 for managing problem behaviors.

EVALUATION

Evaluation of short-term goals centers around physiologic stability and safety and the need for constant reassessment. Are the vital signs stable? Are the patient's skin turgor and urine specific gravity within normal limits?

Evaluation also includes identifying whether long-term outcome criteria have been met, which may include the following:

- Patient will remain safe.
- Patient will be oriented to time, place, and person by discharge.
- Underlying cause of delirium will be treated.
- Patient will return to premorbid level of functioning.

The following vignette illustrates the fear and confusion a patient may experience when admitted to an intensive care unit (ICU). Read the following account and analyze the nurse's approach.

VIGNETTE: A 55-year-old married man, Mr. Arnold, is admitted to the ICU after having triple bypass cardiac surgery. Postoperatively, he arrives in the ICU without further complications. Upon awakening from the anesthesia, he hears the nurse exclaim, "I need to get a gas." Another nurse answers in a loud voice, "Can you take a large needle for the injection?"

During this period, Mr. Arnold experiences the need to urinate and calmly asks the nurse if he can go to the bathroom. She replies: "You don't need to go; you have a tube in." He again complains about his discomfort and assures the nurse that if she will let him go to the bathroom, he will be fine. The nurse informs Mr. Arnold that he cannot urinate and that he has to keep the "mask" on so that she can get the "gas" and check his "blood levels." On hearing this, Mr. Arnold begins to implore more loudly and states that he sees the bathroom sign. In reality, the sign is an exit sign. He assures the nurse that he will only take a minute if allowed to go to the bathroom.

To help present reality, the nurse removes the restraints so that Mr. Arnold's head can be raised to verify that the sign is actually an exit sign. He abruptly breaks away from the nurse's grasp and runs down the hall. He flees into a room and barricades himself behind a locked room. He pulls out his chest tube, Foley catheter, and intravenous lines. Ten minutes later, the nurses and security personnel break through the barricade and escort Mr. Arnold back to bed.

The following day, Mr. Arnold is fully oriented. He tells the nurses that yesterday he thought he had been kidnapped and was being held against his will. When the nurse yelled out about *blood* "gas," he thought she was going to kill him with *noxious* gas through his facemask. All he could think about was escaping his tormentor.

Evaluation of Nurse's Intervention

- The nurses did not assess for or recognize the alteration in Mr. Arnold's mental status.
- The nurses did not recognize risk factors for delirium: postoperative status, misinterpretation of body sensations (needing to void), misinterpretation of environmental cues (exit sign).
- Factors that exacerbated the patient's confusion include the nurses' failure to listen to the patient, the use of medical jargon and loud voices in the ICU setting, and the nurses' failure to introduce themselves and explain their role in the patient's care.

TABLE 18.4 **Potential Nursing Diagnoses for the Confused Patient**

Symptom	Potential Nursing Diagnoses[a]
Purposeless activities Wanting to get out of bed Pulling out catheters, etc. Picking at skin Unsteady gait Forgetting things like turning off the stove or losing things	*Risk for injury* *Risk for fall-related injury*
Wandering behavior	*Risk for injury* *Impaired mobility* *Wandering*
Confused Disoriented Perceptual problems Paranoid ideation	*Delirium* *Impaired cognition* *Acute confusion* *Disorientation* *Impaired perception* *Fear*
Labile mood, catastrophic reactions	*Labile moods* *Anxiety* *Depression*
Too disorganized to complete activities of daily living or feed self or take fluids	*Impaired ability to bath* *Impaired ability to dress* *Impaired ability to groom* *Risk for impaired nutritional intake*
Sleep-cycle disturbances; sundowning	*Impaired sleep*
Hyperactive symptoms: anxiety, fear, agitation	*Agitation* *Anger* *Fear* *Anxiety*
Hypoactive symptoms: dazed, depressed	*Depressed mood* *Impaired cognition* *Impaired volition*
Difficulty expressing needs; trouble with word finding	*Impaired communication*
Does not recognize familiar people or places, has difficulty with short- and/or long-term memory, forgetful and confused	*Impaired cognition* *Impaired memory* *Acute confusion* *Chronic confusion*
Devastated over losing place in life as known (during lucid moments), fearful and overwhelmed by what is happening to him or her	*Spiritual distress* *Hopelessness* *Situational low self-esteem* *Grief* *Impaired coping process*
Family and loved ones overburdened and overwhelmed, unable to care for patient's needs, sadness about loved one's illness	*Impaired family coping* *Impaired family process* *Dysfunctional grief* *Caregiver stress*

[a]The International Classification for Nursing Practice (ICNP) is a product of the International Council of Nurses (ICN). Retrieved from http://www.icn.ch/what-we-do/ICNP-Browser/.

- A lack of adherence to safety protocols also occurred: The nurse removed restraints without careful assessment and sufficient staff present.
- What else could the nurses have done to help orient and comfort Mr. Arnold?

In June 2016, the ANA and the American Delirium Society created a resource-rich website designed to provide nurses with the information needed to prevent, identify, and manage delirium in various patient populations. You can access the website at http://www.nursingworld.org/Delirium-Prevent-Identify-Treat.

TABLE 18.5 Interventions for a Patient With Delirium

Orientation

- Introduce self and role with every interaction; assign same personnel each shift.
- Use calm, short, concise instructions and explanations.
- Use patient's name frequently; maintain face-to-face contact.
- Address reality-based ideas such as the weather outside and time of day when intervening.
- Continually reorient when interacting.
- Encourage family pictures and familiar objects in room.
- Validate feelings and clarify perceptions.
- Encourage family visits and calls.
- Engage in respectful and developmentally appropriate communication (avoid elder speak).

Sensory Stimulation

- Maintain normal schedules and routines.
- Provide sensory aids as needed (hearing aids, glasses).
- Provide adequate and appropriate lighting; this lessens illusions.
- Keep window blinds open during the day and closed during night hours.
- Provide personalized, age-appropriate television and radio options.
- Engage in personalized, meaningful conversation to stimulate memory.
- Consult with occupational and recreational therapy to provide activities such as magazines, puzzles, coloring books, etc.

Pain Control

- Document and treat pain as needed; evaluate relief.
- Individualize the pain management to include pharmacological and non-pharmacological measures.

Implement Early Progressive Mobility

- Avoid restraints; use sitters for safety.
- Mobilize two to four times per day: range of motion, positioning, ambulation.
- Encourage self-care activities and activities of daily living (ADLs).

Maintain Oxygen Saturation

- Assess for hypoxia and intervene when necessary.

Maintain Hydration and Nutrition

- Offer fluids regularly; measure intake and output.
- Offer dentures at mealtimes.
- Assess ability to feed self; diet modification may be required temporarily; feed when necessary.
- Monitor weight.

Elimination Assessment

- Ensure regular toileting.
- Document urinary output and bowel movements; administer medications for constipation.

Promote Sleep/Rest

- Enforce designated sleep period; discourage excessive daytime sleep.
- Reduce environmental noise; turn off phones, computers, and television; dim lights at night to support usual circadian rhythms.
- Use relaxation techniques.
- Cluster evening nursing care activities to lessen sleep interruptions.
- Avoid the use of hypnotics (ANA, 2016a).

Combative Behavior

- Ignore personal insults and acknowledge how upset the person is feeling.
- Set limits on physically abusive behaviors: "Mr. Jones, you are not to hit me or anyone else. Tell me how you feel."

MAJOR AND MILD NEUROCOGNITIVE DISORDERS

The *DSM-5* (APA, 2013) has defined diagnostic criteria for both **major and mild neurocognitive disorders**. In general, for each of these disorders, there is evidence of (1) cognitive decline from the previous level of performance in one or more of the cognitive domains: complex attention, executive function, learning and memory, language, perceptual-motor, and social cognition. The evidence can come from patient self-report, a knowledgeable informant, or a clinician. Standardized neuropsychological testing by a psychologist can also substantiate these deficits.

In **mild neurocognitive disorder**, there is *modest impairment* in cognitive performance, and the symptoms *do not* interfere with the capacity for everyday activity. With mild neurocognitive disorder, greater time or effort may be required to perform tasks that used to be performed without a thought, and the use of compensatory strategies is often employed. With **major neurocognitive disorders**, there is *substantial impairment* in cognitive functioning, and cognitive deficits *do* interfere with independence in everyday activities. For both the mild and major types, the clinician must specify the medical condition that is the probable cause of the cognitive function. See the *DSM-5* box for common *DSM-5* (APA, 2013) subtypes.

There is a syndrome that is not part of the *DSM-5* (APA, 2013) disorders called **mild cognitive impairment (MCI)**. The main symptoms of MCI involve difficulty with memory, language, thinking, and judgment. MCI is considered an intermediate stage between the expected cognitive decline of normal aging and a more serious cognitive decline. In MCI, an individual might forget things more often, such as important events or appointments, or have difficulty following a conversation or a plot in a book or movie. MCI may increase the risk of later progression to dementia, caused by Alzheimer's disease or other neurological conditions (Mayo Clinic, 2017).

In all disorders in which a patient experiences a change in cognitive functioning, a formal mental status exam that includes a specific examination of cognitive functioning is warranted. See Fig. 18.1 for one example. A thorough medical workup that includes a history and physical, neurological exam, lab tests, scans, and x-rays as indicated is also required to help make an accurate diagnosis.

MAJOR NEUROCOGNITIVE DISORDER (DEMENTIA)

Dementia is a general term for a decline in mental ability severe enough to interfere with daily life. The *DSM-5* (APA, 2013) has incorporated dementia within the broader category of **major neurocognitive disorder.** A *major neurocognitive disorder* usually develops more slowly than delirium. There is gradual progressive impairment, and the disorder is characterized by multiple cognitive deficits. These include evidence of "significant decline in the individual's previous levels of cognitive ability, such as complex attention, executive function, learning and memory, language, perceptual-motor, or social cognition" (APA, 2013, p. 602).

Major neurocognitive disorders can be classified as either primary or secondary. More than 80% of dementias are irreversible primary dementias. Dementias that have a reversible component are **secondary** to other pathological processes (neoplasms, trauma, infections, toxin exposure). When the underlying causes are treated, the dementia often improves. However, most major neurocognitive disorders are related to a **primary** encephalopathy (brain damage).

Alzheimer's disease (AD) is one of the *subtypes of* **major neurocognitive disorder** or *dementia* and the most common cause of

Notes on the Use of the Brief Neurocognitive Mental Status Exam

1. *Behavior observations*
   a. Look for signs of drowsiness or fluctuating degrees of alertness.
   b. This may be formally tested by administering a digit span test or by careful observation during the interview.
   c. Make note of slurred speech or word-finding problems.
   d. Watch for unsteady gait and poor gross motor coordination.
2. *Orientation* – Ask: "What is the date (month, day, year), and what time of day is it now?" "Can you tell me where you are right now? Please be specific." Ask the patient to identify relatives who have accompanied him or her.
3. *Recent memory* – Present three items and ask for immediate recall. Then after a period of five minutes, ask the patient to again recall the three items. Most normal adults should be able to recall three items. Inability to do so may suggest recent memory problems. A second trial may be conducted later in the interview.
4. *Calculations* – Ask the patient to begin with the number 100 and subtract 7 from this number, then subtract 7 again, and so forth. This test provides a rough measure of concentration.
5. *Reproduction of cross and cube* – Present stimulus illustrations shown below. You can copy them onto a 3-by-5-inch, unlined, white index card. Allow the patient to copy the designs one at a time onto a blank sheet of paper. Drawing performance can be compared to samples (see below) to derive rough estimates of the patient's constructional ability.

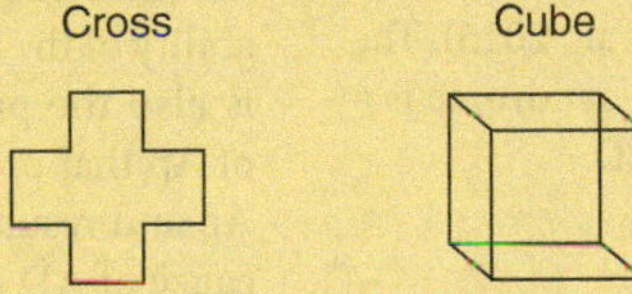

6. *Thinking/Speech* – Note the presence of incoherent or irrelevant speech.

Fig. 18.1 Neurocognitive mental status exam. (From Preston, J., O'Neal, J., & Talaga, M.A. [2010]. *Handbook of clinical psychopharmacology for therapists* [6th ed., pp. 301–302]. Oakland, CA: New Harbinger Publications.)

dementia. AD accounts for 60% to 90% of all dementias in the United States and in 2015 was the sixth-leading cause of death in U.S. adults (Gatchel et al., 2016). Every 65 seconds, someone in the United States develops AD. It is also a leading cause of disability and poor health (Alzheimer's Association, 2018). *Primary neurocognitive disorders* have no known cure, are progressive, and are irreversible. Examples of other *major primary neurocognitive disorders* include vascular dementia, Pick's disease, Huntington's disease, Creutzfeldt–Jakob disease, Lewy body disease, and Parkinson's disease (see Table 18.1).

Because assessments and nursing interventions are similar for all patients with dementia, this section focuses on **major neurocognitive disorder due to AD.**

Theory

Risk Factors

With the exception of the rarer cases of AD caused by genetic abnormalities, experts believe that AD develops as a result of multiple factors rather than a single cause.

Age and Gender. Age seems to be the most important risk factor for AD. The incidence of AD doubles after the age of 65. For those under 65 years of age, the incidence is about 4%. For those 65 to 74 years of age, the risk is 15%; for individuals 75 to 84 years of age, the incidence is 43%; and after 85 years of age, the incidence is thought to be between 38% and 50% (Alzheimer's Association, 2018). AD is *not* a normal part of aging. Almost two-thirds of individuals diagnosed with AD are women.

Family History. Individuals who have a parent, brother, or sister with AD are more likely to develop the disease than those who do not have a first-degree relative with AD. Those who have more than one first-degree relative with AD are at even higher risk. A family history is not necessary for an individual to develop the disease (Alzheimer's Association, 2018).

Other Common Risk Factors. There is good evidence that regular physical activity and management of cardiovascular risk factors reduce the risk of cognitive decline and may reduce the risk of dementia. There is also strong evidence that a healthy diet and lifelong learning/cognitive training may reduce the risk of cognitive decline (Institute of Medicine, 2015).

Brain health is affected by the health of the heart and blood vessels. Cardiovascular disease and factors that increase the risk of cardiovascular disease, such as smoking, obesity, and hypertension, are associated with a higher risk of developing dementia. Impaired glucose processing, a precursor to diabetes, also increases risk. Clinical depression also increases risk. People with less formal educational seem to have an increased risk for AD. This may be related to an increased likelihood of having a less mentally stimulating occupation. People at lower socioeconomic levels appear to be more prone to AD than people with a higher standard of living. This may be explained in part by lack of adequate medical care, poor nutrition, and lifestyle practices that increase the risk of developing chronic diseases that, in turn, increase the risk of developing AD.

Additional studies suggest that remaining socially and mentally active throughout life may support brain health and possibly reduce the risk of AD and other dementias. Sensory deprivation and social isolation play a role in the etiology of dementia. Evidence also indicates that moderate and severe traumatic brain injuries increase the risk of developing certain forms of dementia (Alzheimer's Organization, 2018).

Researchers analyzed data from the *Framingham Heart Study* to identify new combinations of risk factors that are linked to an increased risk of dementia in later life. As expected, greater age was strongly associated with dementia, as was a marital status of widowed, lower body mass index (BMI), and having experienced less sleep at midlife (Boston University School of Medicine, 2018).

Genetic Factors

One genetic risk factor consistently related to AD is the cholesterol-carrying apolipoprotein E gene *(APOE e4)*. There are three possible forms of this *APOE* gene: *e2, e3,* and *e4*. Those who inherent one copy of the *APOE e4* form have three times the risk of developing AD (Alzheimer's Organization, 2018). If two copies of the *e4* form are inherited, the incidence increases up to 12-fold (Alzheimer's Organization, 2018). This gene significantly increases risk but does not automatically lead to the disease.

Genetic factors associated with early-onset AD consist of mutations in three different genes, the gene *APP* (amyloid precursor protein) on chromosome 21, the gene *PS-1* (presenilin-1) on chromosome 14, and the gene *PS-2* (presenilin-2) on chromosome 1. These mutations cause a 95% to 100% chance of developing an early-onset form of the disease. Early-onset AD is relatively rare, develops in people ages 30 to 60, and accounts for only 5% of people with the disease (Zhu et al., 2015). The extra copy of chromosome 21 that characterizes Down syndrome is a genetic mutation that increases the risk of developing AD.

Cultural Considerations

Although the symptom presentation of AD is similar among individuals, there are differences in ethnic/racial incidences. Older African Americans are almost twice as likely to develop AD as their Caucasian counterparts. Hispanic Americans are about 1.5 times as likely to develop AD as older white Americans, with some variation of incidence depending on the specific Hispanic ethnic group studied. Asian Americans as a group have a lower incidence of AD than whites, with Japanese Americans showing the lowest incidence of all ethnic groups (Alzheimer's Association, 2018). It has been suggested that African Americans and Hispanics are more prone to illnesses that increase the risk of developing AD, such as high blood pressure, cardiovascular disease, and diabetes.

Variations in health, lifestyle, and socioeconomic risk factors across racial groups likely account for most of the differences in risk factors associated with AD and other dementias by race, rather than genetic factors. Socioeconomic characteristics, including lower levels of education, higher rates of poverty, and greater exposure to early life adversity and discrimination, may also increase risk in African American and Hispanic communities (Alzheimer's Association, 2018).

Health care workers who are able to assess and understand the cultural aspects of caregiving behaviors may be able to offer services and training that are more congruent with the patient's and caregiver's culture. Culturally sensitive care incudes a recognition that we are all a product of our country, religion, ethnic background, language, and family system. It is also important to understand linguistic, economic, and social barriers to health care and social supports. Because health care workers should never assume there is only one approach to every person in a particular ethnocultural group, an individualized cultural assessment is essential (Alzheimer's Association, n.d.).

Acceptance of AD varies greatly among cultural groups. The emotions of frustration, anger, guilt, anxiety, and conflict are closely tied to the cultural value placed on the ability to maintain control. Cross-cultural research identifies how understandings of dementia as either a "natural part of the aging process" or more accurately as a result of brain disease are culturally shaped. Social class can play a role in how dementia is both experienced and conceptualized (Hillman & Latimer, 2017). A lack of understanding of the symptoms of the disease and the shame associated with cognitive decline in some cultures can significantly impact early recognition, long-term treatment, and the provision of support for the individual and significant others.

Clinical Picture

The main underlying neurobiological mechanisms in AD include amyloid or senile plaque formation, development of intracellular neurofibrillary tangles, synaptic deterioration, and neural cell death.

The two main brain lesions involved in this disease are **senile plaques** and **neurofibrillary tangles**. The pathogenesis of AD is complex and involves multiple theories of causation. No single theory clarifies the pathology of the disease. For the most part, the mechanisms are not fully understood at this time.

The *amyloid cascade hypothesis* of AD states that the disease results from a series of abnormalities of the amyloid precursor protein (APP). APP plays a role in regulating synapse formation (the junction between one neuron and another), neural plasticity (the ability of the brain to change), and iron metabolism in the brain. APP is also the precursor to beta-amyloid (Aβ). It is an overabundance of Aβ that produces beta-amyloid plaques, specifically *senile plaques*. Aβ and resultant plaques are toxic to neurons and thought to be one cause of AD neuropathology.

The *cholinergic hypothesis* looks at several different alterations in cholinergic neural transmission as a cause of cognitive impairment. Beta-amyloid is one of the factors that alters the functioning of cholinergic receptors in multiple areas of the brain. Current drug treatments are based on this hypothesis.

Deficits in the expression of nicotinic and muscarinic receptors and alterations in glutamate neural transmission are also implicated in the neurodegeneration and cell death associated with Alzheimer's dementia.

The **tau (τ) protein** *hypothesis* states there is a secondary biological event that causes neurodegeneration. Microtubules in the brain provide support for structural changes, axonal transport, and neuronal growth. This protein stabilizes these tubules. In AD, the tau protein changes, which results in the development of *neurofibrillary tangles*. As this neural transport system collapses, neural cell death occurs. The clinical result is memory failure, personality changes, problems in carrying out daily activities, and other features of the disease

Neuroinflammation is another important factor involved in the cause of AD. Microglia cells, which are responsible for active immunity, function differently in those with AD. This difference leads to *free radicals,* unstable atoms that can damage cells and cause illness and aging.

Oxidative stress is the total burden placed on organisms by the constant production of *free radicals* in the normal course of metabolism. It is believed that good health relies on a balance between oxidative stress and antioxidant defenses. Excessive oxidative stress can develop due to exposure to environmental toxins and increases with advanced age. An increased number of free radicals is implicated in AD.

Another hypothesis looks at the *regulation of intracellular calcium homeostasis in the brain.* This complex mechanism is vital for several cellular pathways and is involved in cell survival and death. In AD, the ability of neurons to regulate calcium is compromised (Sanabria-Castro, Alvarado-Echeverría, & Monge-Bonilla, 2017).

Anatomical changes also seen with AD include the following:

- Cortical atrophy (shrinking) in areas involved in higher-level functioning: thinking, planning, speech, perception, and remembering

- Damage to the **hippocampus**, an area of the cortex that plays a key role in the formation of new memories
- Increase in the size of ventricles (fluid-filled spaces within the brain) due to loss of brain tissue

Imaging techniques reveal significant loss of cells and loss of volume in multiple regions of the brain devoted to memory and higher mental functioning (Agamanolis, 2016).

Stages of Alzheimer's Disease

AD has been classified according to the stage of the degenerative process. The number of defined stages ranges from three to seven, depending on the source of information. Symptoms can fluctuate between the different stages. This section presents four stages of AD to help illustrate the progression of symptoms. Table 18.6 can be used as a guide to review these four stages of AD and highlights the deficits associated with each stage.

The rate of progression varies individually. The mean age of survival after diagnosis is approximately 3 to 10 years (Anderson & Chawla, 2016). Some individuals can live with AD for as long as 20 years (APA, 2013).

Stage 1: Mild Alzheimer's Disease. The loss of intellectual ability is insidious. The person with mild AD loses energy, drive, and initiative and has difficulty learning new things. Because personality and social behavior remain intact, others tend to minimize and underestimate the loss of the individual's abilities. The individual may continue to work, but the extent of the dementia gradually becomes evident in new or demanding situations. During the mild phases of AD, *apathy* is the most common behavioral problem to appear early and often persists throughout the course of the disease. *Depression* and mood swings may also occur early on, especially if there is a family history of depression. Activities such as grocery shopping or managing finances are noticeably impaired during this phase. Confusion can result when the person is in unfamiliar surroundings.

Word-finding difficulties can become evident. Personality changes and uncharacteristic behaviors, such as suspiciousness, can become part of the clinical picture. Forgetfulness and poor judgment are additional symptoms.

VIGNETTE: Mr. Collins, a 60-year-old lineman for a telephone company, feels that he is getting old. He keeps forgetting things and writes notes to himself on scraps of paper. One day on the job, he forgets momentarily which wires to connect and connects all the wrong ones, causing mass confusion for a few hours. At home, Mr. Collins becomes very upset when his wife suggests that they invite the new neighbors for dinner. It is hard for him to admit that anything new confuses him, and he often forgets names and sometimes loses the thread of conversations. Once, he even forgot his address when his car stopped working on the highway. He is moody and depressed and becomes indignant when his wife finds 3 months' worth of unpaid bills stashed in his sock drawer. Mrs. Collins is bewildered, upset, and fearful that something is terribly wrong.

TABLE 18.6 Stages of Alzheimer's Disease

Stage	Hallmarks
Stage 1 (Mild) Forgetfulness	Shows short-term memory loss; loses things, forgets Memory aids compensate: lists, routine, organization Aware of the problem; concerned about lost abilities Depression common—worsens symptoms Disease is not diagnosable from the symptoms
Stage 2 (Moderate) Confusion	Shows progressive memory loss; short-term memory impaired; memory difficulties interfere with abilities Withdrawn from social activities Shows declines in activities of daily living (ADLs), such as money management, legal affairs, transportation, cooking, housekeeping Denial common; fears "losing one's mind" Depression increasingly common; frightened because aware of deficits; covers up for memory loss through confabulation Problems intensified when stressed, fatigued, out of own environment, ill Commonly needs day care, or in-home assistance is needed at this time.
Stage 3 (Moderate to severe) Ambulatory dementia	Shows ADL deficits: willingness and ability to bathe, grooming, choosing clothing, dressing, gait and mobility, toileting, communication, reading, and writing skills Shows loss of reasoning ability, safety planning, and verbal communication Frustration common; becomes more withdrawn and self-absorbed Depression resolves as awareness of losses diminishes Has difficulty communicating; shows increasing loss of language skills Shows evidence of reduced stress threshold; institutional care usually needed
Stage 4 (Late) End stage	Family recognition may disappear; may not recognize self in mirror Nonambulatory; shows little purposeful activity; often mute; may scream spontaneously Forgets how to eat, swallow, chew; commonly loses weight; emaciation common Has problems associated with immobility (pneumonia, pressure ulcers, contractures) Incontinence common; seizures may develop Most certainly institutionalized at this point Return of primitive (infantile) reflexes

From Hall, G. R. (1994). Caring for people with Alzheimer's disease using the conceptual model of progressively lowered stress threshold in the clinical setting. *Nursing Clinics of North America, 29*(1), 129–141.

Stage 2: Moderate Alzheimer's Disease. Deterioration and worsening of symptoms with less ability to compensate become evident during the moderate phase. Often the person with moderate AD cannot remember a phone number or home address. There are memory gaps in the person's history that may fluctuate from one moment to the next. Hygiene suffers, and the ability to dress appropriately is markedly affected. The person may put on clothes backward, button a shirt incorrectly, or not fasten zippers *(apraxia)*. Often, the person has to be coaxed to bathe.

Mood becomes labile, and the individual may have bursts of paranoia, anger, jealousy, and loss of interest in the outside world. A *catastrophic reaction* may occur. This is an excessive reaction to something that may seem inconsequential to caregivers or others. It can lead to physical acting out and hostile behaviors like hitting, screaming, and sobbing on the part of the person with AD. The abnormal moods, inability to follow through with basic activities of daily living (ADLs), and sleep–wake cycle disturbances cause great caregiver burden and caregiver depression. Activities such as driving can become hazardous. Families are faced with the difficulty of taking away the car keys from their loved one. Care and supervision become full-time jobs for family members. Denial mercifully takes over and protects people from the realization that they are losing control, not only of their minds but also of their lives. Along with denial, people with AD begin to withdraw from activities and from others because they often feel overwhelmed and frustrated when they try to do things that once were easy. They may develop psychotic symptoms of hallucinations and paranoid delusions. They may also have moments of becoming tearful and sad.

As important as it is to recognize all of the deficits during the progression to the moderate phase, it is helpful for caretakers to realize that the patient still retains abilities that influence care.

VIGNETTE: Mr. Collins is transferred to a less complicated work position after his inability to function is recognized. His wife drives him to work and picks him up. Mr. Collins often forgets what he is doing and stares blankly. He accuses the supervisor of spying on him. Sometimes he disappears at lunch and is unable to find his way back to work. The transfer lasts only a few months, after which Mr. Collins is forced to take early retirement. At home, Mr. Collins sleeps in his clothes. He loses interest in reading and watching sports on television and often breaks into angry outbursts, seemingly over nothing. Often, he becomes extremely restless and irritable and wanders around the house aimlessly.

Stage 3: Moderate to Severe Alzheimer's Disease. At the moderate to severe stage, the person is often unable to identify familiar objects or people, even a spouse *(severe agnosia)*. The person needs repeated instructions and directions to perform the simplest tasks *(advanced apraxia)*: "Here is the face cloth; pick up the soap. Now, put water on the face cloth and rub the face cloth with soap." **Agraphia** (inability to read or write) is evident. Often the individual cannot remember where the toilet is and becomes incontinent. Total care is necessary at this point, and the burden on the family can be emotionally, financially, and physically devastating. The world is very frightening to the person with AD because nothing makes sense any longer. Agitation, violence, paranoia, and delusions are commonly seen. The tendency to wander is both a *safety and fall risk*. It is estimated that about 60% of people with AD wander and are at risk of becoming lost.

Disinhibition can be a troublesome symptom. This can include things like urinating in public and sexually inappropriate behaviors.

Institutionalization may be the most appropriate recourse at this time because the level of care is so demanding. Violent outbursts and incontinence may be burdens that the family can no longer handle. The following are some criteria that indicate the need for placement in a skilled nursing facility:

- Wandering
- Danger to self and others
- Incontinence
- Behavior affects the sleep and general health of others
- Total dependence on others for physical care

VIGNETTE: Mr. Collins is terrified. Memories come and then slip away. People come and go, but they are strangers. Someone is masquerading as his wife, and it is hard to tell what is real. Things never stay in the same place. Sometimes people hide the bathroom where he cannot find it. He hides things to keep them safe, but he forgets where he hides them. Buttons and belts are confusing, and he does not know what they are doing there anyway. Sometimes he tries to walk away from the terrifying feelings and the strangers. He tries to find something he has lost long ago, if he could only remember what it is.

Stage 4: Late Alzheimer's Disease. Late in AD, the following symptoms may occur: **hyperorality** (the need to taste, chew, and put everything in one's mouth), blunting of emotions, visual agnosia (loss of ability to recognize familiar objects), and **hypermetamorphosis** (manifested by touching of everything in sight). At this stage, the ability to talk, and eventually the ability to walk, is lost. If not already present, the individual may become incontinent, have difficulty swallowing (dysphasia), and may have seizures. Weight loss, increased sleeping, and moaning/grunting are also evident during the final stage. Toward the end of the late stage, stupor and coma may occur. Death frequently is secondary to infection or choking. This person is at great risk for dehydration, malnutrition, bowel and bladder issues, pressure sores, and injuries from falls. Individuals in this stage may be unable to recognize close relatives and friends. This can be especially distressful to caregivers/significant others.

VIGNETTE: Mrs. Collins and the children keep Mr. Collins at home for a short while until his outbursts become frightening. Once, he is lost for 2 days after he somehow unlocks the front door. Finally, Mrs. Collins has her husband placed in a Veterans Administration (VA) hospital. When his wife comes to visit, Mr. Collins sometimes cries. He never talks and is always restrained in his chair when she comes to see him. The staff explains to her that although Mr. Collins can still walk, he keeps getting into other people's beds and scaring them. They explain that perhaps he wants comfort and misses human touch. They encourage her visits, even though Mr. Collins does not seem to recognize her. He does respond to music. His wife brings him a small CD player and plays the country and western music he has always loved; at those times, Mr. Collins nods and claps his hands.

Mrs. Collins is torn between guilt and love, anger and despair. She is confused and depressed. She is going through the painful process of mourning the loss of the man she has loved and shared a life with for 34 years. Three months after his admission to the VA hospital, and 8 years after the incident of the crossed wires at the telephone company, Mr. Collins chokes on some food, develops pneumonia, and dies.

DSM-5 DIAGNOSTIC CRITERIA

Major or Mild Neurocognitive Disorder Due to Alzheimer's Disease

A. The criteria are met for major or mild neurocognitive disorder.

B. There is insidious onset and gradual progression of impairment in one or more cognitive domains (for major neurocognitive disorder, at least two domains must be impaired).

C. Criteria are met for either probable or possible Alzheimer's disease as follows:

For major neurocognitive disorder:

Probable Alzheimer's disease is diagnosed if either of the following is present; otherwise, possible Alzheimer's disease should be diagnosed.

1. Evidence of a causative Alzheimer's disease genetic mutation from family history or genetic testing.
2. All three of the following are present:
   a. Clear evidence of decline in memory and learning at least one other cognitive domain (based on detailed history or serial neuropsychological testing).
   b. Steadily progressive, gradual decline in cognition, without extended plateaus.
   c. No evidence of mixed etiology (i.e., absence of other neurodegenerative or cerebrovascular disease, or another neurological, mental, or systemic disease or condition likely contributing to cognitive decline).

For mild neurocognitive disorder:

Probable Alzheimer's disease is diagnosed if there is evidence of a causative Alzheimer's disease genetic mutation from either genetic testing or family history.

Possible Alzheimer's disease is diagnosed if there is no evidence of a causative Alzheimer's disease genetic mutation from either genetic testing or family history, and all three of the following are present:

1. Clear evidence of decline in memory and learning.
2. Steadily progressive, gradual decline in cognition, without extended plateaus.
3. No evidence of mixed etiology (i.e., absence of other neurodegenerative or cerebrovascular disease, or another neurological or systemic disease or condition likely contributing to cognitive decline).

D. The disturbance is not better explained by cerebrovascular disease, another neurodegenerative disease, the effects of a substance, or another mental, neurological, or systemic disorder.

Diagnostic Tests for Dementia

A wide range of problems may masquerade as dementia and may be mistaken for AD. Depression and dementia in the older adult present with overlapping symptoms. It is important that health care professionals be able to differentiate depression, dementia, and delirium. Refer to Table 18.3 for important differences among these three phenomena. It is important to emphasize that depression and dementia or depression and delirium can coexist in the same person. A complete and thorough medical examination, including neurological, medical, psychiatric history, review of medications, and nutritional evaluation, must be performed.

Other disorders that mimic a *major neurocognitive disorder* include drug toxicity, metabolic disorders, infections, and nutritional deficiencies. **Pseudodementia** is a syndrome with symptoms that suggest dementia but is actually another diagnosis altogether, usually depression. These individuals may show symptoms suggesting dementia, such as self-care deficits, but do not show evidence of cognitive dysfunction when formally tested. When the depression is adequately treated, many symptoms disappear.

There is no standard single physiological test for dementia. Beta-amyloid proteins can now be detected through brain scans or extracting spinal fluid, but these procedures are costly and expensive. In 2018 a new blood test was introduced in Japan. It is expected to be used for regular screening for those over 50 in the next few years. This test may also be able to detect brain abnormalities before the onset of clinical symptoms (Nakamura et al., 2018). Brian imaging studies, including structural imaging with magnetic resonance imaging (MRI), computed tomography (CT), or positron emission tomography (PET), are primarily used to rule out other conditions that may cause symptoms similar to AD.

Specialized mental status exams are the most common screening tests used as part of the assessment process. Some standard ones used are as follows:

- Mini-Mental State Exam (MMSE): a series of questions designed to test a range of everyday mental skills, including attention and memory and simple psychomotor skills.
- **Montreal Cognitive Assessment (MoCA):** a rapid screening instrument for mild cognitive dysfunction that includes attention and concentration, executive functions, memory, language, visuoconstructional skills, conceptual thinking, calculations, and orientation.
- The **SLUMS** examination: screening tool that can discriminate between MCI and no diagnosis and/or major depressive disorder and *major neurodevelopmental disorders* (dementia) (Shwartz, Morris, & Penna, 2017).
- Mini-cog: a person is asked to complete two tasks:
  - Remember the names of three common objects and repeat them a few minutes later.
  - Draw the face of a clock showing all 12 numbers in the right places and a time specified by the examiner.

These are screening tests used to help determine the need for further evaluation.

Neuropsychological testing by a neuropsychologist is sometimes necessary for a more definitive diagnose of dementia and subtypes of dementia (Ritter et al., 2017).

APPLICATION OF THE NURSING PROCESS: DEMENTIA

ASSESSMENT

Overall Assessment

The earliest cognitive symptom most often observed in the development of AD is impairment in memory and learning. In the early stages of the disease, the affected individual may be able to compensate for the loss of memory. Some people may have superior social graces and charm that give them the ability to hide severe deficits in memory, even from experienced health care professionals. "Hiding" symptoms is actually a form of **denial,** an unconscious protective defense against the terrifying reality of losing one's place in the world. Family members may also deny that anything is wrong as a defense against the painful awareness that a loved one is deteriorating. Over time, symptoms become more obvious, and other defensive maneuvers become evident.

Another defense mechanism is confabulation—the making up of stories or answers to maintain self-esteem when the person does not remember. For example, the nurse addresses a patient who has remained in a hospital bed all weekend:

Nurse: "Good morning, Ms. Jones. How was your weekend?"

Patient: "Wonderful. I discussed politics with the president, and he took me out to dinner."

or

Patient: "I spent the weekend with my daughter and her family." *(less grandiose)*

Confabulation is not the same as lying. When people are lying, they are aware of making up an answer; confabulation is an *unconscious* attempt to maintain self-esteem. It is associated with intermediate dementia symptoms.

Perseveration, the repetition of phrases or behavior, is eventually seen and is often intensified under stress. This repetition of remembered phrases may be associated with the *word-finding problems* evidenced in AD. The avoidance of answering questions is another mechanism by which the patient is able to maintain self-esteem in the face of severe memory deficits. Therefore (1) denial, (2) confabulation, (3) perseveration, and (4) avoidance of questions are four defensive behaviors the nurse might notice during assessment.

Cognitive impairment involves the *four A's*:

- **Amnesia or memory impairment.** Initially, the person has difficulty remembering recent events. Gradually, deterioration progresses to include both recent and remote memory.
- Aphasia (loss of language ability). Progresses with the disease. Initially, the person has difficulty finding the correct word, then is reduced to a few words, and finally in late stages is reduced to babbling or mutism.
- Apraxia (loss of purposeful movement in the absence of motor or sensory impairment). The person is unable to perform once-familiar and purposeful tasks. For example, in apraxia of gait, the person loses the ability to walk. In apraxia of dressing, the person is unable to put on clothes properly (may put arms in trousers or put a jacket on upside down).
- Agnosia (loss of sensory ability to recognize objects). The person may lose the ability to recognize familiar sounds (auditory agnosia), such as the ring of the telephone, a car horn, or the doorbell. Loss of this ability extends to the inability to recognize familiar objects (visual or tactile agnosia), such as a glass, magazine, pencil, or toothbrush. Eventually, people are unable to recognize loved ones or even parts of their own bodies.

Disturbances in **executive functioning** (planning, organizing, and abstract thinking) become evident.

Assessment Guidelines

Dementia

1. Identify and treat any general medical conditions that might contribute to the dementia.
2. Evaluate the potential for suicide, self-harm, or aggression toward others.
3. Review the medications the patient is currently taking, including over-the-counter (OTC) remedies, herbs, complementary agents, and recreational drugs.
4. Evaluate the patient's current level of cognitive functioning.
5. Explore how well the family is prepared for and informed about the patient's illness of dementia.
6. Discuss with family members how they are coping with the patient and their main care issues.
7. Assess for evidence of neglect or abuse.
8. Review the resources available to the family. Ask the family members to describe the help they receive from other family members, friends, and community resources. Determine if caregivers are aware of community support groups and resources.
9. Determine the appropriate safety measures needed by the patient and arrange for them to be implemented.
10. Evaluate the safety of the patient's home environment (with regard to wandering, eating inedible objects, falling, and engaging in provocative behaviors toward others).
11. Identify the needs of the family for teaching and guidance. The behaviors associated with AD can be quite challenging to control.

DIAGNOSIS

One of the most important areas of concern is the patient's *safety. Risk for injury* is always present for those with AD. People with AD may wander and be lost for hours or days. Wandering may result from changes in the physical environment, fear caused by hallucinations or delusions, or lack of exercise and boredom.

Seizures may occur in the later stages of this disease. Injuries from falls and accidents can occur during any stage as confusion and disorientation progress. The potential for burns exists if the patient is a smoker or is unattended when using the stove. Prescription drugs can be taken incorrectly, or bottles of noxious fluids can be mistakenly ingested, which results in a medical crisis.

As the person's ability to recognize or name objects is decreased, *Impaired verbal communication* becomes a problem. As memory diminishes and disorientation increases, *Impaired memory, Impaired cognition, Disorientation,* and *Chronic confusion* occur. As the disease progresses, *Self-care deficits* emerge, such as *Impaired ability to bath, Impaired ability to dress, Impaired ability to groom,* as well as *Impaired nutritional intake and Impaired mobility related to wandering.*

During the course of the disease, people show personality changes, increased vulnerability, and often inappropriate behaviors. Common behaviors include hoarding, regression, and being overly demanding and aggressive. *Impaired coping process, Labile mood,* and *Risk for self-destructive behavior* (suicide, self-harm, harm to others) are potential nursing diagnoses. Family caregivers often experience *Impaired family coping* and *Impaired family process.*

Additional family issues may emerge. Perhaps some of the most crucial aspects of the patient's care are support, education, and referrals for the family. The family loses an integral part of its unit. Family members lose the love, function, support, companionship, and warmth that this person once provided. *Caregiver stress* is always present. Planning with the family and offering community support are integral parts of appropriate care. It can be helpful to assess for *Dysfunctional (anticipatory) grief* and provide supportive counseling when needed. Helping the family grieve can make the task ahead less painful. Refer to Table 18.4 for potential nursing diagnoses for confused patients with dementia.

OUTCOMES IDENTIFICATION

Outcomes for patients with dementia are based on the behaviors presented (Box 18.2).

PLANNING AND IMPLEMENTATION

The planning of care for a patient with dementia is geared toward the patient's immediate needs. Areas of assessment can include ADLs

BOX 18.2 Selected Outcome Criteria for a Major Neurocognitive Disorder (Dementia)[a]

Injury

- Patient will remain safe in all environments.
- With the aid of an identification bracelet and neighborhood or hospital alert, patient will be returned within 1 hour of wandering.
- Patient will remain free of danger during seizures.
- With the aid of interventions, patient will remain burn-free.
- With the aid of guidance and environmental manipulation, patient will not be hurt if a fall occurs.
- Patient will ingest only correct doses of prescribed medications and appropriate food and fluids.

Communication

- Patient will communicate needs.
- Patient will answer yes or no appropriately to questions.
- Patient will state needs in alternative modes when aphasic (will signal correct word on hearing it, will refer to picture or label).
- Patient will wear prescribed glasses or hearing aid each day.

Caregiver Role Strain

- Family members will have the opportunity to express "unacceptable" feelings in a supportive environment.
- Family members will have access to professional counseling.
- Family members will name two organizations within their geographical area that can offer support.
- Family members will participate in patient's plan of care, with encouragement from staff.
- Family members will state that they have outside help that allows them to take personal time for themselves each week or month.
- Family members will have the names of three resources that can help with financial burdens and legal considerations.

Impaired Environmental Interpretation: Chronic Confusion

- Patient will acknowledge the reality of an object or a sound that was misinterpreted (illusion), after it is pointed out.
- Patient will state feeling safe after experiencing delusions or illusions.
- Patient will remain nonaggressive when experiencing paranoid ideation.

Self-Care Needs

- Patient will participate in self-care at optimal level.
- Patient will be able to follow step-by-step instructions for dressing, bathing, and grooming.
- Patient will put on own clothes appropriately, with aid of fastening tape (Velcro) and nursing supervision.
- Patient's skin will remain intact and free from signs of pressure.

[a]Not an exhaustive list.

orientation and affect; ability to complete everyday activities; and changes in personality, interests, and drives. Fig. 18.2 presents the Blessed Dementia Scale. It can be used to quantify the degree of intellectual and personality deterioration to plan interventions and track the progression of symptoms. Identifying the level of functioning and assessing caregivers' needs help the nurse identify appropriate community resources.

The health care staff needs to be proactive in minimizing the stressful effects of caregiving as well as in teaching and providing guidelines to caregivers and loved ones. The following measures may help:

- **Have a realistic understanding of the disease** so that expectations for the individual are realistic.
- **Establish realistic outcomes** for the person and recognize when they are achieved. It is useful to remember that even small achievements, like *feeding self,* can be significant for the impaired individual.
- **Maintain good self-care.** Obtaining adequate sleep and rest, eating a nutritious diet, exercising, engaging in relaxing activities, and addressing spiritual needs are critical for nurses and other caregivers.

The needs of people with dementia are complex and change over time according to the stage of the disease. Care settings include the emergency department, the general hospital, home settings, long-term care settings, and the community.

The nurse's attitude of *unconditional positive regard* is the single most effective tool in caring for individuals with dementia. It facilitates cooperation with care, reduces catastrophic reactions, and increases family members' satisfaction with care. A warm, empathic, and nonjudgmental approach using calm, unhurried, clear communication can help allay confusion and agitation. The nurse and others should always introduce themselves with each encounter. Expectations should be clear and explained in simple, step-by-step instructions. To help patients maintain a sense of self-control, they should be given simple and limited choices in their care ("Do you want to wash your face before or after you brush your teeth?").

Specialized interventions for the secondary behavioral disturbances associated with dementia may be required. For example, a woman who is 78 years old and believes that she is 23 and has babies at home would not be calmed by being told that she is 78 and has no babies. It is more helpful to reflect the feeling expressed and show understanding and concern. For example, "Mrs. Green, you miss your children. This can be a lonely place."

Intervention with family members is critical. The "loss" of the person who is loved is painful, and 24/7 care is exhausting. Nurses can teach families about the progression of the illness and give guidelines for safely caring for their family member. Finding appropriate support for families who are grieving and dealing with profound change is an important intervention.

Communication Guidelines

Appropriate communication strategies by nurses and caregivers help to maintain a person's self-esteem and ability to participate in care. People with dementia often find it difficult to express themselves. They may:

- Have difficulty finding the right words.
- Use familiar words repeatedly.
- Invent new words to describe things (neologisms).
- Frequently lose their train of thought.
- Rely on nonverbal gestures.
- Be unable to communicate basics needs (thirst, pain, need to use bathroom) in an understandable way.

Validation therapy is a type of therapeutic communication that places more emphasis on emotional aspects and less on factual content. This imparts respect to individuals and their feelings and beliefs. This is a strategy that can be used by nurses and family members (Kales, Gitlin, & Lyketsos, 2015).

Example: A woman with AD believes her daughter stole her wedding ring. Instead of arguing, (1) validate the reality, (2) empathize, and (3) help the person connect to feelings. A daughter might respond by stating: "Your wedding ring is gone. You think I've stolen it. It was a beautiful ring. How did you and Dad meet?"

BLESSED DEMENTIA SCALE

Patient Name: ____________

Rater Name: ____________

Date:

Instruction

One point for each correct answer unless otherwise indicated. **Score**

CHANGES IN PERFORMANCE OF EVERYDAY ACTIVITIES

A Inability to perform household tasks ____

A Inability to cope with small sums of money ____

A Inability to remember shortlist of items; for example, in shopping list ____

A Inability to find way about indoors ____

A Inability to find way about familiar streets ____

A Inability to interpret surroundings; for example, to recognize whether in hospital or at home; to discriminate between patients, doctors, nurse, relatives, other hospital staff, etc. ____

A Inability to recall recent events; for example, recent outings, visits of relatives or friends to hospital, etc. ____

* Tendency to dwell in the past ____

CHANGES IN HABITS

D Eating
- (0) = cleanly, with proper utensils
- (1) = messily, with spoon only
- (2) = simple solids (for example, biscuits)
- (3) = has to be fed

____

D Dressing
- (0) = unaided
- (1) = occasionally misplaced buttons, etc.
- (2) = wrong sequence, commonly forgetting items
- (3) = unable to dress

____

D Sphincter control
- (0) = complete control
- (1) = occasional wet bed
- (2) = frequent wet bed
- (3) = doubly incontinent

____

CHANGES IN PERSONALITY, INTERESTS, DRIVE

B Increased rigidity ____

B Increased egocentricity ____

B Impairment of regard of feeling for others ____

B Coarsening of affect ____

B Impairment of emotional control (for example, increased petulance and irritability) ____

B Hilarity in inappropriate situations ____

C Diminished emotional responsiveness ____

* Sexual misdemeanor (arising *de novo* in old age) ____

C Hobbies relenquished ____

C Diminished initiative or growing apathy ____

* Purposeless hyperactivity ____

Fig. 18.2 Blessed Dementia Scale. (From Blessed, G., Tomlinson, B. E., Roth, M. [1968]. The association between quantitative measures of dementia and of senile change in the cerebral grey matter of elderly subjects. *British Journal of Psychiatry 114,* 797-811; Stern, Y., Hesdorffer, D., Sano, M., Mayeux, R. [1990]. Measurement and prediction of functional capacity in Alzheimer's disease. *Neurology 40,* 8-14; and Zillmer, E. A., Fowler, P. C., Gutnick, H. N., Becker, E. [1990]. Comparison of two cognitive bedside screening instruments in nursing home residents: A factor analytic study. *Journal of Gerontology 45,* 69-74.))

When using reality orientation, focus on the concrete facts, such as the date, and use the person's name frequently. It is usually not useful to remind a person of forgotten sad events like the death of a loved one.

Reminiscence therapy involves the discussion of past activities, events, and experiences with another person or group of people. Research indicates little or no effect on cognition, but it may have some small effect on quality of life and possibly mood (Woods et al., 2018).

See Table 18.7 for nursing interventions and guidelines for communicating with a cognitively impaired person. These can be taught to family members.

APPLYING THE ART

A Person With a Severe Neurocognitive Disorder (Dementia)

Scenario

I met 75-year-old Mr. Samson on our geriatric rotation. He had recently moved to the Memory Disorder Unit of the nursing facility. His wife of 50 years, whom he called Darlin' (her name was Darlene), had resided on the assisted living side of the facility until her sudden death 3 weeks earlier. Mr. Samson and I regularly used the pictures in the memory book assembled by his wife to remind him about his life.

Therapeutic Goal

By the end of this encounter, Mr. Samson will focus on good times he and his wife shared together and spend less time asking for her and wanting to know when she is coming to visit.

Student–Patient Interaction	Thoughts, Communication Techniques, and Mental Health Nursing Concepts
Student: "Mr. Samson, what's wrong?"	I knew from the chart that Mr. Samson had attended his wife's funeral.
Mr. Samson: *Crying.* "My Darlin', what's wrong with my Darlin'?" *He gestures toward the sign of the memorial service to be held for "Mrs. Darlene Samson" and one other resident who had died the previous month.*	I should have said my name and reminded him that we had talked a few times before, but I was worried because he was sitting in the lobby sobbing. He is crying like he just discovered "his Darlin'" died. How awful to not be able to hold on to your own life and what matters most in your memories.
Student: "Mr. Samson, I'm ______, your nursing student. You feel worried seeing your wife's name on the sign." *He nods.* "Let's use your memory wallet to remember together about your Darlin'." *I wait until he makes eye contact and takes the wallet out of his hip pocket.*	I introduce myself again and use reflection. Diverting to the task of looking through the memory wallet provides structure to help meet safety needs.
Student's feelings: *I am feeling a little anxious now. I hope I did okay in calling Mrs. Samson Darlin' as he does. I hope he'll remember if I show him the picture the staff put in the wallet showing Mr. Samson standing and looking at his wife in the casket. Seems unkind in some ways.*	
Student: *Smiling encouragingly.* "Tell me about the pictures."	I know that the mental health focus needs to include helping with reality orientation for as long as his progressive dementia will allow.
Mr. Samson: *No longer crying.* "This was our house. Darlin' keeps such a great garden. I used to love her tomatoes the best." *He points to the tall plants beside the house.*	He uses the present tense "keeps … garden," but the past tense for "was our house" and "used to love her tomatoes." He is having trouble sorting out the present from the past.
Student's feelings: *He's trying so hard. I admire him. I never knew either of my grandfathers.*	
Student: "You still love tomatoes! I helped you make the tomato salad for lunch. None tastes as good as Darlin's did, I bet."	I make an observation. I refer to Mrs. Samson's tomatoes in the past tense to reinforce reality.
Student's feelings: *I did well here by reminding him of still liking tomatoes.*	
Mr. Samson: "Right. I wonder if Darlin' picked the tomato salad. We meet in the solarium every day."	
Student's feelings: *I feel frustrated that he's talking about Darlin' like she's alive. Two days ago, he talked like he remembered that Mrs. Samson died 3 weeks ago.*	
Student: "Look at this next picture." *I wait as he absorbs the funeral home picture.*	How nontherapeutic. I sound like I am giving a command. I should have started with, "I have some sad news."
Student's feelings: *Was that too direct? I didn't know what to say when he talked about meeting her in the solarium.*	
Mr. Samson: "Oh God, oh God. She died. She's gone. When did she die? How can I go on without her?" *He buries his head in his hands, sobbing.*	
Student's feelings: *He's experiencing this as though for the first time. I feel ready to cry.*	
Student: "You must've loved her very much. It must be lonely without her. I am with you. May I hold your hand?" *He nods.*	Touch communicates caring. I validate his feelings of longing. I ask permission before touching.
Mr. Samson: "We were married 50 years. She's the love of my life. Darlin' was my soulmate."	I remain silent while he talks about his wife. I cannot imagine 50 years with one person. What an accomplishment.
Student: "You say Darlin' was your soulmate. You miss her so much."	I use reflection. I also carefully restate to emphasize his use of the past tense. I wonder what effect the memorial service will have on him. When he comes to the point of grieving anew every time, we will have to take out the funeral picture and emphasize feelings using validation therapy.
Student's feelings: *I'll talk with the treatment team. He may need some extra support as his memory impairment grows and as he faces the memorial service.*	
Mr. Samson: "I do, every minute of every day." *He makes eye contact as we continue talking until he's calmer and no longer crying.*	
Student's feelings: *I like him, and I feel so sad about his situation.*	
Student: "Are you ready to walk together back to your room so you can get ready for reminiscence group?" *He nods.*	Giving him a choice empowers him.

TABLE 18.7 Intervention Guidelines for Dementia (Major Neurocognitive Disorders): Communication

Intervention	Rationale
1. Always identify yourself and call the person by name at each meeting.	1. Patient's short-term memory is impaired; requires frequent orientation to time and environment.
2. Speak slowly.	2. Patient needs time to process information.
3. Use short, simple words and phrases.	3. Patient may not be able to understand complex statements or abstract ideas.
4. Maintain face-to-face contact.	4. Verbal and nonverbal clues are maximized.
5. Be near patient when talking, one or two arm-lengths away.	5. This distance can help patient focus on speaker as well as maintain personal space.
6. Focus on one piece of information at a time.	6. Attention span of patient is poor and patient is easily distracted; helps patient focus. Too many data can be overwhelming and can increase anxiety.
7. Talk with patient about familiar and meaningful things.	7. Self-expression is promoted and reality is reinforced.
8. Encourage reminiscing about happy times in life.	8. Remembering accomplishments and shared joys helps distract patient from deficit and gives meaning to existence.
9. When patient is delusional, acknowledge patient's feelings and reinforce reality. Do not argue or refute delusions.	9. Acknowledging feelings helps patient feel understood. Pointing out realities may help patient focus on realities. Arguing can enhance adherence to false beliefs.
10. If a patient gets into an argument with another patient, stop the argument and separate individuals. After a short while (5 minutes), explain straightforwardly to each patient why you had to intervene.	10. Escalation to physical acting out is prevented. Patient's right to know is respected. Explaining in an adult manner helps maintain self-esteem.
11. When patient becomes verbally aggressive, acknowledge patient's feelings and shift topic to more familiar ground ("I know this is upsetting for you because you always cared for others. Tell me about your children.").	11. Confusion and disorientation easily increase anxiety. Acknowledging feelings makes patient feel more understood and less alone. Topics patient has mastery over can remind him or her of areas of competent functioning and can increase self-esteem.
12. Have patient wear prescription eyeglasses or hearing aid.	12. Environmental awareness, orientation, and comprehension are increased, which in turn increases awareness of personal needs and the presence of others.
13. Keep patient's room well lit.	13. Environmental clues are maximized.
14. Have clocks, calendars, and personal items (family pictures, Bible) in clear view of patient while he or she is in bed.	14. These objects assist in maintaining personal identity.
15. Reinforce patient's pictures, nonverbal gestures, X's on calendars, and other methods used to anchor patient in reality.	15. When aphasia starts to hinder communication, alternate methods of communication need to be instituted.

Health Teaching and Health Promotion

Families who are caring for a member with AD in the home need to know about strategies for communicating and structuring self-care activities (Table 18.8). Education and support can significantly decrease distress in both the person with dementia and the people providing care. Areas for health teaching and health maintenance include the following:

1. Education about the progression of the illness, especially for caregivers. There are virtual reality programs designed to help caregivers understand individuals with dementia so that they can better serve them.
2. Communication strategies to use with the person with dementia
3. How to handle troubling behaviors (Fig. 18.3).
4. How to plan appropriate activities
5. Information about types of care, including adult day care, in-home care, residential care, respite care, and hospice care
6. Information about other community resources, including transportation, housekeeping, and home health aides
7. Planning for the future: Information about financial and legal issues, including advance directives, durable power of attorney, guardianship, and conservatorship and insurance issues
8. Information about recognition of caregiver stress and strategies to facilitate caregiver health

Guidelines for providing a safe environment and strategies for planning appropriate activities are provided in Table 18.9.

The Alzheimer's Association is a valuable resource that provides information, care, and support for all those affected by AD and other dementias. The Alzheimer's Association website (http://www.alz.org) provides online tools and resources, including the following:

1. Information about symptoms of the disease, care strategies, care options, and financial and legal information
2. Information about local support groups and an online community support group and message board
3. Information about how to maintain caregiver health
4. A 24/7 helpline (1-800-272-3900)
5. MedicAlert + Alzheimer's Association Safe Return: a 24-hour nationwide emergency response service for individuals with Alzheimer's or a related dementia who wander or have a medical emergency. Other tracking technologies to help monitor wandering behavior are also discussed (Alzheimer's Association, 2018).

Milieu Therapy

Agitation and aggression are especially distressing to patients, caregivers, and staff in memory units. Psychosocial interventions should always be tried first. Some interventions that are effective in reducing agitation and aggressive behavior are listed in Fig. 18.3. Environmental factors such as overstimulation and understimulation, a lack of activities and structure, and a lack of established routine can contribute to problematic behaviors (Kales et al., 2015). Providing a physically and emotionally safe environment is critical (Table 18.10).

APPLYING EVIDENCE-BASED PRACTICE (EBP)

Problem

An 81-year-old female diagnosed with stage 3 Alzheimer's disease is living in a skilled nursing facility. She is a fall risk and frequently wanders away from the supervised area and goes outside. There are dangers in the uneven ground outside and traffic in the parking lot and nearby streets. She is no longer able to communicate verbally in a meaningful way.

EBP Assessment

A. **What do you already know from experience?**

1. Wandering behavior presents safety and fall risks.
2. This patient has not responded to verbal redirection and staff.
3. Although the staff has caught her before she gets outside on most occasions, when several patient alarms are going off at the same time, she has been able to make it farther.

B. **What does the literature say?**

1. *Alarm fatigue* can occur when alarms are constantly sounding, causing nurses and other staff to become overwhelmed and desensitized (UT Arlington, 2016).
2. It can be difficult to keep patients who wander safe while providing a satisfying quality of life and avoiding restraint use.

C. **What does the patient want?**

1. The patient is no longer able to make her wishes known verbally in a meaningful way.
2. The patient's daughter revealed that her mother had grown up on a farm and spent as much time as possible in nature throughout the years. This information helped the nurse recognize how important being outside would be to the patient.

Plan

The patient's plan of care was revised to include time outside for daily walks in the garden and eating meals outside when weather permitted. The daughter made a commitment to take her mother to nature settings during their time together whenever possible. When the nurse asked the patient if she would like to go outside, her facial expression changed, her eyes brightened, and she verbalized "yes." When the patient was required to be indoors, she was given a nature-centered coloring activity. Nursing leadership convened a working group to discuss strategies to lessen alarm fatigue on the unit.

QSEN Prelicensure Knowledge, Skills, and Attitudes (KSAs) Addressed

Safety and **Patient-Centered Care** were utilized by finding a way to lessen wandering behavior in this patient while providing enjoyable activities. **Informatics** was addressed in considering the issue of alarm fatigue.

TABLE 18.8 Intervention Guidelines for Dementia: Health Teaching and Health Promotion

Intervention	Rationale
Dressing and Bathing	
1. Always have patient perform all tasks that are in patient's ability.	1. Maintains patient's self-esteem and uses muscle groups; impedes staff burnout; minimizes further regression.
2. Have patient wear own clothes, even if in the hospital.	2. Helps maintain patient's identity and dignity.
3. Use clothing with elastic, and substitute fastening tape (Velcro) for buttons and zippers.	3. Minimizes patient's confusion and eases independence of functioning.
4. Label clothing items with patient's name and name of item.	4. Helps identify patient if he or she wanders and gives patient additional clues when aphasia or agnosia occurs.
5. Give step-by-step instructions whenever necessary ("Take this blouse … put in one arm … now the next arm …").	5. Patient can focus on small pieces of information more easily; allows patient to perform at optimal level.
6. Make sure that water in faucets is not too hot.	6. Judgment is lacking in patient; patient is unaware of many safety hazards.
7. If patient is resistant to performing self-care, come back later and ask again.	7. Moods may be labile, and patient may forget but often complies after short interval.
Nutrition	
1. Monitor food and fluid intake.	1. Patient may have anorexia or be too confused to eat.
2. Offer finger foods that patient can take away from the dinner table.	2. Increases input throughout the day; patient may eat only small amounts at meals.
3. Weigh patient regularly (once a week).	3. Monitors fluid and nutritional status.
4. During periods of hyperorality, watch that patient does not eat nonfood items (ceramic fruit, food-shaped soaps).	4. Patient puts everything into mouth; may be unable to differentiate inedible objects made in the shape and color of food.
Bowel and Bladder Function	
1. Begin bowel and bladder program early; start with bladder control.	1. Establishing same time of day for bowel movements and toileting—in early morning, after meals and snacks, and before bedtime—can help prevent incontinence.
2. Evaluate use of disposable diapers.	2. Prevents embarrassment.
3. Label bathroom door as well as doors to other rooms.	3. Additional environmental clues can maximize independent toileting.
Sleep	
1. Because patient may awaken, be frightened, or cry out at night, keep area well lit.	1. Reinforces orientation; minimizes possible illusions.
2. Maintain a calm atmosphere during the day.	2. Encourages a calming night's sleep.
3. Medications are not recommended for sleep. Use of nonmedical interventions. When medications have been prescribed, give lower doses. Sedatives, antidepressants, neuroleptics with sedative properties like atypical antipsychotics may be used. Benzodiazepines should only be used short term.	3. Helps clear thinking and sedates. However, psychotic medications should be used with extreme care, and other methods should be applied first.
4. Avoid the use of restraints.	4. Can cause patient to become more terrified and fight against restraints until exhausted to a dangerous degree.

Sensory Interventions
Music therapy (listening)
Light therapy
Pet therapy
Multisensory stimulation
Hearing aids
Active Therapy/
Structured Activities
Dancing
Exercise
Social interation
Music therapy
(playing/singing)
Art therapy
Outdoor walks
Psychological/Therapy
Validation therapy
Reality orientation
Reminiscence therapy
Psychosocial therapy
Cognitive behavioral therapy
Relaxation training
Structured support groups

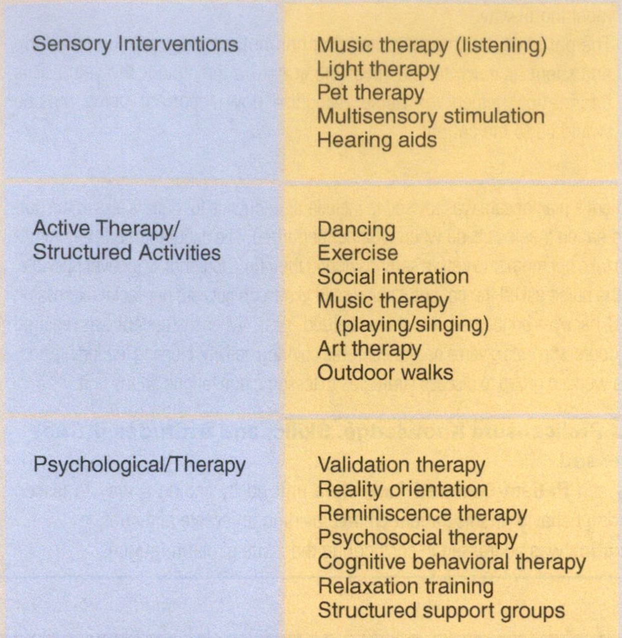

Fig. 18.3 Interventions delivered directly to patients with dementia to reduce agitated and aggressive behavior. (Retrieved from Agency for Healthcare Research and Quality. (2016). *Nonpharmacologic interventions for agitation and aggression in dementia: Executive summary.* Retrieved from https://effectivehealthcare.ahrq.gov/sites/default/files/dementia-agitation-aggression_executive.pdf.)

TABLE 18.9 Dementia (Major Neurocognitive Disorders): Support Services for People and Caregivers

- Referrals to adult day care centers
- Meals on Wheels
- Home health services/homemaker services/personal care services
- Transportation services
- Legal services
- Supervision and care when primary caregiver is out of the home
- Information on support groups within the community
- Information on respite and residential services
- Health care services (geriatric specialists, physical therapy, skilled nursing care)
- Mental health services, social services, protective services if needed
- Hospice
- Telephone numbers for helplines
- The Alzheimer's Association—online education and support services
- Personal emergency response services
- Additional teaching or psychopharmaceutic aids to manage distressing or harmful behaviors when appropriate and safe

Pharmacological, Biological, and Integrative Therapies

Although there is no cure for AD, there are four prescription drugs currently approved by the U.S. Food and Drug Administration (FDA) for individuals with AD. It is hypothesized that the symptoms of AD are associated with low levels of acetylcholine. Medications called cholinesterase inhibitors work by preventing the breakdown of acetylcholine and stimulate nicotinic receptors to release more acetylcholine into the brain. The FDA-approved cholinesterase inhibitors are as follows:

- Galantamine hydrobromide (Razadyne)
- Rivastigmine tartrate (Exelon)
- Donepezil hydrochloride (Aricept)

These agents demonstrate a mild positive effect on cognition, behavior, and ability to function in ADLs for people with *mild to moderate* AD. These medications are effective in slowing down the progression of AD for a limited period, 3 to 6 months only (Burchum & Rosenthal, 2016). The most common side effects are gastrointestinal: nausea, vomiting, diarrhea, loss of appetite, and gastric hemorrhage (rare).

Memantine hydrochloride (Namenda), an N-methyl-D-aspartate (NMDA) antagonist, is an antagonist at the NMDA-glutamatergic receptor, which is associated with memory and learning. The drug works by regulating glutamate and inhibiting the toxic effects of the excess influx of calcium that causes neurodegeneration (Burchum & Rosenthal, 2016). It targets symptoms of AD during the *moderate to severe stages* of the disorder. The main side effects are dizziness, headache, and constipation. The benefits of memantine are time limited and minimal. *Namzaric* is composed of both *donepezil and memantine* and is targeted to treat *moderate to severe* AD.

There are over 100 medications in various stages of development for the treatment and cure of dementia. There are a variety of other therapies in experimental stages. One study shows promising results for *deep brain stimulation,* in which implanted electric wires send electric currents to stimulate the parts of the brain that control executive functioning (Caughill, 2018). See Table 18.11.

Targeting Behavioral Symptoms

Behavioral and psychological symptoms of dementia, sometimes referred to as BPSD, encompass a wide range of behaviors that are unsafe and difficult to manage. The presence of these behaviors frequently results in admission to long-term care facilities. They can fluctuate over time. Behavioral symptoms include physical aggression, loud vocalizations, restlessness, agitation, and wandering. Psychological symptoms include acute anxiety, depressed mood, hallucinations, and delusions.

There are several strategies to help lessen these behaviors. *Music therapy* is the one therapy consistently found to reduce agitation in patients with dementia. *Behavioral management techniques* directed at *enhancing staff communication skills, formal caregiver training,* and *dementia mapping* have been shown to be effective at reducing agitation. *Dementia mapping* is a specialized observation of a person with dementia over a period of time for the purpose of determining *patient-centered care.* A *tailored activities program (TAP)* addresses the abilities of individuals with dementia. *Sensory interventions* include massage, therapeutic touch, and multisensory stimulation. These may help to reduce mild to moderate agitation in the short term (Ijaopo, 2017).

The *DICE approach* can be used to reduce problematic behaviors. It stands for *describe* (the symptoms and possible precipitants), *investigate* (Is there a modifiable cause?), *create* (a plan of revised care), and *evaluate* (Did the new strategy work?). It is a patient-/caregiver-centered approach that uses a thorough assessment to give individualized care (Kales et al., 2015).

When there is a lack of understanding by the caregiver of the behaviors associated with disease progression, there is a potential to worsen the fear and anxiety that underlie BPSD. Caregivers can learn triggers for unwanted behaviors and learn to spot these triggers before the disruptive symptoms fully develop (Kales et al., 2015).

Recognizing possible precipitants to BPSD is the first step for intervention. Signs of agitation, increasing anxiety, and other problematic behaviors may be caused by pain, urinary tract infections, dehydration,

TABLE 18.10 Interventions for a Safe Milieu in the Home

Intervention	Rationale
Safe Environment	
1. Gradually restrict use of the car.	1. Even mild cognitive impairment increases risk of vehicular accident.
2. Remove throw rugs and other objects in person's path.	2. Minimizes tripping and falling.
3. Simplify environment	3. Decreases sensory overload, which can increase anxiety and confusion.
4. Minimize sensory stimulation.	4. Decreases confusion.
5. If patient becomes verbally upset, listen briefly, give support, then change the topic.	5. Goal is to prevent escalation of anger. When attention span is short, patient can be distracted to more productive topics and activities.
6. Use safety locks to prevent leaving the house and opening drawers with harmful objects.	6. May keep patient from wandering into other people's rooms. Increases environmental clues to familiar objects.
7. Label all rooms and drawers. Label often-used objects (hairbrushes, toothbrushes).	7. Prevents accidental harm to self.
8. Install safety bars in bathroom.	8. Prevents falls.
9. Supervise patient when smoking.	9. Danger of burns is always present.
10. If patient has history of seizures, educate family on how to deal with seizures.	10. Seizure activity is common in advanced Alzheimer's disease.
Wandering	
1. If patient wanders during the night, put mattress on the floor.	1. Prevents falls when patient is confused.
2. Have patient wear MedicAlert bracelet that cannot be removed (with name, address, and telephone number). Provide police department with recent pictures.	2. Patient can easily be identified by police, neighbors, or hospital personnel.
3. Alert local police and neighbors about patient wandering.	3. May reduce time necessary to return patient to home or hospital.
4. If patient is in the hospital, have him or her wear brightly colored vest with name, unit, and phone number printed on back.	4. Makes patient easily identifiable.
5. Put complex locks on door.	5. Reduces opportunity to wander.
6. Place locks at top of door.	6. In moderate and late Alzheimer's-type dementia, ability to look up and reach upward is lost.
7. Encourage physical activity during the day.	7. Physical activity may decrease wandering at night.
8. Explore the feasibility of installing sensor devices and web-based GPS system.	8. Sensor provides warning if patient wanders. Global positing system (GPS) can help locate patient.
9. Use a bed monitor.	9. Alerts staff if patient has left his or her bed during the night.
Useful Activities	
1. Provide picture magazines and children's books when patient's reading ability diminishes.	1. Allows continuation of usual activities that patient can still enjoy; provides focus.
2. Provide simple activities that allow exercise of large muscles.	2. Exercise groups, dance groups, and walking provide socialization as well as increased circulation and maintenance of muscle tone.
3. Encourage group activities that are familiar and simple to perform.	3. Activities such as group singing, dancing, reminiscing, and working with clay and paint all help to increase socialization and minimize feelings of alienation.

constipation, sleep disturbances, other unrecognized physiologic needs, feelings of loss, and fear or boredom (Kales et al., 2015). Drug side effects and drug–drug interactions can contribute to patient discomfort and problematic behaviors. Uncorrected problems with hearing or vision can cause additional confusion that can lead to problem behaviors.

The use of physical restraints is no longer sanctioned in those with cognitive deficits.

Medication must be used cautiously when given to control disruptive behavior in patients with dementia. Medication is often associated with falls, worsening cognitive impairment, oversedation, and other adverse drug reactions. All antipsychotics have a Black Box warning of *increased mortality* risk when used for patients with dementia. If used, antipsychotics should be used sparingly and in low doses. Age alters the metabolism, absorption, and elimination of medications, and older adults are more sensitive to all side effects.

In patients with coexisting depression, antidepressants can be considered, although there is no clear-cut evidence of efficacy for dementia. Selective serotonin reuptake inhibitors (SSRIs) have a low side-effect profile and appear to be better tolerated. Antidepressants that are sedating, such as trazodone and mirtazapine, may facilitate sleep and decrease agitation. There is some evidence that citalopram also reduces agitation (Kales et al., 2015). Benzodiazepines are not recommended except for an acute episode because of excessive sedation, tolerance and withdrawal, central nervous system (CNS) depression, and a possible paradoxical disinhibition. The use of non-benzodiazepine sleeping pills has been associated with an increased risk of fractures. With the use of any medication, the risk of side effects must always be considered.

Box 18.3 presents a recent study that demonstrated how certain lifestyle changes may reduce the risk of cognitive decline and dementia.

Neurobiology of Alzheimer's and the Effects of Medication on the Brain

Two essential neurotransmitters implicated in Alzheimer's disease are acetylcholine and glutamate.

Acetylcholine: is involved with learning, memory, and mood. As Alzheimer's disease progresses the brain produces less and less acetylcholine. What little acetylcholine is left is rapidly destroyed by the enzyme acetylcholinesterase.

Cholinesterase: inhibitors keep the acetylcholinesterase enzyme from breaking down acetylcholine, thereby increasing both the level and duration of action of the neurotransmitter acetylcholine.

Glutamate: is involved with cell signaling, learning, and memory. Glutamate binds to cells at the *N*-methyl-D-aspartate (NMDA) receptor and allows calcium to enter the cell. In Alzheimer's disease, excess glutamate from damaged cells leads to chronic overexposure to calcium.

NMDA: antagonists helps reduce excess calcium by blocking some NMDA receptors.

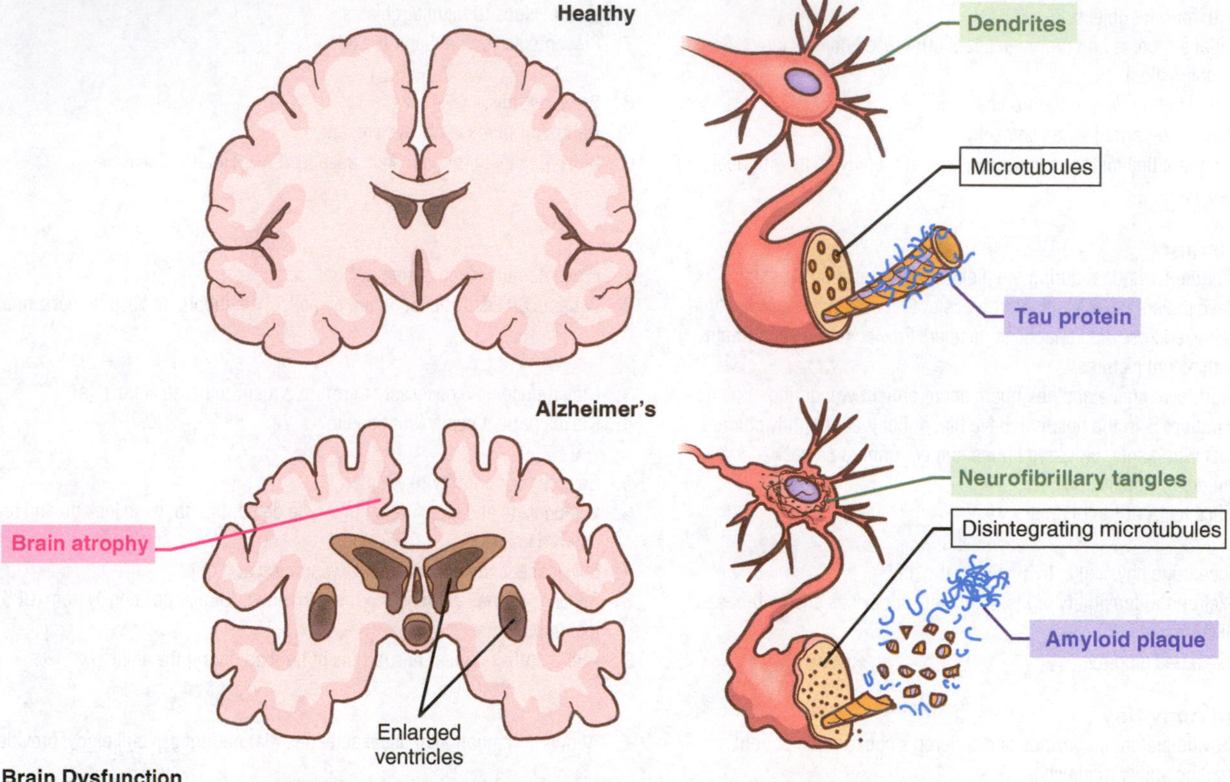

Brain Dysfunction

Amyloid plaques are sticky clumps found between nerve cells that may either cause or be the result of the disease. The clumps block communication at synapses that is normally protected by tau proteins and healthy microtubules. They may also activate immune system cells that trigger inflammation and devour disabled cells.

Neurofibrillary tangles are abnormal collections of protein threads inside nerve cells. They are comprised mainly of a protein called tau. Tangles disrupt the transport of food molecules, cell parts, and other key elements. This disruption results in cell death.

Brain atrophy is the cerebral cortex shriveling up, damaging areas involved in thinking, planning, and remembering. The hippocampus, an area of the cortex that is essential for memory, experiences severe shrinkage. Ventricles, the fluid-filled spaces within the brain, grow larger.

FDA Approved Drugs for the Treatment of Alzheimer's Disease

Drug Name	Brand Name	Classification	Approved for
galantamine	Razadyne	Cholinesterase inhibitor	Mild to moderate
donepezil	Aricept	Cholinesterase inhibitor	All stages
rivastigmine	Exelon	Cholinesterase inhibitor	All stages
memantine	Namenda	Namenda, an NMDA antagonist, helps reduce excess calcium by blocking some NMDA receptors	Moderate to severe
donepezil and memantine	Namzaric	Cholinesterase inhibitor and NMDA receptor antagonist combination	Moderate to severe

TABLE 18.11 Drugs Approved by the U.S. Food and Drug Administration for Alzheimer's Disease

Drug Name	Classification and Indications	How It Works	Adverse Reactions
Memantine (Namenda)	*N*-methyl-D-aspartate (NMDA) antagonist Treats symptoms of *moderate to severe Alzheimer's*	Normalizes and regulates glutamate involved in learning and memory. Excess quantities are thought to contribute to neurodegeneration.	Dizziness, headache, constipation, confusion
Galantamine (Razadyne)	Cholinesterase inhibitor Treats symptoms of *mild to moderate Alzheimer's*	Prevents the breakdown of acetylcholine (ACh), increasing concentration in the hippocampus and neocortex of brain (memory and cognitive functions); stimulates nicotinic receptors to release more ACh in brain	Nausea, vomiting, diarrhea, weight loss, loss of appetite, syncope, gastrointestinal hemorrhage
Rivastigmine (Exelon)	Cholinesterase inhibitor Treats symptoms of *mild to moderate Alzheimer's* disease (comes in patch form)	Prevents the breakdown of ACh and butyrylcholine (similar to acetylcholine) in the brain	Nausea, vomiting, diarrhea, weight loss, loss of appetite, muscle weakness, tremor, syncope bronchospasms, gastrointestinal hemorrhage
Donepezil (Aricept)	Cholinesterase inhibitor Treats symptoms of *mild to moderate and moderate to severe Alzheimer's disease*	Prevents the breakdown of a chemical called acetylcholine in the brain One daily dose at bedtime	Nausea, vomiting, diarrhea, insomnia, fatigue, muscle cramps, gastrointestinal hemorrhage
Namzaric	Combines memantine hydrochloride extended-release (ER) and donepezil hydrochloride Treats *moderate to severe Alzheimer's*	Donepezil: prevents the breakdown of acetylcholine Memantine: regulates glutamate	Same as memantine Same as donepezil

Data from WebMD. (2017). *Treatments for Alzheimer's disease.* Retrieved from https://www.webmd.com/alzheimers/guide/alzheimers-disease-treatment-overview#2

BOX 18.3 Can We Slow the Progression of Cognitive Decline? Potential for the Future

The *Finnish Geriatric Intervention Study to Prevent Cognitive Impairment and Disability* (FINGER study) was a 2-year study completed in 2015. This randomized controlled study examined whether cognitive decline could be prevented in older adults if interventions that addressed modifiable lifestyle risk factors were implemented. It examined the impact of physical activity, diet, vascular risk factors, and brain training. The intervention group underwent a program concentrating on four major areas (Hughes, 2015):

- *Physical exercise* based on international guidelines consisting of individually tailored programs for *regular progressive muscle strength training* and *aerobic exercise*
- *Nutritional advice* based on the Finnish Nutrition Recommendations delivered through individual sessions with a nutritionist
- *Cognitive training* consisting of 10 group sessions with a trained psychologist and 72 individual training sessions involving computer-based training
- *Management of metabolic and vascular risk factors* based on national guidelines. This included regular measurements of blood pressure, weight, BMI, and hip and waist circumference; physical examinations; and recommendations for lifestyle management. Study physicians did not prescribe medication but strongly recommended participants to contact their own physician or clinic if needed.

The 2-year findings indicated a beneficial intervention effect on overall cognitive performance in each of the cognitive domains of memory: executive function and psychomotor speed (Ngandu et al., 2015).

A follow-up study to be completed at a later date will evaluate whether the combined interventions of physical exercise, nutritional counseling and modification, cognitive and social stimulation, and improved self-management of medical comorbidities will demonstrate a benefit in cognitive function in older adults at increased risk of cognitive decline.

From Alzheimer's Association. (2017). *Alzheimer's Association launches $20 million lifestyle intervention trial in the U.S. to prevent cognitive decline.* Retrieved from https://www.alz.org/aaic/releases_2017/AAIC17-Wed-briefing-Developing-Topics.asp.

EVALUATION

Outcomes need to be stated in measurable terms, be within the capability of the patient, and be evaluated frequently. With a progressive disease, outcomes need to be altered to reflect the person's diminished functioning. Frequent re-evaluation of outcome criteria helps to diminish staff and family frustration. Evaluation of short-term goals minimizes the patient's anxiety by ensuring that tasks are not more complicated than the person can accomplish. Promoting the patient's optimal level of functioning and slowing further regression are useful goals to evaluate. Working closely with family members and providing them with the names of available resources may help increase the quality of life for both the family and the patient.

KEY POINTS TO REMEMBER

- *Neurocognitive disorder* (NCD) is a term that refers to disorders marked by disturbances in orientation, memory, intellect, judgment, and affect, resulting from structural changes in the brain.
- *Delirium, major neurocognitive disorders (dementia), mild neurocognitive disorders,* and *mild cognitive impairment* encompass the cognitive disorders discussed in this chapter.
- *Delirium* is marked by acute onset, disturbance in consciousness, and symptoms of disorientation and confusion that fluctuate throughout the day.
- *Delirium* is always secondary to an underlying condition; therefore it is transient, lasting from hours to days until the underlying cause is treated. If the cause is not treated, permanent damage to neurons can result.
- *Mild cognitive impairment (MCI)* is a syndrome in which there is a decline in the previous level of cognition but no significant impairment of functioning. Those with MCI are at greater risk of developing dementia.
- *Major neurocognitive disorders* and *mild neurocognitive disorders* (dementia) demonstrate degrees of functional impairment. These disorders usually have a more insidious onset than delirium. There is global deterioration of cognitive functioning, including memory, judgment, ability to think abstractly, and orientation, which is often progressive and irreversible.
- Dementia may be primary, which includes Alzheimer's disease, vascular dementia, Pick's disease, and Lewy body disease. In this case, the disease is irreversible. Secondary causes of dementia can frequently be reversed with treatment.
- *Alzheimer's disease (AD)* accounts for the majority of the dementias; vascular dementia is the second leading cause (APA, 2013).
- The exact cause of AD is not known. There are a number of risk factors, including advancing age, head trauma, cardiovascular disease, diabetes, lower educational levels, and the presence of apolipoprotein e4 (*APOE e4* allele), among others.
- There are four stages of AD that can overlap: stage 1 (mild), stage 2 (moderate), stage 3 (moderate to severe), and stage 4 (late).
- Major dysfunctional cognitive domains of AD include complex attention, executive functioning, learning and memory, language, perceptual-motor, and social cognition.
- There is no known cure for AD. Drugs that increase the brain's supply of acetylcholine may help slow the progression of the disease for a limited period of time.
- People with AD frequently present behavioral challenges to their families as well as to health care workers.
- Specific nursing, psychosocial, cognitive, and behavioral interventions for neurocognitively impaired individuals can facilitate communication, safety, and self-care, as well as minimize confusion.
- Because AD frequently creates a heavy burden on caregivers, nursing interventions must also address this population. Family teaching and community support are crucial.

APPLYING CRITICAL JUDGMENT

1. Mrs. Kendel is an 82-year-old woman who has progressive Alzheimer's disease (AD). She lives with her husband, who has been trying to care for her in their home. Mrs. Kendel often wears evening gowns in the morning, places her blouse on backward, and sometimes wears her bra backward outside her blouse. She often forgets the location of objects. She makes an effort to cook but often confuses frying pans and pots and sometimes has trouble turning on the stove. Once in a while, she cannot find the bathroom in time, often mistaking it for a broom closet. She becomes frightened of noises and is terrified when the telephone or doorbell rings. At times, she cries because she is aware that she is losing her sense of place in the world. She and her husband have always been close, loving companions, and he wants to keep her at home for as long as possible.
   - **A.** Help Mr. Kendel by making a list of suggestions that he can try at home that might help facilitate (a) communication, (b) activities of daily living, and (c) maintenance of a safe home environment.
   - **B.** Identify at least seven interventions that are appropriate to this situation for each of the areas cited in the question.
   - **C.** Identify possible resources available for maintaining Mrs. Kendel in her home for as long as possible. Provide the name of one self-help group that you would urge Mr. Kendel to join.
   - **D.** Share with your clinical group the name and function of at least three community agencies that could be an appropriate referral for someone in your neighborhood who is living with a family member with AD.

CHAPTER REVIEW QUESTIONS

1. While interacting with a 62-year-old adult diagnosed with a progressive neurocognitive disorder, the nurse observes that the adult has slow responses and difficulty finding the right words. What is the nurse's best initial action?
   - **a.** Suggest words that the adult may be trying to remember.
   - **b.** Ask the adult, "Are you having problems saying what you mean?"
   - **c.** Use silence to allow the adult an opportunity to compose responses.
   - **d.** Discontinue the interaction to prevent further frustration for the adult.
2. An adult diagnosed with stage 2 Alzheimer's disease begins a new prescription for rivastigmine (Exelon). Which nursing diagnosis has the highest priority to add to the plan of care?
   - **a.** Risk for constipation
   - **b.** Impared perception
   - **c.** Impared oral mucous membrane
   - **d.** Risk for impaired nutritional status
3. Which newly hospitalized patient should the nurse monitor closely for the development of delirium?
   - **a.** A 48-year-old who usually drinks a six-pack of beer daily
   - **b.** A 68-year-old who takes aspirin 650 mg twice daily for arthritic pain
   - **c.** A 72-year-old who says, "I have a glass of wine every evening to stimulate my appetite."
   - **d.** A 78-year-old diabetic whose blood glucose levels are consistently greater than 250 mg/dL
4. An 84-year-old tells the nurse, "I do four or five number puzzles every day to keep my brain healthy and sharp." When considering a holistic approach to maintaining mental health, the nurse should respond:
   - **a.** "It is more important for you to have physical activity every day."
   - **b.** "Let's think of some other activities we can add to your daily routine."

CHAPTER REVIEW QUESTIONS—CONT'D

c. "Repetition of the same activity is not helpful for keeping your brain healthy."
d. "There are some herbal preparations that will also help keep your brain sharp."

5. A family member asks the nurse, "I know my uncle's Alzheimer's disease has progressed, but is there any medication that can help him now?" Which response by the nurse is correct?
   a. "I'm sorry, but there are no medications that help with severe Alzheimer's disease."
   b. "Alzheimer's disease sometimes stabilizes. Let's hope that happens in this situation."
   c. "There are a few medications that may help. Let's discuss it with the health care provider."
   d. "It sounds like you're having difficulty accepting that your uncle's disease is irreversible. Would you like to talk about those feelings?"

REFERENCES

Agamanolis, D. P. (updated August 2016). Chapter 9 Degenerative Diseases; Neuropathology An illustrated interactive course for medical students and residents. http://neuropathology-web.org/chapter9/chapter9bad.html.

Alzheimer's Association. (n.d.). Cultural Competence. Alzheimer's Association. https://www.alz.org/Resources/Diversity/downloads/GEN_EDU-10steps.pdf.

Alzheimer's Association. (2017). Behaviors. Alzheimer's Association, RevJan17, 770-10-0021. https://www.alz.org/national/documents/brochure_behaviors.pdf.

Alzheimer's Association. (2018). Alzheimer's disease facts and figures. *Alzheimer's Dementia*, *14*(3), 367–429. Retrieved from: https://www.alz.org/facts/overview.asp.

American Geriatrics Society 2015 Beers Criteria Update Expert Panel. (2015). American Geriatrics Society 2015 updated Beers criteria for potentially inappropriate medication use in older adults. *Journal of the American Geriatrics Society*, *63*(11), 2227–2246.

American Nurses Association (ANA). (2016a). Delirium: A Nurse's Primer. Retrieved from: https://www.nursingworld.org/~4afe6a/globalassets/practiceandpolicy/innovation--evidence/deliriumprimer20160517rev2.pdf.

American Nurses Association (ANA) (2016b). Delirium Prevention Strategies. Retrieved from: https://www.nursingworld.org/practice-policy/work-environment/health-safety/delirium.

American Nurses Association (ANA) (2016c). Delirium: Prevent, identify, treat. Retrieved from: https://www.nursingworld.org/practice-policy/work-environment/health-safety/delirium/.

American Psychiatric Association. (2013). *Diagnostic and statistical manual of mental disorders (DSM-5)* (5th ed.). Washington, DC: APA.

Anderson, H. S., & Chawla, J. (2016). *Alzheimer disease clinical presentation.* Retrieved January 30, 2016, from http://emedicine.medscape.com/article/1134817-clinical#b3.

Boston University School of Medicine. (2018). Age, marital status, BMI and sleep associated with risk for dementia. *ScienceDaily*. Retrieved May 8, 2018 from www.sciencedaily.com/releases/2018/05/180508090715.htm.

Bull, M. (2015). Delirium. *American Nurse Today, 10*(10). Retrieved from https://www.americannursetoday.com/managing-delirium-hospitalized-older-adults/.

Burchum, J. R., & Rosenthal, L. D. (2016). *Lehne's Pharmacology for Nursing Care* (9th ed.). St. Louis: Elsevier.

Caughill, P. (2018). Deep brain stimulation therapy could help treat Alzheimer's. *Fururism*, February 4, 2018, Retrieved from: https://futurism.com/dementia-deep-brain-stimulation/.

Gatchel, J. R., Wright, C. I., Falk, W. E., et al. (2016). Dementia. In T. A. Stern, M. Fava, T. E. Wilens, & J. F. Rosenbaum (Eds.), *Massachusetts General Hospital comprehensive clinical psychiatry* (2nd ed.) (pp. 184–197). St. Louis: Elsevier.

Giddens, J. (2017). *Concepts for nursing practice* (2nd ed.). St. Louis: Elsevier.

Halter, M. (2018) *Varcarolis' foundations of psychiatric-mental health nursing* (8th ed.). St. Louis: Elsevier.

Hillman, A., & Latimer, J. (2017). Cultural representations of dementia. *PLoS Medicine, 14*(3), e1002274. https://doi.org/10.1371/journal.pmed.1002274.

Hughes, S. (2015). *Lifestyle changes can reduce cognitive decline.* Retrieved July 4, 2015, from http://www.medscape.org/viewarticle/842522.

Ijaopo, E. O. (2017). Dementia-related agitation: A review of non-pharmacological interventions and analysis of risks and benefits of pharmacotherapy. *Translational Psychiatry, 7*(10), e1250. http://doi.org/10.1038/tp.2017.199.

Institute of Medicine. (2015). *Cognitive aging: Progress in understanding and opportunity for action.* Washington, DC: The National Academies Press.

Kales, H. C., Gitlin, L. N., & Lyketsos, C. G. (2015). Assessment and management of behavioral and psychological symptoms of dementia. *British Medical Journal, 350*, h369. https://doi.org/10.1136/bmj.h369.

Mayo Clinic. (2017). Mild Cognitive Impairment. April 17, 2017. Retrieved from: https://www.mayoclinic.org/diseases-conditions/mild-cognitive-impairment/symptoms-causes/syc-20354578.

Mayo Clinic. (2018). Delirium. April 18 2018. Retrieved from: https://www.mayoclinic.org/diseases-conditions/delirium/symptoms-causes/syc-20371386.

Nakamura, A., et al. (2018). High performance plasma amyloid-β biomarkers for Alzheimer's disease. *Nature, 554*, 249–254. https://doi.org/10.1038/nature25456.

Ngandu, T., et al. (2015). A 2 year multidomain intervention of diet, exercise, cognitive training, and vascular risk monitoring versus control to prevent cognitive decline in at-risk elderly people (FINGER): A randomised controlled trial. *The Lancet, 385(9984)*, 2255–2263.

Ritter, A. R., Leger, G. C., Miller, J. B., & Banks, S. J. (2017). Neuropsychological testing in pathologically verified Alzheimer disease and frontotemporal dementia: How well do the uniform data set measures differentiate between diseases? *Alzheimer Disease and Associated Disorders, 31(3)*, 187–191. https://doi.org/10.1097/WAD.0000000000000181.

Sanabria-Castro, A., Alvarado-Echeverría, I., & Monge-Bonilla, C. (2017). Molecular pathogenesis of Alzheimer's disease: An update - fulltext. *The Annual Review of Neuroscience, 24*, 46–54. https://doi.org/10.1159/000464422.

Shwartz, S. K., Morris, R., & Penna, S. (2017). Psychometric properties of the Saint Louis University mental status examination. *Applied Neuropsychology: Adult*. https://doi.org/10.1080/23279095.2017.1362407.

UT Arlington. (2016). How the Nursing Industry Is Using Evidenced-based Practice to Reduce Alarm Fatigue. May 11, 2016. Retrieved from: https://academicpartnerships.uta.edu/articles/healthcare/how-the-nursing-industry-is-using-evidenced-based-practice-to-reduce-alarm-fatigue.aspx.

Woods, B., O'Philbin, L., Farrell, E. M., Spector, A. E., & Orrell, M. (2018). Reminiscence therapy for dementia. *Cochrane Database of Systematic Reviews*, 3, CD001120. DOI: 10.1002/14651858.CD001120.pub3.

Zhu, X.-C., Tan, L., Wang, H.-F., Jiang, T., Cao, L., Wang, C., & Yu, J.-T. (2015). Rate of early onset Alzheimer's disease: a systematic review and meta-analysis. *Annals of Translational Medicine*, *3*(3), 38. https://doi.org/10.3978/j.issn.2305-5839.2015.01.19.

19

Substance-Related and Addictive Disorders

Lorraine Chiappetta, Elizabeth M. Varcarolis

http://evolve.elsevier.com/Varcarolis/essentials

OBJECTIVES

1. Identify the 11 diagnostic criteria for **substance use disorder (SUD)** according to the *Diagnostic and Statistical Manual of Mental Disorders,* 5th edition *(DSM-5).*
2. Describe the neurobiological brain changes that occur with addiction. Include the neurotransmitters that enhance the progression of these disorders.
3. Compare predisposing factors associated with the development of an SUD.
4. Identify components of the assessment process that will enable the nurse to provide patient-centered care for an individual with an SUD. **QSEN: Patient-Centered Care**
5. List the signs and symptoms of intoxication, overdose, and withdrawal for alcohol use and opioid use disorders.
6. Identify evidence-based practice interventions that facilitate safe and effective care for individuals with signs and symptoms of intoxication, overdose, and withdrawal. **QSEN: Safety; Evidence-Based Practice**
7. Describe components of interprofessional and intraprofessional teamwork and collaboration that facilitate the short-term and long-term treatment of individuals with an SUD. **QSEN: Teamwork and Collaboration**
8. Identify legal and ethical issues related to SUDs in the nursing profession.
9. Using informatics, identify pharmacological interventions used to facilitate safe withdrawal and to help individuals remain in recovery. **QSEN: Informatics**
10. Identify the principles of the recovery model and how it can be applied to an individual with an SUD.

KEY TERMS AND CONCEPTS

addiction, p. 302
Al-Anon, p. 326
Alateen, p. 326
Alcoholics Anonymous (AA), p. 325
alcohol use disorder (AUD), p. 304
alternative-to-discipline (ADT) programs, p. 320
amotivational syndrome, p. 304
antagonistic effects, p. 309
bath salts, p. 317
blood alcohol concentration (BAC), p. 310
cathinone, p. 317
club drugs, p. 316
cognitive impairment, p. 304
cross-tolerance, p. 307
dual diagnosis, p. 309
e-cigarette, p. 305
enabling, p. 326
flashbacks, p. 309
medication-assisted treatment (MAT), p. 312
motivational interviewing, p. 323
relapse prevention, p. 322
SMART Recovery, p. 325
stigma, p. 303
substance use disorder (SUD), p. 303
substance-induced disorder (SIDs),p. 303
synergistic effects, p. 309
tolerance, p. 306
toxicology screen, p. 318
withdrawal, p. 309

CONCEPT: SPIRITUALITY: *Spirituality* refers to a person's quality of life, health, and sense of wholeness and includes the connection of mind, body, and spirit. Spirituality often includes love, caring, and compassion (Giddens, 2017). For many individuals, *spirituality* is an essential component of recovery from addiction.

INTRODUCTION

Mind-altering substances have been used since ancient times. There is evidence as early as 8000 BC that mead was brewed from fermented honey and was perhaps the first known alcoholic beverage. Today many drugs that are misused are produced in a chemistry lab, making them more toxic, more dangerous, and more addictive.

The use of psychoactive drugs extends across social and economic boundaries. The degree to which drugs are accepted or rejected varies among cultures. Psychoactive substances like alcohol, nicotine, and caffeine are culturally accepted for use by adults in most segments of American society. There are, however, religions and other cultural groups that do not condone the use of alcohol or other drugs as a social practice. Marijuana is another psychoactive drug that is accepted for both recreational and medicinal purposes by some and considered unacceptable and even illegal by other groups.

An unfortunate consequence of the use of psychoactive substances is that it can lead to addiction. **Addiction** is a chronic, relapsing **brain**

disease characterized by compulsive drug-seeking behavior motivated by cravings, despite harmful consequences, and by long-lasting changes in the brain (American Psychiatric Association [APA], 2013).

The treatment of this **brain disorder** is complicated by misconceptions and stigma. Stigma describes the powerful, negative perceptions commonly associated with substance misuse and addiction. These preconceived generalities are rarely based on *factual* information. The most common *myth* is that those who misuse drugs are weak-willed individuals who are lacking morals and self-respect. Addiction isn't a choice about something that is easy to just stop. In a national survey, more than half of those surveyed believed that people with alcohol and drug addiction were likely to be violent toward others, which is another myth (Fletcher, 2015).

Stigma is perpetuated by the continued use of derogatory terms such as *junkie, alcoholic,* or *crackhead* for those with a disease. Thoughts, feelings, and labels can create and perpetuate stigma. Even the term *substance* (drug and alcohol) *abuse* has come to have a derogatory meaning. The current version (5th edition) of the *Diagnostic and Statistical Manual of Mental Disorders* (*DSM-5*; APA, 2013) eliminated the use of this word from its diagnostic categories, but the word persists in the public's mind. In this chapter, a conscious attempt has been made to stop using stigmatizing language like *abuse* so that nurses and other health professionals can move past misperceptions and prejudices to support people with these diseases. An understanding of the neurobiological underpinnings of these brain disorders may also decrease the stigma associated with these diseases.

The *DSM-5* (APA, 2013) has combined multiple related disorders under the heading of "Substance-Related and Addictive Disorders." Substance-related disorders are divided into substance use disorders and substance-induced disorders. The addictive disorders category encompasses non–substance-related disorders.

SUBSTANCE USE DISORDER

The essential features of the diagnosis of substance use disorder (SUD) include "a cluster of cognitive, behavioral and physiological symptoms indicating that the individual continues using the substance despite significant substance related problems" (APA, 2013, p. 483). The diagnosis can be applied to various substances: alcohol, cannabis, hallucinogens (phencyclidine or similarly acting drugs), other hallucinogens (e.g., lysergic acid diethylamide [LSD]), inhalants, opioids, sedatives, hypnotics, anxiolytics, stimulants (including amphetamine-type substances, cocaine, and other stimulants), tobacco, and "other" substances. Caffeine use is not included in the SUD category, but there are caffeine-related disorders listed in the *DSM-5*.

All drugs that are taken in excess share a common direct activation of the brain reward system. This activation, commonly described as feeling "high," is so intense that it can lead to the continued use of these drugs despite negative consequences. Because so many of these drugs lead to physical addiction, another reason there is continued use (especially with addiction to opioids) is to prevent becoming "dope sick" or feeling the disturbing effects of withdrawal. In SUDs, there is an underlying change in brain circuits that may persist beyond detoxification. This accounts for the frequent relapses associated with these disorders (APA, 2013).

Substance-induced disorders (SIDs) can include intoxication (use); withdrawal for some categories of drugs; and other substance-/medication-induced disorders, like psychosis or delirium.

Gambling disorder and Internet gaming disorder are two non–substance-related addictions included in the *DSM-5* (APA, 2013). This reflects the evidence that gambling behavior activates similar reward systems in the brain.

There are certain excessive behaviors that have been described as behavioral addictions, such as Internet gaming addictions, sex addictions, shopping addiction, exercise addiction, and so forth. Currently, there is insufficient evidence to establish a clear diagnostic category for these excessive behaviors (APA, 2013). These *excessive behaviors* can lead to real dysfunction in some individuals.

In 2018 the World Health Organization (WHO) released a new edition of its *International Classification of Diseases,* the ICD-11. It added a new diagnosis of "gaming disorder" under addictive disorders. It is defined as impaired control over digital or video gaming for at least a year, leading to adverse effects on personal health and overall function (Cassoobhoy, 2018). In the *DSM-5,* Internet gaming disorder is identified as a condition for further study (APA, 2013).

Prevalence and Comorbidity

The lifetime prevalence rate of people in the United States who have used illicit drugs is high, with alcohol being the drug most used. Marijuana use has the next highest rate, followed in order by cocaine, LSD, ecstasy, methamphetamine, crack, and heroin. In 2015 alone, almost 500 new psychoactive substances with the potential to be misused were introduced worldwide. The *use* of any psychoactive drug significantly increases a person's risk of developing a substance-related *disorder.*

Statistics on the incidence of SUDs are as follows (American Addiction Centers, 2017):

- Alcohol is the addictive substance most used/misused in America.
- Of American adults, 16.6 million battled an alcohol use disorder in 2013.
- Of Americans aged 12 and older, 586,000 struggled with a heroin use disorder.
- Over 900,000 American adults (over age 11) struggled with a cocaine use disorder in 2014.
- Heroin misuse and addiction have risen in all population and demographic groups in the United States over the past few years.
- Over 2 million Americans over the age of 11 struggled with an opioid pain reliever use disorder in 2014.
- Of American adults (over the age of 11), 4.2 million battled a marijuana use disorder in 2014.

The incidence for specific populations is as follows:

Adolescents (ages 12 to 17):

- Of the American adolescent population, 5% suffers from a substance use disorder; this equates to 1.3 million teens, or 1 in 12.
- Of American adolescents, 700,000 battled an alcohol use disorder in 2013.

Young adults (ages 18 to 25):

- Of American young adults, 1 in 6 battled an SUD in 2014.
- Heroin addiction has doubled in the past 10+ years in this population.

Elderly:

- Up to 15% of elderly individuals suffer from problems with substance misuse and addiction.
- Over 3% of the older adult population struggles with an alcohol use disorder.

Gender:

- In 2013, U.S. adult men struggled with an alcohol use disorder at rates double those of U.S. women.

Ethnicity/Race:

- Native American and Alaska natives: 14.3% in 2014
- Native Hawaiians and other Pacific Islanders: 11.3% in 2014
- Hispanic and Caucasians: 8.5% in 2013
- African Americans: 7.4% in 2013

Other:

- About half of the population of American prisons and jails suffers from addiction.

There is a disconnect between those needing treatment and those who receive treatment (Lipari, Park-Lee, & Van Horn, 2016).

Classified as needing treatment (in 2015)	DID NOT receive treatment in a specialty facility (%)
1 in 20 adolescents (ages 12–17)	93.7
1 in 6 young adults (ages 18–25)	92.3
1 in 14 adults (ages 26+)	87.7

This huge gap in the prevalence of the disease and appropriate treatment for the disease is closely related to both lack of adequate facilities and because many individuals who meet the criteria for SUDs do not perceive themselves as needing treatment.

The consequences of SUDs can be costly because they are often associated with multiple negative outcomes, including involvement with the justice system, increased incidence of chronic health conditions, and poorer health outcomes leading to earlier death. According to the Centers for Disease Control and Prevention (CDC, 2018b), excessive drinking is responsible for 1 in 10 deaths among adults aged 20 to 64 years.

Alcohol use disorder (AUD) is the most common substance use problem in the United States. It involves a "problematic pattern of alcohol use" (APA, 2013, p. 490) leading to some type of impairment or distress. According to the *DSM-5* (APA, 2013), the diagnosis is made if a person has at least 2 of the 11 symptoms listed. AUD can be thought of as a spectrum disorder in which there is a mild (two or three symptoms), moderate (four or five symptoms), and severe (six or more symptoms) level of severity. According to a CDC fact sheet, "binge drinking is the most common pattern of excessive alcohol use in the United States" (CDC, 2018a).

WHO IS A HEAVY DRINKER?: When we really start to think about drinking, we need to know what "too much" actually looks like. "At-risk" drinking is alcohol consumption that exceeds the recommended daily limits:

- **For men:** More than 4 standard drinks on any 1 day, or more than 14 standard drinks in any 1 week.
- **For women:** More than 3 standard drinks on any 1 day, or more than 7 standard drinks in any 1 week.

Psychiatric Comorbidity

There is a high rate of substance use disorders *co-occurring* with a psychiatric disorder. Patients with a mental disorder have a 50% to 60% higher chance of having an AUD than the general population (Black & Andreasen, 2014). And up to 50% of those with an SUD have a co-occurring psychiatric disorder (Sadock, Sadock, & Ruiz, 2015). It is not entirely clear why this occurs. One hypothesis states that the excessive use of drugs brings out symptoms of another mental disorder in vulnerable individuals. Another suggests that mental disorders lead to drug use as a means of "self-medication" to relieve symptoms of that mental disorder. Other hypotheses identify overlapping genetic vulnerabilities; overlapping environmental triggers, such as acute trauma; and abnormalities in similar brain regions as shared risk factors for the development of both types of disorders. A developmental hypothesis suggests that early drug use in the still-developing brain of an adolescent causes dramatic developmental brain changes that increase the risk for mental disorders (McCance-Katz, 2018).

The most common mental disorders associated with SUDs are anxiety disorders, posttraumatic stress disorders, depressive disorders, mania, and schizophrenia. Of individuals with an SUD, 35% to 50% meet the criteria for antisocial personality disorder (Sadock et al., 2015). Other common co-occurring psychiatric disorders include acute and chronic **cognitive impairment**, or changes in the ability to remember, learn, concentrate, or make decisions.

Suicide risk increases significantly among individuals who misuse alcohol and/or drugs and is about 10% higher than in the general population. This may be related to the decreased judgment associated with using psychoactive drugs. There is a 15% higher suicide rate for those who are addicted to alcohol (Sadock et al., 2015).

Marijuana is of particular interest when looking at comorbidity with mental disorders. This drug impairs short-term memory and judgment and distorts perception, which can impair performance in school or at work. Some chronic users of marijuana develop a *loss of motivation* with heavy use. Labeled **amotivational syndrome**, this syndrome is characterized by apathy, loss of achievement motivation, decrease in productivity, difficulty with learning and memory, impaired concentration, lack of personal hygiene, and preoccupation with the drug. It also may negatively affect the still-maturing brain of the adolescent/young adult. It has been suggested that there is a loss of IQ with chronic use. The full extent of the negative and long-lasting effects on cognitive and social development from chronic use by adolescents is still being studied. Several studies have linked early and excessive marijuana use to increased risk for developing psychiatric disorders, including psychosis, in susceptible individuals (National Institute on Drug Abuse [NIDA], 2018c).

There are additional problematic behaviors frequently associated with SUDs. These include an increased risk for harm toward others; increased risk for accidents, including (driving under the influence DUI); and other examples of poor judgment while intoxicated.

Medical Comorbidity

A medical history, physical examination, and laboratory tests are used to gather data about drug-related physical problems. The extent of physical impairment depends on individual susceptibility as well as the amount of drug used, the specific drug used, and the route of administration. All body systems are potentially affected.

Alcohol. Because alcohol use is the most prevalent drug used, *alcohol-related medical problems* are the comorbidities most commonly seen in medical settings. Alcohol-related disorders of the *gastrointestinal system* include esophagitis, gastritis, pancreatitis, alcoholic hepatitis, and cirrhosis of the liver. *Excessive alcohol use* can raise the levels of triglycerides in the blood and lead to stroke, cardiomyopathy, cardiac dysrhythmia, and sudden cardiac death (WebMD Medical Reference, 2017). Communicable diseases like tuberculosis are increased in those who use alcohol.

Excessive alcohol use damages the nervous system and the brain. The **cerebral cortex**, which is responsible for higher brain functions, problem solving, and decision making, is especially vulnerable. The **hippocampus**, which is the center of memory and learning, is also affected, as well as the **cerebellum**, which helps coordinate our movements.

Specific disorders that involve the brain and central nervous system include **Wernicke–Korsakoff's syndrome**, two different constellations of neurological symptoms caused by thiamine (B_1) deficiency. Chronic alcohol use affects thiamine uptake and utilization, leading to the disorder. Although chronic alcohol use is the most common cause of Wernicke–Korsakoff's syndrome, there are other diseases that can lead to this syndrome.

Wernicke's encephalopathy is a neurological disorder marked by *acute/subacute confusional states*, abnormal eye movements (nystagmus), and unsteady gait (ataxia). Wernicke's encephalopathy is a medical emergency that causes life-threatening brain disruption. When treated early it is often reversible, but without treatment, it can lead to chronic dementia and/or death.

Korsakoff's psychosis (Korsakoff's syndrome) refers to *a chronic neurological condition* marked by difficulty/inability to learn new information and remember recent events and the development of long-term memory gaps. Although memory problems are specifically evidenced, other thinking and social skills may be relatively unaffected.

Frequent and excessive alcohol use can also lead to **peripheral neuropathy** resulting from damaged peripheral nerves. Symptoms include sensory (numbness and pain) and motor symptoms (weakness) of the lower extremities.

Central Nervous System Stimulants. **Cocaine** users may experience extreme weight loss and malnutrition, myocardial infarction, brain damage, and stroke. **Methamphetamine** users have an increased risk for hypothermia, seizures, brain damage, kidney damage, stroke, and death. Severe malnutrition, weight loss, and tooth decay are also frequently seen. Long-term use of these stimulants can lead to paranoia, suicidal depression when the drug is stopped, and permanent psychosis.

Nicotine. Cigarette smoking remains the greatest single cause of preventable illness and premature death (Burchum & Rosenthal, 2016). Cigarette smoke contains the psychoactive drug **nicotine** plus more than 7000 chemicals; 70 of those cause cancer (American Cancer Society, 2015; CDC, 2017). Nicotine addiction is high in all groups of people with other SUDs, as well as in those with mental illness. At least 20% of the U.S. population meets the criteria for tobacco use disorder, and nicotine causes 443,000 deaths a year (Burchum & Rosenthal, 2016). In the United States, one in five deaths is caused by tobacco use, and on average, smokers die 10 years earlier than nonsmokers (Jha et al., 2013).

Smoking tobacco can cause chronic lung disease, coronary heart disease, chronic obstructive pulmonary disease (COPD), and stroke, as well as cancer of the lungs, larynx, esophagus, mouth, and bladder. Approximately 50% of Americans who do *not* smoke are exposed to secondhand smoke (SHS), which is also a disease-causing agent. Chewing tobacco increases a person's risk of oral cancer.

Although the rate of cigarette smoking is tapering off, the use of electronic cigarettes (**e-cigarettes**), sometimes called "vaping," is exploding. E-cigarettes contain both nicotine and potentially other toxic ingredients like formaldehyde and acetaldehyde. One study found that high-voltage vaping released enough formaldehyde-containing compounds to increase a person's lifetime risk of cancer 5 to 15 times higher than the risk caused by long-term smoking (Thompson, 2015). In May of 2016, the U.S. Food and Drug Administration (FDA) banned the sale of e-cigarettes to Americans under 18 (United States Food and Drug Administration [FDA], 2020).

Anabolic-Androgenic Steroids. The physiologic effects of chronic *anabolic-androgenic steroids (AASs)* use can be serious and permanent. Disorders include liver damage, renal failure, myocardial infarction, elevated cholesterol levels, and serious depression, especially in withdrawal. Some of the untoward effects of steroid use in men are shrinking of the testicles, infertility, development of breasts, and increased risk for prostate cancer. Women often show male-pattern baldness, changes in menstrual cycle, growth of facial hair, and a deepening of the voice. Stunting of growth attributable to premature skeletal maturation and accelerated pubertal changes can occur in adolescents using AASs (NIDA, 2016a). Research also suggests that users may experience paranoia, jealousy, delusions, and violent mood swings (NIDA, 2016a).

Route of Ingestion. The route of drug administration influences medical complications and affects addictive potential. Drugs such as cocaine, steroids, and heroin can be injected intradermally; subcutaneously, known as "skin-popping"; and intramuscularly. The areas of injection can become scarred, and lesions or abscesses start to form. Local skin and systemic life-threatening infections can result. **Intravenous (IV) drug use** leads to a higher incidence of infections, venous sclerosis, and contraction of human immunodeficiency virus/acquired immunodeficiency syndrome (HIV/AIDS) and hepatitis. Splinter hemorrhages in the fingernails are a sign of endocarditis, which is associated with IV drug use. **Intranasal use** (called **"snorting"**) may lead to chronic sinusitis and a perforated nasal septum. **Smoking** a substance increases the likelihood of respiratory tract problems. Smoked, snorted, and injected drugs all enter the brain within seconds, producing a powerful rush of pleasure that lasts a short period of time, necessitating taking more of the drug more often to recapture the "high." See to Table 19.1 for a description of physical complications associated with various classes of drugs and their routes of administration.

Theory

The individual variation in a person's susceptibility to becoming addicted supports the premise that genetic/biological variations and sociocultural influences all play a role in addiction.

The Neurobiology of Addiction

Three areas of the brain are necessary for life-sustaining functions and at the same time enhance the compulsive drug use that marks addiction (NIDA, 2014):

- **Brainstem**—controls basic functions such as heart rate, breathing, and sleeping.
- **Limbic system**—contains the brain's "reward circuit" that links brain structures controlling feelings of pleasure. It is this phenomenon that motivates us to repeat behaviors that cause pleasure and support survival, such as eating and sex. Along with positive activation for feelings of pleasure, the limbic system is also activated by alcohol and drug use.
- **Cerebral cortex**—includes areas that process information from our senses. One of the most important areas in the cerebral cortex is the forebrain or frontal cortex. The frontal cortex allows us to think, plan, solve problems, and make decisions.

Neurotransmitters

There are many different chemicals in the brain that function as neurotransmitters, but those listed in Table 19.2 do most of the work.

Most psychoactive drugs directly or indirectly target the brain's reward system by flooding the circuit with dopamine. The reward system consists of the ventral tegmental area (VTA), the nucleus accumbens, and part of the cerebral cortex. Dopamine is the neurotransmitter present in regions of the brain that regulate movement, emotion, motivation, and most importantly, feelings of pleasure. When activated at normal levels, this system rewards our natural behaviors, like eating and enjoying sex, so that we repeat these natural and life-sustaining activities by associating them with pleasure. When the system is activated, we *remember* the associated activity as pleasurable and *"learn"* to repeat the behaviors over and over again.

Overstimulating the system with drugs produces an enhanced euphoric effect. We *remember* the effect of the drug, and it *teaches* us to want to repeat use of the drug. Psychoactive drugs tend to release much

TABLE 19.1 Physical Complications Related to Drug Use

Drug	Route	Physical Complications
Heroin	Injected, snorted, or smoked	Chronic constipation Pneumonia Pregnancy: neonatal abstinence syndrome (NAS) From nonsterile technique for any IV drug use: • Endocarditis (infection of the heart lining and valves) • Hepatitis C • Human immunodeficiency virus (HIV) and other blood-borne viruses • Pulmonary complications • Skin infections and abscesses • Scarred or collapsed veins
Marijuana	Smoked, eaten in food	Osteoporosis Respiratory problems (lung infections, acute/chronic chest illnesses) Gynecomastia Impaired immune system Pregnancy: neurological problems in children Increased risk for heart attack and testicular cancer Cannabinoid hyperemesis syndrome—acute severe vomiting
Nicotine	Smoked, chewed	Respiratory problems (lung infections, acute/chronic chest illnesses) Cancers of lungs, mouth, throat Cardiovascular disease and hypertension
Stimulants, including cocaine and methamphetamines	Intravenous Smoked Intranasally	Previously listed IV use complications Respiratory paralysis/arrest Cardiovascular collapse Hyperpyrexia Perforated nasal septum
PCP	Ingested	Respiratory arrest Insensitivity to painful stimuli during use
Inhalants	Sniffed/snorted Huffed (inhaling vapors)	Loss of sense of smell Hearing loss Liver, lung, and kidney problems Tachycardia Neurotoxic symptoms Muscle wasting Accidental suffocation due to method of administration (plastic bag or inhalant-soaked rag over mouth)

Modified from National Institute on Drug Abuse (NIDA). (2017). *Commonly abused drugs.* Retrieved from www.drugabuse.gov/researchers.

more dopamine than natural rewards. The enhanced pleasurable sensation (reward) strongly motivates (teaches) people to want to repeat the use of the drug. This explains the strong desire for repeated use of psychoactive drugs.

With long-term exposure to psychoactive drugs, the brain changes over time. The brain adapts (adjusts) to the surges of dopamine (and other neurotransmitters) by synthesizing less dopamine or by reducing the number of receptors. In fact, with long-term drug use, "natural" dopamine's impact on the reward system can become abnormally low. A person's ability to experience any pleasure is then greatly reduced. Now the person's brain needs a drug to feel "normal," and larger amounts of the drug are needed to get that familiar dopamine "high." The need for larger amounts to get the same effect is called **tolerance**.

Additional changes also occur in neurons and brain circuits. When the concentration of glutamate is altered, adaptations in habit and conscious memory systems can occur. An example of this occurs when *cues* in a person's daily routine, like being in a bar, become associated with the drug experience. Even in the absence of the drug, exposure to these *cues* can trigger uncontrollable cravings. This is why people in recovery are encouraged to stay away from places that remind them of previous drug use (NIDA, 2014). In summary, drug use can change the brain to such an extent that a person can no longer experience (usual) pleasure without the drug. Sometimes the drug is needed to just feel normal again. Even the memory of *using* can trigger an incredible desire to *use* again because of these brain changes. It is these powerful alterations in the brain that make addiction so hard to overcome.

Opioids are chemically similar to naturally occurring *endorphins.* Both opioids and endorphins help reduce pain and produce a euphoric effect by acting upon several different opioid receptors in the brain. The long-term use of opioids can lead to brain changes, including synthesizing less of the naturally occurring endorphins and reducing opioid receptors. The person now needs the opioid to feel "normal." This can lead to addiction. Approximately 80% of current heroin users got started by first misusing prescription opioids (Scholastic, 2016). In addition, 69.5% of more than 67,000 drug overdose deaths in 2018 involved an opioid (CDC, 2020).

Alcohol and other central nervous system (CNS) depressants act on GABA receptors. This finding helps explain the cross-tolerance

TABLE 19.2 Functions Affected by Drugs and Neurotransmitters

Neurotransmitter	Functions Affected	Drugs That Affect Functions
Inhibitory Neurotransmitters		
Gamma-aminobutyric acid (GABA)	Slows neural activity Anxiety Memory Anesthesia	Sedatives, hypnotics, alcohol
Serotonin	Mood Sleep Sexual desire Appetite	MDMA (ecstasy), LSD, cocaine
Acetylcholine	Memory Arousal Attention Mood	Nicotine
Endogenous opioids (endorphins and enkephalin)	Analgesia, sedation Reward/pleasure Mood	Heroin, morphine, prescription painkillers (oxycodone)
Endogenous cannabinoids (anandamide)	Movement Cognition and memory	Marijuana
Excitatory Neurotransmitters		
Dopamine (Dopamine neurotransmitters can be both inhibitory or excitatory.)	Pleasure/reward Movement Attention Memory	All psychoactive drugs directly or indirectly increase dopamine.
Norepinephrine (noradrenaline)	Sensory processing Movement Sleep Mood Memory Anxiety	Stimulants: Cocaine Methamphetamine Amphetamines
Glutamate	Increased neuron activity Learning Cognition Memory	Ketamine Phencyclidine (PCP) Alcohol

Adapted from Sherman, C. (2017). *Impacts of drugs on neurotransmission.* Retrieved from https://www.drugabuse.gov/news-events/nida-notes/2017/03/impacts-drugs-neurotransmission

effects that occur when alcohol use is combined with other CNS depressants like benzodiazepines. **Cross-tolerance** occurs when one builds up a tolerance for one drug while also building up a tolerance for another drug *in the same or a chemically similar class of drugs*.

Cocaine and amphetamines act on the dopamine and serotonin systems, producing an intense rush followed by intense lows, reinforcing compulsive use. These two drugs also share the same receptors and are cross-tolerant.

Genetic Factors

Genetic factors are believed to account for between 40% and 60% of a person's vulnerability to addiction (Black & Andreasen, 2014). AUD is three to four times more likely to occur in children of parents with an AUD. Currently, molecular genetic techniques are being employed to define alcohol-related genes.

Recent research has identified specific gene alleles believed to be risk factors for cannabis dependence (Hand, 2016). There is also some evidence for genetic factors that can link the comorbidity of cannabis dependence with major depression and the risk of developing schizophrenia (Hand, 2016).

Psychosocial and Cultural Risk Factors

Significant risk factors for substance use disorders include the following adverse childhood experiences (ACEs):

- Physical, sexual, or emotional abuse and neglect
- Witnessing violence in the home (partner or parent)
- Substance misuse or mental illness in the home
- Parental separation or incarcerated household member (Substance Abuse and Mental Health Services Administration [SAMHSA], 2017a)

Szalavitz (2015) cites a study that found that those with four or more ACEs have a risk of alcoholism that is seven times greater than those with none. Similarly, boys who have four or more ACEs are nearly five times more likely to inject drugs than those with none.

Neurochemistry of Addiction (e.g. Heroin Use An Epidemic), and the Role of Naloxone

When a person injects, smokes, or snorts heroin/opioid the drug travels quickly to the brain through the bloodstream. In the brain, the heroin is converted to morphine by enzymes. Morphine binds to opiate receptors in certain areas within the reward pathway including the VTA, nucleus accumbens, and cortex. Morphine also binds to areas involved in the pain pathway (including the thalamus, brainstem, and spinal cord).

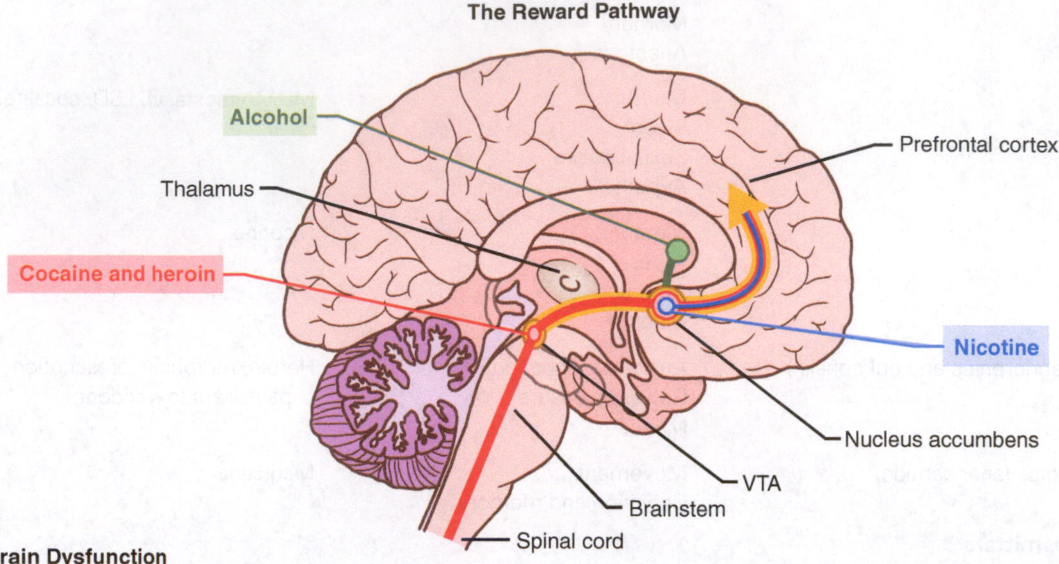

Brain Dysfunction

Tolerance: the analgesic (pain reducing) properties of heroin or morphine no longer respond to the drug in the initial way. Tolerance occurs in the pain passage pathway that includes the thalamus and the spinal cord. These areas are important in sending pain messages and are responsible for the analgesic effects of morphine. However a person does not develop tolerance to the respiratory depressive effects of heroin/morphine.
When morphine binds to opiate receptors, it inhibits an enzyme, adenylate cyclase, that coordinates the firing of impulses. After repeated opiate receptor activation by morphine, the enzyme adapts so that the morphine can no longer cause changes in cell firing.

Addiction: develops when the neurons adapt to exposure of the drug and only function normally in the presence of the drug. Many of the heroin or morphine withdrawal symptoms are generated when the opiate receptors in the thalamus and brainstem are deprived of morphine. Withdrawal can be very serious and the abuser will use the drug again to avoid the syndrome.

Naloxone's Reversal of Opioid Overdose: Overdose is particularly lethal due to respiratory depression. To reduce deaths from overdose naloxone (trade name Narcan) is being increasingly used by both health care providers and the general public. This drug is a pure opioid antagonist with no pharmacological properties. After intravenous, subcutaneous, and intramuscular injection it temporarily (1-2 hours) binds with them. Its binding ability is stronger than morphine's so it can push the morphine off and reverse the effects of morphine. A nasal spray formulation is currently available.

Other risk factors include the following:

- Genetic predisposition to addiction or exposure to alcohol prenatally
- Inadequate parental supervision
- Racism
- Lack of economic opportunity
- Poor self-image, self-control, or social competence
- Lack of employment and neighborhood poverty
- Peer-group behavior

Women are diagnosed with SUDs at lower rates than men, although that trend may be changing. Unfortunately, girls and young women become addicted faster and are apt to suffer the consequences of substance use more rapidly than boys and young men.

In East Asian cultures, the prevalence rate for AUDs is believed to be less. In approximately half of the East Asian population, a response that includes severe flushing and palpitations may occur when alcohol is consumed. The reaction is the result of an accumulation of acetaldehyde, a by-product of the metabolism of alcohol. These individuals have a deficiency of acetaldehyde dehydrogenase, the chemical that breaks down acetaldehyde. This reaction is thought to be effective in preventing many Asians from drinking.

Effects of Substance Use in Pregnancy

Alcohol

Alcohol is a teratogenic (causing birth defects) substance. Drinking alcohol during pregnancy can have physical, mental, and behavioral consequences for the unborn child. Alcohol intake can also cause miscarriage, preterm birth, and stillbirth. Alcohol interferes with the ability of the fetus to receive enough oxygen and nourishment for normal cell development in the brain as well as other organs. The American College of Obstetricians and Gynecologists and the CDC state that there is *no safe amount of alcohol* to drink during pregnancy and recommend total restriction of alcohol during the entire pregnancy (Cohen, 2015). The end of the first trimester is the most vulnerable time for the fetus (Nakhoul et al., 2017). **Fetal alcohol syndrome (FAS)** is the most extreme example of the toxic effect of alcohol on fetal development and is the most common cause of mental retardation (Acharya & Issacs, 2017). Slightly less severe are the fetal alcohol spectrum disorders (FASDs).

The three criteria of FAS are mental retardation, delayed growth and development, and distinctive facial abnormalities. FAS and FASD are lifelong conditions that result in permanent physical disabilities (hearing, eyesight, facial abnormalities, organ deformities, cardiac defects, spinal defects, urogenital defects), mental disabilities (mental retardation, learning disabilities, memory impairment, CNS handicaps), and behavioral problems (hyperactivity, poor impulse control, irritability, criminal behavior) (Acharya & Issacs, 2017).

Nicotine

Women who smoke cigarettes prenatally deliver babies who are twice as likely to be low birth weight and who have increased risk of developmental issues (cerebral palsy, learning disabilities), congenital abnormalities, and respiratory tract problems. Parental prenatal smoking is believed to increase the risk for sudden infant death syndrome (SIDS). *Secondhand smoke* exposure is also thought to increase the risk of SIDS, respiratory tract problems, ear infections, and acute asthma in infants and children (American Cancer Society, 2015).

Opioids

Mothers who take **opiates** during pregnancy are more likely to experience intrauterine fetal and newborn infant death. Infants born to opiate-dependent mothers may also be addicted at birth and experience withdrawal symptoms, called **neonatal abstinence syndrome**. The incidence of this disorder continues to increase.

Common symptoms of the disorder include the following:

- CNS irritability: high-pitched cry, tremors and jitters, convulsions
- Gastrointestinal: loss of appetite, vomiting, diarrhea, dehydration
- Fever, mottled skin, and possible death

Milder cases can last up to 5 days. The long-term effects are variable but may include poor social engagement, shorter attention span, and more difficulty with motor development (Maryland Recovery, 2017).

Phenomena Observed in Substance Use Disorders

The nurse needs to be familiar with the following phenomena when working with patients with substance use problems:

- **Blackouts:** amnesia for the events of any parts of a drinking episode without loss of consciousness.
- **Intoxication:** a transient condition following the administration of alcohol or other psychoactive substance that results in disturbances in the level of consciousness, cognition, perception, affect or behavior, or other psychophysiological functions and responses (WHO, 2018).
- **Tolerance**: the need for higher and higher doses of a substance to achieve the desired effect.
- **Cross-tolerance:** a phenomenon that occurs when tolerance to the effects of a certain drug produces tolerance to another drug (e.g., a person who drinks heavily may require higher doses of a benzodiazepine like lorazepam to obtain sufficient antianxiety effects).
- **Withdrawal** symptoms: these occur after an extended period of continued use and signify *physical dependence.* Withdrawal occurs "when blood or tissue concentration of a substance declines in an individual who has maintained prolonged heavy use of the substance" (APA, 2013, p. 484). When a substance is stopped or reduced, drug-specific identifiable physical and psychological signs and symptoms occur.
- **Synergistic effects**: interactions between two or more *drugs* that cause the total effect of the combined *drugs* to be greater than the sum of the individual effects of each *drug.* For example, taking two CNS depressants together, such as alcohol and benzodiazepines, results in a far greater degree of CNS depression than just the sum of the effects of each. Many unintentional overdose deaths have resulted from this synergistic effect.
- **Cross-dependence:** the substitution of dependence/addiction of one drug for that of another (e.g., methadone, a legal drug, is used to replace heroin, an illegal drug).
- **Antagonistic effects**: these occur when one drug is taken to weaken or inhibit the effect of another drug. For example, a "speedball" is heroin (CNS depressant) that is mixed with cocaine (a CNS stimulant) to soften the intense letdown of withdrawal from cocaine. Naloxone (opioid antagonist) is given to inhibit or reverse the effects of an opioid overdose.
- **Flashbacks**: transitory recurrences of a perceptual disturbance caused by a person's earlier *hallucinogenic drug use.* Flashbacks occur while in a drug-free state. Visual distortions, time expansion, loss of ego boundaries, and intense emotions are reported. Flashbacks can be mild and pleasant or can be a recurrence of frightening images or terrifying ideas from what is labeled a "bad trip."
- **Co-occurring disease**: the coexistence of SUDs along with one or more additional mental disorders. This is sometimes labeled **dual diagnosis**.
- **Codependency**: a type of dysfunctional helping relationship where one person supports or enables another person's compulsive/addictive behaviors to continue. The codependent person may try to "help" the person with an addiction by making excuses for or trying to hide problematic behavior. In this way, the person with a substance/addiction use disorders doesn't experience the negative consequences of his or her maladaptive behavior and will have less incentive to change (Box 19.1).

Clinical Picture

The diagnostic criteria for Alcohol Use Disorder are listed in the *DSM*-5 box on the next page. There are similar criteria for various substances although some do not include withdrawal symptoms. There are no specific withdrawal symptoms for substances such as inhalants, hallucinogens, and phencyclidine

Central Nervous System Depressants

CNS depressant drugs include alcohol, benzodiazepines, and barbiturates. These drugs are cross-tolerant to one another. The signs and symptoms of intoxication are the same, but the treatments and withdrawal are different. The physical and psychological symptoms

BOX 19.1 Codependent Behaviors

- Attempting to control someone else's drug use
- Spending most of your time thinking about the other person
- Finding excuses for the person's continued use
- Covering up or lying about the person's use
- Feeling responsible for the person's use
- Feeling guilty about the other person's behavior
- Avoiding family and social events because of concerns or shame about the member's behavior
- Making threats about substance use behaviors while failing to follow through
- Forcing promises for change
- Feelings of "walking on eggshells" to avoid causing problems
- Allowing own moods to be influenced by the behavior of the person
- Hiding or eliminating drug or alcohol supply
- Assuming duties and responsibilities of the person who is using
- Controlling the family's finances or protecting the person from financial or legal problems

DSM-5 DIAGNOSTIC CRITERIA

Alcohol Use Disorder

A. A problematic pattern of alcohol use leading to clinically significant impairment or distress, as manifested by at least two of the following, occurring within a 12-month period.

1. Alcohol is often taken in larger amounts or over a longer period than was intended.
2. There is a persistent desire or unsuccessful efforts to cut down or control alcohol use.
3. A great deal of time is spent in activities necessary to obtain alcohol, use alcohol, or recover from its effects.
4. Craving, or a strong desire or urge to use alcohol.
5. Recurrent alcohol use resulting in a failure to fulfill major role obligations at work, school, or home.
6. Continued alcohol use despite having persistent or recurrent social or interpersonal problems caused or exacerbated by the effects of alcohol.
7. Important social, occupational, or recreational activities are given up or reduced because of alcohol use.
8. Recurrent alcohol use in situations in which it is physically hazardous.
9. Alcohol use is continued despite knowledge of having a persistent or recurrent physical or psychological problem that is likely to have been caused or exacerbated by alcohol.
10. Tolerance, as defined by either of the following:
    a. A need for markedly increased amounts of alcohol to achieve intoxication or desired effect.
    b. A markedly diminished effect with continued use of the same amount of alcohol.
11. Withdrawal, as manifested by either of the following:
    a. The characteristic withdrawal syndrome for alcohol (refer to Criteria A and B of the criteria set for alcohol withdrawal).
    b. Alcohol (or closely related substance, such as a benzodiazepine) is taken to relieve or avoid withdrawal symptoms.

Specify if:

In early remission: After full criteria for alcohol use disorder were previously met, none of the criteria for alcohol use disorder have been met for at least 3 months but for less than 12 months (with the exception that Criterion A4, "Craving, or a strong desire or urge to use alcohol" may be met).

In sustained remission: After full criteria for alcohol use disorder were previously met, none of the criteria for alcohol use disorder have been met at any time during a period of 12 months or longer (with the exception that Criterion A4, "Craving, or a strong desire or urge to use alcohol," may be met).

Specify if:

In a controlled environment: This additional specifier is used if the individual is in an environment where access to alcohol is restricted.

of intoxication, overdose, and withdrawal, along with possible treatments, are presented in Table 19.3.

Withdrawal reactions to alcohol and other CNS depressants are associated with the most severe morbidity and mortality and are considered a **medical emergency.** The syndrome for alcohol withdrawal is similar for the entire class of CNS depressant drugs. Alcohol is used here as the prototype. The time intervals for the start of withdrawal symptoms are delayed with other CNS-depressant categories of drugs. As patients get older, symptoms of withdrawal continue for longer periods and are more severe than those in younger patients because of slower metabolism and excretion in the elderly.

When a person misuses more than one psychoactive drug, overlapping and simultaneous withdrawal syndromes can present a bizarre clinical picture and may pose problems for safe withdrawal. *It is essential to obtain an accurate history of drug use.*

Alcohol. Moderate use of alcohol is believed to have some positive qualities, including prolonging life, reducing the risk of dementia, and supplying some cardiovascular benefits (Burchum & Rosenthal, 2016).

When alcohol is habitually used to excess over a long period of time, the results are potentially very problematic for the individual and for significant others in that person's life. Disturbances include physiological changes, psychological pain, disruptions in social and family life, and disruptions in education and work life.

Additional cautions associated with alcohol use/misuse include the following:

- **Breastfeeding:** the alcohol concentration in breast milk is equal to the alcohol concentration in the mother's blood.
- Alcohol intake during **adolescence** affects brain functioning in adulthood.
- **Older adults** have lower tolerance for alcohol and can't metabolize alcohol efficiently.

Alcohol Intoxication. An objective measure of intoxication with alcohol is the **blood alcohol concentration (BAC)** level. This laboratory value assists the nurse in determining the level of intoxication and suggests the level of tolerance. It can also help to verify the patient's report of recent drinking. As tolerance develops, a discrepancy can sometimes be seen between BAC and expected behavior. A person with a high tolerance to alcohol may have a high BAC but minimal signs of impairment. *It should be noted that respiratory depression from alcohol use does not build a tolerance. Therefore the higher the amount of alcohol ingestion, the greater the risk for respiratory depression and respiratory arrest, even when there is tolerance to other effects of the drug* (Burchum & Rosenthal, 2016). It is useful to recognize that a person may start to experience withdrawal symptoms even when still intoxicated.

VIGNETTE: Clarence comes to the emergency department with a BAC of 0.21%. He is stuporous and ataxic and has slurred speech. The fact that he is still alive indicates a high tolerance for alcohol. The nursing history reveals an extensive drinking history. When the BAC is this high, assessing for withdrawal symptoms as well as the need for medical intervention is crucial.

Alcohol Withdrawal. Common signs and symptoms of **alcohol withdrawal syndrome (AWS)** include the following (Table 19.4):

- *Autonomic*: Elevated blood pressure (BP), pulse, temperature, diaphoresis, nausea/vomiting, diarrhea
- *Motor*: hand tremor, tremulousness, hyperreflexia, dysarthria, ataxia, seizures
- *Awareness*: agitation, irritability, insomnia, disorientation, delirium
- *Psychiatric*: anxiety, hallucinations, illusions, paranoia and delusions, disinhibition, combativeness

AWS occurs in about 8% of hospitalized patients with AUDs. Sudden cessation of chronic alcohol consumption results in autonomic overactivity and CNS irritability due to decreased synthesis of GABA and increased synthesis of glutamate. An increase in dopamine levels also contributes to this autonomic hyperarousal and may be responsible for the development of hallucinations (Jess et al., 2017).

TABLE 19.3 Central Nervous System Depressants

Drugs	Intoxication Effects	Overdose Effects	Possible Overdose Treatments	Withdrawal Effects	Possible Withdrawal Treatments
Alcohol (ETOH) Barbiturates Benzodiazepines	Physical: • Slurred speech • Unsteady gait • Drowsiness • Decreased vital signs Psychological: • Disinhibition: sexual/aggressive • Impaired judgment and role function • Impaired attention/memory • Irritability	Acute cardio-vascular or respiratory depression Shock Convulsions Coma Death	*Awake:* Induce vomiting. *Coma:* Clear airway; insert endotracheal tube. Other interventions: • Monitor vital signs closely. • Give IV fluids. • Initiate seizure precautions. • Gastric lavage activated charcoal (decrease absorption) • Dialysis • Administer reversal agent flumazenil for benzodiazepines.	Elevated vital signs Nausea and vomiting Tremors Paroxysmal sweats Anxiety and agitation; insomnia Tactile auditory and visual disturbances Seizures Disorientation and delirium	Slow tapering of the substance used For alcohol: Substitution therapy • Use of a benzodiazepine or barbiturate that is then tapered slowly (Alcohol withdrawal is a medical emergency.)

Modified from National Institute on Drug Abuse (NIDA). (2017). *Commonly abused drugs.* Retrieved from www.drugabuse.gov/researchers.

TABLE 19.4 Stages of Alcohol Withdrawal Syndrome (AWS)

Stage	Symptoms
Early/Minor Can occur 2 hr after stopping or reducing use Usually develops within 7-48 hr Symptoms usually peak after 24-48 hr	**Autonomic** Elevated vital signs, diaphoresis, gastrointestinal symptoms, headache **Motor** Hand tremors, feeling shaky inside, jerky movement, ataxia, startle easily, irritability, seizures
Moderate Appears 7 to 48 hr after stopping or reducing use Can continue for 5 to 7 days	Worsening of above autonomic and motor symptoms Continued elevation of all vital signs, including temperature; vomiting; clammy skin **Psychiatric Symptoms** Anxiety, mood lability, combativeness, hallucinations (auditory, visual, and tactile), illusions
Severe Can start in the same time frame as above May progress to delirium tremens (DTs)	All of above symptoms plus seizures **Awareness Symptoms** Disorientation and confusion Agitation and irritability Paranoia and disinhibition

From Jess, S., et al. (2017). Alcohol withdrawal syndrome: Mechanisms, manifestations, and management. *Neurologica,* 135(1), 4–16. Retrieved from https://doi.org/10.1111/ane.12671

Alcohol withdrawal delirium (or delirium tremens [DTs]) is considered a *medical emergency* and can result in death even if treated. The state of delirium usually peaks 48 to 72 hours after cessation or reduction of intake and lasts 2 to 5 days. In addition to anxiety, insomnia, anorexia, and delirium, features can include the following:

- Autonomic hyperactivity (tachycardia, diaphoresis, elevated blood pressure) and fever (temperatures of 100° F to 103° F)
- Severe disturbance in sensorium (disorientation, clouding of consciousness)
- Perceptual disturbances (illusions, visual or tactile hallucinations)
- Fluctuating levels of consciousness ranging from hyperexcitability to lethargy
- Delusions (paranoid), agitated behaviors
- Seizures

There is a growing recognition that there is a second stage of withdrawal from alcohol and drug use called *post-acute withdrawal syndrome (PAWS)*. During this stage, there are fewer physical symptoms but more emotional and psychological withdrawal symptoms.

Post-acute withdrawal occurs because brain chemistry takes time to return to normal. Symptoms of post-acute withdrawal include the following:

- Mood swings, anxiety, irritability
- Tiredness, variable energy, low enthusiasm
- Variable ability to concentration
- Disturbed sleep

Post-acute withdrawal symptoms occur episodically and can last for days to weeks, with episodes occurring up to 2 years following acute withdrawal. These episodes can be uncomfortable and increase the risk of relapse (AddictionAndRecovery.org, 2018).

The Clinical Institute Withdrawal Assessment for Alcohol–Revised (CIWA-Ar) scale provides an efficient (less than 5 minutes) validated and objective means of assessing alcohol withdrawal symptoms that can then be utilized in treatment protocols. The scale is used to assess 10 different categories of symptoms and to rate each symptom on a scale of 0 (not present) to 7 (extreme). A score correlates to the severity of alcohol withdrawal. It can be used in any setting whenever there is a suspicion of AUD and potential alcohol withdrawal. A complete set of vital signs plus the assessment is generally performed every 4 hours or as needed (see http://www.regionstrauma.org/blogs/ciwa.pdf to access the CIWA scale).

Severe levels of withdrawal and DTs require close medical supervision, usually in an intensive care unit. Additional nursing care may include the following:

- Consistent and frequent orientation to time and place should be provided as necessary.
- The use of a sitter or family to stay with the patient can increase orientation and minimize confusion and anxiety.
- A sitter may be required for safety when agitation is present.
- **Presenting reality** may be necessary when visual/tactile hallucinations and illusions are present. A **hallucination** is seeing or feeling things that are not there. **Illusions** are misinterpretations of objects in the environment. These can be terrifying for the patient. If, for example, a person thinks that spots on the wallpaper are blood-sucking ants, it can be helpful to respond, "These are not ants; they are just part of the wallpaper pattern."
- Stay with the patient and reinforce orientation and safety—for example, "I will have a sitter stay with you. You are in the hospital and are safe here."
- A well-lit environment is recommended to decrease shadows and illusions.

Psychopharmacology for Withdrawal. Treatment involves administering a substitute medication that has **cross-tolerance** with alcohol and then gradually tapering the dose. The most common drug class used for alcohol withdrawal is benzodiazepines. These drugs can be given through the oral (per os [PO]), intramuscular (IM), or intravenous (IV) route and are prescribed on a fixed-schedule dose (e.g., lorazepam 2 mg PO every 4 hours) or as symptom-triggered dosing (e.g., lorazepam 1 to 2 mg when the CIWA-Ar score is over 15). This class of medication provides sedation, decreases anxiety and feelings of tremulousness, and decreases the risk of seizures.

Barbiturates, particularly phenobarbital, may be given when the patient is not getting an adequate response to benzodiazepines. **Anticonvulsants** can be used as adjunctive therapy to decrease anxiety and prevent seizures. Elevated vital signs and autonomic symptoms associated with alcohol withdrawal improve with beta-adrenergic–blockade drugs such as **clonidine** but are not useful for other symptoms of withdrawal. Replacement therapy with **thiamine** (vitamin B_1) can prevent Wernicke–Korsakoff syndrome and correct high-output heart failure. **Folic acid** (folate) and **cyanocobalamin** (vitamin B_{12}) can correct megaloblastic anemia, and cyanocobalamin can halt peripheral neuropathy.

These drugs are generally effective for uncomplicated withdrawal symptoms. Severe levels of withdrawal, such as DTs, or other medical complications will require more aggressive and closely monitored treatment, usually provided in a critical care medical unit.

Psychopharmacology for Sobriety/Abstinence. **Medication-assisted treatment (MAT)** is the use of FDA-approved medications in combination with counseling and behavioral therapies to provide a "whole-patient" approach to the treatment of SUDs. Drugs used in helping individuals maintain abstinence from *alcohol* are based on three strategies: making alcohol use unpleasant, reducing psychophysiological symptoms associated with withdrawal, and reducing the reinforcing qualities of drug/alcohol use. The following drugs are FDA approved for the maintenance of sobriety (Burchum & Rosenthal, 2016):

1. **Disulfiram (Antabuse)** is used by individuals who want to stay alcohol-free. Because the effects of the drug are long lasting, it helps prevent *impulsive drinking.* **Patient teaching** includes an explanation that when this drug is mixed with alcohol (as little as a quarter of an ounce) it can cause violent physical reactions such as pounding in the chest, acute hypotension, extreme nausea and vomiting, facial flushing, and potentially death. Patients must also be cautioned not to use products containing "hidden" sources of alcohol. This can include liquid cold and cough medications, vinegar, foods cooked in wine, and mouthwash. Alcohol-based hand sanitizers can also cause an interaction. The drug can only be started when the person has been alcohol-free for weeks. *It takes at least 14 days for the effects of the drug to leave the body.*
2. **Naltrexone (ReVia, Vivitrol)** reduces the desired pleasant feelings ("high") by blocking the release of endorphins related to alcohol and opioid intake. It also helps block drug cravings. Naltrexone seems to be much more effective in those with a family history of AUD. ReVia is the oral form given once a day, and Vivitrol is a long-acting injectable form given once a month.
3. **Acamprosate (Campral)** helps by reducing some of the unpleasant symptoms of abstinence, such as anxiety and dysphoria, which can have the secondary effect of decreasing cravings for the drug.

These drugs work best when they are used as part of a comprehensive treatment plan.

In a randomized clinical trial, **gabapentin** was found to be effective in treating alcohol dependence and relapse-related symptoms of insomnia, anxiety, dysphoria, cravings, headaches, and/or pain in individuals with a co-occurring substance use disorder. Gabapentin has a favorable safety profile (Kantorovich, 2016).

Refer to Table 19.5 for further information about pharmacotherapy for substance use disorders.

Opiates. Opiates belong to the class of *narcotic analgesics*. Opioids produce tolerance, physical dependence, and withdrawal with prolonged use. The most common opiates that are misused are heroin and oxycodone (Burchum & Rosenthal, 2016). Other opiates include hydrocodone, morphine, fentanyl, and codeine. Opiate use often starts when used for pain management. Only a very small percentage of those who have been introduced to opiates for therapeutic reasons develop compulsive drug use (Burchum & Rosenthal, 2016). Misuse of prescription opioids may quickly lead to heroin use because heroin is cheaper and more accessible despite being illegal.

In the United States, more people now die from opioid painkiller overdoses than from heroin and cocaine use combined (NIDA, 2016d). Fentanyl, an opioid that is 50 to 100 times more potent than morphine, and carfentanil, an opioid that is 100 times stronger than fentanyl, have become a big part of the illegal drug trade. The increased use of fentanyl, fentanyl-*laced* heroin, and carfentanil has led to a significant increase in accidental overdoses.

Symptoms of overdose, sometimes called the "*opioid overdose triad,*" are as follows:

- *Pinpoint pupils*
- *Respiration depression*
- *Decreased level of consciousness* (Schiller & Mechanic, 2018)

Immediate emergency care involves administering a reversal agent, then preserving airway and adequate oxygenation.

In an attempt to slow down the epidemic of opioid dependence, the CDC proposed guidelines for primary care physicians who prescribe opiates for chronic pain. The guidelines focus on (1) *when to initiate or continue opioids for chronic pain;* (2) *opioid selection, dosage, duration, follow-up, and discontinuation;* and (3) *assessing risk and addressing harms of opioid use.* These guidelines are not intended for cancer patients, palliative care, or end-of-life treatment (CDC, 2016).

Psychopharmacology for Overdose. Treatment of **opioid toxicity/overdose symptoms** (coma or decreased level of consciousness, pinpoint pupils, respiratory depression) includes administering an opioid antagonist, such as **naloxone (Narcan).** This drug reverses the symptoms of overdose, specifically respiratory and CNS depression. There is a potential for a violent reaction from the patient as he or she gains consciousness. The drug can precipitate withdrawal symptoms. Naloxone is short acting and must be readministered every few hours

TABLE 19.5 Maintenance Drugs for Alcohol and CNS-Depressant Drug Use Disorders

Indications	Patient Teaching
Disulfiram (Antabuse)	
Aversion therapy:	
Ingested in combination with alcohol will cause nausea, vomiting, headache, and flushing (an acetaldehyde reaction).	Patient must be alcohol-free for at least 14 days.
Helps prevent relapse by discouraging impulsive drinking.	Patient must be fully informed about the interaction with alcohol.
	Counsel patient about hidden sources of alcohol that may precipitate a reaction (mouthwash, vinegar, liquid medications, hand sanitizer, wine in food, etc.).
	Adverse effects: metallic aftertaste, dermatitis, hypotension, nausea and vomiting
	Inform health care providers that you are taking this drug.
	Once-daily dosing; effects last up to 2 weeks after discontinuation of disulfiram.
Naltrexone (ReVia)	
Diminishes alcohol cravings	Adverse effects: nausea, abdominal pain; constipation; dizziness; headache; anxiety; fatigue
Blocks the effects of opiates	Can precipitate narcotic withdrawal in patients using opioid drugs or pain medication
Useful in the acute recovery phase of alcohol dependence (first 12 weeks)	
Vivitrol (Naltrexone for Extended-Release, Injectable Suspension)	
Suppresses cravings and pleasurable effects of alcohol	Concurrent use with opioids, such as heroin, can increase the risk of opioid overdose.
	Monthly IM formulation facilitates adherence.
Acamprosate (Campral)	
Decreases longer-term unpleasant effects of withdrawal, including anxiety and restlessness	Reasonably safe in patients with mild to moderate hepatic impairment
Diminishes alcohol cravings	Baseline kidney function labs are required because it is primarily excreted through the kidney.
	Need to have been abstinent at least 7 days
	Adverse effects: diarrhea and decreased libido
	Avoid use in pregnancy.
Buprenorphine Hydrochloride (Buprenex, Subutex); Buprenorphine Hydrochloride and Naloxone Hydrochloride (Suboxone)	
Prevents symptoms of withdrawal in patients addicted to opiates	Adverse effects: dizziness; nausea; respiratory depression
Alternative to maintenance treatment with methadone	Can only be administered from an approved treatment center
Reduces feelings of craving	
Methadone	
Substitution therapy for opioid addiction	Can only be administered from an approved treatment center
Used for withdrawal when slowly tapered	
Used as a maintenance drug for long-term use; dependence on illegal opioid is transferred to methadone	

CNS, Central nervous system; *IM*, intramuscular.

until opioid levels are nontoxic, which may take days (Burchum & Rosenthal, 2016). In November 2015, the FDA approved intranasal naloxone for the emergency treatment of known or suspected opioid overdose. The ready-to-use, single-dose sprayer delivers a 4-mg dose by intranasal administration (Stephens, 2017). Because of the epidemic of overdose and deaths from heroin, this form of naloxone is available to both health care providers and the general public.

More than 30% of overdoses involving opioids also involve the use of benzodiazepines. In one study, overdose deaths for patients receiving both types of medications were 10 times higher than among those only receiving opioids. Both prescription opioids and benzodiazepines now carry FDA Black Box warnings on the label highlighting the dangers of using these drugs together (NIDA, 2018a).

Nalmefene (Revex), a medication typically used to reverse or stop the effects of alcohol poisoning, can also be used to reverse symptoms of an **opioid overdose**. It does have a longer half-life than naloxone but can precipitate a prolonged withdrawal syndrome (NIDA, 2018a).

Psychopharmacology for Withdrawal. Symptoms of withdrawal from opioids include the following:

- *Low energy, irritability, anxiety, agitation, insomnia*
- *Yawning*
- *Flu-like symptoms*
- *Runny nose, teary eyes*
- *Hot and cold sweats, goose bumps*
- *Severe muscle aches and pains*
- *Abdominal cramping, nausea, vomiting, diarrhea*

Acute withdrawal can begin within 1 hour but usually begins about 12 hours after the last opioid use. It peaks at around 3 to 5 days and can last for 1 to 4 weeks. Some addiction specialists describe a *post-acute withdrawal* phase that can last up to 2 years. Symptoms include moods swings, anxiety and depressive symptoms, and insomnia.

The **Clinical Opiate Withdrawal Scale (COWS)** is a useful 11-item scale designed to rate the severity of common acute signs and symptoms of opiate withdrawal and monitor these symptoms. It is usually performed every shift or as needed throughout the detoxification period. A copy of the scale can be found at https://www.mdcalc.com/cows-score-opiate-withdrawal.

Withdrawal management or **detoxification** is the first step in the treatment of opioid addiction. **Methadone,** a long-acting opioid, can be substituted for the specific opioid previously taken by the individual and then titrated downward to help ease the withdrawal symptoms.

Clonidine can assist with the withdrawal effects related to autonomic instability. **Buprenorphine and buprenorphine/naloxone**, agonist/antagonist opioids, can be used for detoxification and longer-term maintenance.

In 2018 the FDA approved Lucemyra, the first nonopioid treatment to facilitate the abrupt discontinuation of opioids by lessening the severity of withdrawal symptoms for those who have developed an addiction to an opioid. Lucemyra is an oral, selective alpha-2-adrenergic–receptor agonist that reduces the release of norepinephrine. The most common side effects are hypotension, bradycardia, and sedation (FDA, 2018).

Psychopharmacology for Maintenance. **Methadone maintenance** is one important element of **medication-assisted treatment (MAT)** for opioid addiction recognized by SAMHSA (2018). With *methadone maintenance,* the drug is taken long term and acts as a substitution drug to initially manage withdrawal symptoms. Staying on the drug also significantly decreases cravings and urges to relapse. Because this maintenance drug does not produce the "high" associated with drug misuse, the individual is better able to more fully participate in therapy and other recovery activities. It also allows the individual to participate more fully in life activities that support continued recovery, such as job training, education, full-time work, and interpersonal relationships. It is a once-a-day dosing because it is a long-acting opioid. By law, methadone can only be dispensed through an opioid treatment program (OTP) certified by SAMHSA.

Buprenorphine (Subutex) is an opioid used to support abstinence. Buprenorphine is less likely to result in overdose because it is a partial agonist. It is longer acting and produces a milder withdrawal syndrome. Less frequent administration, one to three times a week, is required. Buprenorphine tends to alleviate cravings, reduces the use of illicit opioids, has a milder neonatal withdrawal, and increases retention in therapeutic programs (Burchum & Rosenthal, 2016).

Naltrexone, previously identified as a maintenance drug for AUDs, is an opioid antagonist that also blocks the euphoric effect of opioids. This drug will precipitate withdrawal in patients currently taking an opioid.

Suboxone is buprenorphine combined with naloxone. This formulation prevents individuals from misusing buprenorphine as a drug to get "high" because naloxone's antagonist properties prevent that "high."

To facilitate full recovery, participation in a comprehensive treatment program is a usual requirement when these drugs are prescribed.

Table 19.6 lists the signs and symptoms of opiate intoxication, withdrawal, and overdose and possible treatments.

Central Nervous System Stimulants

All stimulants accelerate the normal functioning of the body and affect the CNS. Stimulants are known to increase alertness, heighten sexual arousal, increase behavioral excitement, increase well-being, increase energy, and diminish fatigue (Meyer & Quenzer, 2018). Acute effects include extreme energy; anorexia; possible violence; rambling, incoherent speech; delusions of grandeur; irritability; hostility; anxiety; and fear. Common signs of stimulant use include dilation of the pupils, dryness of the nasal cavity, and excessive motor activity. Some of the consequences of high doses of CNS stimulants are seizures, heart failure, stroke, and integrative hemorrhage (Meyer & Quenzer, 2018). When a person who has ingested a stimulant experiences chest pain or has an irregular pulse rate, the person should be taken to an emergency department immediately. This is especially true if the person has a positive family history of cardiac disease.

Cocaine and Crack. Cocaine is a naturally occurring stimulant extracted from the leaf of the coca bush. Crack is an inexpensive, widely available alkalinized form of cocaine. When crack is smoked, it takes effect in 4 to 6 seconds, producing a fleeting high (5 to 7 minutes) followed by a period of deep letdown that reinforces addictive behavior patterns and guarantees continued use of the drug. Cocaine is classified as a schedule II substance: "high abuse potential with some recognized medical use."

Cocaine exerts two main effects on the body: anesthetic and stimulant. As an anesthetic, it blocks the conduction of electrical impulses within the nerve cells that are involved in sensory transmission, primarily pain transmission. It can be used for nasal surgery to stop bleeding. It also acts as a stimulant for sexual arousal, feelings of euphoria, and violent behavior. Cocaine produces an imbalance of neurotransmitters, dopamine and norepinephrine, which is most likely responsible for many of the physical withdrawal symptoms reported by heavy, chronic cocaine users: depression, paranoia, lethargy, anxiety, insomnia, nausea and vomiting, and sweating and chills.

Drug–drug interaction between **alcohol and cocaine** has been reported by NIDA as one of the most common two-drug combinations that results in drug-related deaths. This is related to how both are metabolized in the liver (Drugs.com, 2018).

TABLE 19.6 Opiates

Drugs	Intoxication Effects	Overdose (OD) Effects	Possible Overdose Treatments	Withdrawal Effects	Possible Withdrawal Treatments
Oxycodone Heroin Morphine Codeine Methadone (Dolophine) Hydromorphone Fentanyl	Physical: • Constricted pupils • Drowsiness • Decreased vital signs • Slurred speech • Psychomotor slowing Psychological: • Initial euphoria followed by dysphoria • Impairment of attention, judgment, and memory	Triad symptoms: 1. Coma 2. Respiratory depression 3. Pinpoint pupils Convulsions Cardiac arrest and death Higher OD risk with benzodiazepine use	Narcotic antagonist, **naloxone** to quickly reverse central nervous system depression May have acute agitation from reversal agent May need to repeat dosage	Yawning Insomnia Irritability Runny nose (rhinorrhea) Panic Diaphoresis Cramps, nausea and vomiting, diarrhea Muscle aches ("bone pain") Fever and chills Lacrimation	Substitution therapy: methadone tapered slowly **Clonidine** for autonomic symptoms (nausea, vomiting, diarrhea) **Buprenorphine:** acts as an opioid substitute that can be tapered

Modified from National Institute on Drug Abuse (NIDA). (2017). *Commonly abused drugs.* Retrieved from www.drugabuse.gov/researchers.

Methamphetamine. Methamphetamine is a highly addictive stimulant related to amphetamines, but it has a longer-lasting and more toxic effect on the CNS. Methamphetamines have neurotoxic (brain-damaging) effects, destroying brain cells that contain dopamine and serotonin. Long-term use of amphetamines can result in visual hallucinations, delusions, and paranoia. The symptoms displayed can resemble the symptoms associated with the psychosis of schizophrenia.

Reduced levels of dopamine from chronic use of methamphetamines can also lead to parkinsonian symptoms. Prolonged use can result in cracked teeth, skin infections, stroke, lung disease, kidney or liver damage, and death.

Table 19.7 outlines the physical and psychological effects associated with intoxication (use) and overdose of amphetamines and other psychostimulants. Emergency treatment for both overdose and withdrawal is also explained.

Nicotine

Nicotine is highly addictive, highly toxic, and used worldwide. Nicotine can act as a stimulant, depressant, or tranquilizer. Nicotine use can result in dependence and development of an "abstinence syndrome" when the drug is abruptly stopped. Major withdrawal symptoms include strong cravings, impaired concentration, nervousness, restlessness, irritability, impatience, and increased appetite, which usually leads to weight gain (Burchum & Rosenthal, 2016).

There are currently seven pharmacological aids approved by the FDA to help people decrease nicotine cravings and suppress symptoms of withdrawal. Five pharmacological aids for smoking suppression are nicotine-based. Nicotine patches, nicotine gum, nicotine lozenges, nicotine nasal sprays, and nicotine inhalers are substituted for smoking and then slowly tapered. Nicotine-free products include varenicline (Chantix) and bupropion (Zyban), an atypical antidepressant. Bupropion is the first choice for smokers with depression.

Marijuana

Marijuana *(Cannabis sativa)* is an Indian hemp plant in which tetrahydrocannabinol (THC) is the psychoactive ingredient. It is usually smoked, but edible options are becoming more popular (Burchum & Rosenthal, 2016).

The use and possession of marijuana are illegal under federal law. Multiple states, however, have sanctioned its use for medicinal and recreational use. The first cannabis-based prescription medication, Sativex, was released in the United Kingdom in 2010 as a mist spray approved to treat spasticity (muscle tightness) in patients with multiple sclerosis. In the United States, the FDA has approved the use of two purified cannabinoids—dronabinol (Marinol) and nabilone (Cesamet). They can be prescribed as antiemetics for the nausea and vomiting associated with chemotherapy. Dronabinol can be prescribed as an appetite stimulant to combat the physical wasting associated with AIDS (Burchum & Rosenthal, 2016). Off label, dronabinol is sometimes prescribed as an adjunctive analgesic medication for neuropathy pain and other chronic pain conditions like fibromyalgia and multiple sclerosis.

THC has mixed depressant and hallucinogenic properties. Marijuana is generally smoked in a pipe or as a "cigarette," inhaled through a vaporizer, or ingested in the form of cannabis-infused foods known as "edibles." Desired effects include euphoria, detachment, and relaxation. Other effects include increased appetite, talkativeness, slowed perception of time, inappropriate laughter, heightened sensitivity to visual and auditory stimuli, and in some cases, anxiety or paranoia. The current forms of marijuana can be very potent, with higher concentrations of THC. This has led to an increase in the incidence of marijuana use disorders and a

TABLE 19.7 Central Nervous System Stimulants

Drugs	Intoxication Effects	Overdose Effects	Possible Overdose Treatments	Withdrawal Effects	Withdrawal Treatments
Cocaine Crack (short acting)	Physical: • Dilated pupils • Elevated blood pressure and pulse • Nausea and vomiting • Insomnia Psychological: • Assaultiveness • Grandiosity • Impaired judgment and role performance • Euphoria	Respiratory distress/arrest Ataxia Hyperpyrexia Convulsions Stroke Myocardial infarction Coma and death	Benzodiazepines: sedation and prevention of seizures Cooling measures for hyperpyrexia IV antihypertensives for elevated BP Supportive measures that treat symptoms: • Maintain airway, breathing, and circulation. • Provide oxygen. • Monitor glucose levels.	Fatigue, lethargy, and sleepiness or Anxiety, agitation, and insomnia Depression and suicide ideation Apathy Disorientation Craving	Medications are given for symptoms relief: • **Modafinil** for excessive lethargy • Diphenhydramine or trazodone for agitation and to facilitate sleep • Analgesics for minor pain • Antidepressants for the symptoms of depression • Short-term use of benzodiazepines as sedatives
Amphetamines Dextroamphetamine Methamphetamine	Increased energy and wakefulness Increased respirations Hyperthermia Euphoria Severe/long term: Paranoia with delusions Visual, auditory, and tactile hallucinations Severe to panic levels of anxiety Potential for violence	Same as above	Same as above	Same as above	Same as above

BP, Blood pressure; *IV*, intravenous.
Modified from National Institute on Drug Abuse (NIDA). (2017). *Commonly abused drugs.* Retrieved from www.drugabuse.gov/researchers.

higher potential for overdose and toxicity. Although marijuana can help ease nausea and vomiting in those with cancer and other conditions, a paradoxical condition, known as cannabinoid hyperemesis syndrome (CHS), can develop in those who have used high-potency marijuana for prolonged periods of time. This syndrome is marked by severe vomiting and acute abdominal discomfort, weight loss, and excessive sweating. Emergency room treatment may be required due to the acute dehydration and potential for kidney toxicity that can result from this syndrome.

Psychoactive Drugs

Club drugs are a group of psychoactive drugs that act on the CNS and can cause changes in mood, awareness, and behavior (Table 19.8). These drugs tend to be used by young adults (age 13 through 20s) in group settings like all-night dance parties, dance clubs, and bars. They include the following:

- *Methylenedioxymethamphetamine (MDMA), also known as ecstasy, XTC, X, E, Adam, Molly, hug beans, and love drug*
- *Gamma-hydroxybutyrate (GHB), also known as G, liquid ecstasy, and soap*
- *Ketamine, also known as special K, K, vitamin K, and jet*
- *Rohypnol, also known as roofies*
- *Methamphetamine, also known as speed, ice, chalk, meth, crystal, crank, and glass*
- *Lysergic acid diethylamide (LSD), also known as acid, blotter, and dots* (NIDA, n.d.)

These recreational drugs produce subjective effects resembling those of both stimulants and hallucinogens. Problematic use of any of these drugs leads to the *DSM-5* diagnosis of "Other Hallucinogen Use Disorders." Alcohol potentiates the effect of all of these drugs and can increase toxicity.

MDMA acts to prolong the effects and increases the amounts of serotonin in the brain. This drug increases norepinephrine, causing an increase in heart rate and blood pressure (NIDA, 2016b). **MDMA** causes euphoria, increased energy, increased self-confidence, increased sociability, and a feeling of closeness to people. Adverse effects such as hyperthermia, heart failure, and kidney failure have occurred. Deaths from acute dehydration have been reported. Chronic heavy recreational use of ecstasy is thought to be responsible for sleep disorders, depressed mood, persistent elevation of anxiety level, impulsiveness, and hostility, as well as selective impairment of episodic memory and attention.

Flunitrazepam (Rohypnol, or "roofies") is a fast-acting benzodiazepine that has been implicated in sexual assault. It produces rapid disinhibition and relaxation of voluntary muscle and unconsciousness. It can also cause the victim to have lasting anterograde amnesia. It is easily mixed with drinks. **GHB, or gamma-hydroxybutyrate,** is a CNS-depressant drug that causes a similar incapacitation due to its sedative effects.

Ketamine is a dissociative anesthetic. This dissociative effect is described as pleasantly floating in space or as the feeling of rising above one's body. For some this sensation is pleasurable and peaceful, but for others it can be terrifying (Burchum & Rosenthal, 2016). Ketamine can cause delirium and respiratory depression that can lead to respiratory arrest and death. It has also been implicated in sexual assault because it produces a generalized anesthesia that lessens the ability to act voluntarily and induces amnesia. Refer to Chapter 22 for more on sexual violence and assault. Refer to Table 19.9.

Multiple club drugs are also sometimes used as "date rape" drugs to make someone unable to say no to or fight back against sexual assault. One in 13 college students said they had been drugged or thought they had been drugged in a 2016 study. Rohypnol is now sold in a form that turns a liquid blue when added to a drink to prevent secretive use. Other products are in development to help keep people safe. One product is a specially treated napkin that can detect if up to 26 drugs have been slipped into your drink (Swaak, 2018).

PCP, piperidine, is an anesthetic structurally similar to ketamine. It is known as angel dust, horse tranquilizer, and peace pill. The signs and symptoms of PCP intoxication range from acute anxiety to acute

TABLE 19.8 Club Drugs

Drugs	Intoxication	Toxic Effects	Toxicity Treatment	Withdrawal Symptoms
Ecstasy (MDMA)	Euphoria, loss of inhibition, a feeling of closeness and/or empathy, increased sensuality	Hyperthermia, dehydration, and hyponatremia Seizures Hypertensive crises Cardiac dysrhythmias Serotonin syndrome Neurological effects (confusion, delirium, paranoia) Cognitive impairment with repeated use	No antidote Activated charcoal to eliminate the drug and prevent further absorption Comprehensive chemistry panel to identify complications (hepatic or renal damage) Treat symptoms: • Monitor airway, breathing, and cardiac system. • Cooling measures • Calm, quiet room • Sedation with benzodiazepines	Profound depression Confusion, sleep problems, anxiety Cravings that can last for weeks
Gamma-hydroxybutyrate (GBH) Rohypnol (benzodiazepine)	Euphoria, reduced inhibitions, reduced judgment Amnesia Loss of control over movements Feeling drunk Unconsciousness Dizziness Confusion Sedation Nausea and vomiting Problems breathing	Cheyne–Stokes respirations Seizures Slow breathing and heart rate Low body temperature Coma Death	No antidote for GHB Activated charcoal to eliminate the drug and prevent further absorption Treat symptoms (as above). Rohypnol reversal agent: Flumazenil	**GHB:** Tremors, insomnia, sweating, anxiety **Rohypnol:** Seizure, headache, muscle pain, anxiety, delirium, cardiovascular distress

Modified from National Institute on Drug Abuse (NIDA). (2017). *Commonly abused drugs.* Retrieved from www.drugabuse.gov/researchers.

psychosis, as well as aggression, violence, and loss of coordination. The use of PCP can also lead to volatile mood swings and bizarre behavior. PCP can produce hypotension, coma, seizures, and muscular rigidity associated with the occurrence of hypothermia (see Table 19.9). Chronic use of PCP can result in long-term effects such as dulled thinking, lethargy, loss of impulse control, poor memory, and depression. Suicide is a significant risk during PCP intoxication. Refer to Chapter 23 for more information on suicide assessment.

LSD (acid), mescaline (peyote), and psilocybin (magic mushroom) are examples of hallucinogens. Mescaline and the mushroom *Psilocybe mexicana* (from which psilocybin is isolated) have been used for centuries in religious rites by Native Americans living in the southwestern United States and northern Mexico. The hallucinogenic experience produced by LSD results in an acute dreamlike state of unreality, and hallucinations. Flashbacks and persistent perception disorders can occur days to weeks later. See Table 19.10 for the signs and symptoms of hallucinogen intoxication and overdose.

Salvia is one of the most potent "natural" hallucinogenic and dissociative drugs available. It produces effects that may include altered perceptions, distorted reality, visual and auditory hallucinations, a loss of control over body movements, and anxiety and fear from a "bad trip." Used in traditional religious rituals among Mexican Indians, it has now become a recreational drug for young adults. It is not regulated. See Table 19.9 for the signs and symptoms of intoxication, overdose, and effects and potential medical interventions when appropriate.

Cathinones

Synthetic **cathinones**, more commonly known as **bath salts**, are human-made stimulant-type drugs. These relatively new mind-altering drugs called new psychoactive substances (NPSs) are unregulated and easily purchased. The number of new cathinones introduced each year is growing, which hinders law enforcement efforts to stop their use. These drugs are marketed as cheap substitutes for other stimulants, such as methamphetamine and cocaine. Symptoms of use include hallucinogenic-delusional properties, dissociation, increased sex drive, extreme agitation, and feelings of superhuman strength and combativeness. These drugs can become addictive, with depression, anxiety, sleep disturbance, and paranoia as withdrawal symptoms (NIDA, 2018b). Synthetic cannabinoids (K2/Spice) also fall into this category. These drugs act like more potent marijuana.

Inhalants

Inhalants are most often used by adolescents and are easily purchased. Inhalant use is also referred to as "huffing" or "backing." Inhalants include volatile solvents such as spray paint, glue, cigarette lighter fluid, and propellant gases used in aerosols. Inhalants starve the body of oxygen and force the heart to beat irregularly and more rapidly. Sudden death can occur from cardiac arrhythmia or arrest and respiratory arrest. Users can experience nausea and nosebleeds and lose their sense of hearing or smell. Chronic use can lead to muscle wasting and reduced muscle tone, with gradual damage to the lungs and the immune system. Long-term use also results in persistent medical and neurological problems, including permanent brain damage and hearing loss (APA, 2013). Those who misuse inhalants are more likely to misuse other drugs (Table 19.11).

TABLE 19.9 Dissociative Drugs

Drugs	Intoxication	Overdose/Toxic Effects	Potential Treatments
Phenylcyclohexyl piperidine (PCP)	Physical: • Impervious to pain • Nystagmus • Increased vital signs • Ataxia • Muscle rigidity • Seizures • Jerking movements • Belligerence, assaultiveness • Impulsiveness • Impaired judgment, and role functioning Severe effects: • Hallucinations • Paranoia • Bizarre behavior (barking like a dog, grimacing, repetitive chanting speech) • Regressive or violent behavior • Labile emotions	Psychosis Hypertensive crisis Cardiovascular accident Respiratory arrest Hyperthermia Seizures	If alert: • *Caution:* Gastric lavage can lead to laryngeal spasms or aspiration. • Acidify urine (cranberry juice, ascorbic acid) to facilitate excretion. • Provide environment with minimal stimuli. • Speak slowly, clearly, and in a low voice. • Administer benzodiazepine. • Administer haloperidol for severe behavioral disturbance (not a phenothiazine). Institute medical intervention for: • Hyperthermia • High blood pressure • Respiratory distress • Hypertension
Ketamine	Varied: • Pleasant floating sensation to out-of-body experiences (peaceful or terrifying)	High doses: amnesia, increased blood pressure, acute respiratory distress	Medical treatment for hypertension and respiratory distress
Salvia	Dissociative experiences Sense of unreality Loss of awareness of sense of body Depersonalization		

Modified from National Institute on Drug Abuse (NIDA). (2017). *Commonly abused drugs.* Retrieved from www.drugabuse.gov/researchers.

TABLE 19.10 Hallucinogens

Drugs	Intoxication Effects	Overdose Effects	Possible Overdose Treatments
Lysergic acid diethylamide (LSD) Mescaline (peyote) Psilocybin	Physical: • Pupil dilation • Tachycardia • Diaphoresis • Palpitations • Tremors • Incoordination • Elevated temperature, pulse, respiration Psychological: • Fear of going crazy • Paranoid ideas • Marked anxiety, depression • Synesthesia (colors are heard; sounds are seen) • Depersonalization • Hallucinations • Grandiosity (e.g., thinking one can fly) • Distorted sense of space and time	Psychosis Brain damage Death	Low-stimuli environment: minimal light, sound, activity. Stay with patient; reassure patient, "talk down" patient. Speak slowly and clearly in a low voice. Give benzodiazepine for extreme anxiety or tension.

Modified from National Institute on Drug Abuse (NIDA). (2017). *Commonly abused drugs.* Retrieved from www.drugabuse.gov/researchers.

TABLE 19.11 Inhalants

Drug	Intoxication Effects	Overdose Effects	Treatment
Volatile solvents (paint thinners, glues, gasoline, dry cleaner fluid) **Gases** (butane, propane, nitrous oxide) **Nitrates** (isoamyl, isobutyl) **Aerosols** (spray paint and others)	Slurred speech Lack of inhibitions Euphoria Dizziness Drunkenness Violent behavior	Liver and brain damage Fatal cardiac rhythm Heart failure Respiratory arrest Suffocation Coma and death Long-term use: deterioration of myelin sheath of nerve fibers; muscle spasms and tremors; difficulty with movements (walking, bending, and talking); hearing loss	Support affected systems. Neurological symptoms may respond to vitamin B_{12} and folate.

Modified from National Institute on Drug Abuse (NIDA). (2017). *Commonly abused drugs.* Retrieved from www.drugabuse.gov/researchers.

APPLICATION OF THE NURSING PROCESS

ASSESSMENT

Assessing the use of substances and problems associated with that use is complex because of the increased use of multiple substances (**multiple drug use/polydrug use**) and the development of chemically engineered designer drugs. Accurate assessment becomes even more complicated in the presence of coexisting psychiatric disorders or physical illnesses, including HIV infection, AIDS, dementia, and encephalopathy.

Sensitivity to multicultural and racial issues is important in interpreting symptoms, making diagnoses, providing clinical care, and designing prevention strategies. Refer to Box 19.2 for areas to be covered in overall substance use assessment.

 Assessment Guidelines

There is a consistent and significant association between alcohol or drug use and injury. Symptoms of acute intoxication and symptoms of injury can sometimes overlap. Therefore the initial assessment must be comprehensive. Assessment related to use must include the following:

- What specific drug(s) have been used?
- For each drug, ask *how much of the drug was used, how often the drug was used, and for how long the drug was used as well as the date of last use.* These questions help the nurse determine the potential for addiction, tolerance, and most importantly, withdrawal.
- Withdrawal management is a priority intervention. A urine and blood **toxicology screen** and **BAC** test should be performed. A breathalyzer test can determine the current level of alcohol intoxication.
- Assess for symptoms associated with toxicity and overdose from a drug or alcohol; this requires immediate medical attention.
- If the patient reveals previous treatment for an SUD and withdrawal, it is important to clarify the symptoms of withdrawal previously experienced. Past experiences with alcohol-related seizures and DTs put the person at greater risk for the development of a more life-threatening withdrawal.
- Assess for level of insight regarding the need for substance use treatment.
- Assessment questions related to possible injury may be important:
  - A description of the accident or physical trauma, especially head trauma
  - A review of all body systems
- A neurological assessment is especially important to rule out other causes for symptoms (e.g., closed head injury).

BOX 19.2 Overall Assessment Guide for Substance Use

History of Patient's Substance Use[a]

1. Age of first use
2. Name of substances used, pattern of use, amount, frequency, and time of last use.[a]
3. Periods of sobriety; previous substance use treatment. What was the outcome?
4. Is there a history of delirium, seizures, or other complications from withdrawal?[a]
5. Is there a history of blackouts, history of overdoses, or other complications from past substance use?
6. Is there a family history of drug or alcohol problems?
7. Does the person have insight about having a substance use problem?

Medical History

1. Coexisting physical conditions
2. Current medications
3. Current medical status

Psychiatric History

1. Current mental status examination
2. History of comorbid psychiatric problems
3. History of treatment for any specific disorder. What medications were prescribed, and what was the outcome?
4. Is there a history of abuse (physical, sexual)? Family violence?
5. Is there a history of suicide? Violence toward others?
6. Does the patient have current suicidal thoughts or thoughts of violence toward others?

Psychosocial Issues

1. Does the patient have a poor work record related to substance use?
2. How has the patient's substance use affected relationships with others?
3. Has the substance use impacted the patient's ability to meet usual role expectations?
4. Are there criminal or legal problems related to substance use?
5. What support system is available to the person. Is the family involved?
6. What lifestyle behaviors contribute to the maintenance of continued drug use?

[a]This information needs to be obtained immediately. It is vital to the evaluation of impending withdrawal, complications of withdrawal, impending overdose, and potential need for medical intervention.

- Assess for comorbid physical and mental disorders.
- Comorbid mental disorders can complicate long-term treatment.
- Assess for risk factors for suicide, injury to others, and self-harm.

Initial Interview

Screening tests can be very helpful in identifying the problems and extent of the substance use. Many standardized screening tools are available. The following are two good examples of screening tools for substance use disorders:

- **Alcohol:** The CAGE questionnaire is a four-question tool used to assess alcohol or drug use. Each positive response is given one point. The score ranges from 0 to 4, with a score of 2 or greater indicating the potential for alcohol or drug use problems (Table 19.12).

TABLE 19.12 Modified CAGE Questionnaire

- ☐ Have you ever felt you should **C**ut down on your drinking or drug use?
- ☐ Have people **A**nnoyed you by criticizing your drinking or drug use?
- ☐ Have you ever felt bad or **G**uilty about your drinking or drug use?
- ☐ Have you ever had a drink or used a drug first thing in the morning to steady your nerves or to get rid of a hangover (**E**ye opener)?

Scoring: Positive responses are given 1 point. A score of 2 or more is considered clinically significant.

From SAMSHA–HRSA Center for Integrated Health Solution. (n.d.). *Screening tools*. Retrieved from https://www.integration.samhsa.gov/clinical-practice/screening-tools

- **Other substances used/misused:** The Brief Drug Abuse Screening Test (B-DAST) can be used to assess the use of other substances (Box 19.3). Each item counts as 1 point, and 6 or more points indicates a serious substance use problem.

Additional screening tools can be found at https://pubs.niaaa.nih.gov/publications/arh28-2/78-79.htm.

Psychological Issues

Denial is an unconscious defense mechanism in which a person refuses to accept reality. Defense mechanisms help us to protect our self-esteem. With denial, people may not even recognize they are refusing to accept reality. Individuals with an SUD are often in denial. They may refuse to accept they have a problem and need help. What is clear to the outside person is not necessarily clear to the person with an SUD. Strong denial may be reinforced by the stigma associated with these disorders (e.g., "I know I am not a 'junkie,' so I must not have that problem").

Closely related to denial is **underreporting**, where the individual is not willing to reveal the full amount of substance use, fearing a negative judgment. **Minimizing** refers to the individual's belief that the pattern of use is not problematic when compared to others (e.g., "Everybody at college drinks"). These defenses are usually associated with protecting the self from feelings of shame or feared consequences.

These psychological concerns negatively affect both an accurate assessment of the problem and successful treatment. Strategies to help the person limit the use of these defenses include approaching the person in a truly nonjudgmental way. It can be useful to avoid labels, such as "You are clearly an alcoholic." A more helpful alternative is to focus on the consequences of the behavior—for example, "You have shared with me that you have experienced a lot of difficulties associated with using. This may be a red flag that there is a problem that needs to be worked on." Offering objective and accurate information about SUDs can also lessen denial—for example, "These liver function blood tests indicate beginning liver damage from the alcohol you have been consuming. Continued use of alcohol may prevent the liver from healing."

Additionally, individuals with an SUD may be **ambivalent** about admitting they have a problem. A part of them may acknowledge that using is causing some problems, but admitting they have a "drinking problem" or considering the idea of never being able to use again is too scary a prospect. They may not feel they have the tools to cope without the use of substances. A full admission by the person that there is a substance use problem is not required to start the treatment process. Offering community resources "if you ever do consider getting help to stop using" can be a good beginning way to help.

BOX 19.3 B-DAST: Brief Drug Abuse Screening Test

Instructions: The following questions concern information about your involvement and abuse of drugs. Drug abuse refers to (1) the use of prescribed or over-the-counter drugs in excess of the directions and (2) any nonmedical use of drugs. Carefully read each statement and decide whether your answer is yes or no. Then circle the appropriate response.

YES NO **1.** Have you used drugs other than those required for medical reasons?
YES NO **2.** Have you abused prescription drugs?
YES NO **3.** Do you abuse more than one drug at a time?
YES NO **4.** Can you get through the week without using drugs (other than those required for medical reasons)?
YES NO **5.** Are you always able to stop using drugs when you want to?
YES NO **6.** Have you had blackouts or flashbacks as a result of drug use?
YES NO **7.** Do you ever feel bad about your drug abuse?
YES NO **8.** Does your spouse (or parents) ever complain about your involvement with drugs?
YES NO **9.** Has drug abuse ever created problems between you and your spouse?
YES NO **10.** Have you ever lost friends because of your use of drugs?
YES NO **11.** Have you ever neglected your family or missed work because of your use of drugs?
YES NO **12.** Have you ever been in trouble at work because of drug abuse?
YES NO **13.** Have you ever lost a job because of drug abuse?
YES NO **14.** Have you gotten into fights when under the influence of drugs?
YES NO **15.** Have you engaged in illegal activities in order to obtain drugs?
YES NO **16.** Have you ever been arrested for possession of illegal drugs?
YES NO **17.** Have you ever experienced withdrawal symptoms as a result of heavy drug intake?
YES NO **18.** Have you had medical problems as a result of your drug use (e.g., memory loss, hepatitis, convulsions, bleeding)?
YES NO **19.** Have you ever gone to anyone for help for a drug problem?
YES NO **20.** Have you ever been involved in a treatment program specifically related to drug use?

Items 4 and 5 are scored in the NO, or false, direction. Each item is 1 point. A score of 6 or more points suggests significant problems.

From Skinner, H. A. (1982). The Drug Abuse Screening Test. *Addictive Behavior, 7,* 363; Substance Abuse and Mental Health Services Administration. (2005). *Substance abuse treatment for persons with co-occurring disorders* (Treatment Improvement Protocol [TIP] Series 42; DHHS Publication No. [SMA] 05-3992). Rockville, MD: Author.

Nurse Self-Assessment

Patients who struggle with addiction can be very difficult to treat. Societal prejudices and stigmatizing attitudes influence the attitudes of health care workers and can negatively affect the care given to these individuals.

It is important for the nurse to examine personal feelings and thoughts about addicted individuals. Are personal attitudes based on accurate information about the *disease* of addiction? Is there an understanding that repeated relapse is not a personal weakness and failure on the part of those with the disorder but, rather, a symptom of a challenging disease? Is there an understanding of *stages of change* and an appreciation for how challenging it is to make the necessary changes to become drug-free? Is there a recognition that relapse is not evidence of treatment failure but, rather, one stage of the change process? For many, each *relapse* can be an opportunity to learn strategies to facilitate longer periods of being drug-free in the future.

Nurses in all specialties must educate themselves about these disorders and current evidence-based treatments. The nurse can use this complex understanding of behavior change to provide individualized, nonjudgmental care.

A patient's slow progress toward recovery can leave the nurse feeling ineffective, helpless, and hopeless. Previous negative experiences with a person with a substance use disorder, such as a family member or a "drunk driver," can consciously or unconsciously influence our thinking about these disorders. Working with a more experienced clinician to help identify transference and countertransference issues that are negatively affecting the provision of care can be helpful.

DIAGNOSIS

The focus of care for patients with SUDs is complex because of the large range of physical and psychological effects of drug use and dependence. Comorbid psychiatric problems must also be addressed. Potential patient problems and nursing diagnoses for people with substance use disorders are listed in Table 19.13.

Substance Use and Health Care Workers

It is believed that health professionals misuse alcohol and other drugs at about the same rate as the general population (10% to 15%). Nursing students are just as vulnerable to addictions. Estimates suggest that 10% to 20% of all nurses in the United States are addicted to some type of illegal or controlled substance (Nauert, 2015). According to the National Council of the State Boards of Nursing (2014), many nurses with a substance use disorder are underidentified, underreported, and untreated, and they may continue to practice. Their impairment may endanger the lives of their patients.

Behaviors that may indicate an impaired nurse include the following:

- Volunteering to work additional shifts to be nearer to the source of the drug
- Spending a lot of time in the bathroom
- Increased patient complaints that pain or sleep medication is ineffective
- Increased inaccurate drug counts and vial breakage
- A tendency to isolate or a preference for working alone
- Irritability, dramatic changes in mood, and decrease in productivity
- Multiple absences and tardiness to work
- The smell of alcohol on the individual's breath while at work

If indicators of impaired practice are observed or suspected, there is an ethical obligation to report, according to the American Nurses Association (ANA) Code of Ethics, Provision 3.6 (ANA, 2015). Intervention is the responsibility of the nurse manager and other nursing administrators. Reporting an impaired colleague is not easy, even though it is our responsibility. Refer to Box 19.4.

A joint position statement of the *Journal of Addictions Nursing*, the Emergency Nurses Association, and International Nurses Society on Addictions presents guidelines relating to SUDs for nurses and nursing students.

Health care facilities should provide education to nurses and other employees relating to alcohol and drug use and should promote safe, supportive, drug-free workplaces. **Alternative-to-discipline (ADT) programs** should be adopted by health care facilities and nursing schools in order to treat nurses and nursing students with SUDs, with the aims of retention, rehabilitation, and reentry into safe, professional practice. Drug diversion should be viewed mainly as a symptom of a serious and treatable disease, not just a crime. Nurses and nursing students should have the responsibility and means to report suspected or actual concerns (Strobbe & Crowley, 2017).

TABLE 19.13 Potential Nursing Diagnoses for Substance Use Disorders

Signs and Symptoms	Potential Nursing Diagnoses[a]
Symptoms indicating withdrawal or overdose	*Withdrawal symptom* *Risk for injury*
Vomiting, diarrhea, poor nutritional and fluid intake (associated with use and withdrawal)	*Impaired nutritional status* *Risk for dehydration*
Audiovisual hallucinations, impaired judgment, memory deficits, cognitive impairments (associated with substance use or withdrawal)	*Impaired cognition* *Risk for delirium* *Risk for confusion* *Distorted thinking process* *Hallucination*
Changes in sleep–wake cycle, from use or withdrawal	*Impaired sleep*
Lack of self-care (hygiene, grooming); failure to care for basic health needs	*Self-care deficit*
Does not perceive dangers of substance use or addiction; minimizes symptoms	*Denial* *Conflicting attitude toward care*
Continued substance use despite negative consequences	*Impaired coping process* *Impaired volition* *Impulse control* *Craving* *Conflicting attitude toward care* *Impaired health-seeking behavior*
Feelings of hopelessness, inability to change, feelings of worthlessness, feeling that life has no meaning or future	*Hopelessness* *Spiritual distress* *Situational low self-esteem* *Chronic low self-esteem* *Risk for suicide* *Shame*
Excessive use negatively affecting all areas of a person's life: loss of friends, poor job performance, increased illness rates, proneness to accidents and overdoses	*Impaired role performance* *Impaired socialization* *Social isolation* *Risk for loneliness* *Anxiety* *Risk for injury*
Family codependent behaviors Family conflict related to continued substance use behaviors	*Impaired family process* *Impaired family coping* *Lack of family support*

[a]The International Classification for Nursing Practice (ICNP) is a product of the International Council of Nurses (ICN). Retrieved from http://www.icn.ch/what-we-do/ICNP-Browser/

OUTCOMES IDENTIFICATION

When planning care for patients with SUDs, the patient's cultural background and values need to be reflected in the plan of care. The following are some examples of desired outcomes:

- Remaining free from injury while withdrawing from the substance
- Beginning to increase insight

BOX 19.4 A Guide for Assisting Colleagues Who Demonstrate Impairment in the Workplace

Nurses and other health professionals impaired by alcohol or other drugs pose a serious risk of harm to patients, colleagues, and themselves. Employers have a duty to protect the patient as well as an ethical obligation to assist their employees. The following guidelines and/or ethical issues should be considered:

- Confidentiality related to information concerning a chemical dependency problem is required by federal law. Each employer should have a policy that includes:
  1. A cause for testing policy
  2. Identification of the person who will interact with the employee concerning their impaired practice
  3. A referral process for evaluation and treatment
  4. Clear consequences associated with refusing treatment
- It is the obligation and responsibility of a colleague or coworker to report an impaired health professional's behavior to the employer or designated supervisor. Workers should not be allowed to give patient care until they have been evaluated and received treatment.
- A health care worker should be offered professional treatment instead of termination. It is more cost effective. Valuable expertise and service history may be lost if the health professional's employment is terminated and he or she is not given the opportunity to get treatment for a progressive medical illness.
- It is important to note that the suicide risk is increased after an intervention or confrontation. It is necessary to ensure the health professional is not left alone after an intervention until a plan is in place.
- The health professional does have the right to refuse treatment. The employer needs to make it clear that if evaluation and treatment are rejected, the health care worker's employment may be terminated.

Adapted from Washington Health Professional Services. (2013). *A guide for assisting colleagues who demonstrate impairment in the workplace.* Olympia, WA: Author.

- Attending programs for treatment and maintenance of sobriety:
  - Self-help groups like Alcoholics Anonymous
  - Group therapy; cognitive-behavioral therapy
  - Other programs associated with recovery
- Attending a relapse prevention program during the active course of treatment
- Identifying cues or situations that pose increased risk of return to drug use (relapse)
- Developing relationships with drug-free supportive persons for socialization
- Recognition that socializing with former substance-using friends can trigger relapse
- Demonstrating at least one or two new coping strategies in dealing with troubling feelings that can increase relapse risk (anger, loneliness, cravings, anxiety)

PLANNING AND IMPLEMENTATION

Planning care requires attention to the patient's social status, income, cultural and ethnic background, gender, age, substance use history, and current condition. One goal of treatment is full abstinence. This may not be the goal of some patients. Abstinence is strongly related to better work adjustment, positive health status, improved interpersonal relationships, and general social stability. Planning must also address the patient's major psychological, social, and medical problems. SUDs are

APPLYING EVIDENCE-BASED PRACTICE (EBP)

Problem

A nursing student was completing her psychiatric nursing rotation at a community hospital. The student's preceptor was an experienced registered nurse (RN) with a history of alcohol addiction who had completed the Chemically Addicted Nurses Diversion Option (CANDO) program in Arizona several years earlier. The preceptor was open with her student about her experiences with addiction and recovery. The student viewed her as a skilled and caring nurse. During the rotation, the preceptor had a grand mal seizure. The student called out for help, then knelt down to assist her preceptor. While in close proximity, she smelled alcohol on her preceptor's breath. The student knows from class that she should report her preceptor, but a friend recently lost her job due to a substance use disorder, and the student is torn and upset.

EBP Assessment

A. **What do you already know from experience?** Alcohol use disorder contributes to poor judgment and errors. It seems reasonable to this student that errors would also occur in caring for patients. The student has seen a punitive response in the workplace to someone she cares about due to alcohol use disorder and does not want to hurt her preceptor.

B. **What does the literature say?**
- Most states have an intervention program for impaired nurses in lieu of discipline.
- The incidence of substance use disorder is nurses is 10% to 20%.
- Relapse can occur as part of the disease.
- The incidence of self-reporting is low due to the nature of addiction and stigma, so most impaired nurses will be noticed first by colleagues.
- Addiction is a treatable disease, and the success rate in impaired nurse programs is good. Early intervention and a nonpunitive approach are essential for recovery.

C. **What does the patient want?**
- The patient in this case is the impaired nurse.
- She has been able to maintain several years of sobriety.
- Relapse is a symptom of the disease.
- She has been an excellent nurse and role model for the student during her psychiatric nursing rotation.

Plan

The student first approached her clinical instructor, who accompanied her to a meeting with the nursing supervisor. The nursing supervisor has experience with the state **alternative-to-discipline (ATD)** program. Recognizing that a substance use disorder is a disease, the supervisor is supportive in helping this preceptor to move toward recovery. The nursing supervisor planned to speak with the preceptor and offer her the ATD program as an option, once she recovers from her seizure. The preceptor would not be allowed to return to work until the issue was decided.

QSEN Prelicensure Knowledge, Skills, and Attitudes (KSAs) Addressed

ATD programs provide greater patient **Safety** because they enable managers to remove nurses from the work environment quickly.

ATD programs provide **Evidence-Based Practice** by providing nonjudgmental support and treatment that encourages nurses to seek help and improve their chances of staying in the profession.

considered a family disease. Involvement of appropriate family members is essential.

The aim of treatment is to facilitate a change in behavior: stopping compulsive drug seeking and use. For many, treatment is a long-term process that involves multiple interventions and regular monitoring. The choice of inpatient or outpatient care depends on cost and the availability of insurance coverage. Outpatient programs work best for those who are employed and who have an involved social support system. People who have no support and structure in their day often do better with inpatient programs.

Communication Guidelines

Communication strategies are designed to address behaviors that are frequently displayed by individuals with an SUD. Problematic behaviors include dysfunctional anger, manipulation, impulsiveness, and grandiosity. Perhaps the best approach is to focus on developing *nonjudgmental and accepting* relationships with individuals so that they feel safe. It is important to communicate in culturally appropriate ways. Anger and manipulative behaviors are best managed with active listening and clear, consistent, and nonpunitive limit setting.

Health Teaching and Health Promotion

Health teaching for substance use disorders includes the same components used for other diseases. These include education about the disease, an accurate understanding of medications used for both withdrawal and maintenance, and self-help strategies. There is a particular emphasis on relapse prevention.

Relapse Prevention

Relapse is a *common symptom* of SUDs. The goal of **relapse prevention** is to help individuals identify "trigger situations" so that periods of sobriety can be lengthened over time. Health teaching should emphasize that *relapse is part of the illness and not a treatment failure.* Recovery is a lifelong process. Refer to Box 19.5 for relapse prevention strategies. Treatment medications facilitate a safe withdrawal and support continued abstinence.

In any health care setting, the nurse can play an important role by recognizing the signs of a substance use disorder, recognizing symptoms of withdrawal, and making appropriate referrals.

VIGNETTE: Bill, a 20-year-old single male, is transported to the emergency department in a coma, accompanied by his mother. Bill lives with his mother. When his mother was not able to wake him up, she dialed 911. A syringe and some white powder were found next to Bill. His breathing is labored, and his pupils are constricted. Vital signs: blood pressure is 60/40 mm Hg, and pulse is 132 beats per minute. Bill's situation is determined to be life-threatening.

Bill's mother reports that Bill had been using heroin for 6 months before entering a methadone maintenance program. Given this history, a narcotic antagonist, naloxone, is given intramuscularly. Within 5 minutes, Bill's breathing improves, and he responds to verbal stimuli. His mother later tells staff that Bill has been in the methadone maintenance program for the past year but has not attended the program or received his methadone for the past week. The mother was encouraged to call the program, and an outreach worker, Mr. Rodriguez, is sent to talk to her and Bill. An appointment is made with this counselor for the following Monday. Mr. Rodriguez talks to Bill regarding how he perceives his situation, where he wants to go, and what he thinks he needs to get there.

After talking to Bill and reviewing Bill's history, the health care team decides that a self-help, abstinence-oriented recovery program might be the most helpful treatment. Bill has not been misusing drugs for a long time, he has a job, and he appears motivated. Naltrexone will be given in conjunction with relapse-prevention training, and Bill will regularly attend Narcotics Anonymous meetings.

BOX 19.5 Relapse Prevention Strategies

Learn About Relapse

1. Relapse is a part of recovery from addiction; 40% to 60% of people relapse. It does not mean failure.
2. Relapse starts with certain cues:
   a. Emotional cues:
      - Increases in anxiety, anger, or depression
      - Increased mood swings
      - Poor eating and poor sleep
      - Feeling restless and bored
   b. Mental response:
      - Glamorizing past drug use
      - Keeping secrets or lying
      - Thinking about using
   c. Physical cues:
      - Stopping counseling and meetings
      - Hanging out with old friends and places where you used

Relapse Prevention Plan

1. Identify potential **triggers** to relapse. These can include:
   a. People who remind you of drug use
   b. Places you used to use
   c. Thoughts that can lead to use
2. Develop a specific plan ahead of time to confront these triggers.
3. Have a plan if you develop **cravings.**
   a. Whom can you call?
   b. How can you distract yourself from the craving?
4. Compile a list of **healthy coping mechanisms.** These can include:
   a. Use relaxation techniques: exercising, deep breathing, meditation.
   b. Make a list of consequences of relapse.
   c. Make a list of what you are grateful for.
   d. Maintain physical and mental health.
   e. Maintain healthy relationships.
   f. Use available supports to maintain abstinence:
      i. Relapse-prevention groups
      ii. Peer-support groups such as Alcoholics Anonymous
      iii. Individual, group, and family therapy

Adapted from Deeds, A. (n.d.). *How to write a relapse prevention plan*: Retrieved from https://www.choosehelp.com/topics/recovery/writing-a-relapse-prevention-plan

Treating Co-occurring Disorders

Co-occurring neuropsychiatric and other mental illnesses may require additional interventions. The nurse needs to be aware of evidence-based clinical practice guidelines that involve individuals with co-occurring diagnoses. The following six principles are applicable in inpatient and outpatient settings:

1. Expect a patient to have at least one co-occurring disorder.
2. Treatment success is increased when providers are empathic, hopeful, and work as a team.
3. Both addiction programs and mental health programs need a dual focus, which requires appropriate training for staff.
4. The SUD and the psychiatric disorder are both considered primary and need concurrent treatment.
5. The recovery process stresses that recovery occurs in stages, and treatment should be matched to the patient's needs, level of motivation, and engagement.
6. Outcomes must be individualized to support progress in small steps over a long period.

Psychotherapy and Therapeutic Modalities

Safe withdrawal and achieving abstinence are only the first steps toward what will be a long and complex recovery. Treatment programs must focus on the many aspects of the person's life that have been altered because of addiction. These include the individual's medical, social, vocational, legal, and psychological needs.

Recovery Model

Recovery experiences are inherently personal, and recovery can be complex and nonlinear. This process occurs via many pathways, and a more individualized approach may be needed.

SAMHSA (2015) established a working definition of *recovery* that is widely accepted by many health professionals, including the U.S. Surgeon General and the Institute of Medicine (IOM). It defined recovery as a *process of change* through which individuals improve their health and wellness, live self-directed lives, and strive to reach their full potential (SAMHSA, 2017b). It has four major dimensions:

- Health—overcoming or managing one's disease
- Home—having a safe and stable place to live
- Purpose—conducting meaningful activities
- Community—having relationships and social networks that provide support, friendship, and hope

Recovery relies on access to evidence-based clinical treatment and recovery support services for all populations.

Psychotherapy assists patients in identifying and using alternative coping mechanisms to reduce reliance on substances. The following therapies have been found to be effective for people on the road to recovery:

- **Cognitive-behavioral therapy** (CBT) helps patients to recognize and avoid old triggers to using substances and offers behavioral strategies to cope with situations that are most likely to induce cravings and abuse of drugs.
- **Motivational enhancement therapy** (MET) is a type of therapy in which a therapist helps a patient to tap into his or her personal motivations to resist drug use. MET can facilitate reduced rates of drug use, fewer arrests, and increased adherence to treatment.
- **Screening, brief intervention, and referral to treatment** (SBIRT) is an evidence-based practice used to identify, reduce, and prevent problematic use and dependence on alcohol and drugs. This is an IOM-recommended strategy for community health care. It consists of three parts:
  1. **Screening:** the patient is assessed for risky substance use behaviors.
  2. **Brief intervention:** the health care professional provides feedback and advice.
  3. **Referral for treatment:** referrals are provided to brief therapy or additional treatment (SAMHSA, 2017c).
- **Motivational interviewing** is an **evidence-based** counseling approach. Based on an understanding of the thoughts and behavior associated with the *stages of change*, it emphasizes the use of a directive, patient-centered style of interaction to promote behavioral change. Therapeutic communication techniques are individualized depending upon the patient's current stage of change. Motivational interviewing is guided by four principles to evoke change:
  1. Express empathy (e.g., "I can understand why using drugs seems appealing in some situations").
  2. Develop discrepancies. *Ambivalence* about wanting help can interfere with seeking treatment. The therapist points out the disparity between what the person is doing versus goals that the person wants to accomplish—for example, "If your goal is to be happy and have a successful career, using heroin daily may get in the way of that." This strategy replaces confrontation and de-emphasizes labels like "alcoholic."

APPLYING THE ART

An Individual With Substance Use Disorder

Scenario

During our previous two encounters, 34-year-old Kristen had repeatedly insisted she would "quit using and take my medication." Kristen, a single mom, has just learned that her own mother has gained legal custody of Kristen's three preschool-aged children related to charges of child neglect. Before each of her two psychiatric hospitalizations in the past year, Kristen chosen heroin over taking her psychotropic medication, which impaired her ability to take care of her children.

Therapeutic Goal

By the end of this interaction, Kristen will show an understanding of the negative consequences of choosing heroin when feeling out of control.

Student–Patient Interaction	Thoughts, Communication Techniques, and Mental Health Nursing Concepts
Kristen: (*Glances my way and motions "come on" as she rapidly paces the hallway.*) **Student's feelings:** *I'm surprised Kristen did not even stop to greet me.*	I had learned in the report about Kristen losing custody of her children. Initially she had cried, but her tears quickly turned to angry pacing. I offer to walk with Kristen.
Student: "Kristen, I'm having trouble keeping up with you. You seem really upset." ***Student's feelings:*** *Addiction makes me angry. Kristen shows such promise and then abandons everything when heroin calls. I know that some people at school see nothing wrong with "recreational" use of drugs. I look around the addictions unit and see pain everywhere.*	Technique: "Sharing observations"
Kristen: "Yes, I'm upset. My so-called mother stole my kids! I never injured my kids. I just asked my 5-year-old whether he wanted new shoes or wanted Mommy to feel better. It's not my fault. So my mother got upset and bought the shoes. She thinks she can buy their love."	Kristen uses projection, blaming her mother for the loss of her children. I remember that sometimes patients use defense mechanisms to prevent anxiety and loss of self-esteem. This includes denial ("I'd never hurt my kids"), rationalization ("It wasn't me who chose heroin over shoes"), and projection.
Student: "Kristen, I'm concerned with what is happening with you, but I'm having trouble keeping up. Could you walk a little slower so that I can hear you clearly?" ***Student's feelings:*** *I really am concerned with her welfare, even though I feel frustrated that she totally denies her addiction.*	Technique: Use of empathy I think Kristen may be ambivalent, not sure if she can tolerate me or anyone.
Kristen: (*Kicks a chair, across the room and yells in my face.*) "Get up here, then, if you care so much!"	She is escalating. I see staff on their way to help. Anxiety is communicated interpersonally. I need to talk her down.
Student's feelings: *I feel unnerved by this incident and want this behavior to stop.*	Okay. I am okay. I need to mindfully breathe and stay calm and in charge of myself.
Student: "Kristen, stop." (*Louder voice, then quieter.*) "Take a deep breath." (*Quietly concerned, trying to make eye contact.*)	I set limits and offer an alternative behavior (give information).
Kristen: (*Meets my eyes. Sarcastically:*) "Here comes the cavalry!" (*Three staff approach but wait as I speak.*) ***Student's feelings:*** *I feel kind of honored that the staff trust that I am doing well enough to wait to see if they're needed.*	Although Kristen uses sarcasm, she nonetheless responds to the staff's arrival by backing away from me.
Student: "Kristen, I trust that you and I can get through this." (*Pauses.*) "Thank you for calming down and backing away from me." (*Looking concerned.*) "I know you're upset. Please back up." (*She does.*) "Thank you, Kristen." (*Staff step back, carefully watching as Kristen slowly walks to the chair. Kristen uprights the chair she kicked over, and then we both sit down.*)	I offer self and use reflection. I treat Kristen with respect as well as model socially appropriate interactions by saying "please" and "thank you" to Kristen for calming down and backing up.
Student's feelings: *I made it through this with no one hurt. I feel more confident, but I'm also really relieved that the staff responded so quickly. I know the staff were ready to intervene if needed.*	Collaborative care is essential to a safe and therapeutic milieu.
Kristen: "I don't know what got into me. I never meant to hurt you."	
Student: (*Making eye contact.*) "It's frightening to see angry behavior and have you screaming in my face. I'm okay now. How about you?"	I assess and also let Kristen know my feelings. Her choices affect others. I nonjudgmentally accept Kristen, but not the hurtful behavior.
Kristen: (*Nods.*) "I'm sorry. Sometimes I feel so out of control." ***Student's feelings:*** *Kristen tries to make things right by apologizing and fixing the chair.*	
Student: "You kicked the chair and screamed in my face, but you were also able to say 'sorry.'"	I name the observed acting-out behavior but also give support by saying, "You were able to . . ."
Kristen: "I meant the 'sorry.' I always mean it. Then the pressure builds and ..." (*Points to the needle tracks on her arms.*)	She uses heroin as a dysfunctional way to cope with anxiety. Unfortunately, the heroin compounds her problems.
Student: "So, when you feel out of control, maybe even overwhelmed, you turn to heroin?"	I am so thankful I have other ways to cope and people who care about me.
Kristen: (*Nods.*) "I am gone. No more Kristen. I forget all the hassles. Then it all crashes down. I lose everything. I've screwed up everything again."	In choosing heroin, she no longer has to deal with any "hassles"; I can see how this may be temporarily attractive.
Student's feelings: *Some days I think how far I still have to go to be a nurse. Then I think of Kristen's long, long road to reach a drug-free life.*	She also sees the downside of using: "I lose everything." The drug erodes her self-esteem and even her sense of self.

APPLYING THE ART—cont'd

An Individual With Substance Use Disorder

Student–Patient Interaction	Thoughts, Communication Techniques, and Mental Health Nursing Concepts
Student: "Everything?"	I use restatement, encouraging her to go on.
Kristen: "Myself, my kids." (*Starts to cry.*)	Kristen shows partial insight but so far avoids attending Narcotics Anonymous.
Student: (*Leans forward, waiting quietly.*)	I use attending behavior.
Student's feelings: *I want to fill the silences, but I contain my anxiety.*	
Kristen: "I miss them so much! They deserve better than me. I need to go lie down." (*Begins to turn away.*)	Kristen uses withdrawal by physically retreating to her room. Kristen feels exhausted by all of the emotions she's experienced.
Student's feelings: *I feel badly for how much she has lost because of heroin.*	
Student: "Okay, I'll check with you after lunch."	I give information and accept Kristen's decision to leave in order to give her control and build trust.
Student's feelings: *I need to debrief in a clinical conference. I'm feeling exhausted too.*	
Kristen: (*Nods, walking toward her room.*)	

3. Roll with resistance. Change is scary. It can be useful to understand the person's point of view first (reflection), then point out alternative ways of thinking for the person to consider.
4. Support self-efficacy. Help the person to believe in the possibility of change by supporting personal strengths (Tan et al., 2015).

Motivational interviewing can be especially helpful in chipping away at the denial associated with SUDs by activating the person's internal motivation. These techniques have also shown effectiveness when helping a person make any type of health-related behavior change.

- **Group therapy** can be an extremely important element of recovery for many individuals with substance use disorders.
- **Family therapy** is a useful adjunct therapy because family members often serve as the core support system for recovering individuals. Psychoeducation helps family members understand the disease. Repairing relationships that were damaged due to addiction is also an important component of family therapy.

The first 6 months of recovery can be the most challenging. Challenges include the following:

- Physical changes occur as the body adapts to functioning without substances.
- The newly sober individual is constantly bombarded with sensory cues that the brain associates with the pleasurable habit. The individual must unlearn habits related to drinking and drug use to prevent triggering cravings and relapse.
- A return of strong emotions previously blunted during drug use can produce anxiety.
- The responses of family members and coworkers to the patient's new behavior must be addressed. Sobriety disrupts a system, and everyone in that system needs to adjust to the change.
- New coping skills must be developed to prevent relapse.

Whatever therapy a person chooses, it needs to be directive, honest, and empathetic. The therapeutic process involves teaching the patient to identify the physical and emotional changes that are currently present. Confidentiality must be maintained throughout therapy *except* when it conflicts with requirements for mandatory reporting (child abuse, danger to self or others).

Self-Help Groups and 12-Step Programs

Alcoholics Anonymous (AA) is a self-help group that is the prototype for all 12-step programs. Three basic concepts are fundamental to 12-step programs:

1. Individuals with addictive disorders are powerless over their addiction, and their lives are unmanageable.
2. Although individuals with addictive disorders are not responsible for their disease, they are responsible for their recovery.
3. Individuals can no longer blame people, places, and things for their addiction; they must face their problems and their feelings.

AA does not work for everyone, but for many, it can be an important part of recovery. It is difficult to study the effectiveness of AA due to the anonymous nature of the program. Evidence does suggest those who become deeply involved in the program usually do better over time. An important aspect of recovery in AA is **spirituality**.

In addition to AA, other 12-step programs include Narcotics Anonymous (NA).

Self-Management and Recovery Training (**SMART Recovery**) is a support program for people with addictions and behavioral disorders (SMART Recovery, 2018). It teaches people how to control their addictive behavior by focusing on underlying thoughts and feelings. The four-point program includes the following:

1. Enhancing and maintaining motivation to abstain
2. Coping with urges
3. Managing thoughts, feelings, and behaviors
4. Lifestyle balance (balancing momentary and enduring satisfactions) (see http://www.Smartrecovery.org)

Residential Programs

Residential treatment programs are best suited for individuals who have a longer history of addiction. The goal of treatment is to effect a change in lifestyle, including abstinence, development of social skills, and elimination of problematic behavior. Follow-up studies suggest that patients who stay in such programs for 90 days or longer exhibit a significant decrease in illicit drug use and recorded arrests. There is also an increase in days of employment. These programs supply a "24/7" drug-free environment for the early days of recovery.

Outpatient Programs

Most treatment for SUDs takes place in the community. Outpatient programs include a variety of psychotherapeutic and pharmacological interventions, along with behavioral monitoring. These programs are popular because they are viewed as flexible, diverse, cost effective, and responsive to the individualized needs of the person. Outpatient programs allow the individual to return home during the recovery period.

This enables the individual to keep in contact with family and sometimes continue working but increases the risk of encountering triggers to sabotage recovery. Outpatient services can include intensive outpatient/partial hospitalization, which provides 4 to 6 hours of treatment each day. It can also include once-per-week counseling services.

Employee Assistance Programs

An employee assistance program (EAP) is a work-based intervention program designed to identify and assist employees in resolving personal problems, including substance/alcohol use, that may be adversely affecting the employee's performance. Some programs deliver short-term crisis counseling and support and referrals, whereas others provide longer-term counseling as an alternative to job termination when the employee's work performance is negatively affected by impairment.

Self-Help Groups for Family Members

An alcohol/substance use disorder is sometimes described as a family disease because all members of the family are affected. *Codependency* defines a relationship in which one partner has extreme physical or emotional needs and the other partner spends most of his or her time responding to those needs. When a person is in a *codependent* relationship with someone who is misusing drugs, both individuals may experience multiple negative effects. Protecting a loved one from the consequences of destructive behavior, labeled enabling, may seem supportive but actually makes it easier for the addicted person to maintain the addiction. The *codependent* individual stops taking care of his or her own needs, leading to poor physical and mental health. (See Box 19.1 for a list of codependent behaviors.) Counseling and support should be encouraged for the family of a person with an SUD to lessen *enabling* and *codependent* behaviors. Al-Anon and Alateen are self-help groups that offer support and guidance for adults and teenagers, respectively. *Al-Anon* believes that together, the families and friends of those with an SUD can provide hope to one another and help solve the various problems they may face. There is a recognition that *AUD* is a family disease, and Al-Anon is committed to helping *family members and friends* cope with a loved one's heavy alcohol (or drug) use.

Breaking Free Online (BFO) is a web-based program that allows individuals to tailor their own substance use and mental health treatment using multiple evidence-based intervention strategies. Currently only available in the United Kingdom, this self-help program was found to result in a significant decrease in weekly alcohol consumption, alcohol dependence severity, depression, and anxiety and significant increases in quality of life as compared to a control group (Ellison, Davries, & Ward, 2015).

Harm Reduction

Harm reduction is a controversial treatment strategy for those with a chronic, relapsing brain disease. It is based on the idea that many people with a substance use problem are not ready to stop using drugs. Ignoring these individuals leads to increased crime, public health problems, and increased community social problems. Harm reduction is described as a set of practices that can reduce the impact of specific drug-using behaviors (Foundations Recovery Network, 2020). The goal is to buffer the community from the full impact of addiction. An example of a harm-reduction strategy might be expanding the availability of methadone maintenance programs. A more controversial harm-reduction practice might include developing a needle-exchange program to reduce the incidence of secondary physical complications associated with drug use. The easy availability of naloxone, a reversal agent for narcotic overdoses, as a tool to prevent overdose deaths is a currently practiced harm-reduction strategy.

EVALUATION

Evaluation is made based on the identified goals of treatment. For some individuals and treatment organizations, **full abstinence** is the goal following a safe withdrawal. Traditionally this has meant abstaining from maintenance medications also. Current thinking encourages the use of maintenance drugs in conjunction with self-help groups and/or therapy.

The *DSM-5* (APA, 2013) recognizes that SUDs range from mild to severe. This suggests that different treatment goals may be useful for different levels of severity. For those with a mild SUD, learning to use substances in moderation may be possible. For others, long-term use of medications that support maintenance may be a preferred treatment. NIDA calls medication an important element of treatment for many patients, especially when combined with counseling and other behavioral therapies (NIDA, 2016c).

Other evaluation measures look at the level of participation in recovery programs, acceptable occupational functioning, improved family relationships, and the ability to relate normally and comfortably to other human beings. The ability to use existing supports and skills learned in treatment is important for ongoing recovery. Continuous monitoring and evaluation increase the chances for prolonged recovery.

KEY POINTS TO REMEMBER

- Substance use disorders (SUDs) are chronic, relapsing brain diseases that present significant public health concerns in adolescents and adults.
- Because the brain doesn't fully mature until the mid-20s, the use of psychoactive drugs in adolescents and young adults can significantly interfere with the brain's ability to function in the future and interfere with psychological and social growth.
- Risk factors associated with the development of an SUD include a combination of genetic, biological, sociological, and environmental factors.
- A comprehensive assessment of individuals with an SUD must include identifying and treating medical and psychiatric comorbidities concurrently.
- The priority nursing assessment for those with an SUD to facilitate a safe withdrawal includes identifying the name of the drug(s) used, the route, the quantity, and the time of last use.
- Individualized treatments following safe withdrawal include psychopharmacology to prevent cravings, individual and group therapies, self-help 12-step groups like Alcoholics Anonymous, and a comprehensive-relapse prevention program.
- Relapse is an *expected complication* in the recovery of addiction.
- An SUD should also be considered a family disease. Family members need support to take care of their own emotional health. Family psychoeducation will help prevent *codependent and enabling behavior,* which tends to prolong the maladaptive behavior of those with an SUD.
- Nurses need to explore their own feelings regarding people who are struggling with an SUD. Strong negative attitudes are common and need to be addressed because they can interfere with the ability to work effectively with a patient.
- *Nurses are at risk for developing an SUD.* When nurses observe signs of impairment in a health care colleague, documentation and reporting are an ethical obligation. *The patient is always the nurse's first responsibility.* There are programs that can provide effective treatment for a colleague while still allowing for an eventual return to work.

APPLYING CRITICAL JUDGMENT

1. Write a paragraph describing your possible reactions to a patient with a substance use disorder.
   A. Would your response be different depending on the substance used (e.g., alcohol vs. heroin, or marijuana vs. cocaine)? Give reasons for your answers.
   B. Would your response be different if the person was a professional colleague? In what way?
2. You have observed a nursing colleague and friend using a psychoactive substance on the unit, exhibiting erratic behavior, and using questionable judgment regarding patient care.
   A. What is an appropriate course of action? What would be your ethical responsibility?
   B. What would be the positive aspects of getting your colleague into an alternative-to-discipline (ADT) program/peer-counseling program?
3. Rosetta Seymour is a 14-year-old teenager who has started misusing oxycodone with her friends. She says that the pills are relatively easy to obtain.
   A. When Ms. Seymour asks you why she needs to take increasing amounts of the drug to get "high," how would you explain the concept of tolerance?
   B. If she had just ingested oxycodone, what physical, behavioral, and psychological signs and symptoms would you expect to see?
   C. If she came into the emergency department with an overdose of oxycodone, what is the priority treatment?
   D. What might be effective long-term care?
4. Tony Garmond is a 45-year-old mechanic. He has a 20-year history of heavy drinking, and he says he wants help to quit.
   A. With a classmate, role-play an initial assessment. Identify essential information to obtain to provide comprehensive care.
   B. Mr. Garmond tried to stop drinking "cold turkey" but is presently in the emergency department with delirium tremens. Which symptoms would you expect to see? What are the appropriate medical interventions?
   C. What are some possible treatment alternatives for Mr. Garmond following detoxification/withdrawal? How would you explain the usefulness and function of self-help recovery programs such as Alcoholics Anonymous or SMART Recovery? What are some additional treatment options?
   D. Identify possible referrals to treatment programs for Mr. Garmond in your community.

CHAPTER REVIEW QUESTIONS

1. A young adult has reported heavy use of alcohol and prescription drugs since mid-adolescence. This individual now has an ataxic gait and uses a cane. Which comment by the nurse presents reality while demonstrating compassion?
   a. "I know you must feel self-conscious about using a cane at your age, but it will help prevent falls."
   b. "Addiction is a fatal disease. If you continue to drink like you have done in past, you will not live another 10 years."
   c. "It's time to face your addiction. You are disappointing your family and must stop drinking for the sake of the people who love you."
   d. "Addiction is powerful. You are young yet cannot walk without a cane. Your health has been significantly affected by your long-term use of drugs and alcohol."
2. The nurse at a local clinic reviews phoned-in requests from patients for prescription refills. As the nurse confers with the health care provider about which prescription refill requests should be authorized, which refill request should be considered first?
   a. Codeine 10 mg PO q4h PRN for an adult with a persistent cough
   b. Hydroxyzine (Vistaril) 25 mg PO TID PRN for an adult who experiences uncomfortable muscle spasms
   c. Lorazepam (Ativan) 1 mg PO BID for an adult who has taken it daily for 3 years for episodes of anxiety
   d. Lomotil 2 mg PO q6h PRN for an adult experiencing severe diarrhea
3. A patient tells the nurse, "After many years, I finally quit smoking. Now I use e-cigarettes only." Which is an appropriate response?
   a. "Using e-cigarettes is now more socially acceptable than using traditional cigarettes."
   b. "Congratulations on quitting, but e-cigarettes contain nicotine and other hazardous chemicals."
   c. "Nicotine is a powerful addiction. Quitting smoking is a big step toward adopting a healthier lifestyle."
   d. "I am glad you have quit smoking. Your loved ones will no longer be exposed to the hazards of secondhand smoke."
4. A young adult tells the nurse, "I have a new prescription for medical marijuana. I use it several times a day for my frequent muscle spasms." What information should the nurse provide first to this patient?
   a. Guidance that the prescription should not be shared with peers
   b. Directions to weigh self once a week and maintain a log of the results
   c. Instructions about safety issues associated with driving or operating machinery
   d. Information about the potential for amotivational syndrome and memory problems
5. A nurse teaches a patient with alcohol use disorder about a new prescription for naltrexone (ReVia, Vivitrol). Which comment by the patient indicates the teaching was effective?
   a. "This medicine will stop my cravings for alcohol."
   b. "I should take this medication only when I feel cravings to drink alcohol."
   c. "This medicine is one part of a bigger treatment plan to help me stay sober."
   d. "I should not use products that contain alcohol, such as cough medicine and aftershave lotion."

REFERENCES

Acharya, K. S., & Issacs, C. (2017). *Psychosocial and environmental pregnancy risks*. Retrieved April 13, 2018, from http://emedicine.medscape.com/article/259346-overview.

AddictionAndRecovery.org (March 21, 2018). Post-Acute Withdrawal (PAWS). Retrieved https://www.addictionsandrecovery.org/post-acute-withdrawal.htm.

American Addiction Centers (December 21, 2017). Statistics on drug addiction. Retrieved from https://americanaddictioncenters.org/rehab-guide/addiction-statistics/#Statistics%20on%20Addiction%20to%20Specific%20Substances.

American Cancer Society. (2015). *Health risks of secondhand smoke*. Retrieved April 13, 2018, https://www.cancer.org/cancer/cancer-causes/tobacco-and-cancer/secondhand-smoke.html.

American Nurses Association (ANA). (2015). *Code of ethics for nurses*. Silver Spring, MD: ANA.

American Psychiatric Association (APA). (2013). *Diagnostic and statistical manual of mental disorders* (5th ed.). Washington, DC: APA.

Black, D. W., & Andreasen, N. C. (2014). *Introductory textbook of psychiatry* (6th ed.). Washington, DC: American Psychiatric Publishing.

Burchum, J., & Rosenthal, L. A. (2016). *Lehne's pharmacology for nursing care* (9th ed.). St. Louis: Elsevier.

Cassoobhoy, A. (2018). *Gaming disorder' is now official*. Medscape. Retrieved from: https://www.medscape.com/viewarticle/899119.

Centers for Disease Control and Prevention (CDC). (2016). CDC Guideline for prescribing opioids for chronic pain — UNITED STATES, 2016. *Recommendations and Reports*, *65*(1), 1–49. March 18, 2016. Retrieved from http://www.cdc.gov/mmwr/volumes/65/rr/rr6501e1.htm.

Centers for Disease Control and Prevention (CDC). (Updated February 2017). *Smoking and tobacco use: Quitting smoking*. Retrieved from https://www.cdc.gov/tobacco/data_statistics/fact_sheets/cessation/quitting/index.htm.

Centers for Disease Control and Prevention (CDC). (Updated March 27, 2018a). *Fact sheets: Binge drinking*. Retrieved from http://www.cdc.gov/ / fact_sheets/cessation/.binge drinkinghttps://www.cdc.gov/alcohol/fact-sheets/binge-drinking.htm.

Centers for Disease Control and Prevention (CDC). (Updated January 2018b). *Fact sheets: Alcohol use and your health*. Retrieved from https://www.cdc.gov/alcohol/fact-sheets/alcohol-use.htm.

Centers for Disease Control and Prevention (CDC). (Updated March 20, 2020). *Drug overdose deaths*. Retrieved from https://www.cdc.gov/drugoverdose/data/statedeaths.html.

Cohen, E. (2015). *No alcohol during pregnancy—ever—lead US pediatricians*. Retrieved from http://www.cnn.com/2015/10/21/health/aap-no-alcohol-during-pregnancy/.

Drugs.com. (2018). Cocaine. Retrieved from https://www.drugs.com/illicit/cocaine.html.

E-medicine. (2015). *Club drugs*. Retrieved from http://www.emedicinehealth.com/club_drugs/article_em.htm.

Elison, S., Davries, G., & Ward, J. (2015). Effectiveness of computer assisted therapy for substance dependence using ratings free online: subgroup analysis of a heterogeneous sample of service users. *Journal of Medical Internet Research Mental Health*, *2*(2). Retrieved from http://www.ncbi.nlm.nih.gov/pmc/articles/PMC4607383/.

Fletcher, A. (2015). *Stereotypes, stigma, and stories of resilience: Changing perceptions of addiction and mental illness*. Retrieved from https://www.rehabs.com/pro-talk-articles/stereotypes-stigma-and-stories-of-resilience-changing-perceptions-of-addiction-and-mental-illness/.

Foundations Recovery Network. (2020). *Addiction treatment alternatives: The way to harm reduction*. Retrieved from https://dualdiagnosis.org/harm-reduction-guide/.

Giddens, J. (2017). *Concepts for nursing practice* (2nd ed.). St. Louis: Elsevier.

Hand, L. (2016). *Researchers identified genetic links to cannabis dependence*. Retrieved from http://www.medscape.com/viewarticle/861695.

Jess, S., et al. (2017). Alcohol withdrawal syndrome: Mechanisms, manifestations, and management. *Neurologica*, *135*(1), 4–16. Retrieved from https://doi.org/10.1111/ane.12671.

Jha, P., Ramasundarahettige, C., Landsman, V., et al. (2013). 21st Century hazards of smoking and benefits of cessation in the United States. *New England Journal of Medicine*, *2013*(368), 341–350.

Kantorovich, A. (2016). Gabapentin for alcohol use disorder: A promising outlook. *Pharmacy Times*. Retrieved from. http://www.pharmacytimes.com/contributor/alexander-kantorovich-pharmd-bcps/2016/08/gabapentin-for-alcohol-use-disorder-a-promising-outlook.

Lipari, R. N., Park-Lee, E., & Van Horn, S. (2016). *America's need for and receipt of substance use treatment in 2015, SAMSHA CBHSQ Report*. Retrieved from https://www.samhsa.gov/data/sites/default/files/report_2716/ShortReport-2716.html.

Maryland Recovery. (2017). *Rates of opioid addicted babies born set to rise again in 2017*. Retrieved from https://www.marylandrecovery.com/blog/rates-of-opioid-addicted-babies-born-set-to-rise-again-in-2017/.

McCance-Katz, E. (2018). *Substance use carries mental health risks—yes, even marijuana, NAMI*. Retrieved from https://www.nami.org/Blogs/NAMI-Blog/March-2018/Substance-Use-Carries-Mental-Health-Risks%E2%80%94Yes-Eve.

Meyer, J. S., & Quenzer, L. F. (2018). *Psychopharmacology, drugs, the brain, and behavior* (3rd ed.). Oxford: Oxford University Press.

Nakhoul, M. R., Seif, K. E., Haddad, N., & Haddad, G. E. (2017). Fetal Alcohol Exposure: The Common Toll. *Journal of Alcoholism and Drug Dependence*, 5(1), 257. Retrieved from https://doi.org/10.4172/2329-6488.1000257.

National Institute on Drug Abuse (NIDA). (n.d.) Club Drugs. Retrieved from https://www.drugabuse.gov/drugs-abuse/club-drugs.

National Institute on Drug Abuse (NIDA). (2014). *Drugs, brains, and behavior: The science of addiction*. Retrieved from https://www.drugabuse.gov/publications/drugs-brains-behavior-science-addiction/drugs-brain.

National Institute on Drug Abuse (NIDA). (2016a). *Drug facts: Anabolic steroids*. Retrieved from http://www.drugabuse.gov/publications/drugfacts/anabolic-steroids.

National Institute on Drug Abuse (NIDA). (2016b). *Drug facts: What is MDMA (ecstasy or molly)*. Retrieved from https://www.drugabuse.gov/publications/drugfacts/mdma-ecstasymolly.

National Institute on Drug Abuse (NIDA). (2016c). Medications for drug addiction. Retrieved from https://www.drugabuse.gov/publications/teaching-packets/understanding-drug-abuse-addiction/section-iv/1-medications-drug-addiction.

National Institute on Drug Abuse (NIDA). (2016d). Most commonly used addictive drugs. Retrieved from https://www.drugabuse.gov/publications/media-guide/most-commonly-used-addictive-drugs.

National Institute on Drug Abuse (NIDA). (2018a). Benzodiazepines and opioids. Retrieved from: https://www.drugabuse.gov/drugs-abuse/opioids/benzodiazepines-opioids.

National Institute on Drug Abuse (NIDA) (2018c). *Drug facts: Synthetic cathinones ("bath salts")*. Retrieved from http://drugabuse.gov/publications/drugfacts/synthetic-cathenones-bath-salts.

National Institute on Drug Abuse (NIDA). (2018d). Marijuana. Retrieved from: https://www.drugabuse.gov/publications/research-reports/marijuana/letter-director.

National Council of the State Boards of Nursing (NCSBN). (2014). *What you need to know about substance use disorder in nursing*. Retrieved from https://www.ncsbn.org/SUD_Brochure_2014.pdfhttp://medicalmarijuana.procom.org/view.resources.php?resourceID=004andthe289&print=true.

Nauert, R. (2015). *New Approach Addresses Substance Abuse Among Nurses. Psych Central*. Retrieved from https://psychcentral.com/news/2011/01/27/new-approach-addresses-substance-abuse-among-nurses/22967.html.

Sadock, B. J., Sadock, V. A., & Ruiz, P. (2015). *Kaplan and Sadock's synopsis of psychiatry: Behavioral sciences/clinical psychiatry*. Philadelphia: Wolters Kluwer.

Schiller, E. Y., & Mechanic, O. J. (2018). Opioid, overdose. StatPearls. Treasure Island, FL: StatPearls Publishing. Retrieved from https://www.ncbi.nlm.nih.gov/books/NBK470415/.

Scholastic Inc. (2016). *Prescription pain medications: What you need to know*. Retrieved from http://headsup.scholastic.com/students/prescription-pain-medications-what-you-need-to-know.

SMART Recovery. (n.d.). New: For healthcare professionals in recovery. Retrieved April 13, 2018 from https://www.smartrecovery.org/new-publication-for-healthcare-professionals-in-recovery/.

Stephens, E. (2017). *Opioid toxicity treatment & management*. Retrieved February 22, 2018, from https://emedicine.medscape.com/article/815784-treatment.

Strobbe, S., & Crowley, M. (2017). Substance use among nurses and nursing students: A joint position statement of the Emergency Nurses Association and The International Nurses Society on Addictions. *Journal of Addictions Nursing, 28*(2), 104–106. Retrieved from https://doi.org/10.1097/JAN.0000000000000150.

Substance Abuse and Mental Health Services Administration (SAMHSA). (2015). Definition of recovery. Retrieved from https://www.ncadd.org/people-in-recovery/recovery-definition/definition-of-recovery.

Substance Abuse and Mental Health Services Administration (SAMHSA). (2017a). Adverse Childhood Experiences. Retrieved from https://www.samhsa.gov/capt/practicing-effective-prevention/prevention-behavioral-health/adverse-childhood-experiences.

Substance Abuse and Mental Health Services Administration (SAMHSA). (2017b). Recovery and recovery support. Retrieved from: https://www.samhsa.gov/recovery.

Substance Abuse and Mental Health Services Administration (SAMHSA). (2017c). SBIRT: Screening, brief intervention, and referral to treatment. Retrieved from https://www.samhsa.gov/sbirt.

Substance Abuse and Mental Health Services Administration (SAMHSA). (2018). Medication-assisted treatment (MAT). Retrieved from https://www.samhsa.gov/medication-assisted-treatment.

Swaak, T. (2018). Date rape-linked drugs could be detected better than ever before thanks to this student's invention. *Newsweek*. Retrieved from http://www.newsweek.com/student-creates-napkin-detects-date-rape-drugs-791350.

Szalavitz, M. (2015). *No, Native Americans aren't genetically more susceptible to alcoholism*. The Verge. Retrieved from https://www.theverge.com/2015/10/2/9428659/firewater-racist-myth-alcoholism-native-americans.

Tan, S. C., Lee, M. W., Lim, G. T., Leong, J. J., & Lee, C. (2015). Motivational interviewing approach used by a community mental health team. *Journal of Psychosocial Nursing and Mental Health Services, 53*(12), 28–37.

Thompson, D. (2015). *High levels of formaldehyde in e-cig vapor*. Retrieved February 18, 2018, from https://www.webmd.com/smoking-cessation/news/20150121/high-levels-of-cancer-linked-chemical-in-e-cigarette-vapor-study-finds#1.

U.S. Food and Drug Administration (FDA). (2018). *FDA News Release: FDA approves the first non-opioid treatment for management of opioid withdrawal symptoms in adults*. Retrieved from https://www.fda.gov/newsevents/newsroom/pressannouncements/ucm607884.htm.

United States Food and Drug Administration. (2020). *FDA News Release: FDA finalizes enforcement polity on unauthorized flavored cartridge-based e-cigarettes that appeal to children, including fruit and mint*. Retrieved from https://www.fda.gov/news-events/press-announcements/fda-finalizes-enforcement-policy-unauthorized-flavored-cartridge-based-e-cigarettes-appeal-children.

Washington Health Professional Services. (2016). *A guide for assisting colleagues who demonstrate impairment in the workplace*. Retrieved from http://www.doh.wa.gov/portals/1/Documents/Pubs/600006.pdf.

WebMD Medical Reference. (2017). *Reviewed by james beckerman*. Retrieved from https://www.webmd.com/heart-disease/guide/heart-disease-alcohol-your-heart.

World Health Organization (WHO). (2018). *Management of substance abuse: Acute intoxication*. Retrieved from http://www.who.int/substance_abuse/terminology/acute_intox/en/.

UNIT IV

Caring for Patients Experiencing Psychiatric Emergencies

Ann Wolbert Burgess, DNSc, APRN, FAAN
Pioneer in Forensic Nursing

Dr. Ann Burgess is a clinical specialist in psychiatric nursing and sexual assault examiner who is an internationally recognized pioneer and researcher in the field of forensic nursing. Dr. Burgess is also a professor of psychiatric nursing at Boston College, where she teaches courses in victimology and forensic studies.

As a prolific author, Dr. Burgess has authored textbooks in psychiatric nursing, crisis intervention, and the treatment of sexual assault victims and offenders. She has coauthored more than 150 professional articles and book chapters, including monographs for the U.S. Department of Justice on child sex trafficking and abduction, among other topics. Her research with victims of abuse began in 1972 when Dr. Burgess and Lynda Lytle Holmstrom cofounded one of the first crisis intervention programs for victims of rape at Boston City Hospital. It was through their research that the diagnosis of rape-trauma syndrome established validity and has been admissible in court decisions. Her research has since included pornography, child eyewitnesses, ethics and sexual assault, exploitation of children, elder abuse, incarcerated women, and cyberstalking. Her work continues in the study of elder abuse in nursing homes, cyberstalking, and Internet sex crimes.

In conjunction with the Federal Bureau of Investigation, Dr. Burgess studied serial perpetrators of sexual abuse and homicide, as well as the connection between child sexual abuse and delinquency and future criminal behavior. She has frequently been an expert witness, including in high-profile cases, and her testimony has been described as "groundbreaking." She has received numerous awards, including Distinguished Professor (Uniform Services University), Inaugural Living Legend Award (American Psychiatric Nursing Association), and Inductee into the Sigma Theta Tau International Nurse Researcher Hall of Fame.

20

Crisis and Mass Disaster

Chyllia D. Fosbre

http://evolve.elsevier.com/Varcarolis/essentials

OBJECTIVES

1. Identify three principles of crisis intervention. How can these be used to provide evidence-based care to a patient in crisis? **QSEN: Evidence-Based Care**
2. Discuss what is meant by primary, secondary, and tertiary crisis intervention. Give a clinical example of the kinds of intervention needed for each phase of crisis intervention.
3. What is a triage team, why is it needed, and what are its responsibilities during an adventitious crisis/mass disaster?
4. Discuss the importance of teamwork and collaboration when identifying the initial needs of people facing an adventitious crisis/mass disaster. **QSEN: Teamwork and Collaboration**
5. Plan patient-centered care for a person who has experienced a situational crisis, and identify the potential cognitive and emotional states likely to be present. **QSEN: Patient-Centered Care**
6. Identify the mental health safety needs that people may face if they do not obtain support during or after a crisis (refer also to Chapter 10).
7. Provide an overview of Critical Incident Stress Debriefing (CISD), including its purpose and process.

KEY TERMS AND CONCEPTS

adventitious crisis/crisis of disaster, p. 333
crisis intervention, p. 331
Critical Incident Stress Debriefing (CISD), p. 337
developmental crisis, p. 332
existential crisis, p. 333
National Incident Management System (NIMS), p. 334
phases of crisis, p. 333
primary care, p. 336
secondary care, p. 336
situational crisis, p. 333
tertiary care, p. 336
triage, p. 334

CONCEPT CAREGIVING: *Caregiving* is made up of actions one does on behalf of individuals who are unable to do those actions for themselves. The realities of caregiving can be very rewarding and provide opportunities for positive change or can produce a negative effect on the caregivers' physical and emotional health (Giddens, 2017). Nurses should be alert to compassion fatigue/secondary traumatic stress. This is the emotional effect that nurses and other health care workers may experience by being indirectly traumatized when helping or trying to help a person who has experienced primary traumatic stress. Nurses need to practice self-care and make a concerted effort to schedule experiences that bring joy, pleasure, and diversion and get medical care to relieve symptoms that interfere with daily functioning.

INTRODUCTION

A child is killed in a drive-by shooting; a husband announces to his wife of 30 years that he wants a divorce; tornadoes rip through cities, leaving devastation, death, and homelessness in their wake. Each of these situations represents a crisis, an event that leaves individuals, families, or entire communities struggling to cope.

Everyone experiences crises. The experience itself is not pathological but rather represents a struggle for equilibrium and adjustment when problems seem unsolvable. A crisis presents both a danger to personality organization and a potential opportunity for personality growth. The outcome depends on how the individual, family, or community perceives and deals with the crisis and what outside supports are available.

Crises are acute, time-limited events experienced as overwhelming emotional reactions. A crisis can be developmental in nature, as described by Erik Erikson, who viewed an individual's progression as a series of developmental crises in stages like trust versus mistrust in infancy or identity versus role confusion during adolescence. A crisis can also be situational, like a terrorist attack, a natural disaster, or being a victim of a crime. Existential crises are inner conflicts, such as a midlife crisis, and usually consist of struggles related to spirituality and life purpose.

Crisis intervention is what nurses and other health professionals do to assist those in crisis to cope and assimilate the experience. Interventions need to be broad, creative, and flexible.

PREVALENCE AND COMORBIDITY

Many factors may limit a person's ability to problem solve or cope with stressful life events or situations. Some of these factors include the overwhelming presence of other stressful life events, mental illness, substance abuse, history of poor coping skills, diminished cognitive abilities, pre-existing physical health problems, limited social support network, and developmental or physical challenges. **Resiliency** is learned through past successful experience with and resolution of crises, and learned coping skills in the family are also germane factors. Resilience can be built through supportive relationships, the ability to make and meet realistic goals, confidence and self-esteem, good communication, problem-solving skills, and the ability to manage strong emotions.

THEORY

Erich Lindemann, an early crisis theorist, conducted a classic study in the 1940s on the grief reactions of close relatives of victims who died in the Coconut Grove nightclub fire in Boston. This study formed the foundation of crisis theory and clinical intervention. Lindemann was convinced that even though acute grief is a normal reaction to a distressing situation, preventive interventions could eliminate or decrease potentially devastating psychological consequences from the sustained effects of severe anxiety (Clark, 2015). He believed that the same interventions that were helpful in bereavement would prove helpful in dealing with other types of stressful events. Lindemann proposed a crisis intervention model as a major element of preventive psychiatry in the community.

In the early 1960s, Gerald Caplan (1964) further elaborated on crisis theory and intervention strategies. Since that time, our understanding of crisis and effective intervention has continued to be refined and enhanced by contemporary clinicians and theorists (James & Gilliland, 2013).

In 1961 a report of the Joint Commission on Mental Illness and Health addressed the need for community mental health centers throughout the country. This report stimulated the establishment of crisis services, which are now an important part of mental health programs in hospitals and communities.

Donna Aguilera and Janice Mesnick (1970) provided a framework for nurses for crisis assessment and intervention, which has grown in scope and practice. Aguilera (1998) continues to set a standard in the practice of crisis assessment and intervention.

Roberts's (2005) seven-stage model of crisis intervention is a more contemporary model useful in helping individuals who have suffered from an acute situational crisis as well as those who are diagnosed with acute stress disorder (Fig. 20.1).

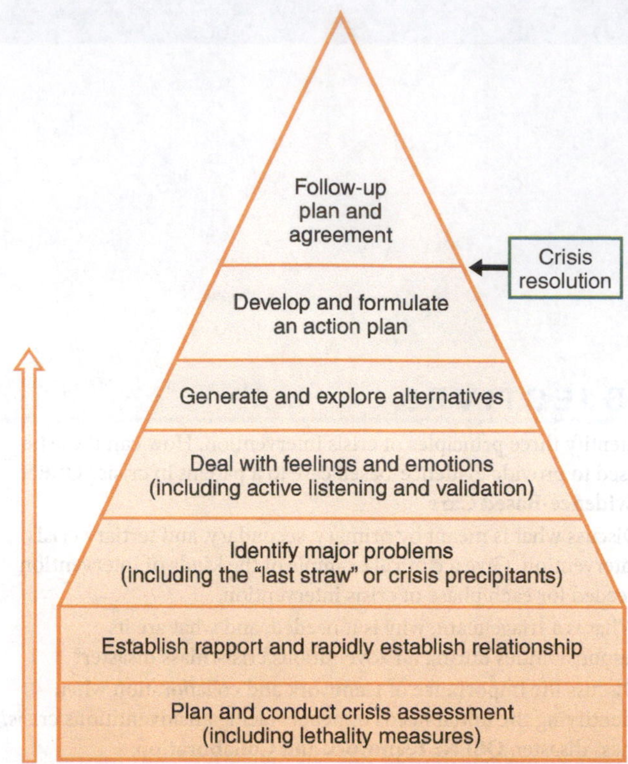

Fig. 20.1 Roberts's seven-stage model of crisis intervention. (From Roberts, A. R. [Ed.]. [2005]. *Crisis intervention handbook* [3rd ed.]. New York: Oxford University Press.)

The devastating effects of the terrorist attacks on September 11, 2001, and the distressing lack of response to the California wildfires that burned over 8,000 acres in 2018 emphasized the need for crisis assessment and intervention by community mental health providers throughout the country to deal with all types of crises and the people who had been traumatized—victims, families, rescue workers, and observers (Kanel, 2015). Crisis theory defines specific aspects of crises that are basic to crisis intervention (Box 20.1).

The ways of assessing crisis described in the following sections are derived from established crisis theory and constitute a sound knowledge base for the application of the nursing process to the treatment of a patient in crisis. An understanding of three areas of crisis theory enables the application of the nursing process: (1) types of crisis, (2) phases of crisis, and (3) aspects of crisis that have relevance for nurses.

BOX 20.1 Foundation for Crisis Intervention

- A crisis is self-limiting and is usually resolved within 4 to 6 weeks.
- The goal of crisis intervention is to return the individual to the pre-crisis level of functioning. Resolution of a crisis may result in return to pre-crisis functioning or to a higher or lower level.
- How a crisis is resolved is unique to the specific crisis, as well as how the individual responds and the interventions of others.
- During a crisis, people are often more open to outside intervention than they are at times of stable functioning. When their normal coping methods have failed, the opportunity exists to learn different adaptive means of problem solving.
- A person in a crisis situation is assumed to be mentally healthy and to have functioned well in the past but is presently in a state of disequilibrium.
- Crisis intervention deals with the person's present problem and resolution of the immediate crisis only, the "here and now." Addressing issues or needs not directly related to the crisis can take place at a later time, and referrals can be provided.
- A nurse must be willing to take a more directive role in intervention, especially initially, which is contrary to the usual therapeutic approach. As anxiety decreases, the patient can assist more in problem solving and planning.
- Early intervention increases the chances of a good prognosis.
- A patient is encouraged to set realistic goals and plan an intervention with the nurse that is focused on the current situation.

CLINICAL PICTURE

Types of Crises

As mentioned, there are three basic types of crises: developmental, situational, and existential. It is possible to experience two types of crisis situations simultaneously. For example, a 51-year-old woman may be going through a midlife crisis (existential) when her husband dies suddenly of cancer (situational). The presence of more than one crisis further taxes the individual's coping skills. People who have pre-existing mental health problems are prone to crisis and more vulnerable to its effects.

Developmental Crisis

A process of maturation through stages occurs throughout life. Erik Erikson (1902–1994) identified eight stages of growth and development in which specific tasks must be mastered to effectively reach maturity. Erikson postulated that each stage constitutes a **developmental crisis**.

When a person arrives at a new stage, previous coping styles are no longer appropriate, and new coping mechanisms have yet to be developed. For a time, the person is in transition. This often leads to increased anxiety, which may manifest as variations in the person's normal behavior until he or she establishes a new equilibrium. Marriage, the birth of a child, and retirement are examples of developmental crises.

Alcohol and drug addiction will interrupt an individual's progression through the maturational stages. As the patient escapes from stressors with substances, he or she is not practicing communication and coping skills that build resilience. When the individual gets clean and sober, he or she will discover that maturation has been halted at about the age that drugs or alcohol began to be used. The good news is that the developmental process can resume and progress through supportive treatment. If individuals do not receive treatment, their coping skills will be compromised. Successful resolution through developmental tasks leads to the advancement of basic human qualities, according to Erikson. The way in which each developmental crisis is resolved becomes a foundation for the next stage and thus affects the ability to pass through subsequent stages. If a person lacks adequate parenting, support systems, and role models, successful resolution of developmental tasks and emotional learning may be difficult or delayed. This can affect the individual throughout the life span. Conversely, successful progression sets the stage for continuing to adjust and mature. When a person is experiencing severe difficulty during a developmental crisis, such as adjusting to retirement, professional intervention may be helpful or needed.

VIGNETTE: A 65-year-old widower is asked to retire from his 40-year career as a city bus driver during company downsizing. Although he had been looking forward to the day when he could spend more time in leisure pursuits, he has spent the first year of retirement rarely leaving his house and becoming progressively more depressed. He finds himself feeling that he is worthless and not a contributing member of society. His sense of self has been impaired. Neighbors and friends encourage him to spend time with his grandchildren or volunteering, but he is unable to accept these activities as important and rejects their suggestions. This gentleman is experiencing both a situational crisis (loss of job) and a developmental crisis (adjustment to retirement and a life stage).

Situational Crisis

A **situational crisis** arises from an external rather than an internal source and is frequently unanticipated. Examples of external situations that can precipitate a crisis include loss of a job, death of a loved one, unwanted pregnancy, a move, change of job, change in financial status, divorce, and severe physical or mental illness. Situational crises are common, and at least some of them will be experienced by all individuals during their lifetime. Response to the situation depends in part on the degree of support available from caring friends, family members, and groups; previous success in navigating life events (resiliency); and the overall physical and emotional health of the individual.

The stressful events that precipitate or constitute the crisis involve a loss or change that threatens a person's self-concept and self-esteem. Successful resolution of a crisis also depends on resolving the grief surrounding the loss.

An **adventitious crisis** (or **crisis of disaster**) is not a common part of everyday life and is similar to a situational crisis but is generally much larger in scale and impacts a community, not just an individual. These types of crises are unplanned and tend to be catastrophic. Adventitious crises may result from natural disasters such as tsunamis, fires, hurricanes, flooding, or earthquakes; national crises such as war, terrorist attacks, airplane or train crashes; or crimes of violence such as shootings in a public venue. These types of incidents leave a wake of devastation, with lives lost, destruction of roadways and utilities, and limited medical services. Mass-casualty incidents can overtax the abilities of first responders, health care systems, and government organizations. Victims are permanently changed and left to mourn, recover from the effects of severe trauma, and rebuild their lives and communities.

Recent studies confirm that the number of natural and geophysical disasters taking place each year is noticeably skyrocketing. Geophysical disasters include earthquakes, volcanoes, dry rock-falls, landslides, and avalanches. Climatic disasters are classified as floods, storms, tropical cyclones, local storms, heat/cold waves, droughts, and wildfires (Borgen Project, 2015).

As this text is being revised, we are experiencing an adventitious crisis of global proportions with the novel conoravirus (COVID-19). Most cities, states, and countries have varying stay-at-home orders, with all but essential businesses being shut down. People in the United States and in many other countries are being asked to maintain at least 6 feet of distance when in public, wear a face mask, and avoid groups of more than 10 people. Weddings have been cancelled, churches closed, and restaurants offering only take-out services. It has caused mass casualties and huge spikes in illness, and hospital systems have been overrun with critically ill patients. At this time we can only speculate on the long-term implications. Nurses across the nation are caring for complex patients, are exposed to illness with lack of personal protective equipment, and stand at rally lines encouraging others to stay safe and stay at home. As you read through this chapter, consider the impact this has had on you and your family, and consider how different individuals in your life have reacted to this incident.

Existential Crisis

As previously discussed, an **existential crisis** is one of questioning life purpose or spirituality. This can be brought on by experiencing a significant event, either positive or negative, such as marriage, death of a loved one, children becoming adults and leaving the home, or reaching an age-related milestone such as turning 40. An existential crisis can lead to newfound motivation or higher goals for self-actualization. It can also cause feelings of isolation, depression, or uncertainty.

Phases of Crisis

Individuals experiencing a crisis will naturally use their normal coping skills to adapt. If the attempts are unsuccessful, the individual will try harder, then expand his or her repertoire of coping skills. As efforts continue to be unsuccessful, the individual will become more frustrated, anxious, and disorganized. According to Lowe and Galea (2015), Caplan identified four distinct **phases of crisis**:

- *Phase 1:* A person confronted by a conflict or problem that threatens the self-concept responds with increased feelings of anxiety. The increase in anxiety stimulates the use of problem-solving techniques and defense mechanisms in an effort to solve the problem and lower anxiety.
- *Phase 2:* If the threat persists and the usual defensive response fails, anxiety and discomfort continue to rise. Individual functioning becomes disorganized. Trial-and-error attempts at solving the problem and restoring a normal balance begin.
- *Phase 3:* If the trial-and-error attempts fail, anxiety can escalate to severe and panic levels, and the person mobilizes automatic relief behaviors such as withdrawal and flight. Some form of compromise, such as redefining the situation or reevaluating needs, may occur in this stage, in order to come to some sort of resolution. An example might be giving in on child visitation in order to end ongoing divorce proceedings.

- *Phase 4:* If the problem is not solved after considerable time and efforts, and coping skills have been ineffective and exhausted, anxiety can overwhelm the person. In this final phase of crisis, serious personality disorganization, depression, confusion, violence against others, or suicidal behavior can develop (Lowe & Galea, 2015).

APPLICATION OF THE NURSING PROCESS

ASSESSMENT

A person's equilibrium may be adversely affected by an unrealistic or skewed perception of the precipitating crisis event or inadequate supports and coping mechanisms (France, 2015). It is crucial to assess these factors when a crisis is evaluated. Data gained from the assessment can assist the nurse and the patient in setting realistic and meaningful goals as well as in planning possible solutions to the crisis situation.

After determining whether there is a need for safety interventions because of suicidal or homicidal ideation or gestures, the nurse then assesses three main areas: (1) the patient's perception of the event, (2) the patient's available supports, and (3) the patient's usual coping skills.

Disaster Response

The **National Incident Management System (NIMS)** "guides all levels of government, nongovernmental organizations (NGO), and the private sector to work together to prevent, protect against, mitigate, respond to, and recover from incidents" during disaster situations (Federal Emergency Management Agency [FEMA], 2018). The increase in natural disasters since 1990 has highlighted gaps and flaws in our ability to respond as a nation. There is still a need for better planning and clearer lines of communication among community, state, and federal disaster agencies in order to be effective in reducing morbidity and mortality.

Efficient response to disaster requires a triage team and an ability to distribute casualties to the most appropriate facility for proper care. The underlying principle of **triage** is to separate those who need rapid medical care from those with more minor injuries. The triage process reduces the acute burden on medical facilities and finite resources, allowing responders to address the greatest number of casualties. The first needs during a disaster include rescue and evacuation efforts, food and shelter, medical attention, and physical safety (FEMA, 2018). Since 2002 the Department of Homeland Security has overseen a variety of agencies that focus on the safety and security of people during disasters in the United States. Nongovernmental agencies such as the International Medical Corps (IMC) and the American Red Cross (ARC) also provide medical care and relief efforts in the United States and around the world. After immediate needs are met, people need help to reconstruct and normalize their lives, including assistance with housing, jobs, and trauma counseling. Victims of a disaster commonly experience *cognitive impairment* such as confusion, difficulty making decisions, and intrusive memories; *behavioral changes* such as substance use, difficulty functioning in work or daily routines, and sleep disturbances; or *emotional issues* such as fluctuating emotions, relationship strain, fear, or withdrawal. Posttraumatic stress disorder (PTSD), anxiety, panic, and depression are common symptoms following a disaster. The importance of crisis intervention and psychological first aid, in addition to physical healing, cannot be overlooked. If individuals are not assisted early on, they are left vulnerable to stress-related disorders and chronic impairment. Disaster nursing is a growing field to address these needs.

Assessing Patient's Perception

Whether an event is perceived as a crisis depends, in part, on the outlook and strengths of the patient. Having a physician's appointment canceled would be viewed as a trivial annoyance to most people, but for someone who is vulnerable to severe schizophrenia, the change could trigger a crisis and lead to worsening of symptoms (decompensation). Therefore it is important to view the event through the eyes of the patient. The nurse's initial task is to assess the individual's and possibly the family's perception of the problem. The more clearly the problem can be understood, the better the chance that an effective solution will be found and followed by the patient. Sample questions that may facilitate the assessment include the following:

- Has anything upsetting happened to you within the past few days or weeks?
- What was happening in your life before you started to feel this way?
- Has anything traumatic happened in the past that is still bothering you?
- What leads you to seek help now?
- Describe how you are feeling right now.
- How does this situation affect your life?
- How do you see this event affecting your future?
- What would need to be done to resolve this situation?
- What type of help do you think you need?

VIGNETTE: A 38-year-old female has gone back to nursing school as a second career. She is currently in her psychiatric nursing course. Normally an excellent student, she had missed two class periods and a clinical day and failed her last exam. Her psychiatric nursing professor calls her in to discuss the situation. The student begins crying and tells her professor that she had been dealing with the loss of her home due to a fire. Even with that severe stressor, she had been coping fairly well by keeping in touch with friends, doing yoga, praying, and focusing on her two young children. She tried to see the relocation as a fresh start with some positive aspects. Recently, however, the student had been unable to complete her yoga routines due to muscle fatigue and pain. It was becoming difficult to even carry her textbooks to and from the car or blow-dry her hair. Her primary care provider (PCP) had initially diagnosed her with stress related to nursing school and the fire, but as the symptoms progressed, she was given the diagnosis of myositis. Myositis is an autoimmune disorder that affects the muscles and produces symptoms of fatigue, weakness, and pain that may be progressive and, at times, fatal (U.S. National Library of Medicine, 2015). The student's normal coping mechanisms had failed with the addition of this diagnosis, and she was now in a crisis situation. She was beginning to display relief behaviors such as panic attacks and withdrawal from life events such as school or socializing with friends. These symptoms are indicative of phase 3 in the phases of crisis. This student is experiencing both situational (medical diagnosis, failing an exam) and adventitious (house fire) crises (Lowe & Galea, 2015).

Assessing the Patient's Perception of the Precipitating Event(s)

The student spontaneously disclosed the upsetting events. What led her to seek help at this time was her failing coping mechanisms and an inability to function in nursing school, as well as the professor calling her in and expressing concern.

Nursing professor: "How are you feeling right now?"

Student: "So overwhelmed. I don't know much about myositis, and I'm so scared. How can I finish school? How can I take care of my children? How bad is it going to get?"

Nursing professor: "What do you see happening in your life right now and in your future?"

Student: "I don't know if I can even finish school. The doctor says I need to start regular medication infusions, which will make me tired."

Nursing professor: "Let's talk and think through this situation together."

Assessing Situational Supports

The patient's support systems are assessed to determine the resources available. Does the stressful event involve important people in the patient's life? Is the patient isolated from others, or are there family and friends who can provide vital support? Family and friends may be asked to aid the individual by offering material or emotional support. If these resources are not available, the nurse or other medical or psychiatric clinicians act as a temporary support system while relationships with individuals or groups in the community are established. The following are some sample questions to ask:

- Whom do you live with?
- Whom do you talk to when you are overwhelmed?
- Whom can you trust?
- Who is available to help you? Do you have a partner or significant other?
- Do you have spiritual beliefs or attend a place of worship?
- Do you attend school or any activities, groups, or clubs?
- During difficult times in the past, who was there to help you?

VIGNETTE

Assessing the Patient's Situational Supports

Nursing professor: "Do you have any family or friends to rely on right now?"

Student: "Yes, I have my best friend, my mother, and my yoga group."

Nursing professor: "Have you been talking to them?"

Student: "Not lately. I've been so overwhelmed and tired that I don't even want to answer my phone."

Nursing professor: "Would it be all right if we called some of your support people together so that they can become more involved? You need to lean on these people again and not isolate so much."

Student: "Yes, I think that's good.... We can call my mom."

Once the student's mother was called, she agreed to come to the school and pick up her daughter. The student, professor, and mother all came up with a plan to help support the student during this time of crisis.

Assessing Coping Skills

In crisis situations, it is important to evaluate the person's level of anxiety. Common coping mechanisms may be overeating, drinking, smoking, withdrawing, seeking out someone to talk to, crying, yelling, sleeping too much, praying, or engaging in other physical activity (Gil & Weinberg, 2015). The potential for suicide or homicide must be assessed. If the patient is thinking of harming self or someone else or is unable to take care of personal needs, hospitalization should be considered (France, 2015). For more about assessing suicide potential, please see Chapter 23.

VIGNETTE: The nursing professor has learned that the student uses yoga, prayer, her children, and friends as support. She has been isolating and not using her support system, partly due to overwhelming stress and partly due to the muscle weakness related to the myositis.

Assessing the Student's Personal Coping Skills

Nursing professor: "Have you been thinking of killing yourself or anyone else?"

Student: "No, I would never do that. But I wish I could just disappear to get rid of all these problems."

Nursing professor: "What do you think we should do in this situation?"

Student's mother: "Maybe I could come and stay with her, or she could stay with me for a while. I could help with the children and driving her to doctor's appointments."

Student: *(begins to cry)* "That would be so wonderful, thank you!"

Nursing professor: "It sounds as if you need more information on your diagnosis as well. You are anticipating the worst scenario, and you need actual facts about what you will be dealing with."

The student, mother, and professor came up with the plan that the student would take a leave of absence from school for a semester, her mother would move in temporarily and help with the children, and the student would seek more information from her PCP about her new diagnosis. In addition, the professor gave the student a referral to a myositis website with information on support groups (http://www.myositis.org).

Assessment Guidelines

1. Identify whether the patient's response to the crisis warrants psychiatric treatment or hospitalization (suicidal behavior, psychotic thinking, violent behavior, or inability to care for self).
2. Determine if the patient is able to identify the *precipitating event.*
3. Assess the patient's understanding of his or her present *situational supports.*
4. Identify the patient's usual *coping skills* and support system and determine what coping mechanisms may help the present situation.
5. Determine whether there are certain religious or cultural beliefs that need to be considered in assessing and intervening in this person's crisis.
6. Assess whether this situation is one in which the patient needs primary intervention (education, environmental manipulation, new coping skills), secondary intervention (crisis intervention), or tertiary intervention (rehabilitation).

DIAGNOSIS

A person in crisis may exhibit various behaviors that indicate a number of problems. See Table 20.1 for signs and symptoms of people in crisis that may be used as a guide for developing nursing diagnoses.

Using the example in the preceding vignettes, the assessment of the nursing student's (1) perception of the precipitating event, (2) situational supports, and (3) personal coping skills provides the nurse with enough data to formulate two patient-centered nursing diagnoses and to work with the student in setting goals and planning interventions.

VIGNETTE

Nursing Diagnoses for the Student

The nurse formulates the following nursing diagnoses for the nursing student:

- *Lack of resilience* related to multiple stressors and new medical diagnosis, as evidenced by social withdrawal and missing school activities
- *Risk for impaired school performance* related to overwhelming stress from school pressures, new medical condition, and parenting responsibilities

OUTCOMES IDENTIFICATION

The planning of realistic patient outcomes is often done in conjunction with the patient or family. Realistic outcomes should consider the person's cultural and personal values. The nurse will document measurable goals that are realistic and include a time estimate. Without the patient's involvement, the outcome criteria may be irrelevant to the patient, leading to a lack of follow-through.

For example, a nurse who suggests that a woman leave her husband because he beats her may be surprised to find that the woman has different thoughts on what she wants as a solution. Thus goals and

TABLE 20.1 Potential Nursing Diagnoses for Crisis Intervention

Signs and Symptoms	Patient-Centered Nursing Diagnoses[a]
Overwhelmed, depressed, nothing in life worthwhile, hopeless, self-hatred	*Depressed mood* *Risk for self-destructive behavior* *Situational low self-esteem* *Spiritual distress* *Hopelessness* *Powerlessness*
Confused, highly anxious, incoherent, crying or sobbing, extreme emotional pain	*Anxiety (moderate, severe, panic)* *Acute confusion* *Labile moods*
Difficulty with interpersonal relationships, isolated, has few or no social supports	*Social isolation* *Lack of social support* *Impaired socialization*
Unable to function at work, school, or home; difficulty completing tasks or concentrating	*Employment problem* *Impaired family process* *Caregiver stress*
Has experienced traumatic, emotionally overwhelming event or loss; feels depressed; insomnia; nightmares; crying; fear	*Risk for post-trauma response* *Rape-trauma response* *Dysfunctional grief* *Impaired sleep*

[a]The International Classification for Nursing Practice (ICNP) is a product of the International Council of Nurses (ICN). Retrieved from http://www.icn.ch/what-we-do/ICNP-Browser/

outcome criteria are always established with the patient and are congruent with the patient's needs, values, and cultural expectations. They may also need to be reviewed and revised over the course of treatment.

VIGNETTE: The nursing student begins treatment in a community mental health clinic. She and her therapist set some outcome goals, and the student shared those goals with her professor:

1. She will attend a myositis support group meeting within 2 weeks.
2. She will learn more about her disorder within 2 weeks.
3. She will call one person daily for support.
4. She will take short walks and stop before reaching the point of fatigue.
5. She will begin medication treatments as prescribed by her provider, scheduled to begin in 1 week.
6. She will attend counseling sessions every 2 weeks.
7. She will return to nursing school next semester.

PLANNING AND IMPLEMENTATION

Nurses may intervene through a variety of crisis intervention modalities, such as disaster nursing, mobile crisis units, group work, health education crisis prevention, victim outreach programs, and telephone hotlines. Crisis situations may present in any setting, including hospitals, clinics, and schools.

The nurse may be involved in planning and intervention for an individual (physical abuse), for a group (students after a classmate's suicide), or for a community (train derailment). In planning after a crisis or disaster, the nurse considers the impact of the event on the patient's life. Is the patient able to continue functioning in work, school, or family responsibilities? Are others close to the patient also affected (France, 2015)? These questions will help guide immediate actions.

Crisis intervention is within the scope of practice of all nurses. Initial goals are patient safety and anxiety reduction.

During the initial interview, the person in crisis first needs to gain a feeling of safety and security. Providing genuine support and hope will begin to decrease the patient's anxiety. The nurse assures the patient in crisis that help is available and that solutions will be found together. The patient's anxiety must be decreased to a level where the patient can hear and absorb potential ideas so that he or she will be able to actively problem solve with the nurse. False reassurance that everything will be all right damages trust and rapport. The nurse will need to be creative and flexible in helping the patient to solve his or her problems. Although the nurse helps guide the patient, it is important to remember that the patient is ultimately in charge of his or her own life and decision making.

See Table 20.2 for crisis interventions and corresponding rationales for patients in crisis.

VIGNETTE: After making a plan with her counselor, the student decides that it is too soon to attend a support group. The patient's right to decide for herself is respected, and the plan is revised to include support groups at a later time.

There are three levels of nursing care in crisis intervention: (1) primary, (2) secondary, and (3) tertiary. As in all areas of nursing, psychotherapeutic nursing interventions in crisis are directed toward these three levels of care.

Primary Nursing Interventions

Primary care *promotes* mental health and reduces mental illness to decrease the incidence of crisis. On this level, the nurse can:

- Work with an individual to recognize potential problems by evaluating the stressful life events the person is experiencing.
- Teach individual-specific coping skills, such as decision making, problem solving, assertiveness skills, meditation, and relaxation skills, to handle stressful events.
- Assist an individual in evaluating the timing or reduction of life changes to mitigate the effects of stress. This may involve working with the patient to plan environmental changes, make important interpersonal decisions, and rethink changes in occupational roles.

Secondary Nursing Interventions

Secondary care establishes intervention during an acute crisis to *prevent* prolonged anxiety from diminishing personal effectiveness and personality organization. The nurse's primary focus is to ensure the safety of the patient. After safety issues are addressed, the nurse works with the patient to assess the patient's problem, support systems, and coping styles. Desired goals are explored, and interventions are planned. Secondary care lessens the time a person is mentally disabled during a crisis. Secondary-level care occurs in hospital units, emergency departments, clinics, or mental health centers.

Tertiary Nursing Interventions

Tertiary care provides support for those who have experienced a severe crisis and are now *recovering* from a disabling mental state. Social and community facilities that offer tertiary intervention include rehabilitation centers, shelter workshops, day hospitals, and outpatient clinics. Primary goals are to facilitate optimal levels of functioning and prevent further emotional disruptions. People with severe and persistent mental problems are often extremely susceptible to crisis, and community outpatient and inpatient facilities provide the structured environment needed for recovery. See Chapter 27 for an extensive discussion of community supports for people with severe and persistent mental problems.

TABLE 20.2 Interventions for Patients in Crisis

Intervention	Rationale
1. Assess for suicidal or homicidal thoughts or plans.	1. Safety is always the first consideration.
2. Take initial steps to make patient feel safe and to lower anxiety, such as providing a quiet environment, building rapport, and acknowledging the crisis experience.	2. When a person feels safe and anxiety decreases, the individual is able to participate in planning.
3. Listen carefully, using eye contact and supportive body language, and provide feedback/summarization to ensure understanding.	3. When a person believes that someone is really listening, he or she feels cared about and supported, and this offers hope.
4. Crisis intervention calls for directive and creative approaches. Initially the nurse may make phone calls to help with tasks such as arranging babysitters and finding shelter.	4. Initially a person may be so confused and frightened that performing usual tasks is not possible.
5. Assess patient's support systems. Rally existing supports (with patient's permission) if patient is overwhelmed.	5. People in crisis are overwhelmed, and nurses need to take a more active role.
6. Identify and mobilize needed social supports.	6. Patients may have concerns regarding shelter, childcare, elder care, medical conditions, food, or psychiatric treatment and support.
7. Identify needed coping skills such as problem solving, relaxation, or job training.	7. Increasing existing coping skills and learning new ones can help with the current crisis and minimize future effects.
8. Collaborate with the patient to plan interventions, as much as he or she is able at given time.	8. Patient's sense of control, self-esteem, and adherence to the plan are increased.
9. Plan regular follow-up to assess patient's progress through clinic appointments, phone calls, or home visits.	9. Plan is evaluated to see what works and what needs adjustment.

Critical Incident Stress Debriefing

Critical Incident Stress Debriefing (CISD) is an example of a tertiary intervention directed toward a group that has experienced a crisis such as a school shooting or natural disaster (Boscarino, 2015). A seven-phase group meeting offers individuals the opportunity to share their thoughts and feelings in a safe and controlled environment. The CISD process can also be effective for staff members who have been exposed to a traumatic event, such as a patient suicide or community violence.

The phases of CISD are the following:

1. *Introductory phase*—The purpose and overview of the debriefing process is presented. Confidentiality is assured, team members are identified, and questions are answered.
2. *Fact phase*—Participants are assisted in discussing the facts of the incident from their perspectives.
3. *Thought phase*—All participants are asked to discuss their initial thoughts about the incident.
4. *Reaction phase*—Participants engage in freewheeling discussion about the worst, most painful parts of the incident.
5. *Symptom phase*—Participants describe cognitive, physical, emotional, or behavioral experiences at the time of the incident and ongoing.
6. *Teaching phase*—The feelings of the participants are affirmed. Guidance is provided regarding future symptoms and stress management techniques.
7. *Reentry phase*—The debriefing process thus far is reviewed, and any new topics are discussed. Team members provide encouragement and resources for additional help, then summarize the experience.

VIGNETTE: The student's ongoing counseling is really addressing all levels of crisis intervention: education and coping skills to prevent future problems, mitigation of symptom severity, and treatment of already-established trauma related to the crisis.

Self-Care for Nurses

Nurses frequently work with people in crisis in all clinical settings—in the emergency department (ED) and on medical, surgical, psychiatric, obstetric, and pediatric units—and also experience crisis in their own lives and with family and friends. Nurses will encounter abused children, burn victims, gang shootings, and numerous other painful situations with their patients. Nurses need to monitor their thoughts and feelings and learn to recognize when they need self-care, support, or professional help. This is especially true in the aftermath of a mass-casualty incident. Nurses often suppress their own feelings in order to effectively handle the immediate situation and may react later with anxiety or shock.

When nurses are unaware of personal feelings or are suppressing them to cope, they may unknowingly prevent the expression of the painful feelings in their patients. Nurses have their own set of life experiences and wounds or sensitive areas. There may be times when the nurse cannot deal effectively with a patient's situation. In these instances, it may be best to ask a colleague to care for the patient. It is crucial that supervision and guidance are available during the training process when working in the area of crisis intervention. Supervisors should be aware of secondary traumatic stress and compassion fatigue and assist nursing staff with identifying and providing support for those at risk. Nurses working with crisis intervention face common problems that must be addressed before they become comfortable and competent in the role. For example, nurses may have difficulty dealing with certain issues such as suicide or child abuse and struggle with personal beliefs that make it difficult to care for their patients. Nurses and other health care workers exposed to disaster situations can become overwhelmed by witnessing the catastrophic loss of human life or mass destruction of homes and communities. Disaster nurses need a supportive network and access to debriefing. Debriefing is an important step for staff in coming to terms with overwhelming situations. Once the crisis is over, debriefing can help staff begin to heal.

EVALUATION

Ongoing evaluation will be performed until the crisis has resolved sufficiently to allow a return to normal pre-crisis functioning. As the patient's anxiety level reduces from severe to moderate to mild through successful interventions, the patient will need less support and will return to independence. Appropriate questions to ask during evaluation(s) are as follows:

- Is the patient safe and feeling secure?
- Is the patient able to use existing coping skills? Has he or she learned new skills?
- Is the patient relying on his or her support system? Have new supports such as groups been put into place?
- Where is the patient's level of functioning in comparison to pre-crisis ability?
- Does the patient need or desire referrals for continued therapeutic work?

Once the process has been started, some patients may choose to explore other areas or issues in their lives.

VIGNETTE: During ongoing counseling, the patient's therapist makes evaluations of her functioning and support. At the end of 6 months, she has started meeting with a support group, her mother is able to move back to her own home, she is receiving regular medication and is feeling strong most of the time, and she is ready to return to nursing school. The patient's therapy frequency has gradually decreased to the current level of one session per month. It is decided to continue the monthly therapy sessions for support as the student returns to college.

APPLYING THE ART

A Person Needing Crisis Intervention

Scenario

A 30-year-old male has brought his young son to the free community health clinic for his allergy shot. The father asked the student nurse working at the clinic to spend some time talking. The father expressed gratitude for being able to obtain health care for his family, despite not having insurance. He also disclosed that his wife is pregnant, and he feels significant stress about caring for his family on a minimum-wage income. He has been having regular panic attacks for the past few months.

Therapeutic Goal

By the end of this interaction, the father will have practiced a deep-breathing technique to use during panic attacks and will be aware of mental health resources available to those with a limited income.

Student–Patient Interaction	Thoughts, Communication Techniques, and Mental Health Nursing Concepts
Father: "How long can a person's heart pound really hard and fast before it gives out?"	I wonder where this is going and if I will know the answer to his question.
Student: "Are you experiencing this now?"	I'm exploring for more information.
Father: "No, just wondering because it happens a lot."	I'm feeling relieved that his panic is not happening now. I'm using my assessment skills to observe his color, breathing, and affect.
Student: "Would you mind telling me what happens?"	I'm continuing to explore, asking closed-ended questions for specific information. I'm hoping my instructor will come around before I run out of questions to ask.
Father: "I start breathing really fast, my heart pounds so I can feel it in my chest, and I feel really scared."	
Student: "How often does this happen and how long does it last?"	
Father: "Almost every day lately, and it lasts about a half an hour."	
Student: "What is happening before it starts?"	
Father: "It happens when I'm thinking about our bills and how I am going to take care of another baby."	
Student: "I can sure understand that, the worry about bills. Have you seen any type of health care provider for this yet?"	Clarifying symptoms Offering self
Father: "I've been to the emergency department a couple of times. They tell me my heart is fine and that it is just stress."	I'm feeling relieved that he has been examined and is okay.
Student: "What have you tried to make it better?"	Leading question, open-ended question
Father: "I try to ignore it and watch TV. I did have some pills from the emergency department doctor, but I ran out."	
Student: "Would you be willing to try a deep-breathing exercise that might help you calm down when you have a panic attack?"	Teaching, modeling Breathing out for one count longer than breathing in combats the tendency to hyperventilate. Deep breathing in this way balances the O_2:CO_2 ratio that is upset by hyperventilation.
Father: "Sure, anything!"	
Student: "Breathe along with me. Breathe in slowly and I will count one … two … three … hold it for a few seconds. Breathe out slowly and I will count one … two … three … four …. hold it for a few seconds." *(Student repeats this through several breathing cycles, also modeling by doing it along with the patient.)* "How do you feel now?"	Exploring
Father: "Very calm and relaxed. Thank you, I think I can try that the next time."	I'm feeling really great that I was able to help him feel better!
Student: "Keep practicing even when you aren't anxious so that you will be ready to use the breathing when you need it. May I give you some resources for counseling on a sliding-income scale?"	Teaching, summarizing Giving information
Father: "Yes, that would be appreciated."	

APPLYING EVIDENCE-BASED PRACTICE (EBP)

Problem

A 62-year-old male presents to a mental health clinic after being referred by his endocrinologist for a psychiatric evaluation and treatment. The psychiatrist meets with the patient and his wife. The patient is tearful, with symptoms of sadness, fatigue, oversleeping, and thoughts of wanting to die. He has recently lost a toe to surgery secondary to diabetes. Since the surgery, his fear and anxiety have increased to a crippling level, and he is afraid of losing his entire leg. He also reports being overwhelmed by the number of doctor's appointments he must attend. The patient's fear is disproportionate to the realistic chance of a leg amputation and is interfering with his ability to manage his diabetes. His high anxiety contributes to forgetting his medications, refusing to exercise, and eating poorly for comfort.

EBP Assessment

A. **What do you already know from experience?** Patients display high anxiety in crisis situations that interferes with their ability to problem solve. Health care providers must take a more directive approach in providing care. The loss of one toe does not translate into a full-leg amputation, especially with proper care. Patients may give up on taking care of themselves if they believe there is no hope or possibility of improvement.

B. **What does the literature say?** Diabetes is associated with increased diagnosis of anxiety disorders. A crisis depends on the patient's perception of the situation. The goal of crisis intervention is a return to at least pre-crisis functioning, but the result may also be a higher or lower level. Patients with depression are less likely to follow through with medical treatment.

C. **What does the patient want?** He wants to feel a lot less anxious and fearful. He wants assurance that his leg won't be amputated and that he will be able to function fully again. He wants to feel like himself, wanting to live again.

Plan

The patient relies heavily on his wife, and she needs to be included for any plan to be successful. The patient is very spiritual, so his minister was asked to visit for support, with the patient's permission, and the patient was encouraged to use his usual coping method of prayer. Rapport is always important but was even more so in this case. The patient was prescribed medication temporarily to help reduce anxiety and depression to a level where other interventions would be possible. The patient was then open to diabetic education, which gave him more realistic information on the possibility of amputation and interventions he could do to prevent that. In the beginning stages, interventions were more directive, but as the crisis abated, the patient was able to independently manage his care. The patient was assessed for suicidal thoughts. He was able to contract for safety not to harm himself, and he was provided with a hotline number and regular counseling.

QSEN Prelicensure Knowledge, Skills, and Attitudes (KSAs) Addressed

Teamwork and Collaboration is evidenced by the interaction between the endocrinologist and psychiatrist, as well as the inclusion of the patient's wife and spiritual leader.

Safety is evidenced by assessing for suicidal thoughts and providing appropriate treatment and by educating the patient to prevent further harm from uncontrolled diabetes.

KEY POINTS TO REMEMBER

- A crisis is not a pathological state but a struggle for emotional balance and equilibrium during a stressful event.
- Crises can lead to high anxiety, loss of functioning, and personality disorganization but can also offer opportunities for positive emotional growth and change.
- There are three types of crises: developmental, situational/adventitious, and existential.
- The National Incident Management System (NIMS) is established to help governmental and private aid groups cooperate seamlessly during a crisis event.
- Situational and developmental crises are usually resolved within 4 to 6 weeks.
- Resolution of a crisis can result in a return to pre-crisis functioning or a higher or lower level of functioning. The goal of crisis intervention is a return to at least the pre-crisis functioning level.
- Social support and intervention can promote successful resolution and help build resilience.
- Crisis therapists take an active and directive approach with the patient in crisis, but as anxiety reduces, the patient becomes more active in planning solutions.
- Crisis intervention is usually provided to a mentally healthy person who is temporarily overwhelmed and unable to function.
- A caring attitude, the ability to be flexible in planning care, the ability to listen, and an active approach help facilitate successful nursing interventions when a patient is in crisis.
- During a disaster, triage helps make the most efficient use of available and limited resources.
- Critical Incident Stress Debriefing (CISD) helps groups of patients or victims, as well as staff or first responders who have been exposed to a crisis, to make sense of the tragedy and to cope.

APPLYING CRITICAL JUDGMENT

1. List the three important areas of crisis assessment once safety concerns have been identified. Give examples of two questions in each area that need to be answered to assist in planning care.
2. A 21-year-old student shares with her college nurse that her father has lost his job. Her father has been drinking heavily for years, and this trend has worsened since his job loss. The patient is having difficulty coping and wants to quit school due to stress and wanting to care for her ill mother and protect her siblings.
   A. How many different types of crises are occurring in this family? Discuss the crises from the viewpoint of each family member: the patient, father, mother, and siblings.
   B. If this family came for crisis counseling, what areas would you assess, and what kinds of questions would you ask to evaluate individual and family needs (perception of events, coping styles, social supports)?
   C. Formulate some tentative goals you might set in conjunction with the family.
   D. Using informatics, identify by name appropriate referral agencies in your community that might be helpful to this family.

APPLYING CRITICAL JUDGMENT—Cont'd

3. Identify an adventitious crisis that you have been aware of and that affected your life or emotions.
   A. If you are among a group of first responders, what would be the initial responsibility of your team?
   B. Identify the needs of the people that would have to be met after safety concerns were addressed.
   C. Discuss what could be done to protect against future mental health issues as a result of the disaster.

CHAPTER REVIEW QUESTIONS

1. While entering the building, an elementary school nurse observes a person in the distance emerging from a forest and approaching the school. The person is dressed in black from head to toe; wearing a backpack; and carrying a long, narrow, dark object. Which action should the nurse take first?
   a. Move to a secure location.
   b. Observe the intruder's features.
   c. Take note of the intruder's location.
   d. Activate the school code for an intruder.
2. An adult has had long-term serious medical problems and has just started a new medication resulting in decreased libido and sexual performance. The adult's spouse privately says to the nurse, "I don't feel loved anymore. I feel sexual urges, but my partner is not interested." Select the nurse's therapeutic response.
   a. "Tell me about how your partner shows love for you."
   b. "You're describing a scenario that many couples face."
   c. "Let's consider some other ways you can satisfy your needs."
   d. "I'm glad you are able to talk about and accept your situation."
3. The nurse in a high school meets with small groups of students the day after a school bus accident resulted in the death of five students. Which comment should the nurse use to begin the session?
   a. "Sometimes life is not fair. Yesterday's tragedy is an example of just how unfair it can be."
   b. "We're grateful that you are safe. Our discussion is to talk about feelings associated with yesterday's tragedy."
   c. "We've had a terrible loss. I also feel your pain. You need to talk about your feelings associated with the event."
   d. "Thank you for coming today. As school leaders, we know it is very important to respond to yesterday's tragedy."
4. A patient on an acute psychiatric unit removed the cap from the ceiling sprinkler, resulting in rapid flooding of the unit. After moving patients to a safe area, which action should the nurse take next?
   a. Conduct individual sessions with patients regarding the experience.
   b. Increase the volume of overhead music to distract patients from the event.
   c. Implement a psychomotor activity to reduce anxiety associated with the event.
   d. Lead a group session with patients to discuss feelings associated with the event.
5. Three weeks after being assaulted by a patient, a nurse develops headaches, insomnia, and gastrointestinal problems. The nurse has had four absences from work over a 2-week period. Which action should the nursing supervisor employ?
   a. Refer the nurse for counseling and support.
   b. Ask the nurse about current personal problems.
   c. Direct the nurse to take paid vacation for the following week.
   d. Schedule the nurse for administrative tasks rather than patient care.

REFERENCES

Aguilera, D. C. (1998). *Crisis intervention: Theory and methodology* (8th ed.). St. Louis: Mosby.

Aguilera, D. C., & Mesnick, J. (1970). *Crisis intervention: Theory and methodology*. St. Louis: Mosby.

Borgen Project. (2015). *Are natural disasters increasing?* Retrieved from http://borgenproject.org/natural-disasters-increasing/.

Boscarino, J. A. (2015). Community disasters, psychological trauma, and crisis intervention. *International Journal of Emergency Mental Health*, *17*(1), 369–371.

Caplan, G. (1964). *Symptoms of preventive psychiatry*. New York: Basic Books.

Clark, E. J. (2015). *Bereavement care for the adult*. Retrieved from http://www.socialworkers.org/pressroom/events/911/clark.asp.

Federal Emergency Management Agency (FEMA). (2018). *National incident management system*. Retrieved from https://www.fema.gov/nims-frequently-asked-questions.

France, K. (2015). *Crisis intervention: A handbook of immediate person-to-person help* (6th ed.). Springfield, IL: Thomas Books.

Giddens, J. (2017). *Concepts for nursing practice* (2th ed.). St. Louis: Elsevier.

Gil, S., & Weinberg, M. (2015). Coping strategies and internal resources of dispositional optimism and mastery as predictors of traumatic exposure and of PTSD symptoms: A prospective study. *Psychological Trauma: Theory, Research, Practice, and Policy*, 7(4), 405–411. https://doi.org/10.1037/tra0000032.

James, K. J., & Gilliland, B. E. (2013). *Crisis intervention strategies* (7th ed.). Pacific Grove, CA: Cengage Learning.

Kanel, K. (2015). *A guide to crisis intervention* (5th ed.). Stamford, CT: Cengage Learning.

Lowe, S. R., & Galea, S. (2015). The mental health consequences of mass shootings. *Trauma, Violence, & Abuse*, 1–21.

Roberts, A. R. (2005). *Crisis intervention handbook: Assessment, treatment, and research* (3rd ed.). New York: Oxford University Press.

U.S. National Library of Medicine. (2015). *Myositis*. Retrieved from http://www.nlm.nih.gov/medlineplus/myositis.html.

21

Child, Partner, and Elder Violence

Chyllia D. Fosbre

http://evolve.elsevier.com/Varcarolis/essentials

OBJECTIVES

1. Differentiate among the four types of family abuse, and give two physical and behavioral indicators for each.
2. Consider how you would communicate with (a) a parent who is suspected of child abuse and (b) a woman who is the victim of intimate partner violence (IPV) while providing patient-centered care. **QSEN: Patient-Centered Care**
3. Identify at least five characteristics of an abusive parent.
4. Evaluate at least three red flags that a nurse might note during a family assessment that could indicate elder abuse is occurring.
5. Incorporating evidence-based practice and safety, identify the most dangerous time in a domestic violence relationship according to the literature. **QSEN: Evidence-Based Practice; Safety**
6. Assess which various professions may be involved in teamwork and collaboration when obtaining forensic evidence from a child or adult victim of abuse. **QSEN: Teamwork and Collaboration**
7. Using a clinical example, describe the factors that make an older adult more vulnerable to abuse and in need of enhanced safety considerations. **QSEN: Safety**
8. Using informatics, research the resources and agencies related to elder abuse, intimate partner violence, and child abuse that are available in your community. **QSEN: Informatics**

KEY TERMS AND CONCEPTS

CONCEPT: INTERPERSONAL VIOLENCE: *Violence* is the intentional use of physical force or power, threatened or actual, against oneself, another person, or a group or community that either results in or has a high likelihood of injury, death, psychological harm, or deprivation (Giddens, 2017). The intergenerational violence theory states that behaviors are developed through role modeling, identification, and human interaction. According to this theory, a child who witnesses abuse or is abused in the family of origin learns that violence is an acceptable reaction to stress and internalizes the violence as a behavioral norm.

INTRODUCTION

Domestic violence (DV) is an extensive public health and criminal justice concern throughout the world. Domestic violence has widespread consequences that affect millions of women, men, and children. Physical and psychological trauma causes long-lasting damage in the lives of the victim, as well as in future generations and communities. In 2017 there were over 4 million referrals to **Child Protective Services (CPS)** involving about 7.5 million children (U.S. Department of Health and Human Services [USDHHS], 2019). The Adverse Childhood Experiences Study (ACES) found significant associations between childhood maltreatment and health and well-being in later life. The greater the number of adverse childhood events, the higher the probability of fetal death, drug and alcohol use, depression and suicide attempts, heart disease, intimate partner violence, early sexual activity and adolescent pregnancy, sexually transmitted infections (STIs), and poorer quality of life (Centers for Disease Control and Prevention [CDC], 2020a). Family violence is prevalent among all ethnic, religious, social, socioeconomic, and age groups. Although the home is supposed to be a safe and secure haven where love and support allow the family members to flourish, it can also be a place where abuse and fear occur. It doesn't matter whether the home is thousands of square feet and professionally decorated or a shanty in a poverty-stricken community; emotional, physical, or sexual abuse or neglect can and does occur (CDC, 2019). Domestic violence is normally thought of as occurring between more powerful (**perpetrator**) and less powerful (**victim**) family members. Examples of this include a grandparent abusing a child or a husband abusing his wife. However, this type of abuse can also be perpetrated by a trusted authority figure such as a religious leader, caregiver, health care provider, teacher, or coach.

The four main categories of abuse are emotional, physical, and sexual abuse and neglect. All abuse can harm the victim's self-esteem and spirit, damaging the ability to form healthy emotional relationships and reach his or her full potential. Recovering from abuse takes a large amount of attention and energy that could better be spent in maturing and progressing through life. The nurse is often the first point of contact for people experiencing domestic violence and is in a position to contribute to prevention, detection, and effective intervention.

Emotional abuse includes name calling, excessive criticism, ignoring accomplishments, yelling and swearing, mocking, isolating, locking the victim in a room, threats and intimidation, and denying abuse and blaming the victim (Vancouver Coastal Health, 2015). **Physical abuse** usually encompasses emotional abuse in addition to physical harm. Types of physical abuse include kicking, hitting, pushing, choking, burning, using weapons, and shoving the victim down stairs. Some physical abuse victims are also tied or locked up for periods of time. Physical abuse has the potential for complications, including deformity, internal damage, fractures, and in some cases death. **Sexual abuse** can occur toward adult or child victims, and both genders can be victims of sexual abuse. Forms of sexual abuse include vaginal or anal rape, oral or manual touching, inappropriate comments, viewing the victim in the shower or while dressing, being made to watch or participate in pornography, and in the most extreme cases being sold to others for sexual favors.

Neglect as abuse includes the inconsistent provision of food, water, shelter, sanitation, or other basic needs. Neglect also encompasses lack of schooling, medical care, or supervision and exposure to violent environments or substance abuse. Economic abuse is a form of neglect and occurs when the dependent person has monetary resources withheld.

Sensitivity is required on the part of the nurse who suspects domestic violence. A person who feels judged or accused of wrongdoing is likely to become defensive, and any attempts to change coping strategies in the family will be thwarted. In some cases, the nurse may be able to recommend resources for solving disagreements or methods of disciplining children, and in other cases the authorities may need to be contacted and involved. Avoiding inflammatory terms such as *abuse* while working with the individuals will be helpful in maintaining rapport and calm. Although there are protective agencies for children and the elderly, in general, most adults may choose to remain in an abusive situation. This can be difficult for the nurse to observe and accept. Potential indicators of domestic violence are listed in Box 21.1.

The victimization of lesbian, gay, bisexual, transgender, and questioning (LGBTQ) individuals is a significant issue because they face higher rates of all abuse and is discussed in Chapter 22.

BOX 21.1 Indicators for Domestic Violence

- Recurrent emergency department (ED) visits for physical injuries attributed to being accident prone
- Somatic symptoms reflecting anxiety or chronic stress, such as hyperventilation, gastrointestinal distress, hypertension, insomnia, nightmares, and even eczema or hair loss in some cases
- Signs of depression, which can include sadness, tearfulness, sleep or appetite disturbance, irritability, loss of interest in usual activities, fatigue, and in some cases thoughts of suicide

THEORY

Most theories of intrafamily violence are related to psychology, sociology, or culture. Most conventional explanations of intrafamily violence are partial and incomplete. Experts advocate for a theory of violence that provides a comprehensive explanation that integrates interpersonal, institutional, and structural aspects of violence. Domestic violence is an extremely complex issue and is most likely an interaction of societal, cultural, and psychological factors and neurobiological influences.

Social Learning Theory

The social learning theory or the **intergenerational violence theory** of family violence purports that behaviors are developed through role modeling, identification, and human interaction (Widom & Wilson, 2015). According to this theory, a child who witnesses abuse or is abused in the family of origin learns that violence is an acceptable reaction to stress, and it becomes a behavioral norm. If the violent acting-out behaviors are condoned in the family or social milieu, the person is rewarded with a sense of power and control over others. Intergenerational abuse is considered a contributing factor in many cases of intimate partner violence (IPV), elder abuse, and child abuse.

Societal and Cultural Factors

According to the CDC (2020a) the following risk factors may be seen:

- Poverty or unemployment
- Communities with inadequate resources and overcrowding
- Social isolation of families
- Substance abuse
- Early parenthood
- Inadequate coping skills
- Family member with chronic health condition

The classic *frustration-aggression hypothesis* proposes that when frustration is high in response to negative societal situations, frustration may lead to aggression. Although these factors do correlate with family violence, they do not cause family violence, and not all frustrated individuals respond with violence. Some people respond to high levels of frustration with despair, depression, and resignation or attempts to change the situation (Widom & Wilson, 2015).

The *patriarchal theory* (often referred to as feminist theory) holds the view that male dominance in our political and economic structure exists to enforce the differential status of men over women. In many subcultures, women are viewed as the property of men, are subservient, and are kept relatively powerless, in part through violence. The World Health Organization (WHO, 2017) identifies "male controlling behaviors towards their partners" as a risk factor for IPV.

Psychological Factors

Psychological theories focus on the abuser having personality traits that cause abusive behaviors. According to psychological theories, the abuser has no control over his or her violence due to genetics, mental illness, or substance, and thus he or she is not at fault. However, it is now known that many abusers and victims do not have a major mental illness according to the results of psychological testing, and many individuals with mental illness are not violent. The use of legal or illegal drugs coexists in some, but not all, cases of domestic violence (Smith & Fazel, 2015).

Other psychological factors correlated with domestic violence include low self-esteem, poor problem-solving skills, history of impulsive behavior, hypersensitivity (sees self as victim), and narcissism (centers on self, lacks compassion for others). People with aggressive traits are usually immature, although some are able to present a mature facade to the outside world. They may report an inability to control physical aggression but may only abuse a partner while being able to restrain themselves from attacking a police officer or boss. See Chapter 24 for neurobiological factors related to violence and interventions for angry and aggressive patients.

CHILD ABUSE

A report of child abuse is made every 10 seconds, and between four and seven children die every day in the United States as a result of child abuse (Childhelp, 2018). **Child abuse** takes place when a child is harmed physically, psychologically, sexually, or through acts of neglect. It is generally believed that the number of child abuse cases is grossly underreported. The vast majority, about 80%, of deaths related to child abuse are in children under the age of 4, with the largest number being infants (CDC, 2020a). Parents are the perpetrators in most cases, although siblings can also abuse one another, or grandparents, aunts, or uncles may be involved. Each state is responsible for providing its own definition of child abuse. Teachers, clergy, nurses, and other health care providers are considered mandated reporters and must report abuse to child protective services. A suspicion and not confirmation of child abuse is all that is necessary to file a report.

An interesting problem in industrialized countries, where financial resources have increased and family size has decreased, is overindulgence of children. Overindulgence can be considered a type of neglect that can result in social and emotional impairment, lack of empathy, and physical problems related to inactivity and obesity. In years of economic recession, stress increases the incidence of child, partner, and elder abuse. Another modern form of emotional abuse is the public shaming of children by posting photos or descriptions on social media (Table 21.1).

TABLE 21.1 Types of Child Abuse and Physical and Behavioral Indicators

Type of Abuse	Physical Indicators	Behavioral Indicators
Physical Abuse		
Intentional physical injury inflicted by a caregiver	Bruises, wounds, injuries in differing stages of healing Patterning of abuse, such as marks in shapes such as coat hangers or cigarette burns, or hidden under clothing where they are harder to discern Bald patches on scalp Subdural hematoma (child younger than 2 years of age) Retinal hemorrhage	Excessive fear of parents or constant effort to please Wary of adult contact Nightmares or anxiety Obvious attempts to hide bruises or injuries Withdrawn, depressed, aggressive, or disruptive behavior at home or school Regressive behavior
Neglect		
Failure to provide for the child's basic needs	*Physical neglect:* Malnourished Underweight, poor growth pattern Inadequately supervised Poor hygiene Unattended physical problems Inappropriate dress *Educational neglect:* School problems or failure Not enrolled in mandatory school for age of child	Soiled clothing, poor hygiene Begging, stealing food Emaciated or has distended belly Arrives early or stays late at school Psychosomatic complaints Delinquency Alcohol or drug abuse Chronic truancy Special educational needs not being attended
Sexual Abuse		
Sexual abuse perpetrated by family or nonfamily member. Some types include exhibitionism; touching; oral, anal, or vaginal penetration; being forced to watch sex acts or pornography. In extreme cases, being sold for sexual favors.	Difficulty in walking or sitting Itching in private areas Urinary tract infections, painful urination Torn, stained, or bloody underclothing Bruises or bleeding in external genitalia, vaginal, or anal areas Sexually transmitted infection, especially in preteens Swollen private areas or discharge Objects or liquid in vagina, rectum, or urethra	Mistrust of adults Abnormal or distorted view of sex Advanced or unusual sexual behavior or knowledge for age Phobias: fear of the dark, men, strangers, leaving the house Delinquency or running away Self-injury or suicidal thoughts or behaviors Mental disorders may develop, including posttraumatic stress disorder, depression, dissociative disorder, eating disorders, conduct disorders, mood swings, and anxiety.
Emotional or Psychological Abuse		
Behaviors that convey to the child that he or she is worthless, flawed, unloved, or unwanted. These include constant criticism, threats, insults, yelling, ignoring, favoritism, and harsh demands.	Speech disorders Lag in physical development	Difficulty in learning and living up to potential Lack of self-confidence Inappropriate adultlike behavior or infantile behavior Poor social skills Dramatic behavior changes such as aggressiveness, drug use, change in friends or clothing, self-harm behaviors, compulsiveness, and a needy pursuit of attention

VIGNETTE: CHILD ABUSE: A 6-year-old Native American male falls on the school playground and goes to the school nurse to have minor abrasions on his knees cleansed and bandaged. While the nurse is taking care of him, she lightly touches his back and he quickly moves away from her. The nurse asks if it hurt, and he quietly nods "yes." She asks a school counselor to come in and has the young boy pull up his shirt. The nurse and counselor see a visible handprint and several welts across his back. The boy quickly starts to say that he was bad, that it was his fault for disrespecting the tribal elders, and that his father was teaching him. The nurse and school counselor know they are mandated reporters. The counselor stays with the child for support while the school nurse calls Child Protective Services (CPS) so that an investigation can be done regarding signs of physical abuse. The counselor and nurse anticipate that the investigation may be taken over by tribal council leaders, and they make sure that CPS is aware that the child is Native American.

APPLICATION OF THE NURSING PROCESS

ASSESSMENT

Child

Often the abused child appears timid or fearful of a parent or caregiver. The child may be disheveled or have a history of absenteeism from school. Even if a parent is abusive, children are very loyal to that parent. They may resist telling about the abuse out of attachment to the parent or fear of retribution later when they are alone. Children tend to believe that the abuse is their fault. If they had caused less trouble, or behaved better, they wouldn't have deserved the punishment or abuse. In general, parents are present for any questioning or examining of their child. In the case of suspected child abuse, however, after the initial interview with the parents, the child should be seen alone, giving him or her a chance to disclose mistreatment. Abusive parents will often find many excuses not to leave their child alone with the nurse. Children should be questioned gently and not pressured and may be better able to express themselves through drawing or playing with dolls. Do not suggest answers to the child. Reassure the child that the situation is not his or her fault. Sitting next to the child may feel supportive. Remember that children are concrete in their thinking. For example, if you ask a child if someone hit him or her, the child may say "no" because the injury occurred through being kicked, not hit. Open-ended questions, such as "How did that happen to you?" "Where do you go after school?" or "What happens when you do something wrong?" may elicit a better response. Do not promise the child that everything said is confidential because abuse must be reported. Avoid showing shock, no matter what the child discloses. The child's privacy must be maintained, including not forcing the child to undress or be examined in front of a group (Ney, 2015).

Parent or Caregiver

Abusing parents vary by degrees of intelligence and education and come from all backgrounds. Specific characteristics are often found either singly or in combination among parents who abuse their children, including a history of being abused themselves, low self-esteem, social isolation or suspiciousness, drug or alcohol abuse, and rigid expectations for the child's behavior (Box 21.2). In interviewing a parent or guardian suspected of child abuse, ensure a private environment. Be direct, understanding, and professional. Be honest about the necessity to report the suspected abuse to CPS. Do not display horror, anger, or a judgmental attitude toward the parent. Again, open-ended questions will elicit the best, most descriptive response. Examples include "What arrangements do you make when you have to leave your child alone?" "How do you punish your child?" "How do you get your infant to stop crying?" and "How are things at home?"

DIAGNOSIS AND OUTCOMES IDENTIFICATION

The most immediate concern is to ensure the child's safety and well-being. Primary nursing diagnoses that can be used to plan care in suspected child abuse include *Physical injury from abuse, Victim of child abuse,* malnutrition, abuse injury, and *Risk for impaired child development.* The outcome of the care plan is that the physical, sexual, or emotional abuse or neglect has stopped. Short-term goals could include receiving medical care within 1 hour, notification of the proper authorities, and maintaining the child's safety until appropriate arrangements have been made.

PLANNING AND IMPLEMENTATION

When child abuse is suspected, persons in authority, including nurses, teachers, spiritual leaders, coaches, counselors, and childcare providers, are *legally* responsible for reporting to the appropriate child protective agency. Each state mandates that a report must be filed when suspected abuse or neglect is encountered. It is not necessary to have proof of the abuse. If there is a suspicion or if the child says something is happening, that is enough grounds to report. It is then up to the CPS agency to investigate and make a determination. For more on reporting child abuse and neglect, go to http://www.childwelfare.gov/ or call 1-800-422-4453.

Child abuse may be first discovered in the emergency department, in an outpatient clinic where the child has been referred for behavioral problems, or at the school. Table 21.2 includes a list of nursing intervention guidelines to be used with the abused child and his or her family, with rationales for the interventions. The physician or nurse practitioner caring for an abused child should incorporate help from a variety of sources to ensure that the child is safe and cared for and that the family receives supportive help. Resources include the hospital social work department, mental health agencies, substance abuse treatment centers, and parenting classes. Counseling and supportive services have been shown to improve life outcomes for abused children. Just the presence of one supportive person and the act of being believed make a significant difference in the child's self-esteem and future success.

Many factors exist in cases of child abuse, often including substance abuse by the parent(s). Additional factors that increase the rate of child abuse include single or teen parenthood, mental illness, a child with a medical or psychological disorder or handicap, and abuse of the parent in childhood or adult relationships.

Societal risk factors also play an important role. Poverty is thought to be among the most frequently and persistently noted risk factors for child abuse. Families that live in communities that are divided, where there are fewer economic opportunities, where norms of society support aggression, and where social isolation occurs are more likely to experience violence within the family (CDC, 2020a).

Early diagnosis of actual or potential child abuse and intervention correlates with a more positive prognosis. Interventions can include strengthening family ties and linking the family with community supports; coordinating services such as parenting skills, anger management, and coping skills; enhancing community awareness of child abuse and healthy parenting concepts; and providing emergency supports such as food and shelter for families (CDC, 2020a).

INTIMATE PARTNER VIOLENCE

Intimate partner violence (IPV) is defined as "a pattern of assault and course of behaviors that may include physical injury, psychological abuse, sexual assault, progressive social isolation, stalking, deprivation, intimidation and threats" between current or former partners of an intimate relationship, regardless of gender or marital status (CDC, 2019).

BOX 21.2 Characteristics of Abusive Parents

- A history of violence, neglect, or emotional deprivation as a child
- Low self-esteem, feelings of worthlessness, depression
- Poor coping skills
- Social isolation, may be suspicious of others
- Few or no friends, little or no involvement in social or community activities
- Involved in a crisis situation such as unemployment, divorce, financial difficulties, abusive relationship
- Rigid, unrealistic expectations of child's behavior
- Frequently uses harsh punishment
- History of severe mental illness, such as schizophrenia
- Violent temper outbursts
- Looks to child for satisfaction of needs for love, support, and reassurance
- Projects blame onto the child for his or her problems
- Lack of effective parenting skills
- Inability to seek help from others
- Perceives the child as bad or evil
- History of drug or alcohol abuse
- Feels little or no control over life
- Low tolerance for frustration
- Poor impulse control

Adapted from Boos, S. C., & Endon, E. E. (2015). Physical abuse in children: Diagnostic evaluation and management. In J. F. Wiley (Ed.), *UpToDate*. Retrieved from http://www.UpToDate.com

The majority of the victims of reported domestic violence are women (CDC, 2019). Domestic violence is the number one cause of emergency department visits by women and is the primary cause of homelessness in women. However, a growing body of research is revealing the prevalence and significance of domestic violence by women against men (CDC, 2019). Actual statistics are hard to ascertain because there is substantial underreporting of IPV by women and even more underreporting by men. Although the exact numbers of abused domestic partners are not known, it is estimated that up to 23% of all U.S. women experience physical assault by an intimate partner, with the worldwide rate reaching 69% (Weil, 2016). Domestic violence by an intimate partner is the leading cause of female homicides and birth defects during pregnancy (CDC, 2019). Attempting to leave the abuser was the precipitating factor in 45% of female murders by their intimate partner. Because of this, it is especially important to educate women on being careful when planning to leave their abusers. If brochures or cards about leaving a partner are discovered, victims may be at greater risk for increased violence, so they are often only given a verbal list of resources instead of printed materials. Domestic violence in intimate partnerships occurs in heterosexual, homosexual, bisexual, and transgendered individuals.

TEEN DATING VIOLENCE

Teen dating violence (TDV) is a disturbing trend, with approximately 25% to 33% of adolescents reporting verbal, physical, emotional, or sexual abuse from a dating partner each year (CDC, 2019). Teen abuse takes many forms, such as extreme possessiveness and jealousy, physical stalking or cyberstalking, manipulation and control of one's partner, demeaning one's partner in front of friends, threatening to commit suicide, or forced intimacy or sex. Depression, posttraumatic stress disorder (PTSD), anxiety disorders, and suicidal thoughts and attempts are potential sequelae to battering for all age groups (President of the United States of America, 2016).

TABLE 21.2 Interventions for the Abused Child and the Child's Family

Intervention	Rationale
1. Adopt a nonthreatening, nonjudgmental relationship with parents.	1. If parents feel judged, they may become defensive and leave without receiving care for the child.
2. Understand that the child does not want to betray his or her parents.	2. Even in an intolerable situation, the parents are the only security the child knows.
3. Provide a complete physical assessment of the child.	3. Allows health care worker to provide care and document evidence.
4. The use of dolls or drawing might help the child to tell how the injury or accident happened.	4. Young children might not have the vocabulary to explain what happened or might be afraid of punishment.
Forensic Issues	
1. Be aware of your agency's and state's policy in reporting child abuse. Contact supervisor or social worker to implement appropriate reporting.	1. Health care workers are mandated to report any cases of suspected or actual child abuse. Suspicion or verbalization is enough to report; you do not have to prove the abuse happened.
2. Ensure that proper procedures are followed and evidence is collected.	2. Appropriate evidence helps protect the child's welfare.
3. Keep accurate and detailed records of incident: • Exact words of what the child or others involved say happened • A body map to indicate size, color, shape, areas, and types of injuries, with explanations • Physical evidence, when possible, of sexual abuse • Use of photos can be helpful. Check hospital policy. Police may be involved for photographing injuries.	3. Accurate records could help ensure the child's safety and support the legal process.
4. Forensic examination of the sexually assaulted child should be conducted according to specific protocols: • Provided by law enforcement agencies • Follows state guidelines (www.childwelfare.gov)	4. Proper collection, handling, and storage of forensic specimens are crucial. Whenever available, a trained team or individual should perform this type of evidence collection for accuracy and sensitivity to the child victim.

Adapted from Varcarolis, E. M. (2015). *Manual of psychiatric nursing care plans: Diagnoses, clinical tools, and psychopharmacology* (5th ed.). St. Louis: Elsevier.

An abusive relationship is all about instilling fear and wanting to have power and control in the relationship. Anger is one way that the abuser tries to gain authority. He or she may also turn to physical, sexual, or psychological violence to maintain control. Psychological abuse may include threats to harm a child, pet, or loved one or displaying weapons. Violence against an intimate partner has effects on not only the victim but also children residing in the home. The children may experience feelings of guilt, depression, and anxiety; behavioral acting-out, including aggression; somatic symptoms; nightmares; detachment from school and friends; and alcohol or drug abuse. In 30% to 61% of IPV cases, the children are also abused (Guy, Feinstein, & Griffiths, 2013) and are unfortunately likely to carry the legacy forward into their adult lives as either the abuser or the abused.

One in five high school students report being bullied by a peer in the past year. Youth violence is connected to future violence toward others, ongoing victimhood, injury, obesity, substance use, depression, and higher rates of dropout and suicide (CDC, 2020b).

> **VIGNETTE: TEEN DATING VIOLENCE/IPV:** A 16-year-old male is brought to the emergency department after passing out at school. The boy admits to taking a handful of unknown pills he bought from another student. When discussing what had happened, the boy explains that 3 days ago his girlfriend posted a message on social media saying that she was breaking up with him because he was a terrible kisser, a horrible date, and worthless as a boyfriend and human being. Since the message was posted, classmates had continued to call him names, and his friends were avoiding him. He tried to tell his parents, who just told him to "handle it like an adult" and "suck it up."

THE BATTERED PARTNER

Intimate partners do not ask to be beaten, nor do they enjoy being battered. The battered partner lives in terror of the next beating. Women do not usually initiate the violence but may retaliate in self-defense. Approximately half of women who were victims of homicide were killed by an intimate partner (CNN, 2018).

The abused woman is often the subject of extreme and irrational jealousy, isolation, and verbal as well as physical abuse. Feelings of powerlessness and low self-esteem are common. After constant belittlement, insults, and degradation, the abused becomes so psychologically destroyed that she (or he) begins to believe her abuser's insults. This phenomenon is also seen in other cases of abuse, such as slavery or prisoners or war. Victims of abuse in general may eventually be brainwashed to the abuser's way of thinking and develop self-hatred. Because of the physical or sexual abuse and threats, the abused lives in a world of terror and fear for her life and the lives of her children. Isolation from family and friends, or even to a remote community, helps to perpetuate the abuse without detection or intervention. The violence and pain that exist inside the home remain secret through threats. Table 21.3 lists characteristics of the abused woman and violent partner.

THE BATTERER

Violence is a learned behavior used by a person to control others. Frequently, violent partners were raised in a home where they themselves were beaten or where they witnessed domestic violence between parents. Abusing someone less powerful or more vulnerable helps the violent partner feel more in control and powerful. Batterers may appear well adjusted from the outside but usually have only superficial relationships with others. They are extremely possessive, are pathologically jealous, believe in male supremacy in relationships, and often have a drug or alcohol problem, which is not a cause of the abuse but often an excuse or something that exacerbates the abuse. Without professional treatment, the behaviors almost always continue to escalate.

CYCLE OF VIOLENCE

Abuse toward a person in a partner relationship is not merely an exchange of blows on an isolated occasion but, rather, a process that increases in intensity and escalates over time. The abusive relationship may start subtly. It may start by the abuser being critical of the way the partner dresses, disciplines the kids, or cares for the home. Or the abuser becomes unreasonably jealous, possessive, and watchful of the partner's activities. The abuse becomes more frequent, intense, and life-threatening over time. In a classic study of 400 women in violent families (Walker, 1979), the cycle of violence was first operationally defined. The **cycle of violence** consists of three phases: (1) tension-building phase, (2) acute battering phase, and (3) honeymoon phase. Fig. 21.1 shows behaviors that characterize the steps in the cycle.

The cycle of violence is a continuing cycle that is hard to break without help. Whatever pattern the violence follows, trust is broken, and shame and fear are constantly underneath the surface of the lives of the victims. Many

TABLE 21.3 Behavioral Characteristics of Intimate Partner Violence

Characteristics of Violent Partner	Characteristics of Battered Partner
Denial and Blame: Denies that abuse occurs, shifts responsibility of abuse to partner; makes statements that the victim caused the abuse or caused the abuser to react that way	Eventually believes that if she does or says the right thing, the abuse will stop. If she does not do anything wrong, abuse will not occur. May be re-creating patterns from abuse during childhood that are familiar.
Emotional Abuse: Belittles, criticizes, insults, uses name calling, undermines	Becomes psychologically devastated and begins to believe partner's words. Lowered self-esteem. Unhealthy bond with the abuser.
Control Through Isolation: Limits family or friends, controls activities and social events, tracks time or mileage on car and activities, stalks at work, takes to and from work or school, may demand permission to leave house	Gradually loses sight of personal boundaries for self, children. Over time becomes unable to accurately assess the situation without validation from a supportive network.
Control Through Intimidation: Uses behaviors to instill fear, such as vile threats, breaking things, destroying property, abusing pets, displaying weapons, threatening children, threatening homicide or suicide, and increasing physical, sexual, or psychological abuse	Results in constant fear and terror that becomes cumulative and oppressive; contemplates suicide, contemplates homicide, occasionally completes suicide or homicide in self-defense. Posttraumatic stress symptoms develop.
Control Through Economic Abuse: Controls money, makes partner account for all money spent; if partner works, calls excessively, forces partner to miss work; refuses to share money	Economic and emotional dependency may result in depression, high risk for secret drug or alcohol abuse. If she works, frequently loses job due to partner stalking and harassing. Is unable to save money to leave.
Control Through Power: Makes all decisions, defines role in the relationship, treats spouse like a servant, takes charge of the home and social life	Continues to lose sense of self, becomes unsure of who she is, defines self in terms of partner, children, job, others; lacks personal power.

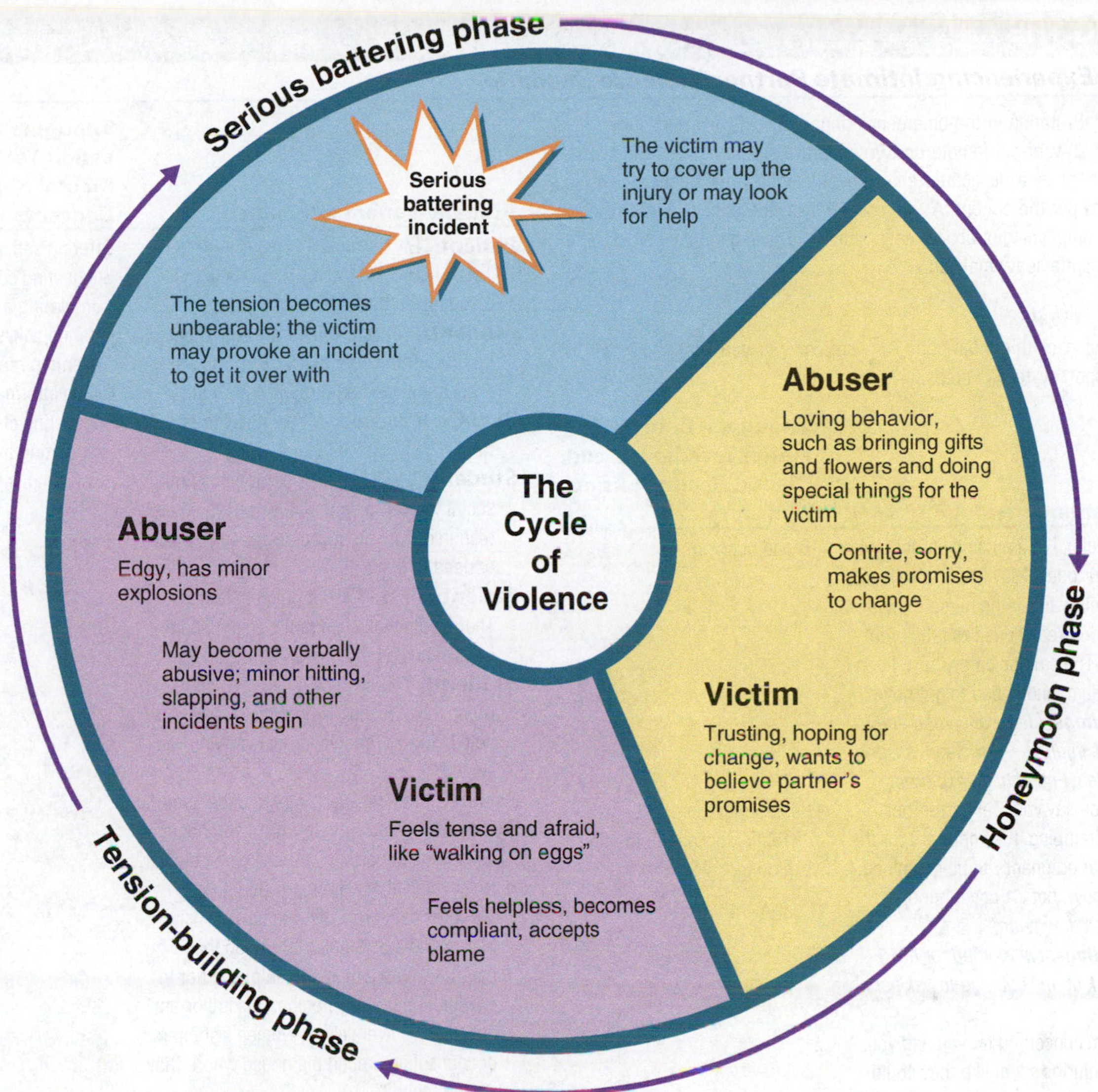

Fig. 21.1 The cycle of violence.

women report that their partners never repent and enter the honeymoon phase but, rather, that the violence is a constant presence in their lives.

WHY ABUSED PARTNERS STAY

There are many reasons women stay in violent domestic situations. Perhaps one of the *strongest* motives for staying is fear that the attacks will become even more violent or that the woman or her children could be murdered if they leave and are found by the batterer. This is a very real concern, and women are at the highest risk of further violence or even death when they threaten to leave or if they leave and are later found by their abuser. Women may end up in an abusive relationship if they were abused as children and abuse seems familiar or normal. The abuse may also start later in the relationship and be slow or subtle. If women have not been exposed to violence in their families, they may not have a frame of reference for early recognition.

Women may not leave an abusive relationship for many reasons. These include lack of financial support, lack of a support system after being isolated, fear or brainwashing developed through the abuse, depression or low self-esteem, religious values against divorce, belief that they deserved the abuse, and staying for the sake of the children. According to one-third of homeless women, many with children, they are homeless as a direct result of DV. Until a woman has experienced a number of abuse cycles, she may believe the honeymoon phase will last and that the abuser has learned his lesson and changed.

APPLICATION OF THE NURSING PROCESS

ASSESSMENT

Abused partners are most often seen in the emergency department, but they may be seen in an urgent care clinic, primary care office, or outpatient psychiatric practice. Although there have been greater recognition of and response to victims of IPV by the health care system, there is room for continued education and improvement. The American Academy of Family Physicians (2018) recommends screening for IPV in women of reproductive age at each visit. As much as we know, some nurses and other professionals still have an attitude of blaming the victim or a lack of understanding as to how the cycle occurs or continues. There has been expanded awareness of military sexual violence against women that was hidden in the past. There are several organizations that offer training for law enforcement and health care professionals to help people leave violent situations.

Some signs of probable IVP include a discrepancy between the injury and the explanation of how it occurred, minimization of the injury or abuse, and fearfulness regarding a partner or other individual. If IPV is suspected, a complete physical examination and appropriate testing

APPLYING THE ART

A Person Experiencing Intimate Partner Violence Scenario

During a clinical rotation in the emergency department (ED), a nursing student encountered a 28-year-old female on two separate occasions. The initial visit was for treatment of a dislocated shoulder sustained after falling down the basement steps per the patient. At the second visit, the patient was 3 months pregnant and complaining of abdominal cramping. Bruising around her left orbit was evident despite heavy makeup.

Therapeutic Goal

By the conclusion of this interaction, the patient will verbalize the intent to access her support system, decreasing her isolation.

Student–Patient Interaction	Thoughts, Communication Techniques, and Mental Health Nursing Concepts
Student: "Hello, I'm a nursing student working in the ED today. May I sit and talk with you while you wait for the nurse-midwife?"	Broad opening
Patient: "I don't really need to talk; I feel better now. The cramps barely hurt. I don't need that exam, and I need to get home."	
Student's feelings: *I feel concerned about the patient's injuries—they seem suspicious or at least need to be explored.*	
Student: "You say you feel better, but you're still cramping. It's important for the safety of your pregnancy to be examined."	Restatement, presenting reality, giving information
Patient: "I know, but ... never mind." *Patient gazes downward.*	Exploring
Student's feelings: *I'm worried for her. I need to work up the courage to ask her about abuse.*	
Student: "I'm concerned for you and your baby. Your injuries seem like they could be related to abuse. Are you being hurt at home?"	
Patient: "Oh no, my husband would never hurt me on purpose."	Restating, exploring
Student: "On purpose. Does he hurt you by accident sometimes?"	Seeking information, suggesting collaboration
Patient: "Well, I deserve it. I don't have the housework done or I am disrespectful to him."	
Student: "Do you have anyone, a friend or family member, you can talk to?"	
Patient: "My husband moved us here to Texas for his job. All my family is in Indiana. I haven't seen them in 3 years."	Offering self/support
Student: "I'm sure you miss them. That can be difficult to be far away when you are pregnant and going through a hard time."	Suggesting collaboration, formulating a plan of action
Patient: *Begins to cry.* "Yes, it is. I'm afraid for the baby. I have to keep calm."	Offering self/support, presenting reality
Student: "I would like to get the hospital social worker for you. She will have some resources for you, if you decide to get help or need to leave."	Giving information
Patient: "Oh no! I'm not going to leave. That would make him really angry, and a family should be together."	
Student: "You don't have to leave; that is your choice. I just want you to have help being so far away from everyone you know."	Suggesting collaboration, formulating a plan of action, offering self/support
Patient: "Yes, please, that would be good."	
Student: "I also want to talk to you about something important. When a woman goes to leave an abusive relationship, that is the most dangerous time to be seriously hurt or killed. It is important to do that carefully, with a plan and help, and not to challenge the angry person. It is important not to leave flyers about women's shelters or counseling around the house where they can be found."	
Patient: "I understand; that makes sense."	
Student: "I'm going to let your midwife and the social worker know about your situation so that we can work together to support you."	
Patient: *(Softly)* "Thank you ... don't say anything to my husband."	
Student's feelings: *I'm relieved that she is getting help and glad I could be part of that.*	

need to be performed. Rape may be part of the abuse, so a gynecological examination, including testing for STIs and evidence collection, should be performed. Approximately 5% of rapes result in a pregnancy, so it is not unusual for the "morning after pill" to be offered (Perry et al., 2015).

Signs of abuse in all ages or genders of victims may include burns; bruises; scars; wounds in various stages of healing, particularly around the head and neck; and fractures of limbs, ribs, or jaw. Physical examination includes assessing for signs of internal injuries (e.g., bleeding), concussions, perforated eardrums, abdominal injuries, eye injuries, and strangulation marks on the neck. An examination might reveal burns from cigarettes, acids, scalding liquids, or appliances. Patterning of injuries can include bruises, lacerations, or contusions in the shapes of objects such as coat hangers, cords, irons, handprints, fly swatters, rope burns, bite marks, or belt buckles. Patterning can also refer to the location of the damage. Abusers often plan the location of abuse so that it cannot be easily noticed, such as on the torso, back, upper arms, and upper legs; inside body orifices; and under the hair. Examination should include attention to these hidden areas.

There are always psychological and emotional scars from abuse. The woman might present with signs of high anxiety and stress and complain of insomnia, chest pain, back pain, dizziness, stomach upset, trouble eating, or severe headache, for example. Signs of posttraumatic stress disorder (PTSD) are often present and should be part of an assessment. A brief history may reveal a series of falls, "accidents," and recent emergency department visits. The victim may be timid or vague in her explanations. A woman with any indication of IPV should always be seen alone, without her partner present, for at least part of the examination time. A reluctance on the part of the partner to leave the patient alone can be a red flag, although other reasons can account for a partner wanting to stay near. While alone, ask the potential victim if someone is hitting or otherwise hurting her—either a current or past partner, or anyone else—and if she feels safe in her current relationship. It is also important to ask if the children are also being harmed by the abuser in any way.

An assessment of the patient's support systems, suicide potential, and coping responses, including learned helplessness, substance abuse, denial, or self-harm, should be included in the assessment. Once the history of abuse has been ascertained, careful documentation, such as verbatim verbal statements and physical findings, should be recorded using a body map (Table 21.4). Ask the woman if she would allow

TABLE 21.4 Interventions for Intimate Partner Violence: Emergency Department

Intervention	Rationale
1. Ensure that medical attention is provided to patient. Document injuries using body map. Ask permission to take photos.	1. If patient wants to file charges, photos boost victim's confidence to press charges now or in the future.
2. Set up interview in private and ensure confidentiality.	2. Patient might be terrified of retribution and further attacks from partner if she reveals abuse.
3. Assess in a nonthreatening manner information concerning: • Sexual abuse • Physical abuse • Emotional abuse • Abuse of children • Drugs of abuse • Thoughts of suicide or homicide	3. These are all vital issues in determining appropriate interventions for depression, anxiety, suicide prevention, and self-medication with alcohol or substances.
4. Encourage patient to talk about the battering incident without interruptions, in a kind and gentle manner, without judgment.	4. When patients share their stories, attentive listening is essential.
5. Ask how patient is faring with the children in the home.	5. In homes in which the mother is abused, children also tend to be abused or traumatized by what they witness.
6. Assess if patient has a safe place to go when violence is escalating. If she does not, include a list of shelters or safe houses with other written information. Some hospitals provide small cards that can fit in a shoe, so that the victim is not endangered by the abuser finding shelter and escape resources.	6. When abused patients are ready to leave their abusers, they need to go quickly. A plan is advised, and it is better to leave when the abuser is not home unless the person is in danger and must flee immediately. Instruct the victim not to confront the abuser when leaving because this may worsen the rage. When a victim leaves, she is at the greatest risk for severe injury or being killed.
Legal Issues	
1. Identify if patient is interested in pressing charges. If yes, give verbal and written information on: • Local attorneys who handle spousal abuse cases • Legal clinics • Battered women's advocates and shelters Call Child Protective Services (CPS) if children are involved. Call law enforcement to make a report and assist the victim.	1. Often the spouse or partner is afraid of retaliation, but when ready to seek legal advice, an appropriate list of lawyers well trained in this specialty area is needed.
2. Know the requirements in your state about reporting suspected spousal abuse.	2. Many states have or are developing laws or guidelines for protecting battered women.
3. Discuss with patient a safety and escape plan during escalation of anxiety before actual violence erupts (see Box 21.3).	3. Document escape plan and include shelter and referral numbers. This can prevent further abuse to children and patient.
4. Throughout work with battered spouses, emphasize that the beatings are not their fault.	4. When self-esteem is eroded, victims often believe that they deserved the beatings.
5. Encourage patient to reach out to family and friends whom they might have been avoiding.	5. Old friends and relatives can make helpful allies and validate that the patient does not deserve to be beaten. The victim will need a lot of support.
6. Know the psychotherapists in the community who have experience working with battered spouses or partners.	6. Psychotherapy with victims of trauma requires special skills.
7. If the patient is not ready to take action at this time, provide a list of community resources: a. Hotlines b. Shelters c. Battered women's groups and advocates d. Therapists e. Law enforcement f. Medical assistance or Aid to Families with Dependent Children (AFDC) g. CPS has resources to support families, in addition to investigating allegations of abuse.	7. It can take time for patients to make decisions to change their life situation. People need appropriate information.

Adapted from Varcarolis, E. M. (2015). *Manual of psychiatric nursing care plans: Diagnoses, clinical tools, and psychopharmacology* (5th ed.). St. Louis: Elsevier.

photos to be taken. Although an adult victim has the right to refuse to report the assault, the nurse can document thoroughly and notify police. This will allow the patient to have contact with law enforcement for future support if needed, even if she chooses not to report at this time. CPS must be notified if there are children in the home because it would be assumed that the violence against the parent could also affect the children.

DIAGNOSIS AND OUTCOMES IDENTIFICATION

The threat to a woman's physical and psychological health, as well as to her life and possibly the lives of her children, as a result of IPV is the immediate concern. Nursing diagnoses that address these areas include *Victim of intimate partner violence, Risk for spiritual distress, Post-trauma response, Lack of social support, Impaired role performance*, and *Physical injury from abuse* (International Council of Nurses [ICN], 2017).

Unfortunately, people who are treated in the emergency department (ED) may admit to IPV but seldom return for treatment. Nurses often have strong reactions when people are the victims of violence. However, in the case of partner abuse, it is up to the abused partner to make the decision to stay in the battering situation or to leave. It is most helpful for the victim if the nurse can accept the person's decision in a nonjudgmental way and support the victim's decision.

The preferred outcome for health care personnel would be to see the victim opt for a safe environment in the form of safe houses, a caring relative, or a friend. The nurse can discuss options and provide the victim with referrals for safe houses and shelters, hotlines, support groups, and legal counseling as well as a **safety plan**. Box 21.3 contains an example of a basic IPV safety plan. Make sure the victim is warned not to leave any literature where the abuser can find it.

BOX 21.3 Basic Intimate Partner Violence Safety Plan

It is important, whenever possible, to work with a domestic violence advocate to develop a safety plan that fits your needs.

- Move to a room with more than one exit, avoiding rooms with potential weapons such as kitchen knives or heavy objects.
- Know the quickest route out of your home.
- Know the quickest route out of your workplace. Determine resources the employer may have to protect employees, such as a security guard escort.
- Keep a bag packed with essentials: clothes, valuables, documents (e.g., passports, Social Security cards, medical records, bank cards, birth certificates), a list of phone contacts, a month's supply of medications, and money. Keep it hidden but make it easy to grab quickly, or consider keeping it with a friend, relative, or at work so that it is not discovered by the abuser.
- Tell your neighbors about your abuse and ask them to call the police when they hear a disturbance.
- Have a code word to use with your children, family, and friends when you need help. Consider some of the new smartphone apps for alerting significant contacts in an emergency.
- Have a safe place selected in case you ever have to leave, such as a friend or relative's home or a shelter.
- Use your instincts, and do not provoke the abuser when considering leaving.
- Unless you are in danger at that moment, try to leave when the abuser is not at home or around you.
- You have the right to protect yourself and your kids.
- Call the National Domestic Violence Hotline at 1-800-799-7233 for further information and guidance.

Adapted from Goodman, P. E. (2006). The relationship between intimate partner violence and other forms of family and societal violence. *Emergency Medical Clinics of North America, 24*(4), 889–903; Office on Women's Health, U.S. Department of Health and Human Services. (2011). *Violence against women: Safety planning for abusive situations.* Retrieved from http://womenshealth.gov/violence-against-women/get-help-for-violence/safety-planning-for-abusive-situations.html

PLANNING AND IMPLEMENTATION

Table 21.4 lists several interventions and their rationales related to the initial ED visit. It is important to help the battered partner begin to understand that no one deserves to be beaten. The victim did not cause the abuse and is not at fault. Years of conditioning that may have started in childhood can take considerable time to heal and relearn. Although a victim may understand these concepts intellectually, it takes time to synthesize them into emotional and visceral understanding.

A Note on Programs for Batterers

Various types of programs have been set up across the country for men and women who batter their partners. Although the focus is on reducing or eliminating domestic violence through self-reflection and skill building, these programs also offer options other than fines or incarceration. Programs vary in their strategies, but usually the first priorities are to protect the victims and to stress that the offender is accountable for the abuse in the relationship (Day, 2015). One study found that the programs help in some ways. For example, the women believed that communication had improved and that most of the men had developed alternate ways of dealing with their angry, impulsive urges other than in physical ways. However, even when the physical violence lessened or abated, the emotional, verbal, or sexual abuse remained or even increased (Day, 2015). The core problem with the aggressor is the need to exert constant and strict control. It is felt by many that in order to change the dynamics of abuse, aggressors need to work at changing their perceptions of themselves and the world, which can reduce the need for violent control. In addition, abusers often were abused or witnessed abuse in their families. Therapy to address the abuser's own personal wounds and emotional issues can also help to break the cycle of violence. Among batterers attending cognitive-behavioral therapy, almost 85% decreased or eliminated their behaviors of perpetrating physical or emotional abuse (Fernandez-Montalvo et al., 2015).

ELDER ABUSE

In the next decade and beyond there will be an overwhelming number of adults 65 years of age and older as the baby boom generation ages and people live longer and healthier lives. However, close to half (45%) of adults ages 65 and older had incomes below twice the poverty thresholds under the Supplemental Poverty Measure (SPM) in 2013 (Cubanski, Casillas, & Damico, 2015). As a result of the growing number of elderly persons, the incidence of **elder abuse** will also increase proportionally, which will translate to more responsibility for the health care system, including nurses. Approximately 10% of older adults are mistreated annually (National Center on Elder Abuse, 2018).

The WHO (2015) considers elder abuse to be a violation of human rights as well as a significant cause of injury, isolation, and despair for the elderly population. As in other age groups, the elderly can be victimized through physical, sexual, or emotional abuse; neglect; and financial exploitation (Box 21.4). Abuse can occur by individuals and

BOX 21.4 Five Types of Elder Abuse

1. **Physical abuse:** The infliction of physical pain or injury through slapping, hitting, kicking, pushing, restraining, overmedicating, or sexually abusing.
2. **Psychological abuse:** The infliction of mental anguish through yelling, name calling, humiliating, or threatening.
3. **Financial abuse or exploitation:** The misuse of someone's property and resources by another person or refusal by a caregiver to provide needed resources.
4. **Neglect:** Failure to fulfill a caretaking obligation to provide nutrition, hydration, shelter, clothing, utilities, medical services, or other basic needs. This category may also include self-neglect.
5. **Sexual abuse:** Nonconsensual sexually molesting, touching, inappropriate comments or exposure to videos or acts, or actual rape.

Adapted from National Center on Elder Abuse Administration on Aging. (2016). *Types of abuse.* Retrieved from http://www.ncea.aoa.gov/FAQ/Type_Abuse/index.aspx

institutions such as skilled nursing facilities (SNFs) or even through self-neglect. Elder abuse is commonly known as "granny abuse" or as "granny dumping" when an elderly family member is left at a medical facility and not picked up by family members. It is estimated that 70% to 80% of elder abuse cases are not reported. The elderly may be hesitant to report family members for a variety of reasons, including intimidation and not wanting to be taken from the family. They may feel their situation is better than the alternatives.

All 50 states have established elder abuse prevention laws and reporting systems, and in all but 6 states reporting is mandatory (Halphen & Dyer, 2015). The **Adult Protective Services (APS)** division of each state receives and investigates reports of suspected elder abuse. To be eligible for APS help in most states, an older adult has to be deemed unable to care for himself or herself. This leaves many older adults who are mentally and physically healthy unprotected in a situation in which they are being abused or exploited by family members. Definitions of elder abuse and APS programs differ among states, making it impossible to know the actual extent of the problem or to conduct sound research. There have been some recent movements at the national level to standardize the approach to the study of elder mistreatment.

THE ABUSED ELDER

Seniors can be especially vulnerable to abuse as well as to other crimes. Age-related syndromes often result in frailty and functional decline, making older adults less able to protect themselves. Abuse of seniors can include rape and sexual abuse. Elder abuse is most often diagnosed in older adults who have depression, alcohol or drug abuse, dementia, or a psychiatric illness, which compounds an older adult's vulnerability and draws attention to the person's situation.

It is estimated that 3% to 27% of the elderly experience some type of abuse or neglect, although the number is believed to be underreported (Halphen & Dyer, 2015). The risk of abuse rises as age advances, with women more often being the victims. People older than 80 years of age are two to three times more likely to suffer abuse and neglect than older adults in the 60- to 80-year-old age group (Halphen & Dyer, 2015).

THE ABUSER

Early studies on elder abuse focused on the caretaker's stress and burden as causative factors in the abuse. More recent research indicates that the characteristics of the elder abuser more closely resemble the characteristics of the abuser in IPV. Most often the abuser is a middle-aged adult child or other family member. Often the caregiver is financially dependent on the older adult. Elder abusers may have a personality profile similar to abusers in other categories (intimate partner, child), such as being abused themselves or using substances. However, the family member inflicting the abuse may not be a cruel or insensitive person but might instead be a caring individual who is under extreme stress. Caregiver stress, caregiver anxiety, and a history of a previously bad relationship are all related to an increased risk of elder abuse (Orfila et al., 2018). The nurse is often the one to observe family interactions and carries some responsibility for assessing and observing family dynamics to determine needs and the potential for abuse. Then the nurse and family must explore possible interventions to lessen family tension, including a change in living situation in some instances.

Abusers can also be staff members or residents in skills nursing facilities or other out-of-home living situations. Contrary to common belief, abuse in nursing homes is most often perpetrated by residents toward other residents rather than by staff members (Halphen & Dyer, 2015).

APPLICATION OF THE NURSING PROCESS

ASSESSMENT

Nurse practitioners, physicians, nurses, and other health care professionals are often the only outside contact an older adult may have. In most states, health care workers are mandated to report elder abuse and neglect to APS (Halphen & Dyer, 2015).

Victims of abuse have twice as many physician and clinic visits as those not subjected to abuse. Because victims of abuse or neglect are most likely to be abused by family members, the abused are often afraid to reveal the abuse. There may be threats about disclosure or retribution, the victim may experience shame, or the abused may want to protect a loved one. There may be fear of being placed in a nursing home, and the known problems may be preferable to an unknown situation or leaving the home and family. It is important that family and friends are allowed to communicate about suspected abuse in a safe and nonjudgmental manner. Health care workers should make a routine evaluation for signs and symptoms of abuse when older adults visit health care facilities. Signs of elder abuse are very similar to those in child abuse or IPV. Some additional red flags more specific to elderly victims (Halphen & Dyer, 2015) include the following:

- Fear of being alone with the caregiver
- Malnutrition or begging for food; dehydration
- Bedsores, skin tears, bruises, swelling, or fractures
- In need of medical or dental care
- Left unattended for long periods
- Reports of abuse or neglect
- Passive, withdrawn, or emotionless behavior
- Appears overmedicated
- Vaginal or rectal pain, tears, or bleeding or STIs
- Concern over finances
- Inability to pay for medications or needed services
- Transfer of property by an elder who lacks the mental capacity to consent
- Valuables missing

When patients with suspected abuse cannot leave the house, home visits may be warranted, allowing the nurse practitioner, physician, or clinician to assess the patient and environment.

TABLE 21.5 Interventions for Suspected Elder Abuse

Intervention	Rationale
1. Check your state for laws regarding elder abuse.	1. All states have adopted laws to help protect elders and support their need for safety.
2. Involve Adult Protective Services (APS) if abuse is suspected.	2. APS can offer many sources to help guard the safety and well-being of abused elders.
3. Meet with other family members to identify stressors and problem areas, including caregiver strain.	3. Other family members may be unaware of the abuser's stress level or the lack of safety available for the abused family member.
4. If there are no other family members, notify other community agencies that might help stabilize the situation, such as: • Support group for elderly patient or for abuser and family members • Meals on Wheels • Day care for seniors • Respite services • Visiting nurse services • Assisted living	4. Minimizes family stress and isolation and increases safety.
5. Encourage abuser to seek counseling.	5. Increases coping skills and social supports.
6. Suggest that family members meet on a regular basis for problem solving and support.	6. Encourages family to learn and solve problems together.

DIAGNOSIS AND OUTCOMES IDENTIFICATION

Nursing diagnoses for abused older adults are much the same as with other cases of abuse. Elderly victims of abuse may be diagnosed with the following: *Victim of elder abuse, Victim of elder neglect, Impaired nutritional status, Impaired protective ability, Impaired socialization,* and *Physical injury from abuse.* The caregiver is an important part of the equation and may also be given a nursing diagnosis, including *Impaired ability to perform caretaking, Conflicting caregiver attitude, Impaired family coping,* and *Financial problem.*

Successful long-term outcomes include the following:

1. Physical, emotional, or sexual abuse has ceased.
2. Neglect or financial exploitation has ceased.
3. Plans are in place to maintain safety.
4. The elder states that he or she feels more comfortable in the home.
5. Follow-up visits reveal less anxiety and tension between the caregiver and the elder.
6. Caregiver strain has been addressed through respite, sharing of responsibilities, and support.

Most hospitals and community centers have protocols that offer guidelines for nurses and other health care workers for suspected elder abuse. Immediate physical safety is always the first concern, as well as referring the patient to APS for evaluation. There are a number of services that APS can offer to address issues of patient neglect, abuse, and other forms of mistreatment. Potential services may include assistance with emergency housing, repairs, or modification for disabilities; help obtaining medical services; resources for food delivery or caretaker services; serving as a patient advocate; and legal referrals. These services are voluntary, and the patient has the right to accept or decline them (Halphen & Dyer, 2015).

PLANNING AND IMPLEMENTATION

In addition to needed compassionate physical care, interventions include providing medical services, implementing APS or law enforcement interventions, and involving social services. Family or caregiver support may be needed, or in some cases alternative housing is necessary. Table 21.5 includes interventions for suspected elder abuse.

EVALUATION

Failures in interventions with abusive families not only are related to personal deficits of the individuals but also involve inadequacies in the social, economic, and political systems in which we all live. Many disadvantaged individuals have limited access to needed services and experience inordinate stressors. Some of the societal attitudes that, in part, support abuse are the acceptance of corporal punishment to discipline children; the unequal caregiving burden placed on women; the lack of education and preparation for parenthood; and the concept of "ageism," in which the elderly are considered to have lesser value. Nurses can be instrumental in altering these perceptions through education in the course of their career.

Evaluation of interventions to stop elder abuse can include the willingness of the victim to acknowledge the abuse and to accept assistance, as well as the success of the plan. Violence is a symptom of a family or health care organization in distress; therefore intervention and evaluation will be a multidisciplinary approach. Follow-up is crucial in ensuring the ongoing safety of the elderly patient and support of the caregiving system, whether that be the family or the skilled nursing facility.

APPLYING EVIDENCE-BASED PRACTICE (EBP)

Problem

A 24-year-old female presents to the emergency department (ED) with complaints of abdominal pain. She is vague about her symptoms and finally explains that she tripped and fell down her front porch steps while carrying groceries. Upon examination, it's discovered that she has bruising on her arms, torso, and left orbit in various stages of healing. Her records indicate several past ED visits for injuries, including a fractured arm. While she is in the examination room, her phone rings constantly with calls from her husband, and she is tense as she answers with short, cryptic responses. She explains that she has to hurry home because she has two young children at home in addition to the toddler who has accompanied her to the ED. The toddler appears pale and shy, quietly holding on to her mother's clothing or hiding behind her.

EBP Assessment

A. **What do you already know from experience?** This patient has been to the ED with several injuries. She presents like other victims of intimate partner violence (IPV) the nurse has treated, being timid, vague, and tense on the phone with her husband. She may or may not be willing to admit the abuse.

B. **What does the literature say?** In cases of IPV, the victim's injuries are often inconsistent with the explanation, and there may be a history of many injuries and ED visits. The victim may appear fearful or intimidated by the abuser. The victim may stay in the relationship for various reasons, including for the children or because she believes it will get better, she thinks she deserves the abuse, or she has nowhere to go. Many homeless women were domestic abuse victims. The highest risk of severe injury or being killed occurs when the victim is trying to leave the abuser. Children may also be abused or traumatized by what they have witnessed.

C. **What does the patient want?** The nurse had another staff member take the toddler for a snack while gently questioning the mother. The patient broke down in tears and admitted she was a victim of IPV by her husband. She was fearful of being harmed and had little support in her life. She was agreeable to speaking with the police, although she was not sure she was ready to leave at this time.

Plan

The patient was examined, including x-rays, and her injuries were treated. Social services was called and met with the patient to give her shelter and safety plan resources. The police took a report and photographs of the abuse. After speaking with everyone, the patient decided to take her children and go to a shelter. A shelter was called, and a representative was dispatched from the shelter to support and assist the patient. Child Protective Services (CPS) was called to remove the two children who were at home with the patient's husband and to initiate an investigation into possible neglect or abuse of the children. The patient was terrified regarding her decision, and the nurse stayed with her during all interviews.

QSEN Prelicensure Knowledge, Skills, and Attitudes (KSAs) Addressed

Safety is evidenced by being aware of potential abuse and taking actions to keep the patient and her children safe.

Teamwork and Collaboration is evidenced by working with social services, law enforcement, an abuse shelter, and CPS to provide needed services for this family.

KEY POINTS TO REMEMBER

- Physical and emotional trauma cause long-lasting damage to individuals and communities and are often passed down in a generational manner.
- Because the incidence of child, partner, and elder abuse is underreported, it is imperative that nurses learn to routinely assess for abuse.
- All states have mandatory guidelines for reporting child and elder abuse. However, in the case of intimate partner violence (IPV), the victim is of a consenting and nonprotected age. Although nurses can provide resources, support, and guidance, it is ultimately the adult victim's choice and responsibility to file any report of abuse.
- When a victim of IPV attempts to leave the abuser, the highest risk of severe harm or homicide exists.
- Abusive parents have characteristics that can be recognized by health care providers.
- Abuse often occurs in a cyclical pattern in which the tension grows, abuse occurs, and then remorse and a honeymoon phase begin. The cycle will almost always continue and escalate without intervention.
- The responsibilities of the nurse and other health care team members in various cases of abuse are discussed.
- Nursing diagnoses, interventions, and outcomes are similar in all abuse cases, although each individual and age group has additional unique needs.

APPLYING CRITICAL JUDGMENT

1. A 6-year-old boy is rushed to the emergency department by a neighbor who found him wandering in the street wearing only a dirty undershirt, seemingly dazed. He is covered in what appear to be cigarette burns, is malnourished, and has bruises on his wrists and ankles. He appears fearful and confused and does not respond to questioning except to say, "I hurt. I don't feel good."
   - A. What is your first priority?
   - B. What would you include in your documentation and on the body map?
   - C. What else could you do to document his injuries besides note them on the body map?
   - D. Which other individuals would you need to involve or notify in this case?

CHAPTER REVIEW QUESTIONS

1. An emergency department nurse assesses a woman suspected of being abused by an intimate partner. Which assessment finding most clearly confirms the suspicion?
   a. Leathery facial tone
   b. Injuries in a bikini pattern
   c. Reluctance to be examined
   d. Lack of eye contact with the nurse
2. An emergency department nurse assesses a child with a fractured ulna. The nurse also observes yellow and purple bruises across the child's back and shoulders. Which comment by the parents should prompt the nurse to consider making a report to Child Protective Services?
   a. "We do not believe in immunization of our children."
   b. "This child is always creating problems for the family."
   c. "Our child would rather play alone than with other children."
   d. "We homeschool our children in order to include religious education."
3. A woman in a relationship characterized by a long history of battering and abuse tells the nurse, "We've had a rough time lately. I admit it: He beat me last night but then said he was sorry." Which event would the nurse expect to occur next in this relationship?
   a. Another beating by the abusive partner
   b. Love, gifts, and praise from the abusive partner
   c. A brief period during which the partners ignore each other
   d. The abusive partner leaving the relationship for a short time
4. The nurse assessed an elderly person who was abused by the caregiver. Afterward, which internal dialogue should prompt the nurse to seek guidance?
   a. "Sometimes I get so discouraged and frustrated with my job."
   b. "It's incredible that anyone could hurt a child or elderly person."
   c. "The abuser was probably a victim of abuse at some point in life."
   d. "I hope the abuser gets victimized so they know what it feels like."
5. A university football coach invites the campus nurse to talk to the team about healthy relationships in the community. Which topic has priority for the nurse to include?
   a. Appropriate behavior with intimate partners
   b. University resources for counseling and support
   c. The importance of role modeling for children and teens
   d. Public recognition of children with life-threatening illnesses

REFERENCES

American Academy of Family Physicians. (2018). *USPSTF draft recommendation: Screen all women of reproductive age for domestic violence.* Retrieved from https://www.aafp.org/news/health-of-the-public/20180504violence.html.

Centers for Disease Control and Prevention. (2019). *Intimate partner violence: Fast facts.* Retrieved from https://www.cdc.gov/violenceprevention/intimatepartnerviolence/fastfact.html.

Centers for Disease Control and Prevention (CDC). (2020a). *Violence prevention: Adverse childhood experiences.* Retrieved from https://www.childwelfare.gov/pubPDFs/canstats.pdf.

Centers for Disease Control and Prevention (CDC). (2020b). *Violence prevention: Youth violence.* Retrieved from https://www.cdc.gov/violenceprevention/youthviolence/fastfact.html.

Childhelp. (2018). *National child abuse statistics.* Retrieved from https://www.childhelp.org/child-abuse-statistics/.

CNN. (2018). *Domestic violence.* Retrieved from https://www.cnn.com/2013/12/06/us/domestic-intimate-partner-violence-fast-facts/index.html.

Cubanski, J., Casillas, G., & Damico, A. (2015). *Poverty among seniors: An updated analysis of national and state level poverty rates under the official and supplemental poverty measures.* Kaiser Family Foundation. Retrieved from http://kff.org/medicare/issue-brief/poverty-among-seniors-an-updated-analysis-of-national-and-state-level-poverty-rates-under-the-official-and-supplemental-poverty-measures/.

Day, A. (2015). Working with perpetrators of domestic violence to change their behavior. *InPsych, 37*(5). Retrieved from https://www.psychology.org.au/inpsych/2015/october/day.

Fernandez-Montalvo, J., Echauri, J. A., Martinez, M., et al. (2015). Impact of a court-referred psychological treatment program for intimate partner batterer men with suspended sentences. *Violence & Victims, 30*(1), 3–15.

Giddens, J. F. (2017). *Concepts for nursing practice* (2nd ed.). St. Louis: Elsevier..

Guy, J., Feinstein, L., & Griffiths, A. (2013). *Early intervention in domestic violence and abuse.* Retrieved from http://www.eif.org.uk/wp-content/uploads/2014/03/Early-Intervention-in-Domestic-Violence-and-Abuse-Full-Report.pdf.

Halphen, J. M., & Dyer, C. B. (2015). *Elder mistreatment: Abuse, neglect, and financial exploitation.* Retrieved from http://www.uptodate.com/contents/elder-mistreatment-abuse-neglect-and-financial-exploitation.

International Council of Nurses. (2017). *International Classification for nursing practice (ICNP).* Retrieved July 7, 2018 from http://www.icn.ch/what-we-do/ICNP-Browser/.

National Center on Elder Abuse. (2018). *Research: Statistics/data.* Retrieved from https://ncea.acl.gov/whatwedo/research/statistics.html.

Ney, T. (Ed.). (2015). *True and false allegations of child sexual abuse: Assessment and case management.* London: Routledge.

Orfila, F., Coma-Solé, M., Cegri-Lombardo, F., Moleras-Serra, A., & Pujol-Ribera, E. (2018). Family caregiver mistreatment of the elderly: Prevalence of risk and associated factors. *BioMed Central Public Health, 18*(167). Retrieved from https://doi.org/10.1186/s12889-018-5067-8.

Perry, R., Zimmerman, L., Al-Saden, I., et al. (2015). Prevalence of rape-related pregnancy as an indication for abortion at two family planning clinics. *Contraception, 91*(5), 393–397.

President of the United States of America. (2016). *Presidential proclamation: National teen dating violence awareness and prevention month 2016.* Retrieved from https://www.whitehouse.gov/the-press-office/2016/01/29/presidential-proclamation-national-teen-dating-violence-awareness-and?platform=hootsuite.

Smith, E. N., & Fazel, S. (2015). Risk factors for violence and suicide in the general population: A meta-epidemiological study. *European Psychiatry, 30*(1), 28–31.

U.S. Department of Health and Human Services, Administration for Children and Families. (2019). *Child maltreatment 2017: Summary of key findings.* Retrieved from https://www.childwelfare.gov/pubPDFs/canstats.pdf.

Vancouver Coastal Health. (2015). *About adult abuse & neglect.* Retrieved from http://www.vchreact.ca/read_psychological.htm.

Walker, L. E. (1979). *The battered woman.* New York: Harper and Row.

Weil, A. (2016). Intimate partner violence: Epidemiology and health consequences. In L. Park (Ed.), *UpToDate.* Retrieved from www.uptodate.com.

Widom, C. P., & Wilson, H. (2015). Intergenerational transmission of violence. In J. Lindert, & I. Levav (Eds.), *Violence and mental health* (pp. 27–46). Netherlands: Springer Netherlands.

World Health Organization. (2015). *Ageing and life course: Elder abuse.* Retrieved from http://www.who.int/ageing/projects/elder_abuse/en/.

World Health Organization (WHO). (2017). *Violence against women.* Retrieved from http://www.who.int/news-room/fact-sheets/detail/violence-against-women.

22

Sexual Violence

Chyllia D. Fosbre, Elizabeth M. Varcarolis

http://evolve.elsevier.com/Varcarolis/essentials

OBJECTIVES

1. Give examples of teamwork and collaboration by identifying the various functions and disciplines that constitute members of the sexual assault response team (SART). **QSEN: Teamwork and Collaboration**
2. Evaluate how sexual assault nurse examiners (SANEs) promote safety by describing the areas of expertise they provide to victims of sexual violence. **QSEN: Safety**
3. Prepare a mock **documentation** of your initial assessment of a victim of sexual assault (including objective and subjective data and a body map).
4. Summarize the characteristics of a perpetrator of sexual assault.
5. Incorporate evidence-based practice by identifying the specific data collected in the forensic component of the assessment that may be used as criminal evidence in court. **QSEN: Evidence-Based Practice**
6. Promote safety by outlining the guidelines for emergency treatment of a woman or man who has been sexually assaulted. **QSEN: Safety**
7. Provide patient-centered care by delineating the symptoms of rape-trauma syndrome that you would include in your teaching to a victim of sexual assault to prepare him or her for the second phase. **QSEN: Patient-Centered Care**
8. Using informatics, write up a list of supports in your community that can be offered to an individual who has been sexually assaulted. **QSEN: Informatics**
9. Identify individual vulnerabilities that might put a person at risk for sexual assault.
10. Using informatics, search the Internet for the April 2013 "A National Protocol for Sexual Assault Medical Forensic Examinations: Adults/Adolescents" (2nd ed.). **QSEN: Informatics**

KEY TERMS AND CONCEPTS

acquaintance rape, p. 356
date rape, p. 356
date rape drug, p. 357
forensic evidence, p. 356
institutional protocol, p. 359
marital/partner rape, p. 356
rape, p. 356
rape kits, p. 359
rape-trauma syndrome, p. 360
sexual assault, p. 356
sexual assault nurse examiner (SANE), p. 359
sexual assault response team (SART), p. 359
survivor, p. 356
victim, p. 356

CONCEPT: SEXUAL VIOLENCE: *Sexual violence* is a public health issue throughout the world and is detrimental to the well-being of an individual, a family, and the community (Giddens, 2017). It is highly important for the nurse to assess the assaulted individual to ascertain if there are any thoughts of suicide or homicide. Crisis counseling should always be available to any person who has been sexually assaulted and should include referrals to the primary care physician, mental health provider, community crisis line, and other resources. Group therapy or support groups can be beneficial for survivors to share experiences with others, are often healing, and can help the survivor break through feelings of isolation, shame, and guilt.

INTRODUCTION

Sexual assault is an act of violence, power, and hate and most often results in devastating severe and long-term trauma. It is often committed in the context of unequal power in order to demonstrate dominance and control. Sexual violence is related to teen pregnancy and the transmission of sexually transmitted infections (STIs), including human immunodeficiency virus (HIV).

In 2012 the U.S. Department of Justice (DOJ) updated the definition of sexual violence by adding: "The penetration, no matter how slight, of the vagina or anus with any body part or object, or oral penetration by a sex organ of another person, without the consent of the victim." Sexual violence occurs when a perpetrator commits sexual acts without a victim's consent or when a victim is unable to consent (e.g., due to age, illness, or while under the influence of drugs or alcohol) or refuse (e.g., due to physical violence or threats) (U.S. Department of Justice, 2018). This updated definition is inclusive for either gender of victim and perpetrator and recognizes that penetration with an object is as violent as penile/vaginal rape.

The term *sexual violence* encompasses any act from sexual harassment to rape. Sexual violence is divided into the following categories (Centers for Disease Control and Prevention [CDC], 2018):

- Completed or attempted forced penetration of a victim
- Completed or attempted alcohol- or drug-facilitated penetration of a victim

- Completed or attempted forced acts in which a victim is made to penetrate a perpetrator or someone else
- Completed or attempted alcohol- or drug-facilitated acts in which a victim is made to penetrate a perpetrator or someone else
- Nonphysically forced penetration that occurs after a person is pressured verbally or through intimidation or misuse of authority to consent or acquiesce
- Unwanted sexual contact
- Noncontact unwanted sexual experiences (e.g., exposure to pornography, harassment, exhibitionism)

Sexual violence among children also includes the following:

- Coercing children to inappropriately touch the molester, often a trusted person
- Showing children pornographic photos and videos
- Initiating inappropriate conversations involving sexual topics

Sexual assault/sexual violence (SV) is an umbrella term encompassing the crimes of **rape**, **date rape**, **acquaintance rape**, gang rape (two or more perpetrators), **marital/partner rape**, sexual molestation, incest, statutory rape, and sexual assault of older adults.

Rape is a legal term rather than a medical diagnosis. Legal definitions of rape vary among states. For example, California defines rape as an offender engaging in sexual intercourse with another person who is not the offender's spouse when the victim is not able to give consent under a variety of circumstances, such as the victim having a mental, developmental, or physical disability; being intoxicated; being unconscious; if there is fear of harm; or if there are threats of retaliation. There are additional definitions of what constitutes rape of a spouse, sexual battery, sodomy, and other types of sexual assault (Rape, Abuse & Incest National Network [RAINN], 2018a).

Date rape is a form of acquaintance rape, but in the case of date rape, the victim has agreed to spend time with the perpetrator but has not given consent for sexual contact.

All individuals who have been the victim of sexual violence suffer severe, deep emotional scars that may stay with them for the rest of their lives. Research has demonstrated that there is a long litany of physical and mental health issues that are more prevalent in people who have been sexually assaulted. Beyond the physical trauma, such as the risk of transmission of STIs or HIV or the risk of pregnancy, long-term psychological trauma can occur. Some of the painful consequences caused by sexual assault are depression, anxiety, difficulties with daily functioning, low self-esteem, eating disorders, self-destructive behaviors, substance abuse, and higher rates of suicide than in the general population. Although the risk exists for both male and female rape victims, male rape victims are more likely to commit suicide and to become infected with HIV through anal tears than are women. Timely and age-appropriate interventions can greatly help to mitigate the devastating psychological sequelae and help **victims** become **survivors**. When emotional symptoms are confronted and addressed, the abused individual has a better chance of leading a full and productive life.

Presently, there is no mandated reporting for crimes of sexual assault unless they involve abuse of a minor or an elder. It is the responsibility of survivors of assault to make the decision to report the crime, and it is the responsibility of health care workers to offer support, to provide information on obtaining legal counsel, and—with the patient's permission—to secure **forensic evidence** (evidence that can be used in court) by a qualified person for future prosecution.

PREVALENCE AND COMORBIDITY

Note that statistics on sexual violence and sexual assault are approximate, are often varied, and only refer to reported cases. It is safe to infer that the actual numbers of sexual assaults are much higher than the quoted statistics. *Both rape and child sexual molestation are among the most underreported crimes.* It is estimated that only one out of three sexual assaults is reported. For victims who are college-age women, only one in five is likely to file a report (RAINN, 2018b).

Children: Child Sexual Abuse

The statistics that we do have for the sexual assault of children are distressing. For example, some estimates indicate that 1 in 9 girls and 1 in 53 boys are sexually molested by the time they are 18 years old. There are estimates that about every 8 minutes, Child Protective Services (CPS) finds evidence supporting a claim for child sexual abuse. For children who experience sexual abuse, 34% are under the age of 12, and 93% of perpetrators are someone the child knows, most often a parent (RAINN, 2018b). The effects of **child sexual abuse** can last a lifetime. Sense of worth, distortion of self-concept, confusion about one's place in the world, and disruption in affective capabilities are common. Unfortunately, people who were sexually assaulted as children are approximately four to five times more likely to be sexually assaulted later in life. Abused children are four times more likely to develop posttraumatic stress disorder (PTSD), are four times more likely to develop a substance use disorder, and are three times more likely to experience major depression (RAINN, 2018b). Child sexual violence that remains untreated may result in mental health issues, drug and alcohol abuse, criminal behavior, higher rates of suicide (either attempted or completed), and (not surprisingly) perpetuation of sexual abuse.

According to Women Organized Against Rape (WOAR, 2015a), common reactions in children who have been sexually abused include the following:

- Fear of being alone, of going to sleep, or of strangers
- Outbursts of anger
- Increased isolation
- Physical symptoms such as headaches, stomach or genital discomfort, and skin rashes in the genital area
- Regression to early behaviors, such as bedwetting or not wanting to sleep alone.
- Inappropriate sexual behaviors, such as sexually acting-out with other children or excessive masturbation

High School

The CDC (2020) states that 8% of high school students reported being hit, slapped, or physically hurt by a boyfriend or girlfriend within the 12 months prior to the survey. Date rape is also reported among high school students, as are physical and emotional abuse. Approximately one in five female high school students reports being physically and/or sexually abused by a dating partner.

Young Adults

Sexual assault is more prevalent in the young adult. Women 18 to 24 years of age who attend college are three times more likely than those who don't attend college to experience sexual assault. Male college students 18 to 24 years of age are five times more likely to be a victim of sexual assault than non–college-attending men.

Among college women, it is estimated that 20% to 25% will experience an attempted or completed rape by the end of their college career, and 90% of those women will know their attackers. The risk of sexual assault for college-age women is greatest during their first and second years of college.

Perhaps the majority of sexual assaults in young adults are acquaintance rapes or date rapes. Alcohol and other drugs often play a part in sexual assault, whether they are taken by the victim, the perpetrator, or both. Contrary to what some young men might think, intoxication by alcohol or drugs is not an excuse for sexual violence; sexual assault is still considered rape under the law. Drugs are often used to facilitate sexual assault. Often these drugs are used for **gang rapes** (two or more

TABLE 22.1 **Drugs Associated With Sexual Assault**

Mechanism of Action	Effect	Additional Information
GHB (γ-hydroxybutyric acid)[a]		
Central nervous system depressant	Onset is within 10 to 20 minutes; duration is dose related and is from 1 to 4 hours *Lower doses:* Produces euphoria, amnesia, hypotonia, and depressed respiration *Higher doses:* Can cause seizures, unconsciousness, nausea and vomiting, coma, and death	GHB needs 12 hours to be excreted from the body Used to treat narcolepsy Rapidly metabolized; difficult to detect in emergency departments and other treatment facilities
Rohypnol (Flunitrazepam)[b]		
Potent benzodiazepine; 10 times stronger than diazepam	Impact is within 10 to 30 minutes and lasts 2 to 12 hours Becomes more potent when combined with alcohol Causes dizziness, amnesia, lack of motor coordination, confusion, nausea and vomiting, respiratory depression, and blackout episodes lasting 8 to 24 hours	Not legal in the United States Detected in urine for up to 72 hours
Ketamine[c]		
Anesthetic frequently used in veterinary practice; also hallucinogenic substance related to PCP (phencyclidine)	Onset is rapid, 20 minutes orally; duration is only 30 to 60 minutes Amnesia effects may last longer Usually administered as a powder that is snorted, smoked, injected, or dissolved in drinks Causes dissociative reaction with a dreamlike state leading to deep amnesia and analgesia and complete compliance of the survivor Later, survivor may be confused, paranoid, delirious, and combative with drooling and hallucinations	

[a]Street names include liquid ecstasy, salty water, scoop, homeboy, and grievous bodily harm.
[b]Street names include "forget" drug, roofies, club drug, roachies, rophies, and Mexican valium.
[c]Street names include special K, vitamin K, bump, kitkat, purple, and super C.

sexual attackers). Although the number of rapes related to date rape drugs seems to be increasing, it is impossible to know the exact statistics. An assaulted woman may not report her abuse because the woman:

- Believes it is her fault
- Does not consider the incident sexual assault
- Does not want to report her abuser for fear of reprisal
- Does not want to get her "friend" or "date" in trouble
- Does not want others to know about the assault
- Cannot remember the incident clearly enough to feel she would be believed by others, especially if she had been drinking and/or taking other drugs
- Does not want to relive the experience by having to talk about the details in a forensic interview

Another consideration is that date rape drugs are cleared from the body fairly quickly, and detecting them in the emergency department or other treatment centers is often difficult. A urine sample must be obtained within a certain period of time to prove the existence of date rape drugs. The date rape drugs γ-hydroxybutyric acid (GHB), flunitrazepam (Rohypnol), and ketamine are used mostly on college campuses (e.g., fraternity houses, bars, raves, clubs, nightclubs). Refer to Table 22.1 for more information on these drugs. Young men as well as women must be cautious about taking a drink that contains a date rape drug. See Applying Critical Judgment at the end of this chapter for ways to minimize the chance of ingesting a date rape drug. However, it is important to remember that the most common drug used to facilitate the crime of rape is still alcohol.

According to WOAR (2015b), common reactions to a sexual assault in adults are as follows:

- Feelings of fear, anxiety, anger, and sadness
- Flashbacks or intrusive thoughts about the assault
- Outbursts of anger
- Eating and sleeping disturbances
- Depression
- Suicidal thoughts or self-harming behaviors
- Increased use of alcohol or drugs
- Changes in relationships with friends, family, and lovers
- Decreased desire for sex

For men and women, other common reactions after a sexual assault include "generalized pain throughout the body, and *emotional reactions* such as anger, fear, anxiety, guilt, humiliation, embarrassment, self-blame, and mood swings" (American College of Obstetricians and Gynecologists [ACOG], 2014).

Men experience the same symptoms women do after being sexually abused. It is just as important for a man to receive counseling for sexual trauma as it is for a woman (WOAR, 2015b). In approximately 10% of sexual assaults, men reported being the victim, and most male rape victims reported being raped by other men (RAINN, 2018b). Gay men are victims of sexual assault slightly more often than are heterosexual men, especially if they are the target of hate crimes. However, heterosexual men are also raped in very large numbers. The vast majority of men who are sexually assaulted are assaulted by men who consider themselves heterosexual, although they may be bisexual. Although a great percentage of male rapes occur in prisons and the military, male rape can happen in cars, restrooms, colleges, and universities; at work; or in the home. The general statistics for male-on-male rapes often do not take into account the large number of unreported male-on-male rapes in prisons and in the military. The incidence of male-on-female rapes in the military is finally being acknowledged; however, male-on-male rapes most often remain unreported. When the number of male-on-male rapes unreported in the U.S. prison system is also considered, the extent and brutality of male-on-male sexual violence are revealed. Although laws addressing male-on-male rape have been established, they are often not acknowledged or enforced, and the culture of blaming the victim persists.

LGBTQ Victims of Sexual Assault

LGBTQ stands for lesbian, gay, bisexual, transsexual (or transgender), and questioning. *Lesbian, gay,* and *bisexual* are sexual orientations, whereas *transsexual* is more of a gender identification. Sexual assault is usually committed by men against women, but it is also committed by women against men and between people of the same gender. The majority of perpetrators are male. Women can force men to have sex, particularly if the male is younger and more vulnerable, and often through blackmail. Women also sexually assault other women, although the statistics are difficult to ascertain.

According to the CDC (2020), the LGBTQ community is at risk for violence in the form of bullying, harassment, physical assault, and increased suicide (attempted or completed) because of the negative way they are perceived and treated in many parts of society. It has been reported that more than 50% of gay men and lesbians recounted at least one incidence of coercion by a same-sex partner. Gay and lesbian sexual survivors may not come forward for fear of facing homophobia and prejudice as well as making their personal lives more public.

THEORY

Vulnerable Individuals

Sexual assault occurs in all age groups, genders, cultures, and socioeconomic backgrounds, but some groups appear to be more vulnerable, and some situations are more conducive to sexual assault. Some of this has been previously stated; however, it all bears repeating.

- **Gender:** Women have a higher vulnerability rate than men (approximately 3 to 1). Both genders are more vulnerable if they are handicapped, have cognitive problems, or have mental disorders.
- **Age:** People 16 to 19 years of age have a higher rate of sexual victimization than any other age group. Children are most vulnerable between 8 and 12 years of age. One in three girls and one in six boys are sexually abused before 18 years of age, which constitutes up to 44% of the total number of sexual assaults or rape.
- **Older adults:** Domestic violence against older adults includes physical and sexual abuse; the perpetrators are most often adult children, especially sons, but can also include spouses, caregivers, health care providers, and other relatives. Although statistics are difficult to ascertain, when an older adult is cognitively or functionally impaired, the likelihood of being sexually assaulted increases.
- **History of sexual violence:** Women who were raped before 18 years of age are two to three times more likely to be sexually assaulted as adults.
- **Drug and alcohol use:** The use of alcohol or drugs by the perpetrator, the victim, or both is related to increased rates of victimization.
- **High-risk sexual behavior:** High-risk sexual behavior is a vulnerability that is often a consequence of childhood sexual abuse.
- **Poverty:** Poverty can make women and children more vulnerable and place them in more dangerous situations. Poor women may be at risk when they need to support themselves or their children and trade sex for food, clothing, money, or other necessary items.
- **Ethnicity or culture:** Sexual violence against indigenous women in the United States is widespread. According to Amnesty International (2015), Native American and Alaskan Native women are more than 2.5 times more likely to be raped or sexually assaulted than other women in the United States. Most of the perpetrators, up to 86%, were non-Native men, as reported by American Indian and Alaskan Native women survivors.

The Perpetrator of Sexual Assault

The causes of violence toward women are multifaceted and involve biological, psychological, and social factors.

Biological Factors

From a *biological* perspective, neurophysiological factors may be risk factors in violent behavior. Alterations in the functioning of neurotransmitters—such as serotonin, dopamine, norepinephrine, acetylcholine, and γ-aminobutyric acid—may interfere with cognition and behavior (see Chapter 24).

Psychosocial Factors

From a *psychosocial* perspective, studies have found a high incidence of psychopathology and personality disorders among sexual offenders. Antisocial personality disorder, in which people are viewed as objects, is one of the most prevalent. The act of rape involves a need for control, power, degradation, and dominance over others rather than sexual satisfaction. It is thought that some sex offenders have difficulty finding willing sexual partners and resort to coercion or rape.

Many characteristics of perpetrators of sexual assault are the same as those found in perpetrators of child abuse, intimate partner violence, and elder abuse (see Chapter 21). Not surprisingly, most perpetrators of sexual abuse report being sexually assaulted as children. Some other characteristics include the following:

- Impulsive and antisocial tendencies
- Association with sexually aggressive and delinquent peers
- Preference for impersonal sex
- Hostility toward women
- Childhood history of sexual and physical abuse or witnessing family violence as a child
- Membership in a gang
- Belonging to a societal group that often refuses to acknowledge acts of sexual assault (e.g., some parts of the military, prisons, and even parts of the Peace Corps to a smaller degree)

Cultural Considerations

Sexual violence occurs in all socioeconomic groups; it occurs in the suburbs, in rural communities, and in large cities; and it occurs in well-educated upper-class families, in middle-class families, and in poor and disadvantaged families. Sexual violence occurs across all ages to men, women, and children.

Cultural and societal factors play a part in forming attitudes, for example, cultural and societal norms that maintain women's inferiority and support male superiority and sexual entitlement may view sexual assault as more acceptable or normal behavior. In such groups, weak laws and policies related to gender inequality and a high tolerance for crimes of violence often coexist. Some college fraternities reflect a societal context that could encourage violence toward women, and sexual assault on campuses is thought to be increasing.

Male-on-male sexual violence in the military seems to be increasing and supports the theory that sexual assault is related to positions of power. Among women, the military is another example of a societal group in which sexual assaults of women result from gender inequality, along with norms that support masculine dominance. Underreporting sexual assaults is rampant in all ages and all groups for both men and women. Mengeling and colleagues (2014) conducted a survey and found that among 205 servicewomen who experienced sexual assault in the military, only 25% reported their assault. The nonreporters stated reasons such as concerns about confidentiality and adverse treatment by peers and the belief that nothing would be done. Interestingly, officers were less likely to report than were enlisted personnel.

Awareness of sexual assault in the military has captured the public's and Congress's attention over the past few years, and changes in military policy are in the process of being implemented. However, in order to instigate substantial change, strong, enforceable laws need to be established, and rape must be recognized as a serious crime for which the perpetrator should be held responsible (Mengeling et al., 2014).

APPLICATION OF THE NURSING PROCESS

ASSESSMENT

Sexual assault response teams (SARTs) are available across the country, most notably in big cities. The purpose of SARTs is to help victims of sexual violence cope with the present situation and aftermath of sexual violence. These teams work in collaboration with a variety of resources, including (1) mental health agencies, (2) rape crisis advocates, (3) law enforcement personnel, (4) detectives or investigators, (5) emergency departments, (6) **sexual assault nurse examiners (SANEs)**, and (7) attorneys. SANEs are forensic nurses who have been certified to work with victims of sexual violence. Some of the functions of the SANE are to perform a physical examination of the survivor, collect forensic evidence, provide expert testimony regarding the forensic evidence collected, support the psychobiological needs of the survivor, be part of the SART, and work closely with law enforcement agencies and the prosecutor's office. Unfortunately, most rural communities don't have certified nurses trained to perform sexual assault kit examinations. Therefore facilities are charged with transferring the victim of sexual assault to the nearest hospital that has a trained forensic nurse or a SANE. Unfortunately, having to travel an hour or two to go through a forensic examination might overwhelm a victim and ultimately allow rapists to reoffend.

Hotlines and Other Sources

If the sexually assaulted individual calls a hotline, a sexual assault and violence prevention center, the police, or a campus medical center, there is certain information the sexually assaulted person needs to know. The assaulted person should have an advocate who can explain more about the person's options and rights (Box 22.1).

Emergency Departments

When an individual who has been sexually assaulted seeks treatment, he or she is most likely seen in the emergency department (ED). People who have been sexually assaulted often go to the ED to find emotional support, help in regaining a sense of control, and reassurance regarding their safety. *A sexual assault victim who arrives at the ED should not be left alone. The staff should provide privacy, and the victim should be a priority in triage.*

The nature of sexual assault carries with it complex implications, and the individual requires psychological support, medical care, documentation of pertinent history, a thorough physical examination, and collection of specimens for use as forensic evidence. Often the physical examination and the collection of evidence are performed by a gynecologist, an ED attending physician, or a SANE. The person who collects the evidence should be forensically trained in the collection of such data. Unfortunately, facilities differ widely in the kind of care they provide, and the ideal is not always the case—care is not always compassionate, comprehensive, or competent. Most hospitals have an **institutional protocol** for evidence collection and use **rape kits**. Correct preservation of body fluids and swabs is essential because DNA (deoxyribonucleic acid; genetic mapping) can help identify the rapist. If a date rape drug is suspected, a urine sample should be collected.

The individual has the right to refuse legal help and medical examination. Sexual assault survivors need to know they have the right to refuse police assistance but still can choose to have forensic evidence collected. To collect evidence, a *consent form must be signed* to take photographs, perform a pelvic examination, and carry out any other procedures necessary to collect evidence and provide treatment. The individual also needs to know that all documentation is confidential—that no one can access the information without permission, unless the case goes to court. Treatment and documentation need to be accurate and meticulous because the documentation may constitute legal evidence if the individual chooses to prosecute.

Caution is advised about the use of pejorative language when documenting the history, findings, and verbatim statements. For example:

- Instead of *alleged*, use *reported*.
- Instead of *refused*, use *declined*.
- Instead of *intercourse*, use *penetration*.
- Instead of *in no acute distress*, describe the behavior.

After the immediate medical issues of the patient have been addressed, it is important that forensically trained personnel perform as many elements of the *forensic examination* as the individual will allow. Once the evidence is collected, it is imperative that providers maintain a "chain of custody" until it is turned over to the authorities.

BOX 22.1 Information to Help a Recent Victim of Sexual Violence in the Aftermath of Rape (Either on the Phone or in Person)

1. Go to a safe place immediately.
2. Consider reporting the rape to the police or to the campus police if it happened on campus.
3. You can report the assault and later choose not to pursue criminal proceedings.
4. If you choose not to report the assault immediately, you can do so at a later time.

Preserve evidence of the rape:

1. Do not wash your hands or face.
2. Do not shower or bathe.
3. Do not brush your teeth.
4. Do not change clothes or straighten up the area where the assault took place.
5. Offer information regarding the location of a sexual assault response team (SART), a violence prevention resource center, a crisis center, or an emergency department in the area.
6. Explain that even if the victim chooses not to press charges, the victim can still have a forensic examination without the rape being reported to the police.

Data from UC San Diego. (n.d.). *What to do if you are raped.* Retrieved from http://www.UCSD.edu/current-students/wellness/_organizations/sarc/if-you-are-raped.html

Assessment Guidelines

Sexual Assault (Follow Unit Protocols)

1. Assess and document the circumstances of the event, including the presence of threats (force, trauma, weapons, resistance, sexual acts), the location of the incident, and the circumstances surrounding the assault. *Document in patient's own words* when possible.
2. Gather data that may be used as criminal evidence in court using the institution's protocol.
3. After consent forms have been signed, forensic evidence (debris) should be obtained from clothing, fingernail scrapings, head hair, and pubic hair; smears for sperm and/or acid phosphatase should be taken from any orifice involved. (*Note:* Elevated prostatic acid phosphatase levels are indicative of the presence of semen.) Permission for any photographs taken during the assessment also needs to be obtained. (Guidelines 3 through 8 are all considered forensic evidence that might be used in court at a later date and should be done by a forensically trained professional [e.g., SANE].)

4. Assess for evidence of any physical trauma (e.g., bites, stab wounds, contusions, gunshot wounds). Use drawings (body map) and photos to identify the areas and size of trauma.
5. Perform pelvic examination to identify vaginal and cervical trauma (perform anal examination in males and sodomized females). Culture for STIs.
6. Perform psychological assessment, noting reactions to the rape event (e.g., crying, fearfulness, agitation, preoccupation, detachment). Describe all behavior in writing.
7. Perform a mental status examination.
8. Determine drug use by either the assailant or the survivor. Assess the situation for the potential involvement of a date rape drug if it occurred in a large gathering (e.g., college campus, bar, party). A urine sample might be useful if timing is correct. Emphasize to individuals that even if they were drinking, they are *not* at fault for being assaulted. (Refer to Table 22.1 for drugs associated with sexual assault.)
9. Identify the victim's support system (e.g., family, friends, others the person trusts), and ask for permission to involve them. Explain possible delayed reactions that might occur.

DIAGNOSIS

Rape-Trauma Syndrome

The nursing diagnosis *Rape-trauma syndrome* is a variant of PTSD and is a common sequela of psychological trauma. Left untreated, psychologically traumatic events can have devastating effects.

There are two phases of rape-trauma syndrome. The acute phase begins immediately after the crisis, followed by the long-term phase, which may begin as long as 2 weeks after the rape and may last years if untreated. *Rape-trauma response* is also a likely diagnosis and includes both the acute phase of disorganization and the long-term recovery phase.

Acute Phase

Typical reactions to a crisis often reflect cognitive, affective, and behavioral disruptions. The most common responses are shock, numbness, and disbelief. A person may appear self-contained and calm. At other times, cognitive function may be impaired, and the person may have difficulty making decisions, solving problems, or concentrating. Or the person may cry, become hysterical, be restless or agitated, or even smile or laugh. The *acute*, or *disorganization, phase* is characterized by physical reactions such as generalized pain throughout the body; eating and sleeping disturbances; and emotional reactions such as anger, fear, anxiety, guilt, humiliation, embarrassment, self-blame, and mood swings (ACOG, 2014). There is no "normal" response to a sexual assault.

Long-Term Phase

The *delayed*, or *organization, phase* may not occur until months or even years after the events and is characterized by flashbacks, nightmares, and phobias as well as somatic and gynecological symptoms (ACOG, 2014). Emotional reactions may include depression, panic disorder, and suicidal ideation and attempts, and substance abuse is more prevalent among survivors of sexual assault. Therefore *Anxiety, Risk for self-destructive behavior, Low self-esteem, Helplessness, Acute confusion*, and *Labile moods*, among others, may also be appropriate nursing diagnoses.

However, PTSD is the long-term consequence of sexual assault. It is important to teach individuals what to expect during this phase so that they will be prepared and not feel as if they are "going crazy" or "losing their mind." It is also important to understand that all sexual assault survivors will deal with the event in their own manner. Common symptoms of PTSD related to sexual assault include the following:

- **Re-experiencing the trauma:** Recurrent nightmares about the rape, flashbacks, or uninvited and intrusive thoughts during the day or night.
- **Social withdrawal:** Called "psychic numbing," involves not experiencing feelings of any kind.
- **Avoidance behaviors and actions:** Avoidance of all places and activities, as well as thoughts or feelings, that could recall events about the rape.
- **Increased psychological arousal characteristics:** Exaggerated startle response, hypervigilance, sleep disorders, or difficulty concentrating.
- **Fears and phobias:** Fear of being alone, fear of sexual encounters, and fear of the indoors or outdoors are just some examples.
- **Nightmares and difficulty sleeping:** Vivid nightmares of the event that wake the individual and cause terror, disturb sleep, and prevent sleep.

OUTCOMES IDENTIFICATION

Short-Term Goals

The patient will:

- Have a short-term plan for handling immediate situational needs before leaving the ED.
- Have a written list of common physical, social, and emotional reactions that may follow a sexual assault before leaving the ED.
- State the results of the physical examination completed in the ED.
- Have written access to information on obtaining competent legal counsel and community supports (individual or group) before leaving the ED.
- Have a follow-up appointment with a rape counselor or crisis counselor.
- Have support from family and friends.
- Have a list with telephone numbers of clinics or rape crisis counselors.

Long-Term Goals

The ideal outcome is that the person eventually will be able to:

- Find ongoing support to help the individual deal with the many confusing and terrifying issues and thoughts regarding the event(s).
- Return to pre-crisis level of functioning with minimal or no residual symptoms (survivor).
- Experience hopefulness and confidence in going ahead with life plans.
- Have comfortable and enjoyable sex (for some, it may take many years for this to happen).

PLANNING AND IMPLEMENTATION

Ensure that examinations are conducted at sites served by examiners with advanced education and clinical experience, if possible (U.S. Department of Justice Office on Violence Against Women, 2013). If a transfer from one health care facility to a designated examination site is necessary, use precautions to protect evidence (U.S. Department of Justice Office on Violence Against Women, 2013).

These patients require compassionate care. **Follow the sexual assault protocol provided in your ED procedure manual. Most protocols will include the following guidelines:** treatment of all physical injuries, STI prophylaxis, pregnancy prevention (if patient agrees), forensic evidence collection, and counseling.

Compassionate care involves approaching the person who has been sexually assaulted in a nonjudgmental and empathic manner. Patients need to hear and understand that the rape is *not* their fault, and confidentiality should be stressed repeatedly. It is important to help survivors and their significant others separate the issues of vulnerability from blame. Although individuals may have made choices that made them more vulnerable to assault, they are *not* to blame for the rape. See Table 22.2 for a list of interventions to be used for the victim of sexual assault.

TABLE 22.2 **Guidelines for Sexual Assault**

Intervention	Rationale
1. Have someone (friend, neighbor, sexual assault advocate, or staff member) stay with the patient while he or she is waiting to be treated in the emergency department (ED).	1. People in high levels of anxiety need someone with them until the anxiety level is down to moderate. *Never leave the individual alone.*
2. **Very important:** Approach patient in a nonjudgmental manner.	2. Nurses' attitudes can have an important therapeutic effect. Displays of shock, horror, disgust, or disbelief can increase anxiety and shame.
3. Confidentiality is crucial.	3. The patient's situation *is not to be discussed* with anyone other than medical personnel involved unless patient gives consent.
4. Explain to the patient the signs and symptoms that many people experience during the long-term phase, for example: a. Nightmares b. Phobias c. Anxiety, depression d. Insomnia e. Somatic symptoms	4. Many individuals think they are going crazy and are not aware that this is a process that many people in their situation have experienced.
5. Listen and let the patient talk. **Do not** press the patient to talk.	5. When people feel understood, they feel more in control of their situation.
6. Stress that the patient did the right thing to save his or her life.	6. Victims of rape might feel guilt or shame. Reinforcing that they did what they had to do to stay alive can reduce guilt and maintain self-esteem.
7. **Do not** use judgmental language: • Reported *not* alleged • Declined *not* refused • Penetration *not* intercourse • Instead of reporting "no acute distress," describe the behavior	7. Pejorative terms often reflect old myths and a lack of knowledge and understanding regarding the rape victim's experience and need for immediate intervention. Words like *alleged, refused,* and *intercourse* all minimize the devastation of the event.
Forensic Examination and Issues	
1. Assess the signs and symptoms of physical trauma.	1. Most common injuries are to the face, head, neck, and extremities.
2. **Explain and get permission from patient to take photos/videos and specimens.**	2. Patient's consent is needed to collect and document evidence, which later may be used in court.
3. Make a body map to identify size, color, and location of injuries. Ask permission to take photos.	3. Accurate records and photos can be used as legal evidence in the future.
4. Carefully explain all procedures before doing them (e.g., "We would like to do a vaginal [rectal] examination and do a swab. Have you had a vaginal [rectal] examination before?").	4. The individual is experiencing high levels of anxiety. Explaining in a matter-of-fact way what you plan to do and why you are doing it can help reduce fear and anxiety.
5. Explain the forensic specimens you plan to collect; inform patient that specimens can be used for identification and prosecution of the rapist, for example: • Debris in head hair and pubic hair • Skin from underneath nails • Semen samples • Blood • Urine sample (if date rape drug is suspected)	5. Collecting body fluids and swabs is essential (DNA) for identifying the rapist.
6. Encourage patient to consider treatment and evaluation for sexually transmitted infections before leaving the ED.	6. Many survivors are lost to follow-up after being seen in the ED or crisis center and will not otherwise get protection.
7. Offer prophylaxis to pregnancy.[a]	7. Approximately 5% to 6% of women who are raped become pregnant.
8. All data must be carefully documented: • Verbatim statements • Detailed observations of physical trauma • Detailed observation of emotional status • Results from the physical examination • All lab tests should be noted	8. Accurate and detailed documentation is crucial legal evidence.
9. Offer support follow-up: • Rape counselor • Support group • Group therapy • Individual therapy • Crisis counseling	9. Many individuals can be burdened with constant emotional trauma. Depression and suicidal ideation are frequent sequelae of rape. The sooner the intervention, the less complicated the recovery may be.

[a]According to the U.S. Department of Justice Office on Violence Against Women (2013, Section C.9), "A victim of sexual assault should be offered prophylaxis for pregnancy, subject to informed consent and consistent with current treatment guidelines. Conscience statutes will continue to protect health care providers who have moral or religious objections to providing certain forms of contraception. In a case in which a provider refuses to offer certain forms of contraception for moral or religious reasons, victims of sexual assault *must* receive information on how to access these services in a timely fashion." From U.S. Department of Justice Office on Violence Against Women. (2013). A national protocol for sexual assault medical forensic examinations: Adults/adolescents (2nd ed.). Retrieved October 5, 2015, from http://www.njrs.gov/pdffiles1./ovw/241903.pdf.

APPLYING THE ART

A Person Experiencing Sexual Assault

Scenario

A neighbor brought 40-year-old Margaret to the emergency department (ED) following her report of a sexual assault by a 20-something male who gained access to Margaret's home by claiming the need to make a phone call because of car trouble. The ED called ahead to a nearby hospital that was set up for sexual assault victims and had a forensic examiner. Margaret was waiting for transportation. My student status enabled me to provide continuity of care so that I could stay with Margaret, never leaving her alone in the ED. I established contact and struggled to hear Margaret, who spoke in a whisper.

Therapeutic Goal

By the close of this interaction, Margaret will allow herself to acknowledge her survival and to express her concerns.

Student–Patient Interaction	Thoughts, Communication Techniques, and Mental Health Nursing Concepts
Margaret: (*Voice tense.*) "I don't want to be alone. Not now. Not ever."	Margaret started our interaction with a whisper, which makes me think she may be reacting with the *controlled style* in this *acute phase of the rape-trauma syndrome.* Yet her tense assertion of not wanting to be alone may indicate the *expressed style.*
Student's feelings: *I would be afraid to be alone, too, if someone attacked me in my own home. But why did she trust a stranger? I struggle with countertransference. I have to be alert to not blame the victim as a way to distance myself; if I make this Margaret's fault, then rape cannot happen to me.*	
Student: "I am staying right here with you. You've been through a terrible ordeal."	I *offer self* and *attempt to translate* into feelings.
Margaret: "I feel so ashamed."	Earlier Margaret asked for water, and I had to say no until all the evidence is collected. I am staying alert and especially careful to follow the rape crisis protocol for this ED for Margaret's sake and for any legal ramifications.
Student: "What happened was not your fault. You don't have anything to be ashamed of."	Reassurance seems supportive but actually discounts the patient's feelings. Margaret feels more alone now.
Student's feelings: *Without thinking, I immediately reassured Margaret that she has no reason to be ashamed. Even as I speak the words, I notice Margaret pulling away. I wonder now if I wasn't really reassuring myself.*	
Margaret: "You don't understand. No one does." (*Looks downward.*)	
Student: "You're right. I don't understand what you went through. Margaret, I care about what happened to you, and I want to understand."	I *offer self* and *give control* to Margaret, acknowledging that only she knows her experience.
Student's feelings: *I do care about Margaret.*	
Margaret: "I don't know how I will ever tell my husband." *(Eyes swell with tears, which she angrily brushes away, then proceeds to rub her temples.)*	
Student: "You feel worried about his reaction."	I *attempt to translate into feelings* by saying "worried." I assess Margaret's *anxiety* to be at least *moderate. Physical signs* arise at the *severe level,* and Margaret is now rubbing her temples, as though she has a headache. Though she did not report a headache at the intake assessment, Margaret's stress and anxiety may be stimulating additional physiological responses.
Margaret: "Why would he even want to be with me—damaged goods."	
Student: "You feel damaged, unlovable."	I use *restatement* and *attempt to translate into feelings.*
Student's feelings: *I feel sad that she has the added burden of dealing with the reactions of loved ones who might not be supportive.*	
Margaret: "Unlovable." *(Eyes again fill with tears. Margaret presses her fists against her eyelids.)*	
Student: "Margaret, it's okay to cry." (*Margaret shakes her head).*	I give permission to lend *support* and *acceptance.*
Student: "I wonder what it would mean to you to cry."	I ask an *indirect question* to assess underlying dynamics.
Margaret: *(Breathing deeply to suppress tears.)* "That I am a weak woman, so weak I couldn't stop that monster."	She uses the word "monster." It must have been such a horrible violation of her personhood.
Student's feelings: *It's kind of scary. This could be me at another time.*	
Student: "You had the strength to stay alive. You did what you had to do to survive. Your instincts acted properly to keep you alive."	I give *support* affirming that Margaret was, in fact, able to stay alive. She survived the assault.
Margaret: "I am alive. Damaged, but alive." *(Eyes water.)*	
Student: "You look close to tears." *(Margaret nods.)* "It's okay to grieve, to let your feelings out."	I *make an observation.* Sharing the pain and allowing the *grief* decrease the intensity of the pain.
Margaret: (*Sobs, accepts a tissue, and holds on to my hand).*	Just then the medical transportation arrived to take her to a hospital with a rape crisis counselor and sexual assault nurse examiner.
Student's feelings: *I feel Margaret's trust that she reaches for my hand.*	

Pharmacological and Psychological Treatment

Emergency Department

The updated U.S. Department of Justice Office on Violence Against Women (2013) protocol emphasizes the following:

- Consider sexual assault patients a priority.
- Perform a prompt, competent medical assessment.
- Then respond to acute injury, the need for trauma care, and the safety needs of patients before collecting evidence.
- Alert forensic examiners (e.g., SANE) of the need for their services.
- Contact victim advocates so that they can offer services to patients, if not already done.
- Assess and respond to safety concerns of victims upon arrival at the examination site (e.g., Are there threats to patient or staff?).
- Assess patients' need for immediate medical or mental health intervention prior to the evidentiary examination, following facility policy.

Physical signs of sexual assault include the following:

- Presence of blood and/or sperm
- Contusions
- Lacerations
- Abdominal trauma
- Joint dislocation
- Mechanical back pain
- Lesions caused by forceful genital penetration
- Abruptio placentae

ED treatment consists of the administration of prophylactic antibiotics for the most common STIs (chlamydia, gonorrhea, trichomoniasis, and bacterial vaginosis [BV]), with the victim's consent. Pregnancy prophylactics include the administration of Ovral tablets if pregnancy tests are negative. *Emergency contraception (EC) is a safe, effective medication that prevents pregnancy after sexual assault. It does not induce abortion or terminate a pregnancy.* In the United States, there are approximately 25,000 pregnancies every year that are a result of sexual assault (Connecticut Alliance, 2018).

The guidelines also recommend updating the individual's tetanus if abrasions or open wounds are present and administration of the hepatitis B vaccine if not already immunized (Ernoehazy, 2013). The ACOG (2014) states that "if the assailant's HIV status is unknown, clinicians should evaluate the risks and benefits of nonoccupational postexposure prophylaxis on a case-by-case basis."

Psychopharmacology

Short-term treatment with a benzodiazepine may help ameliorate the acute anxiety and agitation that follow a trauma. Antidepressants (selective serotonin reuptake inhibitors [SSRIs]) may be helpful for symptoms of PTSD, such as hyperarousal, agitation, and insomnia, and in the treatment of depression and panic attacks.

Psychotherapy

Crisis counseling should always be available to any person who has been sexually assaulted, including referrals to the family physician, community psychologist, or community rape crisis line, for example. The nurse assesses the assaulted individual to ascertain if there are any thoughts of suicide or homicide. If no SART is available, information on support groups, therapists, and attorneys who work with sexual assault survivors should be provided before the person leaves the ED. A list of safe houses should also be available for those involved in intimate partner violence (IPV). Caring for survivors is not completed in a single visit. Their emotional state and other psychological needs should be assessed within 24 to 48 hours by phone after being treated, and actual resolution may take years in some cases.

Group therapy or support groups can be beneficial for survivors. Sharing experiences with others who are going through the devastating physical and emotional aftermath of rape can be healing and break through feelings of isolation, shame, and guilt.

Therapy for Perpetrators

Alterations in thinking and behavior need to be undertaken in order to effect change. Unfortunately, most rapists do not acknowledge the need for change. No single method or program of treatment has been found to be totally effective.

EVALUATION

Most patients eventually will be able to resume their previous lives after supportive services and crisis counseling or therapy. If survivors are relatively free of signs of PTSD and their lifestyles are close to their lifestyles before the rape, the recovery is considered successful. Too often, without counseling of some kind, various sequelae of the assault may remain for years or even a lifetime.

APPLYING EVIDENCE-BASED PRACTICE (EBP)

Problem

A 19-year-old female presents to her college health center. When the registered nurse (RN) is checking her in, the patient asks for the morning-after pill and begins to cry. As the nurse gently talks to her, the patient reveals she was raped while on a date the night before.

EBP Assessment

A. **What do you already know from experience?** Rape victims are often reluctant to talk about what happened and may refuse treatment or to press charges. They may be embarrassed, hoping everything will just go away, or fearful of their attacker. It can be difficult as a nurse to support patient decisions when you feel a different action would be better.

B. **What does the literature say?** Rape is more common than most people realize. Approximately 1 out of every 3 women have had some experience with sexual assault or rape. Of those women, 4 out of 5 were raped before 25 years of age (Office on Women's Health, 2020). About 1 out of every 33 men experience rape or sexual assault (Rape, Abuse, & Incest National Network, 2020). Unfortunately, most rapes are not reported and are even less frequently reported by those who are college-age. The shame and guilt associated with sexual assault can be a barrier to reporting. A sexual assault history should be nonjudgmental and compassionate.

C. **What does the patient want?** The patient is requesting the morning-after pill. She is refusing a forensic examination or to speak with law enforcement. She initially does not want to even talk about the rape anymore with the nurse, but she eventually accepts patient education and resources.

Plan

The nurse supported the patient and followed her wishes. The patient was prescribed the morning-after pill by the clinic physician. The nurse told the patient that she could not and would not force her to do anything she did not want to do but noted that she would like to give her some information. The nurse explained the forensic procedure, sexually transmitted infection testing, and time limits if the patient changes her mind. She discussed how reactions to trauma may appear later as anxiety, depression, isolating behaviors, changes in relationships, decreased self-esteem, suicidal thoughts, flashbacks, or nightmares. The patient was given information on a rape support center, how to contact law enforcement, restraining orders, and counseling services. The clinic is engaged in improving outreach and rape prevention services at the college.

QSEN Prelicensure Knowledge, Skills, and Attitudes (KSAs) Addressed

Quality Improvement was addressed as the clinic worked to improve services. **Patient-Centered Care** was practiced by the nurse as she respected the individual's choices.

KEY POINTS TO REMEMBER

- Sexual assault is an act of violence, control, and hate; it is a criminal offense that often results in severe, long-term psychiatric trauma for the victim.
- To preserve forensic evidence, the victim should be aware of precautions to take before contacting the police, crisis center, or emergency facility.
- Contact with the sexual assault patient usually takes place in the emergency department (ED). Only nurses with special training (e.g., sexual assault nurse examiners [SANEs]) assess the patient, collect data, and provide information and referrals (e.g., to therapists, legal counsel, support groups) for patients before they leave the ED.
- Permission is necessary for collecting forensic data, performing a pelvic examination, and taking photographs. Confidentiality is stressed.
- Following the sexual assault, a forensic examination is conducted and evidence is collected. The patient should be given medications to protect against STIs, evaluated for pregnancy, offered prophylaxis, and if warranted, tested for HIV and syphilis. If abrasions are noted, a tetanus shot may be indicated if not updated in the past 5 years, and inoculation for hepatitis B is needed.
- Careful documentation of findings (diagrams and photos) and observations of emotional status is necessary, and descriptions of the events surrounding the assault should be documented using verbatim statements whenever possible.
- Assessment for date rape drugs should be included if the description of the event (loss of consciousness, vomiting) indicates they are a possibility. In such a case, a urine sample may be obtained.
- To help alleviate anxiety, explanations of all interventions or procedures are provided to the patient before they are performed.
- Before leaving the ED, individuals who have been sexually assaulted are educated about what kinds of reactions are commonly experienced by victims following sexual assault.
- Follow-up counseling, support groups, and referrals to effective legal attorneys who specialize in sexual assault should always be given before discharge from the ED.

APPLYING CRITICAL JUDGMENT

1. Sally M. is brought by a friend to the emergency department (ED). She is dazed, and the friend explains that a few friends went to a bar and met some guy Sally had met at a party on campus. He bought them all drinks. Sally said that after a few drinks, "I felt funny and don't remember much except that I woke up outside the back of the bar with my underclothes off and a number of reddened marks and abrasions on my breasts and arms. I have so much pain and burning in my vagina. I feel like I'm going crazy, I am so frightened." Her friends found her semiconscious and brought her to the ED. Sally appears confused and alternates between crying uncontrollably and staring into space. She repeatedly says she wants to wash up and change clothes, but her friend wanted her to come into the ED as soon as possible.
   A. Chart the objective and subjective symptoms of Sally's physical and emotional trauma using the guidelines from this chapter, and include a body map.
   B. After Sally consents to the forensic examination, how would you describe to her the procedures that will be performed during the forensic and pelvic examinations?
   C. Why might you ask Sally for a urine specimen at this time?
   D. Sally is afraid and does not want her parents or anyone on campus to know what happened, and she especially does not want the event to be reported to the police. What information could you give her that may allay some of her concerns?
   E. Describe the emergency medical treatment that should be offered to all sexually assaulted individuals.
   F. If there is no SART in the ED, what actions should the hospital personnel take in a timely fashion?
   G. You know that Sally may experience devastating sequelae of her sexual assault that can take years to resolve. What kind of supports and referrals should Sally be given before she leaves the ED?
   H. Use the Internet to find resources available in your community to aid rape victims; print a handout with names, addresses, and phone numbers.
   I. Determine if there is a *sexual assault response team* (SART) in your community. Using the Internet, secure the phone number, address, and website URL, and share this information with your classmates.
   J. Determine if there is a sexual assault nurse examiner (SANE) in any of your community clinics or crisis centers, and share this information with your classmates.
2. A friend calls you at 3 AM and tells you that she has been raped and has run out of the man's apartment to a nearby coffeehouse, not knowing what to do. You tell her you will meet her at the coffeehouse and then take her to the ED. You tell her not to go home. What are some other things you would instruct your friend *not* to do to help preserve evidence?
3. Choose five different young people in separate situations with whom to share the following guidelines for diminishing the risk of ingesting date rape drugs when at fraternity parties, large gatherings, raves, nightclubs, or rock concerts:
   - Do not accept open drinks (i.e., alcoholic or nonalcoholic beverages from strangers or others you do not know well or trust; this includes drinks that are in a glass).
   - When in bars or nightclubs, always get your drink directly from the bartender and do not take your eyes off the bartender when you order; do not use the waitress or let somebody else go to the bar for you. At parties, only accept drinks in closed containers like bottles or cans that you open yourself.
   - Never leave your drink unattended or turn your back on your table.
   - Do not drink from punch bowls, pitchers, tubs, or community water/juice bottles.
   - Stay alert; if there is talk of date rape drugs or if your friends seem "too intoxicated" for what they have taken, leave the party or nightclub immediately and do not go back!

CHAPTER REVIEW QUESTIONS

1. An elderly widow tells the nurse, "Since my sister-in-law's death, her husband has been making advances toward me. He tried to come into my home with a bottle of wine. Even though he's family, I'm afraid of what might happen if I let him in." Which action should the nurse take first?
   a. Support the widow to clarify her thoughts and feelings about the situation.
   b. Explain to the widow how to obtain an order of protection (restraining order).
   c. Positively reinforce the widow for addressing the problem with a caring professional.
   d. Educate the widow about sexual assault and violence, including the importance of prevention.
2. An emergency department nurse talks with a newly admitted victim of reported rape. Which communication should the nurse offer to comfort this patient?
   a. "You are safe now. I will stay with you in this private room."
   b. "Would you like your friend to stay with you during your examination?"
   c. "You made a good decision to come to the hospital after you were raped."
   d. "What questions do you have about your examination by the sexual assault nurse examiner?"
3. A patient tells the nurse, "I was raped 8 years ago but never told anyone. Nevertheless, the memories haunt me every day. I should be over it by now." Which comment should the nurse offer next?
   a. "It sounds like you're judging yourself for continuing to struggle with your reaction."
   b. "Rape is criminal behavior. You should have reported the incident to law enforcement."
   c. "Are you now ready to engage in counseling to deal with your reactions to this experience?"
   d. "Although it's important to learn from such life events, it's more important to put things in the past."
4. An emergency department nurse prepares to discharge a victim of reported rape. Which comment by the victim indicates that the nurse's teaching was effective?
   a. "I should bathe frequently over the next week."
   b. "I am required to follow up with law enforcement."
   c. "It's important for me to follow up with counseling."
   d. "I should delay any sexual activity for at least 3 months."
5. A victim of reported sexual assault tells the nurse, "This was entirely my fault. I should never have gone to that party alone." Which response by the nurse is most therapeutic?
   a. "This was a frightening experience for you."
   b. "What do you think you should have done differently?"
   c. "Would you like to tell me more about what happened?"
   d. "It sounds like you're blaming yourself for the assailant's behavior."

REFERENCES

American College of Obstetricians and Gynecologists (ACOG). (2014). *Sexual assault.* Retrieved July 11, 2015, from http://www.agog.org/Resources-And-Publications/Committees-on-Health-Care-for-Underserved-Women/Sexual-Assault.

Amnesty International. (2015). *Maze of injustice: A summary of amnesty international's findings.* Retrieved July 6, 2015, from http://www.amnestyusa.org/our-work/issues/women-s-rights/violence-against-women/maze-of-injustice.

Centers for Disease Control and Prevention (CDC). (2018). *Violence prevention: Materials and multimedia.* Retrieved October 16, 2018, from https://www.cdc.gov/violenceprevention/nisvs/materials.html.

Centers for Disease Control and Prevention. (2020). *Violence prevention: Youth violence.* Retrieved from https://www.cdc.gov/violenceprevention/youthviolence/fastfact.html.

Connecticut Alliance to End Sexual Violence. (2018). *National statistics on sexual violence.* Retrieved from https://endsexualviolencect.org/resources/get-the-facts/national-stats/.

Ernoehazy, W. (2013). *Sexual assault practice essentials updated 2013.* Retrieved July 1, 2015, from http://emedicine.medscape.com/article/806120-overview-treatment.

Giddens, J. F. (2017). *Concepts for nursing practice* (2nd ed.). St. Louis: Elsevier.

Mengeling, M. A., Booth, B. M., Tomer, J. C., et al. (2014). *Reporting sexual assault in the military: Who reports and why most servicemen don't.* Retrieved July 9, 2015, from http://www.sciencedirect.com/science/article/pii/SO749379714001184.

Office on Women's Health. (2020). Sexual assault. Retrieved from https://www.womenshealth.gov/relationships-and-safety/sexual-assault-and-rape/sexual-assault.

Rape, Abuse, & Incest National Network (RAINN). (2018a). *Public policy & action.* Retrieved October 16, 2018 from https://www.rainn.org/public-policy-action.

Rape, Abuse, & Incest National Network (RAINN). (2018b). *Statistics.* Retrieved October 16, 2018 from https://www.rainn.org/statistics.

Rape, Abuse, & Incest National Network. (2020). Victims of sexual violence: Statistics. Retrieved from https://www.rainn.org/statistics/victims-sexual-violence.

U.S. Department of Justice (DOJ). (2012). *An updated definition of rape.* Retrieved from http://www.justice.gov/opa/blog/ updated-definition-rape.

U.S. Department of Justice National Sex Offender Public Website (NSOPW). (2018). *Facts and statistics.* https://www.nsopw.gov/en/education/factsstatistics/?AspxAutoDetectCookieSupport=1.

U.S. Department of Justice Office on Violence Against Women. (2013). *A national protocol for sexual assault medical forensic examinations: Adults/adolescents* (2nd ed.). Retrieved October 5, 2015, from http://www.njrs.gov/pdffiles1./ovw/241903.pdf.

Women Organized Against Rape (WOAR). (2015a). *Child sexual abuse and assault-reactions in children who have been sexually abused.* Retrieved July 5, 2015, from http://www.woar.org/resources/child-sexual-abuse.php.

Women Organized Against Rape (WOAR). (2015b). *Common reactions to sexual assault: Long-term effects of sexual assault.* Retrieved July 5, 2015, from http://www.woar.org/resources/common-reactions-to-assault.php.

23

Suicidal Thoughts and Behaviors

Chyllia D. Fosbre

http://evolve.elsevier.com/Varcarolis/essentials

OBJECTIVES

1. Explain the roles of culture, religion, and socioeconomic status as they relate to suicidal risk.
2. Provide patient-centered care by discussing the implications as well as the risk factors identified in the Modified SAD PERSONS Scale when determining the risk for suicide potential. **QSEN: Patient-Centered Care**
3. Promote safety by discussing the kinds of safety procedures that are followed for an acutely suicidal individual who has been hospitalized. **QSEN: Safety**
4. Describe the need and rationale for postvention for family or friends of an individual who has completed suicide.
5. Discuss how staff psychological postmortem assessment postvention may contribute to improved coordination of care.
6. Identify the needed interventions that might provide quality improvement methods to help identify and prevent suicide for our returning war veterans. **QSEN: Quality Improvement**
7. Summarize the overt, covert, and behavioral clues and the steps in evaluating the lethality of a suicide plan for an individual who is contemplating suicide.
8. Using informatics, make a list of support groups within your community that might help people who are suicidal, such as support groups for veterans, suicide hotlines, crisis centers, and substance use groups (e.g., Alcoholics Anonymous, SMART Recovery). **QSEN: Informatics**
9. Applying communication techniques, identify some of the most important dialogue and questions needed to promote safety. **QSEN: Safety**
10. Contrast and compare the pros and cons of "right to die" physician-assisted suicide (PAS) as outlined in the chapter.
11. Using informatics, go to the Suicide Assessment Five-Step Evaluation and Triage (SAFE-T): Pocket Card for Clinicians (http://store.samsha.gov/product/Suicide-Assessment-Five-Step-Evaluation-and-Triage-SAFE-T-Pocket-Card-for-Clinicians/SMA09-4432). **QSEN: Informatics**

KEY TERMS AND CONCEPTS

CONCEPT: SAFE CARE: *Safe care* is defined as care that maintains a focus on using evidence in clinical decisions to maximize the health outcomes while also reducing the potential for harm (Giddens, 2017). There are a number of tools for ascertaining risk factors for potential suicidal behaviors. However, it is very difficult to predict suicide. Always take an individual very seriously if he or she mentions some form of suicidal ideation. The Suicide Assessment Five-Step Evaluation and Triage (**SAFE-T**) includes guidelines for the assessment and treatment of suicidal behaviors: identify risk factors, identify protective factors, conduct suicide inquiry, determine risk level, and document.

INTRODUCTION

Suicide or **completed suicide** is the act of intentionally ending one's own life. The act of intentionally taking one's own life arouses intense and complex emotions. Completed suicide leaves long-lasting emotional scars with family, friends, and even involved health care providers and spiritual leaders. A **suicide attempt** includes all willful, self-inflicted, life-threatening attempts that have not led to death. **Suicidal ideation** refers to the process of thinking about killing oneself. ***Always*** take an individual very seriously if he or she mentions some form of suicidal ideation. ***Always*** ask, "Are you thinking of killing yourself?" Listen very carefully to what the person does and does not say. Appropriate nursing interventions are outlined later in this chapter.

Another closely related topic is the practice of **physician-assisted suicide (PAS)** or **physician aid in dying (PAD)** for the terminally ill, which operates under very strict guidelines.

The key difference between euthanasia and PAS/PAD is who administers the lethal dose of medication. Euthanasia entails the physician or another third party administering the medication, whereas PAD/PAS requires the patient to self-administer the medication and to determine whether and when to do this (ProCon, 2016).

In the United States, as of July 2019, eight states and the District of Columbia had legislation supporting PAS/PAD (death with dignity laws): California, Colorado, Hawaii, Maine, New Jersey, Oregon, Vermont, and Washington (ProCon, 2019). Of the eight states, all of them require a patient to be a resident of the state, be at least 18 years old, have an estimated 6 months or less to live, and to have made at least two verbal and one written request for PAS/PAD to a physician (ProCon, 2019). A number of states have bills pending legislation. There are seven regions that have legalized PAS/PAD (Belgium, Canada, Finland, Germany, Luxembourg, the Netherlands, and Switzerland) and four that allow euthanasia (Belgium, Colombia, Luxembourg, and the Netherlands; ProCon, 2016). The issue of the "right to die with dignity" is very controversial and complex and one that religious beliefs strongly influence.

PREVALENCE AND COMORBIDITY

Suicide rates differ with gender, age, race, and geography. According to the World Health Organization (WHO, 2018), every year approximately 800,000 people around the world die by suicide. It is a health concern that crosses all borders, all boundaries. It is the second-leading cause of death among 15- to 29-year-olds and is a growing problem in those over 65. The greatest predictor of suicide is a previous suicide attempt; however, there are many other risk factors. In well-developed countries, more suicides are linked with an impulsive decision during a crisis, such as financial problems, the end of a relationship, or a newly diagnosed or worsening health condition. Being a minority also increases the risk and is thought to be linked to those who experience discrimination, such as refugees; indigenous people; lesbian, gay, bisexual, or transgendered people; and prisoners. People who know someone who has committed suicide are also at greater risk (WHO, 2018).

More males complete suicide, but more females attempt suicide. Males tend to use more lethal methods, such as firearms, whereas females more often attempt suicide by overdose. There are also cultural differences that may be seen. For example, in many Native American cultures, suicide by hanging is more frequent than other methods (WHO, 2018).

There are often clusters of suicides, a phenomenon that is often referred to as suicide contagion or copycat suicides. The media play a significant role in suicide contagion, and recommendations on how to report suicide have been issued by the WHO (2017). After the airing of *13 Reasons Why* (a television series that explores the events that led up to the suicide of the main character), mental health professionals saw an increase in suicidal ideation and attempts, and warnings were sent out to schools and parents (American Psychiatric Association, 2018). Some would argue that the show opened up conversations and that more people shared their experiences and thoughts, not that it actually caused an increase in these thoughts or behaviors.

The Centers for Disease Control and Prevention (CDC, 2018) estimates that of those who committed suicide, 22% had a physical health problem, 28% had problematic substance use, and about 46% had a known mental health issue. For those in extreme pain or those with little if any quality of life, intentional death—either physician assisted or self-inflicted—may be a means of escaping from intolerable pain and the extreme limitations imposed by illness.

Certain medications may also contribute to symptoms of depression; these include cardiac mediations, corticosteroids, hormonal medications, chemotherapy, and medications to treat pain. Multiple medications, including nearly all antidepressants, have the adverse effect of inducing suicide ideation, and many come with a Black Box warning. This is why the U.S. Food and Drug Administration (FDA) requires all new drugs to be assessed for the potential to precipitate suicidal feelings.

Traumatic brain injury (TBI) refers to any type of trauma to the head that affects brain functioning. Those who have experienced a TBI are at greater risk for suicide as well as a host of other mental health symptoms and disorders, such as self-harm, impulsive behaviors, anger, depression, and anxiety. It is estimated that between 15% and 23% of returning war veterans have experienced a TBI, which can have a severe impact on a person's functioning (Brenner, 2018). There is also research indicating that older veterans who experienced mild brain injuries during active duty earlier in life are more likely to develop various forms of dementia (Brenner, 2018; Summerall, 2017). Similar findings are being reported with chronic traumatic encephalopathy (repeated concussions, usually from sports), putting athletes in high-contact sports at greater risk for suicide as well (Mayo Clinic, 2018).

Nurses may encounter individuals with suicidal thoughts or active intent in outpatient settings, intensive care units, nursing homes, or medical-surgical units; during home visits; or even among their own family and friends.

THEORY

Psychological Theory

Sigmund Freud (1856–1939) developed some of the first psychological theories of suicide in the early 1900s. Freud described suicide as a murderous attack on an ambivalently loved, internalized significant person, often referred to as "murder in the 180th degree." Building on Freud's theory, **Karl Menninger** (1893–1990) suggested that all individuals who commit suicide experience three interrelated emotions: revenge, depression, and guilt.

Edwin Shneidman (1918–2009) proposed that victims of suicide suffer unbearable psychological pain, a sense of isolation, and the perception that death is the only solution to their situation. In essence, an individual feels "there is no way out." Shneidman identified self-destructive behaviors (compulsive use of drugs, hyperobesity, gambling, self-harmful sexual behaviors, medical noncompliance, and other high-risk behaviors) as **sub-intentioned suicide**.

Herbert Hendin, medical director of the American Foundation for Suicide Prevention, states that Shneidman was the first person in the United States to call public attention to the problem of suicide. Hendin (1996) explains that, in the field of suicide prevention, it borders on malpractice for providers to avoid prescribing medication for patients who have severe depression and suicidal ideation.

Contributing Risk Factors for Suicide

Risk factors for suicide can be broken into three main categories: health, environmental, and historical. Health issues that lead to suicide include comorbid mental health problems; medical problems, especially those that are considered terminal, chronic, or painful; and TBIs. Environmental risk factors include access to means (guns, poison, lethal doses of medication), prolonged stress in relationships, bullying, loss of employment, divorce, and exposure to suicide (either known or through media). Historical risk factors include previous attempts and family history of suicide or adverse childhood events (American Foundation for Suicide Prevention, 2018; CDC, 2018).

Neurobiology of Suicide

Low levels of 5-hydroxyindoleacetic (5-HIAA) in cerebral spinal fluid (CSF) have long been associated with impulsive, suicide-like violence. For example, people who have attempted suicide have lower levels of 5-HIAA serotonin functioning, and those who completed suicide have the lowest levels of 5-HIAA. In fact, low levels of 5-HIAA in the CSF can predict future attempts and future completed suicides (Brendel, Brezing, & Lagomasin, 2016). **Serotonin (5-hydroxytryptamine; 5-HT)** is an important neurotransmitter as it pertains to completed suicide. Studies of the brains of those who have completed suicide show abnormalities of the serotonin system in an area of the brain called the *ventral medial prefrontal cortex*. Changes in both presynaptic and postsynaptic serotonin receptors in the prefrontal cortex are present in some but not all suicide completers (Brendel et al., 2016).

Biological responses to *stress* may also constitute a risk factor for many people. The **noradrenergic system** is a mediator of acute stress responses, and overactivity of that system has been associated with both severe anxiety or agitation and higher suicidal risk, according to Mathews and colleagues' (2013) research of the literature. The **hypothalamic–pituitary–adrenal (HPA) axis** is another major stress response system. The HPA axis is associated with major depression, and suicide victims often exhibit HPA-axis abnormalities (Mathews et al., 2013).

Genetic Factors

Suicide clusters are seen in families. Some of this is attributed to the increase in suicide due to exposure or due to stressful family dynamics, but some researchers also believe there is a genetic component to suicide as well. Recent neuroimaging studies have identified two phenotypes that have a strong connection to suicide (Jollant et al., 2018), lending credence to the belief that there may be a genetic link.

Age

Adolescents and Young Adults

Suicide rates are increasing most rapidly in the 14- to 24-year-old age group in the United States. Native American and Alaskan Native youth have suicide rates at crisis levels and have the highest suicide rate of all youths.

Indigenous populations in the United States have been suffering from a youth suicide epidemic for decades. The epidemic and risk factors associated with it can be connected to the mistreatment of Native Americans throughout history, which has caused their communities to suffer from numerous inequalities, such as poverty, inadequate housing, loss of land, and destruction of culture.

Other strong risk factors for youth are aggression, disruptive behaviors, depression, and social isolation. The following additional factors are related to youth suicide:

- Frequent episodes of running away
- Frequent expressions of rage
- Family loss or instability
- Frequent problems with parents
- Withdrawal from family and friends
- Expression of suicidal thoughts or talk of death or the afterlife when sad or bored
- Difficulty dealing with sexual orientation
- Unplanned pregnancy
- Perception of school, work, or social failure

Older Adults

Surprisingly, although rates were previously much higher, the latest statistics show that suicide is the 17th-leading cause of death of those over 65 years of age, and the percentage increases for those between 75 and 85 years of age and goes up again for those over 85 years of age (American Association for Marriage and Family Therapy, 2018). Risk factors to be assessed among older adults include social isolation, solitary living arrangements, widowhood, lack of financial resources, poor health, and feelings of hopelessness.

Most older adults who complete suicide have visited their primary care physician in the month before the suicide, sometimes on that very day. Recognition and treatment of depression in the medical setting can prevent suicide in older adults.

Cultural Considerations

The meaning of suicide has traditionally reflected the religious beliefs of a culture. For example, in cultures with a Judeo-Christian tradition, life is considered a gift, and to take away one's life is a sin. Cultures historically steeped in Roman Catholic teachings (South America, Spain, Italy, Ireland) often have lower rates of suicide. To the contrary, people who practice the Shinto religion believe in reincarnation; therefore suicide may be seen as an *honorable* solution to life's problems.

BOX 23.1 Modified SAD PERSONS Scale[a]

SAD PERSONS can be modified to remedy the omission of an **available lethal plan.** This modification reminds the clinician to ask about lethal means when assessing suicidality. *If lethal means are available, the clinician can then take whatever action is reasonably indicated to reduce the likelihood of a suicide.*

S	Sex	1 if male
A	Age	1 if <19 or >45 years
D[b]	Depression or hopelessness	2
P	Previous attempts or psychiatric care	
E	Excessive alcohol or drug use	1
R	Rational thinking loss (psychotic or organic illness)	1
S	Separated, widowed, divorced	1
O	Organized plan or serious attempt	2
N	No social support	1
A	Availability of lethal plan	
S[c]	Stated future intent (determined to repeat or ambivalent)	1

Guidelines for Action

Points	Clinical Action
0–5	May be safe to discharge (depending on circumstances). If sent home, have follow-up appointment arranged and discharge patient with family or friend.
6–8	Probably requires psychiatric consultation.
>8	Probably requires hospital admission, voluntary or involuntary. See Chapter 6 for discussion of involuntary hospitalization.

[a]Attempt (A) is also included in this modified scale.
[b]Two points are given for the combination of depression (hopelessness) and previous attempt.
[c]The original SAD PERSONS Scale had "social supports lacking" for the first *S* and "sickness" for the second *S* (which is also a risk factor). In this version, the second *S* stands for "stated future intent."
Data from Patterson, W. M., Dohn, H. H., Bird, J., et al. (1983). Evaluation of suicidal patients: The SAD PERSONS Scale. *Psychosomatics, 24*, 343–349; Wyatt, J. P., Illingworth, R. N., Graham, C. A., et al. (2012). *Oxford handbook of emergency medicine* (4th ed., p. 609). Oxford, England: Oxford University Press. There has been more than one modification to the SAD PERSONS Scale by Patterson et al.

APPLICATION OF THE NURSING PROCESS

ASSESSMENT

There are a number of tools for determining risk factors when assessing for potential suicide. An acronym that can stimulate the health care worker's recall when in a crisis situation is the **Modified SAD PERSONS Scale** (Box 23.1). The SAD PERSONS Scale is commonly used in emergency departments and helps staff to quickly evaluate the urgency of referral to mental health sources or protective care (Wyatt et al., 2012).

The **Suicide Assessment Five-Step Evaluation and Triage (SAFE-T)** for Mental Health Professionals is also very popular (Box

BOX 23.2 SAFE-T: Suicide Assessment Five-Step Evaluation and Triage for Mental Health Professionals

Suicide assessments should be conducted at first contact; with any subsequent suicidal behavior, increased ideation, or pertinent clinical change; and for inpatients, prior to increasing privileges and at discharge.

Risk Factors

Suicidal behavior: history of prior suicide attempts, aborted suicide attempts, or self-injurious behavior

- Current/past psychiatric disorders: especially mood disorders, psychotic disorders, alcohol/substance abuse, ADHD, TBI, PTSD, Cluster B personality disorders, and conduct disorders (antisocial behavior, aggression, impulsivity). Comorbidity and recent onset of illness increase risk.
- Key symptoms: anhedonia, impulsivity, hopelessness, anxiety/panic, insomnia, command hallucinations
- Family history: of suicide, attempts, or psychiatric disorders requiring hospitalization
- Precipitants/stressors/interpersonal: triggering events leading to humiliation, shame, or despair (e.g., loss of relationship, financial or health status—real or anticipated); ongoing medical illness (especially central nervous system disorders, pain); intoxication; family turmoil/chaos; history of physical or sexual abuse; social isolation.
- Change in treatment: discharge from psychiatric hospital, provider or treatment change
- Access to firearms

Protective Factors

Protective factors, even if present, may not counteract significant acute risk.

- *Internal*: ability to cope with stress, religious beliefs, frustration tolerance
- *External*: responsibility to children or beloved pets, positive therapeutic relationships, social supports

Suicide Inquiry

Ask specific questions about thoughts, plans, behaviors, and intent.

- *Ideation*: frequency, intensity, duration—in past 48 hours, past month, and worst ever
- *Plan*: timing, location, lethality, availability, preparatory acts
- *Behaviors*: past attempts, aborted attempts, rehearsals (tying noose, loading gun), nonsuicidal self-injurious actions
- *Intent*: extent to which the patient (1) expects to carry out the plan and (2) believes the plan/act to be lethal versus self-injurious
- *Explore ambivalence*: reasons to die versus reasons to live.
  - For youths: ask parent/guardian about evidence of suicidal thoughts, plans, or behaviors and changes in mood, behaviors, or disposition.
  - Homicide inquiry: when indicated, especially in character-disordered or paranoid males dealing with loss or humiliation. Inquire in four areas listed previously.

Risk Level/Intervention

- Assessment of risk level is based on clinical judgment after completing steps 1 through 3.
- Reassess as patient or environmental circumstances change.

Risk Level	Risks/Protective Factor	Suicidality	Possible Interventions
High	Psychiatric disorder with severe symptoms of acute precipitating event protective factors not relevant	Potentially lethal suicide attempt or persistent ideation with strong intent or suicide rehearsal	Admission generally indicated unless a significant change reduces risk. Institute suicide precautions.
Moderate	Multiple risk factors, few protective factors	Suicidal ideation with plan but no intent or behavior	Admission may be necessary depending on risk factors. Develop crisis plan. Give emergency/crisis numbers.
Low	Modified risk factors, strong protective factors	Thoughts of death; no plan, intent, or behavior	Outpatient referral, symptom reduction. Give emergency/crisis numbers.

Document

- Risk level and rationale; treatment plan to address/reduce current risk (e.g., setting, medication, psychotherapy, ECT, contact with significant others, consultation); firearm instructions, if relevant; follow-up plan. For youths, the treatment plan should include roles for parent/guardian.

ADHD, Attention-deficit/hyperactivity disorder; *ECT*, electroconvulsive therapy; *PTSD*, posttraumatic stress disorder; *TBI*, traumatic brain injury.

23.2). SAFE-T draws upon the American Psychiatric Association Practice Guidelines for the Assessment and Treatment of Patients With Suicidal Behaviors. The five steps are as follows:

1. **Identify Risk Factors.** Note those that can be modified to reduce risk.
2. **Identify Protective Factors.** Note those that can be enhanced.
3. **Conduct Suicide Inquiry.** Note suicidal thoughts, plans, behavior, and intent.
4. **Determine Risk Level/Intervention.** Determine risk. Choose appropriate intervention to address and reduce risk.
5. **Document.** Document the assessment of risk, rationale, intervention, and follow-up.

Verbal Clues

Always take a suicide threat seriously. Whether a person makes one or a thousand threats, take the threats seriously. Assessing verbal clues includes the following:

Overt statements:

- "I can't take it anymore."
- "Life isn't worth living anymore."
- "I wish I were dead."
- "Everyone would be better off if I died."

Covert statements:

- "It's okay now. Everything will be fine."
- "Things will never work out."
- "I won't be a problem much longer."
- "Nothing feels good to me anymore, and probably never will."
- "How can I give my body to medical science?"

Behavioral Clues

Sudden behavioral changes may be noticed, for example:

- Giving away prized possessions
- Writing farewell notes
- Making out a will
- Putting personal affairs in order
- Having global insomnia
- Exhibiting a sudden and unexpected improvement in mood after being depressed or withdrawn
- Neglecting personal hygiene

Assessment Guidelines

Suicide Risk

1. **Identify current feeling states:** feelings of depression, hopelessness, helplessness, anxiety or panic, lack of interest or pleasure, and difficulty sleeping. For example: "Sometimes when I feel ___ (fill in the feeling state identified by the patient), I think about suicide."
2. **Ask directly.** Always ask: "Are you thinking of, or have you been thinking of, killing yourself?" If yes, evaluate the following:
   a. Frequency: How often do these thoughts occur?
   b. Duration: Once they have begun, how long do they persist?
   c. Intensity: On a scale from 0 to 10, how likely are you to act on these thoughts?
3. **Ask if the person has a plan.** "When you think about suicide, do you have a way that you might do this?"
4. **Determine the lethality of the plan in terms of risk.**
   - How detailed is the plan? (The more detailed, the greater its lethality.)
   - How lethal is the proposed method?
     - Guns, hanging, carbon monoxide, and staging a car crash are extremely lethal.
     - Slashing wrists, inhaling natural gas, and ingesting pills are lower risk.
     - A plan that doesn't allow for a last-minute reversal of the action is considered more lethal.
     - Availability of means. Does the person have a gun? Access to a tall building?
5. **Gather information about risk factors**—patient's age, sex, medical problems, psychiatric problems or emotional distress, excessive use of drugs or alcohol, a recent significant loss, unemployment, lives alone, and so forth—that would put the patient at higher risk.
6. **If there is a history of a suicide attempt, assess the following:**
   - Intent: Was there a high probability of being discovered?
   - Lethality: Was the method used highly lethal or less lethal?
   - Injury: Did the patient suffer physical harm (e.g., was the patient admitted to an intensive care unit)?
7. **Consult with one or more professionals and collaboratively develop a safety plan** with the patient. The patient thinks through and writes down ways to cope when feeling suicidal, who can be called, and so forth.
8. **If the patient is to be managed as an outpatient, also assess the following:**
   - Social supports: Is there someone who can stay with the patient?
   - Significant other's knowledge of the signs of potential suicidal ideation (e.g., increasing withdrawal, preoccupation, silence, remorse)
   - Provision of safety resources (knowledge of community resources, telephone numbers)

DIAGNOSIS

The international Classification for Nursing Practice (ICNP) is used in this text for nursing diagnoses. The following may be useful for treatment planning and are patient- and family-centered in their scope: *Risk for suicide, Attempted suicide, Impaired family process, Lack of family support, Risk for dysfunctional family grief, Negative self-image,* and *Risk for self destructive behavior.* Safety should be the highest priority for both the patient and family members because the risk goes up for family members of those who complete suicide.

OUTCOMES IDENTIFICATION

Interventions during the crisis that attempt to accomplish both short-term and long-term outcomes include the following:

Short-term outcomes:

- Will have a family member or friend stay with the suicidal individual overnight
- Will have a follow-up appointment with a counselor or therapist
- Will have a list of telephone numbers of self-help groups, hotlines, organizations, and therapists in the area where the individual lives
- Will seek emergent inpatient care for active suicidal ideation with ongoing safety concerns that cannot be resolved without prompt intervention

Longer-term outcomes:

- Optimizes events and environmental factors to help minimize further self-destructive acts
- Is able to explore alternatives and increase problem-solving skills
- Has shown evidence of increased coping skills
- States that feelings of isolation and loneliness are fewer and less severe
- Is engaged in treatment for co-occurring mental health issues (e.g., depression, substance abuse, posttraumatic stress disorder [PTSD])

PLANNING AND IMPLEMENTATION

Unfortunately, there seems to be a lack of evidence that supports any particular approach to prevention. Often, people who later complete suicide have made their intentions known to a health care worker or physician shortly before the event or have sought nonspecific help. Although restriction of access to means, mental health treatment, assistance with problem-solving skills and other therapies, and prescription of psychotropic medications may be effective, none of these interventions has been systematically investigated.

Some interventions are considered to support a person's resilience and act as protective factors:

- Family and community support
- Effective and appropriate clinical care for mental, physical, and substance abuse disorders
- Restricted access to highly lethal methods of suicide
- Cultural and religious beliefs that discourage suicide and support self-preservation instincts
- Acquisition of learned skills for problem solving, conflict resolution, and nonviolent management of disputes
- Cognitive-behavioral therapy

Nursing interventions during the crisis are outlined in Table 23.1. Nursing interventions after the crisis period are outlined in Table 23.2.

Communication Guidelines

Nurses and other health care providers use communication skills and counseling techniques as one of their most important tools. Communication and counseling skills used by the nurse working with a suicidal person are practiced (1) in the community, (2) in the hospital, and (3) on telephone hotlines. During a suicidal crisis, the following information should be conveyed to the patient in all settings:

- The crisis is temporary.
- Unbearable pain can be survived.
- Help is available.
- The patient is not alone.

The nurse remains nonjudgmental and listens attentively.

Psychotherapy

See Table 23.3 for interventions to be used during follow-up psychotherapy.

APPLYING THE ART

A Person With Suicidal Behaviors

Scenario

I met 55-year-old Raymond on the adult psychiatric unit following a suicide attempt from a self-inflicted gunshot wound. Raymond had damaged the right side of his neck and face and part of his right ear, but he missed every vital vessel and somehow lived. He had shown improvement by participating more actively in group therapy and had progressed from one-to-one observation (no farther than an arm's length away) to close constant observation within continuous visual range. I was meeting with him for the third time.

Therapeutic Goal

By the conclusion of this encounter, Raymond will feel comfortable enough with me to reveal his suicide attempt.

Student–Patient Interaction	Thoughts, Communication Techniques, and Mental Health Nursing Concepts
Student: "Raymond, I'm here after lunch as agreed."	I *offer self.* Being back when I said I would be builds trust.
Raymond: *(Avoids eye contact.)* "You can stay if you want. I don't feel like talking much." *(Glances up briefly, then stares at the floor.)* ***Student's feelings:*** *Although he was reserved, Raymond's voice had more animation earlier. He also made eye contact. Did I do something wrong to impair the relationship?*	Although I need to *evaluate* my *nursing practice,* Raymond's behavior change most likely came from his *mood disorder. Depression* influences his perception of just about everything.
Student: "I'll stay here with you." *(Leans toward him with a concerned expression.)* ***Student's feelings:*** *I have the hardest time waiting. I keep wanting to fill the silence. I sit on the left because Raymond has hearing loss on the right from the gunshot wound.*	I offer *self* with words and with attending behavior. My silence shows nonjudgmental acceptance.
Raymond: *(Silent for 4 minutes.)* "My wife wants a divorce." ***Student's feelings:*** *Divorce. Another loss. I am beginning to pick up his feelings of hopelessness.*	Does this increase his suicide risk further? Such a lethal method … to shoot yourself. I remember that sometimes when a suicide fails, the patient sees himself or herself as a failure once again.
Student: "How devastating. How hurtful." ***Student's feelings:*** *Sometimes when I use reflection, I worry that it sounds fake. Maybe because I'm still having to think about how to ask things. Even if I'm wrong about his feelings, I hope he senses that I care, because I do.*	*Reflection* communicates empathy because I have to really connect to be able to discern his probable feeling.
Raymond: *(Nods.)* "She said she can't take it anymore."	
Student: "You say she can't take it anymore?"	*Restatement* helps him elaborate.

Student–Patient Interaction	Thoughts, Communication Techniques, and Mental Health Nursing Concepts
Raymond: "My depression. Doing this." *(Touches the dressing on his ear, carefully shakes his head from side to side, then stares downward.)* ***Student's feelings:*** *I wonder what his marriage was like before this. When I have trouble with the people I love, I often feel bad about myself too.*	*Suicide* acts as a two-edged sword, hurting the survivors as well as the patient. I remember reading that suicide also acts as an *attempt* to *communicate,* but communicate what?
Student: "You shake your head, like you feel regret."	I *make an observation* and use *reflection.*
Raymond: "About so many things. At my age I should be able to readily name my accomplishments, but all I see are my failures. I can't believe she had an affair. Then I look at how I've screwed up, and it's no wonder. I can't even kill myself right." ***Student's feelings:*** *Where do I start? His despair makes me feel down too.*	At the root of all this rests low self-esteem paired with depression. Was his suicide attempt a way to punish his wife as well as himself for being, as he says, a "screw-up"? His age puts him into *generativity versus stagnation.* To feel he has no accomplishments sounds like stagnation rather than meeting the generativity task.
Student: "You're having trouble finding any reason to choose to live." ***Student's feelings:*** *I should have checked the chart to see if he has attempted suicide before.*	The 3-month period after an attempt remains a high risk for another suicide attempt. I need to actively assess his suicide potential.
Raymond: "Some days more than others." ***Student's feelings:*** *I'm feeling worried that he may attempt again.*	He feels *ambivalent.* I double-check that the staff member assigned to the close, constant observation is indeed watching him.
Student: "So, sometimes you are able to find something in you worth saving." ***Student's feelings:*** *I feel hopeful that he lets himself experience "some days" when he finds a reason to choose life. I need to help him get the feelings out, both the despair and the hope.*	I give *support.* Using the words, "you are able to" reinforces his *self-esteem.*
Raymond: "I guess so, but not today. Not with divorce papers in my hand." ***Student's feelings:*** *He sounds unsure. It's painful to struggle with depression. I know what depression feels like.*	In report this morning, the nurse indicated that Raymond's antidepressant and therapies may be starting to help. I remember that as *depression lifts,* the patient may experience the energy needed to carry through the *suicide plan.*
Student: "Today you're feeling pretty hopeless." *(He nods.)* "So hopeless you're thinking about suicide again?" ***Student's feelings:*** *My anxiety skyrockets. Okay. I am right here in the chair next to him. He and I are both safe right now. I can do this.*	His *suicide risk* suddenly increased with the impact of the divorce papers. He does not have a weapon, but he could rip out his stitches. I stay alert and watch his hands.
Raymond: *(Nods.)*	

Continued

APPLYING THE ART—cont'd

A Person With Suicidal Behaviors

Student–Patient Interaction	Thoughts, Communication Techniques, and Mental Health Nursing Concepts
Student: "Do you have a plan right now?" ***Student's feelings:*** *My heart rate is increasing, but I'm keeping my voice calm.*	I ask a *direct question* to *assess suicide risk.* I need to tell staff as soon as I can. He needs to be on one-to-one observation with staff only an arm's length away.
Raymond: "It'd be easier at home." ***Student's feelings:*** *He's given a lot of thought to this. I'm doing okay with connecting with Raymond.*	Raymond continues to talk, and that is so much healthier than hurting himself.
Student: "So you've thought of suicide while in the hospital, too."	The *current risk* takes precedence over thoughts of suicide at home. I *validate* with him.
Raymond: *(Looks down.)* ***Student's feelings:*** *Is Raymond avoiding eye contact? I don't want to lose the connection.*	He uses *avoidance.* What is he hiding?
Student: "Raymond, I care about you. Have you done or are you planning to do something to yourself right now?" **Raymond:** *(Mumbles.)* **Student:** *(Moving closer.)* "Raymond, I need your help with this. Please. Did you do something?" ***Student's feelings:*** *Part of me prays he will answer me!* **Raymond:** "I saved up all my pills and took them all."	I assess suicidality with a *direct question.* Communicating caring gives support. A *caring* relationship deters suicide.
Student: "When? What? How many?" ***Student's feelings:*** *I feel frantic. Okay, self, breathe mindfully.*	Too many *questions* at once. I will overload him. I need help now.
Student: *I stop asking questions. I call and motion to staff. The nurse comes over to assess and begin emergency intervention with Raymond.* ***Student's feelings:*** *I feel relieved to get help.*	The whole *treatment team* on the psychiatric unit works together. *Confidentiality* always includes the explanation that danger to self or others is always reported.
Student: *(As Raymond is transported off the unit, I walk alongside and hold out my hand.)* "Raymond, you were able to tell me about overdosing. That's a beginning to caring about yourself." ***Student's feelings:*** *By holding out my hand, I nonverbally ask permission to touch.* **Raymond:** *(Squeezes my hand.)* ***Student's feelings:*** *I needed to know that he knows that I care.*	My words and nonverbals give *support.*

TABLE 23.1 Interventions During the Crisis Period

Intervention	Rationale
Inpatient	
1. **Follow institutional protocol** for suicide regarding creating a safe environment (taking away potential weapons—belts, sharp objects; checking what visitors bring into patient's room).	1. Provides safe environment during time patient is actively suicidal and impulsive; self-destructive acts are perceived as the only way out of an intolerable situation.
2. Keep accurate and thorough records of patient's behavior—both verbal and physical—as well as all nursing and physician actions: • Establish frequent rapport with the person. • Assess patient for his or her ability to seek out staff when struggling with suicidal thoughts. If patient is unable to do this, place on close observation.	2. These might become court documents. If patient's needs or requests are not documented, they do not exist in a court of law.
3. *Suicide precaution* (one-on-one monitoring at arm's length away) or *suicide observation* (15-minute visual check of mood, behavior, and verbatim statements), depending on level of suicide potential.	3. Protection and preservation of the patient's life at all costs during crisis is part of medical and nursing staff responsibility. **Follow institutional protocol.**
4. Keep accurate and timely records and document patient's activity—usually every 15 minutes—including what patient is doing, with whom, etc. **Follow institutional protocol.**	4. Accurate documentation is vital. The chart is a legal document regarding patient's "ongoing status" and interventions taken.
5. If accepted at your institution, construct a *safety plan* with the suicidal patient. Use clear, simple language.	5. The *no-suicide contract* helps patients know what to do when they begin to feel overwhelmed by pain (e.g., "I will speak to my nurse/counselor/support group/family member when I first begin to think of harming myself").
6. Encourage patients to talk about their feelings and problem solve alternatives.	6. Talking about feelings and looking at alternatives can minimize suicidal acting-out.

TABLE 23.2 Interventions After the Crisis Period

Intervention	Rationale
1. Arrange for patient to stay with family or friends. If no one is available and the person is highly suicidal, hospitalization must be considered.	1. Relieves isolation and provides safety and comfort.
2. Weapons and pills are removed by friends, relatives, police, or the nurse.	2. Helps ensure safety.
3. Encourage patients to talk freely about feelings (anger, disappointments) and help plan alternative ways of handling anger and frustration.	3. Gives patients alternative ways of dealing with overwhelming emotions and gaining a sense of control over their lives.
4. Encourage patient to avoid decisions during the time of crisis until alternatives can be considered.	4. During crisis situations, people are unable to think clearly or evaluate their options.
5. Contact family members; arrange for individual or family crisis counseling.	5. Re-establishes social ties and mobilizes family support to deal with precipitating event(s) or overwhelming situation.
6. Activate links to social supports in the community (e.g., self-help groups).	6. Diminishes sense of isolation and provides contact with individuals who care about the suicidal person.
7. If anxiety is extremely high or patient has not slept in days, an antianxiety or antidepressant might be prescribed. Only a 1- to 3-day supply of medication should be given. Family member or significant other should monitor pills for safety.	7. Relief of anxiety and restoration after sleep loss can help the patient think more clearly and might help restore some sense of well-being. SSRIs are most commonly given, but they have Black Box warnings, and patient and family/ friends need to be educated.[a]

SSRI, Selective serotonin reuptake inhibitor.

TABLE 23.3 Interventions for Follow-Up Psychotherapy

Intervention	Rationale
1. Identify situations that trigger suicidal thoughts (define the precipitating event).	1. Identifies targets for learning more adaptive coping skills.
2. Assess patient's strengths and positive coping skills (talking to others, creative outlets, social activities, problem-solving abilities).	2. Identifies areas to build on and draw from when planning alternatives to self-defeating behaviors.
3. Assess patient's coping behaviors that are not effective and that result in negative emotional sequelae: drinking, angry outbursts, withdrawal, denial, and procrastination.	3. Identifies areas to target for teaching and planning strategies for supplanting negative behaviors with more effective and self-enhancing behaviors.
4. Encourage patients to look into their negative thinking, and reframe negative thinking into neutral objective thinking.	4. Cognitive reframing helps people look at situations in ways that allow for alternative approaches.
5. Point out unrealistic and perfectionistic thinking.	5. Constructive interpretations of events and behavior open up more realistic and satisfying options for the future.
6. Spend time discussing patient's dreams and wishes for the future. Identify short-term goals that can be set for the future.	6. Renewing realistic dreams and hopes can give promise to the future and meaning to life.
7. Identify things that have given meaning and joy to life in the past. Discuss how these things can be reincorporated in the present lifestyle (e.g., religious or spiritual beliefs, group activities, creative endeavors).	7. Reawakens in patient abilities and experiences that tapped areas of strength and creativity. Creative activities give people intrinsic pleasure and joy and a great deal of life satisfaction.

Postvention

Intervention for family and friends ("survivors") of a person who has completed a suicide—called a **postvention**—should be initiated within 24 to 72 hours after the death. Mourning the death of a loved one who has completed suicide is complicated and painful. Family and friends are often faced with the process of mourning without the normal social supports. Neighbors, acquaintances, and even family and friends are often confused and may be unsure how to help or what to say. They may even blame the family for the death. Families with members who have completed suicide are often stigmatized and isolated (Harvard Women's Health Watch, 2018).

Survivors will often go through the five stages of grief. They will experience denial or have feelings that their loved one will return to them. Anger can be directed at the deceased, at friends of the loved one, at other family members, or even directed toward oneself. In bargaining, the survivors may play out various "what if" scenarios, trying to find the moments when they could have intervened or ways to change the outcome. Depression may come in waves as the reality sets in that the loved one is truly gone. Acceptance comes as survivors begin to acknowledge the loss of their loved one and begin moving forward and planning again (Harvard Women's Health Watch, 2018).

People exposed to traumatic events, such as family and friends of persons who have completed suicide or persons who have experienced the sudden death of a family member or friend, often manifest the following posttraumatic stress reactions: irritability, sleep disturbances, anxiety, exaggerated startle reaction, nausea, headache, difficulty concentrating, confusion, fear, guilt, withdrawal, anger, and reactive depression. The particular pattern of the emotional reaction and the type of response differ with each survivor depending on the relationship to the deceased, circumstances surrounding the death, and the coping mechanisms of the survivor. The ultimate goal of intervention is to reduce the trauma associated with the sudden loss. *Posttrauma loss debriefing* can help initiate an adaptive grief process and prevent self-defeating behaviors.

The American Foundation for Suicide Prevention and Suicide Prevention Resource Center (2018) developed a toolkit for schools to use as a guide for addressing surviving students after a suicide. A school nurse would likely be part of the process of assessing for suicidality of students and providing additional supports.

Self-Care for Nurses

All health care workers who provided care for a person who completes suicide are similarly traumatized. Staff may also experience symptoms of posttraumatic stress disorder, including guilt, shock, anger, shame, and decreased self-esteem. Other patients on the unit who may have suicidal tendencies need to be closely monitored as well. The first 24 hours after inpatient suicide are crucial for both safety and crisis management reasons.

Among the tasks for staff and administrators is a thorough psychological postmortem assessment. The event is carefully reviewed by all members of the treatment team to identify the potential overlooked clues or faulty judgments, as well as to determine changes that are needed to agency protocols. Most facilities have a clear policy about interventions with families after suicide. Although some lawyers advise all health care personnel who had contact with the family to secure legal counsel, others recommend designating a spokesperson who can follow up and provide family and friends with support without discussing the details of the patient's care.

With regard to *documentation*, all staff members need to ensure that the record is complete and entries are completed in a timely fashion. Legal cases have shown that the client should be evaluated periodically for suicide risk, that the treatment regimen should provide high-level security, and that staff members should be informed of the individual's treatment.

BOX 23.3 Guidelines for Survivors of Suicide

- Know you can survive. You may not think so, but you can.
- Know you may feel overwhelmed by the intensity of your feelings, but all your feelings are normal.
- Anger, guilt, confusion, and forgetfulness are common responses. You are not crazy; you are in mourning.
- Having suicidal thoughts is common. It does not mean that you will act on these thoughts.
- Find a good listener with whom to share. Call someone if you need to talk.
- Do not be afraid to cry. Tears are healing.
- Give yourself time to heal.
- Remember, the choice was not yours. No one is the sole influence in another's life.
- Give yourself permission to get help.
- Be aware of the pain of your family and friends.
- Steer clear of people who tell you what or how to feel.
- Know that there are support groups that can be helpful. If you cannot find one, ask a professional to help start one.
- Call on your personal faith to help you through.
- It is common to experience physical reactions to your grief, such as headaches, loss of appetite, and inability to sleep.
- Wear out all of your questions, anger, guilt, or other feelings until you can let them go. Letting go does not mean forgetting.
- Know that you will never be the same again, but you can survive and go beyond just surviving.

Modified from Dunne, E., McIntosh, J., & Dunne-Maxim, K. (1987). *Suicide and its aftermath: Understanding and counseling the survivors.* New York, Norton.

Self-help groups are extremely beneficial for survivors of a suicidal family member or friend. Many people join self-help groups, even if the suicide took place 25 to 30 years ago. Self-help groups for the survivors are similar to all other self-help groups. Essentially, these groups are operated by people who have lost someone through suicide (Harvard Women's Health Watch, 2018).

Box 23.3 gives some guidelines for coping with a suicide loss. Also, the American Foundation for Suicide Prevention (http://www.afsp.org) can provide helpful information.

APPLYING EVIDENCE-BASED PRACTICE (EBP)

Problem

A nurse working on a suicide crisis line receives a call late at night from a 33-year-old male. He reports thoughts of wanting to die and has a plan to shoot himself. As the nurse talks to the patient, she writes down the phone number from caller ID and messages a colleague to dispatch a crisis team. The patient tells the nurse that his father shot and killed himself almost a year ago. He expressed anger that the physician prescribed valium for his depressed and alcoholic father and that he did not receive mental health treatment. The patient also expresses guilt that he had not been aware of his father's despair.

EBP Assessment

A. **What do you already know from experience?** People who have a family member or friend who has committed suicide have increased risk for suicide, especially around anniversary dates. Surviving family members experience a lot of guilt and pain. Depressants such as alcohol and benzodiazepines contribute to depression and suicidal thoughts.

B. **What does the literature say?** Survivors of suicide experience guilt, anger, abandonment, denial, helplessness, and shock. Suicide is the 10th-leading cause of death among Americans, and 800,000 people worldwide die from suicide each year—more than from war and homicide combined. The key to suicide prevention is a collaborative approach (World Health Organization [WHO], 2019).

C. **What does the patient want?** The patient is reaching out for help. Although his suicidal feelings are very strong, he is asking for assistance to control them. He is currently receiving help at a mental health center. He wants the pain to "just go away."

Plan

The nurse immediately obtained contact information from caller ID and the patient and dispatched a crisis team. This procedure was developed in response to quality improvement recommendations because some callers hang up before help could be sent. The nurse obtained the patient's permission to notify his mental health center of his current crisis. The crisis team arrived on the scene, and after assessing the patient's level of suicidality as being high, the team transported him for admission to a psychiatric facility.

QSEN Prelicensure Knowledge, Skills, and Attitudes (KSAs) Addressed

Quality Improvement measures were taken in response to callers hanging up before receiving help.

Informatics was involved by obtaining the patient's information through caller ID, messaging a colleague for help electronically, and emailing the mental health center through a secure portal.

KEY POINTS TO REMEMBER

- People who attempt or complete suicide often share many risk factors, but people who have experienced the same risk factors are not always suicidal.
- Psychosis, substance use disorders, poor problem-solving skills, impulsivity, a low threshold for pain, and feelings of hopelessness place people at high risk for suicide when overwhelmed.
- Adolescents, older adults, white males, Native Americans, and Alaskan Natives have the highest rates of completed suicide. Some cultures play a protective role.
- Always try to identify the precipitating event for clues to areas of intervention.
- Assessment should include verbal clues, behavioral clues, and lethality of the plan as an evaluation of the risk factors.
- The Modified SAD PERSONS Scale gives a quick overview of major risk factors.
- If suicidal risk is assessed, always ask directly: "Are you thinking of killing yourself?"
- During the crisis period when a person is acutely suicidal, specific interventions can prove helpful (in or out of the hospital) and may save lives (see Table 23.1).
- After the crisis period is over, other interventions can prove helpful in increasing coping skills, enhancing problem solving, and minimizing isolation and loneliness (see Table 23.2).
- Recall that intervention for the family and friends of a person who has completed suicide is called *postvention*. Postvention can help lessen the guilt, anger, grief, pain, and myriad emotions that can stay with survivors for years.

APPLYING CRITICAL JUDGMENT

1. Sam T. is a 62-year-old man whose wife recently died of leukemia. His only son moved to California 2 years ago with his two daughters. Sam had been caring for his wife for 3 years before her death and has become withdrawn and despondent since her death. He is now in the emergency department after a "fender bender" and is getting two stitches on his ear; his blood alcohol level is 0.6. He does admit to being very depressed after losing his wife. You ask Mr. T. if he has thought about killing himself, and he says, "Well, there is always a last resort, isn't there?" When you question him about the lethality of his plan, he admits to having a gun in the house for protection.
   A. How many risk factors does Mr. T. have using the Modified SAD PERSONS Scale?
   B. Do you think he needs hospitalization? If not, what should be put in place before he returns home? Explain the rationale behind your answer.
   C. What are Mr. T.'s needs? What kinds of referrals do you think would help him deal with this crisis?
   D. What do you think about the "fender bender"?
   E. Name at least three groups in your community to which you could refer Mr. T.
2. Have you ever known anyone who has completed a suicide? Contemplated suicide? If so, looking back at the risk factors, do you think there were any options open to these individuals? If so, what might have been available for an effective intervention?

CHAPTER REVIEW QUESTIONS

1. A parent tells the nurse about the death of a child 2 years ago. Which comment by this parent warrants the nurse's priority attention?
   a. "I still have some of my child's toys and clothes."
   b. "A parent should never live longer than their child."
   c. "I never returned to church again after the death of my child."
   d. "My child has been dead a long time, but it seems like only yesterday."
2. A patient diagnosed with major depressive disorder was hospitalized for 2 weeks on an acute psychiatric unit. One day after discharge, the patient completed suicide. Recognizing likely reactions among staff, which action should the nursing supervisor implement first?
   a. Assess each staff member individually for suicidal intent and/or plans.
   b. Provide a private setting for staff members to talk about feelings associated with the event.
   c. Remind staff members that suicide is a risk for the patient population and that they are not at fault.
   d. Invite a guest speaker to conduct an educational session for staff members about suicide risk factors.
3. On the sixth anniversary of her spouse's death, a widow says, "Sometimes life does not seem worth living anymore. I wish I could go to sleep and never wake up." Which response by the nurse has priority?
   a. "Are you considering suicide?"
   b. "You still have so much to live for."
   c. "Grief can sometimes last for many years."
   d. "Why do you continue to grieve something from long ago?"
4. A patient who had a stroke 3 days ago tearfully tells the nurse, "What's the use in living? I'm no good to anybody like this." Which action should the nurse employ first when caring for a patient demonstrating hopelessness?
   a. Implement the institutional protocol for suicide risk.
   b. Support the patient to clarify and express feelings of grief.
   c. Educate the patient about the success of stroke rehabilitation.
   d. Offer the patient an opportunity to confer with the pastoral counselor.
5. A single adult says to the nurse, "Both of my parents died several years ago, and my only sibling committed suicide 2 weeks ago. I feel so alone." After determining that the adult has no suicidal ideation, the nurse should:
   a. Explore the adult's feelings of survivor's guilt.
   b. Assess the adult's cultural beliefs and spirituality.
   c. Refer the adult for cognitive-behavioral therapy (CBT).
   d. Refer the adult to a self-help group for suicide survivors.

REFERENCES

American Association for Marriage and Family Therapy. (2018). *Suicide in the elderly*. Retrieved from https://www.aamft.org/Consumer_Updates/Suicide_in_the_Elderly.aspx.

American Foundation for Suicide Prevention. (2018). *Risk factors and warning signs: What leads to suicide*. Retrieved from https://afsp.org/about-suicide/risk-factors-and-waring-signs/.

American Foundation for Suicide Prevention & Suicide Prevention Resource Center. (2018). *After a suicide: A toolkit for schools* (2nd ed.). Retrieved from http://www.sprc.org/sites/default/files/resource-program/AfteraSuicideToolkitforSchools.pdf.

American Psychiatric Association. (2018). *Suicide prevention*. Retrieved from https://www.psychiatry.org/patients-families/suicide-prevention.

Brendel, R. W., Brezing, C. A., & Lagomasino. (2016). This suicidal patient. In T. A. Stern, M. Fava, T. E. Wilens, et al. (Eds.), *Massachusetts General Hospital comprehensive clinical psychiatry* (2nd ed.).

Brenner, L. A. (2018). *Understanding the relationship between traumatic brain injury and suicide*. Retrieved from http://suicideprevention-icrc-s.org/sites/default/files/sites/default/files/events/18_6_19_Brenner%20ICRC-S.pdf.

Centers for Disease Control and Prevention. (2018). *CDC vital signs: Suicide rising across the US*. Retrieved from https://www.cdc.gov/vitalsigns/pdf/vs-0618-suicide-H.pdf.

Giddens, J. F. (2017). *Concepts for nursing practice* (2nd ed.). St. Louis: Elsevier.

Harvard Women's Health Watch. (2018). *Suicide survivors face grief, questions, challenges*. Retrieved July 7, 2018 from https://www.health.harvard.edu/blog/suicide-survivors-face-grief-questions-challenges-201408127342.

Hendin, H. (1996). *Suicide in America: New and expanded edition*. W.W. Norton & Company: New York.

International Council of Nurses. (2017). *International Classification for Nursing Practice (ICNP)*. Retrieved July 7, 2018 from http://www.icn.ch/what-we-do/ICNP-Browser/.

Jollant, F., Wagner, G., Richard-Devantoy, S., Kohler, S., Bar, K.-J., Turecki, G., & Pereira, F. (2018). Neuroimaging-informed phenotypes of suicidal behavior: A family history of suicide and the use of violent suicidal means. *Translational Psychiatry*, *8*. https://doi.org/10.1038/s41398-018-0170-2.

Mathews, D. C., Richards, E. M., Niciu, M. J., et al. (2013). Neurobiological aspects of suicide and suicide attempts in bipolar disorder. *Translational Neuroscience*, *4*(2), 203–216.

Mayo Clinic. (2018). *Chronic traumatic encephalopathy*. Retrieved from https://www.mayoclinic.org/diseases-conditions/chronic-traumatic-encephalopathy/symptoms-causes/syc-20370921.

ProCon. (2016). *Euthanasia & physician assisted suicide around the world*. Retrieved from https://euthanasia.procon.org/view.resource.php?resourceID=000136.

ProCon. (2019). *State-by-state guide to physician-assisted suicide*. Retrieved from https://euthanasia.procon.org/view.resource.php?resourceID=000132.

Summerall, E. L. (2017). *Traumatic brain injury and PTSD: Focus on veterans*. Retrieved from https://www.ptsd.va.gov/professional/co-occurring/traumatic-brain-injury-ptsd.asp.

World Health Organization (WHO). (2017). *Preventing suicide: A resource for media professionals*. Retrieved from http://apps.who.int/iris/bitstream/handle/10665/258814/WHO-MSD-MER-17.5-eng.pdf;jsessionid=1A70F62A2645BDB554E3B32B8B1324B5?sequence=1.

World Health Organization (WHO). (2018). *Suicide*. Retrieved from http://www.who.int/en/news-room/fact-sheets/detail/suicide.

World Health Organization (WHO). (2019). *Suicide: Key facts*. Retrieved from-https://www.who.int/news-room/fact-sheets/detail/suicide.

Wyatt, J. P., Illingworth, R. N., Graham, C. A., et al. (2012). *Oxford handbook of emergency medicine* (4th ed.). Oxford, England: Oxford University Press.

24

Anger, Aggression, and Violence

Chyllia D. Fosbre, Elizabeth M. Varcarolis

http://evolve.elsevier.com/Varcarolis/essentials

OBJECTIVES

1. Discuss the interplay of neurobiology, medical history, past history, and sociological/demographic issues that contribute to risks for violence.
2. Promote safety by demonstrating the physical indicators of a patient who is beginning to escalate out of control. **QSEN: Safety**
3. Provide patient-centered care by comparing and contrasting interventions for a patient who is angry and loud in the pre-escalation phase with those for a patient who is escalating to a more aggressive phase. **QSEN: Patient-Centered Care**
4. Identify specific safety measures you would take when engaged in de-escalating an aggressive individual. **QSEN: Safety**
5. Plan patient-centered nursing care for a patient who is in seclusion. **QSEN: Patient-Centered Care**
6. Incorporate evidence-based practice by describing the use of communication and procedures implemented when placing an individual in restraints. **QSEN: Evidence-Based Practice**
7. Discuss how teamwork and collaboration are vital to applying seclusions or restraints to a patient who is a danger to self or others. **QSEN: Teamwork and Collaboration**
8. Discuss how quality improvement methods can develop from the process of critical incident debriefing. **QSEN: Quality Improvement**
9. Document an example of the areas for which the nurse must provide written information when violence was averted or actually occurred.
10. Incorporate evidence-based practice by identifying calming and reassuring communication and the optimum milieu in managing a patient whose behaviors are escalating. **QSEN: Evidence-Based Practice**

KEY TERMS AND CONCEPTS

CONCEPT: CULTURE: *Culture* is defined as a pattern of shared attitudes, beliefs, norms, roles, and values that can occur among those who speak a specific language or live in a defined region (Giddens, 2017). The different rates of violent crime within cultures emphasize the importance of social factors in the genesis of violence. A culture that supports the use of intimidation and aggression as an acceptable way of problem solving and achieving social status can reinforce the use of violence as acceptable behavior.

INTRODUCTION

Violence is harmful to the health of both the victim and the aggressor. The recipient of violence is susceptible to changes in the brain related to depression, anxiety, and immune-related diseases. Aggressors may suffer the same effects (Society for Neuroscience, 2014).

This chapter discusses how nurses in a variety of health care settings can recognize cues for escalating anger and aggression and how they can learn to de-escalate and intervene when anger is escalating and/or out of control.

ANGER, AGGRESSION, AND VIOLENCE

Universal differentiation among the terms *anger, aggression*, and *violence* is difficult or almost impossible because of cultural perceptions and social backgrounds. **Anger** is a normal—and not always logical—human emotion, and no judgment needs to be passed on it. Anger varies in intensity from mild irritation to intense fury and rage.

Anger is usually a response to something that is happening or has happened. Anger may arise as a response to feelings of hurt, fear, or vulnerability; a threat to one's needs (emotional or physical); or a challenge. Simply put, anger is an unplanned reaction to a stressor. Although we are all familiar with the feelings of anger, not everyone responds to anger with aggression or violence in the same way. When anger is channeled in a constructive manner (e.g., assertive communication, critical reasoning), individual needs can be met in a safe manner. Anger becomes unhealthy if it gets in the way of a person's functioning or relationships or puts others at risk. When anger escalates, the result often leads to aggression or violence. Acting out may meet immediate needs, but it does so at the expense of causing emotional or physical harm to one's self or others.

Aggression is not the same as violence. Aggression may be appropriate or self-protective—as in protecting oneself, one's family, or a person being bullied. Aggression can be defined as "forceful goal directed action that may be verbal or physical; the motor counterpart of the effect of rage, anger, or hostility" (Sadock, Sadock, & Ruiz, 2015, p. 1407). Bresin and Gordon (2013) conducted two research studies based on the catharsis theory of aggression, which implies there is a healing and anger-reducing effect that occurs through aggression. Bresin and Gordon's definition of aggression in these studies was verbal retaliation after participants received negative feedback. This study revealed that there are both adaptive and maladaptive forms of aggression. Maladaptive aggression can include abuse and physical and verbal aggression, whereas adaptive forms tend to have a calming effect. Adaptive aggression can be empowering. Essentially, aggression is used as an attempt to regain control over a stressor or flee the situation.

Violence does not always have anger as its origin, but it does have the underlying intention of doing harm to a specific person or group. Violence is the unjust, unwarranted, or unlawful display of verbal threats, intimidation, or physical force with the intent of causing property damage, personal injury, or even death to another individual (Feinstein & Rothberg, 2014). Acts of violence lead to significant physical and psychological harm to others. *Bullying* is an all too common form of unchecked acts of violence in our schools, workplaces, and health care systems.

Bullying and Violence

Bullying is an intentional display and use of *violence*, as subtle as it might appear in some instances. Bullying can be defined as offensive, intimidating, malicious, condescending behavior designed to humiliate and terrorize. Bullying involves persistent, systemic violence toward an individual or group.

Bullying occurs between persons with different levels of authority (e.g., supervisor or manager to staff nurse, boss to employee, teacher to student, parent to child). **Lateral bullying** refers to bullying among those of equivalent status (e.g., employee to employee, nurse to nurse, child to child, teenager to teenager, sibling to sibling, political opponent to political opponent).

Bullying in Health Care Environments

In an ongoing American Nurses Association (ANA) survey of nurses' health and safety, 21% of respondents reported they were at a "significant level of risk" for violence at work, and 25% to 50% reported experiencing various instances of bullying in their workplace. Specifically, 50% said they had experienced verbal or nonverbal aggression from a peer and 42% from a person with a higher level of authority (ANA, 2015).

Robbins (2015) states that the incidence of bullying in nursing is staggering. Researchers estimate that at least 85% of nurses have been verbally abused by a fellow nurse and that one in three nurses quits his or her job because of bullying; additionally, "bullying—not wages—is the major cause of a global nursing shortage. In the United States, the Bureau of Labor Statistics projects that by 2022, there will be a shortfall of 1.05 million nurses."

The following partial list of bullying behaviors among nurses in the health care setting is consistent with most types of bullying that take place in other workplace environments:

- Providing unwanted or invalid criticism, excessively monitoring another's work
- Gossiping, spreading lies or false rumors, assigning derogatory nicknames
- Taking credit for another person's work without acknowledging his or her contribution, blocking career pathways and other work opportunities
- Publicly making derogatory comments about staff members or their work, including use of body language (eye rolling, dismissive behavior), often in front of others
- Using sarcasm or ridicule, making someone the target of practical jokes
- Blaming someone without factual justification
- Allocating unrealistic workloads and not supporting colleagues
- Being condescending or patronizing
- Using physical or verbal innuendo or abuse, using foul language, raising one's voice and shouting or humiliating someone in front of colleagues
- Breaking confidences

Bullying takes place in all environments. It takes place in politics, workplaces, schools, the home, the military, prisons, among others. In the medical community, bullying behaviors create a toxic environment for staff, patients, and families. School environments, workplace environments, and health care environments should have policies to help eliminate an atmosphere in which bullying and/or violence exists. Those who are bullied are prone to negative feelings about self, humiliation, poor self-concept, and great emotional pain, and many can suffer severe reactions that may last a lifetime, such as depression, posttraumatic stress disorder (PTSD), anxiety disorders, and even attempted or completed suicide.

PREVALENCE AND COMORBIDITY

Anger, aggression, and violence are common aspects of social interaction, occur in all environments, and have become a major public health concern. The incidence of workplace violence in the health care system is notably higher than that found in private-sector industries. Workplace-related violence against nurses is a major occupational health problem. Violence can occur anywhere in the hospital but is most frequent in psychiatric units, emergency departments (EDs), waiting rooms, and geriatric units. Nurses in EDs experienced the highest rate of on-the-job violence.

Specific medical and neurocognitive disorders can result in agitated, aggressive, or violent behavior. For example, certain brain tumors, Alzheimer's disease, delirium, temporal lobe epilepsy, and traumatic brain injury (TBI) can cause changes in personality that include increased aggression or violence. Other medical conditions that may affect an individual's control of violence are infections, subdural hematomas, Tourette's syndrome, degenerative disorders, endocrine-metabolic imbalances, and intoxication.

People with mental health disorders are often perceived as potentially aggressive or violent. It is important to know that psychiatric patients are 2.5 times more often the recipients of violence (e.g., raped, mugged, attacked) than people in the general population (Feinstein & Rothberg, 2014). However, individuals with a chronic psychotic condition (e.g., schizophrenia, mania, substance intoxication/withdrawal) are at a higher risk of perpetrating violence than those who do not have psychotic conditions (Black & Andreasen, 2014). Some individuals with personality disorders (e.g., narcissistic, antisocial, and borderline personality disorders) are also more prone to violent behavior.

THEORY

Environmental and Demographic Correlates of Violence

The strongest predictor of adult violence is *childhood aggression*. Behaviors such as setting fires, performing acts of animal cruelty during childhood, or being diagnosed with conduct disorder are red flags (Black & Andreasen, 2014). Many violent adults were the target of violence in childhood (e.g., physical, sexual, and emotional abuse) and are perpetuating the cycle of violence.

One of the strongest contributing factors to violent behavior in clinical settings is the *abuse of alcohol and other substances* (intoxication or withdrawal), such as amphetamines, cocaine, hallucinogenic drugs, sedative-hypnotics, and other substances that lower inhibitions and impair judgment.

Demographic correlates include risk factors such as male gender, young age (15 to 24 years), and family history of violence. Persons of **lower socioeconomic status** are more likely to be victims and perpetrators of violence. Poorer populations are more apt to experience discrimination, family breakdown, alienation, and a constant fight for survival (Black & Andreasen, 2014). Socially, angry reactions are learned and reinforced through the family and societal norms.

Neurobiological Factors

Brain Structure

There is no one site in the brain responsible for anger, aggression, and violence, although there are many areas of the brain that are believed to contribute in some way to either increasing or decreasing these emotions. The neurobiology of aggression and violence is complex. Our knowledge is incomplete, and much of it comes from animal studies.

As we already know, the limbic system is responsible for our emotional reactions and plays a role in storing our memories. The limbic system is composed of the hypothalamus, hippocampus, amygdala, septum, cingulate, and fornix. Essentially, the *limbic system* mediates primitive emotions and behaviors that are necessary for survival. It has a role in regulating the behavior of aggression in humans and animals, and it judges events as either aversive or rewarding. Specific areas of importance include the hippocampus and *amygdala*. It is thought that the "amygdala is a vital nexus in the neural network supporting aggression and violence" (Victoroff, 2009, p. 2675) and that the amygdaloid cells respond to perceived threats (e.g., emotional facial expressions).

Anger stimulates the *hypothalamus*, causing the body to react to the anticipation of harm (fight-or-flight response). The *temporal lobe* of the brain receives messages from both the limbic system and the hypothalamus. In the temporal lobe, memory is thought to be integrated; memory of previous insults is important in the cognitive appraisal of threat in the face of new stimuli. When the temporal lobe is involved in complex partial seizures, we are more likely to see aggressive behavior. The prefrontal cortex receives messages from both the limbic system and the hypothalamus and appears to play a role in modulating the aggressive impulses in a social context and making judgments of these impulses (Gerken, Gross, & Saunders, 2016). Both magnetic resonance imaging (MRI) studies and positron emission tomography (PET) scans in the prefrontal cortex show changes in violent individuals. MRIs show a reduction in the volume of the prefrontal gray matter. PET scans reveal decreased prefrontal blood flow and metabolism (Gerken et al., 2016).

Neurotransmitters

It seems that most of the neurotransmitters have some connection to aggression and violence. However, to date, the presence or absence of a single neurotransmitter has not been conclusively identified as a contributing factor for violence, although there have been studies and theories.

In numerous studies, low central *serotonin (5-HT, 5-hydroxytryptamine)* function has been correlated with impulsive aggression as well as an impulsive history of suicide, and with low levels of 5-hydroxyindoleacetic acid (5-HIAA), a metabolite of serotonin, in cerebrospinal fluid (CSF). Serotonin is thought to act as a modulator in the central nervous system to lessen impulsive and violent behaviors (Black & Andreasen, 2014). It is unclear, however, if low levels of 5-HIAA in CSF are a marker for impulsivity or a certain pattern of aggression.

As complicated as the catecholamines *(norepinephrine [NE]* and *epinephrine)* are, they are thought to play a role in preparing the body for the fight-or-flight response, both on a peripheral level (preparing muscles and cardiac status for fight or flight) and on a cognitive level. NE may enhance vigilance and play a role in impulsivity and episodic violence in humans (Gerken et al., 2016). The exact effects of NE on violence and aggression are unclear.

It is well accepted that the dopaminergic system is involved in behavioral activation, motivated behavior, and reward processing. It has also been established that dopamine plays an active role in the modulation of aggressive behaviors (Jalain, 2014). A study by Schluter and colleagues (2013) found that higher degrees of dopamine storage in the striatum and midbrain correlated with lower degrees of aggressive responses as identified in PET scans.

Genetic Factors

Twin studies, adoption studies, studies of twins reared apart, and family and molecular genetic studies have long suggested that there is a genetic component in the etiology of violence. However, no specific chromosomal abnormality has been associated with increased risk for aggression (Gerken et al., 2016). Although there seem to be genetic contributions to aggression, most scientists agree that genetic characteristics alone do not account for the complexities of human behavior.

Most likely, the study of the neurobehavioral aspect of violence—particularly frontal lobe dysfunction, altered serotonin metabolism, and the influence of heredity—will lead to a deeper understanding of factors in the genesis of violence. There is little doubt that social and evolutionary factors most likely play a role.

Cultural Considerations

Violence is a complex issue. As mentioned previously, socioeconomic issues, medical issues, and psychiatric issues are all contributing factors. The different rates of violent crime among societies and within subcultures emphasize the importance of social factors in the genesis of violence. For example, race or ethnicity may be a factor.

Males, in general, are far more violent than females. Individuals with the highest prevalence of violence appear to be of lower economic class, are male, have substance abuse disorders, and/or have psychotic or organic medical disorders. A subculture that supports the use of intimidation and aggression as an acceptable way of problem solving and achieving social status can reinforce the use of violence as acceptable behavior. This is particularly true in an environment where healthy, appropriate, and effective ways of dealing with frustration, anger, and aggression are not modeled.

APPLICATION OF THE NURSING PROCESS

ASSESSMENT

Subjective Data

On admission, the nurse completes a comprehensive history of the patient gathered from a variety of sources (using informatics to obtain the patient's history, both medical and psychological), including family, friends, and the patient when appropriate. It is important for the nurse to take an accurate history of the patient's background and usual coping skills, as well as to determine the patient's perception of the issue (if possible). For example, does the patient have a history of previous violence, substance abuse, or psychotic behavior?

The patient should be asked the following questions (Black & Andreasen, 2014):

1. Have you ever thought of harming someone else?
2. Have you ever seriously injured another person?
3. What is the most violent thing you have ever done?

Objective Data

Expressions of anxiety and anger generally look similar. Both may involve increased demands, irritability, frowning, redness of the face, pacing, twisting of the hands, or clenching and unclenching the fists. Changes in mood and behavior from quiet to talkative and loud, from talkative to silent and withdrawn, from calm to angry, or from depressed to elated also may occur. Box 24.1 identifies signs and symptoms that indicate the risk of escalating anger, which may in turn lead to aggressive behavior. Simple observation of these signs, however, does not provide the information necessary to determine the appropriate intervention. Recent history can be invaluable.

VIGNETTE: A male has been admitted to the unit for spouse and child abuse. He is considered at high risk for violent acting-out behaviors. Violence can be anticipated to be toward female authority figures and female staff members. Therefore male staff is assigned to this patient. He is placed in a secure room until his behavior can be assessed more fully. The male nurse conducts the interview with appropriate and unobtrusive staff for backup.

VIGNETTE: An intoxicated, homophobic male is admitted to the unit for detoxification. Violence can be anticipated if an all-male team is brought together to escort the patient to a quiet room. Therefore a female staff member is chosen as the spokesperson, once again with appropriate and unobtrusive staff available for backup.

Assessment Guidelines

Anger, Aggression, and Violent Acting-Out

1. A history of violence is the single best predictor of future violence.
2. Paranoid ideation and frank psychosis (e.g., command hallucinations) are indicators of possible aggression or violence.
3. Patients who are hyperactive, impulsive, or predisposed to irritability are at higher risk for violence.
4. Assess the patient's risk for violence:
   - Does the patient have a wish or intent to harm?
   - Does the patient have a plan?
   - Does the patient have the means available to carry out the plan?
   - Does the patient have demographic risk factors, including male gender, ages 15 to 24 years, low socioeconomic status, and weak support system?
5. Aggression occurs most often in the context of limit setting by the nurse.
6. Patients with a history of inability to control anger and limited coping skills, including the use of intimidation, are at higher risk of using violence.
7. Assess self for personal triggers and responses likely to escalate the individual's violence.
8. Assess personal sense of competence when in any situation of potential conflict; consider asking for the assistance of another staff member.
9. Assess any personal negative thoughts or feelings you may hold toward the patient that could escalate both your anxiety and the anxiety of the patient.
10. Draw on previous knowledge of the policies and procedures for providing care to potentially violent patients.

BOX 24.1 Some Predictive Factors for Violent Outcomes[a]

1. Signs and symptoms that usually *(but not always)* precede violence:[b]
   a. Angry, irritable affect
   b. Hyperactivity: most important predictor of imminent violence (e.g., pacing, restlessness, slamming doors)
   c. Increasing anxiety and tension: clenched jaw or fist, rigid posture, fixed or tense facial expression, mumbling to self (patient may have shortness of breath, sweating, and rapid pulse rate)
   d. Verbal abuse: profanity, argumentativeness
   e. Loud voice, change of pitch, or very soft voice forcing others to strain to hear
   f. Intense eye contact or avoidance of eye contact
2. Recent acts of violence, including property violence
3. Stone silence
4. Suspiciousness or paranoid thinking
5. Alcohol or drug intoxication (withdrawal)
6. Possession of a weapon or object that may be used as a weapon (e.g., fork, knife, rock)
7. Milieu characteristics conducive to violence:
   a. Loud
   b. Overcrowding
   c. Staff inexperience
   d. Provocative or controlling staff
   e. Poor limit setting
   f. Staff inconsistency (e.g., arbitrary revocation of privileges)

[a] Violent outcomes include screaming, cursing, yelling, spitting, biting, throwing objects, and hitting and punching at self or others.
[b] Sometimes violence may seem to "come out of the blue."

DIAGNOSIS

The safety of patients and others is always the first priority. When anxiety escalates to levels at which there is a threat of harm to self or others, *Risk for self destructive behavior, Risk for self mutilation, Impaired impulse control,* and *Risk for violence* are primary diagnoses. If a patient's anxiety is escalating and not amenable to early nursing interventions, and if de-escalating techniques are not effective, psychopharmacological means or restraints may be necessary to ensure the safety of patients and staff.

Initially, when anxiety begins to escalate and there is a potential for aggression, *Difficulty coping* (overwhelmed or maladaptive) is a likely nursing diagnosis. Patients may have coping skills that are adequate for daily events in their lives but are overwhelmed by the stresses of illness or hospitalization. Therefore *Risk for stress overload* might be an appropriate diagnosis. A more long-term nursing diagnosis for patients who have a pattern of maladaptive coping that is marginally effective and consists of coping strategies that have been developed to meet unusual or extraordinary situations (e.g., abusive families) would be *Ineffective family coping.*

Nurses can teach patients methods of coping that will decrease anxiety and distress. However, patient behavior may escalate quickly, or the patient may mask early signs of distress. Nurses may be distracted and may miss those early signs, even when they are visible. Other nursing diagnoses may include *Confusion, Impaired cognition, Risk for compromised dignity,* and *Risk for difficulty with coping.*

OUTCOMES IDENTIFICATION

Short-term or intermediate outcome goals may include the following:

- The patient will display nonviolent behaviors toward self and others by *(date).*
- The patient will recognize when anger and aggressive tendencies begin to escalate and employ at least one new tension-reducing behavior at that time (e.g., time out, deep breathing, talking to a previously designated person, employing an exercise such as jogging) by *(date).*
- The patient will make plans to continue with long-term therapy (individual, family, group, anger management, medication management) to work on violence prevention strategies and increase coping skills by *(date).*

Long-term outcome goals may include the following:

- The patient and others will remain free from injury.
- Hostile and abusive behavior toward others, property, animals, and so on will cease.

TABLE 24.1 Interventions for the Pre-Assaultive Stage: Use of De-Escalation Techniques

Intervention	Rationale
1. Pay attention to angry and aggressive behavior. Respond as early as possible (see Box 24.1).	1. Minimization of angry behaviors and ineffective limit setting are the most frequent factors contributing to the escalation of violence.
2. Emphasize that you are on the patient's side (e.g., "We want to help you, not hurt you.") and that "this is a safe place and you are safe." The clinician should stand at an angle to the patient so as not to appear confrontational.	2. Establish yourself as an ally who wants to help the patient gain control. Never provoke or use threats.
3. Assess personal safety and provide for self-care.	3. Pay attention to the environment. • Leave door open or use hallway. Choose a quiet place but one that is visible to staff. • Have a quick exit available. • If you are uncomfortable, have other staff nearby. • The more angry the patient, the more space is needed to feel comfortable. • Never turn your back on an angry patient. • If on a *home visit*, go with a colleague. • Leave immediately if there are signs that behavior is escalating out of control.
4. Appear calm and in control.	4. The perception that someone is in control can be comforting and calming to an individual who is beginning to lose control.
5. Do not try to speak while the aggressive person is yelling.	5. Loudly arguing with the patient will only escalate anger and violence.
6. Speak softly in a nonprovocative, nonjudgmental manner.	6. When the tone of voice is low and calm and words are spoken slowly, anxiety levels in others may decrease.
7. Demonstrate genuineness and concern. • Do not treat the individual in a humiliating manner. • Ask, "What will help now?"	7. Even the most psychotic schizophrenic individual may respond to nonprovocative interpersonal contact and expressions of concern and caring.
8. Set clear, consistent, and enforceable limits on behavior (see Box 24.2) (e.g., "It's okay to be angry with Tom, but it is not okay to threaten him. If you are having trouble controlling your anger, we will help you.").	8. Gives patient understanding of expectations and consequences of not adhering to those behaviors.
9. If patient is willing, both nurse and patient should sit at a 45-degree angle. Do not tower over or stare at the patient.	9. Sitting at a 45-degree angle puts you both on the same level but allows for frequent breaks in eye contact. Towering over or staring can be interpreted as threatening or controlling by paranoid individuals.
10. When patient begins to talk, listen. Use clarification.	10. Allows patient to feel heard and understood, helps build rapport, and energy can be channeled productively.
11. Acknowledge the patient's needs regardless of whether the expressed needs are rational or irrational, possible or impossible to meet.	11. Contributes to individual's perception that the nurse is trying to understand the core of the aggression. Determine how some of the patient's needs can be met in a productive way.

- The use of assertive and cognitive reasoning behaviors to replace aggressive behaviors is in constant evidence.
- Various healthy anxiety reduction techniques are used to keep anger in check
- Aggressive and violent impulses are controlled.

PLANNING

Planning interventions necessitate conducting a sound assessment, including history (previous acts of violence, comorbid disorders), present coping skills, and willingness and capacity of the patient to learn alternative and nonviolent ways of handling angry feelings. However, one of the most important aspects of planning is consistency of approach by staff. A clear management approach to deal with violent situations and individuals includes staff well versed in unit protocols and well trained in **de-escalation techniques**. De-escalation techniques are outlined and discussed under "Implementation" and in Table 24.1. *Teamwork and cooperation* are paramount in protecting other patients, staff, and particularly the individual who is losing control. The following questions help determine appropriate planning:

Does the patient have:

- Good coping skills but is presently overwhelmed?
- Marginal coping skills?
- A tendency to use anger or violence as a way to cover other feelings and gain a sense of mastery or control?
- A neuropsychiatric or chronic psychotic disorder?
- A tendency toward violence?
- Cognitive deficits (in the form of misinterpretation of environmental stimuli) that predispose to anger?

Does the situation call for:

- Psychotherapeutic approaches to teach the patient new skills for handling anger?
- Immediate intervention to prevent overt violence (de-escalation techniques, restraints or seclusion, or medications)?

Does the environment provide:

- A safe, therapeutic milieu?
- Privacy for the patient?
- Enough space for patients, or is there overcrowding?
- A healthy balance between structured time and quiet time?

Do the skills of the staff call for:

- Additional education in verbal de-escalation techniques?
- Counseling interventions because of punitive and arbitrary approaches to patients?
- Additional training in restraint techniques?

Planning also involves attention to the number of personnel who are available to respond to a potentially violent situation.

BOX 24.2 Setting Limits

1. Set limits in only those areas in which a clear need exists to protect the patient or others.
2. Establish realistic and enforceable consequences of exceeding limits.
3. Make the patient aware of limits and the consequences of not adhering to the limits before incidents occur. The patient should be told in a clear, polite, and firm manner what the limits and consequences are and should be given the opportunity to discuss any feelings or reactions to them.
4. All limits should be supported by the entire staff, written in the care plan, and communicated verbally to all involved.
5. When a decision to discontinue the limits is made by the entire staff, the decision is based on consistent desired behavior, not promises or sporadic efforts.
6. The staff should formulate their own plan to address their own difficulty in maintaining consistent limits.

Adapted from Chitty, K. K., & Maynard, C. K. (1986). Managing manipulation. *Journal of Psychosocial Nursing and Mental Health Services, 24*(6), 8–13.

IMPLEMENTATION

Ensuring Safety

Promoting safety is always a first consideration. **Ensure your safety first.** You must feel safe to be able to communicate in a calm manner. Staff and other personnel should be alerted in case reinforcement is needed. The goals are that no one will become hurt and the patient will experience the least restrictive interventions. The following is a list of specific interventions for working with a potentially angry, aggressive, or violent patient:

1. Move the individual to a calm and quiet place.
2. All patients should be searched for contraband and dangerous objects when admitted to the unit and after visits.
3. Give the patient space. Always minimize personal risks. Stay at least one arm's length away from the patient. Use more space if the patient is anxious or if you want more space. *Always trust your instincts.*
4. Provide adequate space for the patient and staff to ensure easy withdrawal from an escalating situation.
5. Know where panic buttons or alarms are located to be able to call for assistance from other staff quickly. Sometimes it is necessary to wear a body alarm to ensure safety.
6. Exit strategies apply to both the nurse and the patient. The nurse should be positioned between the patient and the door, but not directly in front of the patient or in front of the doorway. Facing the patient can be interpreted as confrontational, and it can also make the patient feel trapped. It is better to stand off to the side and encourage the patient to have a seat.
7. Set limits at the outset using these de-escalation techniques (Box 24.2):
   - Direct approach: "Violence is unacceptable." Describe the consequences (medications, restraints, seclusion). Best for confused or psychotic patients.
   - Indirect approach: Use the indirect approach if the patient is not confused or psychotic. Give the patient a choice. "You have a choice. You can take this medication and go into the interview room (or hallway, for example) and talk, or you can sit in the seclusion room until you feel less anxious."
8. When interviewing a patient whose behavior begins to escalate:
   - Provide feedback about what you observe: "You seem to be very upset." Such an observation allows exploration of the patient's feelings and may lead to de-escalation of the situation.
   - If the patient's behavior continues to escalate, end the interview and assure the patient that the staff will provide for the patient's safety (as well as everyone else's safety); then leave the patient.
9. Having enough staff is essential for a show of strength and is often enough to avert confrontation. One person is chosen as a spokesperson and is the only one who talks to the patient, but staff need to maintain an unobtrusive and nonthreatening presence in case the situation escalates.
10. Give the patient the opportunity to walk to the quiet room voluntarily without assistance when team interventions seem appropriate.
11. Do not touch the patient unless the team is with you and you are ready for a possible restraint situation.
12. In the event of a restraint or seclusion situation, the team functions as a single unit, with each member assigned a limb or a function as previously practiced according to unit protocols and policy.
13. Avoid wearing dangling earrings, necklaces, or ponytails. If wearing a lanyard, ensure it has a safety break-away feature. The patient may become focused on these and grab at them, causing serious injury. This is a serious danger.

Stages of Violence

When interventions to prevent or deal with patient violence are considered, sometimes it is helpful to identify the stage of violence. These stages include the *pre-assaultive stage*, the *assaultive stage*, and the *post-assaultive stage*. See Chapter 11 for nursing interventions for moderate levels of anxiety that escalate to severe and panic levels.

Pre-Assaultive Stage: De-Escalation Approaches

During the pre-assaultive stage, the patient becomes increasingly agitated. Staff members require training in both verbal techniques of de-escalation and physical techniques to restrain without harm. The better trained the staff, the less chance that either staff or the patient will be injured. Verbal interventions are frequently sufficient during this stage. Interventions at this stage are listed in Table 24.1.

Throughout these procedures, maintain the patient's self-esteem and dignity. Linehan (1993) states that respect can be maintained if the nurse operates from the following assumptions:

- Patients are doing the best they can.
- Patients want to improve.
- Patients' behaviors make sense within their world view.

The use of empathic statements—such as "It sounds like you are in pain and confused," "You're here to get help, and we're going to try to figure out what's going on," and "Let us help you, don't be afraid"—can aid in reducing anxiety and anger. These statements reinforce the feeling that the person is in a safe environment and that everyone is there to help in his or her treatment and that staff members have an idea of what the person is going through.

VIGNETTE: A 24-year-old male who was in an automobile accident is bedridden with a pelvic fracture. During his first day of admission, he yells at each nurse who walks by his room, using expletives in his demands that the nurse enter the room.

Intervention

The nurse who is assigned to the patient for the evening stops in his doorway after he yells at her. She asks in a calm manner, showing mild disbelief, "Is this working for you? Do nurses really come in here when you yell at them that way?" The patient responds sullenly, justifying his behavior by complaining about his care. The nurse responds by saying, "It seems to me that you need to feel you can get care when you need it." The patient responds in a loud voice that he has been waiting 20 minutes for a bedpan—how would she like it? The nurse gets him his bedpan, and he calms down somewhat. The nurse's challenge has caught his attention. The nurse then goes on to suggest (i.e., teach) alternative strategies for contacting her and other nurses. The strategies are immediately put to use by the patient.

When health care personnel can teach patients alternate strategies and healthier ways to meet their needs, patients have more choices and thus more control over their situation.

Assaultive Stage: Medication, Seclusion, and Restraint

The American Psychiatric Nurses Association's (APNA, 2000, rev. 2007, rev. 2014) *Seclusion and Restraint Standards of Practice* states:

> *Standard: Any staff providing care to persons at risk for harming themselves or others and who participate in seclusion and restraint shall have received training and demonstrate current competency in all aspects of dealing with behavioral emergencies.*

Be sure to know the unit and hospital protocol for seclusion and restraint in whichever part of the hospital you choose to work.

If the patient progresses to the assaultive stage, the staff must respond quickly. Generally, a team approach with at least five staff members is advisable to restrain a resistant patient, but the team may be larger if the patient requires it. One person is chosen as the spokesperson or leader and is the only one who speaks to the patient and instructs members of the team. The following interventions include the use of medications and seclusion and/or physical restraints.

Seclusion "is the involuntary confinement of a person alone in a room or an area where the person is physically prevented from leaving. It may only be used for the management of violent or self-destructive behavior" (APNA, 2000, rev. 2007, rev. 2014). **Restraint** refers to (1) any manual method or physical or mechanical device, material, or equipment that immobilizes or reduces the ability of a person to move his or her arms, legs, body, or head freely or (2) a drug or medication when it is used as a restriction to manage the person's behavior or restrict the person's freedom of movement and is not a standard treatment or dosage for the person's condition (APNA, 2000, rev. 2007, rev. 2014).

The least restrictive means of restraint is *always* tried first, and seclusion or restraint is used *only after* alternative interventions have been attempted (e.g., trauma-informed approach, verbal interventions, medications, decrease in sensory stimulation, removal of a particular problematic stimulus, presence of a significant other, frequent observation, use of a sitter who provides 24-hour one-to-one observation of the patient).

Seclusion or restraint is used in the following circumstances (APNA, 2000, rev. 2007, rev. 2014):

- The patient presents a clear and present danger to self or others.
- The patient has been legally detained for involuntary treatment and is thought to pose an escape risk.
- The patient requests to be secluded or restrained.

When deciding on whether to use restraints or seclusion, Tasman and colleagues (2015) suggest: "If the patient is an immediate danger to others, restraint is indicated. Yet if a patient is only disruptive and uncooperative, but is not a danger to others, seclusion should be considered. If the patient seems willing to sit in a quiet room, then an unlocked seclusion room may be attempted. If not, then a locked seclusion is indicated. However, if the patient could or does become a danger to self while in seclusion, restraint is appropriate. Even when restrained, a patient will engage."

Before the development of psychotropic medications, seclusion and restraint were extremely common methods of managing aggressive behavior. In the past half-century their use has decreased dramatically as a result of effective medications. *All facilities that use seclusion and restraint have strict regulatory policies that should follow state, federal, and regulatory agency guidelines. Students and all staff members should be familiar with their institution's policies.*

APPLYING THE ART

A Person With Anger and Aggression

Scenario

I'd just attended a group therapy session on the forensic unit, during which the group leader had to set limits with 24-year-old Hector. During our initial one-to-one meeting, Hector had been almost overly polite, in contrast to his abrasiveness with some of the other patients in group. I followed Hector out of the group room.

Therapeutic Goal

By the end of this interaction, Hector will identify at least one incident where a person can demonstrate an act of kindness or caring toward another and still see himself as masculine.

Student–Patient Interaction	Thoughts, Communication Techniques, and Mental Health Nursing Concepts
Hector: *(In harsh, loud voice.)* "Bunch of losers." ***Student's feelings:*** *I was taken aback and intimidated by how lightning-fast Hector's anger arose when some other guys took the seats that Hector had chosen for us during group.*	He went from being friendly with me this morning to this abrupt outburst of anger.
Student: "You're talking about what just happened in group." *(I walk toward the seating area closest to the nurses' station, where I can be observed by the staff, and signal them for help if need be.)* ***Student's feelings:*** *After Hector's bullying episode in group, I feel safer in plain view.*	I validate to make sure I understand his reference. I am beginning to realize that Hector's earlier politeness and charm might have to do with his personality disorder.
Hector: *(In a loud and angry voice.)* "Just because I made those guys get out of those seats. What did you think? You think that's such a big deal?"	
Student: "But why did you have to yell and scream at them? I remember some yelling and swearing." ***Student's feelings:*** *I didn't think this through with all his anger coming out. I am reacting defensively, and I'm feeling like I am in way over my head. I feel like I need a break.*	Asking a "why" question is nontherapeutic for sure. He will take it as criticism. I hope he does not get any angrier.

Continued

APPLYING THE ART—cont'd

A Person With Anger and Aggression

Student–Patient Interaction	Thoughts, Communication Techniques, and Mental Health Nursing Concepts
Student: "What were you feeling when you saw they were in the seats you wanted?" ***Student's feelings:*** *I hope he focuses on his feelings rather than my accusatory "why" question.*	I attempt to translate into feelings. When in doubt, always go for feelings.
Hector: "Look, I always get a raw deal. The leader likes those guys better than me."	After all this, I do not think I will be going with him to occupational therapy. That way, I will get to consult my instructor to check if I am on the right track.
Student: "But when this happened, you were feeling … what?" ***Student's feelings:*** *It really is okay to take care of myself. Knowing I can access my teacher and staff readily if need be allows me to refocus and attend to Hector's needs.*	I again ask him to focus on his feelings.
Hector: "Nothing. Never mind."	I wonder what makes Hector unable to look at his feelings at all. He refers to the leader like he is competing for attention. Almost like sibling rivalry. Perhaps all that macho talk hides low self-esteem.
Student: "I think I'd feel frustrated when directed to give the other patients their original chairs back. Maybe even a little embarrassed."	I give information about self, but really the intent is to reflect Hector's possible feelings.
Hector: *(Avoids eye contact.)* "My dad would've pounded the _____ out of me for letting those guys win."	
Student: "You are able to say how your dad taught lessons with his fists. I'm guessing any little boy would feel enormous pressure when interacting with others in the context of either you win or you get pounded." ***Student's feelings:*** *I'm beginning to see how powerless Hector must feel somewhere inside all that bravado. I am beginning to feel some compassion for him.*	I give support by using the words "you are able to" in order to encourage Hector to recognize a link between his current responses and past abusive experiences.
Hector: "He was just teaching me how to be a man."	He justifies his father pounding on him. A history of violence is the best predictor of violence. Hector defines how to be a man in the same way his father did. Does he know other ways exist?
Student: "I wonder if a person can be a man in other ways besides winning or losing. This morning I saw you help when someone bumped the patient carrying breakfasts back for those who eat on the unit." ***Student's feelings:*** *My belief in my nursing self fluctuates. But I do feel some rapport exists between us.*	I use an indirect question and make an observation of his recent behavior. I know that when a person feels comfortable with you, even if one uses "nontherapeutic techniques," a person will often understand the intent behind the words.
Hector: "What a mess."	
Student: "And you helped anyway. Then, when the patient apologized so much, you told him,' It's okay. Accidents happen.'"	I make observations describing Hector's healthier behaviors, like spontaneously helping another.
Hector: "Others helped too."	Hector excels at generating negative attention. He does not know what to do with positive feedback.
Student: "You also spoke kindly to him."	Again I make an observation and give my attention to positively reinforcing his kind act.
Hector: *(Shrugs.)*	
Student: "Sometimes it seems manliness and kindness might coexist in one person."	I deliberately link Hector's kind words with his earlier idea of manhood.
Hector: *(Nods slightly.)* "I need a drink of water." *(Goes to water fountain.)* ***Student's feelings:*** *I feel glad that he nods even slightly. I find it difficult to make even small changes, like regularly flossing my teeth. What must Hector's world be like? I have people who care about me. Who does he have for support … especially since he's an expert at pushing others away?*	His intermittent explosive disorder is most likely connected to his repeated abusive "lessons" equating any vulnerability or even kindness as weakness. Hector nods, showing partial understanding that demonstrating kindness is okay for a man, although it appears to make him anxious as he uses physical withdrawal (getting a drink) to protect himself (fight-or-flight response).

A patient may not be held in seclusion or restraint without a physician's order (verbal, written, or telephone order). Sometimes this is not possible, and the decision is made by a qualified staff member to initiate seclusion or restraint because of a behavioral emergency. However, either way, the patient must be evaluated within 1 hour by a physician or licensed independent practitioner (LIP). Restraints may be preferred when staff members believe that continued verbal and calming strategies would allow the patient to de-escalate and that restraints could be removed at the earliest possible time. Mechanical restraints are avoided in individuals who have a history of sexual abuse and trauma, and they also are contraindicated in patients who may be at risk for positional asphyxia, sudden cardiac collapse, or other physical and medical conditions.

Once in restraints, a patient must be protected from all sources of harm. *Each team member is trained in the correct use of physical restraining maneuvers and in the use of physical restraints.* The team is organized before approaching the patient so that each team member knows his or her individual responsibility regarding limb securing. The spokesperson explains to the individual in a straightforward and calm manner exactly what the team is about to do and why. If restraints are to be used, the person is informed at this point of the team's intent and the reason for the team's actions. Sometimes the patient is ready to cooperate and moves to the seclusion room on his or her own.

Alternatives to Seclusion and Restraint: The Recovery Model. Sivak (2012) points out that there is no evidence to support the therapeutic value of seclusion and restraint and reports that 150 people die each year as a result of these practices with the mentally ill and that others are left psychologically harmed, physically injured, or traumatized (Substance Abuse and Mental Health Services Administration [SAMHSA], 2011). New approaches that focus on the recovery model are being researched and developed to reduce the use of seclusion and restraint. One potential intervention that came out of the recovery movement is the use of **comfort rooms**, where the psychiatric facility sets aside a "special room" to which a person can go voluntarily to self-manage anxiety and distress (Sivak, 2012).

The use of recovery-model approaches and the "trauma-informed approach" has been reported as helpful to reduce the use of seclusion and restraint (American Psychiatric Association, 2015; APNA, 2000, rev. 2007, rev. 2014). A trauma-informed approach and trauma-specific interventions address reducing the trauma's consequences and facilitate healing. According to SAMHSA (2015), "A program, organization, or system that is trauma-informed:

1. *Realizes* the widespread impact of trauma and understands potential paths for recovery;
2. *Recognizes* the signs and symptoms of trauma in clients, families, staff, and others involved with the system;
3. *Responds* by fully integrating knowledge about trauma into policies, procedures, and practices; and
4. Seeks to actively resist *re-traumatization.*"

SAMHSA (2015) further notes, "A *trauma-informed approach* reflects adherence to six key principles rather than a prescribed set of practices or procedures. These principles may be generalizable across multiple types of settings, although terminology and application may be setting- or sector-specific.

1. Safety
2. Trustworthiness and transparency
3. Peer support
4. Collaboration and mutuality
5. Empowerment, voice, and choice
6. Cultural, historical, and gender issues"

VIGNETTE: A 19-year-old male has a 2-year history of quadriplegia. This patient also has a history of drug abuse that began in grade school, an inability to set or work toward long-term goals, and a primary coping style of anger and intimidation. The patient is admitted to an inpatient psychiatric unit because of increasing suicidal ideation. He clearly communicates to staff that his preferred means of coping with anger is to "cuss people out" and run into them with his wheelchair. However, in the hospital, the consequence of wheelchair assaults is that the patient is secluded in his room, which he finds intolerable. The patient asks the staff to help him manage his anger.

Intervention

The nurse assigned to this young man sets aside time to interview him regarding the triggers for his anger. He identifies several issues that "make him angry." These typically relate to feeling unheard and controlled by the staff. Together, the nurse and patient examine alternative ways for him to deal with these situations, such as telling the staff that he does not feel that they are listening to him and letting them know that he needs to be involved in the planning of his care to increase his sense of control. The patient and nurse role-play a situation in which the patient is told by a staff member that he must attend a group session. Such a situation would usually result in the patient becoming angry and aggressive, but in the role-played situation, he is willing to "try out" alternative communication techniques to communicate his feelings to the staff member and thus to handle his anger. In addition, the patient is willing to enter into a behavioral contract with the nurse, stating that he will not curse at staff or assault anyone with his wheelchair. Instead, he will let the staff know when he is feeling angry and what the triggering issue is so that a nonaggressive resolution can be found.

Response

Because this patient is motivated to gain increased personal control, he responds positively to these suggestions. In addition, once it becomes clear that feeling unheard and out of control underlies most episodes of anger, the patient is able to target these issues for problem solving. He rapidly develops effective and appropriate ways to make himself heard and understood. He also becomes adept at communicating when he feels out of control and at finding ingenious ways of negotiating control on issues that are particularly important to him. The patient's suicidal impulses, which occur when he is frustrated, also diminish.

Once the patient is restrained, the nurse might administer an intramuscular injection of a barbiturate, antihistamine, or antipsychotic depending on the individual's underlying condition and the physician's order. The nurse's role is to provide an explanation to the person for the medication and to make sure that the individual is properly restrained so that the medication can be administered safely. Throughout this time, the spokesperson continues to relate to the person using a calm, steady voice, communicating decisiveness, consistency, and control.

While the patient is restrained and in seclusion, staff closely monitor the patient to determine the person's ability to reintegrate into unit activities. Usually every 15 minutes, face-to-face observation is made through the locked door window. A person 14 years of age or younger should have constant face-to-face observation. Reintegration is gradual and is geared toward the patient's ability to handle increasing amounts of stimulation. If the reintegration proves to be too much for the patient and results in increased agitation, the patient is returned to the room or to another quiet area.

Generally, a structured reintegration is the best approach. For instance, reintegration can begin by reducing four-point restraints to two-point restraints. Once the patient no longer requires the locked seclusion room, the patient may be given specified time-out periods to leave the room and move slowly into the milieu of the unit. The time-out periods are gradually lengthened until the person is able to maintain control within the part of the unit that is quiet, dimly lit, and/or has fewer patients.

Post-Assaultive Stage

Once the patient no longer requires seclusion or restraints, the staff members should review the incident with the patient as well as among themselves. Discussion with the patient is an important part of the therapeutic process. Reviewing the incident allows the patient to learn from the situation, identify the stressors that precipitated the out-of-control behavior, and plan alternative ways of responding to these stressors in the future.

Critical Incident Debriefing

Staff analysis of an episode of violence, referred to as **critical incident debriefing**, is crucial for a number of reasons. *First,* a review is necessary to ensure that quality care was provided to the patient. Staff members need to critically examine their response to the patient. Questions to be answered include the following:

- Could we have done anything that would have prevented the violence?
- If yes, then what could have been done, and why was it not done in this situation?
- Did the team respond as a team? Were team members acting according to the policies and procedures of the unit? If not, why not?
- Is there a need for additional staff education regarding how to respond to violent patients?
- How do staff members feel about this patient? About this situation? Feelings of fear and anger must be discussed and handled. Otherwise, the patient may be dealt with in a punitive and nontherapeutic manner.

Second, the profound effects of workplace violence unfortunately do not disappear after the incident is over, and the harm is not only to the individual assaulted. At times some nurses and staff may internalize (depression, avoidance, withdrawal) or externalize (anger, outbursts, fluctuating mood) their emotional and behavioral responses to the event. These are normal responses to an abnormal event. However, agencies need to provide support and debriefing to prevent long-term psychological sequelae for all types of workplace violence. Employee morale, productivity, use of sick leave, transfer requests, and absenteeism are affected by patient violence, especially if a staff member has been injured. Staff members must feel supported by their peers as well as by the organizational policies and procedures established to maintain a safe environment.

Documentation of a Violent Episode

Most facilities provide standardized seclusion and restraint records. There are a number of areas for which the nurse *must* provide documentation in situations where violence either was averted or actually occurred:

- Reason for seclusion or restraint
- Assessment of behaviors that occurred during the pre-assaultive stage *(time)*
- Nursing interventions and the patient's responses *(time)*
- Evaluation of the interventions used
- Detailed description of the patient's behaviors during the assaultive stage
- All nursing interventions used to defuse the crisis
- Patient's response to those interventions
- Name(s) of person(s) called to assess the patient and order any medications, seclusion, and/or restraints *(time)*
- Time patient put in restraints or seclusion
- Observations of and interventions performed while the patient was in restraints or seclusion (food, toileting, vital signs, verbatim statements, and general behaviors) (15 to 30 minutes depending on state law)
- Any injuries to staff or patient
- The way in which the patient was reintegrated into the unit milieu *(time and behavior)*

See Chapter 6 for more definitive legal and procedural guidelines.

Anticipating Anxiety and Anger

Hospitals can be lonely, scary places for many people. Patients often feel that they are not being heard, and they may feel vulnerable, discounted, frightened, out of control of their situation, and tired. Some patients may have specific vulnerabilities for responding to their increasing anxiety and loss of autonomy with the use of violence. Therefore some patients with poor coping skills or mental or neurological problems may resort to anger, intimidation, or violence to obtain their short-term goals of feeling in control or mastery. For others, the anger occurs when limited or primitive attempts at coping are unsuccessful and alternatives are unknown. For these patients, anger and violence are particular risks in inpatient settings.

This is especially true for hospitalized patients with chemical or alcohol dependency who may be anxious about not having access to their substance of choice; they may have well-founded concerns that any physical pain will be inadequately addressed. Those individuals with marginal coping skills may also have personality styles that externalize blame. That is, they see the source of their discomfort and anxiety as being outside themselves; relief must therefore also come from an outside source (e.g., the nurse, medication).

Interventions begin with attempts to understand and meet the patient's needs. For instance, baseline anxiety can be moderated by the provision of comfort items before they are requested (e.g., decaffeinated coffee, deck of cards); this can build rapport and acts symbolically to reassure the patient. Anxiety also can be minimized by reducing ambiguity. This strategy includes clear and concrete communication. An interaction providing clarity about what the nurse can and cannot do is most usefully ended by offering something within the nurse's power to provide (i.e., leaving the patient with a "yes").

Interventions for anxiety might also include the use of distractions, such as magazines, action comics, and video games. Generally, distractions that are colorful and do not require sustained attention work best, although this varies according to the patient's interests and abilities. Finally, patients with a high level of baseline anxiety and limited coping skills are helped when their interactions with the treatment team are predictable; this might include speaking with the physician at a specific time each day or having the patient see a single spokesperson from the treatment team each day.

Because some patients have limited coping skills, once anxiety is moderated, nursing interventions include teaching alternative behaviors and strategies. With increased tools to deal with anxiety and frustration, patients have the opportunity to have choices and an increased sense of control over their behaviors.

Often, anger may be communicated via verbal abuse directed at the nurse. If attempts to teach alternatives have not been successful, three interventions can be used:

1. The first intervention is to leave the room as soon as the abuse begins; the patient can be informed that the nurse will return in a specific amount of time (e.g., 20 minutes) when the situation is calmer. This is said in a straightforward manner. If the nurse is in the middle of a procedure and cannot leave immediately, the nurse can discontinue conversation and eye contact, completing the procedure quickly and efficiently before leaving the room. Note that the nurse avoids chastising, threatening, or responding punitively to the patient.
2. Withdrawal of attention to the abuse is successful only if a second intervention is also used. This step requires attending positively to, and thus reinforcing, nonabusive communication by

the patient. Interventions can include discussing non–illness-related topics, responding to requests, and providing emotional support.

3. Patients who are regularly verbally abusive may respond best to the predictability of routine, such as scheduled contacts with the nurse (e.g., every 30 minutes or every 60 minutes) as long as the patient's behavior is not abusive. Such a contract works only to the extent that the nurse maintains the scheduled contacts as agreed on, and other staff members must be informed of the contract and remain consistent so that they do not inadvertently sabotage it by responding to incidental requests by the patient. If the patient's illness or injury requires nursing care outside the scheduled contact times, these visits can be carried out in a calm, brief manner. This contract is negotiated with the patient and addresses the patient's anxiety about getting needs met and being heard.

Implementing appropriate interventions can be difficult when the nurse is feeling threatened. Remaining matter-of-fact with patients who habitually use anger and intimidation can be difficult because these people are often skillful at making personal and pointed statements. It is important for the nurse to remember that patients do not know their nurses personally and thus have no basis on which to make accurate judgments. Nurses can also vent their own responses elsewhere, such as with other staff or family members or via critical incident debriefing.

Interventions for Patients With Neurocognitive Deficits

Patients with cognitive deficits are particularly at risk for acting aggressively. Such deficits may result from delirium, dementia (e.g., Alzheimer's disease, multi-infarct dementia), or brain injury. Traditional approaches to disorientation and to the agitation that it can cause have relied heavily on reality orientation and medication. Reality orientation consists of providing the correct information to the patient about place, date, and current life circumstances. For some patients, orientation does not work. Because of their cognitive disorder, they lose touch with reality, and they become frightened and agitated and may become aggressive. Sedating medication may calm agitation, but in some cases the risks may outweigh the benefits. *Sedation only further clouds a patient's sensorium, which makes disorientation worse and increases the risk for falls and injuries. It is better to examine alternative interventions.*

Sometimes the patient with a cognitive disorder experiences such severe agitation and aggression that it is referred to as a **catastrophic reaction**. The patient may scream, strike out, or cry because of overwhelming fear. Adopting a calm and unhurried manner is the best response. The steps for making contact with a patient who is experiencing a catastrophic reaction are listed in Box 24.3.

Patients who misperceive their setting or life situation may be calmed by validation therapy. Some disoriented patients believe that they are young and feel the need to return to important tasks that were a significant part of their earlier years. For example, an older woman may insist that she must go home to take care of her babies. Telling the patient that her babies have grown up and that she no longer has a home is not only cruel but also nontherapeutic and will result in increased agitation. It is often more helpful to reflect back to the patient the feelings behind her demand and to show understanding and concern for her worry.

Rather than attempting to reorient the patient, the nurse asks the patient to further describe the setting or situation referenced by the patient (e.g., the need to return home). During the conversation, the nurse can comment on what appears to be underlying the patient's distress, thus validating it. For example, the woman who believes that she needs to return home to care for her children is asked to tell the nurse more about her children. The nurse may note that the patient misses her children and may be lonely: "Mrs. Green, you miss your children, and the hospital can be a lonely place."

As the nurse shows interest in aspects of the patient's life, the nurse establishes himself or herself as a safe, understanding person who can be trusted. In turn, the patient often becomes calmer and more open to redirection. When patients reminisce in this fashion, they often reorient themselves: "Of course, they're all grown and doing well on their own now." See Chapter 18 for a more extensive discussion of interventions for people with cognitive impairments.

BOX 24.3 Cognitive Deficits and the Catastrophic Reaction: Making Contact

- Cognitive deficits result in:
  - A decreased ability to interpret sensory stimuli
  - A decreased ability to tolerate sensory stimuli
- Striking out represents fear or the feeling that the environment is out of control.
- The presence of a second agitated person (e.g., staff member) leads to increased agitation; therefore:
  1. Face the patient from within 2 feet, remaining as calm and unhurried as possible.
  2. Say the patient's name.
  3. Gain eye contact.
  4. Smile.
  5. Repeat steps 2 through 4 several times if necessary, to gain and maintain eye contact.
  6. Use gentle touch, and keep your voice soft (the person often matches this tone and lowers his or her voice also).
  7. Ask the patient if there is a need to use the bathroom.
  8. Help the patient regain a sense of control—ask what is needed.
  9. Validate the patient's feelings: "You look upset. This can be a confusing place."
  10. Use short, simple sentences. Complex explanations just represent more noise.
  11. Decrease sensory stimulation.
  12. Get the patient to use rhythmic sources of self-stimulation (e.g., humming, a rocking chair).

Adapted from Rader, J., Doan, J., & Schwab, M. (1985). How to decrease wandering, a form of agenda behavior. *Geriatric Nursing, 6*(4), 196–199.

Psychotherapy

Management of chronic aggression requires comprehensive neuropsychological testing and cognitive-behavioral assessment to establish the appropriate treatment approach for each individual. Besides psychopharmacological treatment, individual therapies may include behavioral management, cognitive-behavioral techniques, family interventions, and psychosocial supports (Gerken et al., 2016). The cognitive-behavioral assessment includes determining the psychotherapeutic approach most appropriate for a chronically aggressive patient. Data are obtained regarding the type of aggressive behavior, psychiatric diagnosis, and patient's intellectual ability. Behavioral techniques include limit setting, distraction and redirecting techniques, relaxation, and biofeedback. These techniques have met with limited success.

Gerken and colleagues (2016) suggest that the trauma-informed approach, as well as trauma-informed therapies in combination with medication, is much more successful for diminishing the need for restraint and seclusion.

APPLYING EVIDENCE-BASED PRACTICE (EBP)

Problem

A 60-year-old male diagnosed with schizoaffective disorder had an appointment at a mental health clinic for an outpatient nursing visit. As the patient entered the office, he was gazing downward and seemed tense. He sat down briefly in the chair, then stood up rapidly and jumped on the desk just a few inches away from the registered nurse (RN), shouting, "You all are practicing Voodoo, trying to kill me with the lithium. I'm going to smash your face in!" The RN backed away and stated calmly and firmly, "No, you are not; you are going to leave, or I will call security." The patient rushed out the door and yelled, "I'll leave—you don't have to call security, but when I kill my wife, it's on you!"

EBP Assessment

A. **What do you already know from experience?** Patients with mental illness are not all violent, but there are times when violence and threats occur. Mental health professionals are involved with patients during acute phases of their disorders and must be prepared to react in a safe manner.

B. **What does the literature say?** The duty to warn was developed after a psychiatric patient revealed his plan to kill a young woman to a psychology intern, then followed through with killing her. The duty to warn places limits on confidentiality and requires action on the part of the professional. In some states the duty to warn is mandatory, and in others it is optional or not required at all (National Conference of State Legislatures, 2013). Of psychiatric residents, 40% to 50% will be attacked by a patient during the 4 years of their program (Anderson & West, 2011).

C. **What does the patient want?** When the patient initially came to the clinic, he stated that he wanted to control his anger and was tired of people becoming scared of him. In this moment of acute psychosis, the patient is lashing out. Safety always takes precedence.

Plan

The RN is required in her state to perform a duty to warn. She called the police to report the patient's threat against his wife. Next, she called the patient's wife to let her know a threat had been made against her. The RN also called security to watch the premises for the agitated patient. The police found the patient and completed a report. Eventually, the patient returned to the clinic for future services but was required to have his case manager with him at all times while at the facility.

QSEN Prelicensure Knowledge, Skills, and Attitudes (KSAs) Addressed

Safety was addressed in handling the acute situation and by acting on duty-to-warn guidelines.

Teamwork and Collaboration occurred between the RN, police, security, and the case manager in handling the outburst and threat.

Psychopharmacology

Aggression, hostility, and violent behaviors are usually a result of the underlying psychiatric or medical disorder (Gerken et al., 2016; Preston, O'Neal, & Talaga, 2013).

Medications for Acute Aggression

If treating the underlying condition doesn't work, or if the underlying condition is unknown, the medication prescribed should be the most benign. Benzodiazepines are often the first choice for acute aggressive episodes, especially in episodic dyscontrol and rage episodes.

Benzodiazepines are safe but may have paradoxical reactions in individuals with certain personality disorders (Gerken et al., 2016). Second-generation antipsychotics, particularly ziprasidone (intramuscular) or olanzapine (intramuscular or orally disintegrating), can be useful in emergency situations (Gerken et al., 2016).

Medications for Chronic Aggression

Chronic aggression is a common problem in psychiatry, and aggression can be diminished only after a therapeutic dose of the appropriate medication once a provisional diagnosis is made. Treatment should be geared toward the underlying psychiatric or medical condition. Preston and colleagues (2013) outlined the most effective medications for specific underlying conditions (Table 24.2).

TABLE 24.2 Medications for Chronic Aggression

Medication	Associated Features
Anticonvulsants (e.g., carbamazepine)	Labile mood, poor impulse control, organic illness (e.g., dementia)
Antipsychotics	Disorganized behavior
Beta blockers (propranolol)	Organic illness (e.g., dementia)
Buspirone	Organic illness
Clonidine	Anxiety, agitation
Lithium	Labile mood, impulsivity
Selective serotonin reuptake inhibitors (SSRIs)	Anger "attacks"

Modified from Preston, J. J., O'Neal, J. H., & Talaga, M. C. (2017). *Handbook of clinical psychopharmacology for therapists* (8th ed). Oakland, CA: New Harbinger Publications.

EVALUATION

Evaluation of the care plan is essential for patients who are angry and aggressive. A well-considered plan has specific outcome criteria. Evaluation provides information about the extent to which the interventions have achieved the outcomes. If the outcomes have not been achieved, the plan must be revised. Revision focuses on all aspects of the nursing process:

- Was the assessment accurate and thorough?
- Were the nursing diagnoses applicable to the assessment data?
- Did the nursing diagnoses accurately drive nursing interventions?
- Was the plan comprehensive and individualized?
- Were interventions appropriate?
- Were interventions carried out properly?
- If restraint or seclusion was needed, was the protocol followed correctly, and was safety for staff as well as the patient maintained?
- Were guidelines to improve quality improvement methods found for future use?

For instance, the initial plan may have included an assessment of the environmental stimuli that precede a patient's agitation. Once these are identified, the plan provides interventions that are specific to those stimuli. However, the plan will work only if staff members evaluate the effectiveness of the approach by noting the extent to which agitation is decreased. Evaluation may reveal that the patient's agitation has decreased except in specific situations. The plan is then revised to include these situations.

KEY POINTS TO REMEMBER

- Angry emotions and aggressive actions are difficult targets for nursing intervention.
- Nurses benefit from an understanding of how the angry and aggressive patient should be approached.
- Understanding patient cues to escalating aggression, appropriate intervention goals for individuals in a variety of situations, and helpful nursing interventions is important for nurses in any setting.
- The roles of sociocultural influences and neurobiological vulnerabilities are intertwined in a person's propensity for violence.
- Cues to assess when anger is escalating (verbal and nonverbal, including facial expressions, breathing, body language, and posture) are provided.
- Assess the patient's history. A patient's past aggressive behavior is the most important indicator of future aggressive episodes.
- Many approaches are effective in helping patients de-escalate and maintain control.
- The general hierarchy of interventions for coping with aggression is verbal intervention, trauma-specific interventions, psychopharmacology, seclusion, and then restraint.
- Different interventions are used depending on the patient's level of anger.
- Guidelines for de-escalation of patient behavior are given.
- Specific medications, such as barbiturates, antipsychotics, lithium, selective serotonin reuptake inhibitors (SSRIs), and anticonvulsants, may prove useful for short- or long-term therapy.
- As a last resort, seclusion or restraints may be needed to ensure the safety of the patient as well as the safety of other patients and the staff.
- Each unit has a clear protocol for the safe use of restraints and for the humane management of care during the time the patient is restrained, as well as clear guidelines for understanding and protecting the patient's legal rights.
- Careful documentation of any incidence of escalating violence, especially any violence leading to seclusion or restraints, must be made according to the laws of your state.

APPLYING CRITICAL JUDGMENT

1. Mr. Arnold, a 24-year-old man, is currently in the manic phase of bipolar disorder. He is admitted to an inpatient unit. Staff note that the patient is agitated and irritable and has a history of assault. He shouts at the nurse in a loud, piercing voice, yelling that she is a "slut, a mutt, tut-tut." He is pacing anxiously, invading the staff's personal space, and pointing his finger in the faces of some staff.
   - A. What would be some appropriate nursing diagnoses for Mr. Arnold at this time?
   - B. Describe how you would document his behavior.
   - C. What are some of the interventions you and your colleagues might try first? What interventions might you try next? Explain the rationale for your decision.
   - D. Describe the kinds of objective and subjective data you would document as well as the frequency of documentation according to the protocols of your hospital.
   - E. List the various aspects of interventions of patient care for someone who is in seclusion.
   - F. Role-play verbal techniques you could use during any other interventions being initiated at this time.
2. In the morning 2 days later, Mr. Arnold comes to the nurses' desk and asks for a pass. When told that the physician needs to write an order for his pass and that the physician will not be on duty until the afternoon, Mr. Arnold becomes verbally loud, demanding that the nurse call the physician "right this minute to get that pass."
   - A. What interventions by you and your colleagues would be most appropriate to start at this time?
   - B. Role-play your verbal techniques.
   - C. What are the personal safety measures you and your colleagues would take when treating a patient with escalating aggression?
3. Write a summary of the protocols for intervening with irate patients as found in the hospital procedure manual.
4. Describe a time in your life when you have witnessed bullying or have been bullied by others.
   - A. If you were the one being bullied, describe how you felt. What could be some long-term effects?
   - B. If you were watching a coworker being bullied by a staff member in charge, how might you react today?
   - C. Have you ever witnessed or been involved in a student-to-student, nurse-to-nurse, or colleague-to-colleague incidence of bullying? What would you do today?

CHAPTER REVIEW QUESTIONS

1. Select the completion of the following sentence that demonstrates that an adult is coping in a healthy way: "I am feeling so angry right now …
   - **a.** I'm afraid I'm going to cry."
   - **b.** I would like to punch something."
   - **c.** I want to talk to someone about it."
   - **d.** I want to curl up and sleep for a long time."
2. In a hostile voice, a patient experiencing mania yells at the nurse: "You *will* listen to me and not interrupt. I have some really important stuff to say. I'm tired of you nurses and doctors acting like you have all the answers." To facilitate effective communication, which initial response should the nurse provide?
   - **a.** "You are our patient, so we always listen to you."
   - **b.** "I can talk with you better if you use a calm voice."
   - **c.** "It's our job to help you get through this manic episode."
   - **d.** "Patients have an important role in treatment planning."
3. A female nurse is appointed to a committee with seven men. At the beginning of the meeting, the chairman asks the nurse to be the secretary. The nurse responds, "No. You're just asking me to be secretary because I'm the only woman here." Which response would have been more effective?
   - **a.** "There are others more qualified than I am to be secretary."
   - **b.** "I would be glad to perform another role for our committee."
   - **c.** "I'm probably overreacting, but I find your request offensive."
   - **d.** "Thank you for asking, but your request is sexually discriminatory."

4. An 8-year-old tells a parent, "I like to scare kids at school by showing them pictures of clowns. Some kids are terrified." How should the nurse counsel the parents regarding this behavior?
   a. Recommend family therapy for the child, siblings, and parents.
   b. Suggest the parents enroll the child in an anger management program.
   c. Educate both parents about bullying, including possible origins and long-term effects.
   d. Teach the parents about the developmental phase and tasks for an 8-year-old child.

5. A woman experienced a double mastectomy yesterday. Now she cheerfully says to the nurse, "I didn't need those things anyway. No more wet T-shirt contests for me!" How should the nurse interpret this comment?
   a. The patient is realistically accepting her loss.
   b. The comment is sarcastic, which may reflect anger.
   c. The patient is experiencing a distorted body image.
   d. The comment suggests guilt regarding prior behavior.

REFERENCES

American Nurses Association (ANA). (2015). *ANA panel aims to prevent violence, bullying in health care facilities.* Retrieved July 25, 2015, from http://www.nursingworld.org/MainMenuCategories/WorkplaceSafety/Healthy-Nurse/bullyingworkplaceviolence/ANA-Panel-Aims-to-Prevent-Violence-Bullying.

American Psychiatric Association. (2015). *Psychiatric News Alert: Recovery model helps reduce use of seclusion, restraint and large hospital system.* Retrieved from http://alert.psychnews.org/2014/11/recovery-model-helps-reduce-use-of.html.

American Psychiatric Nurses Association (APNA). (2000, rev. 2007, rev. 2014). *Seclusion and restraint standards of practice.* Retrieved July 12, 2015, from http://www.apna.org.

Anderson, A., & West, S. G. (2011). Violence against mental health professionals: When the treater becomes the victim. *Innovation in Clinical Neuroscience,* 8(3), 34-49.

Black, D. W., & Andreasen, N. C. (2014). *Introductory textbook of psychiatry* (6th ed.). Washington, DC: American Psychiatric Publishing.

Bresin, K., & Gordon, K. H. (2013). Aggression as affect regulation: Extending catharsis theory to evaluate aggression and experiential anger in the laboratory and daily life. *Journal of Social and Clinical Psychology, 32*(4), 400–423.

Feinstein, R. E., & Rothberg, B. (2014). Violence. In J. L. Cutler (Ed.), *Psychiatry* (pp. 403–417). New York: Oxford University Press.

Gerken, A. T., Gross, A. F., & Saunders, K. M. (2016). Aggression and violence. In T. A. Stern, M. Fava, T. E. Wilens, et al. (Eds.), *Massachusetts General Hospital comprehensive clinical psychiatry* (2nd ed.) (pp. 709–717). Philadelphia: Elsevier.

Giddens, J. F. (2017). *Concepts for nursing practice* (2nd ed.). St. Louis: Elsevier.

Jalain, C. I. (2014). *The impact of serotonin and dopamine on human aggression: A systematic review of the literature.* Master's Theses. Paper 6. Retrieved from http://aquila.usm.edu/masters_theses/6.

Linehan, M. (1993). *Cognitive-behavioral treatment of borderline personality disorder.* New York: Guilford Press.

National Conference of State Legislators. (2013). *Mental health professionals' duty to warn.* Retrieved from http://www. ncsl.org/research/health/mental-health-professionals-duty-to-warn.aspx.

Preston, J. D., O'Neal, J. H., & Talaga, M. C. (2013). *Handbook of clinical psychopharmacology for therapists* (7th ed.). Oakland, CA: New Harbinger Publications.

Robbins, A. (2015). *Mean girls of the ER: The alarming nurse culture of bullying and hazing.* May: Marie Claire. Retrieved from https://www.marieclaire.com/culture/news/a14211/mean-girls-of-the-er/.

Sadock, B. J., Sadock, V. A., & Ruiz, P. (2015). *Kaplan & Sadock's synopsis of psychiatry* (11th ed.). Philadelphia: Lippincott Williams & Wilkins.

Schluter, T., Winz, O., Henkel, K., et al. (2013). The impact of dopamine on aggression: An [18F] FDOPA Penn study and healthy males. *Journal of Neuroscience,* 33(43), 16889-16896.

Sivak, K. (2012). Implementation of comfort rooms to reduce seclusion, restraint use, and acting out behaviors. *Journal of Psychiatry & Neuroscience, 50*(2), 24–34.

Society for Neuroscience. (2014). *Aggression on the brain.* Retrieved July 17, 2015, from http://www.brainfacts.org/sensing-thinking-behaving/mood/articles/2008/aggression—the-brain/.

Substance Abuse and Mental Health Services Administration (SAMHSA). (2011). *A seclusion and restraint overview.* Retrieved February 14, 2012, from http://www.samhsa.gov/matrix2/seclusion_matrix.aspx.

Substance Abuse and Mental Health Services Administration (SAMHSA). (2015). *Trauma-informed approach and trauma-specific interventions.* Retrieved July 15, 2015, from http://www.samhsa.gov/nctic/trauma-interventions.

Tasman, A., Kay, J., Lieberman, J. A., First, M. B., & Riba, M. (2015). *Psychiatry: Volume 1* (4th ed.). Hoboken, NJ: John Wiley & Sons.

Victoroff, J. (2009). Human aggression. In B. J. Sadock, V. A. Sadock, & P. Ruiz (Eds.), *Kaplan and Sadock's comprehensive textbook of psychiatry* (9th ed.) (pp. 2671–2702). Philadelphia: Wolters Kluwer/Lippincott Williams & Wilkins.

Zeller, S. L., & Wilson, M. P. (2015). Management of aggression. *Paradigm, 19*(3), 12–15.

25

Care for the Dying and Those Who Grieve

Carol O. Long

http://evolve.elsevier.com/Varcarolis/essentials

OBJECTIVES

1. Discuss and differentiate between palliative care and hospice in terms of (a) purpose, (b) philosophy and goals, (c) settings, and (d) various supports available to families.
2. Compare and contrast the terms *loss, grief, mourning,* and *bereavement.*
3. Identify the behavioral outcomes that indicate healthy bereavement.
4. Delineate at least five symptoms of complicated grief.
5. Discuss and give examples of the various phenomena experienced during the normal grief process (e.g., sensations of somatic distress, changes in behavior).
6. Describe three short-term interventions that can be used to help a person experiencing complicated grief come to terms with his or her loss.
7. Describe and discuss the Four Tasks of Mourning as identified in this chapter.
8. Select at least two patient-centered goals of care at the end of life and discuss how you would address these issues.
9. Identify key communication interventions that support patient-centered goals of care.
10. Explain the interventions you would take to help grieving caregivers in the following areas:
    a. Helping the bereaved caregivers come to terms with their feelings
    b. Helping people say goodbye
    c. Helping families maintain "hope"
    d. Establishing therapeutic presence
11. Describe the importance of self-care interventions for nurses.

KEY TERMS AND CONCEPTS

acute grief, p. 393
ambiguous loss, p. 393
anticipatory grief, 393
bereaved, p. 394
bereavement, p. 394
burnout, p. 403
caring presence, p. 402
compassion, p. 403
compassion fatigue, p. 403
complicated grief, p. 393
disenfranchised grief, p. 393
end-of-life conversations, p. 401
FICA, p. 401
Four Gifts, p. 402
Four Tasks of Mourning, p. 394
grief, p. 393
grief work, p. 394
hospice care, p. 392
loss, p. 393
meaning reconstruction, p. 394
mourning, p. 393
palliative care, p. 392
uncomplicated grief, p. 393

CONCEPT: PALLIATIVE CARE: *Palliative care* is a highly structured and organized system of care intended to address the physical, emotional, social, cultural, and spiritual needs of patients and families experiencing serious, life-threatening, progressive, or chronic illnesses. Palliative care can transform the current disease-focused approach to a patient-centered philosophy, in which the needs of the patient and family goals become essential (Giddens, 2017, pp. 497-498). It is helpful for a nurse to understand the experience of families caring for a terminally ill patient. Encourage family members to express what is important to them, provide a caring presence, and understand that successful bereavement includes a sense that one was able to say goodbye. A nonjudgmental stance, ongoing education, advocacy, and monitoring for complications such as a functional decline of a family caregiver can help.

INTRODUCTION

Over the past 30 years, there have been tremendous advances in end-of-life and palliative care in the United States. The National Palliative Care Registry survey report estimates that more than 75% of all hospitals with 50 or more beds have formal palliative care programs (Center to Advance Palliative Care [CAPC], 2018). Community palliative care fills the gap from hospital care to hospice care. Community palliative care meets the needs of people living at home or in assisted living settings. Palliative care may be available in long-term care facilities. Palliative care, which includes hospice, is widely available across the United States. The National Academy Institute of Medicine (IOM, 2014) *Dying in America* report challenges practitioners and the health care system to improve the quality and availability of palliative care services to support quality of life through the end of life. Five recommendations specify that (1) more and better comprehensive care is needed for people with advanced serious illness, along with (2) improved client–patient communication that includes advance care planning, (3) professional education and ongoing development in palliative care, (4) improved financing to provide quality end-of-life care, and (5) public education and engagement about advance care planning and informed choices.

What is **palliative care**, and how does it improve care for patients with serious, life-threatening illnesses? The National Consensus Project for Quality Care's *Clinical Practice Guidelines for Quality Palliative Care*, 4th edition (2018, p. 2), which is sanctioned by leading hospice and palliative medicine and nursing organizations, provides the following definition:

> Beneficial at any stage of a serious illness, palliative care is an interdisciplinary care delivery system designed to anticipate, prevent, and manage physical, psychological, social, and spiritual suffering to optimize quality of life for patients, their families and caregivers. Palliative care can be delivered in any care setting through the collaboration of many types of care providers. Through early integration into the care plan of seriously ill people, palliative care improves quality of life for both the patient and the family.

These standards and guidelines emphasize collaborative and coordinated care by an interdisciplinary team, services that are available concurrently or independent of curative or life-prolonging care, and support of patient and family hope for peace and dignity until death. **Hospice care** is provided at the end of life and is a part of the palliative care trajectory. A sample of these standards is listed in Box 25.1.

Hospice care is a model for compassionate, holistic, and medically managed end-of-life services. The Medicare hospice benefit was enacted in 1982 and is largely available across all insurance plans. A National Hospice and Palliative Care Organization (2018) report indicates that approximately 4382 Medicare-certified hospices provided care to 1.43 million Medicare beneficiaries enrolled in hospice care for 1 day or more during 2016. The average length of service (ALOS) for Medicare patients enrolled in hospice in 2016 was 71 days. Cancer diagnoses accounted for 27.2% of deaths, followed by heart disease (18.7%), dementia (18%), respiratory disease (11%), stroke (9.5%) and other (15.6%). Most of the care (77%) is provided in the patient's place of residence (e.g., home, nursing home, or residential facility), with 14.6% in a hospice inpatient facility and 7.4% in an acute care hospital.

Hospice care is delivered by an interdisciplinary team of physicians, nurses, chaplains, social workers, home health aides, volunteers, spiritual counselors, therapists, and bereavement counselors. All medications and supplies related to the terminal diagnosis are covered by Medicare reimbursement, and many other insurance providers mimic the Medicare benefit. Individuals are perceived as living fully until they die; their choices and preferences are respected and incorporated in the plan of care. The patient and family are considered the unit of care

BOX 25.1 Selected National Consensus Project Clinical Practice Guidelines, 2018

Domain 3: Psychological and Psychiatric Aspects of Care

Guideline 3.1 Global

The interdisciplinary team (IDT) includes a social worker with the knowledge and skills to assess and support mental health issues, provide emotional support, and address emotional distress and quality of life for patients and families experiencing the expected responses to serious illness. The IDT has the training to assess and support those with mental health disorders, either directly, in consultation, or through referral to specialist level psychological and/or psychiatric care.

Guideline 3.2 Screening and Assessment

The IDT screens for, assesses, and documents psychological and psychiatric aspects of care based upon the best available evidence to maximize patient and family coping and quality of life.

Guideline 3.3 Treatment

The IDT manages and/or supports psychological and psychiatric aspects of patient and family care, including emotional, psychosocial, or existential distress related to the experience of serious illness, as well as identified mental health disorders. Psychological and psychiatric services are provided either directly, in consultation, or through referral to other providers.

Guideline 3.4 Ongoing Care

The IDT provides recommendations for monitoring and managing long-term and emerging psychological and psychiatric responses and mental health concerns.

Domain 7: Care of the Patient Nearing End of Life

Guideline 7.1 Interdisciplinary Team

The IDT includes professionals with training in end-of-life care, including assessment and management of symptoms, communicating with patients and families about signs and symptoms of approaching death, transitions of care, and grief and bereavement. The IDT has established structures and processes to ensure appropriate care for patients and families when the end of life is imminent.

Guideline 7.2 Screening and Assessment

The IDT assesses physical, psychological, social, and spiritual needs, as well as patient- and family preferences for setting of care, treatment decisions, and wishes during and immediately following death. Discussions with the family focus on honoring patient wishes and attending to family fears and concerns about the end of life. The IDT prepares and supports family caregivers throughout the dying process, taking into account the spiritual and cultural background and preferences of the patient and family.

Guideline 7.3 Treatment Prior to Death

In collaboration with the patient and family and other clinicians, the IDT develops, implements, and updates (as needed) a care plan to anticipate, prevent, and treat physical, psychological, social, and spiritual symptoms. The care plan addresses the focus on end-of-life care and treatments to meet the physical, emotional, social, and spiritual needs of patients and families. All treatment is provided in a culturally and developmentally appropriate manner.

Guideline 7.4 Treatment During the Dying Process and Immediately After Death

During the dying process, patient and family needs are respected and supported. Post-death care is delivered in a manner that honors patient and family cultural and spiritual beliefs, values, and practices.

Guideline 7.5 Bereavement

Bereavement support is available to the family and care team, either directly or through referral. The IDT identifies or provides resources, including grief counseling, spiritual support, or peer support, specific to the assessed needs. Prepared in advance of the patient's death, the bereavement care plan is activated after the death of the patient and addresses immediate and longer-term needs.

From National Consensus Project for Quality Palliative Care. (2018). *Clinical practice guidelines for quality palliative care* (4th ed.). Retrieved from https://www.nationalcoalitionhpc.org/ncp/

and receive counseling support around the tasks of anticipatory grief and mourning as well as spirituality and finding meaning and purpose at the end of life.

This chapter focuses on nursing care for those who are dying, care for family members and others who grieve, and self-care for nurses.

LOSS, GRIEF, AND MOURNING

Loss is part of the human experience, and grief and mourning are the normal responses to loss. We grieve on a recurring basis as we face the commonplace losses in our lives, such as the loss of a relationship (e.g., divorce, separation, death, abortion), health (e.g., a body function or part, mental or physical capacity), friendship, status, prestige, or security (e.g., occupational, financial, social, cultural). Some losses may be even more intangible, such as the loss of a projected future or dreams. Normal losses include changes in circumstances, such as retirement, a promotion, marriage, and the aging process.

It could be said that the course of our lives depends on how we adapt to losses and how we use change as a vehicle for growth. Understanding how to support healthy grieving and mourning in oneself and for others is a vital life skill. Unfortunately, contemporary mainstream U.S. culture perpetuates many damaging **myths about grief and mourning,** such as:

- Grief and mourning are the same experience and the same for everyone.
- There is a predictable and orderly stage-like progression to grieving.
- It is best to move away from grief rather than toward it.
- Following the death of someone important to you, the goal is to "get over it."
- Tears are an expression of weakness.

Grief is the individualized response to a loss that is perceived, real, or anticipated. Grief is a normal response to loss at the time of death, and various reactions can occur (Strada, 2016). It is experienced emotionally, cognitively, physically, socially, and spiritually. Normal grief is known as uncomplicated grief. *Uncomplicated grief is anything but uncomplicated,* but it is described as a normal progression through the grief process, as defined by cultural and societal values, and includes reactions such as depressed mood, insomnia, anxiety, poor appetite, loss of interest, guilt, dreams about the deceased, confusion, and poor concentration. Psychological states may include shock, denial, anger, and yearning and searching for the deceased. People with grief may experience isolation and disappointment as their friends and families fail to understand what they are facing. Spirituality is frequently either shaken or strengthened by the experience of profound loss. Acute grief, a term coined by Dr. Erich Lindemann (1994), is the result of an unexpected death of a family member and can result in an exacerbation of any pre-existing medical or psychiatric problems. A history of depression, substance abuse, or posttraumatic stress disorder (PTSD) can complicate grief.

The term anticipatory grief, although far from a perfect term, helps people recognize that grief is a part of the complex process of living with a terminal prognosis (Strada, 2016). During anticipatory grieving, the dying individual and family may display primary emotions such as anger (e.g., protesting that this is happening, anger at the patient for not fighting harder, anger at the medical system, displaced anger at others because of helplessness in the face of suffering, anger at God), sadness (e.g., sorrow and regret for the present and the future), hurt (e.g., pain over what the patient is enduring, the pain of being unable to protect each other, the pain of loss), fear and anxiety (e.g., a pervasive sense that something more should or could be done, dread of what is coming next, loss of control, a sense that time is running out), and bridled grief (e.g., experiencing hits or bursts of grief but keeping it in check as long as the patient is alive). From the moment of diagnosis, patients and families begin to both experience and anticipate losses, and it does *not* become any easier when death occurs.

Disenfranchised grief is a term coined by Dr. Kenneth Doka (1989) to acknowledge losses that are not socially sanctioned, openly acknowledged, or publicly mourned. Grief may be disenfranchised because of the relationship of the griever (e.g., life partner, health care worker, defense attorney, divorced spouse), the nature of the loss (e.g., miscarriages, abortions, war heroes), the type of death (e.g., executions, homicides, suicides, human immunodeficiency virus/acquired immunodeficiency syndrome [HIV/AIDS]), or the grieving style related to gender differences or stage in life. These individuals may not have the opportunity to publicly grieve the loss. Once losses are recognized as disenfranchised, it becomes easier to support them within and among individuals sharing the same experience.

Complicated grief essentially means that the grief work is unresolved and occurs when individuals have difficulty coming to terms with their loss and experience phenomena outside the normal grief reaction, which impairs the individual's ability to function in social or occupational situations or resume previous roles. Thoughts may be intrusive, involving preoccupation with the deceased long after what is felt to be a normal period of mourning coupled with an inability to get away from persistent and painful yearning for the loved one. The bereaved may want to die in order to rejoin their loved one: "Life is empty. I have no interest in anything. I am only half a person now." Complicated grief may be chronic or grief that extends for at least a year after the death; delayed, when normal grief reactions are postponed or suppressed; or exaggerated, when the individual takes drastic measures that are self-destructive (e.g., suicide) or masked; it may be present when the survivor is unaware that behaviors that are interfering with normal activities are a result of the loss. The *Diagnosis and Statistical Manual of Mental Disorders,* 5th edition (*DSM-5*; American Psychiatric Association [APA], 2013) identifies criteria that define complicated grief as a disorder called *persistent complex bereavement disorder*.

Ambiguous loss, a term coined by Dr. Pauline Boss (2011), represents another type of grief and explains losses that are related to presence and absence. Ambiguous loss is a loss that is unclear; it has no resolution and no predictable ending or closure. It occurs in two situations. The first is when the physical body is absent but the person is still psychologically present to family and others, such as individuals who are missing as a result of an airplane or military incident. The second type of ambiguous loss is when the body is physically present but the person is physiologically changed or absent from how he or she once was, as is the case in dementia. For caregivers, the grief that is experienced with ambiguous loss in dementia is confusing and unlike other types of grief. Ambiguous loss in dementia can block the caregiver's ability to cope when engaging in the necessary and important tasks of caring for the person and for themselves. Family members may experience ongoing stress and grief that lead to depression, anxiety, and family discord and, subsequently, dysfunctional relationships. Over time, ongoing dissonance can erode once-positive interactions, leading to isolation for caregivers (Long, Favaro, & Mulder, 2017). Implementing interventions to help caregivers accept the ambiguity of dementia is one strategy, along with measures for self-care.

Mourning refers to all the ways in which a person outwardly expresses grief and the efforts taken to manage grief. This includes culturally determined practices such as wakes, funerals, sitting shiva (a ritual specific to Jewish mourners), or decorating the gravesite. Mourning is influenced by culture, religious or spiritual practices, family traditions, and one's own personality and beliefs. The passage of time alone does not always heal grief; it is what we do with the time that seems to help. Sharing our grief with others seems to relieve some of its effects and allows us to move through it. Social media sites provide outlets for grievers to find understanding and meaningful connections with others. Attending grief support groups and seeing a counselor are also activities of mourning. It is mourning that gradually releases us from the pain of loss.

Grief and mourning occur during the bereavement period. Bereavement refers to the time of sadness after a significant loss through death. The person who is grieving is referred to as the bereaved. Most cultures provide symbols and contexts for bereavement, such as wearing black or a black armband. Bereaved people experience themselves as being set apart from the current of ordinary life. Contemporary society in the United States has left behind the visible symbols of bereavement, with the result that those in mourning often feel isolated and alone. Bereavement counseling includes pre- and post-death bereavement counseling. The hospice benefit provides bereavement counseling for family and others for up to 13 months after the patient's death.

THEORY

Some of the most widely known early grief theorists describe common psychological and behavioral phenomena experienced by those who are grieving a loss. Erich Lindemann (1994), in his classic study about the survivors of Boston's Coconut Grove nightclub in 1942, coined the term grief work, which is used to describe the process of grief recovery or how a person adjusts to the loss. Others postulated various phases of bereavement that proceed in orderly sequences within certain time frames; the best known is from Elisabeth Kübler-Ross's (1969) book *On Death and Dying*. The various frameworks for grieving and phases of grief are useful for helping people to normalize the deeply felt and disturbing phenomena they experience when they confront profound loss. However, these frameworks do not provide the focus of care during the grieving process, nor do they typify the predictability of a person moving through stages. The process of grief work derives from the details of a person's unique experience, and the emotions felt do not always follow a pattern of response by constructing and reconstructing the world around him or her through the experience as a survivor of loss known as meaning reconstruction (Neimeyer et al., 2010). The following are common phenomena a person may experience at some point in the grief process:

1. Shock and disbelief
2. Denial
3. Sensation of somatic distress
4. Preoccupation with the image of the deceased
5. Guilt
6. Anger
7. Change in behavior (e.g., depression, disorganization, panic, restlessness)
8. Reorganization of behavior directed toward a new object or activity
9. Acceptance

Although emotional responses vary from one individual to the next, a common first response is that of **denial**. The person is emotionally unable to accept his or her painful loss. Denial functions as a buffer against intolerable pain and allows the person slowly to acknowledge the reality of death. A death may be accepted intellectually during this stage—"It's just as well, she was suffering"—although the emotional responses are still repressed. Denial is a needed defense that lasts for a few hours or a few days. Denial can also be thought of as disbelief and may recur over the early course of bereavement (e.g., "This morning I picked up the phone to call her and dialed her number before I remembered that she is gone"). However, persistent denial suggests that the mourning may be complicated, making it difficult to move through the process of mourning.

As denial fades, painful feelings begin to surface. The finality of the loved one's death becomes more of a reality. Waves of anguish and pain are experienced and may be localized in the chest or the epigastric area. **Anger** may surface at this time. Awareness by staff that anger is often displaced onto people in the health care environment may decrease defensive staff behaviors. **Guilt** is often experienced, and the bereaved blames himself or herself for taking or for failing to take specific actions. The person who is grieving may need to be supported patiently as he or she gradually comes to terms with a past that cannot be changed by hindsight. Guilt often indicates profound regret that things could not have been different from the way they were.

Crying is a common phenomenon early on (and often within cultural norms) with intense suffering and despair. Crying can afford a welcome release from pent-up anguish and tension. Assessment of cultural patterns is important in understanding crying. Failing to cry can be the result of cultural influences or environmental restraints. The person may cry in private. Inability to cry, however, may be the result of a high degree of ambivalence toward the deceased. A person who is unable to cry may have difficulty in successfully completing the work of mourning. Various phenomena experienced during bereavement are described in Table 25.1.

Other theories that describe how we grieve and the relationship to mourning have emerged. Self-control is valued, and the dominant cultural and familial message is usually "Shape up and get on with your life." In reality, mourning demands that who we are and the world we live in be reconstructed and remodeled in major ways. This requires much talking, working, engaging, writing, feeling, experimenting, and risk taking, supported by others who do not try to fix or rush the griever. Instead of "getting over it" as soon as possible, successful mourning asks us to engage in a complex process of finding a new and durable connection to who we are now and to the person who died. J. William Worden (2009) describes this process as the Four Tasks of Mourning:

1. Accept the reality of the loss.
2. Process the pain of grief while caring for the self.
3. Adjust to a world without the deceased.
4. Find an enduring connection with the deceased in the midst of embarking on a new life.

These tasks indicate a natural movement that results when people actively engage in mourning, rather than fitting one's own experience into someone else's framework. When people "hang in there" with their mourning over time, they instinctively progress toward the final task. Finally, they are able to remember the loved one without so much pain. They have the energy to engage in life and be open to new relationships and activities. They sense that they now carry that departed person with them in an enduring way that no longer requires a physical presence.

Other research focuses on issues such as the relationship between grief and trauma, the grieving process during various developmental periods of life, the advantages of resiliency and adaptability in mourning, interventions appropriate for specific populations, the definition of complicated or intractable grief and its treatment, and many more topics. According to Bonanno (2009), resilient people show no grief, and the absence of grief is a healthy outcome. These individuals have the ability to "bounce back" from adversity and regain health.

APPLICATION OF THE NURSING PROCESS

ASSESSMENT

Often the history of an individual can alert health care personnel to signs or symptoms of potential difficulty that a person may

TABLE 25.1 Phenomena Experienced During Bereavement

Symptoms	Examples
Sensations of Somatic Distress	
The bereaved may experience tightness in the throat, shortness of breath, sighing, mental pain, or exhaustion; food tastes like sand; things feel unreal. Pain or discomfort may be identical to the symptoms experienced by the deceased. Normally, symptoms are brief.	A woman whose husband died of a stroke complains of weakness and numbness on her left side.
Preoccupation With the Image of the Deceased	
The bereaved introduces into conversation, thinks about, and talks about numerous memories of the deceased. The memories are positive. This process continues with great sadness. The idealization of the deceased lets the bereaved relive the gratifications associated with the deceased and helps resolve any guilt the bereaved feels concerning the deceased. The bereaved may also assume many of the mannerisms of the deceased through identification. Identification serves the purpose of holding on to the deceased. Preoccupation with the deceased can continue for many months before it lessens.	A man whose wife has very recently died states, "I just can't stop thinking about my wife. Everything I see reminds me of her. We picked up this seashell on our honeymoon. I remember every wonderful moment we had together. The pain is so great, but the memories just keep coming." His friends notice that when he talks, his hand gestures and expressions are very like those of his recently deceased wife.
Guilt	
The bereaved reproaches himself or herself for real or imagined acts of negligence or omissions in the relationship with the deceased.	"I should have made him go to the doctor sooner." "I should have paid more attention to her, been more thoughtful."
Anger	
The anger the bereaved experiences may not be toward the object at its source. Often the anger is displaced onto the medical or nursing staff. Often it is directed toward the deceased. The anger is at its height during the first month but is often intermittent throughout the first year. The overflow of hostility disturbs the bereaved, resulting in the feeling that he or she is "going insane."	"The doctor didn't operate in time. If he had, Mary would be alive today." "How could he leave me like this ... how could he?"
Change in Behavior: Depression, Disorganization, Restlessness	
A person may exhibit marked restlessness and an inability to organize his or her behavior. A depressive mood during routine activities is common, decreasing as the year passes and the intensity of the grief declines. Absence of depression is more abnormal than its presence. Loneliness and aimlessness are most pronounced 6 to 9 months after the death. Reorganization of behavior directed toward a new object or activity gradually occurs. The person renews his or her interest in people and activities. The grieving thus releases the bereaved from one interpersonal relationship, and new ones are free to take its place.	Six months after her husband died, Mrs. Faye states, "I just can't seem to function. I have a hard time doing the simplest tasks. I can't be bothered with socializing. I feel so down ... so, so empty." Twenty months after her husband's death, Mrs. Faye tells a friend, "I'll be away this weekend. I am going fishing with my brother and his friend. This is the first time I've felt like doing anything since Harry died."

encounter during a time of mourning. The following questions identify risk factors that may complicate the successful completion of mourning:

1. Do any of the following factors relate to the bereaved?
   - Was the bereaved heavily dependent on the deceased?
   - Were there persistent, unresolved conflicts with the deceased?
   - Was the deceased a child (perhaps the most profound loss of all)?
   - Does the bereaved have a meaningful relationship or support system?
   - Has the bereaved experienced a number of previous losses?
   - Does the bereaved have sound coping skills?
2. Was the deceased's death associated with a cultural stigma (e.g., AIDS, suicide, homicide)?
3. Has the bereaved had difficulty resolving past significant losses?
4. Does the bereaved have a history of depression, drug or alcohol abuse, or other psychiatric illness?
5. If the bereaved is young, are there indications for special interventions?
6. Was the deceased a veteran or victim of war?

Prolonged depression is the most common response to unresolved grief. Disturbances in mood are associated with biological changes in the body during stress-related depressive illness. Some examples include electrolyte disturbances, nervous system alterations, and faulty regulation of the autonomic nervous system. Always assess the potential for suicide. Someone who is having difficulty negotiating the work of mourning and is suffering can benefit from counseling, as mentioned earlier.

Assessment Guidelines

Grieving and Complicated Grieving

1. Identify whether the individual is at risk for complicated grieving (see assessment history).
2. Identify the bereaved person's cultural and spiritual beliefs, length of typical grieving, and mourning rituals.
3. Evaluate for psychotic symptoms, agitation, increased activity, alcohol or drug abuse, and extreme vegetative symptoms (e.g., anorexia, unintended weight loss, insomnia).
4. Do not overlook people who do not express significant grief in the context of a major loss. These individuals might have an increased risk of subsequent complicated or unresolved grief reactions.
5. Complicated grief reactions require significant interventions. Suicidal or severely depressed people might require hospitalization. Always assess for **suicide** with signs of depression or other dysfunctional signs.
6. Assess support systems. If support systems are limited, find bereavement groups in the community.

7. When grieving is stalled or complicated, a person is at high risk for major depression or other mental illnesses. There are a variety of therapeutic approaches that have proved beneficial. Make referrals.
8. Grieving can bring with it severe spiritual anguish. Assess whether spiritual counseling or a specific counselor would be useful for the bereaved.

Table 25.2 presents a comparison between the symptoms of a "normal" mourning process and those of a complicated grief reaction.

DIAGNOSIS

Four nursing diagnoses that apply to grief are *Dysfunctional grief, Risk for dysfunctional grief, Grief,* and *Risk for depressed mood.* During the time of grief, especially if the grieving process is prolonged or symptomatic (e.g., profound depression or disorganization), other nursing diagnoses may come into play. *Impaired coping process, Risk for difficulty with coping, Spiritual distress, Lack of social support, and Risk for Social Isolation* are examples.

OUTCOMES IDENTIFICATION

Ideally, successful outcomes would include the following. The individual:

- Can tolerate intense emotions
- Reports decreased preoccupation with the deceased (loss)
- Demonstrates increased periods of stability
- Tends to previous responsibilities
- Takes on new roles and responsibilities
- Has energy to invest in new endeavors
- Expresses positive expectations about the future
- Remembers positive as well as negative aspects of the deceased loved one

PLANNING AND IMPLEMENTATION

Nurses constantly encounter people and families who are faced with loss, although that loss might not be the reason they first entered the medical or psychiatric health care system. In hospital settings, grief is expressed when there is a loss other than death—for example, loss of a limb from amputation or loss of a breast after surgery for breast cancer. Sometimes simple active listening can go a long way in offering comfort and respite from loneliness, or perhaps a referral to a grieving support group is indicated. Still, at other times the nurse may realize that even though individuals present with a medical or emotional problem, they are also undergoing a profound loss; therefore the nurse might suggest the need for a referral for grief counseling or psychotherapy. As mentioned, physical or emotional symptoms may be related to a complicated grief reaction.

The nurse's focus when facilitating bereavement is on helping the bereaved deal with the most important issues emerging at a particular time. Often the nurse or other caregiver can best serve the grieving

TABLE 25.2 Common Responses and Pathological Intensification During Grief

Typical Response	Pathological Intensification
Dying	
Emotional expression and immediate coping with the dying process	Avoidance; feeling of being overwhelmed, dazed, confused; self-punitive feelings; inappropriately hostile feelings
Death and Outcry	
Outcry of emotions with news of the death and turning for help to others or isolating self with self-soothing	Panic, dissociative reactions, reactive psychoses, suicidal ideation
Warding Off (Denial)	
Avoidance of reminders and social withdrawal, focusing elsewhere, emotional numbing, not thinking of implications to self or of certain themes	Maladaptive avoidance of confronting the implications of death through drug or alcohol abuse, promiscuity, fugue states, phobic avoidance, feeling of being dead or unreal
Reexperience (Intrusion)	
Intrusive experiences, including recollections of negative experiences during relationship with the deceased, bad dreams, reduced concentration, compulsive reenactments	Flooding with negative images and emotions; uncontrolled ideation, self-impairing compulsive reenactments, night terrors, recurrent nightmares, distraught feelings resulting from the intrusion of anger, anxiety, despair, shame, or guilt; physiological exhaustion resulting from hyperarousal
Working Through	
Recollection of the deceased and a contemplation of self with reduced intrusiveness of memories and fantasies and with increased rational acceptance, reduced numbness and avoidance, more "dosing" of recollections, and a sense of working it through	Feeling of inability to integrate the death with a sense of self and continued life; persistent warding-off themes that may manifest as anxious, depressed, enraged, shame-filled, or guilty moods; self-injurious behaviors; and psychophysiological syndromes
Resolution	
Reduction in emotional swings and a sense of self-coherence and readiness for new relationships; ability to experience positive states of mind	Failure to negotiate the process of mourning, which may be associated with inability to work or create, or to feel emotion or positive states of mind

From Horowitz, M. J. (1990). A model of mourning: Change in schemas of self and other. *Journal of the American Psychoanalytic Association, 38*(2), 297–303.

TABLE 25.3 Interventions for Helping People in Grief

Intervention	Rationale
1. Use methods that can facilitate the grieving process.	
a. Give your full presence: use appropriate eye contact, attentive listening, and appropriate touch.	a. Talking is one of the most important ways of dealing with acute grief. Listening patiently helps the bereaved express all feelings, even ones he or she feels are "negative." Appropriate eye contact helps to convey the awareness that you are there and are sharing the person's sadness. Human touch can express warmth and nurture healing. Inappropriate touch can leave a person confused and uncomfortable.
b. Be patient with the bereaved in times of silence. Do not fill silence with empty chatter.	b. Sharing painful feelings during periods of silence is healing and conveys your concern.
2. Know about and share with the bereaved information about the phenomena that occur during the normal mourning process, because they may concern some people (intense anger at the deceased, guilt, symptoms the deceased had before death, unbidden floods of memories). Give the bereaved support during the occurrence of these phenomena and a written handout for reference.	2. Although the knowledge will not eliminate the emotions, it can greatly relieve a person who is thinking there is something wrong with having these feelings.
3. Encourage the support of family and friends. If no supports are available, refer the patient to a community bereavement group. (Bereavement groups are helpful even when a person has many friends or much family support.)	3. Friends can help with routine matters. For example: • Getting food into the house • Making phone calls • Driving to the mortuary • Taking care of children or other family members
4. Offer spiritual support and referrals when needed.	4. Dealing with an illness or catastrophic loss can cause the most profound spiritual anguish.
5. When intense emotions are in evidence, show understanding and support (see Table 25.4).	5. Empathic words that reflect acceptance of a bereaved individual's feelings are healing.

Modified from Robinson, D. (1997). *Good intentions: The nine unconscious mistakes of nice people*. New York: Warner Books.

person simply by being present, listening with interest, and encouraging talking and the recounting of meaningful stories. Tables 25.3 and 25.4 provide guidelines for helping people grieve.

Psychotherapy

Grief is a process that most of us manage by receiving help from family and friends and by staying connected to community activities. Some people find comfort and support in grief counseling or support groups. A counselor with spiritual expertise may be helpful for some with existential or spiritual distress. For people at risk for complicated grief reactions (history of mental illness, loss by suicide or homicide, facing multiple simultaneous losses, loss of a child), brief and time-limited psychotherapy may be indicated. According to Zisook and Zisook (2005), the following are essential components of effective short-term therapy:

1. **An educational component:** Helps people learn what to expect and how to normalize their confusing feelings and behaviors.
2. **Encouragement of full expression of emotions and affect:** May include writing letters to deceased, role-playing, and looking at pictures.
3. **An attempt to help the bereaved come to peace with a new relationship to the deceased:** Involves the process of integrating the loss of the deceased into current reality (Box 25.2).

Box 25.3 offers guidelines that can help people and their families cope with loss. More complicated or pathological patterns of grief may require special techniques, such as grief work. When a major depression or other mental health illness is involved, psychotherapeutic techniques geared toward grief work as well as toward addressing the individual's mental health issues can help greatly in improving the person's quality of life. At times, psychobiological interventions may be needed (e.g., antidepressants). Finally, tap into a multitude of resources on end of life and depression from the National Institute on Aging (e.g., see https://www.nia.nih.gov/health/end-of-life and https://www.nia.nih.gov/health/depression-and-older-adults) and other evidence-based materials. These resources can be helpful to your understanding as well as patients in learning more about end-of-life care.

TABLE 25.4 Guidelines for Communicating With a Bereaved Individual

Situation	Sample Response
When you sense an overwhelming *sorrow*	"This must hurt terribly."
When you hear *anger* in the bereaved person's voice	"I hear anger in your voice. Most people go through periods of anger when their loved one dies. Are you feeling angry now?"
If you discern *guilt*	"Are you feeling guilty? This is a common reaction many people have. What are some of your thoughts about this?"
If you sense a *fear* of the future	"It must be scary to go through this."
When the bereaved seems *confused*	"This can be a confusing time."
In almost any *painful situation*	"This must be very difficult for you."

Adapted from Robinson, D. (1997). *Good intentions: The nine unconscious mistakes of nice people* (p. 9). New York: Warner Books.

BOX 25.2 Grief and Recovery: The Lived Experience

My husband died almost 4 years ago after 54 years of marriage, 12 children, and 29 grandchildren. Within 1 year of his death, our youngest child had her first baby. We all feel Bob had a hand in sending us Benjamin. When I lost Bob, it was very difficult. He died peacefully 5 days after he was diagnosed with pancreatic cancer. It was so sudden and unexpected that it left me feeling as though I had been ripped in half with bloody, jagged edges. The pain was so unbearable, I didn't know if I could survive. I could not imagine any way to get through this. With my deep faith in God's love, the unconditional love and support from my family and friends, I managed to cope. I had grief counseling for 1 year. I learned that you heal in time, but time does not heal. I put my whole self into the process of grieving and healing. It is the most difficult job a person can do, and it takes all your energy. Now I live my life on a new level. Each day is a gift. I have grown to recognize it's important to just "be"—to be who I am; the integrated person of me and Bob, to be totally present to where I am and who I am with. My memories are laced with joy and gratitude as well as sadness. I am stronger; more resilient. I have peace.

Lois Kalafut, April 1, 2015
(direct quote)

BOX 25.3 Guidelines for Dealing With Loss

Take the time you need to grieve. The hard work of grief uses psychological energy. Resolution of the numb state that occurs after loss requires a few weeks at least. A minimum of 1 year, to cover all the birthdays, anniversaries, and other important dates without your loved one, is required before you can learn to live with your loss.

Express your feelings. Remember that anger, anxiety, loneliness, and even guilt are normal reactions and that everyone needs a safe place to express them. Tell your personal story of loss as many times as you need to—this repetition is a helpful and necessary part of the grieving process.

Establish a structure for each day and stick to it. Although it is hard to do, keeping to some semblance of structure makes the first few weeks after a loss easier. Getting through each day helps restore the confidence you need to accept the reality of loss.

Do not feel that you have to answer all the questions asked of you. Although most people try to be kind, they may be unaware of their insensitivity. Down the road, you may want to read books about how others have dealt with similar circumstances. They often have helpful suggestions for a person in your situation.

As hard as it is, try to take good care of yourself. Eat well, talk with friends, get plenty of rest. Be sure to let your primary care clinician know if you are having trouble eating or sleeping. Make use of exercise. It can help you release pent-up frustrations. If you are losing weight, sleeping excessively or intermittently, or still experiencing deep depression after 3 months, be sure to seek professional assistance.

Expect the unexpected. You may begin to feel a bit better, only to have a brief emotional collapse. These are expected reactions. Moreover, you may find that you dream about, visualize, think about, or search for your loved one. This, too, is a part of the grieving process.

Give yourself time. Do not feel that you have to resume all of life's duties right away.

Make use of rituals. Those who take the time to say goodbye at a funeral or a viewing tend to find that it helps the bereavement process.

If you do not begin to feel better within a few weeks, at least for a few hours every day, be sure to tell your physician or primary care practitioner. If you had an emotional problem in the past (e.g., depression, substance abuse), be sure to get the additional support you need. Losing a loved one puts you at higher risk for a relapse of these disorders.

From Zerbe, K. J. (1999). *Women's mental health in primary care* (pp. 207–208). Philadelphia: Saunders. Lois Kalafut, April 1, 2015 *(direct quote)*

Patient- and Family-Centered Goals of Care

No one spends as much time at the bedside of those who are dying and with their families than nursing professionals. Thus caring for individuals with serious or life-threatening illnesses through death and supporting their families require special skills, personal awareness, and ongoing self-care. Because of their daily, hands-on care and the mandate of the profession to comfort the patient, nurses have a heightened proximity to the experiences and feelings of their patients. Nurses are affected by cultural myths about grief and mourning in the same way the rest of society is; when they are faced with a person who is grieving or dying, nurses may feel uncomfortable and unequipped to face the loss. They often feel acutely uncomfortable when witnessing expressions of deep grief and pain and try to "fix it" with an intervention. Normal activities of mourning, such as weeping, protesting, or expressing anger or despair, are perceived as "meltdowns" or signs of "losing it," and nurses may feel inadequate in the face of such "breakdowns" and leave the griever, consider medicating the griever, or request a counselor for the griever. This reflects our societal misunderstandings about grief and mourning and may also be a response to the nurse's unmourned losses, difficult memories, and unresolved feelings that are awakened. The following competencies, skills, and interventions assist nurses in understanding their own feelings about loss and grief and ways to enhance caring for terminally ill patients and their families, both of whom may be grieving.

Communication Skills

Communication skills are vital in connecting with dying individuals and their family members and are an essential competency in palliative care. To be comfortable in caring for the terminally ill requires addressing barriers, such as fear of one's own mortality, lack of experience in caring for the dying, the desire to foster hope, and unrealistic societal expectations for cure. Family system changes, financial uncertainties, compromised educational or mental health capacity, physical limitations, and the impact of culture and spirituality are factors that influence communication (Ragan, 2016). Becoming proficient in effective nonverbal and verbal communication is directed at overcoming these barriers and instituting methods or practices that support the patient and family members.

Be genuinely interested without feeling the need to be an expert or have the answers. Ask open-ended questions and listen in a spirit of seeking to understand the dying individual, not to "fix" him or her. This is the person's story. Avoid using the lens of your own belief system. You are there to learn and support, not to change the individual's spirituality or faith, or lack thereof. Seek to hear unspoken questions. Sometimes a patient's existential issues are not communicated in words. These may be unspoken questions, such as: "Do you know what I am hoping for today?" "Can you tell if I am feeling despair?" "Do you know what brings me courage and peace?" "Can you help calm my fears?" *Possessing good listening skills is cited as the most important characteristic needed by a health care worker when talking with a dying individual and his or her family.* Sometimes, by listening to a patient's dreams, these unspoken emotional or spiritual states can also be explored and addressed.

One of the most important skills necessary in caring for the dying and their family members is to be "in the moment," which is also known as **therapeutic presence**. For the health care practitioner, this means that the art of presence needs to be seen as a preferred treatment intervention and not simply as the absence of being able to "do something for them." Effective presence requires that the care provider accept the reality of suffering, helplessness, mourning, and mortality itself. It asks one to slow down, put other demands aside for a while, and simply be there. Watch and listen, tolerate pauses and silences, and use open-ended questions.

Demonstrate presence and caring behaviors. Allow for a review of successes in the patients' lives and their lasting legacy; discuss any suicidal thoughts using a nonjudgmental approach, and make appropriate referrals for care; allow time for patients to express their feelings, and give them as much control over their care as possible; assist in supporting the family in repairing conflicts; help to make the most of things they enjoy (e.g., visits with friends, foods and music, storytelling, living

APPLYING THE ART

A Person Experiencing Grief

Scenario

I met 19-year-old Monica during her brief hospitalization to stabilize her insulin-resistant (type 1) diabetes. Under her veneer of sarcasm, I sensed depression as she talked about her pledging a sorority, too much partying, failing grades, her diabetes raging out of control, and the fact that her mother is dying.

Therapeutic Goal

By the conclusion of this interaction, Monica will make at least one decision to break out of her self-destructive cycle and deal with the issue(s) and feelings she is pushing down.

Student–Patient Interaction	Thoughts, Communication Techniques, and Mental Health Nursing Concepts
Monica: "You're back again. Couldn't find anything better to do?"	
Student's feelings: *Monica's sarcasm tends to disconcert me until I remind myself that fear and loss fuel her anger.*	
Student: "Hi, Monica. I will be working with you again today. How are you?"	I ignored her comment, which *non-reinforces* the sarcasm. I am willing myself to not take it personally.
Monica: "Fine. The doctor just yelled because my right heel has a sore on it that I've ignored. If I fail one more class, I go on academic probation, and finals start next week. Yeah, I'm doing just great."	I forgot that using a social greeting like "How are you?" typically elicits an automatic "fine." Using a *broad opening* like "What's been happening with you since we talked yesterday?" would better let Monica know that I really want her to share.
Student: *(Leaning in.)* "Somehow your 'just great' doesn't sound so great."	I make an observation and then use *attending* body language to show empathy.
Student's feelings: *I feel overwhelmed listening to her. Because I carry a heavy academic load, I identify with her struggles. Yet I feel some frustration that Monica does not seem to take charge of her life.*	Is that countertransference? Is that my own fear that I will lose control of all the pieces I juggle?
Monica: "No use worrying." *(Leaning in and speaking quietly.)*	
Student: "And yet somehow the worry creeps back in. Sometimes the worry looks like sadness or even anger. Sometimes it shows up as a blood sugar that refuses to stabilize."	I refer to "the worry" and "a blood sugar" to depersonalize the reference, yet still allow Monica to choose insight, if possible.
Student's feelings: *I hope I'm not pushing her too much. We have some rapport, and she lets herself vent with me.*	
Monica: *(Nods.)*	
Student: "You feel overwhelmed."	
Monica: "The doctor yelling about my foot! Wish I could hide in some hole where no one could ever find me or tell me what I should be doing."	In *crisis terms,* the doctor "yelling" likely acted as the *precipitating event.*
Student: "I wonder what pressures you the most."	I ask Monica an indirect question to help her identify stress. Should I have instead attempted to translate into feelings? For example, "You're discouraged and having a hard time believing in yourself."
Monica: "The feeling that no matter what I do, it isn't enough. It isn't good enough. I'm not good enough."	
Student: "You say you aren't good enough—for whom?"	I am assessing a *balancing* factor in *crisis* when I help Monica talk about her *perception of the event* and most significantly, her perception of self.
Monica: "Since I was diagnosed when I was 6, my mother insisted I was the same as everybody else. 'The diabetes doesn't change anything, Monica. You can do anything!' So I pledge a sorority, go with the flow, ignoring what I should or shouldn't eat or drink. Then I stay out late and screw up my sleep, and my blood sugar goes haywire. I feel bad, so I don't study."	Monica *projects* the blame for her trouble onto her mother. *What must it be like for a person to deal with diabetes since the age of 6?*
Student: "So in trying to prove the diabetes does not matter, it ends up influencing major areas of your life. What does your mother say now?"	I *clarify* to try to understand Monica's meaning. I also *gather information.*

Continued

APPLYING THE ART—cont'd

A Person Experiencing Grief

Student–Patient Interaction	Thoughts, Communication Techniques, and Mental Health Nursing Concepts
Monica: "Nothing. She doesn't know I'm in here."	Monica independently brought up the subject of her mother, so I will listen to see if her mother is a *situational support, a second balancing factor in crisis.*
Student: "She doesn't know?"	I *restate* to say, "Go on."
Monica: "I thought I could put it off until after finals, but my life is falling apart."	
Student: "Put what off, Monica?"	I still do not understand about "put off," so I ask an *indirect question.*
Student's feelings: *Did I do this the right way? I probably should have helped her talk about her life falling apart, but I am also curious about what she has put off.*	
Monica: *(Sobbing.)* "She's dying. My mother is dying. She's survived the cancer so long that I never thought she'd actually die. She has maybe 2 months."	She has been grieving losing her mother.
Student: "Oh! I'm so sorry. You've been holding this pain inside, trying to put off ...?"	
Student's feelings: *My feelings of sorrow came out without my thinking first.*	
Monica: "No one knows. My friends don't even know."	
Student's feelings: *I feel compassion for her. She must feel so alone.*	
Student: "I wonder what telling others would mean to you."	
Monica: "That I can't make it by myself. That it's real. She's going to die. I can't do my life without her." *(Crying.)*	I wonder if *unconsciously* Monica's nonadherence with her diabetic regimen and doing poorly at school has to do with *acting out* her belief that "I can't do my life without her." I know how devastated I would be to lose my mother.
Student's feelings: *I am picking up some of her feelings of aloneness and powerlessness with the impending death of her mom. I have to watch that I don't get sucked into these feelings but rather focus on Monica's feelings and thoughts.*	
Student: "Monica, what are you saying—that you don't want to live?"	Is she saying she cannot live without her mother? Is this a covert message about suicide?
Monica: "I wouldn't do anything to hurt myself, but I already feel so lonely, like she's gone already."	She describes *anticipatory grief.* However, Edwin Shneidman might refer to her behavior as subintentional suicide.
Student's feelings: *I feel relieved that she chooses to not hurt herself, although her lifestyle choices aren't healthy.*	
Student: "You feel lonely. You miss her already. In what ways have you been able to let your mother know what she means to you?"	I validate to be sure I understand. Again, I need to assess for countertransference and keep the pace at Monica's comfort level, not my own.
Student's feelings: *Helping Monica look at saying goodbye makes me think about telling the people I love how much they mean to me.*	
Monica: "I haven't gone home all semester. I barely talk when she calls. I guess if I go home, I can't pretend that it's not happening anymore."	Monica uses the word *pretend.* The *denial* stage of grief plays a part, too.
Student: "It's natural to feel afraid. It's scary to let yourself experience this pain of saying goodbye." *(She nods.)* "I wonder what you think might happen."	I give *support* and ask an *indirect question.*
Student's feelings: *I feel good that Monica is working with me to think through how she will handle talking to her mother.*	
Monica: "Maybe I won't be strong. I'll break down."	
Student: "And then?"	I help Monica *problem solve* by anticipating what will likely happen with each step, in order to decrease her *anxiety.* Being able to predict meets *safety needs.*
Monica: "My mom will cry, too."	
Student: "You will cry together." *(Monica nods.)*	
Monica: "I need to talk to her. Will you stay with me while I call?"	
Student: "Yes."	Our talking together highlighted the third crisis *balancing factor,* namely, *situational support.* Before we terminate today, I want to help Monica think about who can lend support as she juggles school, her diabetes, and the *grief* of losing her mother.
Student's feelings: *I am honored that Monica is reaching out to me and has at least made a decision to be with her mom and share their losses together.*	Monica's decision to call her mother means she is *working through the denial stage* of the grief process and she is ready to go through the painful process of saying goodbye.

BOX 25.4 Dignity in Caring

"Patient care and caring about patients should go hand in hand. Caring implicates our fundamental attitude towards the dying, and the ability to convey kindness, compassion and respect. Yet all too often, patients and families experience health care as impersonal, mechanical; and quickly discover that patienthood trumps personhood. … Caring is the gateway to disclosure; without it, patients are less likely to say what is bothering them, leading to missed diagnoses, medical errors and compromised patient safety."

From Chochinov, H. M. (2013). Dignity in care: Time to take action. *Journal of Pain and Symptom Management, 46*(5), 756–759.

BOX 25.5 FICA: Taking a Spiritual History

F: Faith and Belief "Do you consider yourself spiritual or religious" or "Do you have spiritual beliefs that help you cope with stress?" If the patient responds "no," the physician might ask, "What gives life meaning?" Sometimes patients respond with answers such as family, career, or nature.

I: Importance "What importance does your faith or belief have in your life? Have your beliefs influenced how you take care of yourself in this illness? What role do your beliefs play in regaining your health?"

C: Community "Are you a part of a spiritual or religious community? Is this of support to you, and how? Is there a person or group of people you really love or who are really important to you?" Communities such as churches, temples, and mosques, or a group of like-minded friends can serve as strong support systems for some patients.

A: Address "How would you like me, your health care provider, to address these issues in your health care?" Often it is not necessary to ask this question but to think about what spiritual issues need to be addressed in the treatment plan. Examples include referrals to chaplains, pastoral counselors, or spiritual directors, journaling, and music or art therapy. Sometimes the plan may be simple—to listen and support the person in his or her journey.

From Puchalski, C. M., & Romer, A. L. (2000). Taking a spiritual history allows clinicians to understand patients more fully. *Journal of Palliative Medicine, 3*(1), 129–137. Reprinted with permission, C. Puchalski, MD, 2015.

in the moment); and assist with spiritual comfort—finding solace in spiritual beliefs and achieving a peaceful death. Convey caring, sensitivity, and compassion. Listen. Be patient; be present (Box 25.4).

People going through intense life experiences report that they do not remember what others said to them but only how others made them feel. The intentional presence of another person makes people feel seen, valued, and important.

Assess and Address Spirituality

Nurses can strengthen their comprehensive care-planning skills by giving additional attention to spirituality and cultural determinants of care near the end of life (Long, 2016). Spirituality goes beyond religious affiliation and practices and can be an important component of how an individual defines hope and healing. Spirituality encompasses questions about how our lives relate to the rest of creation without requiring a specific religious affiliation; for example: What energizes our lives? What will survive our personal death, if anything? How do we explain to ourselves the things that happen in life? When do we feel most peaceful? How have we surmounted life's hardest challenges? Using the FICA tool, nurses can learn about the patient's spirituality and provide a means for augmenting strengths and decreasing distress (Box 25.5). Nurses have a unique opportunity to integrate spirituality into patient care through assessment, planning, and interventions that support the patient and family experiencing life-threatening illness or at the end of life (Puchalski & Ferrell, 2010; Puchalski et al., 2009).

Advance Care Planning

Nurses have an ethical duty to help their dying patients and their families through conversations regarding advance care planning (American Nurses Association [ANA], 2015). What we know is that approximately one in three adults completes any type of advance directive for end-of-life care, and two out of every five Americans age 65 and older have not completed any advance directive (Yadav, Gabler, & Cooney, 2017). There are many documented barriers to **advance care planning** and having end-of-life conversations. As a result, the care people would choose at the end of life may not be the care that they receive. Patients and families may create barriers by concealing the extent of their worry and grief, by feeling confused and fearful about dying, and by adhering to cultural preconditions. Physicians may fear bearing bad news, not fully understand advance directives, view death as the enemy, have medical-legal concerns, and lack training in interpersonal relational processes. Nurses can assist dying patients in clarifying goals and wishes for end-of-life care by exploring values, beliefs, and priorities.

Advance directives provide a person with the right to self-determination and specificity in everyday clinical decisions and actions and affirm choices for treatment options such as cardiopulmonary resuscitation, tube feedings, internal cardiac devices, and comfort care. These written instructions identify the patient's wishes when the patient is no longer able to speak on his or her own behalf. Living wills, durable power of attorney for health care, and programs such as the Five Wishes and Physician Orders for Life-Sustaining Treatment (POLST) specify these decisions; however, when there are no advance directives, these decisions are unknown. Interdisciplinary teamwork is vital to ensure that decisions are documented and that patients have the conversation about their wishes with their durable health care power of attorney to ensure their rights are upheld. Advance care planning conversations and documented advance directives are necessary to ensure that plans are concordant with care at the end of life (Hopping-Winn et al., 2018).

Interdisciplinary Teamwork

Interdisciplinary teamwork is essential in the care of the dying and their family members. Collaboration among colleagues of different disciplines joins members together to create a holistic person and family-centered plan of care. Collaboration requires team member flexibility, collective ownership of goals, and sharing with one another to create tasks and responsibilities and mutual respect (du Pré & Foster, 2016). Similarly, effective teams must learn to overcome conflicts within the team. This requires openness, joint ownership, and respect for one another. For the person who is dying and the family members, this is essential in executing a plan of care that meets the needs of the individual and contributes to a "good death" (Box 25.6).

Caring for Those Who Grieve

Endings matter, not just for the person but, perhaps even more, for the ones left behind. (Gawande, 2014, p. 232)

Needs of family members are a constant focus in palliative care. The transition from thoughts of the person living to thoughts of the person dying or "fading away" evolves during the end of life journey. Adjustments to a "new way of life" redefine family identities and roles. Increasing physical and emotional burdens may ensue, and changes in everyday life may occur daily. A continual search for meaning spawns personal growth, and preparation for death includes meeting the patient's final wishes (Steele & Davies, 2015). Thus nurses can help families during this time with the caring interventions discussed in the following subsections.

Helping Bereaved Caregivers

Once a distressing symptom has been identified as grief, there are many activities of mourning that can bring some relief and improve coping. Actively mourning includes talking about feelings, journaling

BOX 25.6 How Do Nurses Learn About Caring for End-of-Life Patients?

Sponsored by the American Association of Colleges of Nursing and the City of Hope, the End-of-Life Nursing Education Consortium (ELNEC) has been in existence for 18 years. The ELNEC curriculum and supportive materials are evidence-based and targeted at improving end-of-life education in nursing schools and continuing education of practicing nurses employed in health care organizations. To date, more than 22,500 nurses across the globe have learned about palliative care nursing and the care of patients from young to old; pain and symptom management; loss, grief, and bereavement; ethics and goals of care; cultural and spiritual considerations in palliative care; communication methods; and care of the patient and family during the final days and hours. Core themes across all curricula include (1) care of the dying patients and their family members as a unit of care, (2) the importance of culture, (3) the role of the nurse as advocate, (4) the critical need for attention to special populations, (5) end-of-life issues that affect systems of care, (6) critical financial issues that influence end-of-life care, and (7) interdisciplinary care for quality care at the end of life.

Data from End-of-Life Nursing Education Consortium. (2015). *ELNEC fact sheet.* Retrieved from http://www.aacn.nche.edu/elnec/about/fact-sheet; End-of-Life Nursing Education Consortium. (2012). *History, statewide efforts and recommendations for the future: Advancing palliative care nursing.* Retrieved from http://www.aacn.nche.edu/elnec/publications/ELNEC-Monograph.pdf

or writing, emoting, expressing what needs to be said, resolving and forgiving things that hurt, recognizing differences in grieving styles and abilities, using simple ritual, seeking support outside the family, and planning for a changed life. People often rehearse important events in life, such as becoming a parent, moving to a new home or job, or getting married or divorced. It can also help people to rehearse life as it may be after loved ones decline further and ultimately die. Families during these transition phases can be supported by the nurse.

Clinical interventions related to anticipatory grieving can be facilitated by helping family members normalize feelings, listening actively, and helping in the development of supportive relationships. A nonjudgmental stance, ongoing education, advocacy, and monitoring for complications or a maladaptive state such as the functional decline of the family caregiver can help with proactive attention to anticipatory grieving (Shore et al., 2016).

VIGNETTE:

Naming Something Gives Us Options

Julie was the wife, younger by 20 years, of a hospice patient dying of lung cancer. Julie cared for Edward in their home with help from the hospice team. During each home visit, the hospice social worker noticed that Julie seemed more drawn and fatigued. That was understandable because Edward was getting weaker, thinner, and more confined to his room. The social worker asked Julie what was most distressing to her at the present time. In tears, she said that Edward was no longer looking fondly at her or wanting to spend time together. She thought he no longer loved her, and this was deeply painful to her. The social worker described the phenomenon of anticipatory grieving and talked about the many losses they were both experiencing. "You mean Edward is grieving?" Julie said with amazement. "Yes," replied the social worker. "You are too. Just think of all that he will soon be forced to leave, most of all you, the love of his life. One way to deal with that is to withdraw early, to avoid some of the pain of parting." Julie's relief was obvious. She easily grasped that although she wanted to grow closer as she anticipated his death, Edward might need to shut her out. Thereafter, she began to act on her mourning needs by being with him more, even as she supported Edward's needs by letting him know she understood how hard this was for him. Of course, Julie was grief-stricken when he died, but she had been able to express her love, reminisce about their life together, reflect the value of Edward's life back to him, and say goodbye. In addition, she had been spared needless suffering before his death due to prematurely pulling apart from each other.

Helping People Say Goodbye

It is helpful for a nurse to understand the experience of families caring for a terminally ill patient. When bereaved caregivers were asked about their main challenges in a series of interviews (Clukey, 2007), they identified the following:

- *Adjusting to caregiving demands.* This challenge becomes all-consuming and includes physical, emotional, and practical stressors. With the patient getting so much attention, you can help by inquiring of caregivers how they are doing and what they are feeling. Listen and ask open-ended questions. Ask how you can help them.
- *Gathering information.* Most caregivers have a need to understand everything they can about the diagnosis, treatment options, and medical care for their loved ones. Anxiety usually surrounds these topics, and obtaining information may buttress a sense of control. You can help by communicating acceptance of their need to understand things. Encourage them to ask questions as often as necessary. Slow down, repeat instructions, and check in frequently to see if they would like anything clarified.
- *Finalizing the connection to the dying person.* This is often done by spending time with the patient and enjoying things together. Reminiscing, looking at photographs, and visiting are all ways to show appreciation for the person's life. Barriers to this process may be the tendency to protect each other by pretending that time will never run out; loss of energy, alertness, and focus; the effects of medications; and resistance to feeling the pain of grief.

Dr. Ira Byock (2004) provides a simple structure to this process in the **Four Gifts** of resolving relationships. In essence, they invite movement through four phases of communication:

- Forgiveness (I forgive you; please forgive me.)
- Love (I love you; I know you love me.)
- Gratitude (Thank you, and I receive your thanks.)
- Farewell (We will have an enduring connection.)

Each emotional movement opens into the next. Think of these as simple, natural, spontaneous, and creative. When they have taken place, people report a sense of peace and gratification. Encourage family members to express what is important to them, provide a **caring presence**, and understand that successful bereavement includes a sense that one was able to say goodbye. For example, out-of-town family members can speak to a nonresponsive patient through a telephone held to the patient's ear; a card or letter can be read to a dying patient and placed in his or her hands on behalf of a family member who cannot be at the bedside. These simple interventions help satisfy the need to finalize the connection with the loved one.

Helping Families Maintain Hope

Families seem to need to have hope as long as the dying person is present. *Do not think of hope as a form of denial of reality.* Hopefulness can coexist with knowledge that recovery or longevity is not a realistic goal. Forms of hope include the hope that the loved one knows how important he or she is to them, the hope that the caregivers are not falling short in their efforts at providing comfort, and the hope that the dying person knows how much he or she will be missed. Sources of hope for terminally ill patients and families include humor, uplifting memories, setting goals, and maintaining independence and the love and support of family members and friends (Cotter & Foxwell, 2015). Additional ways to foster hope and connectedness can be achieved through reminiscence, encouraging life review for patients, and legacy-building. Dignity therapy is an evidence-based intervention that assists patients to discuss the most meaningful aspects of their lives and to document their legacy (Chochinov, 2012).

VIGNETTE:
Guiding the Family in Saying Goodbye

The plan was for John to move from the intensive care unit (ICU) to home with hospice care, have his ventilator removed at that time, and die peacefully surrounded by his family. A hospice bereavement counselor was consulted to help prepare John's four teenage grandchildren for his death. When the counselor arrived at the hospital late on the afternoon of his impending transfer home, she discovered that John was too fragile to be moved and would be extubated in the ICU instead. His wife, two adult children, and the four grandchildren were gathered in a waiting room, restless and worried. The counselor worked closely with the ICU nurse to help the family with the task of finalizing the relationship. They were invited to gather around John to touch him, tell him what he meant to them, share stories, and connect with him as each one preferred. While he was not able to respond, the nurse suggested that he might be able to hear them anyway. Gradually the family relaxed and expressed many things, crying, laughing, and holding hands. Then the staff asked if anyone wanted time alone with John. His wife immediately stepped forward. After her, each one requested private time. Finally, they were asked to leave the room so that he could be medicated and extubated in private. Each step was carefully explained by the nurse and counselor. Finally, the whole family circled his bed, weeping or silent, as he gradually stopped breathing. The two staff members kept vigil with them in a corner of the room. His death was peaceful and quiet. So was the family, as each person gave him a final kiss before leaving the room.

The message: The dying person, if cognitively intact, often has preferences about where he or she will die, with what level of consciousness, with which people around, and with what level of comfort. Each family member will usually have a sense of how it will be at the time of the death. Some know they want to be present. Others prefer to remember the patient alive. When the hopes of the survivors are not met, people usually need to reconcile themselves with their disappointment during the period of bereavement. You can help by understanding the function of hope during the time of anticipatory mourning. You can listen carefully when hopes are being abandoned or reformulated as conditions change. Be sensitive to the fact that each member of the family, including the dying person, will have differing hopes. Assess hopes by asking open-ended questions, such as "How would you like her to feel about that?" or "Ideally, how would you like this to work out?"

Self-Care for Nurses

One of the hazards and challenges of becoming a professional care provider is that of practicing self-care. First, we must understand why this is so important. Then we must establish habits of good self-care. Finally, we must continually return to these habits as they are pushed into the background by the necessities of life and work. Nursing requires many skills and much knowledge but also a great deal of compassion. **Compassion** is the ability to be with someone who is suffering. Compassion is a relational phenomenon. It is less like a feeling and more like a human capacity that is developed and sustained in relationship to others. Even brief and fleeting expressions of compassion nourish this quality in our self and in others. Truly hearing the suffering of others puts us in touch with our own needs and vulnerabilities, and we may feel like protecting ourselves from that vulnerability. One way to do that is to engage in our own thoughts rather than deeply listening to another's need. Many in helping professions worry that they are not as compassionate as they would like to be and tell themselves that they are "failures." **Burnout**, decreased work performance due to negative behaviors and thoughts, and **compassion fatigue**, or the emotional pain or cost of working traumatized persons, may result in stress responses for nurses (Cross, 2019). Think of compassion and self-care as a practice or a habit of thought and action that connects us meaningfully with others. Discover what practices keep refilling your reservoir of compassion and make them habitual, which will augment job satisfaction.

Sometimes nurses need to mourn the death of a person for whom they have provided care and developed fondness. An entire staff may need to mourn the death of a particular patient or an overload of recent deaths. After patients die, nurses may be faced with managing their own tasks of mourning, such as making sense of the death, dealing with mild to intense emotions, and realigning relationships. Support groups, debriefing sessions, and the ability to attend memorial services are just a few ways that health care organizations can support nursing staff and diminish the potential for compassion fatigue.

To balance a work life that centers on others, create habits that reconnect you with your own life, your well-being, your commitment to work, and your enjoyment of the larger world. Find people you can trust at work and support one another. Accept one another's failings, successes, vulnerabilities, and intentions. Work for systemic changes at your place of employment that will enhance self-care, such as exercise programs and periodic debriefings and memorials when patients die. Review key ethical standards regularly (ANA, 2015). They express the highest and best goals of nursing care. Continue to increase your knowledge base and seek professional certifications. Ask your supervisor to email inspiring or appreciative messages to the staff. Take a few moments to thank and appreciate one another. Use your spiritual belief system to provide a sustaining context for human suffering and human kindness.

EVALUATION

Evaluation addresses whether the goals of care and outcomes have been met. The work of grief is over when the bereaved can realistically remember the pleasures and disappointments of the relationship with the lost loved one. Brief periods of intense emotions may still occur at significant times, such as holidays and anniversaries, but the person or family members have energy to reinvest in new relationships that bring shared joys, security, satisfaction, and comfort. If, after a normal period (12 to 24 months), a person has not been able to find pleasure, satisfaction, and comfort in his or her life, then reassessment and re-evaluation are indicated.

KEY POINTS TO REMEMBER

- The process of dying in the United States is undergoing transformation.
- Palliative care provides holistic interdisciplinary care for people with serious, life-limiting illnesses. Palliative care includes hospice, which is a model of care designed to help patients and family members during the last 6 months of life.
- Grief is everything experienced inside a person in response to a loss, real or perceived, including the loss of a person, security, self-confidence, or a dream.
- Anticipatory grieving describes the complex experience of patients and families during the period following a serious diagnosis. Health care professionals can guide families through some of the tasks of anticipatory mourning while providing much-needed normalization and therapeutic presence.
- Mourning is the social expression of grief. Mourning is what enables people to move through the pain and trauma of major loss as part of the bereavement process.

APPLYING EVIDENCE-BASED PRACTICE (EBP)

Problem

A 76-year-old widow has become increasingly depressed after her husband of 53 years passed away 9 months ago. She has approached a physician in Oregon, where it is legal to prescribe medication for suicide via the Death With Dignity Act. She became aware of this option when a young woman with brain cancer was prominent in the news after choosing her death date rather than enduring prolonged suffering. The widow mentioned her thoughts to her husband's hospice nurse when she visited as part of follow-up care.

EBP Assessment

A. **What do you already know from experience?** Older adult patients who lose loved ones often become depressed and do not care for themselves. Thoughts of wanting to die and join their other family members are common. The grieving process takes considerable time, longer than many people recognize. The longer a couple has been together, the longer this process may take. Hospice programs offer counseling for the surviving family member.

B. **What does the literature say?** It can be difficult to differentiate between grief and depression in older adults. Medications and other physical ailments can further complicate the scenario. Unfortunately, many people, including health care professionals, accept sadness and depressive symptoms as part of old age, but these can be treated. (See National Institute on Aging resources on aging and depression.) Nurses need to examine their feelings and positions on these issues and be prepared to discuss them more often.

C. **What does the patient want?** Although this patient initially says she wants to die, through conversation it becomes evident that she really wants the emotional pain to end and is feeling very overwhelmed and lonely. She is in fairly good health, with the exception of decreased nutrition and hydration since her husband's death. She is willing to accept help and try other avenues rather than pursue assisted suicide.

Plan

The hospice nurse arranges for the patient to see her primary care physician (PCP) and also for delivery of meals. The patient agrees to attend a grief support group. The hospice nurse helps the patient reach out to family and friends and increase her contacts and activities with them. One of the patient's children started leaving a family pet with her on the weekends, to see if that was something she would enjoy and could handle. The hospice nurse will continue to follow up with the patient for up to a year.

QSEN Prelicensure Knowledge, Skills, and Attitudes (KSAs) Addressed

Patient-Centered Care was used in formulating goals and outcomes unique to this individual.

Evidence-Based Care was provided as tenets of grief and depression supported the care plan.

- A spiritual and cultural assessment should be part of every nursing evaluation. It is crucial for health care professionals to avoid imposing their own views, faith, and beliefs on others, especially patients who are facing the vulnerabilities of serious illness and end of life.
- Compassion is a human quality and capacity that occurs and is nourished in relationships. It develops throughout a lifetime.
- Common phenomena are evident during the experience of grief, and people usually show similar patterns of grief and mourning within their cultural norms. Culture greatly affects the patterns of response to death and dying in patients as well as in nurses.
- Developing habits and practices of self-compassion is key to maintaining good self-care.
- Health care workers can use a number of communication skills to help comfort the bereaved and facilitate mourning. Actively listening to a grieving person's story without offering banal or philosophical responses can assist in healing. Short-term grief counseling and support groups are often helpful.
- Indicators of the potential for complicated or unresolved grief include social isolation, extensive dependency on the deceased person, unresolved interpersonal conflicts, loss of a child, violent and senseless death, or a catastrophic loss. A history will often reveal potential risks for complicated grieving.
- Grief work is successful when the relationship to the deceased person has been restructured and energy is available for new relationships and life pursuits. The work of mourning is complete when the bereaved person or persons can realistically remember both the pleasures and the disappointments of the lost relationship. Outcomes for successful grief work have been identified.
- Grief, when experienced by health care workers, can reactivate distressing feelings related to previous losses. It is important to recognize that staff members need psychological support when they work with people who are grieving to avoid burnout or compassion fatigue.

APPLYING CRITICAL JUDGMENT

1. Mr. Hendrix's wife is dying, and she is ready to leave the hospital to go home with the aid of hospice. Mr. Hendrix asks you what hospice can do for his wife: "How can they help me care for her? Everything is so complicated and overwhelming. Who else will be there? I am so scared. I just don't know what to do."
   - **A.** Since you know Mr. Hendrix is very anxious at this point, how would you explain to him clearly and concisely the services hospice can offer both him and his wife?
   - **B.** Mr. Hendrix tells you he does not know what to say to his wife; he says that watching her die is too hard for him and that it is very difficult to be with her, which makes him feel guilty. What guidelines can you give them in helping to say goodbye (consider the Four Gifts)?
   - **C.** If you are the nurse on the hospice team, discuss ways in which you can provide therapeutic presence for Mr. and Mrs. Hendrix.
   - **D.** If Mr. Hendrix has specific spiritual or religious beliefs that you believe might help him and his wife during this time, how could you assess these beliefs?
   - **E.** Discuss the importance *to you* of how a person's spiritual beliefs or religious beliefs (e.g., What gives me strength? What is my purpose for being here? What brings me peace? How am I spiritually connected to other humans?) might help both the person who is dying and his or her loved ones.

2. What are some concrete ways in which you can help another person to cope with a loss? Identify specific components in the following areas:
   A. How can you let the person tell his or her story?
   B. What is the potential therapeutic value of doing so?
   C. Avoiding banal advice, what are some things you might say that could offer comfort? Use the guidelines in Tables 25.3 and 25.4 to describe how you would help a person who is suffering a profound loss.

CHAPTER REVIEW QUESTIONS

1. Sixteen years ago, a toddler died in a tragic accident. Once a year, the parents place flowers at the accident site. How would the nurse characterize the parents' behavior?
   a. Mourning
   b. Bereavement
   c. Complicated grief
   d. Disenfranchised grief
2. A recently widowed adult says, "I've been calling my neighbors often, but they act like they don't want to talk to me. I just need to talk about it, you know?" What is the nurse's best action?
   a. Say to the person, "You may call me anytime you need to talk."
   b. Ask the person, "What do you mean by 'I just need to talk about it'?"
   c. Educate the person about the importance of finding alternative activities.
   d. Tell the person the location and time of a local bereavement support group.
3. A physician informed an adult of the results of diagnostic tests that showed lung cancer. Later in the day, the patient says to the nurse, "My doctor said I have breathing problems, right?" Which nursing diagnosis is applicable?
   a. *Denial* related to acceptance of new diagnosis
   b. *Spiritual distress* related to unresolved life conflicts
   c. *Situational low self-esteem* related to stress of new diagnosis
   d. *Acute confusion* related to metastatic changes to cerebral function
4. A nurse leads a bereavement group. Which participant's comment best demonstrates that the work of grief has been successfully completed?
   a. "Our time together was too short. I only wish we had done more things together."
   b. "I know our life together was a blessing that I did not deserve. I wish I had said, 'I love you' more often."
   c. "Other people knew my loved one as a good and helpful person. I hope people see me in the same way."
   d. "Our best vacations always involved water. When I see pictures of the ocean, those memories come flooding in."
5. A nurse who has worked for a community hospice organization for 8 years says, "My patients and their families experience overwhelming suffering. No matter how much I do, it's never enough." Which problem should the nursing supervisor suspect?
   a. The nurse is experiencing spiritual distress.
   b. The nurse is at risk for burnout and compassion fatigue.
   c. The nurse is not receiving adequate recognition from others.
   d. The nurse is at risk for overhelping, which creates dependency.

REFERENCES

American Nurses Association (ANA). (2015). *Code of ethics for nurses with interpretive statements*. Silver Spring, MD: ANA.

American Psychiatric Association (APA). (2013). *Diagnosis and statistical manual of mental disorders: (DSM-5)*. Washington, DC: APA.

Bonanno, G. A. (2009). *The other side of sadness: What the new science of bereavement tells us about life after a loss*. New York: Basic Books.

Boss, P. (2011). *Loving someone with dementia*. San Francisco: Jossey-Bass.

Byock, I. (2004). *Dying well: Peace and possibilities at the end of life*. New York: Riverhead Books.

Center to Advance Palliative Care (CAPC). (2018). *Growth of palliative care in U.S. Hospitals: 2018 Snapshot (2000-2016)*. Retrieved July 8, 2018, from https://media.capc.org/filer_public/27/2c/272c55c1-b69d-4eec-a932-562c2d2a4633/capc_2018_growth_snapshot_022118.pdf.

Chochinov, H. M. (2012). Dignity therapy. *Final words for final days*. New York: Oxford University Press.

Clukey, L. (2007). "Just be there": Hospice caregivers' anticipatory mourning experience. *Journal of Hospice and Palliative Nursing, 9*(3), 150–158.

Cotter, V. T., & Foxwell, A. M. (2015). The meaning of hope in the dying. In B. R. Ferrell, N. Coyle, & J. Paice (Eds.), *Oxford textbook of palliative nursing* (4th ed.) (pp. 475–486). New York: Oxford University Press.

Cross, L. (2019). Compassion fatigue in palliative care nursing: A concept analysis. *Journal of Hospice & Palliative Nursing*, 21(1), 21-28. doi: 10.1097/NJH.0000000000000477.

Doka, K. (1989). *Disenfranchised grief: Recognizing hidden sorrow*. New York: Lexington Books.

du Pré, A., & Foster, E. (2016). Transactional communication. In E. Wittenberg, B. R. Ferrell, J. Goldsmith, T. Smith, S. Ragan, M. Glajchen, et al. (Eds.), *Textbook of palliative care communication* (pp. 14–21). New York: Oxford University Press.

Gawande, A. (2014). *On being mortal: Illness, medicine and what matters in the end*. London: Profile Books.

Giddens, J. F. (2017). *Concepts for nursing practice* (2nd ed). St. Louis: Elsevier.

Hopping-Winn, J., Mullin, J., March, L., Caughey, M., Stern, M., & Jarvie, J. (2018). The progression of end-of-life wishes and concordance with end-of-life care. *Journal of Palliative Medicine, 21*(4), 541–545.

Institute of Medicine of the National Academies. (IOM). (2014). *Dying in America: Improving quality and honoring individual preferences near the end of life*. Washington, DC: National Academies Press. Retrieved February 13, 2015 from *http://www.nationalacademies.org/hmd/Reports/2014/Dying-In-America-Improving-Quality-and-Honoring-Individual-Preferences-Near-the-End-of-Life.aspx OR https://www.nap.edu/read/18748/chapter/1#xi.*

Kübler-Ross, E. (1969). *On death and dying*. New York: Macmillan.

Lindemann, E. (1994). Symptomatology and management of acute grief. *American Journal of Psychiatry, 151*(6), 156.

Long, C. O. (2016). The spiritual self: Pathways to inner strength for caregivers. *Arizona Geriatrics Society Journal, 22*(2), 14–18.

Long, C. O., Favaro, S., & Mulder, H. (2017). *Elder care A resource for Interprofessional providers: Ambiguous loss*. Portal of Geriatrics Online Education. Retrieved from https://pogoe.org/productid/21972.

National Consensus Project for Quality Palliative Care. (2018). *Clinical practice guidelines for quality palliative care* (4th ed.). Richmond, VA: National Coalition for Hospice and Palliative Care. Retrieved from https://www.nationalcoalitionhpc.org/ncp.

National Hospice and Palliative Care Organization (NHPCO). (2018). *NHPCO's facts and figures: hospice care in America 2017, revised 2018.*

Alexandria, VA: National Hospice and Palliative Care Organization. Retrieved from https://www.nhpco.org/sites/default/files/public/Statistics_Research/2017_Facts_Figures.pdf.

Neimeyer, R. A., Burke, L. A., Mackay, M. M., et al. (2010). Grief therapy and the reconstruction of meanings from principles to practice. *Journal of Contemporary Psychotherapy, 40*(2), 73–83.

Puchalski, C., & Ferrell, B. R. (2010). *Making health care whole: Integrating spirituality into palliative care.* West Conshohocken, PA: Templeton Press.

Puchalski, C., Ferrell, B. R., Virani, R., et al. (2009). Improving the quality of spiritual care as a dimension of palliative care: The report of the consensus conference. *Journal of Palliative Medicine, 12*(10), 885–904.

Ragan, S. L. (2016). Overview of communication. In E. Wittenberg, B. R. Ferrell, J. Goldsmith, T. Smith, S. Ragan, M. Glajchen, et al. (Eds.), *Textbook of palliative care communication* (pp. 1–9). New York: Oxford University Press.

Robinson, D. (1997). *Good intentions: The nine unconscious mistakes of nice people.* New York: Warner Books.

Shore, J. C., Gelber, M. W., Koch, L. M., & Sower, E. (2016). Anticipatory grief: An evidence-based approach. *Journal of Hospice and Palliative Nursing, 18*(1), 15–19.

Steele, R., & Davies, B. (2015). Supporting families in palliative care. In B. R. Ferrell, N. Coyle, & J. Paice (Eds.), *Oxford textbook of palliative nursing* (4th ed.) (pp. 500–514). New York: Oxford University Press.

Strada, E. A. (2016). Grief reactions. In E. Wittenberg, B. R. Ferrell, J. Goldsmith, T. Smith, S. Ragan, M. Glajchen, & G. Handzo (Eds.), *Textbook of palliative care communication.* New York: Oxford University Press.

Worden, J. W. (2009). *Grief counseling and grief therapy: A handbook for the mental health professional* (4th ed.). New York: Springer.

Yadav, K. N., Gabler, N. B., Cooney, E., et al. (2017). Approximately one in three US adults completes any type of advance directive for end-of-life care. *Health Affairs, 36*(7), 1244–1251.

Zisook, S., & Zisook, S. A. (2005). Death, dying and bereavement. In B. J. Sadock, & V. A. Sadock (Eds.), *Kaplan & Sadock's comprehensive textbook of psychiatry* (Vol. 11) (8th ed.) (pp. 2367–2392). Philadelphia: Lippincott Williams & Wilkins.

UNIT V

Age-Related Mental Health Disorders

Shirley A. Smoyak, PhD, ScD, RN, FAAN
Author, Editor, Distinguished Professor, and Living Legend in the Field of Psychiatric-Mental Health Nursing

Dr. Shirley Smoyak is an icon in psychiatric-mental health nursing. She has been a professor at Rutgers University for more than 50 years, teaching in the domains of mental health and illness, psychiatric nursing, family dynamics, health care administration, culture and health, and qualitative research methods. She was in the first class to finish the master's program for psychiatric nurses developed by Hildegard Peplau (the "mother of psychiatric nursing"), whom Smoyak considered to be her professional mentor. Smoyak earned a PhD in sociology, with subspecialties in families, mental illness, and deviance, and received an Honorary Doctorate from Kingston University. The professor who nominated Dr. Smoyak described her as "an inspirational figure and role model for students. She has boundless energy and enthusiasm for her area of expertise and can explain complex concepts in a way that people can relate to ... one of the figureheads of our profession." As a child of immigrants from Austria-Hungary, Smoyak developed a cultural sensitivity that has infused her work. A literature search for Dr. Smoyak's publications returns topics ranging from criminal stalking to the future of psychiatric nursing, writing well for publication, and the dangers of energy drinks. Since 1981, Smoyak has been the editor of the *Journal of Psychosocial Nursing and Mental Health Services,* the only journal dedicated to psychiatric nursing practice, and she is an international lecturer. Additionally, Dr. Smoyak is the founder and a board member of the American Psychiatric Nurses Association and has served on the board of the New Jersey State Nurses Association. She is a Charter member of the New Jersey Society of Certified Clinical Specialists in Psychiatric and Mental Health Nursing and the American Academy of Nursing. She has received numerous awards, including the American Academy of Nursing Living Legend distinction, Excellence in Practice and Roll of Honor from the New Jersey State Nurses Association, and Distinguished Lifetime Professor from the Malta Psychiatric Nurses Association.

26

Children and Adolescents

Chyllia D. Fosbre

http://evolve.elsevier.com/Varcarolis/essentials

OBJECTIVES

1. Discuss the importance of understanding developmental theory when performing an assessment or providing care for children or adolescents. Give examples of developmental information you would gather.
2. Using evidence-based practice and considering holism, formulate a patient-centered care plan for a child or adolescent who is diagnosed with a mental health disorder. **QSEN: Evidence-Based Practice**
3. When considering the disorders of children and adolescents discussed in this chapter, list the symptoms that would raise concern for the patient's safety. **QSEN: Safety**
4. Identify situations and opportunities requiring teamwork and collaboration with staff members, other departments, or parents and family when caring for minor patients. **QSEN: Teamwork and Collaboration**
5. Evaluate the emotional and physical needs of a child with either an autism spectrum disorder or attention-deficit/hyperactivity disorder, and identify evidence-based behavioral interventions. **QSEN: Evidence-Based Practice**

KEY TERMS AND CONCEPTS

attention-deficit/hyperactivity disorder (ADHD), p. 410
autism spectrum disorder (ASD), p. 410
bibliotherapy, p. 415
conduct disorder (CD), p. 412
dramatic play therapy, p. 415
mental status assessment, p. 413
movement and dance therapy, p. 415
music therapy, p. 415
oppositional defiant disorder (ODD), p. 412
play therapy, p. 415
recreational therapy, p. 415
resilience, p. 409
separation anxiety disorder, p. 411
temperament, p. 409
therapeutic drawing, p. 415
therapeutic games, p. 415
therapeutic holding, p. 415
Tourette's disorder, p. 411

CONCEPT: DEVELOPMENT: *Development* is a complex process that involves the integration of a variety of gradual changes that occur across multiple domains and result in an individual's functional abilities. The individual's state of health, environment, and/or life experiences may alter an aspect of development, causing it to stagnate or regress to an earlier stage (Giddens, 2017). About 21% of 9- to 21-year-olds in the United States suffer from a serious mental illness. Only about a fifth of young people receive the needed mental health care each year. Untreated mental illness leads to more serious complications later in life. Treatment of childhood and adolescent disorders requires a collaborative approach that often includes play, art, and bibliotherapy as well as individual, family, and group therapy.

INTRODUCTION

One in five children and adolescents will experience the effects of a mental health or learning disorder before the age of 18, and it is estimated that about 80% of mental health issues begin in childhood and continue into adulthood (Child Mind Institute, 2016). Approximately 6.8% of 3- to 17-year-olds have a diagnosis of attention-deficit/hyperactivity disorder (ADHD), making it one of the most common childhood conditions. This is followed by conduct disorders (3.8%), anxiety disorders (3%), depression (2.1%), autism spectrum disorders (1.1%), and Tourette's (0.2%) (Centers for Disease Control and Prevention [CDC], 2017a).

Children with mental illness often meet the criteria for more than one diagnostic category. Approximately 50% of children diagnosed with ADHD also have another behavioral or mental health condition, such as a disruptive disorder, depression, anxiety, or a learning disorder (CDC, 2017b). A diagnosis of high-functioning autism is linked to a 74% prevalence for another mental health condition (Belardinelli, Raza, & Taneli, 2016). There are also connections between physical health issues and mental health diagnoses. Youth who have asthma are three times more likely to have an anxiety disorder than youth who do not have asthma (Dudeney, Sharpe, Jaffe, Jones, & Hunt, 2017).

THEORY

A child's vulnerability to psychological conditions is the result of complex interactions between biological, psychological, genetic, and environmental variables. Younger children are more difficult to diagnose than older children because the boundaries between normal and abnormal behaviors are less distinct and because young children have more limited verbal skills. Diagnosis may be delayed until the child reaches school age and symptoms become more apparent.

Genetic Factors

Genetic factors have been implicated in a number of childhood mental disorders, including autism, mood disorders, schizophrenia, ADHD, and intellectual developmental disorders (mental retardation). Approximately 75% of children with ADHD have a family member with a mental health disorder (American Psychiatric Association [APA], 2017). Research studies have linked over 1000 genetic changes to autism spectrum disorder, but it is still believed that about 40% of the risk factors are not genetic (National Institutes of Health [NIH], 2017).

Temperament is a combination of personality traits made up of nine different areas: activity level, biological rhythms, sensitivity, intensity of reaction, adaptability, approach/withdrawal, persistence, distractibility, and mood. Temperament is thought to be both genetically influenced and learned through relationships with family members and caregivers (Rymanowicz, 2017). In the case of the difficult-child temperament, if the caregiver is unable to respond positively to the child, there is an increased risk of insecure attachment, developmental problems, and mental disorders. For example, in a large, boisterous family, several children may flourish and enjoy the environment, whereas another child may isolate to avoid the excessive stimulation.

Resilience is a factor associated with temperament. A child who is resilient can adapt to and overcome stressors, and resilience is a trait that can be learned. It includes thoughts, behaviors, and actions that are triggered by a stressor. A child who is resilient will more easily adjust in the face of adversity (American Psychological Association, 2017).

Biochemical Factors

Biochemical factors in childhood psychological conditions, as in adult conditions, include alterations in neurotransmitters. For example, inadequate norepinephrine and serotonin levels are related to depression and suicide. In ADHD, the neurotransmitter affected seems to relate to the subtype of ADHD symptoms. In the inattentive type, the norepinephrine transporter gene is affected. Patients with predominantly hyperactive-impulsive type have a variation in their dopamine transporter gene. In the combined type, the choline transporter gene is affected. This may explain why certain types of ADHD medications are more effective with certain subtypes. Stimulants tend to affect dopamine, whereas nonstimulants such as atomoxetine (Strattera) affect norepinephrine. In addition, serotonin levels play a factor in impulse control and aggression. People who have ADHD with normal serotonin levels seem to be more immune to the self-blame associated with ADHD symptoms (Gromisch, 2018).

Environmental Factors

Environmental factors cause stress to children and adolescents and shape their development. Abuse and neglect of any kind increase a child's risk for developing psychological conditions. Those experiencing emotional abuse are at an even higher risk of developing symptoms of mental illness (Cecil et al., 2017). The brain is more plastic (moldable or malleable) during childhood, with neuronal chains being rapidly connected. These connections are based on environmental input telling the child that the world is good and safe or scary and unpredictable. Without intervention to form more positive neuronal pathways, these early connections can guide thoughts and behaviors for the rest of a person's life. Trauma, including removal from parents, exposure to violence, observation of parental drug and alcohol abuse, and the effects of parental mental illness, increase the risk of physical and mental health conditions. According to the Adverse Childhood Experiences (ACE) study, the greater the number of adverse events, the higher the probability that mental and physical issues will occur. Adverse events include physical, sexual, and emotional abuse; neglect; violence toward mother; substance abuse in the home; mental illness in the home; divorce or separation of parents; and incarceration of a parent. The more events a child experiences, the greater the ACE score. The greater the ACE score, the more likely the person will experience social, emotional, and cognitive impairments; the individual is also more likely to participate in high-risk behaviors and to experience earlier or more severe disease, disability, or social problems. A higher ACE score is linked with a greater risk for depression, substance use as an adult, an increase in suicide attempts, and high-risk sexual behavior and also increases the risk of early heart attacks, respiratory distress, and other medical symptoms (Substance Abuse and Mental Health Services Administration [SAMHSA], 2017a). The ACE study has helped advance and highlight the connection between trauma, mental health, and physical problems.

NEURODEVELOPMENTAL DISORDERS

Neurodevelopmental disorders occur when there is some delay in one or more areas of development. These disorders include intellectual disabilities, communication disorders, autism, ADHD, learning disorders, and motor disorders. It is estimated that about 15% of children ages 3 to 17 have been diagnosed with one of many neurodevelopmental disorders (U.S. Environmental Protection Agency, 2017).

Intellectual Disability

Intellectual disabilities (IDs), previously called mental retardation, affect approximately 0.05% to 1.55% of the population (American Speech-Language-Hearing Association [ASLHA], 2017). This disorder is categorized as mild, moderate, severe, or profound.

Causes may be hereditary factors (Tay–Sachs disease, fragile X syndrome, cerebral palsy), alterations in early embryonic development (Down syndrome, fetal alcohol syndrome, hydrocephalus), pregnancy and perinatal problems (fetal malnutrition, prematurity, maternal age, hypoxia, infections), and other factors such as trauma and poisoning (Krucik, 2015).

IDs are further classified by levels of severity (mild, moderate, severe, and profound). This is based on functional adaptation in conceptual, social, and practical domains (APA, 2013; ASLHA, 2017). In the past, ID was ranked based on IQ scores. This is now only one of many factors considered when determining severity.

The mild form of ID constitutes 85% of cases. These children develop communication and social skills with minimal sensorimotor impairment and are often indistinguishable from children with normal-range IQs. They are able to perform self-care and may be capable of vocational training and independent living. The conceptual domain is at a mid–elementary school level. More than half of these individuals will own a home, marry, and have children (APA, 2013; Pivalizza, 2015).

The moderate form of ID constitutes 10% of cases. These children develop communication, social, and academic skills slowly. The conceptual domain is at an elementary school level, with reading ability commonly at a first- to third-grade level. Although these individuals are able to perform activities of daily living, ongoing assistance is needed for conceptual tasks of daily life. They may have long-term intimate relationships and friends but may not interpret social cues accurately. Support is needed to obtain success in employment and in areas such as transportation and money management skills (APA, 2013; Pivalizza, 2015).

The severe form of ID constitutes 3% to 4% of cases. Speech may be delayed or absent, and individuals often use single-word phrases and gestures. Most individuals in this category require assistance with daily living skills, may perform simple tasks with help, and require significant support and a supervised living environment. In general, these individuals do not marry or have children and have a shortened life span. Maladaptive behaviors, such as self-harm, may be present (APA, 2013; Pivalizza, 2015).

The profound form of ID constitutes 1% to 2% of cases. These individuals are mostly nonverbal and do not learn to read. Some individuals are able to learn simple tasks such as dressing themselves. They tend to have sensory and physical impairments, requiring medical equipment and constant supervision to support functioning. Life expectancy in this group is significantly reduced, usually between 4 and 20 years (APA, 2013; Pivalizza, 2015).

VIGNETTE: INTELLECTUAL DISABILITY: An 8-year-old male is attending second grade. He was held back a year because of his poor reading comprehension and delayed social skills. Despite being with younger children, he is remarkably smaller than his classmates. He was initially diagnosed with ADHD and learning disabilities; however, after discussing his history with his adoptive parents, there was some suspicion that his intellectual disability was due to fetal alcohol syndrome. His physical characteristics, which include small stature, wide-set eyes, and small head circumference, also support this diagnosis.

Communication Disorders

Language Disorders, Speech Sound Disorders, Childhood-Onset Fluency Disorder (Stuttering), and Social Communication Disorder

These disorders include deficits in language, speech, and communication. Assessment should take into account the child's cultural and language context (APA, 2013). It is not uncommon for children growing up in a home of one language to have some language barriers when attending a school where another language is predominant, but the child should be communicating with family at an age-appropriate level. Childhood-onset fluency disorder (stuttering) usually occurs before age 6 and is characterized by broken speech and word substitutions to avoid problematic words. Verbalization causes physical tension and anxiety for the child, which can then exacerbate the speech symptoms. Children who stutter may be teased or bullied and have difficulty performing in the classroom, contributing to self-esteem and socialization issues.

Autism Spectrum Disorder

Autism spectrum disorder (ASD) now encompasses former diagnoses of Asperger's syndrome and pervasive developmental disorders. ASD presents with deficits in social and emotional interactions, as well as repetitive patterns of behavior, interests, or activities. Children may twirl, walk on their toes, flap their arms, or rock. These behaviors are collectively referred to as self-stimulatory or "stimming." Stimming can be mild and barely noticeable (tapping fingers on leg) or severe (banging head on floor or biting) and can cause injury and scarring. People with autism tend to become focused on a particular subject and perseverate on it. They may gain a profound amount of knowledge about their preferred interests but are delayed in most other academic and life domains. A lack of interest in social interaction is often the key symptom that is noticed initially. Children with this disorder are often loners and may dislike physical affection. They tend to get very upset with changes in routine, changes in caregivers, or changes in their environment (CDC, 2016).

The severity of ASD is categorized into levels based on functional ability. In Level 1 there is a noticeable social deficit, but language and speech are normal. Individuals have difficulty switching between activities, and they struggle with organization and planning. In Level 2 there is a noticeable deficit in both verbal and nonverbal social and communication skills. Social impairment and repetitive behaviors are obvious to others. These individuals do not tend to initiate social interactions, and change in routine causes distress. In Level 3 social deficits are severe, with communication being limited and needs-based. Individuals may be nonverbal, speak in few-word sentences, be difficult to understand, make odd noises, echo a word or sentence over and over, or use overly literal language. Repetitive and restrictive behaviors markedly interfere with functioning in all spheres. Changing focus, action, or routine causes great distress. Aggression toward self or others is more common at this level (CDC, 2016).

VIGNETTE: AUTISM SPECTRUM DISORDER: The parents of a 4-year-old toddler notice that their child prefers to play alone when they take her to the park. She spends most of her time in the sandbox spinning the wheels on the cars. When the toddler hears a word, she tends to repeat it over and over and is not using full sentences. She becomes easily overwhelmed in crowds and will start to flap her arms and cry. She resists hugs and physical affection. She is in preschool, and her teachers have suggested that she be evaluated for autism by a developmental pediatrician.

Attention-Deficit/Hyperactivity Disorder

The symptoms of attention-deficit/hyperactivity disorder (ADHD) include problems with concentration, such as making careless mistakes, difficulty remaining focused, being easily distracted, appearing not to listen when spoken to, lack of follow-through, struggling with organizational and time management skills, and forgetfulness. Individuals with ADHD may also avoid tasks that require sustained mental effort, misplace items, and tend to be messy. Children may fidget, squirm, leave their seat at school, run or climb when not appropriate, blurt out answers or comments, interrupt, or talk excessively. As adults, this may present as an internal restlessness more than as physical impulsivity (APA, 2013). The symptoms of ADHD can result in children being disciplined repeatedly in the classroom and at home, and peers may tease them, leading to problems with self-esteem. Schoolwork can fluctuate between excellent projects and poor assignments. Students can be intelligent, but performance is hindered by distractibility and other symptoms (CDC, 2017d). ADHD is one of the most common mental health conditions diagnosed in children.

Specific Learning Disorders

Discovery of learning disorders, which include dyslexia and dyscalculia, occurs during elementary school years. Symptoms include difficulty in learning and using academic skills. Learning disabilities are not related to developmental delays. It is estimated that 5% to 15% of school-age children have a learning disorder, and they are more common in males. Learning disabilities are linked to higher rates of dropping out of school, depression, suicide, unemployment, and underemployment, as well as lower income (APA, 2013).

Motor Disorders

Tourette's disorder, developmental coordination disorder, and several other motor or vocal tic disorders are listed in the *Diagnostic and*

Statistical Manual of Mental Disorders, 5th edition (*DSM-5*; APA, 2013; Sadock, Sadock, & Ruiz, 2015). Two are briefly discussed in this section.

- *Developmental coordination disorder.* The symptoms of this disorder include delayed coordinated motor skills, presenting as clumsiness, slowness, and difficulty with handwriting or riding a bike (Nelson, 2015).
- Tourette's disorder. The symptoms of this disorder include motor as well as vocal tics, with an onset in early childhood. Tics can be mild, such as clearing the throat or jerking a limb, or as severe as loudly yelling out an animal noise or curse word, with spasms intense enough to cause the patient to be flung out of a chair. Tics can be very embarrassing to children and adolescents as they attempt to navigate social and dating relationships.

BIPOLAR AND MOOD DISORDERS

Bipolar disorder is discussed in detail in Chapter 16. The diagnosis of bipolar disorder in children is controversial because children at a young age normally have temper tantrums and some mood lability. Mood lability is also common in teenagers as hormones change during puberty. It is when symptoms are severe and affect the ability to function that diagnosis and treatment are typically recommended. The mean age for the first manic, hypomanic, or major depressive episode is 18 to 20, although it can occur as early as mid-childhood (APA, 2013).

One of the differences with depression in children is that a low or depressed mood may present as anger and irritability. Children may also have somatic symptoms related to depression and anxiety, including stomach aches, nausea, and headaches, that are unexplained by medical conditions. Medical causes should be ruled out for any ongoing physical symptoms. Adolescents have a higher rate of suicide, so it is especially important to be aware of the typical and atypical presentations of depression (National Institute of Mental Health, 2016).

Disruptive mood dysregulation disorder (DMDD) is classified as a depressive disorder and is a new diagnosis with the *DSM-5* update that was released by the APA in 2013. A child with DMDD experiences symptoms before the age of 10 and is not diagnosed until the age of 6. The primary symptoms include an angry or irritable mood, as well as temper tantrums or outbursts that are bigger than would be expected for the child's age and are occurring three or more times a week. Symptoms are severe enough to cause problems in functioning at home, school, or in the community (APA, 2013; National Institute of Mental Health, 2017). This diagnosis was added to reduce the number of children who were being incorrectly diagnosed with bipolar disorder. There is some thought that children diagnosed with DMDD may eventually be diagnosed with bipolar disorder in adulthood; however, because this is a new diagnostic category, there is little research to support the transition from DMDD to bipolar.

VIGNETTE: A 12-year-old student has made daily trips to the school nurse for the past 3 days with complaints of an upset stomach. The school nurse suspects the student is having physical symptoms because of an increase in stress and gently assesses the situation. The student immediately bursts into tears when the nurse asks how things are going at home. The nurse learns the student heard her parents arguing about getting a divorce. She doesn't feel like she can talk to her parents and is embarrassed to talk about it with friends. The nurse helps the student realize her upset stomach is from the stress and anxiety and teaches her a simple guided-imagery technique to help refocus her thoughts and calm her mind.

ANXIETY DISORDERS

Separation anxiety disorder, selective mutism, and specific phobias in childhood are discussed in this section. The symptoms of anxiety are similar in all age groups, with the exception of separation anxiety disorder, which is only diagnosed in children.

- Separation anxiety disorder. The child displays developmentally inappropriate fear or anxiety surrounding separation from the person to whom the child is most attached. The child may worry about losing important people to injury or death or about being lost or kidnapped. The child may refuse to stay with grandparents or friends and insist on sleeping near the parental figure. Nightmares with the theme of separation may occur, as well as somatic complaints such as stomach distress when separation is anticipated. The symptoms are considered normal up to age 1. The prevalence is 4% in children and 1.6% in adolescents.
- *Selective mutism.* The child displays a consistent failure to speak in situations where speaking is an expectation, although the child is able to speak at other times. Symptoms interfere with academic, social, or occupational achievement.
- *Specific phobias in childhood.* Phobias are discussed in Chapter 11. Some phobias often seen with children include fear of the dark, monsters, costumed characters, injections, water, and certain animals. Phobias occur in 5% of children and 16% of adolescents (APA, 2013).

OBSESSIVE-COMPULSIVE AND RELATED DISORDERS

Trichotillomania and excoriation disorder frequently begin in childhood. *Trichotillomania* is the recurrent twisting or pulling out of one's hair, resulting in hair loss or damage. The individual attempts to stop, without success, and the behavior causes distress. The prevalence in the adolescent and adult population is 1% to 2%, and it is more common in females. Excoriation disorder is recurrent skin-picking, resulting in skin lesions, infection, and scarring. The lifetime prevalence is about 1%, and it is more common in females.

TRAUMA- AND STRESSOR-RELATED DISORDERS

Children may also respond differently to trauma and stress and have an increase in complaints of physical symptoms, nightmares, bed wetting, or other regressive symptoms. One trauma- and stressor-related disorders specific to children is *reactive attachment disorder (RAD).* RAD is defined as a consistent pattern of inhibited, emotionally withdrawn behavior. Children with RAD rarely seek comfort or respond to comforting. Symptoms include limited positive affect, irritability, sadness, fearfulness, and minimal social responsiveness. Causes of RAD include inconsistent care, frequent changes in caregivers, and living in foster homes or orphanages.

FEEDING AND EATING DISORDERS

Eating disorders are discussed in Chapter 14. However, there are three feeding and eating disorders that are seen more commonly in children. These three disorders are as follows:

- *Pica.* Pica involves the persistent eating of nonfood substances, such as sand or dirt, chalk, paint chips, ice, cloth, or hair. It is not part of a culturally accepted ritual or practice, and onset is commonly in childhood. There is potential for harm or death, depending on what is ingested.
- *Rumination disorder.* This disorder involves repeated regurgitation of food, which is then re-chewed, re-swallowed, or spit out. The

behavior may be self-soothing and often corrects itself if it occurs in infancy.

- *Avoidant/restrictive food-intake disorder.* With this disorder, there is a persistent failure to meet nutritional or energy needs. It results in weight loss or failure to gain weight, significant nutritional deficiency, or dependence on supplements.

Eating disorders in children and teens can lead to a host of serious physical problems and even death. A child needs treatment right away because the best results occur when eating disorders are treated at the earliest stages.

ELIMINATION DISORDERS

Elimination disorders are often problematic in childhood and can lead to bullying and negatively affect self-esteem. Enuresis is the repeated voiding of urine and can be involuntary or intentional. Enuresis occurring after the age of 5 is abnormal. Encopresis is the repeated passage of feces, and it can also be involuntary or intentional. It is considered abnormal after the age of 4. Encopresis is further categorized into primary, secondary, retentive, and nonretentive, of which 80% to 90% of cases are the retentive type. If not treated, serious complications such as megacolon can occur (Stanford Children's Hospital, 2017).

GENDER DYSPHORIA

This disorder relates to the feeling that a person is in the wrong-gender body; it is discussed in Chapter 27.

Gender dysphoria is being discussed in a more open manner in our society. Caitlyn (formerly Bruce) Jenner, an Olympic medalist, is a recent example of an individual who underwent gender alignment procedures to physically appear like the woman she is inside. Some literature has found that young children can already report feeling like the opposite gender. Parents react in various ways to disclosures of this nature, with some showing acceptance in providing opposite-gender clothing and experiences and others becoming distraught and rigid.

It is a good exercise to think carefully about how you would react if your child were to tell you he or she is transgender. What behaviors would you allow or not allow, and why? How do you think other children at school or family members would react? What practical considerations exist, such as bathroom and locker room issues?

DISRUPTIVE, IMPULSE CONTROL, AND CONDUCT DISORDERS

Oppositional defiant disorder and conduct disorders are two disorders found in the child and adolescent populations presented here. The remaining disorders are covered in Chapter 27.

Oppositional defiant disorder (ODD) goes beyond the normal limit testing typical of children. Symptoms must be displayed with at least one person who is not a sibling and include at least four of the following: often loses temper, easily annoyed, angry, argues with authority figures, defies or refuses rules, deliberately annoys others, blames others for mistakes or misbehavior, vindictive (Cleveland Clinic, 2017).

Conduct disorder (CD) is more severe than ODD. Children diagnosed with CD must display at least three of the following criteria: bullies or intimidates others; initiates physical fights; has used a weapon (bat, brick, knife); physically cruel to people or animals; has stolen while confronting a victim; has stolen nontrivial items; has forced someone into sexual activity; deliberate fire-setting to cause damage; deliberate destruction of property; has broken into a house, car, or building; lies to obtain favors or to avoid obligations; stays out at night despite parental rules; has run away overnight at least twice; often truant from school (American Academy of Child and Adolescent Psychiatry, 2017).

APPLYING EVIDENCE-BASED PRACTICE (EBP)

Problem

A 16-year-old male in a motorized wheelchair arrives at the psychiatrist's office with his parents for a medication management visit. He is able to communicate positive and negative feelings through facial expressions and verbalizations. He is unable to speak in full words or sentences. One of his primary diagnoses is autism spectrum disorder (ASD). He displays repetitive actions and interests, which include wearing masks and hats. He is prone to lashing out at others and biting and hitting himself. As he has grown larger and stronger, it is becoming increasingly difficult for his supportive and loving, but elderly, parents to care for him.

EBP Assessment

A. **What do you already know from experience?** ASD appears in mild through severe presentations. Especially in severe cases, it becomes difficult for patients to remain at home as they mature. Size, strength, and hormones all contribute to additional challenges. Parents can be exhausted and even endangered, yet remain reluctant to place their children outside of the home. Communication can be especially difficult in severe cases of this disorder.

B. **What does the literature say?** The beliefs of elderly parents with autistic children affect their ability to cope. Some parents believe that autism is a punishment, whereas others see it as a manageable situation. Most parents have a positive outlook and see their children as they could have been without the disorder; they realize that there is more to their children than most people see. They also experience guilt and judgment by others for the child's disruptive behaviors. Many parents do not realize that some features of autism can be improved (CDC, 2016).

C. **What does the patient want?** The patients in this example include the young man with ASD and his parents because he cannot fully communicate and they are his guardians. His parents know him very well and are able to interpret a lot of his needs and interests for the provider. Both parents and the patient experience considerable frustration surrounding communication deficits and would like that to improve. All three parties are disappointed that their care aide has left and are displeased with their new aide, feeling there is not a good connection with the patient.

Plan

The psychiatrist worked with the treatment team to arrange for a different care aide. Medications were left the same because the recent exacerbation in behaviors was situational to the previous aide leaving the position and was decreasing. The treatment team contacted disability services and arranged for the patient to receive an electronic communication device, as well as instruction in its use for the patient and parents. The next time the psychiatrist saw this patient, he proudly showed her his progress using the device.

QSEN Prelicensure Knowledge, Skills, and Attitudes (KSAs) Addressed

Safety was addressed by ensuring the aide was a good fit with the family and evaluating medications.

Informatics played a role through the use of an electronic communication device.

SUBSTANCE-RELATED AND ADDICTIVE DISORDERS

Substance use disorders are a significant issue in adolescence and are estimated to occur in 5% of youth between ages 12 and 17 (SAMHSA, 2017b).

One study found that 17.6% of 8th graders and 55.6% of 12th graders had used alcohol within the past year, and 27.2% of high school students had used illicit drugs within the past year (National Institute on Drug Abuse, 2016). It is important for nurses to be aware of the prevalence of substance abuse in child and adolescent populations.

APPLICATION OF THE NURSING PROCESS

ASSESSMENT

Mental Health Assessment

The mental health assessment for children focuses more on developmental stages. Neurodevelopmental issues are usually discovered in childhood and are observed through comparison with normal developmental milestones, such as walking, toilet training, talking, and forming relationships with caregivers. The assessment of a child is holistic and includes the presenting problem, medical and developmental issues, family history, physical examination, and a **mental status assessment**. In adolescents, it is also important to consider substance use, sexual activity, self-harm behaviors, and suicidal thoughts. Depending on the answers and presentation of the patient, additional details and areas of mental assessment may be explored. Although assessing risks is important, assessing strengths and protective factors is key in working with a younger population. Identifying strengths and protective factors can help in treatment planning and allows the treatment team to support and bolster areas of strength (Flacks & Boynton-Jarrett, 2017).

Methods of collecting data include interviewing, screening, testing (neurological, psychological, intelligence), observing, and interacting with the child or adolescent. Histories are taken from parents and caregivers and may include reports or conversations with teachers or other school professionals. Children and adolescents should be included in conversations when possible. It is important to keep in mind that children are concrete and literal in their thinking and may also be afraid to directly disclose problems at home, at school, or within other activity groups. Play therapy can allow the nurse or care professional to gain information in a nonthreatening manner. Observing interactions with parents, siblings, or caregivers can provide insight as well. The child or adolescent should spend some time alone with the interviewer so that the opportunity to disclose abuse is made available (Box 26.1).

Many professionals will likely be involved in the diagnosis and treatment of children. The initial diagnosis may be made by a primary care provider during a well-child examination at which time they are referred to a specialist for further evaluation and treatment. Speech and language therapists may assess a child with speech delays or abnormal speech production. A physical and occupational therapist may assess fine and gross motor skills or identify sensory processing issues. A school psychologist may be involved in learning disorder and IQ testing. Genetic testing may be done to identify genetic abnormalities. A child and adolescent psychiatrist or psychiatric-mental health nurse practitioner may diagnose anxiety or mood-related concerns, whereas a neuropsychologist or developmental pediatrician may conduct more extensive testing to more clearly identify areas of intellectual impairment. In many states, therapists and counselors can also provide a diagnosis.

A nurse may work as a case manager and help connect the different types of specialists involved in caring for the child. A school nurse may also work with the child and family to develop an individualized education plan to identify ways to accommodate the child's developmental, behavioral, or emotional needs.

A nursing assessment should include developmental stages, speech and language patterns, social skills, environment, and interactions within the family. Observation of feeding and elimination patterns may also help clinicians identify childhood-based disorders. Observing social interactions, energy level, eye contact, and characteristics of play may all provide insight into a variety of disorders. The evaluation and assessment of a child will likely be lengthier and more in-depth than what might be seen in an adult assessment.

As with any population, safety is a priority. Impulse control disorders may lead to unsafe actions. Cognitive delays may lead to poor awareness of safety issues, such as the danger of following strangers. Eating nonfood items can cause medical problems. Home visits may help a nurse identify additional safety concerns in the environment.

Once safety is assessed, trauma should then be ruled out as a cause for the behaviors. Children are a vulnerable population that can be exploited and abused, and behaviors are often a form of communication that something is wrong. See Chapter 21 for further discussion on child abuse and neglect.

DIAGNOSIS

The International Classification of Nursing Practice nursing diagnoses that are commonly used with children include *Risk for deficient food intake* for children who have feeding disorders or *Risk for constipation* or *Risk for diarrhea* for children with elimination disorders. For children with developmental delays, a nursing diagnosis might include *Impaired child development* or *Impaired school performance*. When there are breakdowns in parenting, the diagnoses of *Impaired parenting, Impaired child attachment*, or *Risk for caregiver stress* may be used.

PLANNING AND IMPLEMENTATION

Psychopharmacology

Psychopharmacology for children should be implemented only after addressing behaviors and providing any additional supports needed. Medications may be used in children when other approaches have failed. Many of neurocognitive disorders such as communication disorders or intellectual disabilities will respond to medications, and medications may be helpful in treating comorbid symptoms of anxiety, depression, or aggressive behaviors. Attention-deficit/hyperactivity disorder is often treated with stimulant medications such as methylphenidate (Ritalin), amphetamine salts (Adderall), or lisdexamfetamine (Vyvanse). These help improve attention and focus as well as reduce hyperactive behaviors. Children with autism spectrum disorders may take antipsychotic medications such as risperidone (Risperdal) or aripiprazole (Abilify) to reduce aggression and irritability or may take selective serotonin reuptake inhibitors (SSRIs) such as fluoxetine (Prozac) and sertraline (Zoloft) to improve anxiety or obsessive traits.

For anxiety and depression, SSRIs are considered first-line medications. Most antidepressants carry a black box warning that children and young adults may experience suicidal ideation while taking the medication. Suicide assessment should be part of the routine assessment at every patient contact in primary care and in mental health clinics.

BOX 26.1 Child–Adolescent Mental Status Assessment

General Appearance
- Size: height and weight
- General health and nutrition
- Dress and grooming
- Distinguishing characteristics
- Gestures and mannerisms
- Looks or acts younger or older than chronological age

Activity Level
- Hyperactivity or hypoactivity
- Tics, other body movements
- Autoerotic and self-comforting movements (thumb sucking, ear or hair pulling, masturbation, rocking)

Speech
- Rate, rhythm, intonation, pitch
- Vocabulary and grammar appropriate to age
- Mute, hesitant, talkative
- Articulation problems
- Unusual characteristics (pronoun reversal, echolalia, gender confusion, neologisms)

Coordination or Motor Function
- Posture, gait, balance
- Gross and fine motor movement
- Writing and drawing skills
- Unusual characteristics (bizarre postures, banging, biting self, tiptoe walking, hand flapping)

Affect
- Predominant emotions expressed and facial expression
- Feelings appropriate to the situation
- Range and intensity of feelings
- Unusual characteristics (apathy, sulking, oppositional behavior, overly emotional)

Manner of Relating
- Eye contact
- Ability to separate from caregiver, be independent
- Attitude toward interviewer and others, social reciprocity
- Behavior during interview (patience, impulsiveness, aggressive, ability to have fun or play, frustration level)

Intellectual Functions
- Fund of general information
- Ability to communicate (follow directions, answer questions)
- Memory
- Creativity, humor
- Learning and problem solving
- Conscience (sense of right and wrong, accepts limits)

Thought Processes and Content
- Orientation
- Attention span
- Self-concept and body image
- Fantasies and dreams
- Ego-defense mechanisms
- Perceptual distortions (hallucinations, illusions, unusual ideas)
- Sex role, gender identity

Characteristics of Child's Play
- Age-appropriate use of toys, and play with peers
- Themes of play
- Imagination and pretend play
- Role and gender play
- Relationships with peers (empathy, sharing, waiting for turns, best friends)

Children should always be started on a lower dose of medication and monitored more frequently than one might for an adult.

Children with elimination disorders might also receive desmopressin (DDAVP) to reduce bedwetting or may receive stool softeners or laxatives for constipation. A medical cause should be ruled out in any child who is wetting the bed. After ruling out a medical cause, stopping fluids an hour or two before bedtime, waking a child at night to use the bathroom, or using an alarm that sounds if the child wets the bed are usually the preferred treatment options before starting medications. For a child with diarrhea or constipation, a review of diet may identify culprits such as cheese, which is frequently known to cause constipation, or lactose, which can cause diarrhea in someone with a lactose intolerance. Anxiety and trauma can also impact elimination.

Although no medications are specifically approved for conduct disorder, some of the medications used to treat hyperactivity in ADHD can be helpful, or mood stabilizers or antipsychotics may be used to reduce anger and irritability.

As a newer diagnosis, disruptive mood dysregulation disorder has no approved medications. However, improvements are being seen with a variety of medications. Medications such as guanfacine and clonidine are often used to reduce behavioral outbursts. Risperidone and aripiprazole may help both mood and behaviors. Mood stabilizers such as valproic acid, carbamazepine, and oxcarbazepine may also help with mood and behaviors.

Nonpharmacological Interventions

Parental involvement and support are recognized as critical factors in the supportive and educational interventions for the child or adolescent. In addition to therapy with a single family, group therapy with several families facing similar challenges provides support and insight.

Group therapy for younger children takes the form of play. As children get older, more talk therapy can occur. Groups are effective for common issues such as bereavement, abuse, chronic illness, or addiction. One of the challenges of using groups when working with children and adolescents lies in the contagious effect of disruptive behavior.

Milieu therapy is a philosophical basis for structuring inpatient and other long-term treatment programs. The nurse and other team members collaborate to provide a therapeutic environment that facilitates growth, safety, and positive change.

Behavior modification and CBT are based on the principle that rewarded behavior is more likely to be repeated. Connections between thoughts, feelings, and behaviors are identified, and techniques help to develop rational thinking, better choices, and impulse control. Progress is rewarded with attention, praise, or other desired outcomes or privileges. Point systems or behavioral charts are examples. Rehearsing new behaviors and relaxation and guided imagery may be employed.

Restraints and seclusion are dangerous, controversial treatment modalities for children (as well as for adults). Injuries and even death have been associated with seclusion and restraint with children. In recent years, most facilities have become restraint-free in all but the most emergent of situations when a patient is in immediate danger of harming self or others. Seclusion and restraint are closely monitored and allowed only for short periods of time within prescribed and monitored guidelines. Gentle **therapeutic holding**, which is nonpunitive in nature, or helmets to protect a patient during head banging can be used.

Instead of seclusion, a unit may have an unlocked **quiet room** for a youth who needs to be removed from the situation for either self-control or control by the staff. **Time out** is a common method for intervening in disruptive or inappropriate behaviors, both by parents and in mental health settings. The child's individual behavioral goals, developmental stage, and age are considered in setting limits on behavior by using time-out periods. If they are overused or inconsistent, time outs lose their effectiveness. Some professionals argue that using a time out is a form of rejection and urge parents to use a "time-in" approach where parents offer affection through hugs, calm communication, and reassurance that the parents are available when the child is ready to discuss the situation.

Play therapy is based on the notion that play is the work of childhood and the way a child learns to master impulses and adapt to the environment. Play is also the language of childhood and the communication medium for assessing developmental and emotional status, determining a diagnosis, and instituting therapeutic interventions. There are many forms of play therapy that can be used individually or in groups. Playrooms are equipped with art supplies and a variety of toys, including hand puppets, dolls, dollhouses, and action figures. These toys provide the child with opportunities to act out conflicts and stressful situations, to work through feelings, and with the help of the therapist, to develop more adaptive ways of coping. Drawings can be evaluated for inner conflict, family relationships, and other stressors in the child's life.

Dramatic play therapy, also called *psychodrama*, is a treatment modality that uses dramatic techniques to act out emotional problems, examine the experience, develop new perspectives, and try out new behaviors. This modality may be used with groups of older children and adolescents. The dramas can be videotaped for reviewing the experience and facilitating new learning. This type of therapy is not recommended with psychotic youth.

Therapeutic games are an ideal assessment tool for children who may have difficulty talking about their feelings and problems, and they also allow a nonthreatening way to develop rapport with health care workers. The game might be as simple as checkers, but therapeutic games are more effective in eliciting children's fears and fantasies. A well-known game is the *Talking, Feeling, and Doing Game* (Gardner, 2007). The player draws a talking, feeling, or doing card, which gives instructions or asks a question, such as "All the girls in the class were invited to a birthday party except one. How did she feel?" If this game is played with a group, additional responses can be elicited.

Bibliotherapy involves using children's books and literature to help the child express feelings in a supportive environment, gain insight into feelings and behavior, and learn new ways to cope with difficult situations. Children unconsciously identify with the characters in the story, so the books selected should reflect the situation or feeling that is problematic for the child (Pincus, 2012).

Therapeutic drawing allows children to spontaneously express themselves in artwork that captures thoughts, feelings, and tensions they may be unable to express verbally. When drawing any human figure, children leave an imprint of their inner self, including attitudes about the family. The following list notes characteristics that are general indicators of children's emotions or meanings found in a drawing. However, the normal presentation for age groups must be considered; for example, a toddler might not include arms in a drawing because he or she ran out of room on the paper, whereas missing arms in the drawing of an older child would more likely indicate a feeling of powerlessness. It is recommended that the nurse working with children consult an authoritative book on interpreting children's drawings.

- Size of figures: very large (aggression, poor impulse control); very small (shyness, insecurity)
- Omission of body parts: hands (trauma, insecurity), arms (inadequacy, powerlessness), legs (lack of support), feet (insecure, helpless), mouth (difficulty expressing self, not having a voice)
- Facial expressions: personal mood and affect of child or others in the picture
- Integration of body parts: scattered or disorganized parts indicate cognitive or psychological problems or both.
- Placement of the child in relation to other family members: Is the child close to the father, with the mother in a distant corner of the page? This could indicate an emotional distance or be an indication of living arrangements.
- Differences in facial expressions of family members: For example, is one person angry and the rest fearful?
- Colors can indicate a cheerful, angry, or sad mood.

Music therapy instigates changes in both the physiology of the nervous system and social interactions. Music therapy may incorporate recorded music, songs, songwriting, or the use of a musical instrument. Children love to use simple noisemakers for the expression of feelings, for the development of coordination and rhythm, and as an opportunity for social interactions. Music on inpatient units is often used to create a relaxing mood for rest periods and bedtime.

Movement and dance therapy is a direct expression of the self that helps the youth become more aware of feelings and thoughts, dissipate tensions, develop greater body awareness, improve or correct a distorted body image, improve coordination, and increase social interactions. The type of movement used with children can be as simple as a game of "Follow the Leader," or it can be creative, free-form movements to the mood of the music. For older children and adolescents, more formal classes in exercise, karate, or the latest dance craze may be of interest.

Recreational therapy generally takes place off the unit and is often conducted by a recreational therapist with assistance from the nursing staff. Activities are often organized around a game that teaches psychomotor and social skills, such as volleyball or swimming. Special field trips give children the opportunity to be like other children and to act appropriately in public situations, leading to increased self-control and self-esteem.

It is important for the nurse to reassure the parents that various types of therapy are beneficial. When a child says that all he or she does is play games when meeting with the therapist, the parent may not understand the underlying therapeutic purpose of play and become concerned that there will be a lack of progress or that issues are not being addressed.

KEY POINTS TO REMEMBER

- About 20% of children and adolescents are estimated to have mental health problems, and only a small percentage of these youths actually receive treatment.
- Risk factors known to contribute to the development of mental and emotional problems in children and adolescents include genetic, biochemical, developmental, environmental, and cultural factors.
- Resiliency helps protect children and adolescents in stressful situations. Temperament, problem-solving skills, and the support of a nurturing adult contribute to resiliency and successful navigation of stressful events
- The most commonly diagnosed child psychiatric disorders are mood disorders, anxiety disorders, attention-deficit/hyperactivity disorder (ADHD), and conduct and oppositional disorders.
- Treatment of childhood and adolescent disorders requires a collaborative approach.
- In addition to individual, family, and group therapy, play therapy, art therapy, and bibliotherapy are helpful for children. The older the child, the more he or she should be involved in treatment decisions.
- The family is an integral part of the supportive and educational system for the child and adolescent.

APPLYING CRITICAL JUDGMENT

1. A 4-year-old boy has been diagnosed with an autism spectrum disorder (ASD).
   A. Describe the kinds of data you might find on assessment in terms of communication, socialization, behaviors, and activities.
   B. Name at least four realistic nursing interventions and outcomes for this child.
   C. Which treatment modalities and supports do you think would be the most effective for a child with ASD?
2. A 7-year-old girl in second grade has been diagnosed with attention-deficit/hyperactivity disorder (ADHD).
   A. What clinical behaviors might she be exhibiting at home and in the classroom, in the areas of inattention, hyperactivity, and impulsivity?
   B. Identify at least four nursing interventions that you might include in her treatment plan or suggest to the family.
   C. What type of medications might be considered for this client?
3. An 8-year-old boy has been diagnosed with conduct disorder.
   A. What are some of the behaviors you might expect to be reported about this child, in light of his diagnosis?
   B. What are the goals for this child? What is the overall prognosis for children with this disorder? Do further research if necessary.
   C. What are several ways you could support the child's parents in being more effective?
   D. Identify resources within your community to which you might refer this family for guidance.

CHAPTER REVIEW QUESTIONS

1. The nurse interviews the parent of a 7-year-old child diagnosed with moderate autism spectrum disorder. Which comment from the parent best describes autistic behavior?
   a. "My child occasionally has temper tantrums."
   b. "Sometimes my child wakes up with nightmares."
   c. "My child swings for hours on our backyard gym set."
   d. "Toilet training was more difficult for this child than my other children."
2. A nurse plans to lead a group in a residential facility for kindergarten-age, abused children. Which strategy should the nurse incorporate?
   a. Building a house using blocks
   b. Telling a story about a child who felt sad
   c. Drawing pictures of fun activities at a park
   d. Reading and discussing a book about abused children
3. Which scenario presents the highest risk for a pregnancy resulting in offspring with an intellectual developmental disability (IDD)?
   a. 18-year-old mother who received no prenatal care
   b. 32-year-old woman diagnosed with anorexia nervosa
   c. 26-year-old father with a history of episodic alcohol abuse
   d. 38-year-old father diagnosed with generalized anxiety disorder
4. A community mental health nurse talks with a 6-year-old child whose divorced parents have shared custody. Which initial question will best help the nurse explore the child's perception of home life?
   a. "Is your life different from your friends' lives?"
   b. "Are you happiest at your mother's or your father's house?"
   c. "Do you find it hard to move back and forth between two homes?"
   d. "What are some of the good and bad things about living in two places?"
5. The parent of an adolescent recently diagnosed with schizophrenia says to the nurse, "This is entirely my fault. I should have spent more time with my child when he was a toddler." Which response by the nurse is correct?
   a. "Schizophrenia is genetically transmitted, so it was not in your control."
   b. "Your child's disorder is more likely the result of an undetected head injury."
   c. "Environmental toxins are directly implicated in the origins of schizophrenia."
   d. "Lack of prenatal care causes schizophrenia rather than early childhood events."

REFERENCES

American Academy of Child and Adolescent Psychiatry. (2017). *Conduct disorder resource center*. Retrieved November 24, 2017 from http://www.aacap.org/aacap/Families_and_Youth/Resource_Centers/Conduct_Disorder_Resource_Center/Home.aspx.

American Psychiatric Association. (2013). *Diagnostic and statistical manual of mental disorders (DSM-5)* (5th ed.). Washington, DC: APA.

American Psychiatric Association. (2017). *What is ADHD?* Retrieved November 5, 2017 from https://www.psychiatry.org/patients-families/adhd/what-is-adhd.

American Psychological Association. (2017). The road to resilience. Retrieved November 23, 2017 from http://www.apa.org/helpcenter/road-resilience.aspx.

American Speech-Language-Hearing Association. (2017). *Intellectual disability*. Retrieved November 23, 2017 from https://www.asha.org/PRPSpecificTopic.aspx?folderid=8589942540§ion=Incidence_and_Prevalence.

Belardinelli, C., Raza, M., & Taneli, T. (2016). Comorbid behavioral health problems and psychiatric disorders in autism spectrum disorders. *Journal of Childhood & Developmental Disorders*, *2*(2). https://doi.org/10.4172/2472-1786.100019. http://childhood-developmental-disorders.

Cecil, C. A. M., Viding, E., Fearon, P., Glaser, D., & McCrory, E. J. (2017). Disentangling the mental health impact of child abuse and neglect. *Child Abuse & Neglect: International Journal*, *63*, 106–119. https://doi.org/10.1016/j.chiabu.2016.11.024.

Centers for Disease Control and Prevention (CDC). (2006). *Thirteen-month delay between evaluation and autism diagnosis in children*. Retrieved November 24, 2017 from https://www.autismspeaks.org/docs/Press_release_JDBP_autism_diagnosis.pdf.

Centers for Disease Control and Prevention (CDC). (2015). *Tourette syndrome (TS)*. Retrieved from http://www.cdc.gov/ncbddd/tourette/treatments.html#CBIT.

Centers for Disease Control and Prevention (CDC). (2016). *Autism spectrum disorder (ASD)*. Retrieved November 24, 2017 from https://www.cdc.gov/ncbddd/autism/hcp-dsm.html.

Centers for Disease Control and Prevention (CDC). (2017a). *Children's mental health: Data & statistics*. Retrieved November 5, 2017 from https://www.cdc.gov/childrensmentalhealth/data.html.

Centers for Disease Control and Prevention (CDC). (2017b). *Attention-deficit/hyperactivity disorder (ADHD)*. Retrieved November 5, 2017 from https://www.cdc.gov/ncbddd/adhd/conditions.html.

Centers for Disease Control and Prevention (CDC). (2017c). *Autism spectrum disorder (ASD): Screening and diagnosis*. Retrieved November 24, 2017 from https://www.cdc.gov/ncbddd/autism/screening.html.

Centers for Disease Control and Prevention (CDC). (2017d). *Attention-deficit/hyperactivity disorder (ADHD)*. Retrieved November 24, 2017 from https://www.cdc.gov/ncbddd/adhd/.

Child Mind Institute. (2016). *Children's mental health report*. Retrieved November 5, 2017 from childmind.org/2016report.

Cleveland Clinic. (2017). *Oppositional defiant disorder*. Retrieved November 24, 2017 from https://my.clevelandclinic.org/health/articles/oppositional-defiant-disorder.

Dudeney, J., Sharpe, L., Jaffe, A., Jones, E. B., & Hunt, C. (2017). Anxiety in youth with asthma: A meta-analysis. *Pediatric Pulmonology*, *52*(9), 1121–1129. https://doi.org/10.1002/ppul.23689.

Flacks, J., & Boynton-Jarrett, R. (2017). *Strengths-based approaches to screening families for health-related social needs in healthcare settings: Preview of recommendations*. Retrieved November 23, 2017 from https://www.cssp.org/publications/documents/Strengths-based-Screening-Preview-Recommendations.pdf.

Freedman, E. G., & Foxe, J. J. (2017). Eye movements, sensorimotor adaptation and cerebellar-dependent learning in autism: Toward potential biomarkers and subphenotypes. *European Journal of Neuroscience*, 1–7. https://doi.org/10.1111/ejn.13625.

Gardner, R. A. (2007). *Psychotherapy of children with conduct disorders using games and stories*. Washington, DC: American Psychological Association [DVD].

Giddens, J. F. (2017). *Concepts for nursing practice* (2nd ed). St. Louis: Elsevier.

Gromisch, E. S. (2018). *Neurotransmitters involved in ADHD*. Retrieved November 24, 2017 from http://psychcentral.com/lib/neurotransmitters-involved-in-adhd/.

Krucik, G. (2015). *What causes mental retardation? 17 possible conditions*. Retrieved from http://www.healthline.com/symptom/mental-retardation.

Mayo Clinic. (2017). *Bed-wetting*. Retrieved November 24, 2017 from https://www.mayoclinic.org/diseases-conditions/bed-wetting/diagnosis-treatment/drc-20366711.

National Association of Anorexia Nervosa and Associated Disorders (2017). *Eating disorder statistics*. Retrieved November 24, 2017 from http://www.anad.org/get-information/about-eating-disorders/eating-disorders-statistics/.

National Institute for Children's Health Quality and American Academy of Pediatrics. (2002). *NICHQ Vanderbilt assessment scales: Used for diagnosing ADHD*. Retrieved from http://www.nichq.org/childrens-health/adhd/resources/vanderbilt-assessment-scales.

National Institute on Drug Abuse. (2016). *Drug facts: High school and youth trends*. Retrieved from http://www.drugabuse.gov/publications/drugfacts/high-school-youth-trends.

National Institute of Mental Health. (2016). *Risk of suicide*. Retrieved from http://www.nami.org/Learn-More/Mental-Health-Conditions/Related-Conditions/Suicide.

National Institute of Mental Health. (2017). *Disruptive mood dysregulation disorder*. Retrieved November 24, 2017 from https://www.nimh.nih.gov/health/topics/disruptive-mood-dysregulation-disorder-dmdd/disruptive-mood-dysregulation-disorder.shtml.

National Institutes of Health. (2017). *Genetics home reference: Autism spectrum disorder*. Retrieved November 5, 2017 from https://ghr.nlm.nih.gov/condition/autism-spectrum-disorder#genes.

Nelson, S. L. (2015). *Developmental coordination disorder treatment and management*. Retrieved from http://emedicine.medscape.com/article/915251-overview.

Pincus, D. B. (2012). *Growing up brave*. New York: Little, Brown and Company.

Pivalizza, P. (2015). *Intellectual disability (mental retardation) in children: Management; outcomes; and prevention*. Retrieved from http://www.uptodate.com/contents/intellectual-disability-mental-retardation-in-children-management-outcomes-and-prevention#references.

Pomerantz, J. M. (2013). *HAM-A Hamilton anxiety scale*. Retrieved from http://www.psychiatrictimes.

Quinn, P. D., Chang, Z., Hur, K., Gibbons, R. D., Lahey, B. B., et al. (2017). ADHD medications and substance-related problems. *American Journal of Psychiatry*, *174*(9), 877–885. https://doi.org/10.1176/appi.ajp.2017.16060686.

Rymanowicz, K. (2017). *The nine traits of temperament*. Michigan State University Extension. Retrieved November 5, 2017 from http://msue.anr.msu.edu/news/the_nine_traits_of_temperament.

Sadock, B. J., Sadock, V. A., & Ruiz, P. (2015). Child psychiatry. *Kaplan & Sadock's synopsis of psychiatry: Behavioral sciences/clinical psychiatry*. Philadelphia: Lippincott Williams & Wilkins.

Spence, S. H. (1994). *Spence children's anxiety Scale*. Retrieved from http://www.scaswebsite.com/.

Stahl, S. M. (2017). *Prescriber's guide: Stahl's essential psychopharmacology* (6th ed.). New York: Cambridge University Press.

Stanford Children's Hospital. (2017). *Encopresis*. Retrieved November 24, 2017 from http://www.stanfordchildrens.org/en/topic/default?id=encopresis-90-P01992.

Substance Abuse and Mental Health Services Administration (SAMHSA). (n.d.). *SAMHSA-HRSA Center for Integrated Health Solutions: Screening tools* . Retrieved November 24, 2017 from https://www.integration.samhsa.gov/clinical-practice/screening-tools#suicide.

Substance Abuse and Mental Health Services Administration. (2017a). *Adverse childhood experiences*. Retrieved on November 23, 2017 from https://www.

samhsa.gov/capt/practicing-effective-prevention/prevention-behavioral-health/adverse-childhood-experiences.

Substance Abuse and Mental Health Services Administration. (2017b). *Age- and gender- based populations.* Retrieved November 25, 2017 from https://www.samhsa.gov/specific-populations/age-gender-based.

TLC Foundation for Body-Focused Repetitive Behaviors. (2016). *Expert consensus treatment guidelines: Body-focused repetitive behaviors: Hair pulling, skin picking, and related disorders.* Retrieved November 24, 2017 from https://www.bfrb.org/storage/documents/Expert_Consensus_Treatment_Guidelines_2016w.pdf.

U.S. Environmental Protection Agency. (2017). *Health: Neurodevelopmental disorders.* Retrieved November 23, 2017 from https://www.epa.gov/sites/production/files/2017-07/documents/neurodevelopmental_updates_0.pdf.

Zeliadt, N. (2016). *Motor problems in infancy may forecast autism.* Retrieved November 24, 2017 from https://spectrumnews.org/news/motor-problems-in-infancy-may-forecast-autism/.

27

Adults

Lisa M. Baker

http://evolve.elsevier.com/Varcarolis/essentials

OBJECTIVES

1. Discuss ways serious mental illness (SMI) affects individuals, families, and society.
2. Discuss the safety issues and problems experienced by those living with serious mental illness. **QSEN: Safety**
3. Describe evidence-based practice for SMI. **QSEN: Evidence-Based Practice**
4. Role-play a therapeutic interaction designed to improve treatment adherence for an individual with SMI.
5. Describe common sleep disorders, their treatment, and related nursing care.
6. Describe the core characteristics of impulse-control disorders and their societal implications.
7. Role-play a therapeutic interaction with a person who is portraying impulse-control disorders.
8. Describe gender dysphoria and appropriate nursing care.
9. Describe sexual disorders and their implications for society.
10. Discuss the forms of treatment for pedophilia disorder.
11. Role-play a therapeutic interaction with a person who is portraying attention-deficit/hyperactivity disorder (ADHD).

KEY TERMS AND CONCEPTS

any mental illness (AMI), p. 419
Assertive Community Treatment (ACT), p. 423
cognitive-behavioral therapy (CBT), p. 423
continuous positive airway pressure (CPAP), p. 433
deinstitutionalization, p. 422
dialectical behavior therapy (DBT), p. 423
impulse-control disorders, p. 424
mental health courts, p. 422
National Alliance on Mental Illness (NAMI), p. 424
outpatient commitment, p. 421
paraphilias, p. 427
paraphilic disorders, p. 427
peer-support specialist, p. 424
reality testing, p. 422
recidivism, p. 428
recovery model, p. 424
rehabilitation model, p. 424
serious mental illness (SMI), p. 419
sleep apnea, p. 432
sleep disorders, p. 432
sleep hygiene, p. 433
social skills training, p. 424
supported employment, p. 424
transinstitutionalization, p. 422

CONCEPT: SLEEP: *Sleep* is defined as natural and necessary, involving a shift in physiological and neurological activity that is intended to be restorative. Sufficient quality sleep is crucial to metabolic regulation, cognitive functioning, quality of life, mood, and nearly every other aspect of existence (Giddens, 2017, p. 94). Sleep disturbances can both contribute to and be caused by disorders such as depression, characterized by increased sleep or insomnia, or mania, characterized by a decreased need for sleep. Stress reduction and active relaxation reduce anxiety and promote rest. Normalizing sleep patterns is important, along with individual and family therapy to address underlying concerns.

INTRODUCTION

This chapter focuses on mental health issues and needs primarily affecting the adult population. We look at what it is like to have a serious mental illness (SMI), the issues and challenges faced by those diagnosed with these illnesses, and resources and treatment programs available for persons with SMI. Other adult mental health issues examined in this chapter include **gender dysphoria,** disorders involving **impulse control, sexual dysfunction, adult attention-deficit/hyperactivity disorder** (ADHD), and **sleep–wake disorders.** Gender dysphoria is not a disorder; however, this syndrome will be discussed and refers to distress experienced when there is a mismatch between one's assigned gender and one's gender identity and lived experience (Sadock, Sadock, & Ruiz, 2015).

UNDERSTANDING SERIOUS MENTAL ILLNESS

Categorizing mental illness according to levels of severity has significant implications for setting mental health policy, determining insurance reimbursement, and facilitating access to appropriate care. The federal government delineates any mental illness (AMI) and **SMI** (National Institute of Mental Health [NIMH], 2017). AMI is defined as any mild, moderate, or severe serious mental illness and therefore includes SMI. SMI is described as a subset of AMI and comprises those with serious impairment resulting in reduced function in at least one or more of the major domains of life. Each year in the United States, 18% of adults experience AMI, and 4% experience an SMI (NIMH, 2017). In this chapter, the focus is on serious mental illness, such as schizophrenia and bipolar disorder, which affects about half of the people in the SMI group. SMI involves significant continuous or reoccurring impairment of global functioning that creates disability in 30% to 50% of cases. Other SMIs include severe forms of depression, panic disorder, and obsessive-compulsive disorder.

VIGNETTE: You are a 19-year-old nursing student working as a nursing assistant. One night, while studying alone in your dorm, you hear someone call your name. No one is there, and you attribute it to lack of sleep. However, over the coming weeks, this happens repeatedly, and the voices begin to comment on what you are doing, criticize you, and tell you what to do. You have trouble concentrating. Your schoolwork and grades suffer. It seems like people know what you're thinking or hate you; now uncomfortable around others, you begin to avoid friends, skip classes, and quit work.

Distracted by ever-present voices, you step into the street and are struck by a car. A police officer comes to your aid, but you believe he wants to kill you and you run, only to be caught and restrained. The next few days are a confusing, frightening blur of doctors, nurses, injections, and restraints. You are on a psychiatric unit and told that you have something called schizophreniform disorder.

Medications push the voices into the background, but you feel disconnected, like you are wrapped in layers of cotton. Just as you begin to trust some of the staff, you are discharged with an appointment to see a new doctor in a mental health center far from your neighborhood. At the center, people look and act strangely; some mumble to themselves, some get too close to you, and some pull away when you walk by. You think, "This can't be happening," and you wonder what your future will be like.

Individuals with SMI usually have difficulties in multiple areas, including activities of daily living (e.g., cooking, hygiene), relationships, social interaction, task completion, communication, leisure activities, safe movement about the community, finances and budgeting, health maintenance, vocational and academic activities, and coping with stressors. Associated issues for those with SMI include poverty, stigma, isolation, unemployment, poorer health outcomes, law enforcement encounters, victimization, and inadequate housing or homelessness.

Extent of the Problem

Effect on an Individual With Serious Mental Illness

Individuals with SMI often fall well short of their potential, experiencing significantly less academic, vocational, and relational success than they would have otherwise. They are often stigmatized and can experience rejection and discrimination. They are more likely to be victims of crime, have undertreated or untreated illnesses, die prematurely, be homeless, be incarcerated, be unemployed or underemployed, engage in substance abuse, live in poverty, and report a lower quality of life than those without such illnesses.

Effect on Families, Caregivers, and Significant Others

The burden on caregivers is significant and is affected by their own coping abilities, support systems, and financial and other resources. Caregivers may not understand the mental illness, may not know how to cope with it or how to help, and may not have access to their loved one's treatment team, leaving them feeling frustrated and powerless. Chronic caregiving demands can result in burnout, maladaptive coping, withdrawal from the patient, and even rejection or abuse (Leng et al., 2019; Settineri et al., 2014). Caregivers themselves can also be stigmatized simply by being associated with a person with SMI, leading them to keep the problem a secret and reducing access to social support.

Effect on Society

Historically, most treatment for serious mental illness has been financed with public dollars rather than private insurance; however, this may be changing as a result of the Patient Protection and Affordable Care Act, which mandated **parity** for mental illness coverage (e.g., requiring benefits for mental health and substance abuse treatment to be equal to those for medical illness). Medicaid expansion in a number of states represents a greater cost to taxpayers but made more care available to persons with SMI. Social Security Disability Income (SSDI), for disabled persons with a significant work history, and Supplemental Security Income (SSI), for indigents ineligible for SSDI, both provide income to assist people with SMI who meet government criteria; income for an individual, however, is limited (for SSI, the limit is $783 per month) and is reduced based on assets and non-SSI income (Social Security Administration, 2018). Persons with untreated or inadequately treated SMI are more likely to commit criminal offenses and be incarcerated. Finally, these illnesses strike in the prime of life, and they are among the top causes of disability worldwide (World Health Organization, 2019).

Issues Facing Those With Serious Mental Illness

Even with successful treatment, people with SMI often experience **residual symptoms and relapse** (a reoccurring or worsening of one's illness), which can occur even when one adheres to treatment. These can lead to frustration and a fear that one will not get better or that one's treatments are not effective. In turn, the patient may decide to discontinue treatment, ironically worsening the course of the illness and increasing the negative consequences to self and society.

Medication side effects can include a wide range of distressing effects, including sedation, visual blurring, involuntary movements, weight gain, sexual dysfunction, and medical conditions such as metabolic syndrome, which is defined as three of four of the following: hypertension, hyperlipidemia, hyperglycemia, and central obesity. Newer antipsychotic agents tend to have fewer and more tolerable side effects but can be more expensive and can cause metabolic syndrome, increasing the risk of cardiovascular disease and diabetes. Addressing side effects is essential because they may impair one's quality of life or lead to treatment nonadherence. Patient education is important because some side effects respond to treatment (e.g., medications such as benztropine, among others, reducing involuntary movements) or can be counteracted by lifestyle or behavior changes (e.g., changing position slowly to prevent dizziness from orthostatic hypotension). Refer to Chapter 17 for a discussion of antipsychotics and patient and family teaching for these drugs.

Loss, hopelessness, and depression may be experienced. Relapse may lead to feelings of guilt and helplessness. Persons with SMI may experience a profound sense of loss for the future they had anticipated, contributing to major depression or hopelessness. For example, one may have been a pre-med student with hopes of medical school, but a severe mental illness may leave the person unable to perform schoolwork, employed in a minimum-wage job, and living in a group home. This loss of potential, along with the demands and effects of chronic illness on daily life, can lead to despair, substance abuse, or suicidality, especially if the individual has no family or outside supports. Between 5% and 10% of those with SMI commit suicide.

Co-occurring medical illnesses, some a consequence of medication, frequently exist in serious mental illness. *Poverty* and lack of access to quality food can cause poor nutrition. *Anhedonia* (inability to experience pleasure) and *anergia* (reduced spontaneous movement) lead to a sedentary lifestyle. People with SMI may not provide for their own health needs and may not receive adequate care because of costs, difficulty accessing health care, or ill will (e.g., emergency department personnel assuming because a person is psychotic, his chest pain is not real). Presenting complaints may be expressed bizarrely (e.g., describing pain as "demons sticking needles in me") and be misunderstood by staff. People with SMI may also make ill-advised choices regarding substance abuse or sexual activity, risking sexually transmitted infections (STIs) and unplanned pregnancies. The final result is that persons with SMI die 25 years earlier and have a risk of death that is 2.5 times that of the general population (Welsh & McEnany, 2015).

Unemployment and poverty contribute to poor self-esteem and a lack of identity. Of people with SMI, 62% are unemployed, and a person disabled by an SMI on SSI receives less than 50% of the median income (Social Security Administration, 2018; U.S. Census Bureau, 2018). It can be difficult to find an employer open to hiring a person with an SMI, and laws to prevent discrimination do not guarantee a job.

Housing instability can contribute to stress for individuals with SMI. Persons who cannot afford a car need to live near public transportation, reducing their options. Limited affordable housing may require them to live where violence and gunshots are common occurrences—not a good situation for anyone, let alone a person overwhelmed by mental illness. An episode of inappropriate behavior could lead to eviction and difficulty obtaining future housing.

Stigma about mental illness is a significant problem. Stigma is perpetuated by stereotypical images or language in the media, thoughtless comments by everyday people or celebrities, and misperceptions of mental illness. It can cause people to assume that those with SMI are less capable, responsible for their own illness, and even dangerous. It can leave the affected person feeling ashamed or angry, pushing one away from others and reducing access to potential support systems. Many people do not yet realize that calling a mentally ill person "crazy" is equivalent to calling someone with an intellectual disability a "retard." Patients with SMI and their advocates, such as the National Alliance on Mental Illness (NAMI) and other advocacy groups, work to reduce stigma, just as was once necessary for the stigma affecting intellectually disabled persons. Refer to Chapter 2 for more on stigma.

Social isolation and loneliness are increasing overall in the United States, and these negatively affect physical and mental health (Holt-Lunstad et al., 2015). A lack of social contacts and loneliness are risk factors for mortality on par with obesity (Holt-Lunstad et al., 2015). Those with SMI are especially vulnerable to experiencing social isolation and loneliness. Stigma and social stratification reduce social contact with groups that are outside the mainstream, such as individuals with SMI. Poverty (which interferes with participation in social or recreational activities), impaired hygiene, gaps in social skills, and anxiety also reduce interaction and social support. Medication may reduce one's libido or sexual function and interfere with intimate physical relationships. Negative self-image and delusional thinking may create additional barriers to relationships.

Inadequate treatment and treatment nonadherence is another common issue in patients with serious mental illness. Evidence-based practice implementation and quality improvement methodologies have improved care for physical conditions, but improvement is lacking in mental health care services (Kilbourne et al., 2018). Implementing treatment innovations and changing practice standards can be a slow process. The newest medications or other treatments may be excluded from state hospital formularies or unapproved by third-party payers. Reduced public funding for health services during times of economic cutbacks intensifies problems with treatment access and quality. Some medications can cost up to $64,000 per year, and even with Medicaid, co-pays or a spend-down (a need to exhaust one's own funds each month in order to reestablish Medicaid eligibility) may be required. Persons with very limited income may opt to spend it on personal needs instead of treatment. Stigma may lead a person to discontinue treatment so that he or she will not be labeled as mentally ill. Staff turnover and insufficient time to establish therapeutic relationships may reduce trust in staff and increase treatment resistance. Nonadherence increases the risk of relapse by four to seven times.

Anosognosia, the inability of a person to recognize that he or she has an illness because of the illness itself, also contributes to nonadherence. With mental illness, it is the brain itself, the same organ needed for self-awareness, that is sick. It is an extremely frustrating dilemma and one that contributes significantly to treatment nonadherence and all its attendant problems. Consider: Would you take medicine for an illness you do not believe you have?

Substance use disorder co-occurs in 50% of those with an SMI. It may be maladaptive coping or self-medicating, a way of countering the dysphoria or other symptoms of one's illness or the side effects of one's medications. Substance abuse interferes with psychiatric treatment and contributes to relapse, physical health problems, incarceration, and reduced quality of life. Persons with concurrent psychiatric and substance abuse disorders are said to have a **dual diagnosis**. Of persons with SMI, 70% smoke, and they are less likely to reduce tobacco use compared with the general population (Peckham et al., 2017).

The incidence of **victimization** is higher among those with mental illness; one study reported a victimization rate of 46.8% (Albers et al., 2018). Impaired judgment; impaired interpersonal skills (e.g., unknowingly acting in ways that might provoke others, such as standing too close or not responding to commands); poor self-esteem; appearing more vulnerable to criminals; and living in high-crime, transient, and drug-infested neighborhoods all can contribute to victimization. Sexual victimization, such as sexual assault or coerced sexual activity, also occurs (e.g., a person whose boyfriend "loaned" her sexually to peers in return for drugs, compelling her to cooperate in return for housing). Those with certain personality disorders have increased victimization or perpetration of crimes (Albers et al., 2018), depending on the internalizing or externalizing nature of their personality and interactions with others.

Issues Affecting Society and the Individual

Some with SMI cannot be persuaded to accept treatment. **Involuntary treatment** involves treatment mandated by court order and delivered without the person's consent. Outpatient commitment requires that persons with SMI accept outpatient treatment and is designed to provide for mandatory continuing treatment in the least restrictive setting, typically after the patient leaves a hospital or prison. It is a form of assisted treatment that helps people with anosognosia and/or treatment resistance to maintain the best mental health status possible (Kisely, Campbell, & O'Reilly, 2017; Swartz et al., 2017).

Criminalization of the mentally ill refers to persons with SMI being arrested for behavior caused by their illness instead of being treated as ill. Criminal actions may be the result of desperation, impaired judgment, psychotic thinking, or impulsivity. Those who are untreated have more symptoms and impairment and may become disruptive or commit (usually nonviolent) offenses such as trespassing. For example, during the winter, a homeless man with SMI loiters in laundromats and libraries for warmth. He refuses traditional shelters and is at risk for hypothermia, so police who are not aware of other options may jail him for trespassing simply to protect him from hypothermia. Alternately, he might disrupt others at the library and be charged with disorderly conduct. Advocates for persons with SMI strongly support efforts to **decriminalize** behavior caused by mental illness. An important intervention is educating law enforcement officers and first responders (e.g., through crisis intervention training programs sponsored jointly by law enforcement and mental health agencies) to recognize mental illness, to safely de-escalate persons with SMI, and to connect mentally ill citizens with help and treatment instead of jailing them (Parker et al., 2018). **Mental health courts** are designed to intercept persons with SMI after arrest and divert them to treatment instead of incarceration.

Transinstitutionalization is the shifting of a person or population from one institution to another, such as from state hospitals to jails, prisons, nursing homes, or even the street. Although **deinstitutionalization** (moving persons from inpatient psychiatric care, such as state hospitals, to the community) was intended to provide care in less restrictive settings and reduce costs for state hospitals, in many cases the new setting is actually more restrictive, and the costs have simply been transferred to another provider (e.g., prisons or Medicaid). Nearly one-quarter of all persons under correctional control (imprisonment, probation, or parole) have an SMI, and about 15% of male inmates and 30% of female inmates suffer from SMI (Robertson et al., 2014). There are more persons with SMI in jails and prisons than in psychiatric hospitals, and less than half of those incarcerated were arrested for a violent offense (Kim, Becker-Cohen, & Serakos, 2015). Settings such as jails, prisons, and nursing homes often lack the special programming and skilled staff needed to assist persons with SMI, and as a result, their recovery and stability may be compromised.

APPLICATION OF THE NURSING PROCESS

ASSESSMENT

Assessment should focus especially on signs of risk to self or others (including unsafe behavior, suicide risk, and homicidal thinking); depression or hopelessness; substance use or abuse; sleep impairment; impulsivity; diminished **reality testing** (the ability to accurately determine what is or isn't real); delusional thinking; hallucinations; and inadequate attention to proper nutrition, clothing, or medical care. Impaired judgment, paranoia, and psychosis increase the risk of dangerous behavior; such persons may start fires by forgetting pots left on the stove, may hurt self or others in response to command hallucinations, or may hurt a person they perceive as a threat.

It is also essential to observe for signs of impending relapse and treatment nonadherence. Correcting nonadherence helps prevent relapse, and early detection and treatment of relapse reduce its severity and duration. It is also important to assess for physical health problems (e.g., tumors, metabolic disorders) that may cause psychiatric symptoms and be mistaken for mental illness. Monitoring co-occurring illnesses ensures that self-care and health care are satisfactory.

Areas that might need further investigation when planning long-term care for persons with SMI include the following:

- **Problems involving primary support groups** (death, illness, divorce, sexual or physical abuse, neglect of child, discord with siblings, birth of a sibling)
- **Problems related to the social environment** (death or loss of friends; inadequate social support; isolation; difficulty with acculturation, discrimination, adjustment to life changes [e.g., new housing])
- **Educational problems** (illiteracy, conflict with teachers or classmates, need for accommodation due to SMI symptoms)
- **Occupational problems** (unemployment, potential job loss, work stress, difficult work conditions, job dissatisfaction, unmet need for accommodations, conflict with others)
- **Economic problems** (income insufficient to meet essential needs, access to entitlements)
- **Problems with health care services or access** (inadequate care, lack of transportation to health care facilities, unable to afford treatment)
- **Problems involving crime or law enforcement** (arrest, incarceration, victim of crime)

DIAGNOSIS

Nursing diagnoses for persons who have an SMI include *Impaired adjustment, Impaired family coping, Impaired coping process, Impaired health maintenance, Impaired impulse control, Risk for loneliness, Self-care deficit, Low self-esteem, Non-adherence to medication regime,* and *Risk for dysfunctional grief* (International Council of Nurses [ICN], 2019). See Table 27.1 for selected interventions that are appropriate for helping persons who have an SMI.

OUTCOMES IDENTIFICATION

The following are examples of potential long-term outcome measures. The individual:

- Identifies "voices" as hallucinations.
- Distinguishes delusional thoughts from reality.
- Remains free from law enforcement involvement.
- Maintains stable housing.
- Remains free from harm.
- Demonstrates treatment adherence.

PLANNING AND IMPLEMENTATION

Interventions to Promote Treatment Adherence

1. Monitor side effects and provide education and treatment to minimize resulting distress (e.g., for dry mouth, sugar-free lozenges to promote salivation; taking medications earlier in the evening to reduce morning grogginess at work or school).
2. Simplify treatment regimens to make them easier to follow (e.g., once-per-day dosing instead of twice daily).
3. Anosognosia (inability to recognize that one is ill) is a significant factor in nonadherence. Linking treatment adherence to achieving the patient's goals can bypass the patient's lack of insight by motivating the patient with his or her own goals, not the goal of recovering from an illness that he or she cannot perceive (e.g., guide the patient to see that the medications will improve concentration and help the patient keep his or her job).
4. Emphasize and reinforce improvement, connecting this to the patient's treatment adherence.
5. Facilitate access to treatment providers and medication. Inconvenient appointment times, inability to reach prescribers for refills, and similar issues are obstacles to adherence.
6. Facilitate referrals for assistance with treatment costs. Some pharmaceutical companies have special low-cost options for low-income persons, and some persons may be eligible for Medicaid under Medicaid expansion legislation or other state programs.
7. To improve insight and motivation, educate patients about the nature of SMI and the role of treatment in the person's recovery and quality of life.
8. Assign consistent, committed caregivers who have (or are skilled at building) therapeutic bonds with the patient; trusting one's providers is essential for treatment adherence.
9. Encourage involvement in support groups (e.g., NAMI, http://www.NAMI.org). The patient may be more likely to accept support and information from peers who have more insight and experience with SMI and treatment.
10. Provide culturally sensitive care. Appreciating a person's values and beliefs (e.g., suspicious attitudes toward authority figures or valuing of self-sufficiency) may be crucial to promoting treatment adherence.
11. When feasible, consider judicious use of medication decreases, changes, or discontinuation to control side effects and/or improve the therapeutic alliance.

TABLE 27.1 Interventions for Serious Mental Illness (SMI)

Intervention	Rationale
1. Mutually develop short- and long-term, patient-centered goals and interventions that will help the patient achieve the desired quality of life, rather than focus on symptom reduction.	1. Patient involvement in goal setting and treatment selection builds the therapeutic alliance, increases the patient's sense of control over his or her life, and increases the likelihood of treatment adherence and success.
2. Enhance and promote reality testing (e.g., teaching a patient, when he or she hears voices, to scan the immediate environment to see if anyone else seems to be hearing the voices; if not, encourage the patient to label it as a hallucination and to disregard it or distract self from it).	2. Impaired reality testing is common in SMI and contributes to hallucinations and delusional thinking. Training and encouraging the patient to verify whether experiences are real can help the patient meet his or her goals despite residual symptoms.
3. Provide psychoeducation, guidance, support, and reinforcement for actions that the patient can use to manage the symptoms of SMI (see Box 17.3). Include the family in psychoeducational activities as tolerated and possible.	3. Simple auditory distractions such as listening to music can reduce distress caused by auditory hallucinations; gaining mastery over symptoms improves function, reduces disruption, and provides one with a sense of control and confidence.
4. Reduce loneliness and isolation by interacting frequently with the patient, supporting opportunities for interaction (e.g., day programs, social and recreational events), helping the patient to manage social anxiety, helping the patient who does not want to socialize to identify and use alternative means to achieve support or comfort (e.g., pets, stuffed animals, calling support phone lines), and involving the patient in social skills training.	4. SMIs decrease sociability and predispose individuals to isolation as a result of stigma, loss of social skills, and social discomfort. Activities that increase skill and comfort with interaction, especially with supportive people and positive role models, such as other patients who are further along in recovery, contribute to improved functioning and a higher quality of life.
5. Encourage involvement of patient and his or her loved ones in NAMI support meetings and peer-based services.	5. NAMI members and peers "have been there" and can provide support, socialization, and practical suggestions for issues and problems facing patients and significant others; involvement in such groups also instills hope and empowers the patient.
6. Provide education and support regarding making sound decisions about interpersonal relations, STI prevention, and family planning.	6. People with SMI may have impaired judgment, feel isolated, and feel vulnerable to victimization, STIs, and undesired pregnancies; patients seeking to have families may benefit from genetic counseling.
7. Connect the patient with case managers and other personnel who are likely to be able to work with him or her for extended periods and who are skilled at developing and maintaining therapeutic relationships.	7. Trusting and therapeutic relationships are key resources for achieving treatment adherence, and patients with SMI often require extended periods of working with staff to form these connections.
8. Actively promote treatment adherence by tying adherence to the patient's own goals and other motivational and educational approaches.	8. Treatment adherence reduces relapse and improves the long-term prognosis and quality of life.
9. Provide psychosocial support.	9. This aids in maintaining therapeutic rapport and helps the patient to maintain positive self-esteem and to cope effectively rather than maladaptively.
10. Provide regular and frequent contact with the patient, but not so much that it overstimulates the patient or contributes to paranoia.	10. Ongoing contact promotes therapeutic alliances and allows for monitoring so that relapse or nonadherence can quickly be intercepted.
11. Educate, guide, support, and reinforce behaviors that prevent or control actual or potential medical comorbidities; act as an advocate as needed to ensure adequate health care for the patient with SMI.	11. Patients with SMI have higher burdens of physical illness, poorer hygiene and health practices, less access to effective medical treatment, and more premature mortality than the general population.
12. Involve persons with co-occurring substance abuse or addiction with AA or NA and dual-diagnosis SAMI services.	12. Substance abuse rates are high in SMI populations, increase relapse, and interfere with recovery; achieving sobriety is mostly associated with AA and integrated treatment programs.

AA, Alcoholics Anonymous; *NA*, Narcotics Anonymous; *NAMI*, National Alliance on Mental Illness; *SAMI*, substance abuse/mental illness; *STI*, sexually transmitted infection.

12. When medically appropriate, support the use of medication monitoring or long-acting forms of medication (depot injections or sustained-release formats) to maximize the benefits of medication.
13. Never reject, blame, or shame the patient when nonadherence occurs; instead, simply label it as an issue for continuing focus, and understand that adherence often requires numerous attempts.

Evidence-Based Treatment Approaches

The following evidence-based treatment approaches are recommended for use for those with SMI and are available in a variety of settings in many communities.

Assertive Community Treatment (ACT) programs use a treatment-team approach and have been shown to improve symptom management and quality of life while reducing rehospitalization (NAMI, 2019a). Instead of working with multiple departments or agencies, the patient works solely with an established team of professionals who provide comprehensive services and 24/7 access to a team member.

Cognitive-behavioral therapy (CBT) helps patients change thoughts, feelings, and behaviors to decrease symptomatology and improve quality of life. CBT helps patients perceive circumstances more accurately and positively by guiding them to reconsider their perceptions and restructure their thinking to be more realistic. CBT may be an effective intervention for patients with psychotic disorders to reduce anxiety and depression (Opoka & Lincoln, 2017).

Dialectical behavior therapy (DBT) includes aspects of CBT and mindfulness practices, focusing on accepting what cannot be changed and changing what is amenable to change. Patients learn mindfulness techniques, distress tolerance, emotional regulation, and interpersonal effectiveness. DBT may reduce symptoms of mood disorders and reduce the frequency of self-harm (Hawton et al., 2016).

The promotion of family support and partnerships with providers is based on the premise that having sound support systems is one of the strongest predictors of recovery and that treatment is enhanced when treatment providers work as empathic partners with patients and significant others (NAMI, 2019b). An example of this partnership is NAMI's Family-to-Family program, a psychoeducational program focusing on the skills families need to cope with their loved one's illness and to promote recovery (NAMI, 2019b).

Social skills training focuses on teaching a wide variety of social skills. Social deficits cause both direct and indirect functional impairment; people unable to respond assertively, for example, may instead respond aggressively or may fail to meet their needs at all. Complex interpersonal skills (e.g., negotiating or resolving a conflict) are broken down into subcomponents that are then taught in a concrete, stepwise fashion.

Vocational rehabilitation and supported employment enhance self-esteem, improve organizational abilities, and increase socialization and income. Vocational rehabilitation includes prevocational training (skills needed to obtain employment) and initial employment in a sheltered setting (e.g., a patient-managed business), building to competitive employment in the business world. Supported employment focuses on on-the-job training and support, often with job coaches at the employee's side, enabling rapid and continued employment (Frederick & Vanderweele, 2019).

Rehabilitation Versus Recovery

Until recently, the **rehabilitation model** has been the dominant paradigm in mental health care. It focuses on deficits, symptoms, and stability rather than on quality of life and cure. It has been criticized for stabilization over growth and for producing dependence on health care providers, with staff relating to the patient as parents do to children. As a result, mental health patients and advocates led a patient movement that emphasizes choices and empowerment, culminating in the **recovery model** of care. It is promoted by the **National Alliance on Mental Illness (NAMI)**, a leading advocacy organization, along with many other mental health organizations and treatment providers. The recovery model stresses a partnership between care providers and the patient, both working together in planning and directing treatment. It emphasizes hope and empowerment and focuses on strengths rather than limitations, helping the individual to use his or her strengths to achieve the highest quality of life possible.

Other Potentially Beneficial Approaches or Services

The following offer potential benefit to those living with serious mental illness:

- **Advance directives** give the patient the opportunity to direct how future relapses and treatment needs should be managed. The directive is a document signed when the patient's illness is under control and informed decisions are possible. For example, when well, a patient can give consent to hospitalization or forced medications and specify when these responses may be used, maintaining control over treatment and avoiding involuntary admission and related court involvement.
- **Peer support and patient-managed programming** range from informal "clubhouses" that offer socialization, recreation, and sometimes other services to competitive businesses such as snack bars or janitorial services that provide needed services and patient employment while encouraging independence and building vocational skills. **Peer-support specialists** are specially trained individuals who have experienced severe mental illness and are further along in the recovery process and provide supportive services to persons with SMIs; being in recovery themselves, they serve as role models and sources of hope, and their guidance may be perceived as more acceptable and valid than that provided by staff.

IMPULSE-CONTROL DISORDERS

> **VIGNETTE: Kleptomania** Sarah, age 76, is shopping when she notices the lipstick display. She rarely wears lipstick but is drawn to the display and feels an urge to take one. She suppresses the urge, but it grows harder to resist; ultimately, she snatches the lipstick, putting it in her purse. She feels a sense of relief, almost an odd sort of pleasure. Over time, this urge to steal things happens increasingly. Usually Sarah cannot resist, sometimes taking ridiculous chances in taking things that she doesn't even need. She feels ashamed and, consumed with remorse, sometimes returns the items or throws them away. Even though she has been caught and threatened with jail, the irresistible urge to steal continues.

Impulse-control disorders involve a decreased ability to resist an impulse to perform certain acts. In most cases the pattern is one of increasing tension that builds until a particular action is taken, followed by a sense of relief. The actions may be impulsive (e.g., stealing) or involve considerable planning (e.g., fire setting) and may range from benign to potentially harmful to self or others. The tension reduction reinforces the action and makes future resistance more difficult. Except for pathological gambling, these disorders are considered to be relatively rare (Table 27.2).

Theory

Biological Factors

The causes underlying impulse control disorders are not clearly established. Certain disorders or abnormalities of the brain seem to increase impulsiveness or reduce one's ability to resist impulses. Violent people appear to have higher serotonin levels in the brain (Klasen et al., 2019) and may show electroencephalographic differences.

Frontotemporal dementia or tumors (especially those affecting the right hemisphere), Parkinson's disease, dementia, and multiple sclerosis can contribute to impulsivity, as can traumatic brain injury and substance abuse, but the link in these disorders is unclear. Dopamine-receptor agonists (e.g., certain stimulants and antiparkinsonian medications) can also impair impulse control (Grall-Bronnec et al., 2017).

Genetic Factors

A gene associated with impulsive violence is suspected of weakening the brain's impulse-control circuitry (Klasen et al., 2019). Although the incidence of some impulse disorders is greater within families (e.g., trichotillomania), neither this gene nor others have been linked causally to these disorders.

Psychological Factors

Theories regarding psychological causes of these disorders include an impaired ability to manage anxiety, wherein the person might be defending against (coping with) anxiety by subconsciously choosing an action that gives a sense of control over the anxiety. This theory is supported by a pattern of increased impulsive acts during periods of high stress. Some of these disorders may be a variant, or an expression, of disorders such as obsessive-compulsive disorder (OCD) or posttraumatic stress disorder (PTSD). Finally, a person may experience craving for the act and relief upon achieving it, suggesting an addictions-based etiology.

Clinical Picture

The person experiences a recurring and irresistible urge to enact a behavior despite its being illogical, distressing, or potentially harmful. Judgment is intact, and psychotic elements are absent. Descriptions of each disorder can be found in Table 27.2.

People with impulse-control disorders usually realize that the acts are illogical or wrong, but despite their best efforts, the urge to act overwhelms them. They are often confused and troubled by their urges, feeling embarrassment, shame, or guilt as a result of their behaviors; these responses can lead to depression and suicidality (Grant & Leppink, 2015). They may find themselves socially isolated or stigmatized.

Kleptomania can contribute to shoplifting losses. Gambling can cause tremendous personal financial losses; disrupt families; and cause loss of status, housing, possessions, jobs, and marriages. Intermittent explosive disorder and pyromania can cause property damage and injury or death to others and can place the person at risk of being sued or injured by the victim's defensive response. When criminal offenses are involved, society pays the costs of prosecution, incarceration, and forensic treatment, and the individual may subsequently lose civil rights (e.g., the right to vote) or access to private or governmental entitlements (e.g., eligibility for federal housing assistance, ability to hold a professional license or work in a particular field).

APPLICATION OF THE NURSING PROCESS

ASSESSMENT

The diagnosis of impulse-control disorders first requires the elimination of other medical and psychiatric causes for the behavior (e.g., antisocial personality disorder, substance abuse), as well as ruling out other causes, such as seeking profit or attaining revenge.

Information suggesting the presence of an impulse-control disorder is often minimized, withheld, or concealed by the person or overlooked by staff; careful assessment is therefore important. Because the nurse's beliefs and attitudes about the behaviors in question may compromise his or her ability to perceive or remain objective about the disorder, self-awareness is essential. For example, if the nurse believes that setting fires is simply criminal behavior and not related to a mental disorder, the nurse may overlook the impulse-control disorder or fail to help the person obtain care.

Because actions associated with impulse control disorders may be embarrassing or even criminal in nature, building trust and conveying empathy and acceptance are key aspects of helping the person disclose these problems. Significant others who may be less reluctant to share information can also help identify concealed disorders. Nurses should look for patterns of recurrent loss of control in the patient's responses and history and should observe for signs such as fascination with fire, unusual familiarity with gambling terminology, patches where hair is thin, or pulling at one's hair.

TABLE 27.2 Impulse Control Disorder

Disorder	Description
Intermittent explosive disorder	Recurrent, unpremeditated episodes of marked verbal or behavioral aggression or rage. The acts are often severe enough to hurt people or destroy significant property and occur in otherwise normal individuals. The acts are disproportionate to the perceived provocation and can occur in response to ordinarily minor events such as traffic delays. The individual may feel depressed or remorseful afterward and may face recrimination, arrest, civil actions, and loss of relationships and employment as a result of the acts. "Road rage" is sometimes a manifestation of this disorder.
Kleptomania	An uncontrollable and recurrent urge to steal. The thefts produce a sense of psychological gratification and often involve items of little value or use to the person who takes them. Persons often report a buildup of tension before stealing and a sense of relief afterward (APA, 2013). The objects taken may have a symbolic meaning (e.g., power or beauty), but often the person cannot explain the reason and usually perceives the thefts as illogical and wrong. Kleptomania may begin at any age, and two-thirds of people affected are women. The behavior may occur at widely scattered intervals or be more regular and protracted. Prosecution may occur, although mental health advocates distinguish kleptomaniac behavior from criminality.
Pyromania	A reoccurring compulsion to set fires and experiencing a sense of accomplishment or relief when setting fires, often accompanied by a sense of pleasure or release (APA, 2013). The fires are set for sexual or other emotional gratification, not arson for profit or revenge. The person has a fascination with fires and "gains great pleasure from starting them, watching them, helping to put them out, and watching what happened afterwards" (Francis 2013, p. 141) but has little regard for the life or property that may be destroyed in the fire. This disorder may result in criminal prosecution.
Gambling disorder	A preoccupation with gambling and an inability to resist the urge to gamble despite significant disruption of family, finances, work, and other aspects of one's life; it is sometimes known as pathological gambling. The individual feels aroused and positive when gambling and experiences a relief of tension. The gambler can't get enough and finds he or she needs to raise the stakes to feel the same high. When not gambling, the person experiences irritability, restlessness, anxiety, and sadness and can't wait to get back to the action (withdrawal) (Francis 2013, p. 139). Pathological gamblers may lie, rationalize, manipulate others, and conceal their behavior in order to maintain it. Work and social functioning may be disrupted. Most people with this disorder are men, and the lifetime prevalence of this disorder is about 0.5% to 1% (APA, 2013). The *Diagnostic and Statistical Manual of Mental Disorders,* 5th edition *(DSM-5)* categorizes this as an addictive disorder (APA, 2013).
Trichotillomania	Repetitively pulling out one's hair in order to relieve tension. The person may pull out hair only occasionally and for brief periods or regularly and for hours at a time. It tends to worsen under stress but also occurs when the person is calm, sometimes in an almost absent-minded fashion. The hair loss is often noticeable and significantly affects the individual's social comfort and self-esteem, sometimes causing severe distress. It may be self-limited or continue for decades and can involve hair from any location.

Data from American Psychiatric Association. (2013). *Diagnostic and statistical manual of mental disorders* (5th ed.). Washington, DC: Author; Francis, A. (2013). *Essentials of psychiatric diagnoses: responding to the challenges of* DSM-5. New York: Guilford Press.

TABLE 27.3 Interventions for Impulse Control Disorders

Intervention	Rationale
1. Guide the person to understand and practice tension reduction and stress control strategies such as stress avoidance, correction of negative self-talk, and breathing control exercises.	1. Tension usually precedes and contributes to impulsive actions; tension reduction and adaptive tension management can reduce impulsive behavior.
2. Promote the progressive substitution of alternate, less maladaptive responses to tension, such as applying pressure to one's scalp with a thumb rather than pulling out one's hair.	2. Impulse control disorders involve maladaptive behaviors, some of which are criminal offenses; substitution of more adaptive responses can prevent negative consequences.
3. Assist the person to explore feelings associated with the impulses, such as shame, fear, or guilt, and to manage these feelings effectively.	3. Negative emotions contribute to stress and tension, leading to maladaptive impulsive behaviors.
4. Assist the person to identify the consequences of his or her actions (e.g., "How do other people respond when you ______?," "Tell me what things are like the day after you've set a fire," and "Imagine you set the fire: what do you think will happen in the days and weeks that follow?").	4. Identifying consequences can help the person become more empathic to his or her effect on others, and increase motivation to refrain from problematic behaviors. Guide the person to imagine the consequences of behavior and dampen urges to act on impulses.
5. Educate the person that drugs and alcohol may increase impulsiveness through disinhibition or impairment of judgment; educate the person regarding the effect of "triggers," that is, circumstances that evoke tension or impulses (e.g., going to bars).	5. Disinhibiting drugs and exposure to triggers that evoke impulsive behavior increase impulsive actions; reducing disinhibition and exposure to triggers reduces the frequency and intensity of the impulsive actions.
6. Pathological gamblers may respond well to group therapy; organizations such as Gamblers Anonymous (http://www.gamblersanonymous.org) provide significant assistance through support, education, and practical tips on managing gambling impulses and other concerns.	6. Twelve-step programs have been shown to be of significant help in reducing activities that have a compulsive or addictive component; peer support groups are effective for confronting defenses and rationalization used to support the gambling.
7. Persons with trichotillomania can benefit from special hairstyling, hair weaves, or other cosmetology assistance; they may require considerable support in order to access such resources, however, because of embarrassment.	7. Hair loss can create a significant cosmetic defect, resulting in impaired self-esteem and further dysfunctional coping; compensating cosmetically for such defects can enhance the person's self-image and self-esteem.

It is helpful to ask about circumstances that increase tension, as well as ways in which the person reduces this tension. Empathic prompting can be helpful (e.g., "Sometimes people find themselves feeling tense and having urges to do things to release the tension. Can you tell me about times when this may have happened to you?"). Frank, direct questioning can set a tone for openness and prompt more candid responses (e.g., "Tell me about times when you've come close to losing control.").

A person's legal history may also suggest these disorders. Recurrent assaults or any episodes of fire setting merit further assessment. Further, the person may be dealing with concurrent depression or be sufficiently distressed to be considering self-harm. Assessment for these risks is essential. Finally, it is always important to assess how the disorder has affected the patient and significant others, as well as the patient's knowledge of the disorder and ways of reducing or coping with it.

DIAGNOSIS

A variety of nursing diagnoses may apply to people with impulse-control disorders: *Impaired impulse control, Impaired adjustment, Anxiety, Impaired family coping, Difficulty coping, Risk for injury, Low self-esteem, Impaired socialisation,* and *Social isolation* (ICN, 2019). Nursing interventions for these disorders vary with the disorder, but some general interventions likely to fit most are listed in Table 27.3.

OUTCOMES IDENTIFICATION

Expected outcomes vary with the disorder but typically focus on reducing the problematic acts and substituting more adaptive means to reduce tension. Examples include the following: "(Person) does not set fires," "Hair loss is reduced by 20%," "(Person) demonstrates use of three or more tension-reduction strategies," and "(Person) rates anxiety as 5 or less on a 0-to-10 scale."

PLANNING AND IMPLEMENTATION

Treatment for impulse-control disorders may involve a combination of psychotherapy and medication. Because these disorders usually do not create an imminent risk to oneself or others, or present with emergent needs, treatment is usually provided on an outpatient basis.

Psychopharmacology

Medication options for clients with impulse-control disorders may include antidepressants, lithium, mood stabilizers, atypical antipsychotics, and naltrexone (Sadock et al., 2015).

Nonpharmacological Treatments

Hypnotherapy may be of benefit in selected disorders, and cognitive-behavioral approaches, such as habit reversal (identifying and reducing thoughts that trigger undesired actions) and sensitization (imagining negative consequences, such as getting caught, when the urge occurs), are evidence-based practices in disorders such as trichotillomania (Garrett & Giddings, 2014). Biofeedback has been used to reduce habitual and impulsive behaviors (Fielenbach et al., 2017). Group psychotherapy provides for therapeutic confrontation from peers and tends to be particularly helpful for people who have poor insight or difficulty accepting responsibility for their behavior. Gamblers Anonymous, similar to Alcoholics Anonymous, may be an effective intervention for those with compulsive gambling (Sadock et al., 2015).

GENDER DYSPHORIA AND SEXUAL DISORDERS

GENDER DYSPHORIA

Gender dysphoria (GD), previously known as *gender identity disorder,* is now considered in the mental health field to be a *difference,* not a disorder or pathology. GD involves persistent, strong gender identification where a person feels he or she is of a different gender than that indicated by his or her physiology, and the original gender (or that assigned by society in the case of ambiguous genitalia) causes distress. Often the person with gender dysphoria believes that he or she was born in the wrong body. People with GD experience persistent discomfort with their gender-related roles and possess a strong and persistent desire to assume the characteristics (e.g., dress and mannerisms) and roles of the opposite gender, as well as a desire to have the primary and secondary sex characteristics of the other gender (American Psychiatric Association [APA], 2013). Persons with GD may alter their dress, use hormonal medications, and pursue surgery in order to appear as, or become, their identified gender. GD typically first becomes apparent in childhood or adolescence, and the cause is uncertain; theories include alterations in sexual hormones and related neurodevelopment in utero or developmental differences in early life (Sadock et al., 2015). *Cisgender* is the term used for gender identity that matches one's sex at birth, whereas *transgender* or *nonbinary* is the opposite (Boehmer et al., 2019; Nguyen et al., 2019).

People with GD may experience significant embarrassment, shame, discrimination, and social isolation because many people in our society do not understand how one could believe that one is not of the gender previously thought. There is considerable stigma about GD, and others may react with repugnance. GD also raises practical issues: If you feel that you are female, you might prefer to use a restroom labeled for females; however, if you appear to others as a male, women might take exception to your presence in a restroom designated for females and could even assume you are committing criminal behavior such as voyeurism. For people with gender dysphoria, counseling can help patients compare and choose various paths they might take, including sexual reassignment, and cope with their feelings and society's responses to this nonpathological difference. Hormonal agents to alter sexual characteristics may be used.

Persons who choose gender reassignment engage in specific steps to prepare for the transition:

1. Psychotherapy to assist the person in fully considering and preparing for this very involved and long-term process
2. Living for a period (e.g., 1 to 2 years) as a member of the desired gender to ensure readiness. During this time, the person is usually given hormonal therapy to suppress undesired physical characteristics and elicit desired sexual characteristics, such as to diminish facial hair and enlarge breasts, or to alter one's voice; this may be the last step for many people.
3. Surgical intervention to alter the person's secondary sex characteristics to match those of the identified gender

PARAPHILIAS AND PARAPHILIC DISORDERS

Paraphilias are sexual acts or fantasies that involve deviation from conventional, socially acceptable sexual behavior. They are not disorders per se; they are on a continuum with normal sexual interests and practices, and unless the person experiences distress about the sexual differences, they typically do not merit a need for treatment (Holoyda & Kellaher, 2016). The incidence of paraphilias is difficult to measure because stigma, potential for embarrassment, and other concerns cause reluctance to disclose this information. Divergent religious and cultural beliefs have created conflict within our society about how to define appropriate sexual behavior. For example, opinions vary widely in terms of what is an appropriate age to begin sexual relations or whom one should be able to choose as a sexual partner; conflict stemming from such beliefs can result in ostracism, hostility, and even aggression. Education, counseling, and support are helpful both for persons who come to perceive themselves as "perverted" or abnormal as a result of negative societal views and for family members and significant others who are hurt and confused.

In contrast, **paraphilic disorders** are defined in the *Diagnostic and Statistical Manual of Mental Disorders,* 5th edition *(DSM-5)* as paraphilias that cause distress, risk of harm, or actual harm to oneself or others (APA, 2013). Paraphilic disorders involve a preoccupation with sexual fantasies and related urges and behaviors that focus on nontraditional or socially unacceptable sexual "targets," such as children, animals, or objects. Persons with these disorders may or may not act on their fantasies and urges; enacting such fantasies can involve criminal acts.

Theory

Biological Factors

The causes underlying paraphilic disorders have not yet been determined. Some researchers believe pedophilia should be viewed somewhat as a neurodevelopmental disorder because structural and functional differences in the frontal, temporal, and limbic regions of the brain have been observed (Tenbergen et al., 2015). Traumatic brain injuries and dementia may also be associated with impulsive behavior, behavioral disinhibition, and inappropriate sexual behavior (De Giorgi & Series, 2016; Sadock et al., 2015).

Psychological Factors

A failure to develop appropriate attachments in early childhood, resulting in inadequate or inappropriate attachments at later developmental stages, may contribute to paraphilic disorders. Another theory is that the disorders are learned responses to inappropriate sexual role models. One's own sexual victimization may contribute to paraphilic disorders, particularly those associated with sexual offenses; 30% to 60% of pedophiles were themselves sexually abused as children. Funding entities and research institutions, perhaps because of the controversial aspects of these disorders, are sometimes reluctant to support research related to the causes and treatment of paraphilic disorders, limiting our understanding (Tenbergen et al., 2015).

Clinical Picture

The *DSM-5* (APA, 2013) distinguishes multiple types of paraphilic disorders, described in Table 27.4. The diagnosis of these disorders first requires eliminating all other medical and psychiatric causes of the behavior in question (e.g., criminal intent, mania, dementia, substance abuse). Paraphilic disorders do not involve psychotic features, and most have their onset during adolescence. Most people with paraphilic disorders are male, and diagnosis requires that the features must have been present for at least 6 months (i.e., occasional experiences of gratification through paraphilic-like experiences would not meet the diagnostic criteria for a paraphilia).

Although not paraphilic disorders, sexual addiction and other forms of distress or dysfunction related to sexuality can be diagnosed as *sexual disorders not otherwise specified* (NOS). Other disorders related to sexuality, although not covered in this chapter or classified as sexual disorders, include those relating to chromosomal abnormalities (e.g., Klinefelter's syndrome), head trauma or other organic disorder, compulsive use of pornography, and sexual aberrations arising from SMIs that affect impulse control and social and sexual interaction.

Effect on Individuals, Families, and Society

The effect of paraphilias may be relatively minor and limited to the individual with the diagnosis (e.g., a person with transvestic fetishism). When people with paraphilias engage sexually with unwilling partners (e.g., frotteurism or voyeurism), victims are violated and may experience significant and protracted psychological distress.

TABLE 27.4 Paraphilic Disorders

Disorder	Description
Fetish	Any unusual preoccupation or desire for an object, body part, or activity that one needs in order to achieve sexual gratification. The object of the fetish is not one typically associated with sexual gratification by most persons within a given culture. It is a paraphilia (an unusual sexual interest) and not typically a sexual disorder in that it does not cause significant distress or harm.
Exhibitionistic disorder	The achievement of sexual arousal or pleasure by exposing one's genitals, usually to an unsuspecting stranger. Sufferers have strong, recurrent fantasies about exposing genitalia. Upon exhibiting genitalia, one may experience shame and embarrassment and can face criminal charges and loss of relationships and employment. Exhibitionism usually starts in adolescence and seems to taper off by age 40.
Fetishistic disorder (fetishism)	Having difficulty achieving sexual arousal except when using or thinking about an inanimate object or part of the body. The individual experiences significant distress, and the fetish objects are not those usually associated with sexual arousal (e.g., feet, shoes).
Frotteuristic disorder (frotteurism)	Obtaining sexual arousal and gratification from rubbing one's genitals against unsuspecting others in public places. It causes marked distress or interpersonal difficulties, and criminal prosecution can result.
Pedophilia	Pedophilia involves fantasized or actual sexual activity with a prepubescent child, wherein the person has either acted on the fantasies or has experienced significant distress or difficulties as a result of the fantasies (APA, 2013). Pedophiles may focus on children of the same, opposite, or both genders, although most are heterosexually focused. They may focus on children exclusively or may also have a sexual interest in adults. Some with pedophilia focus on relatives (incestual form), others on non–family members, and some on both. The disorder causes revulsion in most adults, and pedophilic actions are often considered the most intolerable of criminal offenses.
Sexual masochism and sexual sadism disorders	Deriving sexual gratification from having pain and/or humiliation inflicted upon oneself (masochism) or creating psychological and physical pain in others (sadism). Masochism can include bondage, verbal abuse, electrical shocks, whipping, being urinated on, or being forced to humiliate oneself. Sadism includes inflicting such acts on a (usually masochistic) partner and often involves dominating one's partner physically and psychologically. The partner may be consenting or nonconsenting.
Transvestic disorder	Deriving sexual gratification by dressing as a person of the opposite gender. Unlike gender dysphoria, which involves a conflict between one's beliefs about true gender and biological gender (or the gender assigned by society), the transvestite does not perceive a conflict with gender but enjoys dressing in a gender-incongruent manner.
Voyeuristic disorder	Also known as voyeurism, this disorder involves deriving sexual gratification from observing unsuspecting persons in sexually arousing situations (e.g., undressing or engaging in sexual activity).

Data from American Psychiatric Association. (2013). *Diagnostic and statistical manual of mental disorders (DSM-5)* (5th ed.). Washington, DC: The Association.

Paraphilic, and especially pedophilic, *offenders* can harm or kill their victims, and even when the victim is physically uninjured, there is often significant, protracted, and sometimes disabling psychological damage. Survivors are at increased risk of disorders such as PTSD, depression, anxiety, deliberate self-harm, dissociation, and substance abuse disorders. Families, loved ones, and the general community are often traumatized and left unable to trust others or feel fully secure (see Chapter 22).

Sexual abuse is a significant problem in our society. However, only a portion of this abuse involves pedophilia. Parents and caregivers commit up to 90% or more of the sexual abuse of children in the United States, whereas strangers are believed to account for less than 5% of child sexual offenses (see Chapter 21). Family members may choose children not because of sexual attraction per se (as would most pedophiles) but because they are readily accessible, often unable to resist, and able to be controlled by the abuser through threat and intimidation. The **recidivism** (repeating of a previous offense) rates for untreated child sexual offenders (both pedophilic and nonpedophilic combined) range from 30% to 50% in offenders under 60 years of age (Harvard Health Publications, 2014).

Persons with these disorders may be distressed by their symptoms, overwhelmed with shame or guilt. Others display more antisocial or narcissistic tendencies and are indifferent or blasé about their sexual offenses or may attempt to justify their actions through rationalization or other means. Some even lobby to decriminalize sexual acts involving children, claiming they are natural or will not harm children (viewpoints not supported by ethics or scientific evidence). Conversely, some pedophiles seek to refrain from harming children directly but may do so indirectly by accessing (and thus supporting) child pornography. Other sexual disorders, such as compulsive sexual behavior (sometimes called sexual addiction), can contribute to guilt, relational discord, low self-esteem, and STIs.

Societal responses to sexual offenders include educating the public, warning potential victims (via sexual offender registries and notification of those residing nearby), correctional monitoring, and restricting access to potential victims (by prohibiting contact with children and restricting residences to areas away from schools and playgrounds). Although intended to prevent sexual offenses, these restrictions may ostracize possibly reformed offenders and create unintended consequences (e.g., isolation, unemployment, homelessness), which may in turn make it more difficult to track and treat offenders. Information on sexual offenses and sexual offender listings can typically be found on the web pages of local law enforcement agencies.

However, because reoffending after incarceration is not rare, some states now hold sexual offenders in inpatient psychiatric treatment settings (usually state forensic hospitals) for extended periods after they have completed their prison sentences. This "preventive psychiatric incarceration" is controversial within the mental health field; some believe it is an abuse of psychiatry to (1) hold a person who does not require inpatient psychiatric care in an inpatient setting or (2) incarcerate a person because of what he or she might do in the future (Weinberger et al., 2018).

TABLE 27.5 Interventions for Sexual Disorders

Intervention	Rationale
1. Use inclusive language, convey acceptance, normalize disclosure pertaining to sexuality, and provide active support.	1. These actions promote free and open discussion of the person's behavior and needs.
2. Assist individuals with gender dysphoria to connect with peers and professionals who are supportive and receptive, and to access helpful resources such as http://www.wpath.org and http://www.transgenderlaw.org.	2. Stigma and discrimination can cause isolation and hopelessness; connecting with others and pursuing educational resources for the person and significant others can enhance understanding and acceptance.
3. Maintain and reinforce appropriate interpersonal boundaries with people with sexual disorders.	3. Role modeling of appropriate boundaries allows the person to identify and adopt more effective ways of relating to others, and maintains professional relationship.
4. Mutually set, track, revise, and reinforce incremental goals, along with related actions that will meet those goals.	4. Mutual goal setting enables the person to "own" the goal; incremental goals are easier to attain, reducing discouragement from unmet goals, and provide a series of successes that reinforce one's efforts.
5. Guide the person to practice tension reduction and stress control strategies such as avoidance of stress, correction of negative self-talk, and use of breathing control exercises.	5. High levels of stress and tension, especially when coupled with a limited or ineffective repertoire of coping strategies, increase the chance of maladaptive behaviors.
6. Educate the person (and any support persons and personnel from the criminal justice system) about the disorder: its causes, treatments, and ways to cope with and control symptoms and maladaptive behaviors.	6. Understanding one's disorder, as well as ways to cope with or reduce symptoms, can decrease guilt and powerlessness, instilling hope and improving the person's sense of control.
7. Assist the person to identify and explore feelings preceding or associated with the target behavior (e.g., excitement, shame, guilt).	7. Unresolved feelings can cause desperation and lead to acting-out or loss of control.
8. Assist the person to identify the consequences of his or her actions (e.g., ask, "How do other people seem to feel about your behavior?" or "What tends to happen when you go where children play?").	8. Insight that develops from within tends to be more accepted than feedback provided externally; covert sensitization—guiding the person to connect an undesired behavior with negative consequences—diminishes unacceptable behaviors.
9. Address comorbid disorders and mental health needs (e.g., substance abuse, sexual victimization during one's youth).	9. Depression and other mental disorders impair problem-solving and coping abilities, draining the person's energy for addressing the target problems.

Adapted from Royal College of Psychiatrists. (2013). *Good practice guidelines for the assessment and treatment of adults with gender dysphoria.* Retrieved from https://www.rcpsych.ac.uk/docs/default-source/improving-care/better-mh-policy/college-reports/cr181-good-practice-guidelines-for-the-assessment-and-treatment-of-adults-with-gender-dysphoria.pdf?sfvrsn=84743f94_2

APPLICATION OF THE NURSING PROCESS

ASSESSMENT

People often conceal or deny paraphilic thoughts and behavior, making careful assessment and validation of the patient's reports important. Written assessment questionnaires can elicit possibly embarrassing information without the tension of a face-to-face interview, forming the basis of a more focused interview thereafter. Significant others who are less reluctant to share information can also help identify concealed issues (e.g., it is not unusual for adult children of individuals with pedophilia to report inappropriate sexual contact during their childhood). In some cases, the person may be dealing with concurrent depression or be sufficiently distressed to be considering self-harm, making assessment for this risk essential; this is especially true for those who recently have been accused of (or publicly exposed in reference to) sexual offenses involving children and who face considerable shame and even hostility within their families and communities as a result (such persons are at especially high risk of suicide in the first 24 to 48 hours after incarceration). Finally, it is always important to assess how the disorder has affected the person and significant others, as well as the person's knowledge of the disorder and ways of coping with it.

DIAGNOSIS

A variety of nursing diagnoses may apply to individuals with paraphilias and paraphilic disorders, including *Impaired adjustment, Anxiety, Impaired family coping, Difficulty coping, Relationship problem, Risk for injury, Low self-esteem, Impaired sexual functioning, Risk for violence, Problematic sexual behavior,* and *Social isolation* (ICN, 2019). Nursing interventions for these disorders vary with the disorder and its expression in a particular person and are affected by any comorbid mental health disorders. Some general interventions likely to fit most related circumstances are listed in Table 27.5.

OUTCOMES IDENTIFICATION

Expected outcomes vary with the disorder but typically focus on reducing the problematic acts and substituting more adaptive means to meet sexual needs. Examples of desired outcomes include "(Person) reports ability to fantasize about adults as well as children," "(Person) does not go to locations where children are likely to be found," and "(Person) rates urge to have contact with children a 5 or less on a 1-to-10 scale."

PLANNING AND IMPLEMENTATION

Psychopharmacology and Nonpharmacological Treatments

Pedophiles and other sexual offenders may seek treatment when sufficiently distressed by their disorder, when compelled to do so by courts, or when necessary to address the concerns of significant others. Except for criminal offenders with comorbid SMIs, treatment is usually on an outpatient basis and appears to be beneficial in some cases.

Treatment of pedophilia usually involves medications and psychotherapy. Pharmacological treatment typically involves medications that reduce impulsive or compulsive behavior, such as antidepressants, naltrexone, antipsychotics, mood stabilizers, or medications that interfere with the production of sexual hormones in order to reduce sexual urges (Holoyda & Kellaher, 2016), in effect producing varying degrees of **chemical castration.** Patients typically receive a monthly injection, and hormonal levels are monitored to ensure effectiveness. Side effects in men include feminization and weight gain. Infrequently, agents for chemical castration are used, and in rare cases, surgical castration may be pursued by the patient in lieu of drugs. Psychotherapy typically involves individual and group therapy focused on improving impulse control and increasing empathy for victims.

Treatment for other paraphilic disorders includes psychopharmacological interventions and psychotherapy. Medication options include naltrexone and antidepressants to reduce compulsive or impulsive behavior. Psychotherapeutic treatments include individual and group psychotherapy and psychoeducational interventions. CBTs in particular are believed to be helpful. Behavioral approaches can include desensitization techniques to reduce sexual responsiveness to undesired stimuli. In some cases, patients are guided to fulfill their gratification needs in non–socially offensive ways, such as via masturbatory reconditioning. Twelve-step programs also have been effective for some, and treatment of comorbid disorders, particularly those that impair impulse control (e.g., substance abuse), can reduce the risk of recidivism or conversion to criminal behavior (Mayo Clinic, 2019).

Self-Care for Nurses

A nurse's beliefs and attitudes about these behaviors may compromise objectivity or create distress. If the nurse is a survivor of sexual abuse, treating perpetrators can be particularly difficult and even traumatic. Therefore self-care and self-awareness are essential when working with persons with these disorders (e.g., clinical supervision to help one recognize and deal with subjective responses to the patient; counseling to help cope with reawakened memories of earlier abuse). If nurses believe they cannot work with the patient appropriately, perhaps reassignment, if possible, while working on reframing thoughts and feelings, is best. Actions associated with paraphilias may be embarrassing or even criminal in nature, making building trust and conveying empathy and acceptance essential but challenging.

ADULT ATTENTION-DEFICIT/HYPERACTIVITY DISORDER

VIGNETTE: Andrea, a 32-year-old graduate student in psychology, presents at the student health center with concerns that she might have attention-deficit/hyperactivity disorder (ADHD). She reports that throughout her life, teachers and others told her she was extremely bright, but that somehow this was not reflected in her grades, which were Bs and Cs. She notes that she has difficulty maintaining concentration, often "tuning out" during lectures and having to regularly reread parts of her assignments.

Andrea has difficulty sitting still and sometimes interrupts others impulsively, then apologizes. When distracted, she has difficulty regaining her train of thought. Disorganization, worry, and irritability trouble her. She often loses track of belongings, spends much time looking for misplaced items, forgets appointments, and frequently overlooks tasks she had intended to do.

Other psychiatric and physical problems are ruled out. After treatment with methylphenidate and counseling, Andrea reports that she was able to finish a major written assignment in one-third the time and with much less stress than before treatment. She is happy with the improvement and hopeful and says that friends have commented that she seems more at ease and less scattered. She agrees to join an ADHD support group on campus to obtain support and practical suggestions for managing the disorder.

Prevalence and Comorbidity

ADHD involves a persistent pattern of inattention, impaired ability to focus and concentrate, and hyperactivity and impulsivity that are more noticeable and more severe than would otherwise be seen at a given developmental level. **Attention-deficit/hyperactivity disorder (ADHD) inattentive type** involves a similar presentation but without the hyperactivity and is common in females with ADHD. ADHD is discussed in detail in Chapter 26; coverage here focuses only on aspects related to its presence in adults.

ADHD appears to have a lower prevalence in adulthood (2.5% vs. 5% in children [APA, 2013]), although this may really reflect inadequate screening and the enhanced ability of adults to compensate or conceal their symptoms. Adult ADHD is associated with a wide variety of interpersonal and social problems, including relational discord and reduced academic and vocational performance. It can limit or disrupt a person's ability to function in any realm and can negatively affect health habits. Psychiatric comorbidity, particularly anxiety and mood disorders, is common in ADHD (Sadock et al., 2015). Co-occurring disorders include Tourette's syndrome and other tic disorders, substance abuse, STIs, traumatic brain injuries, and trauma.

Theory

ADHD is believed to be a neurodevelopmental disorder with multiple contributing factors, including smaller brain volume, white- and gray-matter alterations (Jadidian, Hurley, & Taber, 2015), and alterations in the neurotransmitter dopamine (Sadock et al., 2015). There appears to be a strong genetic and familial component, with an estimated heritability of approximately 74% (Faraone & Larsson, 2019). Social and biological adversity (interpersonal and biological challenges) are possible factors; fetal distress, prematurity, exposure to neurotoxins toxins such as lead, and maternal substance abuse, particularly in the prenatal and early postnatal period when brain development is rapid, are implicated, as are conflict and distress within one's family (Sadock et al., 2015).

Clinical Picture

ADHD tends to be underdiagnosed in adults. The diagnosis is complicated by the complexity and varied presentation of the disorder. Adult ADHD features are similar to those of children but affect adult roles such as postsecondary education, employment, and marriage. Common presentations include impaired focusing and concentration, disorganization, impulsiveness, impaired task completion, irritability and impaired frustration tolerance, labile mood, and impaired social/relational/educational/vocational functioning (Sadock et al., 2015). Because these features can occur for many reasons, it's not unusual for adults to be unaware that they have ADHD or for clinicians to overlook this diagnosis in adults.

Effect on Individuals, Families, and Society

The effect of ADHD is significant. Adults diagnosed with ADHD as children tend to achieve lower socioeconomic status; complete fewer years of school; use nicotine, alcohol, and drugs at higher rates; have more traffic incidents (e.g., road rage, accidents, speeding offenses); have more contact with police; are at greater risk of STIs and trauma; change jobs more frequently; report more interpersonal and relational difficulties; and have higher rates of anxiety and depression than people without ADHD (Franke et al., 2018; Mayo Clinic, 2017; Miranda et al., 2014). ADHD is also significantly more prevalent in incarcerated populations, suggesting ADHD may increase the propensity toward criminal activity.

The effect on society is less well established. ADHD inhibits academic achievement at all ages, and it is believed to reduce work productivity and increase criminal justice system costs significantly, but hard data do not yet exist.

APPLICATION OF THE NURSING PROCESS

ASSESSMENT

ADHD is diagnosed based on the characteristic patterns of behavior and organizational and attentional dysfunction, which are the cardinal features of these disorders, using patient reports, nursing observation, and when available, reports of employers, family members, and other third parties as assessment data. Assessment should also include the person's present knowledge of and ability to cope with the disorder. Support systems play a major role in the person achieving successful outcomes and should be assessed. ADHD can significantly impair parenting ability, so parental role functioning should be assessed as well. Because of the high percentage of co-occurring mental disorders and the complexity of ADHD, a complete mental health assessment (in complicated cases, by an ADHD specialist) is recommended.

Clinicians should use interview areas that are relatively quiet and free of distractions. It is usually helpful to keep comments and questioning concise and concrete. If needed, prompts can help the person organize responses and stay on track. Observe for disorganization; distractibility; irritability; lability; impulsive comments or actions; difficulty processing information or following instructions; difficulty achieving at the expected level in social, educational, and vocational settings; and hyperactivity (excess or nonpurposeful motor activity). Substance abuse can mimic ADHD and should be ruled out.

DIAGNOSIS

Nursing diagnoses for ADHD include *Impaired socialization, Impaired impulse control, Relationship problem, Difficulty coping, Impaired family coping, Impaired adjustment, Anxiety,* and *Impaired cognition* (ICN, 2019). Nursing interventions focus on symptom management and coping with the illness (Table 27.6). Interventions for adults may be different from those for children.

OUTCOMES IDENTIFICATION

Examples of potential outcome measures include the following: "(Patient) demonstrates ability to stay on task by completing one task before starting another," "(Patient) discusses three techniques to reduce environmental distractions," and "(Patient) rates concentration as a 5 or greater on a 1-to-10 scale."

PLANNING AND IMPLEMENTATION

Psychopharmacology

Medications are a well-established treatment for ADHD. In most cases the same drugs used to treat children are also used to treat adults. Stimulants are the most widely used medication for ADHD, and they show a high degree of efficacy, with 75% to 95% of patients reporting improvement. Examples include methylphenidate (e.g., Concerta, Metadate, Ritalin), dextroamphetamine (Dexedrine), dextroamphetamine-amphetamine (Adderall XR), and lisdexamfetamine (Vyvanse); some are available in short- and long-acting forms (Mayo Clinic, 2017). Longer-acting and timed-release forms allow persons to take the medicines only once or twice per day, before and after (rather than during) school or work, a popular feature that helps improves adherence (inattentiveness, disorganization, and distractibility contribute to decreased adherence in ADHD).

Stimulant medications are thought to augment the dopamine and/or norepinephrine neurotransmission that regulates prefrontal cortex activities critical for the modulation of behavior, attention, and cognition. It might seem counterintuitive for stimulants to help hyperactivity, but these medications all promote enhanced dopamine and norepinephrine functioning and do not have the degree of classical stimulant effects seen when used by persons without ADHD. One concern noted in the use of such stimulants is sharing the medicine with others or the medication being diverted by others; although this is a criminal offense, such sharing has been increasing, especially among college students, and should be addressed during patient education; ironically, research suggests that although stimulants may enhance learning in those with ADHD, its effects on learning in those without ADHD is negligible (Benson et al., 2015).

Other medications used to treat ADHD include antidepressants such as bupropion (Wellbutrin) and atomoxetine (Strattera).

TABLE 27.6 Interventions for Adult Attention-Deficit/Hyperactivity Disorder (ADHD)

Intervention	Rationale
1. Educate the person and significant other(s) about ADHD: its causes, treatments, and especially ways to cope with and control its symptoms.	1. Understanding the psychological and psychiatric aspects of one's disorder, as well as ways to cope with or reduce symptoms, can decrease powerlessness, instill hope, and improve the person's sense of control.
2. Guide the person to understand and practice stimulation reduction strategies such as environmental structuring (reducing auditory and visual distractions).	2. Environmental distractions make already-impaired concentration more difficult.
3. Mutually set, track, revise, and reinforce incremental goals, along with actions that will meet those goals.	3. Mutual goal setting increases the person's "buy-in"; incremental goals are easier to attain, reducing discouragement from unmet goals and providing successes that reinforce the person's efforts.
4. Guide the person to identify and use enhanced organizational skills; many techniques exist to increase organization and efficiency in completing tasks, from reminder lists to using personal digital assistants (PDAs) to track appointments. Daily organizers and workbooks for adults with ADHD are available.	4. Enhancements in organization can improve functioning and promote a positive self-image as the person experiences increased task success; Internet resources and print publications can be accessed for this purpose.
5. Guide the person to identify and use enhanced time management skills (e.g., structured priority setting wherein the person asks self, "What will happen if I do not do this task next?" and then uses those responses to determine which task to tackle next).	5. Better time management can improve functioning and reduce stress; Internet resources and published materials on this topic can be readily accessed.
6. Assist the person to identify and explore feelings about ADHD and its effect on his or her life and to correct any distorted self-talk pertaining to self-image.	6. ADHD may contribute to frustration or impaired self-esteem because of daily challenges and one's unmet potential; people with ADHD may be critical of themselves and use negative "self-talk" (e.g., "I am so stupid; why can't I do this? What is wrong with me!").
7. Encourage participation in ADHD support groups and vetted online support resources such as ADHD blogs.	7. Support groups and online resources can provide pragmatic "helpful hints" from peers and support from an "I've been there" perspective.
8. Address comorbid disorders and mental health needs such as substance abuse.	8. Depression and other disorders further impair problem-solving and coping abilities; substance abuse can significantly worsen impulsivity and concentration.

TABLE 27.7 Sleep-Related Disorders

Disorder	Description
Insomnia disorder	Perceived insufficient sleep, or sleep that is perceived as not restful. Generally, 7 to 9 hours of sleep per night is considered normal. Many physical, psychological, and social factors can contribute to insomnia (e.g., shift work, traumatic experiences, poor sleep hygiene).
Hypersomnolence disorder	Perceived excess sleep, either at night and/or falling asleep during the day
Obstructive sleep apnea/hypopnea	A temporary cessation (apnea) or decrease (hypopnea) in breathing during sleep. Usually due to a mechanical obstruction that increases when prone or when muscles relax during sleep, it is more common in obese persons. It sometimes occurs for nonstructural reasons as well. It can impair cognitive function and increases many health risks, including cardiovascular disease and mortality risk.
Narcolepsy	Sudden, irresistible urges to sleep. One may suddenly fall asleep under any circumstance; some continue automatic behavior as if in a mental fog. Episodes are not recalled after awakening.
Circadian rhythm disorders	Dysregulation of the internal circadian rhythms relative to one's usual sleep cycle. The sleep–wake cycle can shift in various ways (e.g., sleeping during the day rather than at night). One variant stems from shift work and involves sleepiness at work and home.
Sleep arousal disorders	Abnormal experiences or behaviors occurring during sleep. In the rapid eye movement (REM) type, the person experiences arousal during REM sleep and may vocalize or enact behaviors as if awake, often in response to what one is dreaming at the time. It can be dangerous (e.g., striking out if dreaming that one is being attacked). In the non-REM form, the behavior is typically sleepwalking, and the abnormal experience is sleep terror, often accompanied by screaming. During sleepwalking, the person is not consciously aware of his or her actions and is difficult to awaken; it can be dangerous depending on the environment in which it occurs.
Restless leg syndrome	An urge to move one's legs, usually in response to an irritating sensation in the legs that improves with movement. It can significantly disrupt sleep.

Antidepressants may take several weeks to take full effect, much longer than stimulants, but are useful for persons who have cardiovascular or other health problems that are contraindications for stimulants (Stahl, 2015). Also, unlike stimulants, antidepressants are not addictive and are less likely to be abused.

Nonpharmacological Treatments

Psychotherapeutic treatments and symptom management skills are also important in managing ADHD. Cognitive therapy is helpful for correcting distortions in self-image and improving focus and concentration, and psychotherapy may address co-occurring issues such as relationship discord and coping with chronic illness. Psychoeducation about the disorder and its treatment, along with instruction in techniques for managing and coping with symptoms, is essential and may be done individually or in a group setting. Support groups, helpful for addressing self-esteem and anxiety issues, can be excellent sources of practical hints for managing the disorder and useful in adjusting to life with ADHD.

SLEEP-RELATED DISORDERS

Sleep-related disorders include a variety of alterations in sleep. They can involve physical illnesses or abnormalities (e.g., restless leg syndrome, obstructive sleep apnea) or psychiatric disorders like anxiety, depression, or PTSD that disrupt sleep. Sleep can also be affected by phenomena such as shift work (night shifts and rotating shifts). Specific sleep-related disorders are described in Table 27.7. Medications and illness can increase or decrease sleep needs and abilities and can disrupt sleep quality.

Prevalence and Comorbidity

Temporary episodes of sleep disruption are universal experiences and often accompany stressful situations such as physical illness, surgery, work or school demands, and grief and loss situations. Some sleep disorders, such as insomnia (difficulty falling or staying asleep), are common, affecting about one-third of all persons (Bhaskar, Hemavathy & Prasad, 2016); others are less common, such as sleep apnea, which affects 9% of women and 24% of men (Garvey et al., 2015). Other conditions are rare, such as narcolepsy (inability to remain awake when needed), which affects 79 out of 100,000 people (Scheer et al., 2019). Physical illnesses ranging from pulmonary insufficiency to restless leg syndrome commonly accompany and contribute to sleep disorders.

Theory

Sleep is vital for life. It is believed to play a major role in memory, moving memories from short-term recall states to longer-term memory. Long known to provide a restorative function, sleep plays a key role in neuro-immune health, increasing the circulation of cerebrospinal fluid and removing damaging by-products of neuronal activity such as beta-amyloid (Hladky & Barrand, 2017). Lack of sleep may contribute to emotional dysregulation.

Sleep can be divided into two phases or types. **REM** (rapid eye movement) sleep is characterized by inhibition of voluntary movement, fluctuating periods of rapid eye movement, and dreaming. **Non-REM** sleep is further divided into four stages that are characterized by specific electroencephalogram (EEG) patterns, and one's ability to be aroused varies with each stage. Both REM and non-REM sleep can be disrupted in sleep disorders (Lubit, 2015).

The suprachiasmatic nucleus in the hypothalamus is believed to be the primary regulator of sleep cycles, affecting sleep cycles by stimulating the pineal gland to release melatonin. The neurotransmitters serotonin and norepinephrine play a role in promoting sleep, whereas dopamine affects wakefulness.

Disorders such as narcolepsy appear to have a genetic component, being more common in identical twins and first-degree relatives, whereas other sleep disorders do not yet have established genetic connections (Lubit, 2015). Bipolar disorder is believed to involve abnormalities in a "clock" gene that result in sleep dysregulation (Schuch et al., 2018).

Psychological states and disorders affect sleep in a variety of ways. Sleep disturbance and dysregulation can both contribute to and be caused by disorders such as depression (characterized by increased sleep or insomnia) and mania (characterized by a decreased need for sleep) (Sadock et al., 2015). Insomnia can signal or contribute to relapse in depression, mania, and schizophrenia. Anxiety and worry are common sources of insomnia. Traumatic experiences and related disorders such as PTSD feature sleep disruptions such as insomnia and nightmares.

Clinical Picture

Sleep disorders often begin in early adulthood and may worsen with age. Persons with sleep-related disorders typically complain of inadequate and/or low-quality sleep or, conversely, excessive drowsiness. They may also report associated symptoms such as grogginess, increased accidents, and impaired concentration or comorbidities such as anxiety, depressed mood, loss or grief, or physical illness. These features range from mildly to severely distressing and disruptive to normal functioning.

Effect on Individuals, Families, and Society

Sleep loss contributes to physical health problems such as obesity, diabetes, cardiovascular disease, and impaired immune system functioning (Schmid, Hallschmid, & Schultes, 2015; Takahashi, 2014). Narcolepsy in middle-age and older adults is associated with a 1.3-fold increase in mortality (Jennum et al., 2017), although the mechanism is not understood. It is estimated that 15% to 30% of persons operate with insufficient sleep (less than 7 hours per night), leading to increased motor vehicle and other accidents; almost 30% of drivers report falling asleep at the wheel, and almost 20% report having near misses due to driving while drowsy (Centers for Disease Control and Prevention [CDC], 2011; Inoue & Komada, 2014; WebMD, 2019).

Daytime drowsiness can reduce alertness and vigilance, impair judgment, and interfere with memory (WebMD, 2019); these are particular concerns for night-shift workers in public safety and health care fields (Reszka et al., 2018), who are at increased risk of accidents and making errors, endangering their patients (and themselves) because of occupational sleep disruptions. Such shift work is also disruptive to the employee's family and social life.

APPLICATION OF THE NURSING PROCESS

ASSESSMENT

Screening for sleep disorders is very important due to their frequency, potential to affect health, and association with other physical and psychiatric disorders. Assessment is by interview pertaining to sleep habits and patterns, subjective quality of sleep, and associated features such as sleepwalking or nightmares. Sleep journals are used to determine actual sleep patterns and duration more objectively, and formal sleep studies (usually involving EEG and respiratory monitoring, along with direct observation during sleep, by specially trained technicians) can also be used for more accurate diagnosis. Respiratory function studies may be indicated as well. Interview the person and those he or she sleeps with for signs of nocturnal hypoxia (e.g., snoring, gasping, choking sensation, periods of apnea, restlessness, frequent arousal) or its later consequences (e.g., headaches, dry mouth in the morning, feeling unrested, daytime sleepiness or fatigue, morning confusion, irritability, or depression).

DIAGNOSIS

Nursing diagnoses for sleep-related disorders include *Anxiety, Difficulty coping, Impaired gas exchange, Impaired sleep, Risk for impaired sleep,* and *Risk for injury* (ICN, 2019).

OUTCOMES IDENTIFICATION

Examples of potential outcome measures include "Patient reports sleeping 7 to 9 hours per night," "Patient discusses three techniques to promote quality sleep," and "Patient rates quality of rest as a 6 or greater on a 1-to-10 scale."

PLANNING AND IMPLEMENTATION

Nursing interventions for sleep disorder focus first on relieving underlying causes of sleep disturbance, such as hospital noise, scheduling procedures during hours of sleep, and impaired **sleep hygiene** practices. Contributing emotional factors, such as pain, grief, and anxiety, are also addressed. Specific interventions related to sleep are discussed in Table 27.8.

Psychopharmacology

Insomnia is sometimes treated with sedative-hypnotic drugs. There are three benzodiazepine-like drugs that are frequently used for insomnia: zolpidem (Ambien), eszopiclone (Lunesta), zaleplon (Sonata). As well, suvorexant (Belsomra), a novel selective dual-orexin-receptor antagonist, may be prescribed. These drugs react quickly, reduce awakenings, increase total sleeping time, and are well tolerated (Burchum & Rosenthal, 2016). Benzodiazepine and benzodiazepine-like drugs can cause grogginess, impaired coordination and reflexes, dizziness, and increased fall risk in susceptible persons, and patients should be educated to use these with caution. Some are potentially addictive, and because tolerance can develop, they are encouraged to be used on a short-term basis. Benzodiazepines may increase the risk for dementia (Tapiainen et al., 2018).

A sleep aid not approved by the U.S. Food and Drug Administration (FDA) and available over the counter that may be helpful for some is *melatonin* (appropriate doses are 0.3 to 1 mg several hours before sleep). It appears safe for short-term use, but long-term safety has not been confirmed. *Kava* products are used by some but have been linked with severe liver damage; persons using these products should consult their physician or nurse practitioner. *L-tryptophan supplements* are also used but should be used with caution due to an association with potentially dangerous eosinophilia-myalgia syndrome. Treating anxiety and depression that contribute to insomnia is often necessary.

Narcolepsy is treated with stimulants like modafinil (Provigil), which has fewer undesired effects on sleep; side effects include headache, irritability, and gastrointestinal complaints.

Nonpharmacological Treatment

Mechanical devices such as ventilation assistance devices (e.g., **continuous positive airway pressure [CPAP]** machines) may be necessary for obstructive sleep apnea. CBT focuses on changing patterns of thinking, especially negative thinking (Sadock et al., 2015), to reduce stress and promote rest. CBT-I is a newer form of CBT for insomnia that focuses on sleep hygiene and changing thoughts, feelings, and behaviors that contribute to poor sleep (Haynes et al., 2018). Stress reduction and active relaxation reduce anxiety and promote rest. Environmental management (e.g., reducing distraction, exposure to stimulation) and normalizing sleep patterns are important interventions. Individual and family therapy to address underlying concerns may be needed.

TABLE 27.8 Interventions for Sleep Dysregulation

Intervention	Rationale
1. Educate the person and significant other(s) about proper sleep hygiene—practices that promote restful sleep such as those noted here.	1. Understanding one's disorder and the rationale for ways to cope with it can increase motivation and instill hope that the condition will improve.
2. Keep a sleep diary to track patterns related to sleep: time going to bed, time arising, awakenings during the night, and activities or anxieties occurring just before bed.	2. Tracking sleep and factors that affect it can help one recognize sleep disorders and identify causes that can then be addressed.
3. Mutually set concrete sleep-related goals and develop actions that will meet those goals (e.g., set a target time to be in bed and to wake). Tie these goals to other goals that the person is motivated to attain (e.g., note that adequate rest will promote healing and speed recovery or improve concentration and help with success at work or school).	3. Mutual goal setting is motivating and increases the person's commitment to achieving the goals. Concrete goals are easier to target and measure and provide a sense of success that reinforces the person's efforts and motivates adherence to the plan.
4. Engage in exercise or other physical activity in the evening, 2 hours prior to bedtime, to increase tiredness.	4. Exercise increases tiredness and promotes sleep but is initially stimulating and should be avoided just before bedtime.
5. Guide the person to identify and use stress avoidance (e.g., assertive communication, time management), cognitive interventions (e.g., changing negative thoughts, distracting oneself from worries, making expectations of oneself more realistic), and relaxation techniques (e.g., deepening and slowing breathing, calming music, relaxing physical activity) to reduce anxiety.	5. Stress and worry contribute significantly toward insomnia.
6. Reduce stimulation such as background noise (e.g., use sound generators that produce white noise or calming environmental sounds) and exposure to bright light or blue light from electronic screens before sleep (e.g., dim lights and refrain from using any screen-based device for 1 hour before bed, or at least while trying to fall asleep). Use the bedroom only for sleep or sex, not for television viewing.	6. Stimulation promotes wakefulness and is useful for daytime drowsiness and narcolepsy, but it interferes with sleep.
7. Establish a routine to stabilize sleep times wherever possible, finding and sticking to a consistent sleep pattern. Go to bed at least 8 hours prior to when one needs to awake. Maintain this pattern on days off.	7. A regular sleep pattern helps the body synchronize sleep with circadian rhythms and promotes sleep because the body does not have to adjust to a varying schedule.
8. If unable to sleep for more than 30 minutes, leave the bedroom and engage in relaxing and distracting activities, returning to bed again when feeling tired.	8. Sleep is unlikely if one is still awake after 30 minutes; getting up to engage in activities that promote sleep is more likely to cause sleep than staying in bed.
9. Adhere to treatment recommendations for any physical or psychiatric disorders that interfere with sleep.	9. Depression and other disorders further impair sleep regulation.
10. Minimize the use of all stimulants (e.g., caffeine, nicotine) and do not use these for at least 4 hours before bedtime. Also refrain from the use of alcohol for sleep.	10. Stimulants are useful for narcolepsy but may interfere with sleep; stopping them well before bedtime allows them to be at least somewhat metabolized before bedtime.
11. Never go to bed hungry or eat just before bedtime.	11. Hunger and digestive activity can both interfere with sleep.
12. If having trouble sleeping, consider refraining from napping, even if tired.	12. Naps can be helpful to promote alertness for shift workers or those who cannot get a full night's sleep but can cause initial grogginess on awakening and can interfere with sleep at night.
13. Darken your sleeping space as much as possible.	13. Light can disturb sleep and disrupt sleep cycles.
14. Arrange your room and bedding for maximum comfort based on your personal preferences.	14. Uncomfortable bedding and room temperatures cause restlessness and interfere with sleep quality.
15. Persons doing night-shift work should expose themselves to bright light at night and keep all lighting dim during the day.	15. This lighting pattern simulates the normal day–night light levels usually experienced and promotes better sleep during night-shift workers' sleep time.

APPLYING EVIDENCE-BASED PRACTICE (EBP)

Problem

A 34-year-old transgender (female-to-male) patient approaches the nurse at his primary care physician's (PCP's) office after an appointment. He reveals that he has not taken his male hormones for about 4 months since moving from a large city in California to a small rural town in Idaho, noting that his current PCP has been unwilling to order them. At first, a slight elevation in liver enzymes was the reasoning, but as time has gone on, the patient feels that the PCP does not understand or agree with his transgender transition. The patient is beginning to grow breasts again, and his mood has been irritable at home with the family.

EBP Assessment

A. **What do you already know from experience?** There is still considerable stigma and lack of understanding in the general population and even among health care professionals regarding transgender patients. Transgender patients can cross-dress, take hormones, or have surgery as part of their transition.

B. **What does the literature say?** Lesbian, gay, bisexual, transgender, and queer (LGBTQ) patients experience health care disparities and barriers and may avoid treatment because of real or perceived discrimination (Glick et al., 2018). Homophobia in medical practice is real; research reports that 7% of physicians have discomfort treating gay and lesbian patients, and 22% feel uncomfortable treating transgender patients (Marlin et al., 2018). Bias against LGBTQ patients is prevalent among heterosexual nurses and is highest among heterosexual female nurses against male patients who are gay (Sabin, Riskind, & Nosek, 2015). Nursing students' attitudes toward LGBTQ patients have improved, but homophobia is still prevalent (Lim & Hsu, 2016). Recommendations to improve care include providing a welcoming environment; using gender-neutral terminology; adding a transgender option to gender checkboxes; screening for gender dysphoria; and addressing the patient using the preferred name, pronoun, or gender. Be open to discussing gender-related issues, and train staff in sensitivity. A gender-neutral or inclusive restroom is helpful (Gay and Lesbian Medical Association, n.d.).

C. **What does the patient want?** The patient wants to get back on his hormones as soon as possible and wants to be supported by his health care team. He feels guilty for the stress his moodiness has inflicted on his family.

Plan

The nurse obtained contact information from the patient for his doctor in California. She recommended that the patient attempt to contact his former doctor for assistance in getting hormones in the interim. She also performed online research regarding transgender transitioning and issues in health care and approached the PCP she works with to learn more information together. She also asked colleagues for recommendations for providers in the area with experience with transgender treatment. Her PCP appreciated her assistance and was open to consulting with these providers and to possible referral if needed.

QSEN Prelicensure Knowledge, Skills, and Attitudes (KSAs) Addressed

Patient-Centered Care was provided by additional learning and possible referral.

Teamwork and Collaboration was addressed by contacting other providers and by the PCP and nurse learning together.

KEY POINTS TO REMEMBER

- Serious mental illnesses (SMIs) are recurrent or long-lasting and often disruptive or disabling conditions.
- Stigma and chronicity present many challenges to coping with an SMI and contribute to a variety of other social, physical health, and mental health problems: substance abuse, poverty and unemployment, comorbid physical illnesses and premature mortality, arrest and incarceration, homelessness, depression, powerlessness, and suicide risk.
- Assertive community treatment and peer-based services (e.g., clubhouses, peer-support specialists) are evidence-based practices shown to benefit persons with SMIs.
- Impulse-control disorders involve impulsive behaviors that are disruptive and serve to relieve psychological tension. These disorders include impulsive thefts, fire setting, sudden assaults or property destruction, hair pulling, and pathological gambling.
- Impulse-control disorders are treated primarily through psychotherapy and sometimes with medications.
- A person with gender dysphoria believes his or her biological gender is incorrect and that he or she should be the opposite gender.
- People with gender dysphoria may be subject to ridicule and harassment and may experience significant distress related to their gender dissatisfaction. One intervention is gender reassignment, which involves counseling, experiencing life for 1 or 2 years as the opposite gender, using hormones, and being surgically reassigned.
- Paraphilic disorders are disorders in which sexual gratification is obtained in atypical and often socially unacceptable ways.
- Pedophilia includes having sexual fantasies or contact with children. This disorder stirs strong feelings in health care staff and society.
- The causes of paraphilic disorders are not clearly established, but neurological dysfunction may be a contributing factor.
- Psychotherapy and medications that reduce sexual drive may reduce offensive sexual behavior in pedophiles.
- Attention-deficit/hyperactivity disorder (ADHD) is associated with childhood but may continue into or first be diagnosed in adulthood. In adults, it is characterized by difficulty maintaining focus and organization and can be disruptive to task completion, employment, relationships, and other areas of functioning.
- ADHD often goes undiagnosed in adults, who may try to compensate for its symptoms. It is treated with a combination of psychotherapy and stimulants (or sometimes other drugs).
- Sleep disorders can have physical, psychological, or social causes. Physical and psychiatric disorders, stress, and shift work can disrupt sleep.
- Impaired sleep can affect one psychologically and physically, contributing to disorders such as depression, bipolar disorder, obesity, and neuro-immune system dysfunction.
- Sleep loss due to shift work can increase the risk of errors and accidents, a particular concern for health care and public safety workers.
- Sleep disorders are treated by correcting underlying conditions and promoting sound sleep hygiene practices.

APPLYING CRITICAL JUDGMENT

1. You are working with a person who has recently been diagnosed with adult ADHD. He is very impulsive and frequently makes comments to you and others that are inappropriate and rude. You find yourself avoiding him and feeling angry toward him. Describe or role-play what you would say in response to help reduce such comments.
2. The parents of a 37-year-old man with an SMI ask you for help; they are becoming frightened of their son, who is increasingly hostile in response to their efforts to get him to take showers, accept medication, and get a job. They report that they have not often been able to talk with those treating their son because of regulations restricting the sharing of private health care information. Discuss how you might address both the issues of confidentiality and the conflicts experienced when the parents attempt to change their son's behavior.
3. Debate the pros and cons of the proposition that sexual offenders who harm children should be held indefinitely in preventive detention for the greater good of society.
4. A patient with SMI is about to begin outpatient services at your community mental health center after years of institutionalization in state hospitals and prisons. Discuss the major issues he will likely face and the services that ideally would be available in your community.

CHAPTER REVIEW QUESTIONS

1. A nurse leads a milieu meeting in an outpatient program for adults diagnosed with serious mental illness. Four patients complain that another patient is "always begging us for money." Which comment by the nurse is therapeutic?
   - **a.** "If you can afford to help each other, it is reasonable to do so."
   - **b.** "Let's review what we have learned about being assertive with others."
   - **c.** "No one needs to bring money to our program. Lunch is provided at no charge."
   - **d.** "Let's show understanding of each other. Money management is a problem for everyone."
2. An outpatient nurse has lunch with a group of patients diagnosed with serious mental illness. The nurse observes an obese adult ask a malnourished adult, "If you aren't going to eat your apple, will you give it to me?" What is the nurse's best action?
   - **a.** Remind both adults that sharing food with each other is not permitted.
   - **b.** Remind the malnourished adult of treatment goals related to weight gain.
   - **c.** Reseat the patients at two separate tables for the remainder of the meal.
   - **d.** Overlook the remark. Both adults are permitted to make their own decisions.
3. A nurse plans a psychoeducational group about physical health in an outpatient program for patients diagnosed with serious mental illness. Which topic has priority?
   - **a.** Heart-healthy living
   - **b.** Living with diabetes
   - **c.** ABCDEs of skin cancer
   - **d.** Breast and testicular self-examination
4. A nurse working in the county jail assesses four new inmates. The nurse should direct officers to place which inmate under suicide watch?
   - **a.** An inmate charged with breaking and entering
   - **b.** An inmate charged with criminal solicitation (prostitution)
   - **c.** An inmate charged with a lewd and lascivious act perpetrated on a minor
   - **d.** An inmate charged with assault and battery of an elderly person
5. A person diagnosed with serious mental illness has been homeless for 8 years and says, "I don't have any money because I've never had a job. I can't afford a place to live." Which intervention should the outpatient mental health nurse add to the plan of care?
   - **a.** Requisition the patient's legal record of arrests and convictions.
   - **b.** Help the patient to apply for Supplemental Security Income (SSI).
   - **c.** Assist the patient to apply for Social Security Disability Income (SSDI).
   - **d.** Seek to have the patient adjudicated *non compos mentis* (incompetent).

REFERENCES

Albers, W., Roeg, D., Nijssen, Y., van Weeghel, J., & Bongers, I. (2018). Profiling of victimization, perpetration, and participation: A latent class analysis among people with severe mental illness. *PLOS One, 13*(11).

American Psychiatric Association (APA). (2013). *Diagnostic and statistical manual of mental disorders* (5th ed.). Washington, DC: APA.

Benson, K., Flory, K., Humphries, K., et al. (2015). Misuse of stimulant medication among college students: A comprehensive review and meta-analysis. *Clinical Child and Family Psychology Review, 18*(1), 50–76.

Bhaskar, S., Hemavathy, D., & Prasad, S. (2016). Prevalence of chronic insomnia in adult patients and its correlation with medical comorbidities. *Journal of Family Medicine and Primary Care, 5*(4), 780–784.

Boehmer, U., Clark, M. A., Lord, E. M., & Fredman, L. (2019). Caregiving status and health of heterosexual, sexual minority, and transgender adults: Results from select U.S. regions in the behavioral risk factor surveillance system 2015 and 2016. *Gerontologist,* 59(4), 760-769.

Burchum, J., & Rosenthal, L. (2016). *Lehne's pharmacology for nursing care* (9th ed.). St. Louis: Elsevier.

Centers for Disease Control and Prevention (CDC). (2011). Unhealthy sleep-related behaviors. *Morbidity and Mortality Weekly Report, 60*(8), 234–266.

Mayo Clinic. (2017). *Adult attention-deficit/hyperactivity disorder.* Retrieved May 14, 2019, from http://www.mayoclinic.org/diseases-conditions/adult-adhd/basics/symptoms/con-20034552.

Mayo Clinic. (2019). *Compulsive sexual behavior.* Retrieved May 8, 2019 from https://www.mayoclinic.org/diseases-conditions/compulsive-sexual-behavior/diagnosis-treatment/drc-20360453.

De Giorgi, R., & Series, H. (2016). Treatment of inappropriate sexual behavior in dementia. *Current Treatment Options in Neurology, 18*(9), 41.

Faraone, S. V., & Larsson, H. (2019). Genetics of attention deficit hyperactivity disorder. *Molecular psychiatry, 24*(4), 562–575.

Fielenbach, S., Donkers, F. C., Spreen, M., & Bogaerts, S. (2017). Neurofeedback as a treatment for impulsivity in a forensic psychiatric population with substance use disorder: Study protocol of a randomized controlled trial combined with an n-of-1 clinical trial. *JMIR Research Protocols, 6*(1).

Francis, A. (2013). *Essentials of psychiatric diagnoses: Responding to the challenges of DSM-5*. New York: Guilford Press.

Franke, B., Michelini, G., Asherson, P., Banaschewski, T., Bilbow, A., Buitelaar, J. K., et al. (2018). Live fast, die young? A review on the developmental trajectories of ADHD across the lifespan. *European Neuropsychopharmacology: The Journal of the European College of Neuropsychopharmacology, 28*(10), 1059–1088.

Frederick, D. E., & Vanderweele, T. J. (2019). Supported employment: Meta-analysis and review of randomized controlled trials of individual placement and support. *PLOS One, 14*(2), e0212208.

Garrett, K., & Giddings, K. (2014). Improving impulse control: Using an evidence-based practice approach. *Journal of Evidence-Based Social Work, 11*, 73–83.

Garvey, J. F., Pengo, M. F., Drakatos, P., & Kent, B. D. (2015). Epidemiological aspects of obstructive sleep apnea. *Journal of Thoracic Disease, 7*(5), 920–929.

Gay and Lesbian Medical Association. (n.d.). *Guidelines for care of lesbian, gay, bisexual, and transgender patients*. Retrieved from http://www.glma.org/_data/n_0001/resources/live/GLMA%20guidelines%202006%20FINAL.pdf.

Giddens, J. F. (2017). *Concepts for nursing practice* (2nd ed). St. Louis: Elsevier. Glick, J. L., Theall, K. P., Andrinopoulos, K. M., & Kendall, C. (2018). The role of discrimination in care postponement among trans-feminine individuals in the U.S. national transgender discrimination survey. *LGBT Health, 5*(3), 171–179.

Grall-Bronnec, M., Victorri-Vigneau, C., Donnio, Y., Leboucher, J., Rousselet, M., Thiabaud, E., et al. (2017). Dopamine agonists and impulse control disorders: A complex association. *Drug Safety, 41*(1), 19–75.

Grant, J. E., & Leppink, E. W. (2015). Impulse-control and conduct disorders: Limited evidence, no approved drugs to guide treatment. *Current Psychiatry, 14*(1), 29–35.

Harvard Health Publications. (2014). *Pessimism about pedophilia*. Retrieved May 19, 2019, From http://www.health.harvard.edu/newsletter_article/pessimism-about-pedophilia.

Hawton, K., Witt, K. G., Salisbury, T. L. T., Arensman, E., Gunnell, D., Hazell, P., et al. (2016). Psychosocial interventions following self-harm in adults: A systematic review and meta-analysis. *Lancet Psychiatry*, 3, 740 –750).

Haynes, J., Talbert, M., Fox, S., & Close, E. (2018). Cognitive behavioral therapy in the treatment of insomnia. *Southern Medical Journal*, 111, 75–80.

Hladky, S. B., & Barrand, M. A. (2017). Metabolite clearance during wakefulness and sleep. *Handbook of Experimental Pharmacology*, 253, 385-423.

Holoyda, B., & Kellaher, D. (2016). The biological treatment of paraphilic disorders. *Current Psychiatry Reports, 18*, 19.

Holt-Lunstad, J., Smith, T. B., Baker, M., Harris, T., & Stephenson, D. (2015). Loneliness and social isolation as risk factors for mortality: A meta-analytic review. *Perspectives on Psychological Science, 10*(2), 227–237.

Inoue, Y., & Komada, Y. (2014). Sleep loss, sleep disorders and driving accidents. *Sleep and Biological Rhythms*, 12, 96–105.

International Council of Nurses (ICN). (2019). *International classification for nursing practice*. Retrieved May 10, 2019 from http://www.old.icn.ch/what-we-do/ICNP-Browser/.

Jadidian, A., Hurley, R. A., & Taber, K. H. (2015). Neurobiology of adult ADHD: Emerging evidence for network dysfunctions. *Journal of Neuropsychiatry and Clinical Neuroscience, 27*(3), 173–178.

Jennum, P., Thorstensen, E. W., Pickering, L., Ibsen, R., & Kjellberg, J. (2017). Morbidity and mortality of middle-aged and elderly narcoleptics. *Sleep Medicine*, 36, 23–28) .

Kilbourne, A. M., Beck, K., Spaeth-Rublee, B., Ramanuj, P., O'Brien, R. W., Tomoyasu, N., et al. (2018). Measuring and improving the quality of mental health care: A global perspective. *World Psychiatry: Official Journal of the World Psychiatric Association (WPA), 17*(1), 30–38.

Kim, K., Becker-Cohen, M., & Serakos, M. (2015). *The processing and treatment of mentally ill persons in the criminal justice system*. Washington, DC: Urban Institute. Retrieved May 15, 2019, from http://www.urban.org/sites/default/files/alfresco/publication-pdfs/2000173-The-Processing-and-Treatment-of-Mentally-Ill-Persons-in-the-Criminal-Justice-System.pdf.

Kisely, S. R., Campbell, L. A., & O'Reilly, R. (2017). Compulsory community and involuntary outpatient treatment for people with severe mental disorders. *Cochrane Database Systematic Review, 17(3)*, CD004408. doi:10.1002/14651858.CD004408.pub5.

Klasen, M., Wolf, D., Eisner, P. D., Eggermann, T., Zerres, K., & Zepf, F. D., et al. (2019). Serotonergic contributions to human brain aggression networks. *Frontiers in Neuroscience, 13*, 42.

Leng, A., Xu, C., Nicholas, S., Nicholas, J., & Wang, J. (2019). Quality of life in caregivers of a family member with serious mental illness: Evidence from China. *Archives of Psychiatric Nursing, 33*, 23–29.

Lim, F. A., & Hsu, R. (2016). Nursing students' attitudes toward lesbian, gay, bisexual, and transgender persons: An integrative review. *Nursing Education Perspectives, 37*(3), 144–152.

Lubit, R. (2015). *Sleep disorders*. Retrieved May 19, 2019, from http://emedicine.medscape.com/article/287104-overview.

Marlin, R., Kadakia, A., Ethridge, B., & Mathews, W. C. (2018). Physician attitudes toward homosexuality and HIV: The PATHH-III Survey. *LGBT Health, 5*(7), 431–442.

Miranda, A., Berenguer, C., Colomer, C., et al. (2014). Influence of the symptoms of attention deficit hyperactivity disorder (ADHD) and comorbid disorders on functioning in adulthood. *Psicothema, 26*(4), 471–476.

National Alliance on Mental Illness (NAMI). (2019a). *Family-to-Family program*. Retrieved May 11, 2019 from https://www.nami.org/Find-Support/NAMI-Programs/NAMI-Family-to-Family.

National Alliance on Mental Illness (NAMI). (2019b). *Psychosocial treatment*. Retrieved May 15, 2019 from https://www.nami.org/Learn-More/Treatment/Psychosocial-Treatments.

National Institute of Mental Health. (2017). *Mental illness*. Retrieved from https://www.nimh.nih.gov/health/statistics/mental-illness.shtml.

Nguyen, H. B., Loughead, J., Lipner, E., Hantsoo, L., Kornfield, S. L., & Epperson, C. N. (2019). What has sex got to do with it? The role of hormones in the transgender brain. *Neuropsychopharmacology, 44(1), 22–37*.

Opoka, S. M., & Lincoln, T. M. (2017). The effect of cognitive behavioral interventions on depression and anxiety symptoms in patients with schizophrenia spectrum disorders: A systematic review. *Psychiatric Clinics of North America, 40*, 641–659.

Parker, A., Scantlebury, A., Booth, A., MacBryde, J. C., Scott, W. J., Wright, K., et al. (2018). Interagency collaboration models for people with mental ill health in contact with the police: A systematic scoping review. *British Medical Journal Open, 8*(3), 2.

Peckham, E., Brabyn, S., Cook, L., Tew, G., & Gilbody, S. (2017). Smoking cessation in severe mental ill health: What works? An updated systematic review and meta-analysis. *BMC Psychiatry, 17*(1), 252.

Reszka, E., Wieczorek, E., Przybek, M., Jablonska, E., Kaluzny, P., Bukowska-Damska, A., et al. (2018). Circadian gene methylation in rotating-shift nurses: A cross-sectional study. *Chronobiology International, 35*(1), 111–121.

Robertson, A., Lin, H., Frisman, L., et al. (2014). Mental health and reoffending outcomes of jail diversion participants with a brief incarceration after arraignment. *Psychiatric Services, 65*(9), 1113–1119.

Sabin, J. A., Riskind, R. G., & Nosek, B. A. (2015). Health care providers' implicit and explicit attitudes toward lesbian women and gay men. *American Public Health Association, 105*(9), 1831–1841.

Sadock, B., Sadock, V., & Ruiz, P. (2015). *Kaplan & Sadock's Synopsis of psychiatry* (11th ed.). Philadelphia: Wolters Kluwer.

Scheer, D., Schwartz, S. W., Parr, M., Zgibor, J., Sanchez-Anguiano, A., & Rajaram, L. (2019). Prevalence and incidence of narcolepsy in a U.S. Health Care Claims Database, 2008-2010. In *Sleep*. United States: Sleep Research Society. Oxford University Press.

Schmid, S., Hallschmid, M., & Schultes, B. (2015). The metabolic burden of sleep loss. *Lancet Diabetes and Endocrinology, 3*(1), 52–62.

Schuch, J. B., Genro, J. P., Bastos, C. R., Ghisleni, G., & Tovo-Rodrigues, L. (2018). The role of CLOCK gene in psychiatric disorders: Evidence from human and animal research. *American Journal of Medical Genetics. Part B, Neuropsychiatric Genetics, 177*(2), 181–198.

Settineri, S., Rizzo, A., Liotta, M., et al. (2014). Caregiver's burden and quality of life: Caring for physical and mental illness. *International Journal of Psychological Research, 7*(1), 30–39.

Social Security Administration. (2018). *Understanding supplemental security income SSI eligibility requirements*, 2015 edition. Retrieved from https://www.ssa.gov/ssi/text-benefits-ussi.htm.

Stahl, S. (2015). *Stahl's essential psychopharmacology prescriber's guide* (5th ed.). New York: Cambridge University Press.

Swartz, M. S., Bhattacharya, S., Robertson, A. G., & Swanson, J. W. (2017). Involuntary outpatient commitment and the elusive pursuit of violence prevention: A view from the United States. *Canadian Journal of Psychiatry, 62*(2), 102–108.

Takahashi, M. (2014). Assisting shift workers through sleep and circadian research. *Sleep and Biological Rhythms, 12*, 85–95.

Tapiainen, V., Taipale, H., Tanskanen, A., Tiihonen, J., Hartikainen, S., & Tolppanen, A.–M. (2018). The risk of Alzheimer's disease associated with benzodiazepines and related drugs: A nested case–control study. *Acta Psychiatrica Scandinavica, 138*(2), 91–100.

Tenbergen, G., Wittfoth, M., Frieling, H., Ponseti, J., Walter, M., Walter, H., et al. (2015). The neurobiology and psychology of pedophilia: Recent advances and challenges. *Frontiers in Human Neuroscience, 9*, 344.

U.S. Census Bureau. (2018). *Income and poverty in the United States, 2017*. Retrieved May 11, 2019 from: https://www.census.gov/data/tables/2018/demo/income-poverty/p60-263.html.

WebMD. (2019). *Ten things to hate about sleep loss*. Retrieved May 8, 2019 from https://www.webmd.com/sleep-disorders/features/10-results-sleep-loss#1.

Weinberger, L. E., Sreenivasan, S., Azizian, A., & Garrick, T. (2018). Linking mental disorder and risk in sexually violent person assessments. *Journal of the American Academy of Psychiatry and the Law*, 46, 63–70.

Welsh, E., & McEnany, G. (2015). Approaches to reduce physical comorbidity in individuals diagnosed with mental illness. *Journal of Psychosocial Nursing, 53*(2), 33–37.

World Health Organization (WHO). (2019). *Mental disorders affect one in four people*. Retrieved May 11, 2019 from https://www.who.int/whr/2001/media_centre/press_release/en/.

28

Older Adults

Chyllia D. Fosbre

http://evolve.elsevier.com/Varcarolis/essentials

OBJECTIVES

1. Identify facts and myths about aging.
2. Describe the negative effects that "ageism" and "elderspeak" can have on older adults.
3. Identify ways you can challenge ageism and increase the awareness of those who care for older adults.
4. List group interventions commonly used with older adults, and describe how implementing teamwork and collaboration plays a part. **QSEN: Teamwork and Collaboration**
5. Using a comprehensive geriatric assessment, identify guidelines for assessing an older adult, including safety promotion.
6. Discuss how you might apply communication strategies during an interview or assessment with an older adult.
7. Identify differences between an older adult and younger adult in the approach to patient-centered care for a patient with depression and suicidal ideation and identify risk factors for elder suicide. **QSEN: Patient-Centered Care**
8. Using evidence-based research, identify differences in the physiological effects of alcohol use on an older individual compared with those on a younger adult. **QSEN: Evidence-Based Practice**
9. Identify quality improvement methods you can use to address the use of physical and/or chemical restraints. **QSEN: Quality Improvement**
10. Discuss institutional requirements related to the Patient Self-Determination Act of 1990.
11. Use informatics to determine laws and regulations in your state for the rights of older adults who are also lesbian, gay, bisexual, or transgender (LGBT). **QSEN: Informatics**
12. Contrast and compare living wills, health care directives, and durable powers of attorney as used in health care settings.

KEY TERMS AND CONCEPTS

advance directive, p. 448
age discrimination, p. 440
ageism, p. 440
chemical restraints, p. 448
directive to physician, p. 449
durable power of attorney for health care, p. 449
elderspeak, p. 441
geropsychiatric nurses, p. 440
living will, p. 449
Patient Self-Determination Act (PSDA), p. 448
physical restraints, p. 448

> **CONCEPT: CLINICAL JUDGMENT:** *Clinical judgment* is an interpretation of or conclusion about a patient's needs, concerns, and problems and the decision to take action or not. Noticing is critical to making an effective judgment to address a patient issue. The factors behind the nurse's eyes are as important as what is in front. Knowing the older adult allows the home health nurse to understand the patient's baseline mental status and to notice subtle changes in cognition or affect (Giddens, 2017). Nurses need to be concerned with and sensitive to possible alcohol abuse among older patients. The older person with alcohol use disorder may display vague symptoms of contusions, malnutrition, self-neglect, depression, and falls. Assessment is necessary to differentiate the normal physiological changes of aging from those attributable to excessive drinking.

INTRODUCTION

The older adult population is one of the most vulnerable populations in the United States. The baby boom generation (individuals born between 1946 and 1964) is aging and is predicted to strain the health care system with a rapid increase in the older adult population. The medical and mental health access of this population is an issue that will have to be addressed by all aspects of society (e.g., socioeconomic condition, legal system, and most profoundly, our health care system). This chapter discusses some of the concerns related to the growing numbers of older adults and health care issues unique to this population.

According to the World Health Organization (WHO, 2017), about 15% of the older adult population (60 years and older) has some form of mental health disorder. These problems are often unidentified. Among the stressors unique to older adults is a decline in physical functioning. They are also more likely to face many losses of close relationships as friends and loved ones pass away. It is also important to understand that those with physical health conditions like heart disease, which are more common in older age, put people at higher risk for developing mental health conditions like depression (WHO, 2017). The increasing number of older adults is altering the socioeconomic conditions and health care focus in the United States. By 2030, 20% of the U.S. population will consist of individuals older than 65 years of age, which translates into an increase in health care spending and a shrinking workforce. Among older adults, the fastest-growing subgroups are minorities, the poor, and those ages 85 years and older (National Council on Aging [NCOA], 2018).

About 65% of older adults have at least two chronic health conditions, and over 40% have three or more (Health in Aging, 2016). After age 85, there is a one in three chance of developing dementia, immobility, incontinence, or another age-related disability.

Women generally outlive men by an average of 7 years. Husbands typically die before their spouses, so they benefit from the support of their wives to help with health-related issues. Older women are more likely to be widowed, to live alone, or to be institutionalized. Women tend to have less support at the end of life because they outlive their spouses. In Western society, families often live apart—in separate homes, states, or even countries. There is less of a community surrounding individuals as they age.

There are noticeable differences between individuals in their 60s and people in their 80s. Those in the younger group are relatively healthy, whereas those in the older group are much more vulnerable, frail, and at risk for visual problems, cognitive impairment, and falls. Persons in the older age group also have more limited economic resources and community supports and are more affected by the chronic diseases and disorders of aging (*Healthy People 2020*, 2016). At the end of 2019, Social Security payments were under $1500 a month (Van De Water & Romig, 2020). Considering the average one-bedroom apartment is over $1000 a month (Temple, 2019), it is easy to see how finances can become a significant barrier to care.

AGEISM

Ageism refers to deeply rooted negative attitudes or bias toward people because of their age. In this section we are looking specifically at the bias toward the elderly. In American culture, there is a general dislike of the older adult by the younger generations (Bergman & Bodner, 2015). *Age prejudice* is based on the notion that aging makes people increasingly unattractive, unintelligent, asexual, unemployable, and senile. **Age discrimination**, on the other hand, includes actions and outcomes that reflect the bias toward the elderly. An example of this is hiring a younger, inexperienced person over an older, seasoned employee with years of experience.

Ageism is not limited to the way the young may look at the old. It can also be perpetrated by those in the older population when they become critical of themselves and their peers. The threat of social disgrace by association with the frail and infirm may prevent strong social groups. Age proximity raises feelings of vulnerability. This may explain why older adults often do not like to be referred to as "old." By seeing themselves as young, they adjust better to their advancing years (Gendron et al., 2015).

Ageism differs from other forms of discrimination in that it cuts across gender, race, religion, sexual orientation, and national origin. In our culture, old age does not award a prestigious status, recognizing the value of wisdom. Rather, it is a social category with negative connotations. Today, a new form of ageism puts the older adult in a no-win situation: those who are wealthy are envied for their economic success (even though it was earned), those who are middle class are blamed for straining the Social Security system, and those who are poor are resented for being tax burdens.

The results of ageism can be observed throughout every level of society. Even health care providers are not immune to its effects. Negative values can surface in myriad ways in the health care system: difficulty in obtaining insurance and support programs, caring for younger patient groups first, and personal beliefs and attitudes of the nurse that can infiltrate care.

Ageism Among Health Care Workers

Health care personnel do not always share medical information, recommendations, and opportunities with the older adult. Studies show that older adults receive less information and sometimes less care than those who are younger. Ageism is also reflected in public policy, which leads to discrimination against older adults.

Health care workers who deal on a daily basis with confused, ill, and frail older adults may tend to develop a somewhat negative and biased view of them. The negative attitudes of most health care workers are often a reflection of the stereotypical views of society. The rendering of medical care to older adults has been burdened with pessimism and professional aversion. In Western culture, there is an underlying belief that health care dollars should be spent on the younger and that the older adult has lived a good life and is no longer contributing financially to the pool (Kagan & Melendez-Torres, 2015). In Eastern or Native American cultures, the wisdom of the elderly is valued above the strength and stamina of the young, and past contributions are rewarded (North & Fiske, 2015).

Negative views of the older adult have significant implications for practice, education, and research. Positive attitudes toward older adults and their care need to be instilled as part of basic nursing education (Coleman, 2015). If the overall goal of nursing programs is to prepare students to practice in the future, then preparing students to care for older adults in a wide variety of settings is mandatory because that *is* the future. One of the ways institutional ageism is expressed is through length-of-stay averages that reflect a younger population's time frame and ability to heal (Kydd & Fleming, 2015). With the growing baby boom population, there is an even greater need for health care professionals who can work with the older adult. The present health care system is unprepared to care adequately for the number of elderly persons with medical or mental health needs already in the system. According to the literature, an increased understanding of ageism leads to greater patient satisfaction (Ouchida & Lachs, 2015).

The Institute for Healthcare Improvement (2018) recommends identifying the "4 M's" when caring for the elderly:

- Identify what **m**atters.
- Consider **m**entation and provide appropriate supports.
- Encourage **m**obility within the individual's physical limitations.
- **M**edication should be optimized to reduce polypharmacy and overmedication.

Box 28.1 lists some facts and myths about aging.

ASSESSMENT AND COMMUNICATION STRATEGIES

Nurses who work with older adults require specific knowledge about normal aging, drug interactions, chronic disease, treatment modalities, cultural influences, and the effect on loved ones. **Geropsychiatric nurses** work with older adult patients who have mental health problems and may be employed in a variety of settings, including nursing homes, assisted living facilities, community centers, inpatient units, prisons, and homeless shelters. One challenge is that this population still has medical issues in addition to psychiatric concerns, which must be ferreted out and addressed.

The National Institutes of Health (NIH) recommends a comprehensive geriatric assessment to evaluate and manage the care and progress of all older adult patients. A comprehensive geriatric assessment takes into consideration the various aspects of functioning. These areas can include mental status, general physical health, ability to address health care needs, ability to manage finances, socialization, home maintenance and safety, nutrition and hydration, mobility, and a thorough review of medications and potentially negative interactions. Fig. 28.1 provides an example of a comprehensive geriatric assessment. Younger patients may be comfortable discussing personal issues such as family conflicts, feelings of sadness, sexual practices, finances, and bodily functions, whereas older adults may view these topics as private or taboo. Older generations were raised to keep personal matters private and were not taught to process emotions in the same way as younger generations have been. One of the gifts nurses can give their older patients is an understanding of this generational difference and some gentle education guided by patient comfort level. A private and quiet setting is essential to a thorough assessment that touches on many personal topics, including sex and abuse. Additional measures include asking patients what they would like to be called, positioning self at the same level, using touch (per patient comfort level), body language, and eye contact to convey warmth and interest. Summarizing and inviting feedback are helpful.

Elderspeak is a term that refers to the unnecessary use of simple, childlike phrases; slow speech; high volume; and collective pronouns (Do "we" want to take a bath?) when communicating with older adults. The intention behind it is typically aimed at creating a sense of caring; however, it can inadvertently imply that the older adult is incompetent. Studies are finding that these interactions can be perceived as insults, whether intentional or not, and contribute to poorer health outcomes.

Another related communication problem occurs when health care workers dismiss the presence of older adults in the room and speak *about* them rather than *to* them. Nursing students should consciously avoid using elderspeak. Address the older adult when asking a question, and when necessary, ask the family member or other health care worker(s) if they have anything to add. Box 28.2 provides helpful communication and interview techniques.

Pharmacology and the Aging Adult

Pharmacology becomes increasingly complicated as adults age. One major factor is that the pharmacokinetics (absorption, distribution, metabolism, and excretion) of any drug change as we age. As the metabolism slows, drugs last longer, and levels build up in the body. In addition to metabolism issues, older people frequently do not drink adequate fluids or move as much. Approximately 50% of accidental drug-related deaths occur in the older population (*Healthy People 2020*, 2016). Factors contributing to medication nonadherence include complicated directions in small print, hearing and visual impairments, cognitive and memory deficits, child-resistant packaging, and inability to pay for medication.

BOX 28.1 Facts and Myths About Aging

Facts

- The senses of vision, hearing, touch, taste, and smell decline with age.
- Muscular strength decreases with age. Muscle fibers atrophy and decrease in number.
- Regular sexual expressions are important to maintain sexual capacity and effective sexual performance.
- At least 50% of restorative sleep is lost as a result of the aging process.
- Older adults are major consumers of prescription drugs because of the high incidence of chronic diseases in this population.
- Older adults have a high incidence of depression.
- Many individuals experience difficulty when they retire.
- Older adults are prone to becoming victims of crime.
- Older widows appear to adjust better than younger ones.

Myths

- Most adults past the age of 65 years are demented.
- Sexual interest always declines with age.
- Older adults are not able to learn new tasks.
- As individuals age, they always become rigid in their thinking and resistant to change.
- Older adults are financially secure and no longer impoverished.
- Most older adults are infirm and require help with daily activities.
- Most older adults are socially isolated and lonely.
- All older adults are significantly hard of hearing and should be spoken to in a loud voice.

APPLYING EVIDENCE-BASED PRACTICE (EBP)

Problem

A parish nurse visits an elderly member of the church community after she had not attended church in a few weeks. The nurse finds her patient weak and confused. As part of her nursing assessment, she reviews all of the patient's medications. She finds some inconsistencies, including taking older prescriptions and newly ordered prescriptions together, taking similar class blood pressure medications from a primary care physician (PCP) for hypertension and from a psychiatric nurse practitioner for anxiety and sleep, and taking 3 units of insulin glargine (Lantus) instead of 30 units. The patient had become confused when changing from an insulin bottle and syringe to using an insulin pen several months previously. Her fluid intake was also inadequate.

EBP Assessment

A. **What do you already know from experience?** Elderly patients are vulnerable to medication interactions, polypharmacy, confusion, and dehydration. Many elderly patients resist drinking adequate fluids due to increased trips to the bathroom. Elderly patients may be hard of hearing and have memory impairments, which contribute to misunderstanding or forgetting provider instructions. This population may also lack a support system to help with these issues.

B. **What does the literature say?** Polypharmacy is a serious issue in the elderly, with daily pill burdens of up to 60 pills per day. A "cascade" effect sometimes occurs when a medication is prescribed to treat side effects from the first medication. Most individuals over 65 years of age take between 5 and 10 medications, and the number is significantly higher in long-term residents. Farrell and colleagues (2013) suggest a monitored medication taper, or even an inpatient stay, during which medications are weaned over several weeks to evaluate what is still needed. Being aware of pharmacological interactions and nonadherence in older adults is imperative for nurses (Wooten, 2015).

C. **What does the patient want?** She wants to feel better so that she can attend church again. She is confused about her medications and wants help organizing them.

Plan

The parish nurse carefully reconciled the medications and disposed of older medications. She made the patient a chart of her current medications and times. She purchased four weekly medication sets and loaded them with the morning and evening dosages. She spent time on patient education about the medication uses and side effects. She discussed the importance of hydration in metabolizing the medications safely. She made an appointment with the PCP and attended with the patient to discuss the incorrect medication usage, as well as to obtain a titration schedule for the insulin based on Accu-Chek readings. Once the patient was feeling better, she happily returned to her church activities and friends.

QSEN Prelicensure Knowledge, Skills, and Attitudes (KSAs) Addressed

Safety was addressed through medication reconciliation and patient education.

Teamwork and Collaboration was apparent as the parish nurse worked with the PCP to assist the patient.

Comprehensive Geriatric Assessment

Name: ______________________ Date of birth: __________ Gender: ________

Physical Health				
Chronic disorder				
Vision	Adequate	Inadequate	Eyeglasses: Y N	Needs evaluation
Hearing	Adequate	Inadequate	Hearing aids: Y N	
Mobility	Ambulatory: Y N Falls: Y N		Assistive device:	Needs evaluation
Nutrition	Albumin: ______ Weight: ______		TLC: ______ Weight loss or gain: Y N	HCT: ______ Needs evaluation
Incontinence	Y N		Treatment: Y N	Needs evaluation
Medications	Total number: Adverse effects/allergy: ______		Reviewed & revised: Y N	
Screening	Cholesterol: ______ Mammogram: ______ Osteoporosis: ______ Pap smear: ______ PSA: ______	TSH: ______ Date: ______ Date: ______ Date: ______ Date: ______	B_{12}: ______ N/A N/A N/A N/A	Folate: ______
Immunization	Influenza: ______ Pneumonia: ______ Tetanus: ______	Date: ______ Date: ______ Date: ______	Booster: ______	
Counseling	Diet Smoking	Exercise Alcohol	Calcium Driving	Vitamin D Injury prevention
Mental Health				
Dementia	Y N	MMSE score: ______	Date: ______	Cause (if known):
Depression	Y N	GDS score: ______	Date: ______	Treatment: Y N
Functional Status				
ADL	Bathing: I D Transferring: I D		Dressing: I D Feeding: I D	Toileting: I D Continence: I D

KEY: *ADL*, Activities of daily living; *B_{12}*, vitamin B_{12}; D, dependent; *GDS*, Geriatric Depression Scale; *HCT*, hematocrit; *I*, independent; *MMSE*, Mini-Mental State Examination; *N*, no; *PSA*, prostate-specific antigen; *TLC*, total lymphocyte count; *TSH*, thyroid-stimulating hormone; *Y*, yes.

Fig. 28.1 Comprehensive geriatric assessment.

Previous studies have found that anticholinergic activity, which is a side effect of many commonly used drugs, has been linked with reduced brain function and early death in elder adults (Brooks, 2016). A recent study on anticholinergic drugs that featured neuroimaging in users and nonusers demonstrated increased brain atrophy and hypermetabolism in users, thus explaining the increased risk for cognitive decline, poor memory, and diminished executive function (Brooks, 2016). Antihistamines and antidepressants are commonly prescribed medications with anticholinergic effects. This class also includes medications like nifedipine, codeine, hypertensive drugs, and drugs taken for congestive heart failure. Anticholinergics typically decrease saliva and cause sedation, leading to dry eyes, reduced fluid for body processes, and fall risk. The nurse needs to review all prescription and over-the-counter medications the patient is taking, be alert to the anticholinergic side effects, and keep in mind the delayed metabolism in elderly patients. It is best to avoid anticholinergic drugs in the elderly whenever possible. The prescriber needs to be notified if the patient is taking one or two medications that have this potential because anticholinergic effects are cumulative.

PSYCHIATRIC DISORDERS IN OLDER ADULTS

Not only are older adults with mental disorders less likely to be accurately diagnosed, but they are also more likely to receive inappropriate or inadequate treatment compared with younger adults (NCOA, 2018). It is important to keep in mind that presentations of mental disorders vary substantially with age. This is especially true for individuals with depression and anxiety. Mental illness is sometimes misinterpreted as normal aging, and as a result, patients are not provided with treatment that could improve their quality of life. Solid evidence-based literature and studies dealing with geriatric anxiety disorder, bipolar disorders, geriatric schizophrenia, or geriatric alcohol use disorders are in short supply (NCOA, 2018). Common mental health issues affecting older adults discussed in this chapter are depression, suicide, memory impairment, and alcohol and drug use. In addition to mental health diagnoses, elder abuse and caregiver role strain are significant concerns in this population. These issues are discussed in Chapter 21. Cognitive symptoms affecting the elderly adult are discussed in Chapter 18.

BOX 28.2 Communication Guidelines for Interviewing the Older Adult

1. Gather preliminary data before the session, and keep questionnaires relatively short.
2. Ask about often-overlooked problems, such as difficulty sleeping, incontinence, falling, depression, dizziness, sexual activity, alcohol or drug use, or loss of energy.
3. Pace the interview to allow the patient to formulate answers; resist the tendency to interrupt prematurely.
4. Use simple choice questions if the older patient has trouble coping with open-ended questions.
5. Begin with general questions, such as, "How can I help you most at this visit?" or "What's been happening?"
6. Be alert for information on the patient's relationships with others; thoughts about family or co-workers; typical responses to stress; and attitudes toward aging, illness, occupation, and death.
7. Assess mental status for deficits in recent or remote memory, and determine if confusion exists.
8. Note all medications the patient is taking and assess for side effects, efficacy, possible drug interactions, and if the patient is taking them regularly and correctly.
9. Determine how fast the condition of the patient has been changing, and assess the extent of the patient's concerns.
10. Include the family or significant other in the interview process for added input, clarification, support, and reinforcement, with the patient's permission.

From National Institute on Aging. (2011). *Working with your older patient: A clinician's handbook.* Bethesda, MD: Author.

Depression

Depression is the most common, the most debilitating, and also the most treatable psychiatric disorder in the older adult (Robinson, Smith, & Segal, 2016). Depression in later life creates pain, suffering, poor quality of life, and spiritual anguish. Depression can be dangerous when the older person is also experiencing a chronic illness, loneliness, or losses (e.g., spouse, job, independence, home, finances, or health), and depression is the biggest risk factor for suicide (Robinson et al., 2016).

Health care providers frequently misinterpret clinical depression in older adults as a normal part of aging, especially if the older adult is experiencing neurological symptoms (dementia) or other physical illnesses (Robinson et al., 2016). Symptoms of depression, such as memory loss, intellectual impairment, asocial behavior, or agitation, may be misinterpreted as dementia or other cognitive disorders. As a result, older adults may miss out on treatment that would improve quality of life significantly.

A careful assessment is needed to distinguish among delirium, dementia, and depression because presenting symptoms can be similar, or two or more may co-occur. (Table 28.1 presents a comparison of delirium, dementia, and depression.) Chapter 18 gives thorough assessment guidelines and interventions for a patient experiencing delirium or dementia.

In making an assessment, the nurse needs to be familiar with the symptoms of depression in general and how symptoms may differ in the elderly. Besides the core symptoms we recognize regarding depression (see Chapter 15), depression in the elderly may be expressed as physical symptoms or negative behaviors such as forgetfulness, agitation, combativeness, constant complaining, irritability and anger, treatment-resistant aches and pains, fatigue, apprehension, unwarranted suspicion or paranoia, and low self-esteem.

A variety of biological and psychosocial risk factors for depression have been identified. These include medical illness, functional disability, social isolation, accumulation of life stressors, losses, and genetic vulnerabilities. Depression can be caused by a wide variety of drugs, including steroids, beta blockers, weight loss medications, opioids, benzodiazepines, and varenicline (Chantix), and by medical disorders such as hepatitis, cardiac disease, and cerebrovascular accident as well as respiratory, endocrine, and thyroid disorders. Depression contributes to suicide potential. A thorough assessment for any medical- or drug-induced side effects should be performed in addition to the psychosocial assessment. (Fig. 28.2 presents the Geriatric Depression Scale.)

Depression in later life increases the risk for medical comorbidities, suicide, disability, and family caregiving burden. Undiagnosed depression also increases the risk for unhealthy behaviors to compensate for mood, such as substance abuse or gambling, and contributes to the progression of other chronic illnesses (NCOA, 2018).

Depression in later life responds well to (1) *psychosocial treatments* that relieve loneliness, such as group aerobic exercise sessions; (2) *talk therapies* such as psychotherapy or cognitive behavioral therapy, which may be effective with or without the use of medications; and (3) *establishment of social support systems* such as group meals, scheduled visitors, and volunteer work (Robinson et al., 2016). These psychosocial and cognitive interventions can be critical in treating late-life

TABLE 28.1 Comparison of Delirium, Dementia, and Depression

	Delirium	Dementia	Depression
Onset	Sudden, over hours to days	Slowly, over months	May have been gradual with exacerbation during crisis or stress
Cause or contributing factors	Hypoglycemia, fever, dehydration, hypotension; infection, other conditions that disrupt body's homeostasis; adverse drug reaction; head injury; change in environment (e.g., hospitalization); pain; emotional stress	Alzheimer's disease, vascular disease, human immunodeficiency virus (HIV) infection, neurological disease, chronic alcoholism, head trauma	Lifelong history, losses, loneliness, crises, declining health, medical conditions
Cognition	Impaired memory, judgment, calculations, attention span; can fluctuate throughout the day	Impaired memory, judgment, calculations, attention span, abstract thinking; agnosia	Difficulty concentrating, forgetfulness, inattention
Level of consciousness	Altered	Not altered	Not altered
Activity level	Can be increased or reduced; restlessness, behaviors may worsen in evening (sundowning); sleep–wake cycle may be reversed	Not altered; behaviors may worsen in evening (sundowning)	Usually decreased; lethargy, fatigue, lack of motivation; may sleep poorly and awaken in early morning
Emotional state	Rapid swings; can be fearful, anxious, suspicious, aggressive, have hallucinations and delusions	Flat; delusions	Extreme sadness, apathy, irritability, anxiety, paranoid ideation

Geriatric Depression Scale (Short Form)

	Yes	No
1. Are you basically satisfied with your life?	○	○
2. Have you dropped many of your activities and interests?	○	○
3. Do you feel that your life is empty?	○	○
4. Do you often get bored?	○	○
5. Are you in good spirits most of the time?	○	○
6. Are you afraid that something bad is going to happen to you?	○	○
7. Do you feel happy most of the time?	○	○
8. Do you often feel helpless?	○	○
9. Do you prefer to stay at home, rather than going out and doing new things?	○	○
10. Do you feel you have more problems with memory than most?	○	○
11. Do you think it is wonderful to be alive now?	○	○
12. Do you feel pretty worthless the way you are now?	○	○
13. Do you feel full of energy?	○	○
14. Do you feel that your situation is hopeless?	○	○
15. Do you think that most people are better off than you are?	○	○

Fig. 28.2 Geriatric Depression Scale (Short Form). (From Sheikh, J. I., & Yesavage, J. A. [1986]. Geriatric Depression Scale [GDS]: Recent evidence and development of a shorter version. In T. L. Brink (Ed.), *Clinical gerontology: A guide to assessment and intervention* [pp. 165–173]. New York: Haworth Press.)

depression because fewer than 50% of older adults on antidepressants achieve full symptom remission.

In addition to the therapies, antidepressants and electroconvulsive therapy (ECT) may be appropriate for more severe depression, especially for those persons who have suffered a lifelong battle with this disorder. Elderly persons with severe depression respond similarly to middle-aged adults with depression in terms of both psychopharmacology and ECT; however, the relapse rates are higher in older adults. Intractable depression may be treated with ECT, which is effective in 80% of cases (Kellner, 2015). However, this treatment is time consuming, usually requiring a course of around a dozen treatments, and carries unwanted side effects, including memory impairment and regular exposure to strong intravenous medications, including anesthesia. These untoward effects may be especially risky in elderly patients.

Antidepressant Therapy

In choosing a drug to treat depression in the older adult, the primary emphasis is placed on avoidance of side effects rather than on efficacy. Lower dosages are initiated, often half of a usual adult dosage, and the medication is advanced gradually. Practitioners often remember the adage "start low, go slow" for young and elderly patients (Ruscin & Linnebur, 2014). The patient and caregivers must be aware that the onset of or an increase in suicidal thoughts is a potential side effect of antidepressant medication. Although this does not occur in the majority of patients, it is important to provide patient education and monitoring for this serious potential side effect.

The choice of which class of antidepressants to use for older adults is complex. Selective serotonin reuptake inhibitors (SSRIs) have traditionally been the first-line antidepressants for older adults because of their more benign side effects and their lack of toxicity when taken in overdose. However, SSRIs may also cause an increased risk of bone fractures and place older adults at risk for hip fractures (Zhou et al., 2018) as well as increased bleeding. Some studies rate the risk of morbidity with SSRIs as higher than with tricyclic antidepressants. Fractures are twice as common when patients are using SSRIs, through falls or even minor activity such as walking. Tricyclic antidepressants have more cardiac and anticholinergic side effects, as well as more interactions with other medications. Studies have found a higher rate of stopping treatment with tricyclics due to the side-effect profile (Espinoza & Unutzer, 2016). The risks and benefits, medical profile, and medication list must be assessed carefully in choosing the best antidepressant for a particular patient. Discontinuation symptoms may occur when stopping a medication, which may lead to an increase in symptoms that were previously well controlled, such as depressed mood or anxiety, or make a person feel physically ill. Antidepressants should be decreased slowly to prevent undue stress on the patient and limit discontinuation effects.

Psychotherapy

Clinicians, including nurses, nurse practitioners, therapists, and psychologists, may provide individual or group psychotherapy to the depressed patient. As previously mentioned, groups can diminish social isolation and loneliness and help the members understand that they are not alone in their situation. Mixed-age groups can be beneficial for a variety of energy and insights, whereas same-age groups can help provide support from others in similar situations. Group members can learn creative ways to raise their mood and increase quality of life within various types of groups (Table 28.2).

Cognitive-behavioral therapy (CBT), problem-solving therapy (PST), interpersonal therapy (IPT), and supportive therapy are often used alone or as an adjunct to psychopharmacology. Most research shows a combination of therapy and medication to be the most effective approach.

Suicide

According to the Centers for Disease Control and Prevention (CDC, 2015), the suicide rate for those over 65 has dropped considerably, and it is now the 17th-leading cause of death among those 65 and over. That being said, nursing assessments and interventions for suicidal ideations and the treatment of depression need to be thorough for elderly patients. Early identification of risk factors needs to be made in all settings, especially the emergency department, primary care, and mental health settings. As many as 70% of elderly patients visited their primary care provider within a month of committing suicide (American Psychological Association, 2016).

Even though the suicide rate among older adults has decreased from previous levels, it is likely underreported. Suicide is not always listed on the death certificate when suspected, and passive behaviors such as alcoholism, starvation, overmedicating, or losing the will to live may

TABLE 28.2 Useful Group Therapy Modalities for Older Adult Patients

Remotivation Therapy	Reminiscence Therapy (Life Review)	Psychotherapy
Purpose of Group		
Resocialize regressed and apathetic patients Reawaken interest in the environment	Share memories of the past Increase self-esteem Increase socialization Increase awareness of the uniqueness of each participant	Alleviate psychiatric symptoms Increase ability to interact with others in a group Increase self-esteem Increase ability to make decisions and function more independently
Format		
Groups are made up of 10 to 15 people Meetings are held once or twice a week Meetings are highly structured in a classroom-like setting Group uses props Each session discusses a particular topic	Groups are made up of 6 to 8 people Meetings are held once or twice weekly for 1 hour Topics include holidays, major life events, birthdays, travel, and food	Group size is 6 to 12 members Group members should share similar: Problems Mental status Needs Sexual integration Group meets at regularly scheduled times (certain number of times a week, specific duration of session) and place
Desired Outcomes		
Increase participants' sense of reality Offer practice of health roles Realize more objective self-image than older adult can	Alleviate depression in institutionalized older adult Through the process of reorganization and reintegration, provide avenue by members Achieve a new sense of identity Achieve a positive self-concept	Decrease sense of isolation Facilitate development of new roles and re-establish former roles Provide information for other group Provide group support for effecting changes and increasing self-esteem

From Matteson, M. A., & McConnell, E. S. (Eds.). (1988). *Gerontologic nursing: Concepts and practice* (p. 80). Philadelphia: Saunders.

not be recognized as suicidal behaviors (CDC, 2016a). Elderly individuals have many risk factors that can lead to suicide, such as feelings of hopelessness, uselessness, and despair; medical issues; functional loss and pain; financial distress; and a variety of losses. A history of suicide attempts is always a risk factor. Suicidal gestures in the elderly may be desperate cries for help or serious attempts at dying, as in other age groups. An inverse relationship between economic conditions and suicide rate has been identified.

Assessment of Suicide Risk

The assessment of elderly individuals must include attention to the high-risk factors that potentially contribute to suicide, such as widowhood, acute illnesses and intractable pain, status change, chronic illness, family history of suicide, chronic sleep problems, alcoholism, depression, and other losses (see Chapter 23). Losses may be personal (death of a family member or close friend), economic (loss of job or home), social (loss of prestige or position), or functional (loss of health or mobility). Multiple losses accompany the aging process, increasing stress at a time when the older adult may be the most vulnerable and least able to cope with stress, thus precipitating a depressive state. According to Erik Erikson's stages of development, the elderly must find meaningful activities in their lives to replace the jobs and successes they have lost in order to successfully transition to a fulfilling older life (ego integrity vs. despair) (Heffner, 2015). Nurses can assist patients with this transition toward wisdom, reviewing their lives with a sense of completeness, and ultimately acceptance of death.

In assessing suicide risk, the health care provider must consider previous suicidal behavior, the seriousness of the intent, the presence of active plans, the availability of the means to commit the act, and the lethality of the method chosen. Compared with those in younger age groups, older adults are less likely or able to communicate their suicidal thoughts and plans. Nurses play a vital role in the prevention of older adult suicide because of their presence in every care setting and the trust that patients place in them. Talking about suicide should not be avoided, but as with all age groups and even more so in the elderly due to generational differences in communication, the subject of suicide must be approached gently. Just the word *suicide* can be upsetting and stigmatizing, and people have differing definitions of that word. Examples of a beginning approach may be to ask the person if he or she is wishing to not to be alive, or to be with deceased loves ones, or to no longer experience all of the stressors. If the person answers affirmatively, the conversation can be continued. Helping the patient to remember and talk about what he or she has to live for or what he or she would want to see in the future is helpful in alleviating suicidal thoughts. See Chapter 23 for more detailed information on this subject, including the newly Modified SAD PERSONS Scale and the **Suicide Assessment Five-Step Evaluation and Triage (SAFE-T) for Mental Health Professionals**. Attention must be focused on building awareness, routine screening, and the use of community resources in the high-risk elderly population (Substance Abuse and Mental Health Services Administration [SAMHSA], 2009).

Alcoholism, Substance Use, and Addiction

The American Medical Association has called alcohol and substance abuse among older adults a hidden epidemic. Rates of alcoholism and prescription drug abuse may increase in the older population because the baby boom generation, which had greater lifetime rates of drug use, is now aging. Identifying alcohol and substance abuse is often difficult because personality and behavioral changes may be unrecognized or attributed to medications, dementia, or medical issues. As with other generational communication differences previously discussed, such as processing emotions or discussing suicide, older patients may have a different definition or understanding of alcohol and substance use. Cocktail hours were common among older generations, as was the generous prescribing of benzodiazepines. Many older adults do not recognize their substance use patterns as a problem until they go into withdrawal when their medication is left behind while on vacation or they do not have access to alcohol while hospitalized.

Alcoholism

Elderly patients with substance use issues may have a long-term problem or a newly developed addiction in response to life stressors. The loss of a spouse and distance from family may contribute to alcoholism. The lack of structure from work or raising a family may be the impetus for a social drinker to advance to a problematic level of use.

Alcohol and Aging. Excessive consumption of alcohol can create problems for older adults. They have an increased biological sensitivity to (i.e., decreased tolerance for) the effects of alcohol. The decreased tolerance is related to a slower emptying of stomach contents; a slower metabolism, including hepatic function; and an increased sensitivity to alcohol in the brain. As people age, there is a decline in lean muscle mass and an increase in fatty tissue that can contribute to increased blood alcohol levels (BALs) (Yeager & Stepko, 2020). Age-related changes such as decreased dexterity, balance, and flexibility can increase the likelihood of falls, burns, or other accidents when under the influence of alcohol or other substances. Injuries sustained while under the influence tend to heal more slowly than in younger years.

Some drinkers, as they get older, note changes in their response to alcohol, such as the occurrence of headaches, reduction in mental abilities with memory losses or lapses, and feelings of malaise rather than well-being. These problems start to occur at lower levels of consumption than was the case in earlier years, which can indicate liver damage or slowed metabolism in general. Older adults are likely to drink more frequently but in lesser quantities than younger individuals, who tend to drink larger amounts less often. Thus, the possibility of alcohol use in cases of only moderate levels of use by older adults often is not recognized by friends or family as a problem.

Alcohol and Medication. The interaction of drugs and alcohol in the older adult can have serious consequences. Alcohol may prolong, potentiate, or accelerate the metabolism of various drugs. Some drugs, such as benzodiazepines or opiate pain medications, in combination with alcohol can be lethal or contribute to suicidal thoughts and suicide completion.

Older individuals can expect to reach higher BALs than younger people with an equivalent intake of alcohol. Even a moderate intake of alcohol can impair the cognition and coordination skills that are already decreased with age. Extreme care is required when treating the older alcoholic with medication. Central nervous system toxicity from psychiatric drugs increases with aging. Ingestion of antidepressants or tranquilizers can be particularly harmful because their effect is further potentiated by alcohol, and the hepatotoxic effects of medications such as acetaminophen can be compounded.

Compared with younger individuals, older adults take longer to fall asleep and do not sleep as restfully. Although alcohol may help decrease the time it takes to fall asleep, this benefit is offset by frequent awakenings during the night caused by alcohol. Alcohol-related insomnia may encourage an older person to ask a health care provider for a sleeping medication, which can be dangerous in combination with alcohol or other medications. This is another example of why assessing substance use in the elderly population is important.

Symptoms of Elder Addiction. Health practitioners need to be concerned with, and sensitive to, possible alcohol abuse among their older patients. Signs of long-term alcohol abuse, such as pancreatitis or liver disease, blackouts, or major trauma, may not be present in adults who begin drinking later in life. Instead, the older alcoholic may display vague geriatric symptoms of contusions, malnutrition, self-neglect, impaired cognition, sleep disturbances, depression, and falls (Kelly et al., 2018). Also present may be symptoms of diarrhea, urinary incontinence, a decrease in functional status, failure to thrive, and apparent dementia. Symptoms of poor coordination or visual changes may mimic the normal aging process but actually may be a result of excessive drinking. Assessment is necessary to differentiate the normal physiological changes of aging from those attributable to excessive drinking.

Whenever there is a suspicion or indication that an older adult is abusing alcohol, the health care provider should conduct a screening test. The Short Michigan Alcohol Screening Test—Geriatric Version (SMAST-G; http://vtspc.org/wp-content/uploads/2016/12/SMAST-G.pdf) is commonly used to assess alcohol problems (Agency for Healthcare Research and Quality [AHRQ], 2012).

Treatment of the Older Adult. Because many older adults do not live in big families or have work-related contacts, they are less likely to be referred for treatment than are younger drinkers. Too often, by the time the older adult alcoholic is noticed by any treatment agencies, the patient's support systems and resources are severely decreased or depleted. Older patients may also hide their drinking out of shame, feeling sinful, or feeling that they can or should handle it themselves (Kelly et al., 2018).

Treatment plans for the older patient with an addiction should emphasize social therapies. Older adult alcoholics tend to be more passive than younger alcoholics and may need more encouragement from health care professionals to participate in groups such as Alcoholics Anonymous and individual and family therapy. The prognosis for the patient who develops a drinking problem later in life is excellent because the individual has lived most of his or her life without this habit. Brief treatment is often successful, and nurses can be instrumental in educating the patient and encouraging the development of resources for the elderly. For those elderly adults with long histories of alcohol use who meet the criteria for alcohol dependence, a more rigorous treatment plan is required, including detoxification, often a few days in an inpatient unit (USDHHS, 2014). Medications to curb cravings, such as naltrexone, an opiate agonist, may also play a part in longer-term treatment (Johnson, 2015). Recent studies show that gabapentin is very helpful in reducing cravings as patients become sober.

Substance Use

Illegal Drug Use. For adults 65 and older, the Substance Abuse and Mental Health Services Administration (SAMHSA) reports a projected rise in substance use disorders from 2.2% to 3.1% between 2001 and 2020. The most common drugs leading to emergency room visits in older adults are prescription and nonprescription pain medication, followed by benzodiazepines, then alcohol, psychotropics, cocaine, heroin, and marijuana. Some signs of substance misuse may include change in cognition, blackouts, increased tolerance to medications, unexplained injuries or injuries that do not fit the reported cause, and frequently losing medication that is abused when other medications are filled on time, as well as psychiatric symptoms like changes in sleep, mood, and appetite (SAMHSA, 2017).

Acquired Immunodeficiency Syndrome and AIDS-Related Dementia

Human immunodeficiency virus (HIV) infection and acquired immunodeficiency syndrome (AIDS) remain a growing problem among the elderly. People 55 years of age and older accounted for one-quarter of all Americans living with HIV in 2012. Older Americans are more likely to be diagnosed with HIV infection later in the course of their disease (CDC, 2016b). Of the 6955 deaths related to AIDS in 2013, 2588 (37%) were among people 55 years of age and older (CDC, 2016b).

Blood transfusions are no longer the main cause for the spread of AIDS in the older adult, unless the transfusion occurred before 1985. Research shows that older adults remain sexually active and thus are at risk for HIV and AIDS because of failure to understand and practice safe sex. Men who have been treated for erectile dysfunction are also considered at risk for HIV/AIDS. Diagnosis and treatment of HIV and AIDS in the older adult may be delayed because health care providers believe that this population is not sexually active, another aspect of ageism. Lack of adequate knowledge about HIV and AIDS, other sexually transmitted infections, and safe-sex practices among older adults increases the risk for HIV infection and AIDS in this age group.

Older women who are sexually active are at higher risk for HIV and AIDS from an infected partner than are older men. Changes in vaginal tissue caused by the aging process can lead to tears in the vaginal mucosa during intercourse, allowing HIV to penetrate more easily. In addition, because pregnancy is no longer a threat, the use of condoms in this age group is uncommon.

Dementia is often a sequela in people with HIV infection and AIDS. Dementia caused by AIDS and dementia caused by Alzheimer's disease can be easily confused. Therefore a careful assessment and workup are required, including testing for HIV/AIDS.

LEGAL AND ETHICAL ISSUES THAT AFFECT THE MENTAL HEALTH OF OLDER ADULTS

Among the most important of many legal and ethical issues for practicing nurses to be familiar with are the following:

1. Use of restraints
2. Decision making about health care
3. Elder abuse (a serious problem for the older adult discussed in Chapter 21)
4. End-of-life care (addressed in Chapter 25)

Right to Die

One ethical dilemma in nursing is the question of whether older adults have the right to end their lives themselves or by way of physician-assisted suicide (PAS). Suicide raises spiritual and moral issues. Some in society believe that older adults with terminal illnesses or those who suffer intractable pain should be able to control their own deaths. Others believe that suicide is never a correct option. If an alert older adult patient is confronted with an intractable, lingering, and painful illness, with no hope of relief except through death, is suicide justifiable?

According to the American Nurses Association (ANA), nurses are prohibited from participating in assisted suicide or euthanasia, as a direct violation of the ANA's *Code of Ethics for Nurses* and its covenant with society to provide humane, comprehensive, and compassionate care. The withholding or withdrawal of life-sustaining treatment (ventilation, cardiopulmonary support, chemotherapy, dialysis, medications, nutrition, and hydration) is ethically acceptable. This is considered as allowing the patient to die from the underlying condition and does not involve direct action to end a life. Administering medications with the intent to promote comfort is not the same as the intent to end life. A common example is giving morphine with the intent to reduce pain in terminal illness, although this medication also depresses the respiratory center. Nurses are expected to care for their patients despite any philosophical differences with decisions regarding treatments and death (ANA, 2016). Assisted suicide is now legal in California,

Colorado, Hawaii, Maine, New Jersey, Oregon, Vermont, Washington, and Washington DC. If a nurse works in a state where assisted suicide is not legal and participates in helping a patient to end his or her life, the nurse is at risk for legal action and loss of licensure. The Oregon Nurses Association has developed guidelines for nurses, stating they can explain assisted suicide law, discuss options, and provide resources (ANA, 2016). Conversely, the American Public Health Association supports allowing a competent adult to obtain a prescription to self-administer and to control the time and manner of his or her own death (ANA, 2016). As the population ages, end-of-life discussions will become more common and pressing.

The Netherlands has historically been pro-PAS, with rates of PAS there progressively increasing through the years. The topic is explored by Richard Fenigsen (2011). In one vignette, a lonely and depressed widow repeatedly asked her physician for a lethal dose of medication, and he finally complied. After the woman's death, when the physician was reviewing the case, a colleague queried, "Did you think of buying her a cat?" This scenario raises poignant questions and stimulates thought about the multiple aspects and concerns surrounding this issue.

Although suicide is discussed in Chapter 23, specific factors that concern older adults, such as retirement-related difficulties, physical illness, economic problems, loneliness, social isolation, multiple losses, and the concept of ageism, have been illuminated here. Education of the public and health care providers will become increasingly important as the general population ages.

Use of Restraints

The use of restraints encompasses ethical, legal, and safety concerns. Restraints can be both physical and chemical. **Physical restraints** are any manual methods, materials, or equipment that inhibits free movement. Examples include tightening a bedsheet to limit movement, raising side rails, applying wrist or waist restraints, or positioning a wheelchair to restrict movement. Devices on clothing that trigger an alarm to notify staff that an older adult is leaving a room or an area are not considered restraints. **Chemical restraints** are drugs given for the specific purpose of inhibiting a certain behavior or movement that are not part of the normal treatment plan. Although common in past decades, restraint use is becoming increasingly rare as facilities adopt restraint-free policies and train staff in advanced de-escalation and communication techniques (National Alliance on Mental Illness [NAMI], 2016).

Physical Restraints

Whether health care providers have the right to restrain another individual physically has always been debated. Surveys undertaken by the state and federal authorities in the United States in the 1970s and 1980s revealed levels of physical restraint use as high as 75% in some facilities (NAMI, 2016). Physical restraints were traditionally used with confused or medicated hospitalized patients, primarily to prevent disruption of medical therapies and to prevent falls. Although meant to enhance safety, they are often perceived as abusive by patients and families.

Research beginning in the 1980s has shown more harm than benefit with the use of restraints (NAMI, 2016). Physical restraints can pose a risk of death through strangulation or asphyxiation and lead to muscle loss, incontinence, pressure sores, agitation, and bone weakness when used for prolonged periods of time. In elderly patients, restraints can contribute to cognitive impairment, physical weakness, fall risk, anxiety, feelings of humiliation, and emotional withdrawal and should only be used as a last resort.

More facilities are using electronic sensing systems to alert staff if a resident is about to stand up or try to get out of a bed or wheelchair, adjusting staffing patterns, and providing enhanced training of staff. Other efforts that replace the practice of restraint use include strength training for the patient, the use of mobility devices and hearing aids, lower beds, reduction of obstacles, improved lighting, and door alarms.

Physical restraints should be used for emergency purposes only when there is a threat to the safety of the resident or others, never as a means of controlling behavior or as punishment. According to The Joint Commission (Joint Commission on Accreditation of Healthcare Organizations [JCAHO], 2015), restraint use now has very specific and time-limited guidelines, requiring a provider order, constant monitoring, rotation of the restraints to rest the limbs, offering water and toileting, and documentation of alternative methods tried.

Nurses can avoid liability by knowing the laws in their state, adhering to the policies and procedures of the institution at which they work, and using good nursing judgment. All nursing homes and hospitals should have written restraint procedures and policies. If restraints are used, the nurse is responsible for the patient's safety, and creative nursing skills and interventions are frequently more beneficial.

Chemical Restraints

Unfortunately, with restrictions on physical restraints, there has been an increase in off-label use of certain medications (particularly second-generation antipsychotics) as chemical restraints to control the behavior of elderly patients. In 2008 the U.S. Food and Drug Administration (FDA) issued Black Box warnings for the use of antipsychotics in controlling behavioral symptoms in elderly patients with dementia. The Centers for Medicare and Medicaid Services (2017) monitor long-term antipsychotic use and report a decrease in the use of antipsychotics in the elderly, from 30% down to 19%.

CONTROL OF THE DECISION-MAKING PROCESS

Patient Self-Determination Act

Since the 1960s, individuals' desire to participate in decision making about their own health care has increased. Congress passed the **Patient Self-Determination Act (PSDA)** in 1990, requiring that health care facilities provide clear, written information to every patient regarding his or her legal right to make health care decisions, including the right to accept or refuse treatment. The PSDA also establishes the right of a person to provide written treatment directions for clinicians in the event of a serious illness. Increasing numbers of older adults are creating written directives.

Advance Directive

Advance directive is a term used to describe living wills, durable powers of attorney for health care, and health care surrogate appointments. Health care institutions that receive federal funds are required to provide each patient with written information regarding his or her right to execute advance directives and must inquire whether such directives have been made by the patient. The patient's admission records should state whether such directives exist.

Such a directive indicates preferences for the types of medical care desired. The directive comes into effect should physical or mental incapacitation prevent the patient from making health care decisions. These wishes can be communicated through one or more of the following: (1) a living will, (2) a directive to physician, and (3) a durable power of attorney for health care. These documents must be in writing, and the patient's signature must be witnessed and, in some states, notarized.

Living Will

A **living will** is a personal statement of how and where one wishes to die, and it can be changed at any time by the individual. It is activated only when the person is terminally ill and incapacitated. Executing a living will does not always guarantee its application.

Directive to Physician

In a **directive to physician**, a physician is appointed by the individual to serve as a proxy. Many of the features of a directive to physician parallel those of a living will, and designating the physician as surrogate can be particularly useful in cases of terminal illness when an individual has no family. Unlike the living will, the directive to physician can be revoked orally at any time, without regard to patient competency.

Durable Power of Attorney for Health Care

The **durable power of attorney for health care** differs from a living will in that a person is appointed to act as the patient's agent. Individuals do not have to be terminally ill or incompetent to allow the empowered individual to act on their behalf.

Older adults who are lesbian, gay, bisexual, or transgender (LGBT) often have many conflicts within state or federal facilities such as nursing homes. Many states have adopted laws that allow gay and lesbian couples to marry, and in 2013 the Supreme Court ruled that married same-sex couples were entitled to federal benefits, thereby allowing the rights of all spouses in a marriage. In states that have not adopted laws for gay and lesbian marriages, there is sometimes a cruel bias of not allowing visitation rights or power of attorney for LGBT patients' partners. These trends have been changing, and the recent Supreme Court ruling in favor of same-sex marriage should alleviate most of the prejudice and differential treatment between heterosexual and homosexual couples.

Nursing Role in the Decision-Making Process

The nurse explains the ethics and legal policies to both the patient and the family and helps them understand the concepts behind advance directives. The family need not feel morally obligated to provide for all possible medical care when such care will only extend the suffering of a loved one. This is especially true when such extraordinary measures *do not represent the person's values and beliefs*. The nurse serves as an *advocate* and a knowledgeable resource person for the older adult patient and family. The patient is encouraged to verbalize his or her feelings and thoughts during this sensitive time of decision making. Maintaining an open and continuing dialogue among patient, family, nurse, and primary care provider (physician or nurse practitioner) is important. The nurse supports the patient and person(s) appointed to act on the patient's behalf and seeks consultation for any ethical issues the nurse feels unprepared to handle.

The law does not specify who should talk with patients about treatment decisions, but in many facilities, nurses are being asked to discuss this issue with the patient. If the advance directive of a patient is not being followed, the nurse intervenes on the patient's behalf. Although nurses, especially in nursing homes, may discuss options with their patients, they may not assist patients in writing advance directives because this is considered a conflict of interest. The existence of an advance directive serves as a guide for the older adult patient's rightful wishes in this process.

KEY POINTS TO REMEMBER

- The older adult population continues to increase as the baby boomers start reaching 65 years of age.
- The increase in the number of older adults poses a challenge to the entire health care system. There is much to be done to prepare and respond to the special needs of this population.
- Attitudes toward the older adult are often negative and stereotypical, reflecting an ageism bias common in our society. Health care providers can hold biased views of the elderly that affect caregiving.
- Nurses should be knowledgeable about the process of aging, including the differences between normal and abnormal aging changes.
- Older adults face increasing problems of alcoholism, illicit drug use, abuse and misuse of prescription and over-the-counter drugs, and suicide.
- The current philosophy of care mandates that patients be free from unnecessary use of drugs and physical restraints.
- Nurses working with mentally ill patients should study psychotherapeutic approaches relevant for older adults, such as remotivation and reminiscence therapy, and offer psychotherapy groups geared toward the special needs of this population.
- When it comes to dying and death, older adults' wishes and those of their families may differ and are frequently ignored. The implementation of the Patient Self-Determination Act (PSDA), passed in 1990, can afford patients autonomy, choice, and dignity in their death process.

APPLYING CRITICAL JUDGMENT

1. A 70-year-old male has been admitted to the intensive care unit with a diagnosis of alcohol withdrawal delirium. He is confused and combative and threatens to strike the nurse who is trying to render care to him unless he is allowed to leave the unit. The nurse applies wrist restraints to prevent him from striking her and from leaving the room.
   - **A.** What are the mandates of The Joint Commission regarding the use of restraints? What were the reasons restraints were found to be dangerous?
   - **B.** What other actions besides applying restraints could the nurse employ in this situation, consistent with a restraint-free philosophy?
   - **C.** What are the possible legal repercussions for the nurse?
   - **D.** What potential harmful consequences, physical and psychological, could occur with this patient?
2. The same patient as in the first scenario has received treatment for alcohol withdrawal. He appears very quiet, refuses to eat, does not sleep at night, and admits to thoughts of desperation and wishing that he could die. He also confides that he started drinking heavily and attempted suicide when his wife died 5 years earlier.
   - **A.** Choose specific assessment tools to use in assessing the patient's depression, suicide risk, and alcohol use.
   - **B.** What kinds of supports would you suggest be available to the patient upon discharge? What types of information might you need to know about this patient to best plan his discharge care?

APPLYING CRITICAL JUDGMENT—Cont'd

3. A 57-year-old woman is admitted to the hospital after a heart attack exacerbated by the chemotherapy used to treat metastasized liver cancer. Her son says that she does not want anyone to resuscitate her. Acting both as a nurse and as a patient advocate, explain to the patient and her son what an advance directive is and what needs to be done to make the patient's wishes known.
4. Think about an example of ageism you may have noticed in your family or in your role as a nursing student or that you may have participated in yourself toward an elderly person without recognizing it. Discuss your example with a classmate and listen to his or her example.
5. Briefly interview someone older than 70 years of age about the changes he or she has noticed in his or her own life and health and the world. Also, ask for examples of ageism the person has noticed.

CHAPTER REVIEW QUESTIONS

1. An 85-year-old woman says to the nurse, "I raised three children, but now two of them barely speak to me. I did not do a good job of instilling a family spirit." Which response should the nurse provide?
   a. "Do you think this situation is likely to change?"
   b. "If you could relive those earlier years, what would you do differently?"
   c. "There's no guidebook for parenting. Your children have made their own choices."
   d. "Your children are likely to regret their behavior. I hope you can find it in your heart to forgive them."
2. The nurse asks an 87-year-old, "How are you doing?" The patient replies, "I have good days and bad days." Select the nurse's therapeutic response.
   a. "How is your sleep?"
   b. "Tell me more about that."
   c. "Are you feeling depressed?"
   d. "We expect that from people your age."
3. A 92-year-old lives alone, but family members assist with transportation and home maintenance. This adult tells the nurse, "They mean well, but sometimes my family treats me like a child." What is the nurse's best action?
   a. Encourage the adult to overlook these behaviors from family members.
   b. Role-play with the adult ways to share these feelings with family members.
   c. Contact family members privately and educate them about the harmful effects of ageism.
   d. Reinforce family members' good intentions and say, "It's fortunate your family is so helpful."
4. A nurse assesses a 78-year-old patient who lives alone at home and is beginning three new prescriptions. Which question by the nurse will best provide for the patient's safety?
   a. "How do you store your medications at home?"
   b. "What is your usual bowel elimination pattern?"
   c. "Who usually helps you with your medications?"
   d. "How much alcohol do you drink on a normal day?"
5. Which scenario presents the most risk factors for suicide?
   a. 64-year-old black female whose husband died 3 months ago
   b. 72-year-old white female scheduled for hip replacement in 2 weeks
   c. 82-year-old widowed white male recently diagnosed with pancreatic cancer
   d. 92-year-old black male who recently moved into the home of his adult children

REFERENCES

Agency for Healthcare Research and Quality (AHRQ). (2012). *Screening, behavioral counseling, and referral in primary care to reduce alcohol misuse-Comparative effectiveness review*. No. 64. Retrieved from http://www.ncbi.nlm.nih.gov/books/NBK99199/pdf/Bookshelf_NBK99199.pdf.

American Nurses Association. (2016). *Position statement: Nurse's roles and responsibilities in providing care and support at the end of life*. Retrieved June 9, 2018 from https://www.nursingworld.org/~4af078/globalassets/docs/ana/ethics/endoflife-positionstatement.pdf.

American Psychological Association (APA). (2016). *Mental and behavioral health and older Americans*. Retrieved from http://www.apa.org/about/gr/issues/aging/mental-health.aspx.

Bergman, Y. S., & Bodner, E. (2015). Ageist attitudes block young adults' ability for compassion toward incapacitated older adults. *International Psychogeriatrics, 27*(9), 1541–1550.

Brooks, M. (2016). *Imaging shows basis for anticholinergic harm in elderly*. Retrieved from http://www.medscape.com/viewarticle/862299.

Centers for Disease Control and Prevention (CDC). (2015). *Suicide facts at a glance, 2015*. Retrieved from http://www.cdc.gov/violenceprevention/pdf/suicide-datasheet-a.pdf.

Centers for Disease Control and Prevention (CDC). (2016a). *Study looks at suicide rates from 1928–2007*. Retrieved from http://www.cdc.gov/ViolencePrevention/suicide/index.html.

Centers for Disease Control and Prevention (CDC). (2016b). *HIV among people 50 or over*. Retrieved from http://www.cdc.gov/hiv/group/age/olderamericans/index.html.

Centers for Medicare and Medicaid Services. (2017). *Data show national partnership to improve dementia care achieves goals to reduce unnecessary antipsychotic medications in nursing homes*. Retrieved June 9, 2018 from https://www.cms.gov/Newsroom/MediaReleaseDatabase/Fact-sheets/2017-Fact-Sheet-items/2017-10-02.html?DLPage=2&DLEntries=10&DLSort=0&DLSortDir=descending.

Coleman, D. (2015). Does ageism still exist in nursing education? *Nursing Older People, 27*(5), 16–21.

Espinoza, R. T., & Unutzer, J. (2016). *Diagnosis and management of late-life unipolar depression*. Retrieved from http://www.uptodate.com/contents/diagnosis-and-management-of-late-life-unipolar-depression.

Farrell, B., Shamji, S., Monahan, A., et al. (2013). Reducing polypharmacy in the elderly. *Canadian Pharmacists Journal, 146*(5), 243–244.

Fenigsen, R. (2011). Other people's lives: Reflections on medicine, ethics, and euthanasia, part two: Medicine versus euthanasia. *Issues in Law & Medicine, 26*(3), 239–279.

Gendron, T. L., Welleford, E. A., Inker, J., et al. (2015). The language of ageism: Why we need to use words carefully. *Gerontologist [online]*, 1–10.

Giddens, J. F. (2017). *Concepts for nursing practice* (2nd ed). St. Louis: Elsevier.

Health in Aging. (2016). *Many older adults have both chronic illness and "geriatric syndromes."* Retrieved from http://www.healthinaging.org/resources/resource:many-older-adults-have-both-chronic-illnesses-and-geriatric-syndromes/.

HealthyPeople2020. (2016). *Older adults*. Retrieved from https://www.healthypeople.gov/2020/topics-objectives/topic/older-adults.

Heffner, C. (2015). *Erikson's stages of psychosocial development*. Retrieved from http://allpsych.com/psychology101/social_development/#.Vdo5E_lVikp.

Institute for Healthcare Improvement. (2018). *Initiatives: Age-friendly health systems*. Retrieved June 9, 2018 from http://www.ihi.org/Engage/Initiatives/Age-Friendly-Health-Systems/Pages/default.aspx.

Johnson, B. A. (2015). *Pharmacotherapy for alcohol use disorder.* Retrieved from http://www.uptodate.com.

Joint Commission on Accreditation of Healthcare Organizations (JCAHO). (1999). *Standards for behavioral health care.* Oakbrook, IL: JCAHO.

Kagan, S. H., & Melendez-Torres, G. J. (2015). Ageism in nursing. *Journal of Nursing Management, 23*(5), 644–650.

Kellner, C. (2015). *Unipolar major depression in adults: Indications for and efficacy of electroconvulsive therapy (ECT).* Retrieved from http://www.uptodate.com.

Kelly, S., Olanrewaju, O., Cowan, A., Brayne, C., & Lafortune, L. (2018). Alcohol and older people: A systematic review of barriers, facilitators and context of drinking in older people and implications for intervention design. doi.org/10.1371/journal.pone.0191189.

Kydd, A., & Fleming, A. (2015). Ageism and age discrimination in healthcare: Fact or fiction? A narrative review of literature. *Maturitas, 81*(4), 432–438.

National Alliance on Mental Illness (NAMI). (2016). *NAMI calls for major reforms in use of physical restraints in psychiatric facilities.* Retrieved from http://www.nami.org/Press-Media/Press-Releases/1998/NAMI-Calls-For-Major-Reforms-In-Use-Of-Physical-Re.

National Council on Aging. (2018). *Economic security for seniors facts.* Retrieved June 9, 2018 from https://www.ncoa.org/news/resources-for-reporters/get-the-facts/economic-security-facts/.

North, M. S., & Fiske, S. T. (2015). Modern attitudes toward older adults in the aging world: A cross-cultural meta-analysis. *Psychological Bulletin, 141*(5), 993–1021.

Oaklander, M. (2015). Your attitude about aging may impact how you age. *Time.* Retrieved from http://time.com/4138476/aging-alzheimers-disease/.

Ouchida, K. M., & Lachs, M. S. (2015). *Not for doctors only: Ageism in healthcare.* Retrieved from http://www.asaging.org/blog/not-doctors-only-ageism-healthcare.

Robinson, L., Smith, M., & Segal, J. (2016). *Depression in older adults and the elderly.* Retrieved from http://www.helpguide.org/articles/depression/depression-in-older-adults-and-the-elderly.htm.

Ruscin, J. M., & Linnebur, S. A. (2014). *Drug-related problems in the elderly.* Retrieved from http://www.merckmanuals.com/professional/geriatrics/drug-therapy-in-the-elderly/drug-related-problems-in-the-elderly.

Substance Abuse and Mental Health Services Administration (SAMHSA). (2009). *Suicide assessment five-step evaluation and triage.* Retrieved from https://store.samhsa.gov/sites/default/files/d7/priv/sma09-4432.pdf.

Substance Abuse and Mental Health Services Administration (SAMHSA). (2017). *A day in the life of older adults: Substance use facts.* Retrieved June 9, 2018 from https://www.samhsa.gov/data/sites/default/files/report_2792/ShortReport-2792.html.

Temple, S (2019). *America's 2019 rental market in review: Did renters pay more?* Retrieved from https:///www.abodo.com/blog/2019-annual-rent-report/.

U.S. Department of Health and Human Services. (2016). *2020 topics and objectives: Older adults.* Retrieved from https://www.healthypeople. gov/2020/topics-objectives/topic/older-adults.

U.S. Department of Health and Human Services. (2014). *NIH SeniorHealth: Prescription and illicit drug abuse.* Retrieved from http://nihseniorhealth.gov/drugabuse/treatingsubstanceabuse/ 01.html.

U.S. Food and Drug Administration (FDA). (2008). *Antipsychotics are not indicated for the treatment of dementia-related psychoses.* Retrieved from http://www.fda.gov/drugs/drugsafety/postsmarketdrugsafetyinformation-forpatientsandprovider.

Van De Water, P. N., & Romig, K. (2020). *Social Security benefits are modest.* Retrieved from http://www.cbpp.org/research/social-security/social-security-benefits-are-modest.

Wooten, J. M. (2015). Pharmacotherapy considerations in elderly adults. *Southern Medical Journal, 105*(8), 437–445. Retrieved from http://www.medscape.com/viewarticle/769412_1.

World Health Organization. (2017). Mental health of older adults. Retrieved June 9, 2018 from http://www.who.int/news-room/fact-sheets/detail/mental-health-of-older-adults

World Health Organization. (2018). Suicide: Key facts. Retrieved June 9, 2018 from http://www.who.int/en/news-room/fact-sheets/detail/suicide.

Yeager, S., & Stepko, B. (2020). *How alcohol affects us as we age: Why it matters that older adults are drinking more than ever.* Retrieved from https://www.aarp.org/health/healthy-living/info-2020/increased-drinking-among-65plus.html.

Zhou, C., Fang, L, Chen, Y, Zhong, J., Wang, H., & Xie, P. (2018). Effect of selective serotonin reuptake inhibitors on bone mineral density: A systematic review and meta-analysis. *Osteoporosis International, 29(2018),* 1243–1251. doi: 10.1007/s00198-018-4413-0.

APPENDIX A

Complementary and Alternative Treatments

Christina Fratena

Disorder	Therapy	Description
Anxiety	Natural products/herbs	Supplements, vitamins, minerals, and herbs/botanicals are used to reduce anxiety Examples: • **Kava**: rare cases of hepatotoxicity • **L-theanine:** increases GABA and alpha activity • **5-HTTP**: may be used for panic attacks
	Aromatherapy	Essential oils are used to enhance physical and mental well-being and for healing Guidelines for safe use include dilution rates, avoiding ingestion and use around eyes, and obtaining training for use in pregnancy, lactation, and with children (National Association for Holistic Aromatherapy, n.d.) Examples: • Roman chamomile • Clary sage • Lavender • Mandarin • Neroli • Vetiver
	Exercise	Physical activity is used to reduce symptoms of anxiety Exercise alters dopamine, serotonin, and norepinephrine; increases brain-derived neurotrophic factor; and reduces oxidative stress levels (Hamilton & Rhodes, 2015)
	Mind-body therapies: yoga, mindfulness-based stress reduction	Techniques such as yoga and mindfulness are used to enhance the mind's positive impact on the body A specific yoga breathing technique may also reduce symptoms of obsessive-compulsive disorder
	Expressive therapies	Music is used to promote relaxation, decrease autonomic arousal, and calm the body
	Virtual reality–graded exposure therapy	Computer images in a virtual world stimulate anxiety while the patient practices relaxation training
	Electroencephalogram (EEG) or electromyography (EMG) biofeedback	Scalp sensors measure brain activity, and patients learn how to regulate the body's responses to stress
	Heart rate variability biofeedback	The variability of intervals between heartbeats is measured, and feedback promotes increased variability, lowers stress levels, and improves overall well-being
Attention-Deficit/Hyperactivity Disorder (ADHD)	Diet/nutrition	Food colorings, additives, sugar, and certain food allergens are avoided to help decrease symptoms of ADHD
	Natural products/herbs	Supplements, vitamins, minerals, and herbs/botanicals are used to decrease symptoms of ADHD Examples: • **Omega-3 fatty acids:** high doses may decrease symptom severity • **Zinc:** may decrease hyperactivity • **Acetyl-L-carnitine**: may decrease symptoms of inattention

Continued

Disorder	Therapy	Description
	EEG biofeedback	Scalp sensors measure brain activity, and patients learn how to regulate body responses Symptoms of inattention, impulsivity, and hyperactivity are decreased
	Mind-body therapies	Techniques such as yoga, mindfulness, and massage are used to enhance the mind's positive impact on the body and decrease symptoms of ADHD
	Exercise	Physical activity is used to lessen the symptoms of ADHD
Bipolar	Natural products/herbs	Supplements, vitamins, minerals, and herbs/botanicals are used to help stabilize mood Example: • **Omega-3 fatty acids**: decreased mood swings when taken with a mood stabilizer
	Exercise	Physical activity is used to decrease symptoms of mania
Depression	Natural products/herbs	Supplements, vitamins, minerals, and herbs/botanicals are used to improve mood Examples: • **St John's wort:** used in mild to moderate depression • **Omega-3 fatty acids:** used in conjunction with antidepressants • **SAMe:** used for moderate to severe depression with or without antidepressants; risk of serotonin syndrome
	Exercise	Physical activity is used to improve depressive symptoms
	Bright light therapy	Light boxes are used to decrease melatonin, reducing the symptoms of depression
	Mind-body therapies: yoga	Yoga is an effective treatment for major depressive disorder
	Diet/nutrition	Regular meals consist of fish, fruit, raw or cooked vegetables, and omega-3 fatty acids (Le Port, et al., 2012) Vitamin D supplementation reduces depressive symptoms (Sepehrmanesh et al., 2015)
	Massage therapy	A broad group of medically valid therapies involving rubbing or moving the skin are used to reduce depressive symptoms (Hou et al., 2010)
	Repetitive transcranial magnetic stimulation (rTMS)	Stimulation of the brain using a magnet on the scalp is used to help improve refractory depression (Rachid, 2018)
	Intermittent theta-burst stimulation (iTBS)	A more intense form of rTMS has shown promising results in reducing refractory depression (Williams et al., 2018)
Posttraumatic Stress Disorder (PTSD)	Virtual reality–graded exposure therapy	Virtual environments are used for progressive exposure therapy Virtual environments may be even more effective than medication in PTSD and decrease symptoms by 30% (McLay et al., 2011)
	Acupuncture	Needles are inserted in the skin at key points (meridians) to modulate the flow of qi Acupuncture may be as effective as cognitive behavioral therapy
	Eye movement desensitization and reprocessing (EMDR)	Patients explore disturbing memories while simultaneously focusing on external stimuli such as eye movements or hand-tapping
Schizophrenia	Natural products/herbs	Supplements, vitamins, minerals, and herbs/botanicals are used to alleviate symptoms of schizophrenia Examples: • **Omega-3 fatty acids** • **Folic acid**: reduces positive and negative symptoms • **Thiamine**: used in conjunction with an antipsychotic • **Glycine**: improves functioning and decreases negative symptoms • **Ginkgo biloba**: used in conjunction with an antipsychotic
	Acupuncture	Needles are inserted in the skin at key points (meridians) to modulate the flow of qi Auditory hallucinations may be decreased similar to antipsychotics
	Mind-body therapies: yoga	Yoga enhances the positive interaction between the mind and body, which helps to decrease agitation and anxiety
	Avatar therapy	Patients converse with an avatar that represents the hallucination Avatar becomes less derogatory and more submissive over time, reducing the severity of the auditory hallucinations (Craig et al., 2018)

Disorder	Therapy	Description
Substance Use	Diet/nutrition	Relapse is reduced with diets low in sugar and caffeine and high in omega-3 fatty acids
	Natural products	Supplements, vitamins, minerals, and herbs/botanicals are used to help reduce cravings, withdrawal, and the effect of substances on the body Examples: • **Amino acids** such as taurine and L-tryptophan decrease cravings and help with withdrawal • **SAMe** may decrease the risk of liver damage • **Kudzu** decreases cravings and can help prevent relapse
	EMG, thermal EMG, and EEG biofeedback	Patients are able to view the activity in the muscles and brain and learn how to self-regulate the body's response to stress Biofeedback may decrease the relapse rate of alcohol use disorders (Lake, 2009; Markiewicz, 2017)
	Exercise	Physical activity may decrease the relapse rate of alcohol use disorders
	Mind-body therapies: yoga	Yoga enhances the positive interaction between mind and body, which helps to decrease agitation and anxiety and reduces relapse
	Cranioelectrotherapy stimulation (CES)	A weak electrical current in the head and neck reduces the severity of withdrawal for alcohol and opiates

REFERENCES

Craig, T. K. J., Rus-Calafell, M., Ward, T., Leff, J. P., Huckvale, M., Howarth, E., & et al. (2018). AVATAR therapy for auditory verbal hallucinations in persons with psychosis: A single-blind, randomized controlled trial. *Lancet Psychiatry*, *5*, 31–40.

Hamilton, G. F., & Rhodes, J. S. (2015). Exercise regulation of cognitive function and neuroplasticity in the healthy and diseased brain. *Progress in Molecular Biology and Translational Science*, *135*, 381–406.

Hou, W. H., Chiang, P. T., Hsu, T. Y., Chiu, S. Y., & Yen, Y. C. (2010). Treatment effects of massage therapy in depressed people: a meta-analysis. *Journal of Clinical Psychiatry*, *71*(7), 894–901.

Lake, J. (2009). *Integrative mental health care. A therapist's handbook*. New York, NY: W.W. Norton & Company, Inc.

Le Port, A., Gueguen, A., Kesse-Guyot, E., Melchior, M., Lemogne, C., Nabi, H., & et al. (2012). Association between dietary patterns and depressive symptoms over time: A 10-year follow-up study of The GAZEL cohort. *PLoS One*, *7*(12), 1–8.

Markiewicz, R. (2017). The use of EEG biofeedback/neurofeedback in psychiatric rehabilitation. *Psychiatria Polska*, *51*(6), 1095–1106.

McLay, R. N., Wood, D. P., Webb-Murphy, J. A., Spira, J. L., Wiederhold, M. D., Pyne, J. M., & et al. (2011). A randomized, controlled trial of virtual reality-graded exposure therapy for post-traumatic stress disorder in active duty service members with combat-related post-traumatic stress disorder. *Cyberpsychology, Behavior, and Social Networking*, *14*(4), 223–229.

National Association for Holistic Aromatherapy. (n.d.). *Most commonly used essential oils*. Retrieved from http://www.naha.org.

Rachid, F. (2018). Maintenance repetitive transcranial magnetic stimulation (rTMS) for relapse prevention in depression: A review. *Psychiatry Research*, *262*, 363–372.

Sepehrmanesh, Z., Kolahdooz, F., Abedi, F., Mazroii, N., Assarian, A., Asemi, Z., & et al. (2015). Vitamin D supplementation affects the beck depression inventory, insulin resistance, and biomarkers of oxidative stress in patients with major depressive disorder: A randomized, controlled, clinical trial. *The Journal of Nutrition and Disease*, *146*(2), 243–249.

Williams, N. R., Sudheimer, K. D., Bentzley, B. S., Pannu, J., Stimpson, K. H., Duvio, D., & et al. (2018). High dose spaced theta-burst TMS as a rapid-acting antidepressant in refractory depression. *Brain*, *141*, 1–5.

B APPENDIX

Answer Key

Chapter 1

1. **Answer: b.** Although all of the scenarios present opportunities for a nurse to intervene, the correct response presents an imminent danger to the patient's safety and well-being.
2. **Answer: c.** Trauma occurs in many forms, including physical, sexual, and emotional abuse; war; natural disasters; and other harmful experiences. Trauma-informed care provides guidelines for integrating an understanding of how trauma affects patients into clinical programming.
3. **Answer: d.** The patient's report suggests that depression is occurring. With the increased understanding of the biology of psychiatric illnesses, treatment approaches have evolved rapidly into more scientifically grounded methods, particularly psychopharmacology.
4. **Answer: d.** The correct response recognizes the recovery model, which has the following tenets: Mental health care is consumer and family driven, with patients being partners in all aspects of care; care must focus on increasing the consumer's success in coping with life's challenges and building resilience; and an individualized care plan is at the core of consumer-centered recovery.
5. **Answer: a.** Caring is evidenced by empathic understanding, actions, and patience on another's behalf; actions, words, and presence that lead to happiness and touch the heart; and giving of self while preserving the importance of self. Comforting is a part of caring, which includes social, emotional, physical, and spiritual support.

Chapter 2

1. **Answer: c.** Stigma refers to the array of negative attitudes and beliefs regarding mental illness. Bias, prejudice, fear, and misinformation contribute to stigma.
2. **Answer: c.** In the correct response, the nurse answers rather than evades the question, provides accurate information, and uses terminology a 9- or 10-year-old child can understand. Many of the most prevalent and disabling mental disorders have been found to have strong biological influences, including genetic transmission.
3. **Answer: d.** Resiliency is the ability to recover from or adjust successfully to trauma or change. A successful transition through a crisis builds resiliency for the next difficult trial. In the correct response, the person demonstrates acceptance of the paralysis and a focus on his or her abilities and assets.
4. **Answer: a.** Diagnoses classify disorders that people have, not the person. For this reason, it is important to avoid use of expressions such as "a schizophrenic" or "an alcoholic." The nurse has a responsibility to educate the coworker.
5. **Answer: c.** Many biological, cultural, and environmental factors influence mental health. Persons who are normal also may experience dysfunction during their lives. The death of a spouse is a difficult experience, so crying is expected.

Chapter 3

1. **Answer: b.** A therapeutic milieu provides a healthy social structure within an inpatient setting or structured outpatient clinic. Groups aim to help increase patients' self-esteem, decrease social isolation, encourage appropriate social behaviors, and educate patients in basic living skills, such as good hand washing. Coping with grief and loss (Option a) would be more appropriately provided by a therapist or advanced practice nurse.
2. **Answer: b.** Maslow's hierarchy of needs is placed conceptually on a pyramid, with the most basic and important needs on the lower level. The higher levels, the more distinctly human needs, occupy the top sections of the pyramid. When lower-level needs are met, higher-level needs are able to emerge. Self-actualization and esthetics are the highest-level needs.
3. **Answer: c.** The goal of CBT is to identify the negative patterns of thought that lead to negative emotions. Once the maladaptive patterns are identified, they can be replaced with rational thoughts. A person must be able to engage in meaningful dialogue to benefit from CBT.
4. **Answer: c.** Rapid, unthinking responses are known as automatic thoughts. Often these automatic thoughts, or cognitive distortions, are irrational because people make false assumptions and misinterpretations. Once the negative patterns of thought that lead to negative emotions are identified, they can be replaced with rational thoughts.
5. **Answer: a.** Rigid or disengaged boundaries are those in which the rules and roles are followed despite the consequences.

Chapter 4

1. **Answer: a.** The cerebellum is critical in both motor and cognitive functions. Alterations in cerebello-thalamo-cortical circuits may manifest as disturbances of coordination, balance, and gait. Safety is the nurse's first concern.
2. **Answer: c.** Risperidone blocks α_1- and H_1 receptors. It can cause orthostatic hypotension and sedation, which can lead to falls.
3. **Answer: b.** Olanzapine (Zyprexa) has metabolic side effects, particularly weight gain. Metabolic monitoring for all patients receiving atypicals is recommended, although risperidone (Risperdal) and quetiapine (Seroquel) have lower weight gain. Ziprasidone (Geodon) and aripiprazole (Abilify) are considered weight neutral. Metabolic monitoring usually includes measurements of body weight, BMI, waist circumference, fasting plasma glucose level, and fasting lipid profile.
4. **Answer: c.** At lower doses, trazodone loses its antidepressant action while retaining hypnotic effects through histamine-receptor antagonism; therefore, it is useful for insomnia. Fifty milligrams is a low dose. High doses of trazodone are required for the serotonergic action to relieve depression.
5. **Answer: d.** Executive functions occur in the cerebrum. Loss of cortical tissue has been associated with schizophrenia as well as with

treatment involving haloperidol and other typical antipsychotics. In contrast, newer atypical antipsychotics and antidepressants have been found to increase brain volume and structural synaptic/neuronal plasticity.

Chapter 5

1. **Answer: a.** The patient's comments indicate problems with the use of leisure time. Recreational activities improve emotional, physical, cognitive, and social well-being. A recreational therapist is the best member of the treatment team to provide these services. Asking the patient about program preferences (Option b) may give the nurse more information but does not provide any action to improve well-being.
2. **Answer: c.** The plan of care begins with a medical assessment to rule out or consider co-occurring/comorbid conditions.
3. **Answer: d.** Safety is a key consideration in the selection of activities. The correct response identifies an activity likely to appeal to the population but without physical contact between patients or equipment, which may be associated with injury.
4. **Answer: a.** Mental health parity refers to third-party (insurance) coverage of care for mental illness and addictions similar to the coverage of the care for physical illness. Federal and state legislation apply, but coverage varies by state. Some states offer full parity for mental illness insurance coverage.
5. **Answer: c.** The nurse's skills from the medical unit will be valuable, but this nurse will need to expand his or her skill set to effectively care for a psychiatric population. Working with an experienced psychiatric nurse will provide opportunities for learning.

Chapter 6

1. **Answer: d.** Despite personal misgivings, the nurse must maintain the fiancé's confidentiality.
2. **Answer: b.** The scenario offers no indication that the patient is dangerous or out of control; therefore, less restrictive interventions should be employed. The nurse has a responsibility to provide guidance to the certified nursing assistant.
3. **Answer: a.** Fidelity is the ethical principle of maintaining loyalty and commitment to the patient. The nurse in this situation is not maintaining commitment to patients by refusing to work the shift. It is not, however, illegal for a nurse to call off for personal reasons, making this an ethical decision.
4. **Answer: d.** Institutional policies and practices do not absolve an individual nurse of responsibility to practice on the basis of professional standards of nursing care. State nurse practice acts specify that assistive personnel must work under a nurse's supervision.
5. **Answer: d.** Sleep deprivation causes impaired practice, which jeopardizes patient safety. The colleague's comments indicate that impairment is likely. The nurse should confer with the supervisor to determine the appropriate action.

Chapter 7

1. **Answer: c.** The patient's thyroid problems may have reemerged and can mimic depression.
2. **Answer: d.** The focus of the question is the caregiver. The demands associated with the care of three elderly persons who live at a distance have the potential of overwhelming the caregiver. Because there is no evidence of role strain, a risk diagnosis is formulated.
3. **Answer: b.** Hypnosis is not within the scope of practice of a staff-level registered nurse. The state nurse practice act details regulations regarding scope of practice. Hypnosis is an advanced practice intervention.
4. **Answer: c.** Outcomes, as well as interventions, must always be individualized to the patient and should reflect the patient's multidimensional needs. Although it is important to confer with the patient about which outcomes are desirable, a patient experiencing panic is unable to engage in decision making or learning activities.
5. **Answer: b.** It is important to document the events and actions taken in both patients' records; however, confidentiality must be maintained. Using the initials of the patients involved is one way to ensure that confidentiality is maintained.

Chapter 8

1. **Answer: b.** The correct response encourages description and helps the patient to express feelings related to this experience.
2. **Answer: c.** The correct response demonstrates the therapeutic technique of presenting reality. Giving advice, disagreeing, and changing the subject are nontherapeutic communication techniques.
3. **Answer: a.** The correct response demonstrates the therapeutic technique of reflection.
4. **Answer: c.** Therapeutic use of touch is a basic aspect of the nurse–patient relationship and is often perceived as a gesture of warmth and friendship, but the response to touch is culturally defined. Many Hispanic Americans are accustomed to frequent physical contact and perceive it in a positive way.
5. **Answer: a.** Telehealth is a live, interactive mechanism used to track clinical progress and provide access to people who otherwise might not receive good medical or psychosocial help. The nurse should provide accurate education about this mechanism and ensure the patient's rights to privacy.

Chapter 9

1. **Answer: d.** The correct response is respectful and recognizes that trust between the nurse and patient needs to be developed. The correct response is also open ended, which is an appropriate communication technique to begin a new relationship.
2. **Answer: b.** The nurse has a responsibility for self-care and must set limits on the neighbor's intrusive calls. Specifying the frequency and time allotment for calls shows compassion for the neighbor while preventing infringement on the nurse's personal life.
3. **Answer: d.** Preparing and analyzing a process recording provides an opportunity for clinical supervision of the experienced nurse. The nurse and the supervisor examine the nurse's feelings and reactions to the patient and the way in which they affect the relationship.
4. **Answer: c.** It's important for the nurse to continue to assess the adult, respect the adult's individuality, and delay judgment regarding whether the person is experiencing illness. Avoiding crowds may be an effective coping technique for this patient.
5. **Answer: c.** Countertransference refers to the tendency of the nurse to displace onto the patient feelings related to people in his or her past. Frequently, the patient's transference to the nurse evokes countertransference feelings in the nurse.

Chapter 10

1. **Answer: b.** Eustress is beneficial stress that will help the couple to focus, problem solve, and successfully plan their wedding.
2. **Answer: a.** Yoga and other physical activities can be effective ways to manage stress. These activities deepen breathing, relieve muscle tension, and can elevate levels of the body's own endorphins, which induces a sense of well-being.
3. **Answer: d.** The scenario suggests that the spouse has experienced the effects of long-term stress. When stress is prolonged, the body stays alert. Chemicals produced by the stress response can have damaging effects on the body, causing physical diseases. Although

all of the actions may be indicated, obtaining a health assessment from the primary care provider has the first priority.

4. **Answer: a.** The veteran has high risk for posttraumatic stress disorder (PTSD). When PTSD is untreated or undertreated, painful repercussions often occur, particularly marital problems, unemployment, heavy substance abuse, and suicide. The highest priority is an assessment of suicide risk.
5. **Answer: c.** Although dissociative identity disorder can be a very interesting diagnosis, the nurse should avoid focusing more on one patient at the expense of others.

Chapter 11

1. **Answer: b.** Rationalization refers to justifying an action to satisfy the listener.
2. **Answer: b.** Although all of these situations may produce some level of fear or anxiety, the correct response presents a scenario of imminent, specific danger.
3. **Answer: d.** The student is demonstrating projection, as evidenced by not taking responsibility for his or her own behavior and blaming the instructor for a perception of failing. In the correct answer, the instructor avoids a defensive response and reinforces that the responsibility belongs to the student.
4. **Answer: c.** Altruism is a health defense mechanism in which emotional conflicts and stressors are addressed by meeting the needs of others. With altruism, the person receives gratification either vicariously or from the response of others.
5. **Answer: d.** People who have just experienced a disaster such as a tornado will most likely be experiencing severe or panic levels of anxiety. People at this level would benefit most from short, clear instructions. The other options are more appropriate for someone with mild to moderate anxiety.

Chapter 12

1. **Answer: a.** Safety is the nurse's first concern. One serious risk associated with doctor-shopping is medication interactions and duplicate medications.
2. **Answer: b.** It's important for the nurse to convey compassion and support to the patient but without reinforcing the symptoms. Case management can help to limit health care costs. Seeing the patient at regular intervals can instill security and avoid frantic and frequent demands. The patient who establishes a relationship with the case manager often feels less anxiety because he or she has an advocate and feels that someone is managing and aware of his or her care.
3. **Answer: b.** A paresthesia is a tingling or pricking sensation. Conversion disorder (functional neurobiological symptom disorder) usually involves weakness or paralysis, abnormal movement, swallowing or speech difficulties, seizures or attacks, and sensory problems. Patients may be distressed or show *la belle indifference* (a lack of emotional concern). Despite the diagnosis, the patient's complaints must be taken seriously. Further evaluation is needed.
4. **Answer: b.** Nurses should avoid emphasizing feelings but should continue to show interest in the patient. Ignoring feelings or symptoms completely could result in missing a serious medical issue. Frequent use of benzodiazepines is not recommended, but patients may benefit from other anxiolytic medications. When somatic symptom disorders are suspected, a nurse may be assigned as a main contact point, but the patient should still be encouraged to discuss care his or her providers.
5. **Answer: c.** People with factitious disorder imposed by another may do things to cause symptoms or illness in another person. They will often go from provider to provider or hospital to hospital. The motivation is for the attention, caring, and sympathy they receive as the caregiver of the victim.

Chapter 13

1. **Answer: a.** The persons exhibits callousness, entitlement, lack of remorse, and disregard for the rights of others. These characteristics are common in persons diagnosed with antisocial personality disorder.
2. **Answer: c.** People diagnosed with narcissistic personality disorder consider themselves special and expect special treatment. Their demeanor is arrogant and haughty. They have a sense of entitlement.
3. **Answer: a.** People diagnosed with borderline personality disorder frequently use the defense of splitting, which strains personal relationships. Splitting is the inability to integrate both the positive and the negative qualities of an individual into one person.
4. **Answer: c.** Genetics seems to play a significant role in the development of schizotypal personality disorder, which is more common in families with a history of schizophrenia.
5. **Answer: b.** Alcohol abuse is a commonly occurring problem in persons diagnosed with antisocial personality disorder.

Chapter 14

1. **Answer: b.** People with eating disorders may perceive themselves as overweight and place unrealistic value on being thin. Losing 15 pounds is not likely to alter all aspects of someone's life.
2. **Answer: c.** Thought processes that accompany anorexia nervosa include a terror of gaining weight, viewing oneself as fat even when emaciated, and judging one's self-worth by one's weight or size.
3. **Answer: c.** The comment by the psychiatric technician trivializes the patients' problems. Low self-esteem and self-doubts about personal worth are characteristic features of persons who have eating disorders. The comment contributes to these aspects of self-perception.
4. **Answer: c.** Cognitive distortions with underlying emotions of anxiety, dysphoria, low self-esteem, and feelings of lack of control are often present in persons with eating disorders. In this instance, the adolescent is catastrophizing. The nurse should first help the patient to identify the fears. Cognitive distortions are consistently confronted by all members of the interdisciplinary team in preparation for carefully planned challenges to the patient later in treatment.
5. **Answer: d.** The laboratory results show hypokalemia and hypocalcemia, which are likely to affect cardiac function, producing bradycardia, arrhythmias, and/or murmurs.

Chapter 15

1. **Answer: c.** The stress–diathesis model explains depression from an environmental, interpersonal, and life-events perspective combined with biological vulnerability or predisposition (diathesis). Psychosocial stressors and interpersonal events, such as abuse, trigger certain neurophysical and neurochemical changes in the brain. Early life trauma is a significant component in the stress reaction.
2. **Answer: d.** The correct response accomplishes two results: the nurse can further assess the patient's complaint, and the nurse uses clarification, a therapeutic communication technique.
3. **Answer: c.** Helplessness is sometimes a finding in major depressive disorder. The nurse has a responsibility for patient advocacy. Helping the patient to advocate for self is empowering.
4. **Answers: b, c.** The possibility that antidepressant medication might contribute to suicidal behavior, especially in children and adolescents, has been a long-time concern, and all antidepressants include a Black Box warning. The use of selective serotonin reuptake inhibitors shows a strong association with a reduction in suicide. All

treatments have potential risks; each patient should be considered individually when antidepressants are prescribed. All consumers of antidepressants should be observed carefully for worsening of depression and suicidal thoughts.

5. **Answer: d.** ECT is safe and effective and can achieve a 70% to 90% remission rate in depressed patients within 1 to 2 weeks. ECT is especially indicated when there is a need for a rapid, definitive response when a patient is suicidal or homicidal as well as in selected other circumstances.

Chapter 16

1. **Answer: c.** The nurse has responsibility for advocacy. In view of the patient's long history of problems, a legal guardian should be considered.
2. **Answer: b.** Numerous posts on a social network page indicate hyperactivity, which is a hallmark of mania.
3. **Answer: a.** Patients should stop taking lithium if excessive diarrhea, vomiting, or sweating occurs. These problems can lead to dehydration, which can raise serum lithium to toxic levels.
4. **Answer: d.** The correct response shows use of the therapeutic communication technique of verbalizing the implied. Gaining insight contributes to relapse prevention.
5. **Answer: a.** Safety is a priority. Mania impairs the person's judgment and impulse control, which may result in harm to self. The correct response identifies potential dangers and shows care for the patient.

Chapter 17

1. **Answer: b.** Concrete thinking refers to literal interpretations, with an inability to comprehend abstract concepts.
2. **Answer: a.** The daily experience of negativity creates a scenario in which the risk for suicide is high. Depressive symptoms occur frequently in schizophrenia. Suicide is the leading cause of premature death in this population.
3. **Answer: c.** Neuroleptic malignant syndrome (NMS) occurs in persons who have taken antipsychotic agents and usually begins early in the course of therapy. It is characterized by a decreased level of consciousness; greatly increased muscle tone; and autonomic dysfunction, including hyperpyrexia, labile hypertension, tachycardia, tachypnea, diaphoresis, and drooling. Treatment consists of early detection, discontinuation of the antipsychotic agent, management of fluid balance, reduction of temperature, and monitoring for complications. Treatment of this problem should occur in a medical unit.
4. **Answer: b.** The patient's comments suggest that akathisia, which is an extrapyramidal symptom, is occurring. The nurse should assess the patient for other indicators of this side effect of antipsychotic medication.
5. **Answer: c.** Paranoia causes an inability to trust the actions of others. Therapeutic strategies should focus on lowering the patient's anxiety and decreasing defensive patterns. The application of principles for dealing with paranoia is helpful for establishing trust and rapport.

Chapter 18

1. **Answer: c.** Silence is a therapeutic communication technique. It is respectful and provides an opportunity for the adult to compose responses.
2. **Answer: d.** Side effects of rivastigmine (Exelon) include nausea, vomiting, diarrhea, weight loss, loss of appetite, and muscle weakness.
3. **Answer: a.** Withdrawal from alcohol, anxiolytics, opioids, and central nervous system stimulants presents a significant risk for the development of delirium. The correct response identifies a patient who is likely to have tolerance to alcohol and is thus at risk for alcohol withdrawal delirium.
4. **Answer: b.** Important considerations for promoting mental health in the older adult include the need for older adults to continue to include social, intellectual, and physical activities in their routines. Older adults can continue to learn and contribute even when physiological changes occur.
5. **Answer: c.** Memantine (Namenda), an *N*-methyl-D-aspartate (NMDA) antagonist, and some cholinesterase inhibitors may be prescribed to treat symptoms of moderate to severe Alzheimer's disease.

Chapter 19

1. **Answer: d.** The correct response recognizes the power of addiction but presents the reality of the consequences of continued use.
2. **Answer: c.** Lorazepam is a benzodiazepine. Sudden withdrawal from this class of medications has medical complications, including the possibility of death; hence this refill request has priority.
3. **Answer: b.** The nurse should educate the patient. E-cigarettes are advertised as safe; however, they contain nicotine as well as other hazardous chemicals.
4. **Answer: c.** All of the options are correct, but safety is the nurse's first concern. Marijuana is a psychoactive substance. Effects include euphoria, sedation, perceptual distortions, and hallucinations; therefore, driving or operating machinery may be hazardous.
5. **Answer: c.** Naltrexone (ReVia, Vivitrol) reduces the desired pleasant feelings related to alcohol or opioid intake and helps to reduce drug cravings. It is part of a total program for maintaining sobriety.

Chapter 20

1. **Answer: a.** This scenario presents a potential adventitious crisis in phase 1. The nurse must first consider safety. After moving to a secure location, the nurse can activate the school's code for an intruder and describe the intruder to law enforcement.
2. **Answer: c.** The scenario presents a maturational crisis. Helping the spouse to consider other options is the nurse's most therapeutic action.
3. **Answer: b.** In phase 1 of a crisis, a person faces a conflict or problem that threatens the self-concept and responds with increased feelings of anxiety. The nurse should first assure students that they are safe and then specify the reason for the session.
4. **Answer: d.** After addressing safety concerns, the nurse should take steps to help patients feel safe and lower anxiety, such as providing a quiet environment, building rapport, and acknowledging their crisis experience. A group session will allow patients who are unable to articulate their feelings to hear from patients who are able to discuss it.
5. **Answer: a.** Nurses need to monitor their thoughts and feelings and learn to recognize when they need self-care, support, or professional help. This is especially true in the aftermath of violence. Nurses often suppress their own feelings in order to effectively handle the immediate situation and react later with anxiety.

Chapter 21

1. **Answer: b.** The majority of the victims of reported intimate partner violence are women. Intimate partner violence is the number one cause of emergency department visits by women. Patterns of damage are often in locations that cannot be noticed easily, such as the torso, back, upper arms, upper legs, inside body orifices, and under the hair.
2. **Answer: b.** The acute injury, coupled with bruises of different ages, suggest that the child may be abused. Abusive parents may perceive the child as bad or evil or project blame. The nurse is required to report suspicions of abuse to child protective services.

3. **Answer: b.** The cycle of violence consists of three phases: (1) tension-building phase, (2) acute battering phase, and (3) honeymoon phase. The question scenario shows acute battering, so a period of loving calm is likely to follow.
4. **Answer: d.** Nurses must be self-aware, particularly in highly charged situations. Wishing harm on an abuser may be understandable, but it is an indicator of the nurse's need for guidance.
5. **Answer: a.** Although the nurse may include any of the topics, the topic of appropriate behaviors with intimate partners has priority. The characteristics of the game of football, the physical power required to be a player, and the risk for drug or alcohol misuse among this age group are factors that increase the risk for intimate partner violence.

Chapter 22

1. **Answer: c.** The scenario presents a risk for sexual assault. Many people are sensitive about sexual matters, so the nurse should first give recognition to the widow for her willingness to share the problem. The most common drug used to facilitate the crime of rape is alcohol. Sexual violence occurs across all ages and is perpetrated against men, women, and children. Cultural and societal factors play a part in forming attitudes about sexual violence.
2. **Answer: a.** A sexual assault victim who arrives at the emergency department needs compassionate, supportive care and should not be left alone.
3. **Answer: a.** The correct response demonstrates the use of reflection, a therapeutic communication technique. The consequences of rape can cause serious, long-term psychological trauma. Rape-trauma syndrome is a common sequela. Later in this interaction, the nurse should encourage the patient to consider professional counseling.
4. **Answer: c.** Prior to leaving the emergency department, the patient should have a scheduled follow-up appointment with a rape counselor or crisis counselor.
5. **Answer: d.** Common emotional reactions after a sexual assault include anger, fear, anxiety, guilt, humiliation, embarrassment, self-blame, and mood swings. Compassionate care involves approaching the person who has been sexually assaulted in a nonjudgmental and empathic manner. Patients need to hear and understand that the rape is not their fault. It is important to help survivors separate the issues of vulnerability from blame.

Chapter 23

1. **Answer: b.** The correct response represents a covert message and suggests possible suicidal thinking by the parent. The nurse should further assess the meaning of the comment.
2. **Answer: b.** All health care members who provided care for a suicide victim, including medical staff, nursing staff, and ancillary staff, are at risk of being traumatized by suicide. Staff also may experience symptoms of posttraumatic stress disorder with guilt, shock, anger, shame, and decreased self-esteem. To reduce the trauma associated with the sudden loss, posttrauma loss debriefing can help to initiate an adaptive grief process and prevent self-defeating behaviors.
3. **Answer: a.** The nurse should always take an individual very seriously if he or she mentions some form of suicidal ideation and ask directly about suicide.
4. **Answer: a.** The patient's comment suggests hopelessness, helplessness, and worthlessness. Physical illnesses play a role in increasing suicide risk. Suicide precautions should be initiated.
5. **Answer: d.** Referrals need to be made available to family members and friends to assist them in dealing with and addressing the many emotional reactions and problems that easily may develop after the suicide of a family member or friend. Self-help groups are extremely beneficial for survivors.

Chapter 24

1. **Answer: c.** Talking about one's feelings is healthier than violence or avoidance.
2. **Answer: b.** The patient's behavior is aggressive. Aggressive behaviors reflect rage, hostility, and the potential for physical assault or verbal destructiveness and can be directed at others or oneself. Aggression is a hostile reaction that occurs when control over anger is lost. It is used in an attempt to regain control over the stressor or flee the situation. By suggesting an appropriate behavior, the nurse offers an opportunity for the patient to regain control.
3. **Answer: b.** In the original response, the nurse personalized the request and responded in an aggressive manner. The correct answer demonstrates an assertive response, which would have been more effective.
4. **Answer: c.** Bullying is an intentional display and use of violence, although it may appear mild in some instances. Bullying can be defined as an offensive, intimidating, malicious, condescending behavior designed to humiliate. The scenario identifies an instance of lateral bullying. All kinds of bullying behaviors create a toxic environment. Those who are bullied are prone to negative feelings about self, humiliation, poor self-concept, and great emotional pain, and many can suffer severe, long-term reactions. After educating the parents about bullying, the nurse should assist them in setting limits with the child.
5. **Answer: b.** Sarcasm is a veiled form of anger.

Chapter 25

1. **Answer: a.** Mourning refers to all of the ways in which a person outwardly expresses grief and the efforts taken to manage grief. It does not have a designated time frame and may continue for many years. A once-a-year ritual is an adaptive coping technique to recognize the parents' loss.
2. **Answer: d.** This person is mourning. A grief or bereavement support group is indicated and can provide comfort.
3. **Answer: a.** Although emotional responses to grief vary from one individual to the next, a common first response is that of denial. The person is emotionally unable to accept his or her painful loss. Denial functions as a buffer against intolerable pain and allows the person to acknowledge the reality of a loss slowly.
4. **Answer: d.** The work of grief is over when the bereaved can realistically remember the pleasures and the disappointments of the relationship with the lost loved one. Brief periods of intense emotions may still occur at significant times, but the person or family members have energy to reinvest in new relationships that bring shared joys, security, satisfaction, and comfort.
5. **Answer: b.** The nurse's comment suggests a negative self-judgment. Burnout, decreased work performance, and compassion fatigue (the emotional pain or cost of working with traumatized persons) may result in stress responses for nurses.

Chapter 26

1. **Answer: c.** Prominent behavioral characteristics of ASD include motions repeated over and over (flaps hands, rocks body, spins self in circles, repeatedly turns light on and off), playing with toys the same way every time, getting upset by minor changes (furniture rearranged, changed route to someplace familiar), and obsessive interests.
2. **Answer: b.** Therapeutic interventions should be matched to the developmental level of the child. Abused children are likely to have problems with anxiety or depression. Storytelling is a form of bibliotherapy likely to appeal to kindergarten-age children. Children unconsciously identify with the characters in the story, allowing self-expression in a safe environment to occur. Reading and

discussing a book about abused children may be too charged and would likely increase anxiety.

3. **Answer: b.** IDD may be a result of hereditary factors, alterations in early embryonic development, pregnancy and perinatal problems, and other factors such as trauma and poisoning.
4. **Answer: d.** Developmental level is an important part of the assessment with children, so the nurse should select terms the child will understand. A semistructured interview provides an opportunity for the child to express perceptions about life at home and life at school with teachers and peers. Severe marital discord is a factor that may contribute to mental illness in children.
5. **Answer: a.** Genetic factors have been implicated in a number of childhood mental disorders, including autism, bipolar disorder, schizophrenia, attention-deficit hyperactivity disorder (ADHD), intellectual developmental disorders, and some others.

Chapter 27

1. **Answer: b.** Individuals with severe mental illness (SMI) usually have difficulties in multiple areas, including finances and budgeting. Psychoeducational programming builds interpersonal skills, including assertiveness.
2. **Answer: b.** The consumer has an active role in treatment and quality of life. Poverty and lack of access to quality foods can cause poor nutrition. The recovery model stresses a partnership between care providers and the patient, both working together to plan and direct treatment. Empowering the patient and focusing on strengths rather than limitations helps the patient to use his or her strengths to achieve the highest quality of life possible.
3. **Answer: a.** Although all of the topics are important, heart-healthy living encompasses diet, exercise, lifestyle or behavior changes, and management of hypertension. Persons who take antipsychotic medications are particularly at risk for heart disease and metabolic syndrome as a result of weight gain and hyperlipidemia.
4. **Answer: c.** Pedophilia involves lewd or lascivious (sexual) acts perpetrated on a minor. Perpetrators are at especially high risk of suicide, especially in the first 24 to 48 hours after incarceration.
5. **Answer: b.** Issues for those with severe mental illness (SMI) include poverty, stigma, isolation, unemployment, poorer health outcomes, law enforcement encounters, victimization, and inadequate housing or homelessness. Supplemental Security Income (SSI) provides a modest income for indigent persons ineligible for Social Security Disability Income (SSDI).

Chapter 28

1. **Answer: b.** The developmental task of late life is integrity versus despair. The patient's comment shows feelings of hopelessness and loss, which contribute to despair. The correct response assists the patient to find meaning in life.
2. **Answer: b.** The patient's comment may relate to physical or mental concerns. The nurse should first clarify and explore the meaning of the comment.
3. **Answer: b.** As an advocate, the nurse can help to empower the patient to address the problem. Role-playing provides an opportunity to safely practice different responses.
4. **Answer: d.** The interaction of drugs and alcohol in the older adult can have serious consequences. Alcohol may prolong, potentiate, or accelerate the metabolism of various drugs.
5. **Answer: c.** The highest suicide rate is among white males age 65 and older. Depression can be dangerous when the older person is also experiencing illness, loneliness, or other life losses.

INDEX

Note: Page numbers followed by "b" indicate boxes, "f" indicate figures, and "t" indicate tables.

S

T